NANDA DIAGNOSES

Activity intolerance
Activity intolerance, risk for
Adaptive capacity, decreased: intracranial
Adjustment, impaired
Airway clearance, ineffective
Anxiety
Aspiration, risk for
Body image disturbance
Body temperature, altered; risk for
Bowel incontinence
Breastfeeding, effective
Breastfeeding, ineffective
Breastfeeding, interrupted
Breathing pattern, ineffective
Cardiac output, decreased
Caregiver role strain
Caregiver role strain, risk for
Communication, impaired verbal
Community coping, ineffective
Community coping, potential for enhanced
Confusion, acute
Confusion, chronic
Constipation
Constipation, colonic
Constipation, perceived
Coping, defensive
Coping, family: potential for growth
Coping, ineffective family: compromised
Coping, ineffective family: disabling
Coping, ineffective individual
Decisional conflict (specify)
Denial, ineffective
Diarrhea
Disuse syndrome, risk for
Diversional activity deficit
Dysreflexia
Energy field disturbance
Environmental interpretation syndrome, impaired
Family processes, altered: alcoholism
Family processes, altered fatigue
Fear
Fluid volume deficit
Fluid volume deficit, risk for
Fluid volume, excess
Gas exchange, impaired
Grieving, anticipatory
Grieving, dysfunctional
Growth and development, altered

Health maintenance, altered
Health-seeking behaviors (specify)
Home maintenance management, impaired
Hopelessness
Hyperthermia
Hypothermia
Incontinence, functional
Incontinence, reflex
Incontinence, stress
Incontinence, total
Incontinence, urge
Infant behavior, disorganized
Infant behavior, disorganized: risk for
Infant behavior, organized: potential for enhanced
Infant feeding pattern, ineffective
Infection, risk for
Injury, perioperative positioning: risk for
Injury, risk for
Knowledge deficit (specify)
Loneliness, risk for
Management of therapeutic regimen, community: ineffective
Management of therapeutic regimen, families: ineffective
Management of therapeutic regimen, individuals: effective
Management of therapeutic regimen, individuals: ineffective
Memory, impaired
Memory, impaired physical
Noncompliance (specify)
Nutrition, altered: less than body requirements
Nutrition, altered: more than body requirements
Nutrition, altered: potential for more than body requirements
Oral mucous membrane, altered
Pain
Pain, chronic
Parent/infant/child attachment, altered; risk for
Parental role conflict
Parenting, altered
Parenting, altered; risk for
Peripheral neurovascular dysfunction, risk for
Personal identity disturbance
Poisoning, risk for

Post-trauma response
Powerlessness
Protection, altered
Rape-trauma syndrome
Rape-trauma syndrome: compound reaction
Rape-trauma syndrome: silent reaction
Relocation stress syndrome
Role performance, altered
Self-care deficit, bathing/hygiene
Self-care deficit, dressing/grooming
Self-care deficit, feeding
Self-care deficit, toileting
Self-esteem disturbance
Self-esteem, chronic low
Self-esteem, situational low
Self-mutilation, risk for
Sensory/perceptual alterations (specify) (visual, auditory, kinesthetic, gustatory, tactile, olfactory)
Sexual dysfunction
Sexuality patterns, altered
Skin integrity, impaired
Skin integrity, impaired, risk for
Sleep pattern disturbance
Social interaction, impaired
Social isolation
Spiritual distress (distress of the human spirit)
Spiritual well-being, potential for enhanced
Suffocation, risk for
Swallowing, impaired
Thermoregulation, ineffective
Thought processes, altered
Tissue integrity, impaired
Tissue perfusion, altered (specify type) (renal, cerebral, cardiopulmonary, gastrointestinal, peripheral)
Trauma, risk for
Unilateral neglect
Urinary elimination, altered
Urinary retention
Ventilation, inability to sustain spontaneous
Ventilatory weaning process, dysfunctional
Violence, risk for: self-directed or directed at others

From North America Nursing Diagnosis Association (1994): NANDA nursing diagnoses definitions and classification, 1995-1996. Philadelphia: Author.

Comprehensive Psychiatric Nursing

Comprehensive Psychiatric Nursing

FIFTH EDITION

Judith Haber, PhD, RN, CS, FAAN
Visiting Professor
Division of Nursing
New York University
New York, New York
Private Practice
Stamford, Connecticut

Barbara Krainovich-Miller, EdD, RN, CS
Visiting Professor
Division of Health Sciences
Felician College
Lodi, New Jersey
Private Practice
Garden City, New York

Anita Leach McMahon, EdD, RN
Professor
Division of Nursing
Pasco Hernando Community College
New Port Richey, Florida

Pam Price-Hoskins, PhD, RN, CNAA
Associate Professor
College of Nursing
University of Oklahoma
University Center at Tulsa
Private Practice
Tulsa, Oklahoma

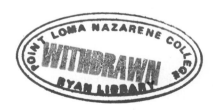

with 32 illustrations and 13 color plates

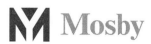
Mosby

St. Louis Baltimore Boston Carlsbad Chicago Naples New York Philadelphia Portland
London Madrid Mexico City Singapore Sydney Tokyo Toronto Wiesbaden

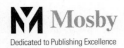

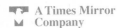

Vice President and Publisher: Nancy L. Coon
Editor: Jeff Burnham
Developmental Editor: Linda Caldwell
Project Manager: Deborah L. Vogel
Production Editor: Mamata Reddy
Layout Artist: Jeane Genz
Designers: E. Rohne Rudder and Frank Loose Design
Manufacturing Manager: Linda Ierardi
Cover Art: Frank Loose Design
Photographer: Patrick Watson

A NOTE TO THE READER:
The author and publisher have made every attempt to check dosages and nursing content for accuracy. Because the science of pharmacology is continually advancing, our knowledge base continues to expand. Therefore we recommend that the reader always check product information for changes in dosage or administration before administering any medication. This is particularly important with new or rarely used drugs.

Fifth Edition

Printed in the United States of America
Composition by Graphic World, Inc.
Lithography/color film by Graphic World, Inc.
Printing/binding by Von Hoffman Press

Mosby-Year Book, Inc.
11830 Westline Industrial Drive
St. Louis, Missouri 63146

Library of Congress Cataloging in Publication Data

Comprehensive psychiatric nursing / Judith Haber . . . [et al.]. —5th ed.
      p.   cm.
     Includes bibliographical references and index.
     ISBN 0-8151-4179-3 (alk. paper)
     1. Psychiatric nursing.   2. Nurse and patient.   I. Haber, Judith.
     [DNLM: 1. Psychiatric Nursing.   WY 160 C737 1996]
RC440.C58   1996
610.73'68—dc21
DNLM/DLC
for Library of Congress
                       96-46940
                       CIP

96 97 98 99 00 / 9 8 7 6 5 4 3 2 1

Contributors

Sharon Bidwell-Cerone, PhD, RN, CS
Clinical Associate Professor of Nursing
School of Nursing
State University of New York at Buffalo
Buffalo, New York

Anicia S. Biglow, RN, MN
President
HUG, Inc.
Atlanta, Georgia

Carolyn Veronica Billings, MSN, RN, CS
Psychiatric-Mental Health Clinical Nurse Specialist
Private Practice
Raleigh, North Carolina

Josepha Campinha-Bacote, PhD, RN, CS, CTN
President, Transcultural C.A.R.E. Associates
Cincinnati, Ohio
Adjunct Assistant Professor
College of Nursing
Ohio State University
Columbus, Ohio

Jeanne Ryan Botz, MS, ARNP, CS
Advanced Registered Nurse Practitioner
The Harbor Behavioral Health Care Institute
New Port Richey, Florida

Melissa Hedinger Cottrell, MSN, RN
Program Director
Eating Disorders Unit
Laureate Psychiatric Clinic and Hospital
Tulsa, Oklahoma

Beverly J. Farnsworth, PhD, RN, CS
Associate Professor and Coordinator, RN/BSN Program
School of Nursing
Kennesaw State College
Marrietta, Georgia
Clinical Nurse Specialist
HUG, Inc.
Atlanta, Georgia

Joy Feldman, Esq., JD, MA, RN
Vice President and General Counsel
The Park Associates, Inc.
East Aurora, New York

Claire Griffin-Francell, MS, APRN
President
Southeast Nurse Consultants, Inc.
Dunwoody, Georgia

Beth Harris, MA, RN, CS
Patient and Family Education Coordinator
New York Hospital-Cornell Medical Center
White Plains, New York

Norine J. Kerr, PhD, RN
Clinical Specialist
Partial Hospitalization Service
Menninger Clinic
Topeka, Kansas

Joyce Larson-Presswalla, PhD, RN
Assistant Professor
University of South Florida
Tampa, Florida

Suzanne Lego, PhD, RN, CS, FAAN
Private Practice
Kent, Ohio; Pittsburgh, Pennsylvania

Stanley J. Matek, MS
President
Professional Ethics Resources
Milwaukee, Wisconsin

Carolyn Maynard, PhD, RN
College of Nursing
University of North Carolina at Charlotte
Charlotte, North Carolina

Madeline A. Naegle, PhD, RN, FAAN
Associate Professor
Division of Nursing
New York University
New York, New York

Elizabeth C. Poster, PhD, RN
Dean and Professor
School of Nursing
University of Texas at Arlington
Arlington, Texas

Karen Howell Richardson
Professor and Program Director
Division of Nursing
Pasco Hernando Community College
New Port Richey, Florida

Ann Robinette, MS, RN, CS
Psychiatric Clinical Nurse Specialist
Private Practice
Glenville, North Carolina

Mary Rosedale, MS, RN,C
Regional Director
Mental Health and Addictions Nursing
US HomeCare Corporation
Manhattan, New York
Assistant Professor
Department of Health Care Programs
Iona College
New Rochelle, New York

Carole A. Shea, PhD, RN, CS, FAAN
Associate Dean and Graduate Director
College of Nursing
Northeastern University
Boston, Massachusetts

Sara Torres, PhD, RN, FAAN
Associate Professor and Chair
Department of Community Nursing
College of Nursing
University of North Carolina at Charlotte
Charlotte, North Carolina

Mary Walker, MA, RN
Psychiatric Clinical Nurse Specialist
Veterans Administration Medical Center
Knoxville, Iowa

Michele L. Zimmerman, MA, RN, CS
Private Practice
Avery Finney Associates
Associate Professor of Psychiatric Nursing
School of Nursing
Old Dominion University
Norfolk, Virginia

"THE CONSUMER'S VOICE" WRITERS

Will Brady
Pat Guerard
Marc Jacques
Steven Caplan

Gabrielle Kitchener
Michael Lonergan
and those who wish to remain anonymous

Reviewers

Carole-Jean Adkisson, MSN, RN
Assistant Professor of Nursing
Tennessee Technological University
Cookeville, Tennessee

Susan Alden, ND, ARNP, CS
Assistant Professor
Teikyo Marycrest University
Davenport, Iowa

Deanah Alexander, MSN, RN, CS
Instructor
West Texas A & M University
Canyon, Texas

Cynthia Hoppe Allen, MPH, RN, MN
Assistant Professor
Charity School of Nursing
Delgado Community College
New Orleans, Louisiana

Janette P. Arblaster, MSN, RN
Nursing Instructor
TriCounty Technical College
Pendleton, South Carolina

Carole A. Auvil, DNSc, MSN, RN
Clinical Assistant Professor
College of Nursing
University of Illinois at Chicago
Chicago, Illinois

Patricia Hentz Becker, EdD, RN
Associate Professor
School of Nursing
La Salle University
Philadelphia, Pennsylvania

Verolyn Barnes Bolander, MS, RN,C
Associate Professor
School of Nursing
University of Texas Medical Branch
Galveston, Texas

Patsy Britting, MSN, RN
Instructor
Psychiatric Mental Health Nursing
West Texas A&M University
Canyon, Texas

Barbara A. Broome, MSN, RN, CNS
Assistant Professor of Nursing
Kent State University
Kent, Ohio
Kent State University-Trumbull Campus
Warren, Ohio

Sharon L. Carlson, PhD, RN
Associate Professor
Department of Nursing
Otterbein College
Westerville, Ohio

Lory Clukey, MSN, RN
Assistant Professor
School of Nursing
University of Northern Colorado
Greeley, Colorado

Emily A. Cook, PhD, RN
Associate Professor
Life College
Marietta, Georgia

Betty J. Craft, PhD, RN, CS
Assistant Professor
College of Nursing
University of Nebraska Medical Center
Omaha, Nebraska

Mary B. Davies, RN
Resource Nurse-Triage Line
Healthfront Education Services, Inc.
Woburn, Massachusetts

Patricia R. Dean, MSN, RN
Associate Professor
School of Nursing
Florida State University
Tallahassee, Florida

Jacqueline K. Dunn, MS, RN, CS-P
Associate Professor
Catonsville Community College
Staff Nurse
Sheppard Pratt Health Systems
Baltimore, Maryland

Ginger W. Evans, MS, MSN, RN, CS
Assistant Professor
College of Nursing
University of Tennessee-Knoxville
Knoxville, Tennessee

Marlene Farrell, MS
Professor of Nursing
California State University
Los Angeles, California
Academic Coordinator, Center for International Nursing
California State University-Dominguez Hills
Carson, California

Edna M. Fordyce, EdD, RN, CS-P
Professor Emeritus
Department of Nursing
Towson State University
Towson, Maryland

E.A. Furlong, PhD, RN, C
Coordinator
Community Health/Community Mental Health Nursing
School of Nursing
Creighton University
Omaha, Nebraska

Rauda Gelazis, PhD, RN, CS, CTN
Associate Professor
Ursuline College
Pepper Pike, Ohio

Rebecca Crews Gruener, MSN, RN
Associate Professor of Nursing
Louisiana State University at Alexandria
Alexandria, Louisiana

Brigitte F. Haagen, MSN, RN, CS
Coordinator, Mental Health Nursing
School of Nursing
Pennsylvania State University
Hershey, Pennsylvania

Bonnie M. Hagerty, PhD, RN, CS
Assistant Professor
School of Nursing
University of Michigan
Ann Arbor, Michigan

Nelda Jeane, MSN, RN, C
Associate Professor of Nursing
Louisiana State University at Alexandria
Alexandria, Louisiana

Gladys C. Keidel, EdD, RN, CN
Educator
Clinical Specialist in Psychiatric Nursing
Shepherdstown, West Virginia

Jeanne B. Kozlak, MSN, RN, CS
Professor of Mental Health Nursing
Department of Nursing
Humboldt State University
Arcata, California

Mary Kunes-Connell, PhD, RN
Associate Professor
Coordinator, Psychiatric/Mental Health Nursing
School of Nursing
Creighton University
Omaha, Nebraska

Sarah Steen Lauterbach, RN, EdD, MSPH
Associate Professor
School of Nursing
La Salle University
Philadelphia, Pennsylvania

Joanne Lavin, EdD, Rn, CNS
Associate Professor of Nursing
Kingsborough Community College
Brooklyn, New York

Barbara H. Lentner, MA, RN
Assistant Professor
Department of Nursing Education
Coe College
Cedar Rapids, Iowa

Melissa Lickteig, MSN, RN
Faculty
Jefferson School of Nursing
Pine Bluff, Arkansas

Kenyann Lucas, MS, RN, CNS
Associate Professor
Associate Degree Nursing Program
Texarkana College
Texarkana, Texas

Linda Nance Marks, EdD, RN
Associate Professor
Director
Learning Resources Center
School of Nursing
The University of Texas at Arlington
Arlington, Texas

Geoffry W. McEnany, PhD, RN, CS
Postdoctoral Fellow
Agency for Health Care Policy and Research
School of Nursing
University of California, San Francisco
San Francisco, California

E. Hope Mena, MS, RN, CNS
Associate Professor of Nursing
Beth-El College of Nursing Health Sciences
Clinical Specialist, Pikes Peak Mental Health Center
Colorado Springs, Colorado

Vicki A. Moss, DNSc(c), MS
Associate Professor
Viterbo College
LaCrosse, Wisconsin

Cindy A. Peternelj-Taylor, RN, BScN, MSc
Associate Professor
College of Nursing
University of Saskatchewan
Saskatoon, Saskatchewan

Anita H. Rhodes, RN, MSN
Instructor
Auburn University
Consultant
East Alabama Regional Inservice Center
Auburn, Alabama

Clementine Hinsperger Rice, MSN, RN, PhD(c)
Assistant Professor
School of Nursing
Oakland University
Rochester, Michigan

Betty W. Ross, PhD, RN, CS
Assistant Professor, Retired
School of Nursing
Fairleigh Dickinson University
Teaneck, New Jersey

Carol A. Sherwood, MSN, RN, CS
Assistant Professor
Simmons College
Boston, Massachussetts

Jane Smith, MSN, RN, CNS
Assistant Professor of Nursing
Lamar University
Beaumont, Texas

Marcy J. T. Smith, MSN, RN, FATS
Professor
Department of Nursing
Cape Cod Community College
West Barnstable, Massachusetts
Stress Concepts—Research-Based Education and
    Consultation
Osterville, Massachusetts

James C. Sorensen, EdD, RN
Associate Professor
Department of Nursing
College of Professional Studies
University of the Incarnate Word
San Antonio, Texas

Lee Anne Xippolitos, PhD, RN, NPP, CARN, CS
Clinical Associate Professor
State University of New York at Stony Brook
Stony Brook, New York
Nurse Practitioner in Psychiatry
Pederson-Krag Continuing Day Treatment Program
St. James, New York

Marylou Yam, PhD, RN, CS
Assistant Professor
Saint Peter's College
Jersey City, New Jersey

For my wonderful family, Lenny, Laurie, and Andrew Haber, whose ever-present love and support are my inspiration.

Judith Haber

For my loving husband, Russell, and granddaughter, Amber, who inspired and supported me in every way throughout the process of writing this book.

Barbara Krainovich-Miller

For R.J., who teaches me love, and for my father, Bill Leach, who taught me that psychiatric nursing is about caring, respect, genuineness, and hope.

Anita Leach McMahon

To Mark, who has taught me how to have fun, to Whitney, who has helped me grow fully into personhood, and to Raegen Siegfried, who encouraged me.

Pam Price-Hoskins

Preface

The publication of the fifth edition of *Comprehensive Psychiatric Nursing* marks another milestone for this textbook and the practice of psychiatric-mental health nursing. The fifth edition of *Comprehensive Psychiatric Nursing* will span the end of the twentieth century and the beginning of the new millennium, the twenty-first century—an awesome event to contemplate.

The challenges of the 1990s have been synonymous with health care redesign and workplace restructuring, which have led to transformation of the delivery of mental health care. The advent of changes created by the knowledge explosion in biological psychiatry and a mandate to provide a full spectrum of health promotion, illness prevention, acute care management, and rehabilitative activities provide a springboard for the delivery of seamless, community-based collaborative care for consumers with neurobiological disorders. Psychiatric nurses are invited to assume new and creative clinical roles that reflect their contributions to the care they provide to the individuals, families, and communities who are consumers of mental health services. Similarly, psychiatric nurses are asked to demonstrate their expertise in organizing and integrating mental health delivery systems. These big changes have challenged the authors to create an exciting and useful text to meet student and provider needs for a biopsychosocial knowledge base that guides practice into the twenty-first century.

Comprehensive Psychiatric Nursing, first published in 1978, was the first comprehensive psychiatric-mental health nursing textbook to use a holistic framework that addressed the biological and psychosocial domains of the person. It was also the first textbook to apply the nursing process to psychiatric-mental health nursing phenomena.

The conception of the original project by Anita Leach McMahon was based on the belief that psychiatric nurses provide essential therapeutic experiences through their relationships with clients and that nurses must engage in an ongoing journey of self-awareness if they are to maximize their therapeutic use of self with clients. The second edition of the text expanded and strengthened the biopsychosocial framework and further operationalized the nursing process while continuing to emphasize the nurse's therapeutic use of self. The third edition reflected the knowledge explosion of the 1980s. It refined and emphasized the significance of the interactional nature of human phenomena by stressing family and community content. The fourth edition reaffirmed the biopsychosocial nature of mental disorders and practice of psychiatric-mental health nursing.

Wide acceptance of the text and professional recognition through two *American Journal of Nursing* Book of the Year Awards and translation of *Comprehensive Psychiatric Nursing* into Spanish and French provide evidence of the contribution this text has made to the art and science of psychiatric-mental health nursing.

OVERVIEW OF THE FIFTH EDITION

The publication of the fifth edition represents another pioneering adventure into the future. Transformation of health care delivery, exploding scientific knowledge, and demand for professional accountability highlight the challenge to target crucial theoretical and clinical issues that will be essential to the practice of psychiatric-mental health nursing in the twenty-first century. In many ways, this looks like a completely new textbook. In some ways it is, since the organization and content have been reconfigured to reflect the most current knowledge in the field. For example, this edition contains 14 new chapters. However, it also retains and builds on the strengths of the previous four editions. The holistic biopsychosocial framework has been expanded to reflect the full spectrum of mental health care delivery and operationalizes the theoretical basis for psychiatric nursing practice.

Our commitment to viewing clinical practice through a psychiatric nursing lens is reflected by the incorporation of the 1994 *Standards of Psychiatric-Mental Health Clinical Nursing Practice* throughout this edition, as well as two of the most current nationally approved taxonomies, North American Nursing Diagnosis Association (NANDA) nursing diagnoses and the Nursing Interventions Classification (NIC). Equally important is a commitment to interdisciplinary collaboration that is reflected by use of the 1994 *Diagnostic and Statistical Manual of Mental Disorders, Fourth Edition* (DSM-IV) medical classification for mental disorders and the inclusion of interdisciplinary treatment plans.

Acknowledgment of the knowledge explosion in psychobiology and its important contribution to providing biopsychosocial care is recognized by a new chapter devoted to psychobiology, including a four-page *full-color* insert that illustrate related psychobiological concepts. In addition, psychobiology is integrated throughout each clinical chapter. The expanded chapter on psychopharmacology reflects the latest psychopharmacology guidelines and also contains a four-page *full-color* insert.

Recognition of the importance of the active participation of the consumers of mental health care, the individuals and families with whom psychiatric nurses collaborate, is reflected by several new features designed to meet consumer needs. A unique new feature, *The Consumer's Voice*, is a vignette written by a mental health consumer that lends credibility to the lived experience of psychiatric clients. Other consumer-focused features include *Cultural Highlights, Consumer/Community Resources, Teaching Points,* and *Medication Tips.*

Finally, our belief in the importance of research-based practice is operationalized by the inclusion of the most current research in the field, a chapter on outcomes management, research-based practice guidelines, and *Research Highlights.* Tools for operationalizing research-based nursing practice include *Interdisciplinary Treatment Plans* and *Nursing Care Plans* that are incorporated in selected (critical paths) chapters.

ORGANIZATION

The book has been organized into six parts that reflect the conceptual framework and the current standards of psychiatric-mental health nursing practice. Part One, *Delivery of Mental Health Care to the Consumer,* an entirely new section, presents cutting-edge issues that reflect contemporary psychiatric-mental health nursing practice and mental health care delivery. The first chapter addresses current and future trends in the delivery of mental health services, followed by a chapter that introduces students to contemporary psychiatric nursing roles and functions. The third chapter focuses on legal and ethical issues related to consumer advocacy, psychiatric nursing practice, and the larger mental health delivery system. A chapter on outcomes management is then presented that reflects the importance of outcome-based clinical practice and the ability of psychiatric nurses to document how they make a difference.

Part Two, *Power Tools for Psychiatric-Mental Health Nursing* contains five revised chapters that focus on psychiatric nursing principles, which are fundamental to operationalizing clinical practice. The first chapter, *The Nursing Process,* provides an organizing framework for applying the ANA *Standards of Psychiatric-Mental Health Clinical Nursing Practice* in a holistic, client-centered manner in chapters throughout this book. The second chapter presents a model for delivering culturally competent nursing care to clients from culturally diverse backgrounds. The third chapter promotes understanding of developmental issues across the life cycle. The fourth and fifth chapters provide essentials of therapeutic communication and a framework for developing nurse-client relationships with consumers of mental health services across the continuum of treatment from one setting to another.

Part Three, *Nursing Interventions,* includes seven chapters that address biopsychosocial intervention modalities. Separate chapters devoted to intervention with individuals, groups, and families are *Crisis Intervention, Working With Groups,* and *Working with Families.* A new chapter, *Psychobiology,* provides the biological framework for the revised and expanded *Psychopharmacology* chapter and another new chapter, *Stress Theory and Interventions.* The psychobiology and psychopharmacology chapters are the foundation for the biological correlates and psychobiological interventions addressed in each clinical chapter, and each contains a four-page full-color insert. A final new and innovative chapter in this section addresses health teaching, an essential psychoeducational nursing intervention.

Part Four, *Continuity of Care,* includes five chapters that address the continuum of care including *Psychiatric Case Management, Health Promotion and Maintenance and Preventive Interventions,* and *Psychiatric Home Care.* These topics, new in this textbook, and separate chapters on psychiatric nursing in inpatient settings and community settings, are more important than ever before, since transformation in the delivery of mental health services now focuses on the integrated delivery of services in traditional and nontraditional settings using a wide range of treatment strategies.

Part Five, *Nursing Management of Mental Health Disorders,* contains 10 chapters that feature consistent organization focusing on the nursing management of specific clinical disorders. The six-step nursing process, each step of which reflects an ANA standard of psychiatric-mental health clinical nursing practice, and NANDA diagnoses provide the organizing framework for new or extensively revised content in each chapter that reflects current thinking and practice. The information in this section has also been reorganized to conform more closely to the DSM-IV classification. As a result, there are separate chapters on the disorders of anxiety; dissociation; post-traumatic stress; impulse-control; personality; substance use; eating; schizophrenia and other psychoses; mood; and delirium, dementia, and other cognitive disorders.

Part Six, *Populations at Risk,* concludes the book with a focus on the unique issues and concerns in the psychiatric treatment of special populations including the completely new chapters of *Psychosocial Problems of Physically Ill Persons, Infants and Children,* and *Homeless Persons.* Significantly revised chapters related to adolescents, elderly persons, victims and victimizers, and persons with severe and persistent mental illness join with the new chapters in this section to round out a clinical focus related to population-based health care, a clinical focus of emerging importance in the field.

Appendixes contain the *Standards of Psychiatric-Mental Health Nursing Clinical Practice,* the *Standards of Addictions Nursing Practice,* the *DSM-IV Classification,* and the *Canadian Standards of Psychiatric and Mental Health Nursing Practice.*

SPECIAL FEATURES

The visionary quality of this edition is also reflected in the special features that reflect "cutting edge" trends in the delivery of mental health care. They have been designed to promote critical thinking in our readers, yet provide a "user-friendly" approach to learning. The special features challenge our readers to apply theory-based psychiatric nursing principles to clinical practice, yet accumulate a wealth of practical clinical tips and resources. Special features include full-color inserts in the psychobiology and psychopharmacology chapters, more boxes, tables, and figures than in previous editions, and a visually stimulating two-color design. All of the following special features are highlighted by a specific design format or icon to guide the reader's attention to their locations within chapters.

The Nursing Process

The discussion of the six steps of the nursing process are highlighted with the following unique title headings as they are operationalized in Parts Five and Six:

Assessment

Nursing Diagnosis

Outcome Identification

Planning

Implementation

Evaluation

CRITICAL THINKING QUESTIONS, derived from a thought-provoking case study that reflects the chapter focus, are located at the end of each chapter. The questions are designed to challenge students, promote independent clinical reasoning, and encourage students to integrate the content in a way that helps them develop a philosophy about psychiatric-mental health nursing.

CULTURAL HIGHLIGHTS provide greater awareness and sensitivity to the relationship among cultural diversity, culturally related mental health issues, and providing culturally competent nursing care.

TEACHING POINTS underscore the importance of the idea that consumers are active participants in their care. Health teaching, an essential health promotive, preventive, acute care, and maintenance psychiatric nursing intervention is presented from a psychoeducational perspective based on the teaching/learning process.

MEDICATION TIPS highlight important psychopharmacological information intended to help consumers develop medication self-management strategies and promote maximum adherence to the psychobiological plan of care.

CONSUMER/COMMUNITY RESOURCES provide practical sources of consumer-oriented information available within the community. These community resources may provide health relevant information, skills development opportunities, and psychosocial support for clients and their families.

THE CONSUMER'S VOICE vignettes, which appear in each chapter in Part Five, provide students with actual experiences of clients (told in their own words) who have specific psychiatric disorders. They also tell students how these individuals learned to live with their disorders and manage them effectively, thereby offering nurses consumer wisdom about how to intervene, support, and advocate for clients with mental health disorders.

INTERDISCIPLINARY TREATMENT PLANS, also called critical paths, clinical pathways, or Care Maps, are included as a special feature in the nursing process and case management chapters, as well as in the chapters of Part Five. This feature highlights the importance of interdisciplinary collaboration in the attainment of cost-effective and quality client outcomes. Each treatment plan has been developed by and is borrowed from a particular health care organization.

NURSING CARE PLANS present concise, relevant nursing care plans for a significant nursing diagnosis based on the major disorders discussed in the text. The care plans include assessment data, DSM-IV diagnoses, nursing diagnoses, expected outcomes, short- and long-term goals, interventions with rationale, and evaluation. They provide a guide for students, to the "whys," as well as the "hows," of effective nursing intervention.

RESEARCH HIGHLIGHTS underscore the importance of research-based nursing practice by incorporating a research summary in all chapters of Part Five. Students are exposed to a concise, readable summary of a research study relevant to psychiatric nursing practice, as well as a series of bullet points related to the study's "real world" implications for clinical practice.

VIDEO RESOURCES at the end of appropriate chapters refer students to specific Mosby videos as a multimedia supplement to the information in the textbook.

NIC interventions
Numerous *Nursing Interventions Classification* (NIC) protocols developed by McCloskey and Bulechek are used to introduce students to this nationally accepted research-based classification system of nursing interventions. NIC clinical practice guidelines have been selected for their relevance to psychiatric nursing practice and to illustrate the emerging trend of using standardized practice guidelines in both inpatient and outpatient clinical settings.

Focused assessment
These guides, featured in clinical chapters, target appropriate assessment categories, highlight relevant assessment questions, and provide examples of possible client responses. Another feature of each assessment section is a listing of specific assessment tools that facilitate data collection and promote critical thinking essential to the diagnostic process.

Clinical examples
Descriptive samples of client situations based on actual clinical experiences are highlighted throughout the text to reinforce exposure to real-life clinical practice.

Learning outcomes
Learning outcomes are provided at the beginning of each chapter to help students identify key content that will guide their systematic mastery of chapter content.

Key terms
Important terms are highlighted for the student in a list of key terms at the beginning of each chapter. Each key term is boldface and the definition is italicized within each chapter. The term is also highlighted in the index.

Key points
Each chapter is summarized with key points that review and reinforce important content areas to assist student integration of new material in a "user-friendly" manner.

TEACHING-LEARNING PACKAGE

Instructor's Resource Manual and Test Bank
This supplement is designed to help faculty develop lectures and reinforce teaching and learning through classroom and clinical activities. Most important is the use of the manual to promote the development of critical thinking in students. This important resource follows the text chapter by chapter and includes learning objectives, suggested course outlines, psychiatric nursing teaching strategies, answer guidelines for textbook critical thinking questions, student worksheets, transparency masters, classroom handouts, and multimedia resources. A test bank containing more than 680 test items in the N-CLEX format is also provided, which includes an answer key, the rationale for each answer, and the applicable nursing process step and cognitive level of each question.

Computerized Test Bank
ESATEST, a computerized version of the test bank, is available in both IBM and Macintosh programs. Users can create tests, modify and add questions, print tests and answer keys, and do on-line testing.

Mosby's Psychiatric Nursing Transparency Acetates, 2/e
This second edition offers 48 *full-color* and two-color transparency acetates covering a variety of psychiatric nursing topics to visually enhance lecture and textbook concepts.

Mosby's Psychiatric Nursing Study Guide
This study guide offers over 100 worksheets with learning activities to supplement textbook use. The worksheets present exercises about the major topics of psychiatric nursing including basic concepts, treatment modalities, nursing management of psychiatric disorders, and lifespan and special populations issues. The exercises can be used as in-class or homework assignments, or can be used by the students in an independent, self-paced manner. A variety of exercises and activities are provided to promote interest and accommodate students' different learning styles.

Mosby's Psychiatric Nursing Video Series

These videos, covering six of the major psychiatric disorders, present nursing care issues and methods for the disorder through clinical vignettes and within an interdisciplinary care format.

Mosby's Nursing Care of Clients with Substance Abuse Video Series

These videos present information about treating various clients with substance abuse in different settings through clinical scenarios and interviews with substance abuse experts.

Mosby's Communication in Nursing Video Series

These videos address communication in nursing in a wide range of health care settings and situations using clinical case studies and interviews with practicing nurses and nurse experts.

ACKNOWLEDGMENTS

We are grateful for the loving support, patience, nurturing, understanding, and sacrifices of the many people who helped us through the challenging and sometimes arduous preparation of the fifth edition.

The value and quality of this edition has been enhanced by the talents of the diverse professionals in nursing education and practice who have participated with us in this effort. In particular the contributions of Barbara Flynn Sideleau to the first four editions as an editor and author is gratefully acknowledged. The addition to the editorial board of Barbara Krainovich-Miller enhanced the development and implementation of this project. Her expertise and her commitment have been valuable contributions to the editorial board.

The authors thank the contributors whose clinical expertise provided a "cutting-edge" knowledge base that strengthened the quality of this edition. We also thank Vickie D. Pflueger, RN,C and Darla Belt, RN, Senior Consultants at Strategic Clinical Systems, Inc. in Granbury, Texas for generously providing the treatment plans that illustrate "state of the art" interdisciplinary care. We are also deeply indebted to Dr. Karen Kangas and the Connecticut Mental Health Consumer Movement, without whose courageous voices the unique Consumer's Voice special feature would not have been possible. We also thank our many students and clients whose collective voices are heard in the clinical examples generously threaded throughout the book, examples that make psychiatric nursing come alive in an exciting manner.

A project of this scope would not be possible without the efforts of many behind-the-scenes people. We wish to express our appreciation to Mosby-Year Book, the publishers of this text. We are especially grateful to Jeff Burnham, Linda Caldwell, and Mamata Reddy who were our ever-present partners in this challenging venture.

The editors of *Comprehensive Psychiatric Nursing* hope that our readers find the fifth edition as exciting to read, use, and teach from as it has been for us to write. We believe that it will be a critical resource in developing clinically knowledgeable and competent psychiatric nurses for the twenty-first century.

Judith Haber
Barbara Krainovich-Miller
Anita Leach McMahon
Pam Price-Hoskins

Contents

Part One

Delivery of Mental Health Care to the Consumer

Chapter 1

Delivery of Mental Health Services

Judith Haber

LEARNING OUTCOMES

After studying and applying the concepts of this chapter, the learner will be able to:
- Describe the paradigm shift in the delivery of mental health services in the United States.
- Identify driving forces influencing change in the delivery of mental health services.
- Discuss how economic forces such as workplace redesign and restructuring of mental health service delivery, managed care, and changes in reimbursement influence changes in the delivery of mental health services.
- Discuss how reconceptualizing health care delivery in relation to community-based primary care influences changes in the delivery of mental health services.
- Discuss how consumer accountability issues, including stigmatization, race and poverty, differential mental health benefits, and outcomes, influence changes in the delivery of mental health services.
- Discuss how the knowledge explosion in areas such as psychobiology and technology influence changes in the delivery of mental health services.
- Evaluate the impact of changes in the delivery of mental health services on the future of psychiatric-mental health nursing practice.
- Specify a biopsychosocial vision for the delivery of mental health services in the year 2000 and beyond.

KEY TERMS

Behavioral managed care
Capitation
Managed care

Managed care programs
Population-based care
Primary care

Vertically integrated delivery systems (VIDS)

You are beginning your study of psychiatric-mental health nursing at an exciting crossroad in the delivery of mental health care. We invite you to join us in exploring the challenge of providing quality mental health care in partnership with clients, their families/significant others, and the communities in which they live.

Perhaps more than any other nursing specialty, the practice of psychiatric-mental health nursing will change because science, technology, and health care restructuring are revolutionizing the way we think about our clients, ourselves as clinicians, and the way in which mental health services are delivered. Developments in psychobiology, which provide amazing insights into the biological dimensions of mental illness, could "medicalize" our treatment perspective as we live through the current "Decade of the Brain." These developments will challenge us to integrate the biological, psychological, spiritual, and sociocultural dimensions of people into an integrated and holistic biopsychosocial reality that represents a futuristic vision for the practice of psychiatric-mental health nursing.

The purpose of this chapter is to examine the rapid advances in health care that present immediate challenges and that speculate about the challenges associated with creating an exciting future for the delivery of mental health services and the practice of psychiatric-mental health nursing.

CREATING THE PARADIGM SHIFT: THE DELIVERY OF MENTAL HEALTH SERVICES FOR 2000 AND BEYOND

Driving forces creating a paradigm shift that contribute to a revolution in the delivery of mental health services and the practice of psychiatric-mental health nursing include the following: economic forces, reconceptualization of health care delivery, consumer accountability, and developments in scientific knowledge. See Table 1-1 for traditional and emerging health care paradigms.

Economic Forces

In the 1990s a dramatic increase in the cost of health care, which now accounts for 14% of the U.S. budget dollar, has provided the driving force for rethinking how the health care dollar is spent. Although the cost of mental health care has remained relatively stable at 8% to 10% of each health care dollar spent, the delivery of mental health services also is being revolutionized in the frenzy to control health care costs while achieving quality client outcomes (Lowery, 1992; McGihon, 1994).

TABLE 1-1

Forces driving the paradigm shift in the delivery of mental health services

TRADITIONAL PARADIGM	EMERGING PARADIGM
Fee-for-service reimbursement	Capitated reimbursement
Unmanaged care	Managed care
Episodic care	Continuous care
Fragmented health care delivery systems	Integrated delivery systems
Inpatient services	Community-based services
Specialty care	Primary care
Cure (high-tech)	Care (low-tech)
Disease focus (illness model)	Wellness focus (prevention model)
Individual-based care	Population-based care
Provider focus	Consumer focus
Paternalism	Egalitarianism
Authoritarian	Collaborative
Physician focus	Diversity of providers
Process	Outcomes

Workplace redesign and restructuring of mental health service delivery

One approach to cost containment includes reorganization of mental health services through workplace redesign, restructuring, and budget reductions in both public and private sector settings. Shifting the focus to the hospital for stabilization and to the community for treatment has resulted in a shortened length of stay for inpatient episodes that decreases mental health costs. In addition, many clients formerly considered candidates for inpatient services are now treated in intensive community-based settings such as day treatment programs, home care, psychoeducation, and case management programs (Division of Social and Community Psychiatry, 1993; Hellwig, 1993; Moller, 1994). Assertive risk reduction and relapse prevention, and crisis intervention programs contribute to promoting maximum client functional status and addressing emerging signs of relapse through the effective use of outpatient mental health services (Murphy and Moller, 1993).

Cost consciousness that drives out inefficiency and waste is a positive force. However, cost consciousness also contains inherent incentives for undertreatment that may put nurses in positions that threaten to compromise their roles as client advocates. Psychiatric nurses must monitor quality initiatives to make sure that downsizing, restructuring, and work redesign are not at the expense of the mental health care consumer. They must also recognize that in a cost containment environment, restructuring will continue and acute psychiatric hospitals will downsize, close, or shift to outpatient programming. Traditional psychiatric hospital nursing positions will be greatly reduced. This trend creates an urgent need for psychiatric nurses to expand their concept of where, when, and how psychiatric nursing care is delivered. Psychiatric nurses of the future will define major career opportunities in community-based primary care and psychiatric settings (Bell, 1993). Emerging role opportunities for psychiatric nurses will be discussed in depth in Chapter 2 and incorporated throughout this textbook.

Managed care

Managed care is another approach to cost containment and the delivery of quality care. *Managed care is a system for delivering a prepaid health-centered benefit package to a defined population or membership. Managed care programs deliver comprehensive health care services to a defined population of consumers for an annual capitated (fixed price per person per year) fee.* It involves integration of services between and among service providers and seeks appropriateness in the type and intensity of care provided to people who are enrolled in a particular managed care plan. Health care services are provided by managed care organizations

such as health maintenance organizations (HMOs) in comparison with preferred provider organizations (PPOs) or the traditional indemnity (fee-for-service) health insurance programs. *Behavioral managed care programs deal with the mental health "carve out" benefits that represent one component of a managed care program.* This means that mental health benefits may be managed by provider organizations that specialize in mental health and substance abuse services (Mechanic, Schlesinger, and McAlpine, 1995). The objectives of behavioral managed health care programs are highlighted in Box 1-1. Managed care programs contain costs through (1) managing benefits, (2) managing care, and (3) managing health:

1. Managing benefits contains cost by establishing mental health benefit restrictions, exclusions, limits, penalties, and incentives. For example, by defining annual or lifetime maximum mental health benefits, deductibles, outpatient copayments, inpatient coinsurances, coverage exclusions, and precertification requirements, managed care companies have created short-term cost savings and cost shifting to the benefit of the employer rather than the consumer (Freeman and Trabin, 1994; Marion, 1996). In general, health insurance packages have usually had differential benefits for mental health versus physical health. Lifetime or annual limits on mental health coverage have had a catastrophic financial impact on families with a relative who has a serious and persistent mental illness. Moreover, limits on or lack of long-term benefits for outpatient mental health treatment has created no financial incentive for development of innovative community-based programs.

2. Managing care focuses on containing costs and ensuring quality of mental health services. This approach limits authorization of benefit expenditures to necessary and appropriate care delivered in the least restrictive, least intrusive treatment setting by qualified providers. Many believe that this approach delivers the right care, to the right client, at the right time, and in the right way at considerable savings when compared with unmanaged care. Man-

Box 1-1

Objectives of Behavioral Managed Health Care

- Facilitating easy access to care
- Taking responsibility for a defined population of clients
- Assigning clients to the least restrictive care that is effective for the client
- Providing care within a well-coordinated and complete continuum of care system
- Using multidisciplinary treatment providers and teams

aged care companies often assign case managers who collaborate with the mental health consumer and family to organize the most appropriate and effective combination of treatment resources to achieve both cost-effective and quality client outcomes (Freeman and Trabin, 1994).

3. Managing health, a long-term approach to cost containment, strives to reduce the demand for mental health services by improving the health status of defined populations and high-risk subgroups of individuals.

Adult high-risk populations include those with severe and persistent neurobiological disorders (see Chapter 38), the homeless mentally ill (see Chapter 37), persons with chemical dependence (see Chapter 27), older adults (see Chapters 7 and 35), and individuals with stress-related disorders such as post-traumatic stress disorder (PTSD) (see Chapter 24) and the psychosocial correlates of the human immunodeficiency virus (HIV) and acquired immunodeficiency syndrome (AIDS) (Krauss, 1993) (see Chapter 32). As vulnerable populations, children and adolescents are, by definition, considered high-risk groups. Extrinsic factors that are part of the environment include living in foster care or homelessness; exposure to violence and physical or sexual abuse; parents who are mentally ill, substance abusers, or both; and chronic medical illness. These represent risk factors for children and adolescents that increase their risk for mental health problems. Intrinsic factors related to biological or genetic variables may be the result of poor prenatal care, chronic physical illness, or brain injury. They include low birth weight, developmental delay, brain damage, addiction as a result of maternal prenatal substance abuse, mental retardation, and early difficulties with temperment (see Chapters 33 and 34).

Methods to manage health include providing health advisors, individual health-risk assessments, health education programs, preventive intervention programs, financial incentives for meeting personal health goals, self-help groups, crisis debriefing services, outreach programs to high users of health care services, and wellness programs that employ strategies to periodically assess the health status of the defined population they target. See Chapter 18 for an in-depth discussion of health promotion and preventive intervention.

Although public funding for these programs is not plentiful and the private sector has yet to widely implement them within the insured population, capitated financing mechanisms have the potential to encourage population-based health. This focus is expected to increase in the managed behavioral health care of the future (Freeman and Trabin, 1994; Institute of Medicine [IOM], 1994; Mrazek and Haggerty, 1994).

Managed care will be an inevitable feature of any new mental health care delivery system. Psychiatric nurses must devote energy to understanding the economic principles of managed care and their relationship to providing cost-effective, quality mental health care that is continuous and comprehensive and addresses client, family, and community mental health needs (Haber, 1996). Psychiatric nurses are perfectly positioned to function within managed care organizations as case managers and utilization review coordinators, or as case managers in mental health agencies. In these roles they will be challenged to balance ethical issues related to providing quality care within a stringent cost containment environment. Client advocacy issues related to confidentiality and obtaining appropriate mental health services will test the commitment of psychiatric nurses to the consumers of mental health care. Understanding how managed care systems work creates a foundation for being able to advocate for clients in an articulate manner. The ability to teach clients how to negotiate within their own managed care system is another benefit derived from developing this knowledge base. Learning how to work within and with managed care organizations will clarify new and emerging career opportunities for psychiatric nurses.

Reimbursement mechanisms

The essence of health care reform is the rapid transition from retrospective, fee-for-service indemnity insurance toward prospective, capitated models of health care financing that characterize HMOs (Sharfstein, 1994). Millions of Americans, including recipients of Medicare and Medicaid, are moving away from traditional health insurance reimbursement mechanisms and, through federal and state programs or through their employers, are individually enrolling in HMOs.

Similar to other prospective payment models like Medicare diagnosis-related groups (DRGs), *capitation* reimbursement models *offer a preset fee for each client in exchange for the delivery of health care services during a given time period* (Reed et al., 1994). Typically, a managed care company such as U.S. Healthcare will contract with a provider organization, that is, a network of mental health providers and/or mental health care treatment facilities, to provide comprehensive mental health care to a defined population of consumers (e.g., 9,000 employees of a corporation or 50,000 Medicare recipients in a single county).

Capitation creates financial incentives to carefully manage care. If care can be provided inexpensively, the provider profits. This health care financing mechanism has been suggested as a vehicle for improving the flexibility and responsiveness of care (Cole et al., 1994). Capitation offers potential advantages to mental health consumers including the following:

• Focused provider responsibility and accountability

- Increased provider flexibility to deliver comprehensive and coordinated services
- Clinical decisions based strictly on clinical requirements
- Consolidation of responsibility that reduces fragmentation of care by permitting one agency to provide, purchase, and coordinate all mental health services
- Increased client advocacy through case management services

The ability of capitation to control costs depends in part on substitution of outpatient care for inpatient care and use of preventive and early intervention to avoid more costly intensive care later (Reed et al., 1994). Historically, inpatient care has provided for all of a client's needs in one setting. The ability to create a comparable network of services in the community cannot be assumed (Cole et al., 1994). Capitated financing of health care is not a guaranteed winner. Among the potential disadvantages for mental health consumers are the following:

- Incentives to contain costs might promote client status quo versus growth resulting in a decrease in quality of client outcomes
- Access to highly trained specialists and more expensive services might be restricted
- Emphasis on cost containment may stifle innovation
- Clients viewed as expensive may be excluded from care
- Preset funds will be inadequate to cover needed client services, thereby jeopardizing delivery of client services

Psychiatric nurses must familiarize themselves with capitated financing mechanisms. This will be the future funding stream for the majority of public and private sector mental health programs and client populations. Program planning and implementation will be a function of being able to demonstrate the cost-effectiveness and quality outcomes of an intervention program for a defined client population within a capitated budget framework. For example, to obtain funding for a community-based psychiatric rehabilitation program, the interdisciplinary team, including psychiatric nurses, would use the findings of research studies that demonstrated both cost-effective and quality clinical outcomes for serious and persistently ill client populations enrolled in similar capitated programs (Reed et al., 1994).

Reconceptualizing Health Care Delivery

The need for a new focus on health in the United States is influencing the reconceptualization of health care delivery, as well as mental health care delivery. As

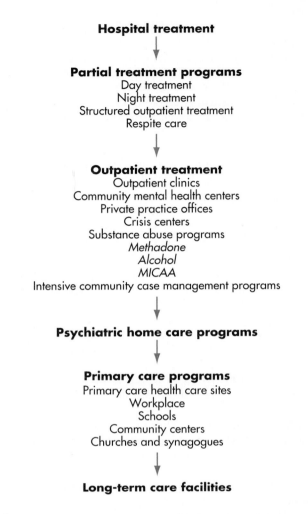

Fig. 1-1 Vertically integrated mental health delivery system.

illustrated in Table 1-1, a special emphasis on emerging paradigm terms such as prevention, wellness, population-based care, continuous care, and community-based primary care. This has provided direction for the shift from a traditional paradigm focus, which supports episodic care, is disease-focused and cure-oriented, and promotes a high-tech system of specialty care that has been located largely in inpatient health care delivery organizations (Aiken and Sage, 1993; IOM, 1994; Marion, 1996). Moreover, ***vertically integrated delivery systems,*** illustrated in Fig. 1-1, *will link all levels of care that are needed by a defined population,* such as those with severe and persistent neurobiological disorders.

The nation is now grappling with how to create systems of care that are consistent with what it values in health care delivery. It does so within changing realities related to access, concern about costs of health care, the growth of managed care, and integrated delivery systems. For psychiatric nurses to understand trends in mental health care delivery, assumptions about and the definition of primary care must be considered.

Primary care

Primary care is regarded as the foundation of an effective health care system because:

1. Primary care is proposed to address a large majority of the health problems (physical, mental, emotional, and social) present in the population.
2. Primary care will be essential to achieving a stronger emphasis on health promotion and disease prevention, as well as care of the chronically ill and providing for a comfortable and dignified death.
3. Personal interactions that include trust and partnership between clients and clinicians will remain an essential component of primary care.
4. Primary care will be concerned with providing continuous, coordinated, collaborative, community-based care.
5. Primary care will be essential to achieving the objectives that constitute value in health care (i.e., quality outcomes, client satisfaction, and efficient use of resources).

Primary care is defined as:

> *The provision of integrated, accessible health care services by clinicians who are accountable for addressing a large majority of personal health care needs, developing a sustained partnership with patients, and practicing in the context of family and community* (IOM, 1994).

This definition suggests that primary care will address a mixture of health problems along a disease spectrum as they occur singly or in combination within a single individual. Ideally, primary care clinicians (physicians, advanced practice nurses, and physician assistants) elicit a full range of client concerns, whether physical or psychosocial. These providers generally will be the first point of contact for clients entering the health care system. It is proposed that primary care providers will manage 80% of the health care needs of their client population (IOM, 1994). Approximately 20% of client problems, based on a particular individual's needs, on safety, or on efficiency, may require the expertise of other health professionals, specialists, or subspecialists such as psychiatrists, advanced practice psychiatric nurses or psychologists, social workers, or occupational therapists. Montano (1994) supports this perspective by noting that historically 50% to 60% of clients with mental illness in the United States are treated exclusively in primary care settings, whereas only 20% visited a mental health professional.

Psychiatric nurses and other mental health professionals must consider how their specialty practice will interface with a primary care delivery system that will become an essential consumer pathway to mental health services (Krauss, 1993). Currently, U.S. health policies treat physical and mental disorders as separate and unrelated phenomena, even though, in reality, there are biopsychosocial determinants of virtually every health problem. The holistic philosophy proposed to be embedded in the primary care approach requires a fundamental revision of this dichotomous perspective.

Studies of primary care practices find a substantial amount of psychiatric morbidity among people who consult their provider for nonpsychiatric health services. It has been estimated that between 11% and 50% of health problems presenting in primary care settings involve diagnosable psychiatric disorders (Worley, Drago, and Hadley, 1990; Eisenberg, 1992; National Institute of Mental Health [NIMH], 1993). Many, if not most, primary care providers fail to recognize and treat psychiatric disorders appropriately or at all (Hoff, 1993). Similarly, the general health needs of clients with severe and persistent mental illness often go undetected and/or untreated as a result of gaps in assessment practices of mental health professionals.

In addition to reforms within the mental health delivery system, basic reforms in primary care mental health services must take place. Such settings must be prepared to provide mental health promotion and prevention services, case finding, mental health assessments, routine treatment, and referral. The nursing profession has a historical commitment to the community-based, client-centered, holistic, prevention-focused, and caring philosophy embedded in the primary care approach. This seems to be a perfect opportunity for psychiatric nurses to conceptualize and define how the biopsychosocial specialty practice of psychiatric nursing will articulate with primary care.

Krauss (1993) proposes the integration of mental health promotion and mental illness prevention programs into existing primary care settings, using nursing professionals, such as psychiatric nurses, who are already well-versed in conducting such programs. Routine primary care mental health assessments of certain risk groups could prevent more serious disorders through casefinding, education, and early support (Dashiff, 1991; Gilbert, 1992; Opie et al., 1992). An increasing emphasis on such *population-based care in which problems (diagnoses) are identified and solutions (interventions) are proposed for defined populations or subpopulations,* in contrast to the individual level, is congruent with this philosophy (Williams, 1996). For example, school-based primary prevention programs for children, adolescents, and their parents, using pediatric nurse practitioners, as well as child and adolescent psychiatric clinical nurse specialists, have proved effective in promoting positive self-concept, increased self-esteem, and a decrease in conduct disorders in youth at risk and in early identification of those at risk for suicide and depression (Lamb and Puskar, 1991; McClowery, 1995).

Psychiatric nurses at the basic and advanced levels of practice should also identify other opportunities to expand the psychiatric nursing intervention role in primary care settings. As interdisciplinary provider networks that provide comprehensive health care increasingly become the norm expected by managed care companies, psychiatric nurses can also market themselves to primary care practices as those specially qualified to deliver reimbursable primary mental health care services such as crisis intervention, stress management, health teaching, medication monitoring and education, individual, group, and family therapy, and bereavement counseling in primary care settings (Haber and Billings, 1995). With their broad biopsychosocial education, psychiatric nurses are well-positioned to collaborate with their primary care and specialist colleagues to meet the psychosocial needs of clients with physical health problems or address the intervention needs of clients with mental health problems. Primary mental health care is discussed in depth in Chapter 2.

Stigmatization

The relative invisibility of mental health in the national health care debate can be linked in part to the traditional mind/body dichotomy that still influences many health and mental health practices and policy decisions. This dualistic perspective seems to result in a continuing bias against those who have mental disorders, especially those who have serious and persistent neurobiological disorders (Hoff, 1993; Krauss, 1993; Thompson, 1994). A recent study concluded that although there is more knowledge, interest, and tolerance about mental illness than existed 25 years ago, there continues to be strong resistance to locating community-based treatment and residential facilities in local neighborhoods—the "not-in-my-backyard" syndrome. There is also a punitive societal attitude toward substance abuse and substance abusers, as exemplified by the "War on Drugs," in which 70% of the money spent on substance abuse goes to law enforcement and criminal justice systems, and only 30% goes to prevention, treatment, and interventions.

The outcome for the consumer of mental health services is feelings of shame, embarassment, alienation, and "second-class citizenship." It is unclear whether this societal attitude springs from ignorance, prejudice, or simple indifference to the plight of the disadvantaged in a society increasingly polarized along class lines (Hoff, 1993). The net effect, especially for public sector clients who are "have nots," is a client population that is easily disenfranchised in terms of stigmatization, poverty, race, differential mental health benefits, lack of comprehensive and community-based care, and reduction in services (see Chapter 18).

Consumer accountability

Consumers of mental health services have been instrumental in creating a shift from a provider-driven to a consumer-driven mental health delivery system that is best exemplified by the political force exerted by the National Alliance for the Mentally Ill (NAMI), a consumer organization that educates, advocates, and lobbies on behalf of individuals and families who have a relative with a mental disorder (see Chapter 18). NAMI has state-level chapters around the country that distribute educational materials related to mental illness that are used to develop public education campaigns to educate and sensitize consumer families, educators, legislators, and policy-makers about the realities of mental illness, especially serious and persistent neurobiological disorders. They also sponsor local support groups for those with mental health problems and their families that help this consumer group feel less alone, isolated, and stigmatized. Support groups also provide a vehicle for teaching families how to manage and cope effectively with the symptoms of mental illness.

Members of NAMI and other mental health consumer organizations also have worked diligently to destigmatize the whole concept of mental illness in light of the explosion of knowledge about the neurobiological basis of such disorders. As an example of consumer power, NAMI members lobby to have these disorders, especially the serious and persistent disorders such as schizophrenia, depression, bipolar disorder, and many of the anxiety disorders, regarded as neurobiological disorders rather than mental illness or mental disorders. The term *neurobiological disorder* signifies the need to regard these disorders in an equal manner with other physical health problems that are neurobiological in nature. The economic implication of this shift would then be to lobby on behalf of parity in reimbursement for these neurobiological disorders with other "physical" neurobiological disorders such as epilepsy or multiple sclerosis. As such, you will often note the term *neurobiological disorder* or *serious and persistent neurobiological disorder* being used throughout this text, as well as more traditional labels such as mental illness and mental disorders.

Mental health consumer organizations also lobby on behalf of developing consumer partnerships with providers of mental health services. As knowledgeable consumers of mental health services, they meet with academic decision makers to define and influence change regarding the content of curricula used to educate mental health professionals in a more futuristic manner. They also meet with providers and provider organizations to influence changes and increase provider accountability in the delivery of mental health services. For example NAMI representatives meet with national and state officials who control allocation of public sector mental health funding streams to highlight the importance of community-based intensive case management programs for people with neurobiological disorders, the majority of whom use public sector mental health resources. Outcome data regarding reduction in number of annual hospital days, improvement in functional status, and quality of life are used to support the cost-effectiveness and quality of such programs for this client population and demonstrate consumer accountability (see Chapter 4).

Psychiatric nurses must be knowledgeable advocates of mental health clients who join with consumer organizations to educate the public, as well as legislators and policymakers, about neurobiological disorders so that the stigma associated with mental illness decreases. As members of interdisciplinary mental health teams, they must also role model how to develop consumer-provider partnerships that shape the creation of ethical and relevant mental health services.

Poverty and race
Poverty and race interact in a variety of ways that create access barriers for consumers to appropriate mental health services. Members of certain racial and ethnic populations, along with the poor, require flexible, culturally sensitive service systems that are tailored to consumer need rather than ones that demand that the consumer fit the system.

Studies assessing the effect of poverty on psychiatric status have shown that people who live in a climate of poverty have a twofold increased risk for an episode of at least one psychiatric disorder. Effects of poverty do not differ by gender, age, race, or history of psychiatric episode (Krauss, 1993). Poor people are more likely to develop the diseases of despair such as alcoholism, drug addiction, child abuse, and violence in the home. It is not surprising that children born into homes where these health problems are present are two to three times more likely to develop emotional or behavioral problems (McClowery, 1995). In 1991 the poverty rate in Caucasian families was 11.3%, an increase from 10.7% in 1990. Among African-American families, the poverty rate rose to 32.7%, up from 31.9% in 1990. For Hispanics the poverty rate increased to 28.7% from 28.1% in 1990. The rate of poverty for Asian Americans rose to 13.8% from 12.2% in 1990 (U.S. Bureau of the Census, 1994). As consumers of mental health care, poor families have difficulty accessing appropriate mental health services and the care provided may be of lower quality.

Use of mental health services is found to differ based on race and ethnicity. Asian Americans have a lower probability than caucasians of using emergency, inpatient, and case management services, and a higher probability of using individual and outpatient services. Their psychiatric problems are often couched as physical health problems because of the shame associated with having a mental health problem, and only as a last resort, do they seek out and use mental health services. African Americans are less likely than caucasians to use case

management and individual outpatient services, but are more likely to use emergency services. This is particularly problematic because this group tends to rely less on more continuous outpatient and case management services. Hispanic Americans have a higher probability of using case management and a lower probability of using emergency services (Briones et al., 1991; Bruce, Takeuchi, and Leaf, 1991; Hu et al., 1991).

According to a major public health document, *Healthy People 2000 Review 1994* (U.S. Department of Health and Human Services, 1995). Progress toward developing a healthier nation will depend on improvements for culturally diverse, poor, federally designated special populations that are at particular risk for developing mental health problems. These specially designated population groups are in need of targeted interventions that must be tailored to meet their unique needs and cultural experience. This issue presents a special challenge for psychiatric nurses to provide accessible, culturally sensitive, and competent care to clients of varied economic and cultural backgrounds (see Chapter 7).

Differential mental health benefits
Historically, reimbursement for mental health care has been limited and unequal to benefits for physical illnesses. Consumers of mental health services find that private insurance benefits for inpatient and outpatient mental health treatment are far less comprehensive than for physical illness. Coverage for acute treatment of mental disorders is far less than what is available for general medical treatments of clients with serious physical illness. Adequate coverage for serious and persistent, catastrophic neurobiological disorders is nonexistent, which exacerbates the public health crisis of severe mental illness in the community (Sharfstein and Stoline, 1992).

Maximum annual or lifetime benefits are lower, deductibles and copayments are higher, the percentage reimbursed is lower, and there are annual or lifetime limits on outpatient services (monetary limits or number of session limits, or limitations in types of services) that are reimbursable (Freeman and Trabin, 1994). Reimbursement for alternatives to hospitalization, such as partial hospital and day treatment programs, is variable. Many consumers with insurance pay for mental health services out-of-pocket for fear they will be denied health insurance if they change jobs and their use of mental health benefits is disclosed.

As many as 40 million Americans have no health insurance and an estimated 50 million are underinsured (Norquist, 1991). In response to inadequate coverage, some states have passed "basic benefits" legislation requiring insurance companies to include certain benefits in all insurance packages. These plans have the same high discriminatory deductibles and, in some cases, absolutely no coverage for mental disorders (Thompson, 1991).

Unlike general health care, mental health care is financed primarily through public funding streams at federal and state levels through programs such as Medicare and Medicaid. As acute mental disorders become serious and persistent, consumers lose their jobs, insurance runs out, available family financial resources are exhausted, and they switch to publicly funded resources and often, public services. Medicaid, supplemental social security income (SSSI), social security disability insurance (SSDI), and Medicare are major sources of funding for psychiatric consumers living in the community. It is estimated that eight types of mental health organizations, including state mental hospitals, private psychiatric hospitals, specialized psychiatric units in general hospitals, Veterans' Administration mental health services, residential treatment centers for emotionally disturbed children, freestanding psychiatric partial-care services, psychiatric clinics, and multiservice mental health organizations such as community mental health centers, currently receive more than $23 billion from all sources. Medicare and Medicaid contribute 20% of these funds (Mechanic and Surles, 1992). Unfortunately, up to 75% of funding for mental health services has been allocated to support inpatient treatment.

As discussed earlier in this chapter, the delivery of health care and mental health care across the nation is being remodeled as a community-based primary care delivery system. This philosophical position coupled with objectives about delivering cost-effective and quality care through capitated managed care systems will result in increased closing of inpatient public and private sector beds and reallocation of funding streams to develop and/or revitalize community-based mental health services. There will also be a need to systematically retrain and redeploy private sector, federal, and state employees, including psychiatric nurses who have spent the majority of their careers working in inpatient settings (see Chapter 20).

In general, psychiatric nurses believe that their accountability to the consumer in a reformed health care system is based on inclusion of the following in relation to mental health benefits:

- Equal availability and quality of treatment based on clinical needs, for both mental and physical health conditions
- Parity of insurance benefits for mental and physical health problems
- Access to appropriate mental health care at any point along the continuum of care in the least restrictive setting
- Risk protection for out-of-pocket expenses associated with long-term or catastrophic care
- Reimbursement to all qualified providers for appropriate care and setting, based on service, not provider

- Emphasis on consumer involvement in all aspects of mental health care delivery (Kneisl, 1994; Krauss, 1993)

As consumer advocates, psychiatric nurses enact professional role responsibilities integral with *Nursing's Social Policy Statement* (American Nurses Association [ANA], 1995) and *A Statement on Psychiatric-Mental Health Clinical Nursing Practice and Standards of Psychiatric-Mental Health Clinical Nursing Practice* (ANA, 1994). In subsequent chapters, this publication will be referred to as psychiatric-mental health nursing's *Standards.* At the local, state, and national levels, they advocate for and lobby on behalf of mental health consumers as change agents who develop relevant consumer mental health services and through political action that strives to obtain available and equitable community-based mental health services (see Chapters 2 and 3).

Outcomes

In this time of dramatically increased accountability, consumers of health care are demanding that reimbursable health care services demonstrate their effectiveness from a quality perspective, as well as their cost-effectiveness. Outcome data about mental health care and psychiatric nursing care demonstrate how these services "make a difference" in the lives of the consumers of mental health care—the clients. Such "hard evidence" about the effectiveness of psychiatric nursing treatment can be presented to consumers, employers who purchase health insurance for their employees, public and private third party payers, including managed care companies, and legislative bodies.

Outcome management programs are designed to assess (evaluate) the effectiveness of health care delivery programs and support data-based decision-making models. Goals of outcomes assessment are as follows:

- Enhancing informed decision making by providers, clients, government, and payers
- Assessing the effectiveness of different treatment interventions
- Developing standards of care and research-based treatment protocols
- Making decisions about utilization of resources

Besides measuring the utilization rates of mental health services and morbidity and mortality, mental health-related outcomes assessment is now being used to measure other aspects of client care that have always been important to psychiatric nursing, such as functional status, quality of life, cognitive functioning, social role functioning, and client satisfaction. Outcomes assessment includes both the professional's evaluation of the client and the client's assessment of his or her own well-being. It is important to include measures of the client's experience. Treatments that claim effectiveness without including the client's perspective are paternalistic (Olsen, 1995).

Evaluation of outcomes benefits consumers by providing information that helps them choose treatment methods. It constrains providers to supply ethical treatments demonstrated to be effective, protecting consumers from ineffectual or harmful treatment (Olsen, 1995). Mental health institutions will use the results of outcome assessments to guide the establishment of treatment policies, practice guidelines, and programs, and to meet the requirements of external agency reviews such as the Joint Commission on the Accreditation of Healthcare Organizations (JCAHO) and the National Committee on Quality Assurance (NCQA).

In this time of dramatically increased accountability, organizations and providers at every level are being asked to demonstrate their effectiveness with outcome data. Given that there are little outcome data about how psychiatric nurses "make a difference," psychiatric nurses will be challenged to conduct outcome research studies. They will also be challenged to develop outcome management programs that use quality assurance and quality improvement data, as well as the findings from outcome research studies, to make informed decisions about improving practice. One of the major consumer complaints about managed care programs is restricted approval of benefits or reimbursement for mental health services such as hospitalization, day treatment, home care, psychoeducation, psychotherapy sessions, and alternative healing strategies. Generation of outcome data about mental health treatment modalities and psychiatric nursing interventions would provide the basis for demonstrating and justifying the quality and cost-effectiveness of one approach versus another (see Chapter 4).

Scientific Knowledge Explosion

Major developments in the growth of scientific knowledge about neurobiology and psychoneuroimmunology have transformed our knowledge base about the biological basis of mental illness. Through advances in the neurosciences, scientists and clinicians are beginning to understand and treat biochemical, psychoneuroendocrinological, and psychoneuroimmunological dysfunctions of the brain and central nervous system that, in the past, have been viewed as disorders of the "mind" (Lowery, 1992).

Psychobiological changes

Biological psychiatry emerged with the birth of psychopharmacology in the 1950s. In the 1970s the synapse became the focus of attention, and in the 1980s, brain research grew to include the role and function of neurotransmitters in emotions and mental illness (McEnany, 1991). In the 1990s the "Decade of the Brain" was initiated by a congressional joint resolution, signed by

President George Bush in 1989, that called for the demystification of brain disorders, commonly referred to as mental illness. Supported by increased funding, psychobiological research is striving to unfold the interrelatedness of mind and body (Hayes, 1995). Psychiatric nursing, as is true of all other mental health disciplines, is entering an age of psychobiological discovery that will change its course. An in-depth presentation of psychobiological content is found in Chapters 13, 14, and 15.

Advancement in understanding the role of neurotransmitters and neuronal receptors in the formation of behavior; the psychobiology of emotions; correction of erroneous beliefs about the brain being unchangeable or irreparable after birth, or unresponsive to the environment, known as brain plasticity; and the molecular genetics of neurobiological diseases such as mood disorders are major research achievements influencing contemporary approaches to the treatment of psychobiological disorders. For example, advances into the molecular genetics of illness and gene therapy hold substantial promise for enhancing our knowledge and treating those neurobiological disorders that have been shown to be familial, such as schizophrenia, bipolar disorder, depression, and anxiety disorders. Growing evidence about the relationship between stress and immunocompetence is providing insights about the link between psychological responses to life events, depression, anxiety, and physical health problems following those events. Just as we are finding that some illnesses have a genetic *and* environmental component that puts a person at risk and influences the expression of the health problem, so too will be the case with mental disorders.

Technological changes

A growth in technology has accompanied these scientific discoveries. These discoveries enable us to examine with greater precision, the structure and function of the brain. Magnetic resonance imaging (MRI) allows access to the brain with increasing sophistication to detect structural abnormalities. Positron emission tomography (PET) and single photon emission tomography (SPEC) scans have begun to provide information about brain function that increases understanding about human behaviors and holds promise for guiding interventions with targeted client populations (Lowery, 1992; McEnany, 1991).

Just as we point to structural and functional abnormalities of the heart to explain symptoms of heart disease, so too will we be able to point to structural or functional abnormalities in the brain to explain the symptoms of mental disorders. As we move toward the twenty-first century, it will become increasingly difficult to separate mental illness as a special phenomenon from other illnesses. Because of the greater sophistication in technology involved in diagnosis and treatment of neurobiological disorders, clients will increasingly be treated in general hospitals, perhaps on neurological or neuropsychiatric units, which use many of these same technologies in the diagnosis and treatment of other illnesses. Not all parts of the mental health specialty system will disappear. Just as a need developed for specialty hospitals for cancer, some hospitals devoted to the care of those with neurobiological disorders may continue to be needed. However, they will likely take on the same high-technology characteristics as the general hospitals (Lowery, 1992).

Impact on psychiatric-mental health nursing

Interestingly, mental health professionals, generations of whom have "cut their therapeutic teeth" on psychodynamic and psychosocial approaches to the treatment of mental disorders, have been slow to accept the science and technology that began to emerge as early as the 1970s. Perhaps the dizzying speed with which so many of these discoveries occurred in the 1980s created a knowledge gap about how to fit the biological dimension with the psychosocial dimension to achieve biopsychosocial integration and usefulness in clinical practice. Clearly, psychobiological discoveries will continue to unfold and influence clinical practice as we move toward the twenty-first century.

For over 40 years, the specialty of psychiatric nursing has demonstrated leadership in developing clinical practice, professional autonomy, political activism, and nursing theory development (McBride, 1990). At a time of dramatic change in the health care and mental health care landscape and a decrease in the percentage of nurses employed in psychiatric settings, we must ask what direction psychiatric nurses at the basic and advanced levels of practice must take to thrive in the 1990s and beyond. It is a given that a holistic approach to psychiatric nursing practice is integral with defining that direction. Essential to that process is a quest to examine and acquire a psychobiological knowledge base that can be integrated into a biopsychosocial practice-education-research framework that can be used to define a cutting-edge role for psychiatric nursing.

Pragmatically, this means that psychiatric nurses must do the following:

- Recognize the value and importance of the psychobiological knowledge domain
- Demonstrate a willingness to acquire a psychobiological knowledge base through undergraduate and graduate education programs, and staff development and continuing education offerings
- Demonstrate competence in physical assessment
- Acquire a psychopharmacological knowledge base and competence in medication administration, monitoring, and client education
- Demonstrate prescribing competence as an advanced practice psychiatric nurse to exercise prescriptive authority

- Synthesize psychobiological knowledge with psychopharmacological knowledge
- Use psychobiological data about neurobiological disorders to guide the development and/or selection of intervention strategies
- Integrate psychobiological knowledge and intervention strategies with psychosocial knowledge and intervention strategies to create a holistic philosophy about psychiatric nursing practice
- Demonstrate biopsychosocial competence as an interdisciplinary team member
- Obtain appropriate professional credentialing

Psychiatric nursing is on the threshold of an exhilarating biopsychosocial future that incorporates the psychobiological knowledge explosion. Although the biological knowledge explosion is exciting, psychosocial competence must remain valued in psychiatric nursing. Psychiatric nurses and their interdisciplinary mental health colleagues must become knowledgeable psychobiological clinicians. However, they must also renew their commitment to communicating therapeutically with clients and their families while attending to the biological and nonbiological contributors to mental disorders and their expression. We must ensure that the quality and human side of mental health treatment is not ignored or sacrificed by psychiatric nursing in the name of cost-effectiveness (Pollock, 1995). It is the belief of the editors of this textbook that a comprehensive biopsychosocial approach should be the hallmark of psychiatric nursing.

SPECULATIONS ABOUT THE TWENTY-FIRST CENTURY AND BEYOND

As we move toward the year 2000 and beyond, psychiatric-mental health nursing will have to take stock of itself, as well as its practice, education, and research, if it is to successfully prepare to meet the challenges of changes in the delivery of mental health care. Psychiatric-mental health nursing will need to rethink its agendas in light of new science and technology and transformational change in the mental health delivery system. In the next century, we will need to rethink the basics of psychiatric-mental health nursing care and the leadership roles of psychiatric nurses as we unfold a prevention-oriented, community-based primary care health care delivery system. Psychiatric-mental health nurses will need to be at the forefront in defining and advocating for a delivery system that values psychobiology, yet listens to clients and families, and that understands the importance of technology in providing diagnostic and treatment insights, yet respects the significance of comprehensive and continuous mental health care that includes prevention, education, and community support systems (Sharfstein, Stoline, and Koran, 1995). Above all, we must respect the judicious allocation of mental health resources but not compromise our ethical commitment to quality. Those are the challenges before us. . . . As you read each chapter of this book, you *will* discover how to make this challenge a reality.

KEY POINTS

- Driving forces creating a paradigm shift that contribute to a revolution in the delivery of mental health services are as follows: economic forces, conceptualization of health care delivery, consumer accountability, and developments in scientific knowledge.
- Economic forces contributing to restructuring of mental health service delivery include workplace redesign, managed care (managing benefits, care, and health), and changes in reimbursement mechanisms from individual fee-for-service models to population-based capitation models.
- Remodeling health care delivery is exemplified by a shift to a wellness-focused, prevention-oriented, community-based primary care system that delivers continuous, coordinated health care addressing the majority of personal health needs of individuals within a family and community context.
- Vertically integrated delivery systems will link all levels of care that are needed by a defined population.
- Consumer accountability is a broad concept that is addressed by examining issues such as stigmatization, poverty and race, differential mental health benefits, and outcomes. Measurement of outcomes involves the conduct of outcomes research as well as establishment of outcomes management programs.
- The scientific knowledge explosion is exemplified by a cascade of discoveries in the neurosciences that are manifested by psychobiological insights that guide the development and targeting of clinical interventions. Technological growth enables us to examine with greater precision, the structure and function of the brain leading to more accurate assessment, diagnosis, and treatment planning.
- Psychiatric-mental health nurses are challenged to become knowledgeable psychobiological clinicians who are equally challenged to renew their commitment to the psychosocial dimensions of client care. A comprehensive biopsychosocial approach should be the hallmark of psychiatric-mental health nursing.

 CRITICAL THINKING QUESTIONS

June, a student nurse, is at the beginning of a 7-week clinical rotation in psychiatric-mental health nursing. She is currently on an inpatient psychiatric admitting unit in a large public sector city hospital for 2 weeks. June overhears the nurses on the unit complaining about the very brief length of stay for clients, the overuse of somatic treatments such as medications and along with the short length of stay, the lack of time to develop a trusting nurse-client relationship using therapeutic communication. She hears the nurses "blame" these changes on managed care, changes in reimbursement, and all of this science coming out of the NIMH. As a student nurse, June is concerned about the forces creating those changes the nurses were talking about. She wonders whether clients, as mental health consumers, are receiving ethical treatment. June also worries about the future of psychiatric-mental health nursing, a career path she is seriously considering.

1. How would June determine the accuracy of the comments she overhears the nurses discussing?
2. How would June articulate the major forces shaping the delivery of mental health services?
3. How could she view these forces as opportunities rather than threats?
4. What strategies would June use to determine whether clients in a managed care system that used capitated reimbursement mechanisms were receiving ethical treatment?
5. For June to have a state-of-the-art image of psychiatric nursing practice, what other kinds of clinical settings would be helpful for the rest of her clinical experience?
6. How would June conceptualize the value/role of psychobiology in psychiatric nursing practice?

REFERENCES

Aiken, L.H., & Sage, W.M. (1993). Staffing national health care reform: A role for advanced practice nurses. *Akron Law Review, 26,* 1-30.

American Nurses Association (1995). *Nursing's social policy statement.* Washington, DC: American Nurses Publishing.

American Nurses Association. (1994). *A statement on psychiatric-mental health nursing practice and standards of psychiatric-mental health nursing practice.* Washington, DC: Author.

Bell, C.C. (1993). The new community psychiatry in 2000 AD. *Hospital and Community Psychiatry, 44,* 9, 815.

Briones, D., Heller, P., Chalfant, H.P., Roberts, A., Aguirre-Hauchbaum, J., & Farr, W. (1990). Socioeconomic status, ethnicity, psychological distress, and readiness to utilize a mental health facility. *American Journal of Psychiatry, 147,* 10, 1333-1339.

Bruce, M., Takeuchi, D., & Leaf, P. (1991). Poverty and psychiatric status. *Archives of General Psychiatry, 48,* 470-474.

Cole, R.E., Reed, S.K., Babigian, H.M., Brown, S.W., & Fray, J. (1994). A mental health capitation program: I. patient outcomes. *Hospital and Community Psychiatry, 45,* 11, 1090-1096.

Dashiff, C. (1991). Marital strife, social support, and the development of mentally retarded toddlers. *Journal of Child and Adolescent Psychiatric and Mental Health Nursing, 4,* 3, 90-95.

Division of Social and Community Psychiatry. (1993). *Hospital without walls,* Durham NC: Department of Psychiatry, Duke University Medical Center.

Eisenberg, L. (1992). Treating depression and anxiety in the primary care setting. *Health Affairs, 11:3,* 149-156.

Freeman, M.A., & Trabin, T. (1994). *Managed behavioral healthcare: History, models, key issues, and future course.* Washington, DC: U.S. Center for Mental Health Services, Department of Health and Human Services.

Gilbert, C. (1992). Sibling incest: A descriptive study of family dynamics. *Journal of Child and Adolescent Psychiatric and Mental Health Nursing, 5:1,* 5-9.

Haber, J. (1996). Managing managed care. *Journal of the American Psychiatric Nurses Association, 2:3,* 101-103.

Haber, J., & Billings, C.V. (1995). Primary mental health care: A model for psychiatric-mental health nursing. *Journal of the American Psychiatric Nurses Association, 1,* 5, 165-174.

Hayes, A. (1995). Psychiatric nursing: What does biology have to do with it? *Archives of Psychiatric Nursing, IX:* 4, 216-224.

Hellwig, K. (1993). Psychiatric home care nursing: Managing patients in the community. *Journal of Psychosocial Nursing, 31:* 12, 21-24.

Hoff, L.A. (1993). Health policy and the plight of the mentally ill. *Psychiatry, 56,* 11, 400-419.

Hu, T., Snowden, L., Jerrel, J., & Nguyen, T. (1991). Ethnic populations in public mental health: Services choice and level of use. *American Journal of Public Health, 81,* 11, 1429-1434.

Institute of Medicine (1994). *Defining primary care: An interim report.* Washington, DC: National Academy Press.

Kneisl, C.R. (1994). On the brink of health care reform: Vital issues for psychiatric-mental health nurses. *Capsules & Comments in Psychiatric Nursing, 1,* 2, 4-17.

Krauss, J.B. (1993). *Health care reform: Essential mental health services.* Washington, DC: American Nurses Publishing.

Lamb, J., & Pusker, K. (1991). School-based adolescent mental health project survey of depression, suicidal ideation, and anger. *Journal of Child and Adolescent Psychiatric and Mental Health Nursing, 4,* 3, 101-104.

Lowery, B.J. (1992). Psychiatric nursing in the 1990s and beyond. *Journal of Psychosocial Nursing, 30,* 1, 7-13.

Marion, L.N. (1996). *Nursing's vision for primary health care.* Washington, DC: American Nurses Publishing.

McBride, A.B. (1990). Psychiatric nursing in the 1990s. *Archives of Psychiatric Nursing, IV,* 1, 21-28.

McClowery, S.G. (1995). The prevention of mental disorders in children. *Capsules and Comments in Pediatric Nursing, 1,* 1, 13-19.

McEnany, G. (1991). Psychobiology and psychiatric nursing: A philosophical matrix. *Archives of Psychiatric Nursing, V,* 5, 255-261.

McGihon, N.N. (1994). Health care reform: Clinical implications for inpatient psychiatric nursing. *Journal of Psychosocial Nursing, 32,* 10, 31-33.

Mechanic, D., & Surles, R. (1992). Challenges in state mental health policy and administration. *Health Affairs, 11,* 3, 34-50.

Mechanic, D., Schlesinger, M., & McAlpine, D.D. (1995). Management of mental health and substance abuse services: State of the art and early results. *Millbank Quarterly, 73,* 1, 19-74.

Moller, M.D. (1994, October). *The three R's program: Relapse, recovery, and rehabilitation.* Paper presented at the 8th Annual American Psychiatric Nurses Association Meeting, San Antonio, TX.

Montano, C.B. (1994). Recognition and treatment of depression in a primary care setting. *Journal of Clinical Psychiatry, 55:* 12, 18-34.

Mrazek, P.J., & Haggerty, R.J. (1994). *Reducing risks for mental disorders.* Washington, DC: National Academy Press.

Murphy, M.P., & Moller, M.D. (1993). Relapse management in neurobiological disorders: The Moller-Murphy symptom management assessment tool. *Archives of Psychiatric Nursing, 7,* 4, 226-235.

National Institute of Mental Health. (1993). *Health care reform for Americans with severe mental illness: Report of the national advisory mental health council.* Rockville, MD: Author.

Norquist, G., & Wells, K. (1991). Mental health needs of the uninsured. *Archives of General Psychiatry, 48,* 475-478.

Olsen, D.P. (1995). Ethical cautions in the use of outcomes for resource allocation in the managed care environment of mental health. *Archives of Psychiatric Nursing, IX,* 4, 173-178.

Opie, N., Goodwin, T., Finke, L., Beatty, J., Lee, B., & Van Epps, J. (1992). The effect of a bereavement group experience on bereaved children's and adolescents' affective and somatic distress. *Journal of Child and Adolescent Psychiatric Mental Health Nursing, 5,* 1, 20-26.

Pinsof, W.M., & Wynne, L.C. (1995). The effectiveness and efficacy of marital and family therapy: Introduction to the special issue. *Journal of Marital and Family Therapy, 21,* 4, 341-343.

Pollock, E.J. (1995, December 1). Managed care's focus on psychiatric drugs alarms many doctors. *The Wall Street Journal,* pp. 1, 23.

Reed, S.K., Hennessy, K.D., Mitchell, O.S., & Babigian, H.M. (1994). A mental health capitation program: II. cost-benefit analysis. *Hospital and Community Psychiatry, 45,* 11, 1097-1103.

Sharfstein, S.S. (1994). Capitation versus decapitation in mental health care. *Hospital and Community Psychiatry, 45,* 11, 1065.

Sharfstein, S.S., & Stoline, A.M. (1992). Reform issues for insuring mental health care. *Health Affairs, 11,* 3, 84-97.

Sharfstein, S.S., Stoline, A.M., & Koran, L. (1995). Mental health services. In A.R. Kovner (Ed.), *Jonas's Health Care Delivery in the United States.* New York: Springer.

Shore, M., & Dickey, B. (1991). The dimensions of the challenge. In *Mental health services in the United States and England: Struggling for change.* Princeton, NJ: Robert Wood Johnson Foundation.

Smoyak, S.A. (1991). Psychosocial nursing in public versus private sectors: An introduction. *Journal of Psychosocial Nursing, 29,* 8, 6-12.

Strickland, D. (1994). The future of guidelines. *Business and Health Special Report, 22,* 3, 27-30.

Thompson, C.P. (1991, July 29). *Statement of the American Psychiatric Association on State-Mandated Benefits and Mental Health Coverage.* Testimony to Subcommittee on Health, Committee on Ways and Means, U.S. House of Representatives, Washington, DC: U.S. Government Printing Office.

Thompson, J.W. (1994). Trends in the development of psychiatric services, 1844-1994. *Hospital and Community Psychiatry, 45:* 10, 987-992.

U.S. Bureau of the Census. (1994). *Current population reports.* Washington, DC: U.S. Government Printing Office.

U.S. Department of Health and Human Services. (1995). *Healthy people 2000 review 1994.* (DHHS Publication No. (PH5) 95-1256-1). Washington D.C.: Author.

Williams, C.A. (1996). Community-based population-focused practice: The foundation of specialization in public health nursing. In M. Stanhope & J. Lancaster (Eds.), *Community Health Nursing: Processes and Practice for Promoting Health* (3rd ed.). St. Louis: Mosby.

Worley, N., Drago, L., & Hadley, T. (1990). Improving the physical health-mental health interface for the chronically mentally ill: Could nurse case managers make a difference? *Archives of Psychiatric Nursing, 4,* 2, 108-113.

Chapter 2

Psychiatric-Mental Health Nursing: 2000 and Beyond

Carolyn Veronica Billings

LEARNING OUTCOMES

After studying and applying concepts of this chapter, the learner will be able to:

- Differentiate the unique aspects of psychiatric-mental health nursing that distinguish it from other mental health care professions.
- Describe the roles and functions of the basic and advanced psychiatric-mental health nurse.
- Identify the advances and developments in the field of mental health that directly affect psychiatric nursing practice.
- Discuss the relationship between changes in society and the need for changes in mental health service delivery.
- Discuss the anticipated changes in psychiatric nursing practice as mental health services evolve into the twenty-first century.
- Identify future challenges for psychiatric nursing.

KEY TERMS

Advanced practice registered nurse	Prevention interventions	Psychiatric-mental health nurse
Holism	Primary mental health care	State Nurse Practice Act

The psychiatric-mental health nursing literature sparkles with the pride, dedication, and excitement that psychiatric nurses feel about their specialty. It is not difficult to speculate why these nurses are so passionate and sentimental about their practice—perhaps it is the sense these nurses have that they truly *can* make a difference or the strong sense of intimacy that comes with working so closely with people's private thoughts and emotions. Perhaps it is because so many psychiatric nurses have gone on to become recognized leaders in health care and in the nursing profession as a whole. Perhaps it is because the opportunity to study human emotions, thoughts, and actions provides each of us with an opportunity to become the best we can be. Perhaps it is because psychiatric nursing has always been on the cutting edge of change—and no less now than before. The shifting sands of health care are creating new pathways—pathways with danger and excitement, crises and opportunities. For psychiatric nurses, these pathways open up possibilities for a journey into a future that means more hope for those with mental illnesses, more options for ways to express ourselves through our practice, more alternative locations where we can bring our services directly to the consumers, and an even greater potential for being all that we can be and doing all that we can do.

The purpose of this chapter is to help the learner appreciate the core values of psychiatric nursing, and how psychiatric nurses make a difference in the lives of the people they serve. Based on the rapidly occurring changes in health care delivery systems, it discusses some of the changes expected to influence psychiatric nursing in the future, and features, roles, functions, and resources that psychiatric nurses have to offer as mental health care in this country continues to evolve.

AN UNDERSTANDING OF NURSING

When Florence Nightingale, the founder of modern nursing, wrote *Notes on Nursing* in 1859, she expressed her belief that nursing is in charge of the personal health of somebody. "What nursing has to do", she stated, "[is to] put the patient in the best condition for nature to act upon him" (Nightingale, 1859). Hildegard Peplau, often referred to as the "mother of psychiatric nursing," defined nursing as a "human relationship between an individual who is sick, or in need of health services and a nurse especially educated to recognize and to respond to the need for help." She referred to nursing as a significant therapeutic, interpersonal process (Peplau, 1952). In 1966, Virginia Henderson wrote a definitive text on nursing entitled, *The Nature of Nursing*. In it she stated, "The unique function of nursing is to assist the individual, sick or well, in the performance of those activities contributing to health or its recovery (or to a peaceful death) that he could perform unaided if he had the necessary strength, will, or knowledge. And to do this in such a way as to help him gain independence as rapidly as possible" (Henderson, 1966). Henderson's definition was so widely embraced that it currently is used as the international definition of nursing. In the words of Martha Rogers, a noted nursing theorist, "Nursing's story is a magnificent epic of service to humankind. It is about people: how they are born, and live, and die; in health and in sickness; in joy and in sorrow. Its mission is the translation of knowledge into human service" (Rogers, 1966). In 1995 the American Nurses Association (ANA) defined nursing as "the diagnosis and treatment of human responses to actual or potential health problems" (ANA, 1995). Echoing the ideas already expressed in the nursing literature, this definition calls attention to a focus on *how persons respond to conditions of health and illness,* not just to the illnesses themselves.

Nursing is a practice discipline. It becomes as it is being done. It is ever-evolving and changes as scientific discovery opens up new avenues for the prevention and treatment of health problems. Thirty years ago, nurses did not draw blood or start intravenous (IV) lines, and no nurse had the legal authority to prescribe medications. Today, nurses routinely carry out activities that were not regarded as nursing functions in the past. Tomorrow's nurses also will experience increased privileges and a even wider range of intervention capabilities.

What Makes Psychiatric Nursing Unique?

Perhaps the most significant difference between psychiatric nursing and the other mental health care disciplines is the consistent emphasis on holism. Psychiatric nursing's philosophical stance is to take into account the biological, psychological, sociological, spiritual, and cultural dimensions of humans in interaction with their physical and social environment (Feild and Winslow, 1985). This commitment to the whole person in psychiatric nursing is drawn directly from the holistic perspective, which is a hallmark concept for the nursing profession in general. Fig. 2-1 illustrates the manner in which nursing's comprehensive approach provides the horizontal thread that brings into focus the individual person as a multifaceted human being.

Psychiatric Nursing as We Know It

Psychiatric nursing is nursing, as it has been defined, practiced in application to populations at risk for, experiencing, or recovering from mental health problems. It incorporates knowledge of the many characteristics that constitute mental health and seeks to help optimize those characteristics in individuals and in their societies. In its first *Statement on Psychiatric Nursing Practice* the ANA (1967) described psychiatric nursing as a spe-

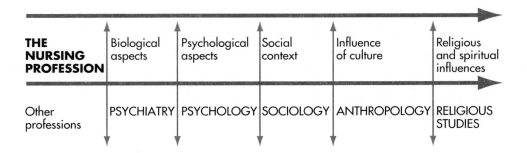

Fig. 2-1 Nursing's holistic perspective of human health and illness.

Box 2-1

Phenomena of Concern in Psychiatric-Mental Health Nursing

These phenomena include actual or potential health problems of clients pertaining to:
- The maintenance of optimal health and well-being and the prevention of psychobiological illness
- Self-care limitations or impaired functioning related to mental and emotional distress
- Deficits in the functioning of significant biological, emotional, and cognitive systems
- Emotional stress of crisis components of illness, pain, and disability
- Self-concept changes, developmental issues, and life process changes
- Problems related to emotions such as anxiety, anger, sadness, loneliness, and grief

- Physical symptoms that occur along with altered psychological functioning
- Alterations in thinking, perceiving, symbolizing, communicating, and decision making
- Difficulties in relating to others
- Behaviors and mental states that indicate that the client is a danger to self or others or has a severe disability
- Interpersonal, systemic, sociocultural, spiritual, or environmental circumstances or events that affect the mental and emotional well-being of the individual, family, or community
- Symptom management, side effects/toxicities associated with psychopharmacological intervention and other aspects of the treatment regimen

From American Nurses Association. (1994). A statement on psychiatric-mental health clinical nursing practice and standards of psychiatric-mental health clinical nursing practice. *Washington, DC: American Nurses Publishing.*

cialized area of practice in the science and art of nursing. The landmark document further observed that the *science* of psychiatric nursing is applied as new and complex theories of human behaviors are developed, and the performance of the art occurs in the purposeful use of self. It was stressed that psychiatric nursing uses a broad spectrum of knowledge in a variety of settings with different psychiatric approaches to care (ANA, 1967). In keeping with the current ANA definition of nursing, in 1994 the Coalition of Psychiatric Nursing Organizations defined psychiatric-mental nursing as "the diagnosis and treatment of human responses to actual or potential *mental* health problems" (ANA, 1994b). Box 2-1 shows the phenomena of concern for psychiatric nursing.

The Holistic Perspective in Action

It is nursing's focus on **holism,** or *the belief that the human being is a unified whole possessing individual in-*

tegrity and manifesting characteristics that are more than and different from the sum of the parts (Rogers, 1970), that offers so much opportunity and so much excitement to psychiatric nursing in the twenty-first century. Although the holistic paradigm has been a hallmark of nursing since the beginning, until recently, psychiatric nursing has not always recognized the biological aspects of health and illness with the same level of interest and involvement as it has the psychological and social perspectives (Drew, 1988). This tendency to be concerned primarily with psychosocial behavior also has been consistent with trends in the field of mental health. Theory in modern psychiatry has shifted from the intrapersonal (within the person) to the interpersonal (within the family/societal system) to the current emphasis on neuroscience, endocrinology, immunology, biochemistry, and genetics. This surge of interest in the biological perspective comes as a result of scientific advances that demon-

Box 2-2

Psychiatric Nursing's Multifaceted Approach to Mental Health Problems

- Analytical and psychodynamic approaches, therapeutic communication
- Art, music, drama, laughter, poetry, pet therapy
- Case management, psychoeducational approaches, bibliotherapy, relapse management
- Cognitive-behavioral, solution-focused, problem-oriented, and brief therapies; crisis intervention; counseling; critical incident stress debriefing
- Genetic, nutritional, and health counseling
- Exercise, dance movement, rolfing

- Healing crystals, therapeutic touch, light therapy
- Hypnosis, trance, neurolinguistic programming, metaphors, relaxation, visual imagery, meditation, reminiscence
- Interactional, transactional, milieu, environmental approaches
- Monitoring effects of psychoactive medication using biobehavioral, pharmacokinetic, and psychopharmacological knowledge
- Prescribing psychoactive medications (advanced practice)

strate the interrelationship between brain, behavior, emotion, and cognition (Abraham, Fox, and Cohen, 1992).

In the field of mental health, the 1990s have been referred to as the "Decade of the Brain," as fast-breaking discoveries are linking biochemistry with human behavior and conditions of mental health and illness. Nevertheless, there are competing opinions about the current movement to "medicalize" mental disorders with those from competing schools of thought who continue to emphasize the importance of psychological, sociological, spiritual, environmental, and/or cultural influences (Peplau, 1995). Some psychiatric nurses have cited the dangers of a wholesale endorsement of the biological aspects of psychiatry to the exclusion or diminishment of the relevance of psychosocial influences (Lego, 1992; Liaschenko, 1989). These and other authors, (McBride, 1990; Abraham, Fox, and Cohen, 1992) stress the importance of maintaining a holistic perspective on mind-body interaction, which highlights the art of psychiatric nursing, as well as the science. With the mental health treatment pendulum swinging from an almost exclusive concentration on psychosocial origins and approaches to mental disorders to an almost exclusive concentration on psychopharmacological remedies, psychiatric nursing has much to offer in advocating a reasoned balance that takes the total person into consideration (Pothier, 1990). One of the most exciting aspects of psychiatric nursing today is the continuing steady stream of creative and innovative interventions that are part of nursing's multifaceted approach to understanding and treating mental health problems (Box 2-2).

GUIDANCE FOR PRACTICE

What exactly is nursing practice, and what exactly can nurses do? The answer to this question can be found in the legal definition and rules and regulations specific to

each state and in professional statements about the scope of nursing practice, the code of ethics, and the general and specialty standards that guide and direct the nurse with regard to practice. These materials form what is sometimes described as a kind of social contract between nurses and consumers of nursing services.

The ***State Nurse Practice Act*** *is the legal document that defines nursing and regulates nursing practice in each state.* Practice acts vary from state to state and the legal scope of nursing practice may differ from one to another. Some state practice acts address nursing practice in general, whereas others address the boundaries of basic and advanced practice separately. In addition, the current elements of nursing practice are defined by certain professional documents published by the American Nurses Association (ANA), which direct, guide, or inform clinical practice. These include nursing's *Social Policy Statement* (ANA, 1995) the *Code for Nurses,* (ANA, 1985) and the *ANA Standards of Clinical Nursing Practice* (ANA, 1991). A significant publication, that applies to psychiatric nursing in particular, is *A Statement on Psychiatric-Mental Health Clinical Nursing Practice* and *Standards of Psychiatric-Mental Health Clinical Nursing Practice* (ANA, 1994a). This publication is the collaborative work of the national organizations representing the specialty (Box 2-3) and as such reflects the combined thinking of recognized leaders in the field of psychiatric-mental health nursing.

A PORTRAIT OF PSYCHIATRIC-MENTAL HEALTH NURSING PRACTICE

Levels of Psychiatric-Mental Health Nursing Practice

Psychiatric-mental health nurses are registered nurses who are educationally prepared in nursing, have recog-

Box 2-3

National Psychiatric Nursing Organizations

American Psychiatric Nurses Association (APNA)
1200 19th Street, N.W., Suite 300
Washington, DC 20036-2401

Association of Child and Adolescent Psychiatric Nurses (ACAPN)
1211 Locust Street
Philadelphia, PA 19107

International Society of Psychiatric Consultation-Liaison Nurses (ISPCLN)
237 Twin Bay Drive
Pensacola, FL 32534-1350

Society for Education and Research in Psychiatric-Mental Health Nursing (SERPN)
237 Twin Bay Drive
Pensacola, FL 32534-1350

nized experience in the specialty, and are licensed to practice in their individual states. Psychiatric nursing is practiced at two levels: basic and advanced. These levels of practice are determined on the basis of education, knowledge, and experience in the specialty, and professional certification.

Basic level

Psychiatric-mental health nurses are the largest group of mental health care providers. They bring specialized knowledge, skills, and abilities to the care of individuals, families, groups, and communities with mental health needs. They assess mental and emotional functioning, develop diagnoses, and formulate plans of care. They provide direct care services and coach, instruct, counsel, and guide their clients toward mental health goals. They su-

pervise other mental health workers, provide comprehensive case coordination, and establish and maintain links with other health services. They work in diverse settings with a wide range of populations to promote mental health and prevent mental illness. Their nursing background prepares them to understand the biological and psychosocial components of health and illness and to monitor physical status and emotional well-being. They are qualified to intervene in health crises and to evaluate the effects and the effectiveness of prescribed pharmacological agents.

The title used to describe the nurse who is certified to practice at the basic level in the specialty is *psychiatric-mental health nurse. These registered nurses (RNs) are educationally prepared in nursing with a baccalaureate degree and have demonstrated through a certification process that they have met the profession's stated requirements, including knowledge about psychiatric-mental health nursing and experience caring for clients with mental health problems.* Certification requirements for the psychiatric-mental health nurse are listed in Box 2-4. The letter "C" placed after the RN (RN,C) is the designation that demonstrates that the nurse is certified at the basic level. Although employers do not always require certification or experience to work as a nurse in a psychiatric setting, completion of the certification process is the profession's way of validating an individual nurse's qualifications, knowledge, and practice in a designated specialty area of nursing. Nurses who work in psychiatric settings and who are novices in the specialty, are entry-level RNs, or are not yet certified, practice in conjunction with psychiatric-mental health nurses and are equally accountable to the specialty practice nursing standards.

Advanced level

The term *advanced practice registered nurse (APRN)* is an *umbrella category used to describe nurses with graduate-level education who may be separately recognized in the practice acts of their states and who are prepared to function in advanced nursing roles with a high degree of autonomy.* This category generally

Box 2-4

Eligibility Requirements for Certification as a Psychiatric-Mental Health Nurse

- Licensure as a registered nurse in the United States or its territories
- A specified amount of direct practice experience in psychiatric-mental health nursing
- Current involvement in direct psychiatric-mental health nursing practice for a minimum time period within a stated time frame

- Access to clinical consultation/supervision with an experienced mental health colleague
- Endorsement from a nurse colleague
- Completion of a specified number of contact hours of continuing education directly related to the psychiatric-mental health field
- Successful completion of a national certifying examination

Box 2-5

Eligibility Requirements for Certification as a Specialist in Psychiatric-Mental Health Nursing

- Current licensure as a registered nurse in the United States or its territories
- A master's degree or higher in nursing with a specialized focus in psychiatric-mental health theory and practice
- Current involvement in direct patient contact in psychiatric-mental health nursing for a specified minimum number of hours per week
- Current, ongoing clinical consultation/supervision with an experienced, qualified mental health colleague

- A specified number of hours of direct advanced clinical practice of psychiatric-mental health nursing during and/or after the master's program of study
- Documented designated number of hours of clinical consultation/supervision by an approved consultant/supervisor with an endorsement from the supervisor (the majority of the consultation/supervision must have been with a qualified nurse peer)
- Successful completion of a national certifying examination

includes clinical nurse specialists, nurse anesthetists, nurse midwives, and nurse practitioners.

Advanced level *psychiatric* nurses are licensed RNs educationally prepared at the master's level. The title used to refer to the certified advanced practice registered nurse within the specialty is *certified specialist in psychiatric-mental health nursing (RN,CS)*. (In some states, these advanced practice registered nurses are referred to in the practice act of their states as psychiatric nurse practitioners.) The requirements for certification as a specialist are listed in Box 2-5.

The certifying body for psychiatric-mental health nurses at both levels of practice is the American Nurses Credentialing Center, a subsidiary of the ANA (American Nurses Credentialing Center, 1996). Certification is renewed on a periodic basis through demonstration of appropriate contact hours of continuing education in the specialty or by reexamination.

Psychiatric-Mental Health Nursing Roles and Functions

According to the *Statement on Psychiatric-Mental Health Clinical Nursing Practice* (ANA, 1994a) as a primary mental health care provider, the psychiatric-mental health nurse works with clients to:

- Maintain health and prevent illness
- Screen for physical and mental health problems, and evaluate the need for additional health care services
- Provide case management to assist the clients in using available resources and monitor their effectiveness
- Encourage and assist clients in activities of daily living (ADLs) such as personal hygiene and feeding or the development of community living skills such as using public transportation or locating appropriate housing

- Teach clients about those aspects of living that influence wellness such as self-care, or specific information about mental illness, relapse, and methods of treatment including medications
- Employ psychobiological interventions such as nutrition/diet regulation, exercise/rest schedules, somatic treatments like light therapy or relaxation and monitor the effects of treatment regimens like psychoactive medication or electroconvulsive therapy
- Initiate direct crisis intervention services
- Offer counseling about health problems
- Follow clients in other settings such as the home to assist with or to monitor their health-related needs
- Use the therapeutic potential in the client's environment or milieu in designing or providing care services
- Act within the community to assure appropriate resources and to instigate changes that address the mental health needs of the population
- Continually advocate for the needs of individual clients and for the population of those with mental disorders and their families

The role of the psychiatric-mental health advanced practice registered nurse also incorporates additional psychobiological and psychotherapeutic interventions involved in the diagnosis and treatment of mental disorders. In an increasing number of states, this will include the authority to prescribe psychoactive medications and adjunctive pharmacological agents, which reduce side effects, and to order diagnostic and laboratory tests. Prescriptive practice authority is designated by state statutes or state agency rules and regulations. The arrangement for nurses to prescribe may be "complementary." This means that the nurse is accountable to a physician, and there are defined mechanisms for supervision of the prescriptive activities (or "substitutive," in which the nurse prescribes) under the authority of the State Board of

Nursing, without requirements of responsibility to any other discipline (Talley and Brooke, 1992).

Advanced practice psychiatric-mental health nurses also have expertise in various psychotherapy modalities and are qualified on the basis of their education and experience to offer individual, couple/family, and group psychotherapy. The standards of practice in the specialty identify the psychotherapies as advanced practice nursing interventions (ANA, 1994a).

The clinical practice of the advanced practice psychiatric-mental health nurse is distinguished by an increased depth of knowledge and a more refined ability to apply such knowledge to the anticipation, identification, and resolution of mental health problems in either individuals or for society at large.

Advanced practice psychiatric-mental health nurses are prepared to conduct comprehensive health and illness assessments and demonstrate competence in the diagnosis and treatment of responses of individuals, families, groups, and communities to actual or potential health problems. They possess a high degree of proficiency in therapeutic and interpersonal skills, and deal with a wide range of complex mental health problems in a variety of settings. The roles of the advanced practice registered nurse include consultation, education, leadership, management, and research, in addition to clinical nursing practice.

THE PROSPECT OF CHANGE: NEW POSSIBILITIES

Certain trends are already beginning to influence the delivery of mental health care. In response to criticisms about the philosophy and cost of health care, the 1990s have witnessed an almost revolutionary upheaval in the delivery of health care and mental health services. This includes a reassessment of the populations in need of services (for whom?); a turnabout in the locations for service delivery (where?); and an adjustment with regard to the types of services (what?).

Psychiatric-Mental Health Nursing: For Whom?

The need for psychiatric and mental health services in this country persists. It is believed that one in three American adults meets the diagnostic criteria for a mental disorder at some point in life (National Institute of Mental Health [NIMH], 1991) and at least 12% of children under age 18 suffer one or more mental disorders (National Advisory Mental Health Council, 1990).

Demographic and societal changes in the United States have brought about dramatic differences that severely affect general and mental health services. Among the most notable population shifts is a rapid expansion of the numbers of older adults, ethnic minorities, the economically deprived, and the educationally disadvantaged. There is an increase in the occurrence of chronic illnesses such as acquired immunodeficiency syndrome (AIDS) and Alzheimer's disease. There is a widespread outbreak of social problems related to mental health such as homelessness, poverty, substance abuse, and violence. In addition, consumer advocacy groups such as the National Alliance for the Mentally Ill (NAMI) and concerned provider groups like the ANA have vigorously advocated for greater access to essential mental health services for underserved populations, especially those adults and children with, or at risk for, severe, persistent mental illnesses (Pothier, 1988; Krauss, 1989; Krauss, 1993). Responsiveness to these developing populations, and special needs, will significantly influence the future of psychiatric nursing.

Psychiatric-Mental Health Nursing: Where?

The introduction of managed care, a second look at the cost of health care benefits, and a questioning of the emphasis on illness care has contributed to fewer inpatient psychiatric hospitalizations and shorter hospital stays. During recent years the majority of psychiatric nurses has worked primarily in public or private acute care institutions or hospitals. The traditional approach to the treatment of mental illnesses has been repeated admissions to an acute care facility, where symptoms are stabilized with medications and clients are often discharged without follow-up care in the community. This fragmented and symptomatic treatment has been referred to as the "revolving door" of the mental health system (Betrus and Hoffman, 1992). Although the majority of those with long-standing mental illnesses are actually in the community, a successful pattern of continuing care outside of a hospital has not yet been achieved for most of this population.

Community-based care

In the last 10 years, there has been a tremendous surge of appeal for a major redesign of mental health services in this country, centering around a concentrated effort to provide them in community-based locations. Attention has focused, for example, on the need for integration of mental-health promotion and mental-illness prevention programs, as well as early case finding into existing primary care settings (Krauss, 1993) (see Chapter 1). The development of new service settings such as group homes, nursing homes, and other residences; nontraditional locations such as churches, clubs, shelters, jails, bus or train stations; and soup kitchens for disenfranchised persons in need of mental health services (Aiken, 1987) has been emphasized. Day care and school-based prevention and early intervention programs to meet the needs of children (Opie and Slater, 1988), depressed youths, and adolescents at risk for suicide (Lamb and Puskar, 1991) are being implemented.

There also is renewed emphasis on community-based outreach treatment for those with severe and persistent mental illnesses. One such program is called Programs for Assertive Community Treatment, or PACT. The PACT concept began as an intensive approach for training in community living targeted to clients with multiple episodes of mental illness and a high use of psychiatric hospitals and other mental health services (see Chapters 18 and 38).

Psychiatric home care has emerged as another viable treatment option, particularly for the homebound elderly or physically ill with coexisting mental disorders. These services minimize or eliminate the need for active treatment in an inpatient setting and represent significant savings in health care costs while offering beneficial help in an at-home setting (Kozlak and Thobaben, 1992). Psychiatric nurses providing home care are experienced in assessing the likelihood of being able to offer appropriate services in the home environment, formulating a treatment plan that takes both psychiatric and medical problems into account, and facilitating efforts to engage family members in the support of progress (Peplau, 1995).

Innovations at the worksite include the addition of prevention, early intervention, and health promotion services in occupational settings (Burgel, 1993). Forward-thinking industries are recognizing the benefits of work-based health promotion programs integrating physical and mental health concepts into on-site primary care service delivery models (O'Donnell and Harris, 1994). This is an ideal work setting for psychiatric-mental health nurses who can do health risk assessments, teach health concepts, do relaxation and stress management training, screen for depression and other mental illnesses, conduct health-focused counseling sessions, and assist employees in altering smoking and eating behaviors associated with heart disease, cancer, and other health problems. Successful worksite health promotion has been demonstrated to reduce health risks and positively affect costly work absenteeism (Pelletier, 1993).

The potential for creative programs and diverse settings is unlimited. The development of outreach mental health service settings will be a major thrust for the twenty-first century. Psychiatric nurses, with their background in the physical sciences, their knowledge of pharmacology, their sensitivity to psychosocial concerns, and their focus on caring, bring the necessary qualifications to the mission of a comprehensive continuum of care in a seamless delivery system without walls. In addition to their already established contributions to inpatient care, psychiatric nurses will move into the community as primary mental health care providers, case managers, program directors, entrepreneurs, and dozens of other creative, innovative roles.

Psychiatric-Mental Health Nursing: What?

The turbulent environment and rapid advances in today's psychiatric health care field are prompting psychiatric nurses to reassess their practices and reevaluate their options. This will result both in a modernization and advancement of traditional practice and some radical shifts in practice as improved program designs, innovative roles and fresh interventions are explored. A renewed focus on case management, integration of physical and mental health concepts, and the prevention of illness and promotion of health offer exciting opportunities for nurses in the specialty. The introduction of trends of managing care, fresh approaches and new models for psychotherapy intervention, and the expansion of roles and functions for advanced practice nurses will most certainly influence significant shifts in the practice of psychiatric-mental health nursing. Setting the tone for the future is reconceptualization of the psychiatric nurse as a provider of primary mental health care.

Primary mental health care

In keeping with the national movement toward primary care mentioned in the previous chapter, psychiatric nurses already are functioning as primary mental health care providers (Haber and Billings, 1993).

> *Primary mental health care is that care which is provided to those at risk for, or already in need of, mental health services.* It begins prior to or at the first point of contact with the mental health care delivery system. It involves all of the continuous and comprehensive services necessary for the promotion of optimal mental health, prevention of mental illness, and health maintenance, and includes the management (treatment) of and/or referral for mental and general health problems, and rehabilitation. Because of its scope, it is comprehensive, holistic health care which considers the needs and strengths of the whole person (Haber and Billings, 1995).

In Fig. 2-2 the professional role responsibilities of psychiatric-mental health nurses as designated in the statement on practice (ANA, 1994a) are featured in the shaded outside circle, and the intervention activities of psychiatric nursing are illustrated in the second concentric circle. The inner circle highlights the health focus central to primary mental health care, whereas the intersecting arrows signify the full range of services essential to the delivery of primary mental health care (Haber and Billings, 1995). This model illuminates the "fit" between the evolving need for primary mental health care services and the traditional roles and functions of psychiatric nurses.

Case management

Psychiatric nurses have served as case managers in the past and will continue to do so in the future. In today's climate of cost-control, the emphasis on case manage-

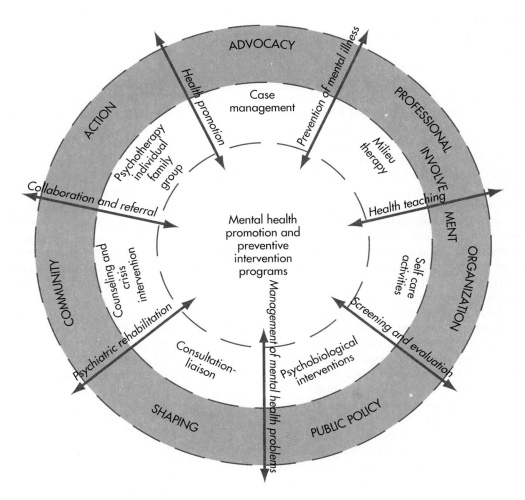

Fig. 2-2 Primary mental health care model. (From Haber J., & Billings C.V. (1995). Primary mental health care: A model for psychiatric-mental health nursing. *Journal of the American Psychiatric Nurses Association, 1,* 154-163.)

ment is to provide the link between quality and cost of care for clients who are in high-cost or high-risk categories. Case management is an essential component of cost-effective care because it minimizes fragmentation and disruption of services while maximizing the coordination of care activities by all involved disciplines and providers within the health care team (Bower, 1992). Nurses, with their broad-based knowledge and skills and their substantial clinical knowledge and judgment are ideally suited to the case manager role. Psychiatric nurses, who understand signs and symptoms associated with mental illnesses, have experience recognizing and managing the effects of psychotropic medications, and have the essential communication skills central to the care of clients with mental illness and their families, bring a wealth of talent and expertise to psychiatric case management (see Chapter 17).

Integrated care

In both inpatient and outpatient settings, psychiatric nurses will pay far more attention to the physical aspect of care, closely integrating their nursing identity with their psychiatric-mental health specialization. In keeping with discoveries in the field, there will be a more pronounced emphasis on the biological aspects of mental disorders, and current information from the neurosciences, particularly psychopharmacology, will be further incorporated into the nursing approach. The ANA, in published psychopharmacology guidelines for psychiatric-mental health nurses, notes that the inclusion of physical, psychiatric, pharmacological, and environmental health dimensions in the clinical management of patient care, in company with the psychosocial orientation long associated with psychiatric nursing, is the essential futuristic model for psychiatric nursing (ANA, 1994b).

Illness prevention intervention

It is hoped that the renewed focus on prevention will result in the development of an improved system of care for at-risk populations in the community (Mrazek and Haggerty, 1994). *Prevention interventions are intended to identify and reduce recognized health risk factors* (Caplan, 1993). Examples of mental health prevention intervention programs that can be carried out by psychiatric nurses include routine screening for mental health problems such as depression, anxiety or potential for suicide, screening for developmental delays in children and adolescents, and early recognition and intervention for individuals and families in circumstances such as disaster recovery, disruption of personal support systems through separation, death, and divorce, and situations of family violence and abuse that place them at high risk for developing mental or emotional disorders.

Managed care

Managed care involves a financial contract arrangement that promises a certain quality of care to the consumer and a guarantee of payment to the provider, while "managing" the cost efficiency of the service. Managed care spans a broad continuum of entities, from the simple requirement of prior authorization for a service in an indemnity health insurance plan to the assumption of all legal, financial, and organizational risks for the provision of a set of comprehensive benefits to a defined population (Hicks, Stallmeyer, and Coleman, 1992). The popularity of managed behavioral health care or managing mental health care has come about as a result of a reimbursement system that has been accused of rewarding lengthy, costly inpatient treatment while neglecting the possibilities inherent in alternative outpatient approaches. The emphasis on managing mental health care is believed by many to be a superior approach that will help control costs and turn the focus of care to quality outcomes (Bryant, 1991).

The proliferation of managed behavioral care agencies, health maintenance organizations, preferred provider organizations, and assess/refer options such as employee assistance programs will call on qualified psychiatric nurses to function as resource and risk managers, benefits interpreters, liaisons to providers, and quality improvement auditors, in addition to more traditional roles of triage nurse and care provider (American Academy of Nursing, 1993; Hicks, Stallmeyer, and Coleman, 1993).

New psychotherapies

Concurrent with advances in biological psychiatry and emphasis on cost-effectiveness, brief approaches to psychotherapy have been introduced as additional treatment options. These approaches emphasize solutions, competence, and capabilities with an eye toward the future over explanations, problems, and pathology, which focus on the past (O'Hanlon and Weiner-Davis, 1989). Cognitive, narrative, strategic, problem-oriented, and solution-focused therapy, neurolinguistic programming, crisis intervention, and single-intervention techniques (Wylie, 1990), in addition to more traditional psychodynamic and psychoanalytical methods, provide a wider range of treatment options for the advanced practice psychiatric nurse therapist.

Expanded functions for advanced practice

Advanced practice psychiatric nurses (clinical nurse specialists and psychiatric nurse practitioners) with expanded practice privileges such as prescriptive authority and hospital admitting privileges, will increasingly function as substitutes for higher cost providers (psychiatrists and psychologists). They will offer services to inner city, rural, and underpriviledged populations through community agencies, to the insured through contracts with managed care companies and health maintenance organizations, and in private practices. In addition, there is potential in the prospect of a truly collaborative practice between physician psychiatrists and psychiatric-mental health clinical nurse specialists functioning in a complimentary and egalitarian relationship to provide quality cost-effective, psychiatric treatment (Saur and Ford, 1995).

CHALLENGES FOR THE FUTURE

Professional Preparedness

Ongoing professional development is an individual responsibility. Changes in the focus of services, the points-of-services, and the types of services in addition to scientific advances in the field will require psychiatric-mental health nurses to reaffirm their status as lifelong learners. New times and new tasks demand new tools. The information explosion and rapidly expanding field of discovery brings special challenges to keep current. Nurses will choose to meet these challenges through additional formal education, credentialing, continuing education, peer association, professional memberships, self-directed studies, literature review, additional training, and other approaches. The availability of computer technology and access to networks of information should facilitate the achievement of the current base of knowledge, skills, and abilities essential to meet the role responsibilities of the future.

Political/Legislative Involvement

Some nurses were astonished when the national debate on health care reform turned out to be more about politics than about health care (Fox, 1993). Nevertheless, the experience was an awakening one. More than ever before, psychiatric nurses recognized that they can indeed play a significant role in health care considerations and perhaps for the first time truly appreciated the importance of active, visible, unified nursing involvement in public policy reform (Shea, 1993). In the aftermath of this experience, it has become obvious that the future of professional nursing, particularly advanced practice nursing, will be profoundly affected by national and state legislation. Currently, for example, many state boards of nursing are revising their practice rules and regulations to specify advanced practice nursing categories. In addition, changes in national health-related entitlement laws such as Medicare and Medicaid could either include or exclude reimbursement for the services of psychiatric nurses. It is imperative for the future of the specialty, and for providing health care access for the citizenry, that psychiatric nurses track and analyze proposed changes in state and national law, which could either limit or expand their practice, and be prepared to speak in favor of, or against, these changes.

Responsiveness to the health care needs of the population is in large part, determined by public policy. With a long history of neglect for those with mental illness and mental health concerns, this nation needs its psychiatric nurses to be politically astute and politically active (Billings, 1993a; Brooks et al., 1993). From membership in their professional and specialty organizations, to informed advocacy with regard to mental health and nursing issues, to seeking seats and offices on policy-making bodies, to providing testimony to legislative bodies, to writing letters to elected representatives, the psychiatric nurses of the future are already and must continue to be "on the move" at the state and national level, keeping nursing's agenda alive.

Emphasis on Outcomes

The crisis of the rising cost of health care has spawned increased pressure to justify the use of nursing resources (Simpson, 1995) and an intense interest on the part of nurses to demonstrate the effectiveness of their care (Brooten and Naylor, 1995) (see Chapter 4). Consequently, there is heightened emphasis on the importance of documenting the results of various models of client care and the impact of nursing practices on targeted outcomes such as safety, functional status, symptom control, utilization of service, quality of life, and client satisfaction (Lang and Marek, 1992). Psychiatric nurses in particular have fallen behind in the areas of specifying what it is they actually do, and what value or usefulness it represents in terms of actual client outcomes. Few studies have focused on elaborating the outcomes of psychiatric nursing care (Burdick, Stuart, and Lewis, 1994; or build

Box 2-6

Just Imagine...

Relax, lean back, take a deep breath, and imagine yourself, the psychiatric nurse of the future. It is late afternoon and you are getting ready to drive to the community center where you will be offering a class on conflict resolution for couples. This project is a part of a family violence project, which was funded by a national grant. As you get behind the wheel of your car, you roll down the window to appreciate the fresh air, cool breeze, and warm sunshine.

You can hear the sounds of children playing in the schoolyard where you are parked. You have just finished working with a group of teachers who are concerned about the children's reaction to the death of a classmate. This Teacher Support Program is a part of the new focus on mental health in the schools.

You spent this morning checking on clients in the community outreach program. As case manager for a group of 10 clients, you do home visits, medication checks, supportive counseling, make referrals as they are needed, and touch base with the family members. As you sit there, letting the sun shine in through the car windows, you think about how great you felt when you saw how well Mr. Lopez was doing, and how pleased his daughter was that he was able to spend time with her and her children yesterday without getting too anxious and overwhelmed.

Tomorrow is depression screening day at the Golden Age Club, and a team meeting at the mental health center. Two days each week, you are part of the rural clinic service, which involves on-site outpatient care in your county.

You took this position because you knew it would be challenging and rewarding. It allows you the right amount of direct client contact and enough opportunity to do health teaching as well as illness care. Some of your "psych" nursing colleagues would rather work on the inpatient unit at the hospital or in the community mental health center, but this flexibility and mobility fits your need for variety and autonomy. " The neat thing about psychiatric nursing," you think, "is that there are so many options and opportunities. And this is good; this is definitely good. . . ."

on prior research in the field (Merwin and Mauck, 1995). Although some psychiatric nurse authors have studied clinical outcomes, client satisfaction, and cost savings related to the services of clinical specialists in psychiatric-mental health nursing (Baradell, 1994; 1995; Murphy and Moeller, 1993), psychiatric nursing has more work to do to remain viable in tomorrow's market.

Psychiatric nursing diagnoses (Loomis et al., 1987) must be fully integrated into the taxonomy of the North American Nursing Diagnosis Association (NANDA), and psychiatric nursing interventions (McCloskey and Bulecheck, 1996) must be specified and entered into national unified data bases in the National Library of Medicine (Billings, 1993b). Clinical research focusing on the outcomes of psychiatric nursing care must be conducted and the results published.

These *are* exciting times to be involved in psychiatric-mental health nursing. Box 2-6 is a short journey that helps a learner be part of this excitement as a psychiatric nurse of the future.

KEY POINTS

- Emphasis on the biological and behavioral interface opens up dynamic possibilities for psychiatric nursing practice.
- The potential for collaborative and multidisciplinary contributions to the understanding of mental disorders and their treatment is greatly enhanced by biobehavioral linkages.
- The artificial barrier between physical and mental illnesses can finally be broken and psychiatric nurses can work far more closely with their colleagues in other specialties to provide a full spectrum of care.
- New integrated approaches applied to the care of people with severe and persistent mental illnesses will most likely stimulate a resurgence of interest and involvement with this previously abandoned population.
- A heightened awareness of the multifaceted components influencing emotional problems will call

 ## CRITICAL THINKING QUESTIONS

Gayle is a psychiatric-mental health nurse who has been working on the inpatient unit of her community hospital for 6 years. She really enjoys her work and the close contact she has with clients and families. She is up for promotion to assistant head nurse and is not sure she would enjoy staff management activities as much as she likes her clinical assignments. Recently, the hospital administrator announced the development of a new hospital outreach service that would provide "seamless" care delivery. This would mean integrating community services such as home health and outpatient clinic with full or partial hospitalization and following assigned patients in all care settings. When she inquired, Gayle was told that the concept of mental health outreach services is currently being developed. Gayle expressed an interest and was asked to serve on an interdisciplinary committee that would determine qualifications, roles, responsibilities, and functions for psychiatric-mental health outreach nurses.

1. What are some of the fundamental differences between inpatient nursing and outreach services?
2. What knowledge, skills, and abilities that are an integral part of psychiatric-mental health nursing can be transferred from inpatient care to community nursing?
3. What additional capabilities might need to be developed by a nurse who has been working exclusively in inpatient psychiatric nursing to successfully bridge the transition to care of psychiatric clients in the community?
4. What services might be added to already existing programs in either setting that would more accurately reflect the concept of primary mental health care?
5. What challenges would you expect the psychiatric nurses who move to outreach services to face, and what resources would you predict they will need to meet them?
6. Think about the potential for the development of collaborative relationships in this new program of care:
   a. How do you see psychiatric-mental health nurses, advanced-practice psychiatric-mental health nurses, physicians, psychologists, social workers, and unlicensed assistive personnel working together to provide the full continuum of care across all settings?
   b. What services are appropriate for each category of worker to perform?
   c. What services are unique to each discipline?
   d. What services overlap?
   e. What laws, rules, regulations, and/or standards will govern the boundaries of their care?
   f. How can quality mental health outreach care be delivered in the most cost-effective and efficient manner?

attention to the need for more socially and culturally sensitive care.

- Increased focus on seamless care delivery will shift psychiatric nursing from hospital-based to a wide variety of settings and new practice opportunities.
- Emphasis on the biological origins of mental illnesses and psychopharmacological treatment will challenge the nurse to keep current in knowledge of the dynamics and kinetics of psychoactive medications and the adjunctive pharmacological agents that ameliorate their side effects (ANA, 1994).
- Cost-consciousness and an effort to avoid duplicate services and waste of resources is expected to open opportunities for psychiatric nurses to expand their practices and to be more fully used as substitutes for and in collaborative practice with physician providers.
- Psychiatric nurses of the future must prepare themselves to work closely with other disciplines to better identify and meet the diverse and complex needs of a wide range of consumers in a large assortment of settings.

REFERENCES

Abraham, I.L., Fox, J.C., & Cohen, B.T. (1992). Integrating the bio into the biopsychosocial: Understanding and treating biological phenomena in psychiatric-mental health nursing. *Archives of Psychiatric Nursing, 6,* 296-305.

American Academy of Nursing. (1993). *Managed care and national health care reform. Nurses can make it work.* Washington, DC: Author.

American Nurses Association. (1967). *Statement on psychiatric and mental health nursing practice.* Kansas City, MO: Author.

American Nurses Association. (1985). *Code for nurses with interpretive statements.* Kansas City, MO: Author.

American Nurses Association. (1991). *Standards of clinical nursing practice.* Washington, DC: Author.

American Nurses Association. (1994a). *A statement on psychiatric-mental health clinical nursing practice and standards of psychiatric-mental health nursing practice.* Washington, DC: American Nurses Publishing.

American Nurses Association. (1994b). *Psychiatric-mental health nursing psychopharmacology project.* Washington, DC: American Nurses Publishing.

American Nurses Association. (1995). *Nursing's social policy statement.* Washington, DC: Author.

American Nurses Credentialing Center. (1996). *ANCC 1996 certification catalog.* Washington, DC: Author.

Baradell, J.G. (1994). Cost effectiveness and quality of care provided by clinical nurse specialists. *Journal of Psychosocial Nursing and Mental Health Services, 32* (3), 21-24.

Baradell, J.G. (1995). Clinical outcomes and satisfaction of patients of clinical nurse specialists in psychiatric-mental health nursing. *Archives of Psychiatric Nursing, 9,* 240-250.

Betrus, P.A., & Hoffman, A. (1992). Psychiatric-mental health nursing: Career characteristics, professional activities, and client attributes of members of the American Nurses Association Council of Psychiatric Nurses. *Issues in Mental Health Nursing, 13,* 39-50.

Billings, C.V. (1993a, February). The possible dream of mental health reform. *The American Nurse, 5,* 9.

Billings, C.V. (1993b). Psychiatric-mental health nursing professional progress notes. *Archives of Psychiatric Nursing, 7,* 174-181.

Bond, G. R., Miller, L.D., Kriumwied, R.D., & Ward, R. (1988). Assertive case management in three CMHCs: A controlled study. *Hospital and Community Psychiatry, 39,* 411-418.

Bower, K. (1992). *Case management by nurses.* Washington, DC: American Nurses Publishing.

Brooks, A.M., Clement, J.A., Billings, C.V., & Gilbert, C.M. (1993). New partnerships: Creating the future. *Journal of Psychosocial Nursing, 31* (8), 37-40.

Brooten, D., & Naylor, M.D. (1995). Nurses' effect on changing patient outcomes. *Image: Journal of Nursing Scholarship, 27,* 95-99.

Bryant, M. (1991). Are rising mental health costs driving you crazy? *Business and Health,* January, 36-43.

Burdick, M.B., Stuart, G.W., & Lewis, L.D. (1994). Measuring nursing outcomes in a psychiatric setting. *Issues in Mental Health Nursing, 15* (2), 137-148.

Burgel, B.J. (1993). *Innovation at the work site: Delivery of nurse managed primary health care services.* Washington, DC: American Nurses Publishing.

Caplan, G. (1993). Organization of preventive psychiatry programs. *Community Mental Health Journal, 29,* 367-395.

Drew, B. (1988). Devaluation of biological knowledge. *Image: Journal of Nursing Scholarship, 20,* 25-27.

Feild, L., & Winslow, E.H. (1985). Moving to a nursing model. *American Journal of Nursing, 85,* 1100-1101.

Fox, J.C. (1993). The role of nursing in public policy reform. *Journal of Psychosocial Nursing, 31* (8), 9-12.

Haber, J., & Billings, C.V. (1993). Primary mental health care: A vision for the future of psychiatric-mental health nursing. *ANA Council Perspectives, 2* (2), 1-2.

Haber, J., & Billings, C.V. (1995). Primary mental health care: A model for psychiatric-mental health nursing. *Journal of the American Psychiatric Nurses Association, 1,* 154-163.

Henderson, V. (1966). *The nature of nursing.* New York: MacMillan.

Hicks, L.L., Stallmeyer, J.M., & Coleman, J.R. (1992). *Role of the nurse in managed care.* Washington, DC: American Nurses Publishing.

Kozlak, J., & Thobaben, M. (1992). Treating the elderly mentally ill at home. *Perspectives in Psychiatric Care, 28* (2), 31-35.

Krauss, J. (1989). The three Cs and the chronically mentally ill. *Archives of Psychiatric Nursing, 3,* 59-60.

Krauss, J. (1993). *Health care reform: Essential mental health services.* Washington, DC: American Nurses Publishing.

Lamb, J., & Puskar, K. (1991). School-based adolescent mental health project survey of depression, suicidal ideation, and anger. *Journal of Child and Adolescent Psychiatric and Mental Health Nursing, 4* (3), 101-104.

Lang, N.M., & Marek, K.D. (1992). Outcomes that reflect clinical practice. National Institute of Health, *Patient outcomes research: Examining the effectiveness of nursing practice.* (DHHS Publication No. 93-3411, pp. 27-38). Washington, DC: Department of Health and Human Services.

Lego, S. (1992). Biological psychiatry and psychiatric nursing in America. *Archives of Psychiatric Nursing, 6,* 147-150.

Liaschenko, J. (1989). Changing paradigms within psychiatry: Implications for nursing research. *Archives of Psychiatric Nursing, 3,* 153-158.

Loomis, M., O'Toole, A., Brown, M., Pothier, P., West, P., & Wilson, H. (1987). Development of a classification system for psychiatric/mental health nursing: Individual response class. *Archives of Psychiatric Nursing, 1,* 16-24.

McBride, A.B. (1990). Psychiatric nursing in the 1990s. *Archives of Psychiatric Nursing, 4,* 21-28.

McCloskey, J., & Bulechek, G. (1996). *Nursing interventions classification (NIC)* (2nd ed.). St. Louis: Mosby.

Merwin, E., & Mauck, A. (1995). Psychiatric nursing outcome research: The state of the science. *Archives of Psychiatric Nursing, 9,* 311-331.

Mrazek, P.J., & Haggerty, R.J. (1994). *Reducing risks for mental disorders.* Washington, DC: National Academy Press.

Murphy, M.P., & Moller, M.D. (1993). Relapse management in neurobiological disorders: The Moller-Murphy symptom management assessment tool. *Archives of Psychiatric Nursing, 7,* 226-235.

National Advisory Mental Health Council. (1990). *National Plan for Research on Child and Adolescent Mental Disorders.* (DHHS Publication No. 90-1683). Rockville, MD: National Institute of Mental Health.

National Institute of Mental Health. (1991). *Caring for people with severe mental disorders: A national plan of research to improve services* (DHHS Publication No. 91-1762). Washington, DC: U.S. Government Printing Office.

Nightingale, F. (1859). *Notes on nursing.* London: Harrison.

O'Donnell, M.P., & Harris, J.S. (Eds.). (1994). *Health promotion in the workplace* (2nd Ed.) Albany, NY: Delmar.

O'Hanlon, W.H., & Weiner-Davis, M. (1989). *In search of solutions: A new direction in psychotherapy.* New York: W.W. Norton.

Opie, N., & Slater, P. (1988). Mental health needs of children in school. Role of the child psychiatric mental health nurse. *Journal of Child and Adolescent Psychiatric and Mental Health Nursing, 1* (1), 31-35.

Pelletier, K.R. (1993). A review and analysis of the health and cost-effective outcome studies of comprehensive health promotion and disease prevention programs at the worksite: 1991-1993 update. *American Journal of Health Promotion, 8,* (1), 50-62.

Peplau, H.E. (1952). *Interpersonal Relations in Nursing.* New York: G.P. Putnam's Sons.

Peplau, H.E. (1995). Some unresolved issues in the era of biopsychosocial nursing. *Journal of the American Psychiatric Nurses Association, 1,* 92-96.

Pothier, P. (1988). Child mental health problems and policy. *Archives of Psychiatric Nursing, 2,* 165.

Pothier, P. (1990). Toward a bio/psycho/social synthesis. *Archives of Psychiatric Nursing, 4,* 77.

Rogers, M.E. (1966, June). *The education violet,* New York University.

Rogers, M.E. (1970). *The theoretical basis of nursing.* Philadelphia: F.A. Davis.

Saur, C.D., & Ford, S.M. (1995). Quality, cost-effective psychiatric treatment: A CNS-MD collaborative practice model. *Archives of Psychiatric Nursing, 9,* 332-337.

Saxe, J.G. (1985). The blind men and the elephant. In D. Hall, (Ed.), *The Oxford book of children's verse in America.* New York: Oxford University Press.

Shea, C.A. (1993). Mental health care reform: A historic meeting of psychiatric nurses. *Journal of Psychosocial Nursing, 31,* (8), 30-33.

Simpson, R. (1995). Ammunition in the board room: The clinical nursing data set. *Nursing Management, 2* (6), 16-17.

Swanson, B., Cronin-Stubbs, D., Zeller, J.M., Kessler, H.A., Bieliauskas, L.A. (1993). Characterizing the neuropsychological functioning of persons with human immunodeficiency virus infection, Part I. Acquired immunodeficiency dementia complex: A review. *Archives of Psychiatric Nursing, 7,* 74-81.

Talley, S., & Brooke, P. (1992). Prescriptive authority for psychiatric clinical specialists: Framing the issues. *Archives of Psychiatric Nursing, 6,* 71-82.

Wylie, M.S. (1990). Brief therapy on the couch. *The Family Therapy Networker, 14* (2), 26-35, 66.

Chapter 3

Legal/Ethical Issues

Joy Feldman
Stanley J. Matek

LEARNING OUTCOMES

After studying and applying the concepts of this chapter, the learner will be able to:
- Explain what it means to be ethical and why the study of ethics is indispensable to every professional.
- Interpret core values of psychiatric nursing.
- Discuss safeguards against deficiencies in ethical judgment.
- Identify the key principles that ground ethical judgment.
- Execute an ethical analysis.
- Define standard of care.
- Define the types of tort most commonly used in suits against psychiatric nurses.
- Explain the relationships among autonomy, privacy, and confidentiality.
- Discuss the distinctions between informed consent and competency, incompetency, and incapacity.
- Identify rights of clients in mental health settings.
- Discuss nurses' obligations as they relate to voluntary and involuntary admission, the right to refuse treatment, the right to participate in formulating the treatment plan, and the use of restraints and seclusion.

KEY TERMS

Autonomy	Informed consent	Principles
Beneficence	Integrity	Profession
Breach of duty	Involuntary admission	Professionalism
Commitment	Least restrictive environment	Restraint
Competency	Malpractice	Rule
Confidentiality	Moral values	Standard of care
Duty of care	Morals	Tort
Ethics	Nonmaleficence	Value
Fidelity	Outpatient commitment	Values clarification
Incapacity	Paternalism	Voluntary admission
Incompetency		

The practice of psychiatric nursing is not exempt from national trends that shift the care of clients from "in-hospital" to "out-of-hospital" settings. The serious and persistent nature of mental illness, the use of chemical and physical restraints, and the discriminatory use of mental health benefits create but a few of the ethical issues facing psychiatric nurses. Historically, the mental health care system violated the human rights of persons with mental disorders. Today, consumerism promotes increased participation of clients in their care and often leads to protection of their rights with legal action.

This chapter presents the interaction among legal issues, professional values, and ethics as they pertain to the responsibilities of psychiatric nurses. It discusses rights conferred by the federal and state courts upon consumers of health care, and identifies the key values and how they have become part of the duties of nurses, and the rights of clients. It reviews the usual grounds for legal action against mental health professionals. It summarizes professional values and ethics relative to nursing practice and highlights those legal and ethical tensions between competing rights or values that most often arise in psychiatric care.

PROFESSIONALISM

There is a long and honorable history to professionalism. The word *profession* comes from the Latin term, *professio,* which denotes a vow, consecration, or formal dedication, usually made in public and for life. In ancient times, such commitments were made for religious reasons. This same sense of commitment carries over to the modern concept of professionalism of psychiatric nurses though not in such directly religious ways. A *profession is defined as a calling that requires (1) specialized knowledge, (2) continuing study, (3) the maintenance of high standards in achievement and conduct, and (4) commitment to a kind of work, which has, as its prime purpose, the rendering of a public service.*

Nursing has met the fourth criterion since time immemorial, and the third since it became institutionalized in modern society, first through religious orders, and later through the formal establishment of secular training programs, certification, and licensure. The refinements represented by the first two criteria and the emergence of a fifth—independence in judgment and action—are matters of social processes more than principle and are thus more subject to the pressure of politics. Even so, "self-regulation" and "independence" have become core features of modern professionalism. One sign of nursing's success as a profession is its ability to formulate and enforce, directly and indirectly, high standards in ethics and performance.

Professionalism is the process through which, over time, an organized occupational group gains the usu- *ally exclusive right (1) to perform a particular kind of work, (2) to control training for such work, and (3) to evaluate the way that work is performed.* The concept of a profession is the basis on which ethical considerations are developed. The process of professionalization is the basis on which certification, licensure, and thus legal obligations have evolved. This interaction between principle and process is important to remember, because it is a point of constant exchange and creative tension between ethics and law in professional life.

The professional practice of psychiatric nursing is guided by the American Nurses Association (ANA) *Statement on Psychiatric-Mental Health Clinical Nursing Practice and the Standards of Psychiatric-Mental Health Clinical Nursing Practice* (ANA, 1994) (see Appendix A). A competent level of care requires professional role behaviors related to quality of care, performance appraisal, education, collegiality, ethics, collaboration, and resource utilization. Activities that maintain the psychiatric nurse's competency as a professional include membership in such professional organizations as American Psychiatric Nurses Association (APNA) and Society for Research and Education in Psychiatric Nursing (SERPN). Certification in the psychiatric nursing specialty or for advanced practice, continuing education, and further academic preparation are all means of maintaining and advancing as a professional psychiatric nurse.

VALUES

Moral and ethical judgments begin with a sense of basic values. *Value* (from the Latin term, *valere,* to make strong, to have worth) is *the importance one places on something.* *Moral values are convictions about character attributes and standards to which one makes personal commitments, and according to which one habitually chooses to act.* However, values do not suddenly spring full-blown into or out of a person's head or heart. They develop gradually as a person matures, forming value sets to be used in the various roles and relationships of life. At some point these sets are expanded and integrated into a relatively stable value system, which is applied habitually. *This habitual way of judging and acting is what constitutes integrity.* What changes a person from a technician into a true professional is commitment to values and priorities. Most essentially, it is commitment to altruistic service and high standards of performance that make the difference—a commitment so complete that, to the professional person, actualizing these values ranks above self-interest, or even better, becomes seen as embodying true self-interest. A true professional can be trusted to meet these high standards day in and day out, regardless of whether anyone else is watching or will ever know.

TABLE 3-1

A framework of moral and ethical values

THE 10 BASIC REALITIES OF HUMAN NATURE	THE 12 PRIMARY MORAL IMPERATIVES	THE SECONDARY (QUALIFIABLE) MORAL IMPERATIVES	THE 22 STRENGTHS OF PERSONAL CHARACTER	PROFESSIONAL VALUES
As human beings we are...	*These facts of human nature require that we...*	*These facts of human nature require that we...*	*The qualities and habits needed personally are...*	*The values to be expressed vocationally are:*

Corporeal:
  Mortal
  Sexual
	Respect life and accept death.
	Be caring.
		Do not kill.
		Do no harm.
		Reduce suffering.
		Reproduce responsibly.
			Respect
			Hygiene
			Enjoyment
			Gentleness
				Nonmaleficence
				Protection
				Advocacy
				Support

Empirical	Acknowledge limits.	Be thorough. Be honest with yourself.	Studiousness Humility	Lifelong learning Specialized skills Research
Rational	Be accountable.	Be consistent. Maintain balance. Respect priorities.	Prudence Temperance	Accountability
Developmental (integrative)	Be open-minded.	Be patient. Seek wisdom.	Tolerance INTEGRITY	INTEGRITY (trustworthiness)
Imaginative	Seek improvement.		Optimism Creativity	Advancement
Free-willed	Be responsible.	Respect the freedom and responsibility of others.	Honor Courage	Autonomy (privacy, confidentiality, informed consent)
Communicative	Be honest.	Communicate precisely.	Honesty	Truthfulness (disclosure) Education

Socially dependent	Be fair.	Respect the rights of others.
		Fulfill obligations.
		Be loyal.
			JUSTICE
			Duty
			
			Loyalty
				JUSTICE:
				  Individual
				  Social
				Fidelity

	Be compassionate.	Prevent suffering. Be peaceful.	Compassion Forgiveness	Compassion
	Contribute to the common good.	Obey just laws.	Citizenship Altruism	Service Beneficence
Environmentally dependent	Be frugal (nonwasteful).	Prevent damage. Repair damage.	Moderation Stewardship	Resource access Conservation

© *1995 Stanley J. Matek,* Professional Ethics Resources, *Milwaukee, WI.* Reprinted with permission.

Persons of honesty and intelligence have long argued over the basis and priority of moral values. Do they rest on something innate (nature) or only on cultural factors (nurture)? Is the best criterion for evaluation, the character and quality of an act, or its results? Is it better to seek the greatest good for the greatest number, or to respect the subjective conscience of the person choosing? Many impressively named schools of ethical thought have emerged over the centuries: hedonism, scholasticism, deontologism, consequentialism, utilitarianism, libertarianism, pragmatism, and dozens more. Each school can usually trounce the others (by pointing out logical flaws) more easily than it can build a flawless rationale for its own point of view. Almost all schools in nearly all cultures agree on the core aspects of human nature and on the direct implications of these attributes for what constitutes good character, good conduct, and the common welfare. Table 3-1 summarizes these commonalities and offers a framework for identifying the most elementary values, norms, and qualities of character agreed on by the world's major religions, philosophies, and cultures.

Values Clarification

Values clarification is a term used by educators to describe the process of personal decision making about conflicting moral values. Individual value systems arise out of a complex mix of inputs from family, school, religion, environment, and peer communications. The process of focusing and organizing personal moral commitments and priorities was described by Kohlberg (see Chapter 7). The ways in which professional values relate to personal character, to more general social values, and to universal human characteristics is presented in Table 3-1. Even the most lofty discussion of values, personal or professional, will be complicated by two unavoidable factors: disagreements over priorities (justice or loyalty, truth or compassion, etc.) and differences in perception based on age and experience.

The problem of priorities can be addressed by developing principles for evaluation, but because evaluative judgments are directly influenced by age and experience, the impact that individual maturity level can have on moral judgment needs to be considered. The need to clarify one's values usually comes from one of the following three situations:

- Exposing oneself to new information or experiences that are inconsistent with the present value system
- Being forced to behave in ways that are inconsistent with one's present value system
- Recognizing, either internally or externally, inconsistencies in one's value system

Nurses therefore need to identify for themselves personal mentors or organizationally sponsored advisors on whom they can confidently call for guidance. Ultimately, each young professional is legally responsible for his or her own actions, and therefore must *personally* find, cultivate, and maintain mentoring relationships with wiser, older peers chosen for their wisdom and integrity.

ETHICS

Morals are habits of judgment and behavior that center on the quality of an action as good or bad. When moral values are refined, organized, and validated through consistent analysis, they rise to the level of *ethics, which has the status of a formal intellectual discipline.* Ethics covers entire value systems, and ethics focuses itself on moral dilemmas—where one must choose between competing goods or different evils. Being ethical means being skillful at maximizing the rationality and optimizing the integrity of complicated or ambiguous moral decisions.

In the world of ethics, principles are few and rules are many. The term *rule* comes from the Latin term *regula,* which means a bar, staff, or measuring stick; hence it suggests also a rule, model, or pattern. In ethics, a **rule** *is an established guide or fixed decision determining conduct* (or what administrators would call policies). Rules are helpful because they are relatively clear, specific, and easy to apply, but rules, unlike principles, have exceptions.

Nursing is deeply rooted in religious tradition, and many nurses base their primary motivations on religious beliefs. Even so, professional ethics are grounded essentially in the core characteristics of humanity and society, and in reason-based discourse or discussion. Only by reasoned dialogue can nurses hold themselves accountable to their fellow members of civil society. This point is crucial because faith exists beyond reason. Faith ought not to be used, especially in a pluralistic society, as a required element in professional culture. However, such faith enhances one's personal motivations; it does not exempt a person from the duties of reason or from respect for the moral autonomy of other people.

In the resolution of ethical dilemmas, it is the accountability of reasoned discourse that makes possible the benefits of mutual understanding, education, and respect. This remains true even and especially amid moral disagreements—exactly at the point where the explicitness of the ethical enterprise enriches and expands the dialogue, and solidifies the grounds for choosing.

Principles of Ethical Reasoning

The most fundamental and universal guidelines in ethics are called principles. The word comes from the Latin

Fundamental Ethical Principles

INTEGRITY

The moral goodness of an act depends on its integrity. The integrity of any action is the product of (1) good intention, (2) good motive, (3) the character of the act, (4) the circumstances affecting the act, and (5) its foreseeable consequences.

MORAL AUTONOMY

Every person has the right to self-determination in choices and actions, and the obligation to avoid exerting undue influence or interference in the choices and actions of others.

RECIPROCITY

Do not to others what you would not want them doing to you.

SUBSIDIARITY

Keep responsibility vested as close to the individual as is reasonable.

PROPORTIONALITY

Seek in every choice or action to achieve balance or due proportion between competing benefits, or between benefits and harms.

(NOTE: The guidelines for priority also express proportion).

PRIORITY

The greater value overrides the lesser.

CORRELATIVITY

In every right there are responsibilities; in every privilege are obligations.

© *1995, Stanley J. Matek,* Professional ethics resources, *Milwaukee, WI.* Reprinted with permission.

term *principium,* which means *beginning;* it in turn derives from *princeps* (ruler, leader, founder). **Principles** *are primary criteria on which other guidelines are based. They are the most fundamental general standards of judgment; they do not themselves change or allow for exceptions.* Box 3-1 presents definitions of the major principles in ethics. Note that they are not rules that tell a person what to do, rather, they address the nature of things, or relationships between them. The principles provide no absolutes but give rise to values. Values

operationalized in the context of a professional role find specific expression in obligations.

These basic obligations generate supplemental obligations: *truthfulness, confidentiality, respect for privacy,* and *fidelity (promise-keeping, nonabandonment, maintenance of trust).* The obligations are usually expressed in the form of professional or institutional codes, operating rules, or state laws and regulations. Although obligations also arise situationally and depend on good judgment, rules alone are never enough. Beyond obligations there are also aspirational ideas especially appropriate for health care providers: *conscientiousness, compassion, kindness, mercy, generosity.* These qualities complete and support those directly required for the nurse and constitute the integrity of conduct and character, which fulfill nursing as a vocation.

For psychiatric nurses, the moral foundation of the nurse-client relationship and thus the nurse's constant overall goal are best summarized in a word—*trustworthiness*—because the nurse has what, to the client, are usually complex knowledge and rare skills. The client has no real choice but to trust the provider, and the nurse must reciprocate by respecting and protecting the trust. Trustworthiness is the integrating element in the nurse-client relationship.

Ethical Competence

The objective of ethics as a formal part of psychiatric nursing education is to produce professionals capable of judging and acting with balance, responsibility, and integrity. These qualities are prerequisites for public trust, because status as a professional gives the nurse so much power over the lives and welfare of clients (Mohr, 1996). Ethical competence as a nursing professional requires the following elements:

- A personal commitment to an adequate base of moral values, and to accountability for how those values are interpreted and applied
- An understanding of how the psychiatric nursing role intensifies and changes normal moral values and applications
- A command of the principles and rules used in resolving dilemmas
- A proficiency, practiced and demonstrated among one's peers, in the use of ethical skills

Ethical Analysis Process

Moral values are matters of personal conviction and responsibility. Moral choices may not always be easy, but they are nearly always simple: good versus bad, right versus wrong. Ultimately, they are always matters of individual conscience.

Ethics, on the other hand, is a matter of ability—skills acquired for use in discerning, defining, distinguishing, deducing and deciding in situations where rights or good objectives conflict. Ethical choices involve dilemmas, which are the need to choose one good or right thing over another. Several forms of ethical conflict may exist. These include the following:

- *Conflict between ethical principles.* A nurse may not personally believe in the use of mind altering drugs but may work in a clinic where holistic care involves prescribing such medications.
- *Conflict between two possible actions.* A nurse who does not believe professionals should strike may need to decide whether to join colleagues on strike or cross the picket line to care for clients.
- *Conflict between the need for reflection and the need for action.* A nurse may act in an emergency before the team has met to discuss a plan of care for a client.
- *Conflict between two unsatisfactory alternatives.* A nurse may have to choose between using sedatives or arm restraints as an emergency procedure when a client is out of control and does not respond to verbal calming.
- *Conflict between role obligations and personally held values.* A director of nursing values fairness and equality for all people but is told by an administrator to transfer a person the administrator does not like.

The process of analyzing an ethical dilemma is outlined in Box 3-2. It involves five steps for applying the values and principles presented in this chapter to actual ethical problems. It may seem difficult at first, because the elements are not familiar. As the nurse grows in exposure and experience, however, these considerations should become habitual, and movement through them should become swift and almost instinctive. The nurse will find this process a rewarding exercise in sensitivity and convictions, a source of satisfaction and peace of mind. The importance of the process lies both in promoting sound decisions by the nurse and in assuring accountability. Matters of conscience are usually personal, but matters of ethics are essentially social, and both peers and the social systems that employ and license nurses have a right to ask them at any time to justify their professional conduct. This therefore represents an obligation for the practicing nurse. Professionals in the mental health field face challenges of exceptional intensity. The honor of professional commitments can become obscured by the sometimes unattractive or unmanageable realities of the clients, the problems, and the limitation of resources. Extra measures of personal conviction and collaborative team support are needed to maintain service levels and patterns that meet acceptable standards of care.

Box 3-2

How to Make A Responsible Ethical Analysis

ANALYZE THE ACTION (FACT FINDING, CLARIFICATION)

- What is the act at issue?
- Who is/should/should not be involved?
- What are/should be the motives?
- What conditions or circumstances affect the situation now? Later?
- Who will/might be significantly affected (the "stakeholders")? How?
- Who is/is not/should/should not be responsible? To what extent?

SPECIFY THE VALUE CONFLICT

- What imperatives and values are at issue? (see Table 3-1, columns 2, 3, and 5)
- Where are the conflicts?
- What qualities of personal character are most needed to deal with this situation? (see Table 3-1, column 4)

APPLY ETHICAL GUIDELINES (SEE TABLE 3-1 AND BOX 3-1)

- What principles, doctrines and rules apply?
- What tensions, conflicts, or needs for exceptions emerge?
- What choices exist? Do they qualify as true dilemmas or not? (A choice between good and bad is no dilemma; it is simply a moral decision—need courage, perhaps, but not analysis.)
- Can a legitimate "middle way" be found?
- If not, what values or norms must be favored, and why?
- How will you resolve the dilemma(s)?

ACT AND DOCUMENT

- Consult as necessary or opportune.
- Make the decision.
- Explain your rationale as needed or helpful.

MONITOR OUTCOMES AND CONSEQUENCES

- Be prepared to amend as needed.

© 1995, Stanley J. Matek, Professional ethical resources, Milwaukee, WI. Reprinted with permission.

PSYCHIATRIC NURSING PRACTICE AND THE LAW

Ethics is about integrity, responsibility, and balance, which are realized in self-directed behavior. The law is about rules and regulations, which represent other-directed behavior. The goal of law is conformity, or at least the defining of acceptable limits of conduct. The intervention of civil law in professional affairs *expresses standards below which practitioners may not perform.* As the nurse begins to explore the interrelatedness of ethics and law, it becomes clear that social policy is embodied in the law.

The law provides a resource for developing a professional sense of duty, standards, and even analysis. The rulings of law ultimately rest on the principles and values as evolved through social consensus. Ethics expresses what *ought* to be, whereas the law guides what *must* be done. That consensus about law must come first from the professions themselves, and thus necessarily from the individual professionals who embody the values from which the consensus arises. The sources of law include the state and federal constitutions, statutes, administrative agencies, and court decisions.

Duty of Care

A legal relationship exists when one individual takes on the status of "patient" or "client" and another individual is employed as a "nurse." When the relationship begins the client implicitly conveys consent to be treated. Legal rights are attached to the status of being a client, and the relationship obligates the nurse to maintain a duty of care. Just as trustworthiness is the ongoing moral foundation of the nurse-client relationship, "duty of care" is its legal foundation.

The *duty of care is the legal standard that applies to every nurse-client relationship.* Violation of the standard of care can result in license suspension or revocation, or in a finding of negligence (for which money damages can be owed to the injured party), or both. Malpractice is a type of negligent tort, which is alleged when a health care professional is accused of violating duty under the standard of care. A *breach of duty is any error or omission committed in the course of duty, regardless of intent.* Liability may be found when the standard is not met and injury to the client results. Nursing malpractice claims arise from harm or injury to a client resulting from a breach in the standard of nursing care. The functions inherent in psychiatric nursing care that are most often breached, giving rise to claims of negligence, are described in Box 3-3. For a claim of malpractice to succeed against a nurse, the following elements must be proven:

- There must be a nurse-client relationship.
- By virtue of the relationship, a duty of care exists.
- The nurse must have breached the standard of care by act or omission.
- The client must have sustained an injury that was proximately related to the error or omission (breach of duty) of the nurse.

Civil law violations are not the only legal consequence of a nurse's breach of duty. Every state has an office of professional licensure and standards, to which incidents of unacceptable professional practice are reported. Most states maintain toll-free numbers to which a consumer complaint may be made to state departments of health or professional licensure. Every complaint is investigated to determine whether practice standards have been violated. License suspensions or revocations are made accordingly. In addition, state law and professional ethics impose on professionals the duty to report a fellow professional for patterns of substandard performance or flagrant misconduct. For example, a nurse legally and ethically is obligated to report a colleague she knows is chemically impaired while caring for clients. Most hospitals have established protocols that guide nurses' actions in such situations.

Torts

Under U.S. law, *interference that harms a person intentionally or accidentally is called a tort.* A *tort* (from the Latin word for "twisted") *is a wrongful act, which results in injury, loss, or damage.* If a client claiming harm proves by a preponderance of evidence that injury resulted from the nurse's wrongdoing, that client is entitled to compensation. Torts are the usual basis for legal action against health professionals. Separately or in combination, the circumstances most often giving rise to tort-based lawsuits against health professionals are negligence, assault and battery, trespass, invasion of privacy, defamation, slander, and false imprisonment. Table 3-2 defines each term and gives an example of each.

Standard of Care

Standard of care describes the minimal level of care that may be delivered to the client under state and federal law. Standards embody the expected competent level of behavior of professional nurses. The standard of care is set internally within the profession and externally by the law. Standards of care develop from the following:

- State nurse practice acts
- Federal agency guidelines and regulations
- Hospital policy and procedure manuals
- Nurses' job descriptions
- Published standards of the professional organization and specialty practice groups

Box 3-3

Bases of Negligence Claims Against Psychiatric Nurses

- *The duty to reasonably recognize suicidal preoccupation or to supervise such patients at risk for suicide.* If omissions are shown in a claim for wrongful death based on failure to prevent suicide, liability can be found.
- *The duty to monitor drug effects and side effects, and to report observations that indicate the need for intervention.* For example, tardive dyskinesia (TD) can be minimized or prevented through careful monitoring and timely intervention.
- *The duty to accurately diagnose, treat, and/or evaluate the intervention(s) selected.* Errors in diagnosis lead to inappropriate treatment. Harm is compounded by the delay and obscured further by overlaying inappropriate medication, making diagnosis even more difficult. Careful observation and sensitive interaction with the patient are ongoing requirements of responsible nursing care. Nurses play a critical role in these team functions in inpatient settings, since they are uniquely positioned to observe patients around the clock.
- *The duty to protect rights.* This duty includes the obligation to avoid any conduct that takes advantage of the patient's vulnerability in relation to the caregiver. Initiating or permit-

ting sexual overtones and/or contact in the relationship is construed by courts as taking unfair advantage of the dependency patients typically experience in therapeutic relationships. Such conduct is gravely improper and subject to liability.
- *The duty to preserve confidentiality and patient privacy.* The duty of confidentiality prohibits disclosure outside the treatment setting of any information obtained in the professional relationship, unless the patient waives the right or it is overridden by a higher duty, such as the *duty to warn.* Violation can result in liability for negligence or invasion of privacy or breach of various statutes protecting confidentiality. (For example, the *Comprehensive Alcohol Abuse and Alcoholism Protection, Treatment and Rehabilitation Act* of 1970, and the *Drug Abuse Offense and Treatment Act* of 1972 require that patient records and information must be kept strictly confidential. They prohibit even answering a telephone request for confirmation that a person is in treatment. State public health and mental health laws universally provide a shield of confidentiality for all medical records.)

TABLE 3-2

Examples of tort law

TORT LAW	DEFINITION	EXAMPLE
Negligence	Involves causing harm through failure to do what a reasonably prudent person would do under similar circumstances	A nurse neglects to use constant observation of a suicidal adolescent in seclusion resulting in an additional attempt with consequent disabilities
Assault and battery	Consists of unwanted touching or other bodily contact, or the threat of same, with the apparent ability to carry it out	A nurse threatens an elderly client with seclusion if she does not eat
Trespass	Invasion of personal territory or space without consent	A male employee rapes a female client
False imprisonment	Involves intentionally confining another within boundaries, with the confinement maintained against the individual's will, if that person is either conscious of it or harmed by it	A client is forced to remain in restraints well beyond what is a reasonable time because she was verbally abusive to the nurse
Invasion of privacy, defamation, and slander	Involves unauthorized release of information or photographs in medical records	A nurse allows a family member to read a client's chart without the client's written permission to do so

The standard of care guarantees the human rights of clients. Historically, the rights of clients with mental disorders, guaranteed under the U.S. Constitution, were violated. Since the 1960s, safeguards have been established so that all clients retain their constitutionally guaranteed rights. Psychiatric-mental health nursing's *Standards* (see Appendix A) outline the unique responsibilities of psychiatric nurses and reflect the standard of care as a whole.

Record Keeping

A key responsibility of psychiatric nurses is accurate record keeping. Medical records are the best, and possibly only, means to later prove that the standard of care was (or was not) followed. Medical records are accepted under the law as objective, reliable proof of the matters documented. Everything contained in the record is accepted as fact and admissible in court. Care that was given but not documented in the record will not be assumed and cannot be proven. From the legal perspective, "if it isn't charted, it was not done." Accordingly, the most helpful record is one that is timely, complete, accurate, unambiguous, factual, objective, and legible.

CLIENT RIGHTS

The standard of care requires protecting client's rights under federal law. The history of care of the mentally ill before 1960s is fraught with violations of human rights. In 1973 the American Hospital Association (AHA) issued a Patient's Bill of Rights, and in 1980 the Mental Health Systems Act (MHSA) adopted into law what had previously been a recommended Bill of Rights for the Mentally

Ill (*MHSA*, 1980) (Box 3-4). People retain the freedom to exercise or not exercise their rights. Numerous federal and state statutes exist to protect the human rights of clients with a mental illness. Most states mandate that a statement of clients' rights be prominently displayed and be given to every person voluntarily or involuntarily admitted.

Federal law imposes liability for depriving someone of federal rights while acting under authority of state law (Social Security Act, 42 U.S.C. 1993). Thus mental health workers employed by a state entity may incur liability if their work-related conduct or indifference results in obstruction of a person's federal rights.

The rights of clients with mental illness are now protected by law. The rules of law establishing client rights include the following:

- Once admitted, a person has a right to appropriate treatment and related services in a setting and under conditions that support the client's real personal liberty and that restrict liberty only to the extent required by treatment needs, requirements of law, and specific judicial orders (if any have been issued).
- Under federal law a client has the right to an individualized, written treatment plan, a right to revision of that plan, and the right to participate in the planning. (Social Security Act, 42 U.S.C. 9501 (c) and 10841 (1) (C)).
- Mental health clients have the right to refuse any treatment modality except when it is (1) ordered by a responsible mental health professional during an emergency, or (2) it is a procedure permitted under

---

Box 3–4

Mental Health Systems Act

Recommended Bill of Rights for Clients

1. The right to appropriate treatment in settings and under conditions most supportive of and least restrictive to personal liberty
2. The right to an individualized, written treatment plan, periodic review to treatment, and revision of plan
3. The right to ongoing participation in the planning of services, and the right to a reasonable explanation of general mental condition, treatment objective, adverse effects of treatment; reasons for treatment, and available alternatives
4. The right to refuse treatment except in an emergency or as permitted by law

5. The right not to participate in experimentation
6. The right to freedom from restraint or seclusion
7. The right to a humane treatment environment
8. The right to confidentiality or records
9. The right of access to records except data provided by third parties or unless access would be detrimental to health
10. The right of access to telephone use, mail, and visitors
11. The right to know these rights
12. The right to initiate grievances when rights are infringed
13. The right to referral when discharged

From Mental Health Systems Act. *(1980). 96th Cong., Pub. L. L96-398, Sec. 9501, Amendment to Senate Bill 1177, September 23, 1980.*

applicable law for a person committed by a court to a treatment program or facility (Social Security Act, 42 U.S.C. 9501 (c) (1) (D) and 10841 (1) (D)).

Right to Autonomy

Autonomy means health care professionals must respect individual clients' decisions and their right to self-determination. It involves such issues as informed consent, competency, commitment for psychiatric care, and care in least restrictive environments.

Informed consent

Informed consent means that clients must receive adequate information about their illnesses and proposed treatments. It is viewed not only as a legal mandate but also as an educational process. For consent to be "informed," the client must understand the following:

- His or her existing condition
- The purpose and advantages of undergoing the proposed treatment(s) or test(s)
- The risks to health or life accompanying the proposed course
- The risks of not proceeding as proposed
- The available alternative options (including doing nothing) with their risks, disadvantages, and benefits

Informed consent in inpatient mental health settings is often complicated by the very symptoms for which the client entered treatment. Belief systems of everyone involved in the admission process affect whether or not the clients are meaningfully informed of their condition or included in treatment planning (Trudeau, 1994). Team members are not without their own needs, motivations, and ability to comprehend possibilities. Add to this the presence of family members who may assert their perspectives and requirements with regard to the client's needs. Also, socioeconomic variables can decisively affect available options. To the extent these forces reduce the client's involvement in treatment planning and informed consent, they infringe on the clients' right to autonomy.

Informed consent for treatment as an outpatient is the right of every client in the system. The growing trend toward outpatient commitment of clients with serious and persistent symptoms has created ambiguity in community-based treatment that needs clarification through legal guidelines to guarantee client's rights.

Because of the nature of mental disorders, several issues about the consent process must be considered. Clients need to be informed of their DSM-IV diagnosis and how such a label relates to the symptoms they are experiencing. The total treatment plan for the client must be explained. Treatments such as individual, group, and family therapy, as well as behavior modification need to be described. Of particular importance is a complete explanation of medications and their side effects. Treatments such as electroconvulsive therapy and psychosurgery require specific consents that outline the risks and intended benefits. Available options for treatment, including the legalities of voluntary and involuntary admission and least restrictive care, must be discussed.

Involving the client in treatment planning and informed consent are basic to ethical performance of professional duties. The presumption of competence is key to responsibly engaging the client in decision-making and respecting the client's rights. In mental health care, it is vital to determine the client's capacity to participate in the cognitive and affective aspects of the decision-making process, and to monitor that capacity on an ongoing basis.

Competency

Under the law, everyone is presumed competent, unless a court proceeding has occurred resulting in judicial determination of incompetence. A *competent* person (18 years of age or more) *is considered legally qualified to enjoy the full range of constitutional rights, such as freedom to enter contracts, marry, vote, own and use property, and obtain or refuse any or all medical or surgical treatment.* It is immaterial whether or not the client's choices are grounded in wisdom, sound judgment, or normal intelligence. The nurse is obligated to treat a competent person within the limits of the client's own consent. The law does not, and could not, apply different standards based on an individual's ability to exercise liberty wisely; it simply guarantees an equal right to liberty.

Differences in individual ability are without legal consequence until the person is sufficiently impaired that forced restriction of his or her liberty becomes necessary. Two such legal avenues are available: incompetency proceedings and involuntary commitment. Both are governed by state mental health laws.

Incompetency

A petition may be made to a court to declare a person *incompetent when self-management abilities are so impaired that the person or persons are at risk for foreseeable harm.* A court declaration of a person as incompetent is an extreme and permanent step, which strips the individual of constitutional liberties resulting from an inability to exercise freedom in a responsible manner. The court appoints a guardian to oversee the welfare of the incompetent person and to protect the person's civil rights as a substitute decision maker. The guardian is given the authority to act on behalf of the incompetent person (the "ward") in all matters on which the person could act if still competent, including informed consent and participation in treatment planning. For example, a client in the late stages of dementia of the Alzheimer's type (DAT) who is no longer able to safely manage activities of daily living (ADLs) may be declared incompetent and may have a guardian appointed by the court to oversee his or her affairs and to manage health care needs.

Incapacity

An attending physician determines after examination that a client with a mental illness is not capable of giving informed consent, that is, the client cannot comprehend the explanations discussed earlier, the client is considered **incapacitated,** *or lacking decision-making capacity.* Such determination must be noted in the medical record, or competence is presumed under the law. For example, a client's level of consciousness and reality orientation may fluctuate, creating an ambiguous situation. The client retains legal competence and the corollary constitutional right to make treatment decisions. Yet the client's clinically diminished decision-making capacity effectively nullifies his or her ability to exercise autonomy. The result is that the client's rights are not reliably preserved.

The absence of a consistent line of demarcation between the ability to make informed decisions and a clinically induced loss of that ability because of psychiatric symptoms makes the determination of incapacity a less than perfect solution. Only physicians are licensed to determine a client's loss of capacity. Such a determination modifies the requirement of informed consent, and enables a transfer of decision-making authority to a substitute authorized by the state law where the client resides. No treatment may be lawfully undertaken that requires the client's consent, except in cases of emergency without a legally appointed substitute, such as a person with a health care power of attorney (previously appointed by the client).

When a client has lost decision-making capacity without having advance directives or a legally appointed decision maker, uncharted ground is left in which the only legal guideline for the professional is the standard of care. The standard of care allows the nurse to provide that care which a reasonable professional with the same training would provide under the same or similar circumstances.

Entry Into Mental Health Treatment

The right to autonomy, as it applies to admission to an inpatient psychiatric treatment facility, is protected by due process of law. Clients are admitted voluntarily or *committed* involuntarily.

Voluntary admission

A **voluntary admission** to a treatment setting *occurs when a client willingly enters and consents to treatment. Clients who are in treatment voluntarily retain all of their civil rights and may discontinue treatment whenever they choose.* If the treatment team disagrees with the wisdom of the client's decision to discontinue treatment, he or she is usually required to sign a form acknowledging that they have been discharged against medical advice, or "AMA."

Voluntary admission is preferred because it indicates that the client recognizes his or her problems in living and willingness to participate in treatment to achieve relief. Psychiatric disturbances, however, sometimes impair the person's ability to recognize or accept the need for institutional admission, making involuntary or emergency admission necessary.

Involuntary admission

Involuntary admission, or **commitment,** *is institutionalizing a person against his or her will and constitutes a deprivation of liberty.* The constitution guarantees that no citizen will be deprived of liberty without due process of law. A citizen may be deprived of liberty based on presenting psychiatric symptoms only under extreme circumstances. Each state has established statutes and regulations that include medical determinations that must be met to justify institutionalizing a person against his or her will.

Involuntary commitment is appropriate for the following persons:

- Clients posing a threat to their own safety or that of others
- Clients who lack sufficient capacity to attend to their own basic needs for shelter, food, and safety
- Clients who are severely mentally ill and judged to be in need of treatment but fail to seek it voluntarily

Involuntary commitment is not necessarily permanent; individuals may later be released from commitment if the deficits for which they were committed diminish or disappear. The rights of involuntarily committed individuals were first recognized legally in two court cases, *Rogers v. Okin* (1979) and *Rennie v. Klein* (1978). The long-standing assumption of both law and psychiatry was that people admitted involuntarily had no capacity to give informed consent or to participate in treatment decisions. Involuntary commitment was assumed to be synonymous with involuntary treatment, designed to impose mandatory care and intervention for those who could not care for themselves. These landmark cases radically changed these assumptions and established that such individuals are presumed to be competent and retain their liberty and privacy interests under the 14th Amendment.

Outpatient commitment

Outpatient commitment *is a form of involuntary treatment and involves a specific outpatient treatment* *program ordered by the court.* The use of outpatient commitment has grown in response to deinstitutionalization initiatives and mandates to treat in the least restrictive environment. Commonly, clients who are committed as outpatients are those who have serious and persistent disorders, have little resources of their own, or have legal issues compounding their illnesses. Substance-impaired individuals, homeless mentally ill persons, and sex offenders are examples of clients who are committed for outpatient treatment.

Little is known about the outcomes of outpatient-mandated treatment. Issues such as decreasing resources for care of those with mental disorders and what to do with noncompliant individuals remain unresolved. The National Alliance for the Mentally Ill (NAMI) has conducted a national survey to assess the extent of the use of outpatient commitment (Torrey and Kaplan, 1995).

Emergency admission

Emergency admission is permitted in almost all states, to enable the community to confine a person with acute symptoms for purposes of nonconsensual emergency evaluation and treatment. Specifics vary among state laws but each requires the client's family, a physician, and/or an agent for the state, to seek the emergency admission and to have a supporting evaluation by a psychiatrist (or designated nurse practitioner in some states) justify the admission. Emergency admissions are limited by state law to 2 to 3 days, after which, if continued confinement is considered necessary, but is refused by the client, court commitment proceedings are required.

Least Restrictive Environment

Clients in the mental health care system are guaranteed the right to treatment in the *least restrictive environment, that setting that least restricts a client's rights.* Federal statutes specifically protect mental health clients' rights to freedom from restraint or seclusion. The meaning of *restraint has expanded over the years to include any physical or chemical measure that impedes freedom of movement.* Fixed lap trays and siderails on beds are now included in the range of traditional devices considered "restraints." Psychotropic medications are included because their powerful mind-altering effects can fulfill the purpose formerly served by straightjackets. In 1982 the U.S. Supreme Court ruled that even involuntarily committed clients are entitled to retain certain liberties protected under the 14th Amendment. These include reasonably safe conditions of confinement, freedom from unreasonable bodily restraints, and the right to receive training and "habilitation," maintaining safety and freedom from restraints. (*Youngberg v. Romeo*, 1982).

Seclusion can offer therapeutic benefit but must be used with caution and recognition that it fundamentally deprives clients of liberty and is a form of false imprisonment. The rights of a client to be free from restraint or seclusion must be weighed against the rights of others to be safe from violence and physical harm. Courts presume the validity of decisions made by qualified professionals, and liability will only be found when decisions depart substantially from accepted professional standards of care. Decisions to use restraint or seclusion must be guided by recognition of the strong liberty interests at stake. The least restrictive means to achieve the desired outcome are required under the law.

Whenever possible, the client should be consulted as to a preference among forms of medically advisable restraint (including medication). Informed consent remains an issue, unless the client has been found to be incompetent or has previously appointed a health care power of attorney, who can give informed consent. Where the client persists in poor impulse control, is subject to violent outbursts, and is resistant to treatment, an involuntary commitment proceeding is indicated to justify nonconsensual restrictive treatment. Chapter 25 discusses the responsibility of the nurse when restraints are used as part of the client's treatment plan.

Right to Privacy/Confidentiality

Every client has the right to privacy. The right to privacy is an individual's right to keep personal information secret. *Confidentiality is an extension of the right to privacy. It surrounds medical care, treatment, and records, and is specifically protected under state law. The duty of confidentiality prohibits a professional from disclosing information obtained as a result of the treatment relationship, except to fellow professionals involved in the client's care.* Violation of this duty can result in liability for negligence, invasion of privacy, and/or breach of statutes protecting confidentiality. Monetary damages may be awarded for each of those bases, determined from the extent of economic and sociopsychological injury caused by the breach of confidentiality.

The stigma that has historically been associated with mental disorders increases the obligation to honor the sacred trust implicit in the nurse-client relationship. Information about clients may be shared with treatment team members, supervisors, students, and faculty who are directly involved in the client's care. Family members, lawyers, outside therapists, and students who are not directly involved in the client's care are excluded from the information loop unless explicit written permission from the client authorizes release of information.

Although the right to privacy requires confidentiality, exceptions are permitted in specific situations. Court-ordered evaluations and reports must be submitted to the court as ordered. Other legitimate reasons for court orders to release information include criminal proceedings, or child abuse and child custody proceedings. If the client is competent, consent is obtained but is not required. Reports required by state law, such as reports of suicide attempts, gunshot wounds, or child abuse are exempt from the confidentiality obligation. In all situations, nurses *must* consult administrative policy related to release of records.

Confidentiality may be violated in an emergency situation when the professional is acting on the client's best interest. For example, a therapist may reveal to an adult family member that an adolescent client is severely suicidal. This is generally done in the presence of the client.

Another situation when a break in confidentiality is permitted involves acting to protect a third party. The courts have found (*Tarasoff v. Board of Regents of University of California, 1976*) that a therapist must warn others when a client poses a serious danger or threat to them.

Right to Refuse Treatment

Psychotropic drugs, electroshock therapy, and psychosurgery are among the mental health treatment modalities to which clients most often object. Today, there is no legal controversy over the right to refuse any of these treatments.

The U.S. Supreme Court declared antipsychotic drugs to be restraint by chemical means (*Washington v. Harper, 1990*). The Court noted that the serious and often permanent side effects of medication threaten client autonomy. Court findings noted that forced administration of medication infringes client's right of refusal and constrains their liberties by chemical means. The Court also ruled that committed clients were presumptively competent, since the state's commitment proceedings had not determined otherwise, and therefore such clients were entitled to rights of autonomy and privacy.

Only when a state can show a compelling interest in administering treatment against the client's will may forced treatment be considered permissible. This ruling extends to treatment of involuntarily committed clients and leads to where there are no clear signposts or easy answers. Each client situation requires careful weighing of the costs and benefits for both the individual and the community and raises ethical questions with legal ramifications. Collaborative decision making by health care personnel, clients, and their families and legal advisors best serves the interests of the client.

Some states have enacted laws in an attempt to provide clear guidelines. Iowa, for example, has adopted laws specifying that hospitalization by itself is not proof of incompetency. At least six states (Arizona, California, Colorado, Illinois, Indiana, and New York) have enacted legislation to protect involuntarily committed clients'

rights to refuse psychotropic or neuroleptic medications. Since the late 1970s, common law in six states has rejected the notion that an involuntarily committed client is incompetent to give informed consent regarding treatment. Thus even where a client's liberty is restricted through commitment, there is no automatic justification for intrusive treatment.

KEY POINTS

- A profession is defined as a calling that requires specialized knowledge, continuing study, the maintenance of high standards in achievement and conduct, and commitment to a kind of work that has as its prime purpose the rendering of public service.
- Value is the importance one places on something. Moral values are convictions about character attributes and standards to which one makes personal commitments and according to which one habitually chooses to act.
- The study of ethics encourages people to determine what they believe, why they believe it, and how to act on their beliefs.
- A value system is formed according to what a person judges as important. From values a person develops value sets that are used in decision making in life roles and relationships. Value sets are expanded over time into habitually applied value systems.
- Values clarification describes the process of personal decision making about conflicting moral values.
- Moral conflict for nurses may occur when two or more opposing ethical principles, possible actions, or unsatisfactory alternatives are available; when the need for reflection vies with the need for action; and when role obligations interfere with personal ethical principles.
- The duty of care is the legal standard that applies to every nurse client relationship. A breach of duty is any error or omission committed in the course of duty, regardless of intent.
- A tort is a wrongful act that results in injuries, loss or damage. Tort-based legal actions against nurses involve negligence, assault and battery, trespass, and false imprisonment.
- Standard of care describes the minimal level of care that may be delivered to the client. Standards involve the expected competent level of behavior of professional nurses.
- Clients in the mental health care system are protected by a "Bill of Rights." Several landmark legal decisions have guaranteed the human rights of clients.

CRITICAL THINKING QUESTIONS

Mr. Smith, a tall fierce-looking homeless man, was brought to the hospital emergency room by three policemen. He muttered, "Kill...kill," and reported voices telling him to kill people—just any people. A resident prescribed Haldol. A nurse brought him his dose, while the police continued to hold him forcibly in the chair. The man insisted he did not want it and would not take it.

1. What are Mr. Smith's rights in this situation?
2. What would you do in this situation?
3. What ethical dilemma is created by this situation?
4. What legal action is required of the nurse?

As the nurse talked to Mr. Smith asking him questions and offering him reassurance, a crowd of staff members began to gather. Mr. Smith relented and took the medication. He was admitted to the locked psychiatric emergency (PE) unit and reluctantly complied with taking the medication for 3 days. His symptoms improved. Then he began to develop side effects and rejected further medication, demanding release. He had no family or surrogate, no job, no address, and no Medicaid or Medicare coverage. The PE Unit was overcrowded and understaffed, and unit policy required referral and release within 3 days of admission. All long-term units in the city were full. (Long-term units had been closed during the community mental health movement days; the governor and mayor had enacted reductions in health social service and police budgets). At a team meeting the nurse supervisor was given the responsibility of finding a solution for Mr. Smith.

5. What feelings do you have about forcing a client to take medication against his will?
6. What suggestions do you have for the care of this client?
7. If you were in charge, what would you do?
8. If the client is discharged, whose human rights are being violated, the clients or those of others?
9. How did the larger society, as described in the situation, have an impact on the care of this client?
10. What can nurses do to promote care of clients like Mr. Smith?

On the fifth day of Mr. Smith's stay, he overpowered a female nurse as she entered the locked unit, escaped, and disappeared. Thirty days later, he pushed the mother of three small children to her death onto the railway of a subway station, was apprehended on site, and jailed for homicide. A high-profile liability lawyer took the case on contingency on behalf of the victim's family.

11. Who is responsible for the death of the woman in this situation?
12. If you were the nurse who was overpowered, what do you think your feelings would be?
13. What could have been done by the nurse, the hospital, and the community to prevent the death of the woman in this situation?
14. Should Mr. Smith have been jailed or returned to the hospital?
15. If you were selected to be a juror in this case, who would you find guilty?

REFERENCES

42 U.S.C. § 1983.

42 U.S.C. 9501 (c) and 10841 (1)(C).

42 U.S.C. 9501 (1)(D) and 10841 (1)(D).

42 U.S.C. 9501 (1)(F) and 10841 (1)(F).

American Nurses Association. (1994). *Statement on psychiatric-mental health clinical nursing practice and standards of psychiatric-mental health clinical nursing practice.* Washington, DC: Author.

Matek, S.J. (1995). Professional Ethics Resources, 1626 North Prospect Avenue, Suite 2004, Milwaukee, Wisconsin, 53202. 1-800-55ETHICS.

Mohr, W. (1996). Ethics, nursing and health care in the age of "re-form." *Perspectives on Community, 17,*(1), 16-21.

Patient Self Determination Act, Public Law No 101-508, 104 Stat. 1388.

Rennie v. Klein 462 F. Supp. 1131 (D.N.J. 1978).

Rogers v. Okin 478 F. Supp. 1342 (D. Mass. 1979).

Tarasoff v. Regents of the University of California, 17 Cal. 3d 425; 131 Cal. Rptr. 14 (1976).

Torrey, E.F., & Kaplan, R.J. (1995). A national survey of the use of outpatient commitment. *Psychiatric Services, 46*(8), 778-784.

Trudeau, M.E. (1994). Informed consent: The patients right to decide. *Journal of Psychosocial Nursing and Mental Health Services, 31*(6), 9-12.

Washington v. Harper, 110 S. Ct. 1028 (1990).

Youngberg v. Romeo, 457 U.S. 307 (1982).

 ## VIDEO RESOURCES

Mosby's Legal and Ethical Issues in Nursing Video Series:
Ethical Dilemmas and Decision Making
Legal Aspects of Nursing Documentation
Introduction to Legal Issues and Terminology
Minimizing Legal Liability
Patient Self-Determination
The Nurses' Rights As an Employee

Chapter 4

Outcomes Management

Elizabeth C. Poster

LEARNING OUTCOMES

After studying and applying the concepts of this chapter, the learner will be able to:
- Describe the evolution from quality assurance to continuous quality improvement and total quality management.
- Identify three characteristics of outcomes management.
- Define the term *indicator* according to the Joint Commission on the Accreditation of Healthcare Organizations (JCAHO).
- Differentiate among structure, process, and outcome indicators.
- Describe three differences between outcome research and outcome evaluation.
- Identify four criteria to be used in selecting outcome evaluation instruments.
- Discuss the role of the psychiatric nurse in identifying expected client outcomes as described by the American Nurses Association (ANA) *Standards of Psychiatric-Mental Health Clinical Nursing Practice.*

KEY TERMS

Indicator

Outcome

Outcome evaluation

Outcome indicator

Outcomes management

Process indicator

Structure indicator

Outcomes management and evaluation are critical functions of all mental health care settings. There is a growing emphasis on the provision of quality care as measured and documented in terms of the effectiveness of care. As we move into the next century, managed care, accrediting organizations, and consumers will increasingly demand access to information, on which they will make decisions that will directly affect the health care institution and its health care providers. Evaluation of the effectiveness of nursing interventions as they relate to clinical client outcomes will therefore become an even more important component of the nursing role. The goal of psychiatric nursing in all types of practice settings is to influence health outcomes and improve the client's health status. Knowledge of the resources, methods, and tools of outcome evaluation provide psychiatric nurses with the ability to demonstrate that these goals are achieved.

HISTORICAL EVOLUTION OF QUALITY ASSURANCE, TOTAL QUALITY MANAGEMENT, AND CONTINUOUS QUALITY IMPROVEMENT

The concept of quality assurance in hospitals dates back to 1917, when the American College of Surgeons (ACS) was the first group to monitor and evaluate the clinical activities of medical staff. The Joint Commission on Accreditation of Hospitals (JCAH) was founded in 1951 and published standards for hospitals to follow, including quality assurance standards. These early standards were general regarding the assessment and improvement of the quality of care. Hospitals performed primarily morbidity and mortality reviews, and the emphasis was on specific problems with medical care.

From these early beginnings to the 1980s, the focus of quality assurance was primarily on problems in the delivery and documentation of care. There were two shortcomings of this problem-focused approach. First, information obtained regarding existing problems was not systematically used to improve care. In addition, it was the process of care, as documented by staff, rather than the outcome of the care from the clients' perspective, that was emphasized.

Other driving forces occurred in the mid-1980s, which reinforced interest in the evaluation and measurement of quality. Hospitals had to respond to changes in reimbursement based on diagnosis-related groups (DRGs), which are preset fees determined by the client's diagnosis, regardless of the actual cost. It also became important to measure quality of care, particularly as it related to cost. Consumers were increasingly demanding information and accountability from health care providers. Finally, private insurance groups were following the government's lead, resulting in more cost constraints on health services delivered. The push was on for quality care that was efficient and effective, and resulted in positive client outcomes.

In the 1990s the Joint Commission on the Accreditation of Healthcare Organizations (JCAHO) introduced the concepts of total quality management and continuous quality improvement (CQI). These terms are often used interchangeably. CQI incorporates many of the elements of quality assurance, broadening its scope to include the principles advocated by industry leaders such as W. Edward Demming, Joseph M. Juran, and Philip B. Crosby (JCAHO, 1991). CQI focuses on systems, rather than individuals; emphasizes multidisciplinary collaborative relationships; and promotes problem solving by teams and the use of statistical tools for the measurement of client outcomes (Decker, Moore-Greenlaw, and Strader, 1994).

Opportunities and challenges for health care in the 1990s include the need to define and track clinical effectiveness through the analysis of clinical data. Competition in the marketplace is becoming more severe and increasingly requires that hospitals demonstrate the effectiveness of their services balanced with cost. The allocation of limited resources is being determined by the proven effectiveness of various services, procedures, and treatment modalities. The goal of managed health care is to provide quality care in a cost-effective way (Hicks, Stallmeyer, and Coleman, 1993). The only way to know if this is occurring is by evaluating the results of this care on clients through outcome evaluation. The demand for health care organizations and providers requires a clear understanding of the definition of quality, as well as the knowledge and tools to quantify the delivery of care, quality-related costs, and the outcomes of care.

Outcome evaluation is an integral part of the larger concept of outcomes management. According to Ellwood (1988), *outcomes management is a technology of client experience consisting of three components: (1) research-based guidelines and standards of practice; (2) measurement of functioning, well-being, and disease-specific clinical outcomes; and (3) access to national data bases of clinical, financial, and health outcomes for comparison (benchmarks) and decision-making purposes.* The goal of outcomes management is to help clients, payers, and providers make rational health care-related choices (Ellwood, 1988).

A Review of Current Forces

Traditionally, health-related thinking was based on a disease model and the medical model rather than on the current wellness and health-promotion models. Based on a wellness model, measures of functioning, well-being, and quality of life are being added to the traditional pathophysiological parameters. Nurses have traditionally emphasized health promotion and are now acknowledged for their expertise in this area of practice. These newer views of health are not only influencing practice but also are shaping public policy. For example, *Healthy People 2000* (U.S. Department of Health and Human Services, 1991) emphasizes that a central purpose of health care is to increase the proportion of Americans who live long, healthy lives. Health means a full range of functional capacity at each stage allowing for the ability to enter into satisfying relationships with others, to work, and to play. Federal legislation has mandated agencies to explore medical effectiveness. The Agency for Health Care Policy Research (AHCPR) has, as its primary responsibility, the implementation of a Medical Effectiveness Program (AHCPR, 1990). This federal agency is awarding grants for research to answer fundamental questions about the medical effectiveness of health care, such as: Do patients benefit? What treatments work best? Are health care resources well-spent? In addition to answering these questions, the development of "practice guidelines" will assist practitioner and client decisions about appropriate health care for specific clinical conditions such as depression (AHCPR, 1990).

Ways are being developed to measure a client's health status and to assess the quality and appropriateness of care. For example, the Rand Corporation's Medical Outcomes Study (MOS) has helped develop instruments that measure the traditional biological parameters and symptoms of client illness and also in developing new methods for obtaining reliable, valid, and efficient information on how clients with chronic disease feel, function, and perform in their natural environment (Rand, 1991). The availability of brief yet reliable and valid measurement tools enables hospitals to conduct outcome evaluation studies that are scientifically sound, as well as feasible, within a busy practice setting.

PSYCHIATRIC NURSING OUTCOMES

Although nursing care is a major component of the treatment of all clients admitted for inpatient psychiatric care, evaluating the direct impact of this care is difficult. In most psychiatric settings in which a multidisciplinary team provides multiple interventions, a direct relationship between client outcome and the quality of care provided by a single discipline is hard to identify and measure. Thus a major challenge facing psychiatric nursing today is to conduct ongoing program evaluation that investigates the relationship between nursing care and desired client outcomes. For example, it is important to know the relationship between staffing mix and maintenance of client safety in the milieu. Is client violence prevented or controlled when the unit is staffed with more highly educated and experienced nurses? Do client's feel

safer when there is a higher or lower ratio of registered nurse (RN) to non-RN staff?

Outcome measurement in nursing has a long history beginning with Florence Nightingale. Although there was renewed interest in the 1970s, the emphasis heightened in the 1980s with new national requirements focusing on outcomes: requirements proposed by the JCAHO, the Health Care Financing Administration (HCFA), the National Association of Private Psychiatric Hospitals (NAPPH), and the Omnibus Reconciliation Act (OBRA). In reviewing nursing services, these organizations have viewed **outcome** *as a measurable change in a client's health status related to the receipt of nursing care.*

Indicators of Quality

As integral members of the multidisciplinary team, nurses need to understand and be involved in the entire process of CQI from assessment to evaluation of client outcomes. One of the ways that psychiatric nurses contribute to their hospitals' CQI programs is by identifying and developing clinical indicators (Podgorny, 1991).

The JCAHO defines **indicators** *as quantitative measures that can be used to monitor and evaluate the quality of important governance, management, and clinical and support functions that affect client outcome* (JCAHO, 1990). Categories of outcome measures range from mortality to quality of life as identified in Box 4-1. A client fall is an example of a clinical indicator. Other examples are medication error rates, episodes of seclusion/restraint, and the number of suicides. Indicators focus attention on what happens to clients as a consequence of how well staff or the organizational system functions.

Structure, process, and outcome are the dimensions of care for which clinical indicators can be developed (Donabedian, 1992). **Structure indicators** *include hospital resources and systems such as staffing requirements, continuing education, and monitoring of licensure of the clinical staff.* **Process indicators** *focus on events, actions, or steps that occur during the course of client care and are usually evaluated according to the documentation in the client's medical record. An* **outcome indicator** *reflects the status of the client as a result of the process of care.* Outcomes are evaluated by both the client and the nurse at discharge and postdischarge according to changes in symptoms, quality of life, and client satisfaction with care received (Bernstein and Hilborne, 1993). Over the years, indicators have evolved with use and changes in emphasis. Historically, indicators focused on structure and process. Recently, interest has shifted to outcome indicators, since outcomes are the ultimate measure of quality care.

The selection of the most important outcome indicators for any TQM/CQI program is a difficult task. In psy-

Box 4-1

Categories of Outcome Indicators

1. Physiological status
2. Psychosocial status
3. Functional status
4. Goal attainment
5. Knowledge
6. Behavior
7. Safety
8. Symptom control
9. Quality of life
10. Satisfaction
11. Re-hospitalization
12. Mortality

TABLE 4-1

Outcome movement today

OUTCOME RESEARCH	OUTCOME EVALUATION
Randomized controlled trials	Routinely delivered care
Tracks clients with one condition	Tracks all clients
Evaluates specific intervention	Evaluates "episode" of care
Evaluates "hard" physiological indicators and laboratory tests	Includes client's perspective
Results narrowly distributed	Information used as a part of ordinary medical care and in making program decisions

chiatry and psychiatric nursing the development of precise, meaningful criteria that describe both negative and positive client outcomes is especially challenging.

The challenge for nurses is to incorporate outcome evaluation into their practice within a busy clinical setting. Outcome evaluation differs from outcome research in a number of important ways (Table 4-1). *Outcome evaluation focuses on routinely delivered care and tracking all the clients within a program or a setting.* As such, these data become an integral part of the setting's TQM/CQI program, evaluating an "episode of care" such as a single hospitalization rather than the effectiveness of a specific intervention like group therapy. The client's perspective in terms of satisfaction and beliefs about his or her own improvement are included in the evaluation. The information that is collected is used as part of the ordinary nursing and medical care and is integral in making program decisions. The primary commonality between outcome research and outcome evaluation is the use of valid and reliable measurement tools in both types of programs. A major difference is that evaluation can be ongoing, whereas research is a more in-depth snapshot of a larger whole. For example, a research question would try to answer the question, "Is group therapy more effective when clients have homework assignments than when there is no homework assignment? An outcome evaluation question related to group therapy would be, "Do clients believe that their conditions have improved as a result of the group therapy intervention?"

COMPONENTS OF OUTCOME EVALUATION

Although the term *outcome* may appear simple at first, it is actually a complex construct made up of many com-

ponents. Three major components are usually included in the measurement of outcomes: (1) the client perspective, (2) multidimensionality of outcomes, and (3) timing of evaluation. Both the practitioner's and the client's perspectives need to be included, since research has shown that there can be significant differences between their views (Mintz et al., 1979).

The Client Perspective

With the increasing emphasis on client-centered care (Gerteis et al., 1993), it is even more important today to evaluate clients' opinions about the care they received. Self-report data from clients with psychiatric symptoms have historically been criticized because of the potential for bias. Yet despite concerns related to validity and reliability of the findings, it is critical to include the client perspective in psychiatric outcome evaluation, not only to demonstrate a respect for clients' views, but also to gain information that only the client can provide. Additionally, perceptions about services are just as important as the clinical features of the program. For all providers and clients alike, perception is reality. A review of the literature by Eisen, Grob, and Dill (1991) provides a thorough overview of both the value, as well as the limitations of self-report methods of clients with mental illness in program evaluation studies. In addition to client satisfaction surveys described in Table 4-2, a number of other questionnaires completed by clients are commonly used in psychiatric outcome evaluation programs such as Symptoms Checklist-90 (Derogatis, 1970). The data ob-

TABLE 4-2

Satisfaction questionnaires

NAME	AUTHORS	CHARACTERISTICS
Consumer Satisfaction Questionnaire	Larsen, et al (1979)	Eight items
		4-point scale
Group Health Association of America (GHAA's) Consumer Satisfaction Survey	GHAA (1991)	63 items
		5-point scale
Patient Satisfaction Questionnaire (PSQ-III)	Hays, Davies, and Ware (1987)	50 items
		5-point scale

tained from these questionnaires are used in conjunction with the data from provider-completed questionnaires.

Multidimensionality of Outcomes

The second component is multidimensionality of outcomes. To comprehensively determine the outcomes of health care or hospitalization on the client's life, it is common practice to evaluate social, work, or school functioning; symptom management; and overall quality of life. This is especially the case with clients who have a chronic medical and/or psychiatric illness. General health measures allow for the assessment of general health outcomes in quantitative terms. For nurses the information is especially relevant in understanding client's responses to their illnesses and the impact of care on these responses. For example, it is important to know not only that the client's symptoms such as hallucinations have diminished but also that he or she has become more involved in the community and with friends as a result of the improved symptoms. The nurse's interventions to help clients plan for reentry into society are critical for successful client outcomes related to overall quality of life.

Selection of the appropriate instruments to evaluate functioning and quality of life need to be based on a number of factors. Most important is the consistency between the conceptual framework of the instrument and the measurement approaches that are used (Strickland, 1991). Another factor to evaluate is the population for whom the instrument was designed. If evaluation is intended to be disease-specific (e.g., depression), then generic tools may not be adequate to determine the affect of the care on a client's specific symptoms of depression. Instead, a specific depression survey such as the Hamilton or Beck would allow for more in-depth assessment of signs and symptoms of this condition. Cul-

tural experience and ethnic background also need to be considered. For example, if the wording of a questionnaire has not been adequately tested with a specific ethnic group, individuals could misinterpret the meaning of words and the answers might not be valid. To ensure that questions are culturally and ethnically appropriate, a number of questionnaires, such as the SF36 Quality of Life Survey (Stewart, Hays, and Ware, 1988), are being translated into languages other than English. Practicality is also important. Instruments need to be client friendly and not require a great deal of staff and client time to complete.

Timing of evaluation

Another component to be considered in any outcome program is the timing of the evaluation. It has been shown that the timing of the evaluation can influence the findings in many areas such as work and social functioning (Mintz et al., 1992). Most outcome evaluation studies conducted with psychiatric clients time the evaluations at three points in time: (1) admission, to develop a base line of information; (2) discharge, to evaluate short-term results; and (3) at a 6-month or 1-year follow-up to evaluate long-term results.

Because of the time interval between discharge and follow-up evaluation, many variables need to be considered in the long-term outcome evaluation. The following are a few of the questions to consider: Did the client seek additional health care in another setting? How many visits? What were the treatments received? Did the client develop another medical or psychiatric condition after discharge? Does the client have social support? Did the client adhere to the prescribed treatment regimen?

To determine the outcome of care even during the acute care episode like inpatient hospitalization, factors such as severity of illness, resource utilization, and demographic variables also need to be taken into consideration. The client's medical record is an excellent source of information. Many hospitals are computerizing medical records in an attempt to more easily gather information and link it to the hospital's quality management and outcome evaluation programs.

THE TOOLS OF OUTCOME EVALUATION

It is important to use a quantitative approach in answering the question: How did hospitalization make a difference? "Guesstimates" based on subjective observation and qualitative assessment methods are no longer acceptable. The increasing sophistication of computer-based information systems makes it possible for nurses to use their hospitals' resources in a cost-effective way for data collection, storage, analysis, and reporting. Many hospitals are also beginning to hire biostatisticians and purchase statistical software packages as part of their quality management and outcome evaluation programs. These resources are also available to psychiatric nurses to assist in the planning and implementation of outcome evaluation studies.

Thousands of instruments are available to measure client outcomes. To select appropriate tools the following criteria can be used as a guide. The instrument should:

- Be reliable and valid
- Be cost-effective to use
- Reflect the dimensions of concern for the specific population
- Include both provider and client self-report measures
- Be brief and simple to administer and score
- Be widely recognized and used
- Be responsive to changes (range of possible values of scores)

Many instruments are in the public domain and can be used without paying a fee (e.g., the 36-item self-report Health Status Survey that measures quality of life). Others that are used currently in many psychiatric settings can be obtained from the authors and may require a fee (e.g., the 21-item self-report Beck Depression Inventory [Beck et al., 1961]). Additionally, there are a number of national organizations dedicated to supporting psychiatric outcome evaluation, which are listed in the Community Resources box below. For example, the Health Outcomes Institute has 18 condition-specific data collection tools, including depression, called Technology of Patient Experiences (TyPEs). This system can:

1. Measure a client's functional status and quality of life over time, using terms readily understandable by and relevant to the client, payers, and providers.
2. Document changes over time in a client's clinical condition as a result of therapeutic interventions.
3. Ensure that data are collected in a common format using widely understood protocols across a large number of sites.
4. Maintain data collected from multiple sites in a single repository, allowing comparison of client outcomes across sites, therapeutic regimens, providers, and others.
5. Incorporate standardized and valid methods of accounting for health care organizations' effects on quality of life.

APPLICATION OF OUTCOME EVALUATION
Inpatient Psychiatric Settings

The following section provides an example of a typical outcome evaluation program that has been developed in

COMMUNITY RESOURCES

National Organizations Supporting Psychiatric Outcome Evaluation

- **Medical Outcomes Trust,** 20 Park Plaza, Suite 1014; Boston, MA 02116; Fax: (617) 426-4131. There is no fee for the *Bulletin* and the SF36 Quality of Life Instrument.
- **Health Outcomes Institute** (formerly Interstudy), 2001 Killebrew Drive, Suite 122; Bloomington, MN 55425; (612) 858-9188. Eighteen condition-specific data collection tools including depression are available; there is a fee for tools.
- **Institute for Health Care Improvement.** One Exeter Plaza, 9th floor; Boston, MA 02116; (617) 424-4800; Donald Berwick, M.D., President.
- **The Human Services Research Institute,** 2336 Massachusetts Ave.; Cambridge, MA 02140; (617) 876-0426; Fax: (617) 492-7401; e mail: tecenter@HSRI.org. Tool kits, consultation, mini-grants are available.
- **State University of New York at Buffalo,** Functional Independence Measure, (1990); (716) 831-2076. There is no fee.
- **University of Connecticut,** Psych Sentinel; (203) 679-3276; Hal Mark, PhD; Severity of Illness measure is based on DSM-IV.
- **Agency for Health Care Policy and Research** (AHCPR), (800) 358-9295; Clinical Practice Guidelines-Depression.

an academic medical center psychiatric hospital, the UCLA Neuropsychiatric Hospital (NPH). The NPH admits severely ill clients from ages 2 to 100 years who have medical and psychiatric comorbid conditions. The outcome evaluation program is an integral part of the hospital's quality management program and is jointly administered by the director of nursing research and education and the director of quality management.

Based on a comprehensive review of the literature and analysis of the needs of the institution, a number of evaluation measures were selected to provide the following types of client information:

- Physical and social functioning, which includes relationships with others and daily activities, work, and school
- Psychiatric symptoms such as depression, anxiety, psychosis, impulsive/addictive behavior, eating disorders, and other condition-specific behaviors
- General health and well-being, including energy, fatigue, pain, physical health
- Changes in health in the past year and use of health care resources
- Client satisfaction with components of the hospital stay and perceptions of improvement

Volunteers who are carefully screened and extensively trained collect the data. Every client who is admitted is asked to complete questionnaires on admission, at discharge, and at 6 months postdischarge. The findings of the evaluation are distributed to providers and hospital administrators. The data base is available to hospital staff for research, education, administrative, clinical, and marketing purposes. In addition, the data highlight many opportunities for the achievement of continuous quality improvement goals.

Community Psychiatric Settings

As inpatient settings are attempting to document client outcomes, so are outpatient, community, home health care, and various psychiatric rehabilitation centers. A report from the National Institute of Mental Health (NIMH), *Caring for People with Severe Mental Disorders: A National Plan for Research to Improve Services* (1992), proposed that mental health services researchers need to improve and expand their efforts to better understand the effectiveness and outcomes of mental health services nationwide. In response to this call for action, three significant papers (Cook, 1992; Lehman, 1992; McGlynn, 1992) were written that reviewed the current state of mental health services research and the measurement tools available to health care professionals and researchers.

These three papers clarified existing measures that could effectively be used for outcome evaluation in a wide variety of nonacute care psychiatric settings. Since the current trend is a decrease in admissions to inpatient psychiatric hospitals and more community-based settings, these papers are especially helpful in understanding the scope of the challenge of outcome evaluation in these settings.

THE ROLE OF THE PSYCHIATRIC NURSE IN EVALUATING THE OUTCOMES OF CARE

According to psychiatric-mental health nursing's *Standards* (ANA, 1994) outcome evaluation is an integral aspect of the role of the professional nurse. Professional nurses are accountable for client outcomes in all psychiatric settings. According to these standards, theory and research guide the professional nurse's evaluation of client outcomes. (See Appendix A of this text.)

The ultimate goal of nursing care is to improve the client's health status. This goal is broad and takes into consideration the client's functional status and quality of life, and reflects current scientific knowledge and conceptualization of health.

One of the ways in which nurses can meet this standard in everyday practice is by adhering to each component of the nursing process and documenting the care provided in a retrievable form. The medical record is a document that can be used as a data base and is especially useful if it has been computerized. The charting of the client's diagnosis, nursing interventions, and achievement of measurable goals can provide useful outcome information to be used in conjunction with other quantifiable client information documented by members of the multidisciplinary team.

Indicator: Client Safety/Fall Outcomes

One of the roles of psychiatric nurses, regardless of the type of setting, is to ensure the safety of the clients. One outcome of care related to this function is that clients are discharged from the hospital without falling. Protection from falling is especially important in a psychiatric setting because of the influence of high-risk factors such as labile mental status that can influence judgment and lead to maladaptive behavior, the use of medications that can affect gait and proprioception, and disorders that alter awareness of the safety hazards in the environment. Additionally, most psychiatric clients are not restricted to their beds but are ambulatory.

Using the hospital's unusual occurrence (U/O) reports as a data base, nurses can collect, analyze, and track the effectiveness of their care. If the U/O report does not include an adequate amount or type of information, a coding guide can be developed to ensure that client outcomes are documented. The essential information includes: type of fall, reason for fall, treatment postfall, time and location of treatment, and severity of outcome. Demographic information about the client, such as age, gender, diagnoses, and others, can be obtained from the hospital's information system. Quantifying the severity of client outcome is essential. A Likert scale, which includes four levels of severity from "none" to "death," is a typical scale (Poster and Pelletier, 1990). The results of monitoring client fall outcomes can be used as an opportunity for improvement if the fall rates increase or to demonstrate the effectiveness of nursing care in the area of fall prevention and client safety.

Outcome and process indicators are monitored on a specified basis so that nursing staff are able to track unexpected variations in the frequency and immediately take corrective action if needed. At the UCLA NPH, client falls are monitored by the Nursing Quality Improvement Committee on a monthly basis. The U/O data are quantified, and a fall rate is calculated based on a national standard of the number of falls per 1,000 patient-days (Morse and Morse, 1988). Data from each of the six inpatient units are analyzed separately because of differences in the ages and other risk factors of the client population. A review of the literature did not locate a benchmark for falls in similar psychiatric settings. However, a report of 25 falls per 1,000 patient-days was documented in one study of geropsychiatric clients in a Veteran's Administration Medical Center (Hernandez and Miller, 1986).

It was clear from this review that UCLA NPH needed to analyze its own data, which would then be used as a benchmark against which future fall rates would be evaluated. A total of 494 falls occurred in a group of 4,156 clients admitted to the hospital over a 34-month period of time (Poster, Pelletier, and Kay, 1991). Additionally, it was found that the fall rate was the highest on the geropsychiatric unit. Although not as high as the 25 falls per 1,000 clients reported elsewhere, this was viewed as an opportunity for improvement. A fall prevention protocol was developed, which could be implemented on any of the inpatient units but was most useful for the geriatric clients who were at the highest risk for falls. Using the study data as a base line, postintervention data were also collected on an ongoing basis. The effectiveness of this nursing intervention on client outcomes was demonstrated using information that was documented and collected as a routine part of nursing practice. The savings in costs to clients can be determined using these same data. Costs can be determined in terms of decreased lengths of stay of clients who do not fall compared with those who fall, as well as in the savings to the hospital by prevention of legal claims.

Indicator: Predicted Client Outcomes

Another example of demonstrating the effectiveness of nursing care on client outcomes is quantifying the achievement of short-term goals or predicted client outcomes at the time of discharge. Since nurses plan for changes in client behavior as a consequence of nursing interventions, the level of intensity of behaviors, as well as the presence or absence of behaviors, can be scored to show change. For example, at the time of discharge, the client will be able to state three side effects of his or her medication. Data related to each of the following statements can be used to present the data collected from the nursing records:

- Total number of predicted outcomes/short-term goals
- Number of predicted outcomes/short-term goals met by discharge
- Number of predicted outcomes/short-term goals not met by discharge
- Percentage of goals met and not met based on the total number
- Number of predicted outcomes/short-term goals for which there was no documentation found

These basic findings can be used to support the effectiveness of the nursing care or to highlight documentation problems. If clients are not meeting the goals, it might also be the case that the goals are not realistic for the length of client stay or other reasons. Additionally, a review of the appropriateness of the goals based on the client's condition, age, and other factors will need to be made as part of the evaluation.

KEY POINTS

- Three characteristics of outcome management are as follows:

  1. Research-based guidelines and standards of practice.
  2. Measurement of functioning, well-being, and disease specific clinical outcomes.
  3. Access to national data bases of clinical, financial, and health outcomes for comparison (benchmarks) in decision-making purposes.

- Indicators or qualitative measures can be used to monitor and evaluate the quality of important government, management, clinical, and support functions that affect client outcomes.
- Structural indicators include hospital resources and systems such as staffing requirements, continuing education, and monitoring and licensure of clinical staff.
- Process indicators include events, actions, or steps that occur during the course of client care and are usually evaluated according to the documentation in the client's medical record.
- Outcome indicators reflect the status of the client as a result of the process of care.

• The three components of outcome evaluation are as follows:

1. The clients perspective as well as the clinician's
2. Mutlidimensionality of outcomes (quality of life, signs and symptoms, and satisfaction with care)
3. Timing of evaluation.

• The following four criteria are to be used in selecting outcome evaluation instruments:

1. Reliability and validity
2. Cost effectiveness
3. Inclusion of the dimensions of concern for the specific population
4. Both practitioner and client self-report measures

• ANA's (1994) *Statement on Psychiatric-Mental Health Clinical Nursing Practice and Standards of Psychiatric-Mental Health Clinical Nursing Practice* includes outcome evaluation as an integral aspect of the role of the psychiatric nurse.

 CRITICAL THINKING QUESTIONS

The nursing staff on one of the hospital's inpatient adult units has been asked by the director of the quality improvement department to conduct an outcome evaluation study related to their client teaching activities. During the nursing meeting, the staff agreed that they would focus their study on the outcome of their client teaching related to medication education. The unit has a program which includes the following:

• Provision of booklets to clients that contains basic information about the classification of medication that they are prescribed (i.e. antidepressants, psychotropic medications, antimanic medication, lithium)
• Group education that focuses on general content such as side effects and self-administration strategies
• Individualized teaching by nursing staff and physicians.

1. Discuss your plan to design an outcome evaluation study to determine the impact of medication teaching on clients' knowledge.
2. How would you determine whether clients have gained knowledge as an outcome of the education program?
3. How would you consider clients' varying length of stay and severity of illness factors in the study?

REFERENCES

Achenbach, T., & Edelbrock, C. (1981). Behavioral problems and competencies reported by parents of normal and disturbed children aged four through sixteen. *Monographs of the Society for Research in Child Development, 46,* (1, Serial No. 188).

Achenbach, T., & Edelbrock, C. (1983). *Manual for the child behavior checklist and revised child behavior profile.* Burlington, VT: Department of Psychiatry, University of Vermont.

Agency for Health Care Policy and Research. (1990, March). *Medical treatment effectiveness research.* Rockville, MD: Author.

American Nurses Association. (1994). *Statement on psychiatric-mental health clinical practice and standards of psychiatric-mental health clinical practice.* Washington, DC: Author.

Beck, A., et al. (1961). An inventory for measuring depression. *Archives of General Psychiatry, 42,* 667-675.

Bernstein, S.J., & Hilborne, L.H. (1993). Clinical indicators: The road to quality care? *Journal on Quality Improvement, 19*(11), 501-508.

Cook, J.A. (1992). Outcome assessment in psychiatric rehabilitation services for persons with severe and persistent mental illness. Unpublished manuscript. The Rand Corporation.

Davies, A.R., Doyle, M.A., Rutt, W., Orsolits, S.M., & Doyle, J.B. (1994). Outcomes assessment in clinical settings: A consensus statement on principles and best practices in project management. *Journal on Quality Improvement, 20*(1), 6-16.

Decker, P.J., Moore-Greenlaw, R.C., & Strader, M.K. (1994). Functional Standards: The walls come tumbling down. *Journal of Nursing Administration, 24* (7/8), 18-20.

Derogatis, L.R., (1970). SCL-90. *Administration, scoring, and procedures manual-revised version.* Baltimore, MD: John Hopkins Hospital.

Donabedian, A. (November, 1992). The role of outcomes in quality assessment and assurance. *Quality Review Bulletin,* 356-360.

Eisen, S.V., Dill, D.L., & Grob, M.C. (1989). *BASIS-32: A self-report measure for evaluating patient progress.* (Evaluative Service Unit Report NO. 76). Belmont, MA: McLean Hospital.

Eisen, S.V., Grob, M.C., & Dill, D.L. (1991). Outcome management: Tapping the patient's perspective. In S.M. Mirin, J.T. Gossett, & M.C. Grob (Eds.). *Psychiatric treatment advances in outcome research.* Washington, DC: APA Press.

Eisen, S.V., Grob, M.C., & Klein, A.A. (1986). BASIS: The development of a self-report measure for psychiatric inpatient evaluation. *The Psychiatric Hospital, 17,* 165-171.

Ellwood, P.M. (1988). Outcomes management: A technology of patient experience. *New England Journal of Medicine, 318,* 1549-1556.

Endicott, J., Spitzer, R.L., Fleiss, J.L., & Cohen, J. (1976). The global assessment scale: A procedure for measuring overall severity of psychiatric disturbance. *Archives of General Psychiatry, 33,* 766-771.

Gerteis, M., Edgman-Levitan, S., Daley, J., & Delbanco, T.L. (1993). *Through the patient's eyes: Understanding and promoting patient centered care.* San Francisco: Jossey-Bass.

Goodman, W.K., et al. (1989). The Yale Brown obsessive-compulsive scale I: Development, use, and reliability. *Archives of General Psychiatry, 46,* 1006-1011.

Group Health Association of America, Inc. (1991). GHAA's Consumer Satisfaction Survey. Washington, DC: Author.

Guy, W. (1976). *ECDEU assessment manual for psychopharmacology.* Washington, DC: National Institute of Mental Health.

Hamilton, M. (1960). Rating depressed patients. *Journal of Clinical Psychiatry, 41,* 21-24.

Hays, R.D., Davies, A.R., & Ware, J.E. (1987). Scoring the Patient Satisfaction Questionnaires: PSQIII. MOS Memo No. 866, *Medical outcomes study.* Santa Monica, CA: Rand Corporation.

Hernandez, M., & Miller, J.A. (1986) How to reduce falls. *Geriatric Nursing, 7*(3), 97-103.

Hicks, L.L., Stallmeyer, J.M., & Coleman, J.R. (1993). *The role of the nurse in managed care.* Washington, DC: American Nurses Association.

Joint Commission on Accreditation of Healthcare Organizations. (1991). *The transition from QA to CQI: An introduction to quality improvement in health.* Oakbrook Terrace, IL: Author.

Kessler, R.C., et al. (1994). Lifetime and 12 month prevalence of DSM-III-R psychiatric disorders in the US: Results from the National Comorbidity Survey. *Archives of General Psychiatry, 51,* 8-19.

Kiresuk, T.J., & Sherman, R.E. (1968). Global attainment scaling. *Community Mental Health Journal, 4,* 443-453.

Larsen, D.L., Attkisson, C.C., Hargreaves, W.A., & Nguyen, T.D. (1979). Assessment of client/patient satisfaction: Development of a general scale. *Evaluation and Program Planning, 2,* 197-207.

Lehman, A.F. (1992). Measures of humanistic outcomes (quality of life) among persons with severe and persistent mental illness. Unpublished manuscript. The Rand Corporation.

Linn, M.W., & Linn, B.S. (1982). The Rapid Disability Rating Scale-2, *Journal of the American Geriatric Society, 30,* 378-382.

McGlynn, E.A. (1992). A review of measures in the clinical domain for research with persons with severe and persistent mental disorders. Unpublished manuscript. The Rand Corporation.

Mintz, J., et al. (1979). Patient's therapist's and observers' views of psychotherapy: A "Rashomon" experience or reasonable consensus? *British Journal of Medical Psychology, 46,* 83-89.

Mintz, J., Mintz, L.I., Arruda, M.J., & Hwang, S.S. (1992) Treatments of depression and the functional capacity to work. *Archives of General Psychiatry, 49,* (10), 761-786.

Morse, J., & Morse, R.M. (1988, December). Calculating fall rates: Methodological concerns. *Quality Review Bulletin,* 369-371.

National Institute of Mental Health. (1992). *Caring for people with severe mental disorders: A national plan for research to improve services.* Washington, DC: Author.

Overall, J., & Gorham, D. (1962). The brief psychiatric rating scale. *Psychology Report, 10,* 782-812.

Podgorny, K. (1991). Developing nursing focused quality indicators. *Journal of Nursing Care Quality,* 47-52.

Poster, E.C., Pelletier, L.R., & Kay, K. (1991). A retrospective cohort study of falls in a psychiatric inpatient setting. *Hospital and Community Psychiatry, 42*(7), 714-720.

Poster, E.C., & Pelletier, L.R. (1990). *Fall outcome coding guide.* Los Angeles: Authors.

Rand Corporation. (1991). *The health sciences program.* Santa Monica, CA: Author.

Roy-Byrne, P. (1995). A psychiatrist-rated battery of measures for assessing the clinical status of psychiatric inpatients. *Psychiatric Services, 46*(4), 347-352.

Speilberger, C., Gorsuch, R., & Lushen, R. (1970). *Manual for the state-trait anxiety inventory.* Palo Alto, CA: Consulting Psychologist Press.

Stewart, A.L., Hays, R.D., & Ware, J.E. (1988). The MOS short-form general health survey: Reliability and validity in a patient population. *Medical Care, 26,* 724.

Strickland, O.L. (1991, September 11-13). Measures and instruments in patient outcomes research: Examining the effectiveness of nursing practice. *Proceedings of the State of the Science Conference,* 143-153.

U.S. Department of Health and Human Services. (1991). *Healthy People 2000* (DHHS Publication No. 91-50213). Washington, DC: U.S. Government Printing Office.

Yesavage, J., et al. (1983). Development and validation of a geriatric depression screen scale: A preliminary report. *Journal of Psychiatric Research, 17,* 37-49.

Part Two

Power Tools for Psychiatric-Mental Health Nursing

Chapter 5

The Nursing Process

Barbara Krainovich-Miller

LEARNING OUTCOMES

After studying and applying the concepts of this chapter, the learner will be able to:

- Compare the nursing process with the definition of nursing and the ANA's psychiatric-mental health nursing's *Standards.*
- Describe the relationship of the nursing process to diagnostic reasoning as a critical-thinking process.
- From a cognitive, affective, and behavioral functioning perspective, determine the appropriate standardized assessment tools to use for assessing individuals who are potentially experiencing a mental health disorder.
- List the commonly occurring North American Nursing Diagnosis Association (NANDA) nursing diagnoses experienced by clients with mental health disorders.
- Explain the relationship among the planning stage of the nursing process, measurable outcomes, and interventions for derived nursing diagnoses.
- Implement the evaluation stage of the nursing process.
- Explain the differences and similarities among individualized and standardized nursing care plans, interdisciplinary treatment plans, and clinical pathways.
- Compare and contrast nursing interventions classification (NIC) interventions and nursing care plans.
- Discuss the relationship between research-based protocols and nursing interventions.
- List the differences and similarities of the nursing process, the ANA's psychiatric and mental-health nursing's *Standards,* and the standards of the Joint Commission on Accreditation of Hospital Organizations (JCAHO).

KEY TERMS

Assessment	Nursing diagnosis	Phenomena of concern
Diagnostic reasoning	Nursing process	Subjective data
Multiaxial assessment system	Objective data	

s a nursing student, you are familiar with the nursing process as a framework for practice. The purpose of this chapter is to explain its use by basic level psychiatric nurses who work in a variety of settings. In addition, the use of nursing process by nurses in advanced practice is discussed. At this point, you might be thinking, "Why is it necessary to go over the steps of the nursing process? Does it change when dealing with psychiatric client populations?" The answer to your questions is that it does not change, but clients with mental health disorders do present situations that require the nurse to reframe how and what type of data are collected. This phenomenon will become clearer as you review the specific examples presented in this chapter to illustrate the use of nursing process with this type of client. In addition, subsequent clinical chapters (Part Five) and chapters on populations at risk (Part Six) will provide relevant examples for clients with specific mental health disorders.

DEFINITION OF NURSING AND THE PSYCHIATRIC-MENTAL HEALTH NURSING *STANDARDS*

ANA's (1995) *Social Policy Statement* definition of nursing is reflected in the latest description of psychiatric-mental health nursing as "the diagnosis and treatment of human responses to actual or potential mental health problems" (ANA, 1994). *Human responses of actual or potential mental health problems are referred to as **phenomena of concern.*** Examples of psychiatric nursing's phenomena of concern are presented in Chapter 2.

Nurses who practice psychiatric nursing, regardless of the health care setting, must meet the competency level standards of professional nursing care and performance as described in ANA's (1994) psychiatric-mental health nursing's *Standards.* These standards reflect ANA's (1991) *Standards of Clinical Practice.* Psychiatric-mental health nursing has six professional standards of care and eight standards of professional performance (see Appendix A).

The psychiatric-mental health professional standards of care (ANA, 1994) present nursing process as the six standards of care: (1) assessment, (2) diagnosis, (3) outcome identification, (4) planning, (5) implementation, and (6) evaluation.

The standards of care and professional performance will be discussed throughout Parts Five and Six of this text. Chapter 2 discusses the major reasons for differentiating basic and advanced levels of psychiatric-mental health clinical nursing practice. This differentiation reflects the complex nature and change in scope of psychiatric-mental health clinical nursing practice. The student is encouraged to read this primary ANA (1994) document to more fully understand the reasons for differentiating basic and advanced levels of practice.

THE NURSING PROCESS AND DIAGNOSTIC REASONING

The framework for the ***nursing process*** for this text is ANA's (1994a) psychiatric-mental health nursing *Standards.* The six standards of care are as follows: *assessment, diagnosis, outcome identification, planning (selecting therapeutic interventions to achieve outcomes), implementation (documenting interventions according to the nurse's level of basic or advanced practice, education, and certification), and evaluation (documenting client attainment or nonattainment of expected outcomes).*

In psychiatric-mental health clinical nursing, the steps of this clinical decision-making process (nursing process) are a demonstration of the nurse's critical thinking abilities and related actions with individuals experiencing mental health disorders. A psychiatric nurse uses diagnostic reasoning to carry out the nursing process. It is especially evident in the steps of assessment and diagnosis. ***Diagnostic reasoning*** *is defined as:*

> *"... a process that enables an observer to assign meaning and to classify phenomena in clinical situations by integrating observations and critical thinking. This information processing involves sensory, working, and [long-term] memory. It is a series of clinical judgments made during and after data collection, culminating in informal judgments [inferences] or formal diagnoses ..."* (Carnevali and Thomas, 1993).

Diagnostic reasoning begins as soon as the nurse becomes aware of the client. It is used to collect the appropriate nursing/psychiatric/psychosocial health and physical data during nursing assessment, as well as in subsequent interactions, and to recall related theory and research. This is done to validate subjective and objective findings so that accurate nursing diagnoses can be made.

The nurse-client relationship (see Chapter 9) is essential to carrying out the nursing process within psychiatric nursing practice. Accurate and clear documentation of nursing process provides for continuity of care among nurses and members of the health team for clients with mental health disorders. Students are probably most familiar with the documentation of nursing process in the format of a written nursing care plan. Documentation provides evidence that psychiatric nurses meet national standards of the profession related to care and performance. It also offers measurable evidence that psychiatric nurses' care and performance brings about realistic quality client outcomes.

Assessment

Assessment is the first standard and refers to the systematic collection of objective and subjective data on a client. Assessment of the psychiatric client is an ongoing process, from the initial assessment, throughout the episode of treatment, whenever the nurse is in contact with the client (e.g., in a community program, in the home, or in a street environment). Evaluation of these data is also an ongoing process that occurs simultaneously during assessment and subsequent stages of the nursing process.

Direct data sources: subjective and objective data

The psychiatric nurse collects subjective and objective data by directly observing and formally interviewing the client. *Subjective data include reports or experiences described by the client; these descriptions are exactly what the person states are his/her thoughts and feelings and are referred to as symptoms. Objective data are behaviors observed in the client or findings of diagnostic tests; these are considered objective indicators of health or deviations of health or human responses to problems and are referred to as signs* (Gordon, 1987; Kaplan, Sadock, and Grebb, 1994).

Table 5-1 provides common examples of subjective and objective data. In nonpsychiatric settings the nurse and physician often consider subjective reports of the client to be tentative until they are verified through objective data (diagnostic tests). In psychiatry, symptoms may be "put together" and a diagnosis made without objective data such as diagnostic tests to verify or confirm the symptoms. For example, a client may state, "I am going to kill myself," and along with other objective data,

the diagnosis of major depression will be made. The diagnosis is made despite the fact that there is not an objective diagnostic test to confirm that the client really means to act on this threat of suicide. Although there is more of an emphasis on the role of neurobiological antecedents and consequences in psychiatric disorders, there are not specific test findings to confirm a diagnosis. Therefore subjective findings are essential to the diagnostic process for determining mental health disorders.

Indirect data sources

Indirect data collection in the psychiatric setting is similar to other areas of nursing practice. It refers to the review of the overall information contained in the client's chart. In some psychiatric settings and situations the nurse may not be the person who directly collects some of the subjective and objective data. For example, the psychiatrist may be the one to administer a mental status examination (MSE) rather than the nurse. Box 5-1 outlines the important indirect sources of subjective and objective client data that need to be reviewed when completing a comprehensive nursing assessment. It is extremely important for the nurse to compare the data directly collected during the nursing assessment with similar data collected by others. If these data were collected during a similar period and there were great variations, then the differences between these situations should be discussed with the other involved professionals before drawing any conclusions or finalizing a nursing diagnosis.

Nursing assessment guide

During the initial nursing interview of the client, the nurse uses multiple nursing and non-nursing models and theories to guide the collection and evaluation of the data. The main outcome of a comprehensive nursing assessment is the formulation of one or multiple nursing di-

TABLE 5-1

Direct observation data sources

SUBJECTIVE DATA (SYMPTOM) SOURCES	OBJECTIVE DATA (SIGNS) SOURCES
Client states: "I feel sad, angry, and upset" "Where am I?" "There is nothing wrong with me" "I feel depressed" "I have no energy" "My heart is pounding" "I don't believe in my religion any more" Family member: "I am so tired, I can't sleep because my son paces all night"	Nurse observes the client to assess the following: • Constricted affect • Slow speech • Psychomotor retardation • Pale facial color • Turned down mouth Nurse palpates a radial pulse of 112 Nurse obtains a blood pressure (BP) reading of 160/80

Box 5-1

Indirect Data Sources

The psychiatric nurse reviews the following data:
I. Psychiatric interview and/or psychiatrist's history and physical including:
   a. DSM-IV Diagnostic Label(s)
   b. MSE results
   c. Physical examination: biological/neurological assessment results
   d. Behavioral, emotional, and social history
II. Interviews of client by other mental health team professionals
III. Psychological testing results
IV. Other diagnostic tests
V. Prior medical records

agnoses. A typical comprehensive nursing assessment form, sometimes referred to as a nursing history health assessment, collects data related to biopsychosocial information regarding a client's:

- Spiritual/philosophical beliefs
- Emotional and biological gender/growth and developmental stages
- Sociocultural background
- Psychological and biological aspects of current and/or previous psychiatric history

Box 5-2 presents an example of a comprehensive nursing assessment form; each category lists questions that might be asked when assessing these multiple categories.

An example of a nursing theory that is used as a framework for assessment and also commonly used by psychiatric nurses is Peplau's psychodynamic theory of nursing. In this case the nurse would initiate the nurse-client relationship expecting to first help the client recognize and understand his or her problem and determine how much help is needed during the first phase (Peplau, 1987). To meet this nursing goal, the nurse would use multiple intellectual and interpersonal skills such as observation, interviewing, self-reflection, recording, and data analysis (Peplau, 1987).

Another commonly used framework for psychiatric nursing assessment guides is Gordon's functional health patterns. Assessment of a client's functional health patterns results in the formulation of more accurate nursing diagnoses (Levin and Crosley, 1986).

A commonly used non-nursing model is Erikson's stages of emotional growth and development. Nurses use this model as a guide to determine if the person is functioning at an expected or appropriate level of emotional

functioning. This model is particularly helpful for age-related developmental assessment (see Chapters 33, 34, and 35).

Although there are various nursing assessment forms for the collection of data regarding the client's psychiatric and physical health patterns and status, almost all guides assess, in one way or another, the client's psycho/social/spiritual/biological functioning. The first assessment standard lists these similar dimensions and recommends the use of a systematic interview guide, as well as various standardized tools, for assessing risk factors and that the data are documented (see Appendix A).

Comprehensive psychiatric nursing history/health assessment

The assessment of the client in the psychiatric setting is quite complex. The client's psychosocial and mental status are extensively and systematically assessed. A physical assessment is also conducted but its depth and breadth varies from client to client, and setting to setting. The dimensions that are assessed help the nurse make a judgment or nursing diagnosis regarding the emotional, cognitive, and behavioral status of the client (ANA, 1994).

The direct collection of subjective and objective data of the client refers to the nurse actually performing a comprehensive psychosocial/mental/physical history and health assessment. During the structured interview of the client, the nurse directly asks questions, and documents verbal and behavioral responses to the questions, makes observations, and/or performs a physical inspection, auscultation, and palpation of the client's body systems. In addition, the nurse may need to interview the family/significant others, as well as review multiple indirect data sources (see Box 5-1). An example of this type of comprehensive nursing assessment is given in Box 5-2.

The depth and breadth of the assessment performed by the psychiatric nurse depends on two factors: (1) the philosophy, protocol, and type of the health care/mental health/psychiatric agency, and (2) whether the nurse is functioning at the basic or advanced level of psychiatric-mental health clinical nursing practice. Although assessment is discussed in relation to the initial interview, data collection is a continual process.

Physical assessment component

The physical assessment aspect of a comprehensive assessment (see Box 5-2) is now more in-depth than was performed in previous years (Dunn, 1993). The use of the multiaxial assessment categories of the American Psychiatric Association (APA) *Diagnostic and Statistical Manual of Mental Disorders, Fourth Edition* (DSM-IV), (see Appendix C) reflects the complexity of today's client

Box 5-2

Comprehensive Psychiatric-Mental Health Nursing History/Health Assessment Form

BASIC STATISTICS

Client's Name_____Age_____Name preference_____
DOB_____Date of admission_____Date of Assessment_____Admitting Dx:_____Axis I:_____
Axis II:_____Axis III:_____Axis IV:_____Axis V_____

Psychosocial Assessment

SPIRITUAL/PHILOSOPHICAL

- What is your religious preference?
- How often do you practice your religion?
- Does your religion offer you a source of hope, comfort, or strength?
- Do you want to speak to a priest, rabbi, or other religious leader?
- If you have no religious preference, what are your sources of hope, comfort, or strength?

RACIAL, CULTURAL, AND ETHNIC BACKGROUND (INSERT Y OR N WHERE APPROPRIATE)

- What is your cultural heritage?
- Do you practice many _____ some _____ or none _____ of your cultural customs?
- Were you born in the United States?
- Were your parents _____ your children _____ your spouse _____?
- How well does the client understand the questions?
  -Not at all _____; needs a translator _____
  -Somewhat, rephrasing _____ and pictures help _____
  -Understands most of the time _____
  -Understands English _____
- What made you come for help?
- What kinds of things help when you are ill in your country?
- In your country, who do people go to when they are sick?
- Is it customary in your country for people to stay in the hospital?
- If you are hospitalized, what can we do to help you with some of your cultural practices? (E.g., Are there any special foods you want to have or avoid?)

EDUCATIONAL AND EMPLOYMENT BACKGROUND (INSERT Y OR N WHERE APPROPRIATE)

Elementary _____ High School _____ College (yrs) _____
Degrees _____
Occupation _____ Currently working? _____
How long? _____
- Do you like the work you are (were) doing?
- How stressful is (was) your job on a scale of 1 to 5, 1 being least stressful, 5 most stressful?
- Will this hospitalization threaten your job security?
- What have you told or will you tell your employer about your hospitalization?

RELATIONSHIPS WITH FAMILY AND SIGNIFICANT OTHERS

Marital status: S _____ M _____ D _____ How long? _____
Remarried _____ How long? _____
Number of children _____ M _____ F _____ Living with you _____
- Who are the members of your family?
  -Names and ages _____
  _____
  _____
- How would you describe your relationship with each of them?
- Who are your close friends?
- How would you describe your relationship with them and they with your family?
- Who shares the family activities or tasks of daily living?
- Which family member is most supportive during times of stress?
- Do family members respect each other's point of view?
- Have you lost a member of the family or a friend?
  -How recent?
- What have (will) you tell your family members regarding your hospitalization?
- How can we help you and your family during this hospitalization?

NORMAL COPING ABILITY

Ability to Discuss Current, Known Health Problems
- What is the reason for this hospitalization?
- Have you experienced a crisis or loss?
  -How recent?
- How did you handle these situations?
- During the interview, does the client ask any questions regarding his or her problem or request information about his treatment?
- Any evidence of problem solving?

Behavioral Changes Resulting from Stress
- Does the client's affect (emotional response), mood, or behavior reveal anxiety (e.g., restlessness, difficulty sleeping, poor eye contact, trembling, facial tension) or depression (e.g., blunt affect, expressions of helplessness, guilt, apathy, low self-esteem, slow speech)?
- Have there been any changes in the following, and if so, what?
  -Eating habits
  -Sleeping habits

Box 5-2—cont'd

Comprehensive Psychiatric-Mental Health Nursing History/Health Assessment Form

-Exercise
-Work habits
-Physical complaints
-Sexual activity
• Do you have trouble concentrating on tasks or completing projects?
• Have you had any unprovoked emotional outbursts? (E.g., Do you start crying for no reason, yell, or throw things?)

COPING RESOURCES

• During the interview, has the client asked for help?
• What works best for you during times of stress? If no answer, then ask the following and have the client describe if it helps:
  -Talking with others _____ Who? _____ Does it help? _____
  -Sleeping _____ Does it help? _____
  -Eating _____ What type of food? _____ Does it help? _____
  -Smoking _____ What type? _____ How often? _____ Does it help? _____
  -Drinking alcohol _____ Wine _____ How much? _____ How often? _____ Does it help? _____
  -Taking medication _____ What type? _____ Does it help? _____
  -Any other drugs _____ What type? _____ Does it help? _____
• What type of problem solving works best for you?

UNDERSTANDING THE HEALTH PROBLEM

Client's Perception
• Who is your usual physician or medical/family doctor?
• Have you ever gone to a psychiatrist, psychologist, or nurse therapist, or for any type of group or individual counseling?
• Have you ever attended self-help group sessions? If so, which ones?
• Tell me what you think is your psychiatric health problem?
• What type of treatment was discussed with you?
• Do you think the client understands the severity of the illness and the proposed treatment?
• What is your usual BP? _____ Pulse? _____ Respiratory rate? _____
• What type of diet do you usually eat? _____

Attitude Toward Health Care Providers
• Who is your physician?
• Do you know that I am a nurse?

Compliance with Previous and Current Therapies
• Have you begun medication? If so, when?
• Have you ever taken psychiatric medication before? If so, when?
• Any reactions?
• Are you allergic to any medications?
• Have you attended any therapy or activity?

Physical Assessment (as needed)
• Inspect and/or auscultate, palpate, or percuss appropriate body systems:
  -Pulse _____
  -Apical _____
  -R _____
  -BP _____
  -T _____
  -Breath sounds _____
  -Integumentary system: skin, nails, hair, and scalp _____
  -Unusual marks, scars, etc, on torso (front and back), legs, arms, feet, hands, face, neck, hair
  -Head, eyes, ears, nose, sinuses, mouth, pharynx, throat, lungs, heart, vascular system, breasts, abdomen, gastrointestinal tract, and genitourinary tract
  -Musculoskeletal, neurological, nutritional
• Does client wear glasses? _____ Contacts? _____ Bifocals? _____ Hearing aid? _____
• Does the client have any significant diseases, surgeries, or previous hospitalizations? _____
• Recent blood transfusions: How many? _____ When? _____
• Sexual partners: How many and when? _____ Frequency and satisfaction _____

Mental Status Assessment

GENERAL APPEARANCE AND BEHAVIOR

• Is the person dressed appropriately for age, weather, occasion, and social norms?
  -Female: Makeup _____ N _____ Y _____ appropriate?
  -Hair: Clean _____ Neat _____
  -Skin (color, turgor, clean odor)
  -Posture
• Describe behavior and psychomotor activity?
• Describe the client's attitude toward you?

MOOD AND AFFECT

• What is the client's mood?
• Does the affect fit the content and overall body language?
  -Is it appropriate?

Continued.

Box 5-2—cont'd

Comprehensive Psychiatric-Mental Health Nursing History/Health Assessment Form

SPEECH

- Is the client's speech understandable (normal, pressured, slow, fast, monotone, dramatic, have an accent)?

PERCEPTUAL DISTURBANCE

- Does the client demonstrate evidence of hallucinating (verbally, nonverbally)?
- With what does the client respond?
- Does the client verbalize feelings of depersonalization and derealization?
  -What are the content and context?
- Is there any evidence of illusions? If so, what?
- Ask the client: have you ever heard voices or sounds, or seen things that others do not see?

THOUGHT

- Does the client have difficulty expressing self in an organized and easy-to-follow manner?
- Does the client jump from one subject to another (flight of ideas)?
- Is the client hesitant or slow in expressing ideas?
- Ask the client: how would you describe your ability to think?
- Ask the client: are you experiencing any difficulty in your ability to think?
- Is there any evidence of delusions? If so, are they bizarre, paranoid, or grandiose?
- Are there any ideas of reference?

SENSORIUM AND COGNITION

Use the Mini-Mental State Examination (MMSE) and/or assess the following.

Alertness and Level of Consciousness

- Is the client oriented times three? Date/time _____
  Place _____ Person _____
- Is the client alert?
- Memory: _____

-Immediate recall and retention: ask the client to repeat a series of numbers
-Recent memory: ask the client his or her name, or what time it is.
-Recent past memory: ask the client what day it was yesterday.
-Remote memory: ask the client what year he or she was born.
- Is the client able to read or write a sentence?
- Ask the client to explain a simple proverb.
- Ask the client to make change or to estimate a distance.

IMPULSE CONTROL

- During the interview, does the client demonstrate any difficulty controlling verbal or physical impulses (sexual or toward self) against person or property?
- Ask the client if he or she is having thoughts about harming self or others?

JUDGMENT AND INSIGHT

Ask the client the following:
- How does your behavior affect your activities of daily living (ADLs) or social functioning?
- What would you do if you smelled smoke where you live?
- What do you think contributed to your getting ill?

RELIABILITY

- Do the client's statements coincide with your observations, history, or what has been reported to you?

SAFETY

Select data from current assessment to determine level of risk.

SUMMARY: PRIORITY DIAGNOSIS AND RELATED FACTOR AND DATA

Nursing diagnosis #1 _____

Supporting data: _____

Nursing diagnosis #2 _____

Supporting data: _____

Nursing diagnosis #3 _____

Supporting data: _____

Outcomes for client's hospitalization:

Potential discharge needs:

Additional comments

Nurse's signature _____ Date _____

Box 5-3

Contents of a Written Psychiatric Report

1. Psychiatric interview
2. General physical/neurological examination
3. Diagnostic tests results
4. Social worker's interviews
5. Tentative multiaxial DSM-IV diagnoses (see Appendix D)
6. Prognosis
7. Etiologies

with mental illness, who is not as medically stable as once thought (APA, 1994).

A few factors that contribute to this issue include the following: (1) An increasingly older adult population with psychiatric and multiple medical problems, (2) a high rate of substance abusers with multiple medical problems, and (3) an epidemic rate of clients with the human immunodeficiency virus (HIV) or acquired immunodeficiency syndrome (AIDS), who are not only medically ill but who also experience multiple psychiatric problems (Krainovich-Miller et al., 1995).

The physical assessment is done systematically, although not necessarily from head to toe. The ability of the psychiatric client to tolerate the closeness necessary for a physical examination varies greatly. This part of the examination may need to be conducted in parts, with or by another member of the health team. It might cause less anxiety for the client if the physical examination starts with the less personal aspects of the body, such as the hands and feet, then proceeds to the more intimate aspects like the torso and head, and then to the eyes, ears, and mouth. In some situations, when a client has psychiatric and medical diagnoses, it is best for one nurse to conduct the personal interview and another nurse to perform the physical examination, especially if sensitive or sexual body parts are to be examined. It also depends on other factors, including the comfort levels of both client and nurse, the stage of the therapeutic relationship, and the practice level and experience of the nurse. For example, with a highly agitated client, unless it is a critical medical situation, it is best to wait until the agitation decreases to complete the examination.

Whenever possible, it is important that the nurse perform his or her own physical assessment of the client's physical functioning to determine normal and deviation baseline data. Some of the data collection may seem redundant because some of the physical examination includes documentation that was assessed during the MSE

(e.g., observation of gait, asymmetry, movements, tremors, physical weight, skin). However, it still must be assessed and documented in a formal manner for the purpose of completing a typical comprehensive physical and neurological assessment. Data collected by various health professionals should be compared before final conclusions are drawn. Chapter 13 discusses content related to the physical/neurological assessment.

Discharge assessment
Because clients spend less time in the inpatient psychiatric setting, it is imperative that discharge planning begin with the first encounter the nurse has with the client. The comprehensive assessment form in Box 5-2 illustrates this point.

Research and the Joint Commission
Regardless of the specific nursing assessment form used, research supports that a structured assessment results in better clinical judgments and nursing care planning. In addition, the Joint Commission on Accreditation of Healthcare Organizations (JCAHO) *Mental Health Manual* (1995) indicates that if a psychiatric inpatient setting chooses "safety risk" as one of its outcome criteria, then it must demonstrate that it has in place a systematic way of assessing all psychiatric clients for suicidal risk factors and potential for violence or falls.

Questions that directly assess and document this information would demonstrate nursing's contribution to meeting this criterion. For example, the information obtained from the questions on the comprehensive nursing assessment form (see Box 5-2) related to the dimensions of normal coping, mood and affect, perceptual disturbance, thought, sensorium and cognition, and impulse control, as well as documenting the collected data as risk factors in the safety section demonstrate that these risks were systematically assessed on admission and appropriate nursing diagnoses, outcomes, and plans were developed.

The mental health team: other sources of client assessment data
The psychiatric nurse at the basic level, whether in inpatient or community psychiatric health care settings, functions collaboratively. Overall, it is similar to the role of the nurse in nonpsychiatric settings. The following are the usual staff members of the mental health team: advanced practice psychiatric nurse, activity assistant, basic-level psychiatric staff nurse, clinical psychologist, nutritionist, activity therapist, physician's assistant, psychiatrist, psychiatric assistant or technician, psychiatric social worker, recreational therapist, and/or religious advisor. In addition, there are many auxiliary personnel (housekeepers, unit clerks, secretaries) that keep the environment clean and running smoothly.

Data collection is a collaborative effort; data from all mental health team members are used in the formulation of the interdisciplinary treatment plan for a particular client. The importance of documenting the nursing process and the need for collaborative relationships among mental health team members is discussed in Chapter 8.

Psychiatric interview and psychiatric report

Whether in an inpatient or community-based setting, the initial psychiatric interview is usually conducted by the psychiatrist. Box 5-3 lists the major components of a typical psychiatrist's psychiatric report. The psychiatrist writes the report but does not necessarily collect all the data. For example, nurses and other members of the professional mental health team may formulate the treatment plan recommendation. In turn, each member of the team may use the psychiatric report's information in their respective plans of care.

In some settings the nurse may initiate the psychiatric interview. In other instances the client is admitted to the unit from the emergency room, where a psychiatric interview was initiated by the psychiatrist. In other cases the psychiatric interview is conducted by the program's psychiatrist or the client's private psychiatrist. However, in almost every setting or situation, the psychiatric staff nurse conducts a separate nursing history/health assessment in the development of a nursing care plan for the client. The psychiatric report is one of the primary documents for the nurse to review.

Multiaxial system The DSM-IV uses a multiaxial assessment for arriving at the client's axis diagnosis. A ***multiaxial assessment system*** *facilitates a comprehensive evaluation of multiple factors, and is a more systematic way of communicating complex clinical information regarding an individual experiencing a mental health disorder.*

The multiaxial system of DSM-IV is used by psychiatrists, psychologists, social workers, and advanced practice nurses for determining a client's diagnosis and is used for reimbursement purposes. The basic level psychiatric nurse needs to be familiar with the DSM-IV's taxonomy to communicate with all members of the team. For example, knowing the DSM-IV terminology assists in understanding the psychiatric report and progress notes. Table 5-2 lists the five axes and their foci. The clinical and population chapters of this text use the DSM-IV classification of disorders and refer to multiaxial assessment and dual diagnoses. See Appendix C for an explanation of each of these axes.

The mental status examination The client's mental status is usually assessed by a number of different health care professional team members, the depth and perspective is different for each team member. An MSE may be initiated or conducted by the psychiatrist, psychologist, or advanced-practice nurse; most often it is completed by the psychiatrist. The MSE is an assessment of the mental status of the individual and provides a comprehensive view of the client during the interview process. Box 5-2 indicates the essential components of an MSE. Table 5-3 includes examples of the type of data collected for each of these categories.

Evaluation of cognitive impairment is a highly formal assessment usually conducted by experts in psychological testing. However, a practical and clinically useful way of quickly assessing the sensorium and cognition category is to use a mini-mental status examination (MMSE). An example of a question used to assess this area is to ask the client to name the year, season, date, day of the week, and month. One point is given for each correct answer. A maximum score for each area is five, with 30 for the overall score.

Physical and neurological assessment

Many psychiatric disorders have a neurobiological risk factor, etiologic factors, or an organic cause or consequences. Although the psychiatrist may perform the complete physical/neurological examination, if deviations are assessed, a consult by an internist, neurological physician, or specialist is usually requested.

TABLE 5-2

Multiaxial system of the DSM-IV classification

Axis I	Clinical disorder and other conditions that may be a focus of clinical attention
Axis II	Personality disorders and mental retardation
Axis III	General medical conditions
Axis IV	Psychosocial and environmental problems
Axis V	Global assessment of functioning

From American Psychiatric Association. (1994). Diagnostic and statistical manual of mental disorders, fourth edition, *Washington, DC: Author.*

Diagnostic tests   Table 5-4 lists common psychological assessment tools (see also Tables 4-2); Box 5-4 lists intelligence, personality, and memory tests, which are usually medical and neurological tests. Many routine laboratory tests are administered in an attempt to collect data that assist in determining or verifying the initial DSM-IV diagnosis, and/or rule out any physiological, medical, and/or neurological disorder, antecedents, or consequences. In addition, these tests are usually ordered at selected intervals to monitor for desired therapeutic medication levels, as well as undesired effects. For example, routine laboratory blood tests may determine if any major organ was affected by the client's substance abuse and/or if psychotropic medication treatment was reached.

TABLE 5-3

Examples of data documented on a comprehensive mental status examination

ASSESSMENT CATEGORY	EXAMPLES OF DATA COLLECTED
General description of client	Tense posture; bizarre clothing, short, thin, childlike appearance; combative; restless; wringing of hands
Affective	Angry mood but affect blunt, inappropriate emotional response while discussing delusions of persecution
Language	Talkative, slow speech, mumbles at times, no accent
Perceptual	Hallucinations evident (e.g., "I know they are going to get me"); denies hearing voices before this incident
Thought process	Paranoid themes, ideas of reference (e.g. "The radio is talking to me.")
Sensorium and cognition	Alert and oriented to day, time, and year but unable to keep focused; unable to explain similarities between a peach and nectarine; able to make change and approximate a distance
Impulse control	Client states, "I want to hurt someone."
Judgment and insight	Unable to state what effect current behavior has on ADLs; cannot explain what he or she would do if smelled smoke in home environment; some awareness of problem, but blames others (e.g., "I know I am ill, but my mother made me crazy.")
Reliability	Denies using drugs but has a history of trouble with the law over drug use

TABLE 5-4

Psychological assessment tools

INSTRUMENT	MAIN PURPOSE
Global Assessment of Functioning (GAF) Scale	Considers psychological, social, and occupational functions
Mini-Mental Status Examination (MMSE)	Sensorium and cognition evaluation
Beck Depression Inventory, Hamilton Depression Rating Scale, or Manic State Rating Scale	Mood disorders
Hamilton Anxiety Rating Scale or Anxiety States Inventory	Anxiety states and disorders
Schedule for Affective Disorders and Schizophrenia (SADS), or Thought Disorder Index (TDI)	Used to validate presence of schizophrenia and psychosis
Structured Clinical Interview for DSM-IV Dissociative Disorders (SCID-IV)	Dissociative disorders
Systematic Assessment for Treatment of Emergent Events (SAFTEE)	Adverse effects of drugs

Box 5-4

Psychological Tests

INTELLIGENCE

- Stanford-Binet
- Wechsler Intelligence Scale (WAIS) for adults and children (WISC)

PERSONALITY AND OTHER MEMORY TESTS

- Rorschach Test
- Thematic Apperception Test (TAT)
- Minnesota Multiphasic Personality Inventory (MMPI)
- Draw a Person Test
- Sentence Completion Test
- Bender-Gestalt Test
- Blacky Test (usually with children)
- Wechsler Memory Scale
- Word Association Test

Chapters 13 and 15, offer additional explanations on the role of laboratory tests in the assessment of psychiatric clients.

Nursing Diagnosis

As discussed, the nursing assessment data are formally documented on a comprehensive psychiatric nursing history/assessment (see Box 5-2). The data are used to formulate a nursing diagnosis and should be documented at the end of a completed nursing assessment on a nursing care plan (see the nursing care plan on pp.70-71) and can be placed on an interdisciplinary treatment plan.

The ANA's (1994) psychiatric-mental health Standard II, *Diagnosis*, indicates the use of diagnoses from a recognized classification system such as NANDA (see Appendix A). Other taxonomic classification systems are also approved for psychiatric nursing, such as the International Classification of Diseases (ICD) or the DSM-IV (see Appendix C). The advanced-practice psychiatric-mental health clinical nurse specialist usually uses the DSM-IV classification system, as well as NANDA nursing diagnoses.

Through the use of diagnostic reasoning, the psychiatric nurse critically evaluates the assessment data from all relevant sources. The collected data are formally analyzed and synthesized. This critical thinking process results in selecting the data that best represents the defining characteristics, relations to, and risk factors of a selected nursing diagnosis; it results in an accurate clinical judgment or nursing diagnosis. A *nursing diagnosis* refers to *a clinical judgment about individual, family, or community responses to actual and potential health problems and life processes. Nursing diagnoses provide the basis for selection of nursing interventions to*

BOX 5-5

Components of a Diagnosis

LABEL

Provides a name for a diagnosis; it is a concise term or phrase that represents a pattern of related cues and may include qualifiers (see below)

DEFINITION

Provides a clear, precise description, delineates its meaning, and helps differentiate it from similar diagnoses

DEFINING CHARACTERISTICS

Observable cues/inferences that cluster as manifestations of a nursing diagnosis; these are listed for actual and wellness diagnoses.

- A defining characteristic is described as "critical" if it must be present to make the diagnosis and is described as "major" if it is usually present when the diagnosis exists.
- It is described as "minor" if it provides supporting evidence for the diagnosis but may not be present. Critical and major defining characteristics need to be substantiated by research.

RELATED FACTORS

Conditions/circumstances that contribute to the development/maintenance of a nursing diagnosis

RISK FACTORS

Environmental factors and physiological, psychological, genetic, or chemical elements that increase the vulnerability of an individual, family, or community to an unhealthful event

From North American Nursing Diagnosis Association. (1994). NANDA nursing diagnoses: Definitions & classification, 1995-1996. Philadelphia: Author.

achieve outcomes for which the nurse is accountable (NANDA, 1994).

The nursing diagnosis of moderate anxiety related to threat to or change in role functioning (see the nursing care plan on pp. 70-71) is an example of a nursing diagnosis that meets the NANDA criteria. The two-part statement of the diagnosis provides the basis for the selection of nursing interventions listed in the second column that would bring about the outcomes listed in the first column. In other words the nursing interventions address not only the "moderate anxiety," but also the source of the anxiety ("related to" factors) of threat to or change in role functioning. The definitions for the two-part statement are presented in Box 5-5. For the purpose of understanding this feature, briefly stated rationales for the interventions are listed in the third column. In clinical practice the rationales for nursing interventions are not written; for academic purposes they are usually written in great detail.

Along with NANDA (1994), ANA also approved three other taxonomic classification systems for general use and testing (McCormick et al., 1994). They are the nursing interventions classification (NIC) and two other taxonomies for home health nursing, the Omaha System and the Home Health Care Classification. NIC interventions address a number of common problems or phenomena that psychiatric clients experience. NIC interventions are research-based practice guidelines. For the purposes of this text, related NIC interventions (McCloskey and Bulechek, 1996) are used in conjunction with selected nursing interventions for the NANDA-approved nursing diagnoses highlighted in a chapter's nursing care plan. The NIC intervention for anxiety reduction is listed in Box 5-6, and it is referred to in the second column of the nursing care plan on pp.70-71). This will be discussed further in the next sections.

NANDA taxonomy

NANDA (1994) nursing diagnoses are at various levels of refinement. Although NANDA's taxonomy places the approved diagnostic categories into nine human response patterns—exchanging, communicating, relating, valuing, choosing, moving, perceiving, knowing, and feeling—for ease of use in the clinical setting, most nurses use the al-

phabetical list (see inside front cover). Each diagnostic label can be given a qualifier, for example, adding the term *acute* to the diagnostic category of anxiety (Table 5-5). Nursing diagnoses can be actual, risk, or wellness diagnoses. Each of the clinical chapters focuses on NANDA diagnoses that are found most commonly with clients experiencing a particular DSM-IV disorder.

The psychiatric nurse, when evaluating assessed client data, compares the data with all components of the selected label or diagnosis. If none or few of the assessed client data match the selected diagnosis, as defined by the components of NANDA, then different labels should be reviewed.

This is especially important if the "critical" or major defining characteristics were not observed in the client. For example, a nurse may have assessed the following data about the client: unable to meet basic needs, high rate of accidents, difficulty establishing relationships, inability to problem solve, and inability to ask for help. The nurse decides that the person is experiencing the nursing diagnosis of defensive coping. Yet after careful examination of this diagnostic label, it is determined that none of the major defining characteristics (e.g., of denial, obvious problems and weaknesses, projection of blame or responsibility, rationalizes failures, hypersensitive to slight criticism, or grandiosity) were assessed (NANDA, 1994). On further review of closely related diagnostic labels, it was determined that the nursing diagnosis of ineffective individual coping was a better clinical

Box 5-6

Anxiety Reduction

DEFINITION

Minimizing apprehension, dread, foreboding, or uneasiness related to an unidentified source of anticipated danger

ACTIVITIES

Use a calm reassuring approach.

Clearly state expectations for patient's behavior.

Explain all procedures, including sensations likely to be experienced during the procedure.

Seek to understand the patient's perspective of a stressful situation.

Provide factual information concerning diagnosis, treatment, and prognosis.

Stay with patient to promote safety and reduce fear.

Encourage parents to stay with child as appropriate.

Provide objects that symbolize safeness.

Administer back rub or neck rub as appropriate.

Encourage noncompetitive activities as appropriate.

Keep treatment equipment out of sight.

Listen attentively.

Reinforce behavior as appropriate.

Create an atmosphere to facilitate trust.

Encourage verbalization of feelings, perceptions, and fears.

Identify when level of anxiety changes.

Provide diversional activities geared toward the reduction of tension.

Help patient identify situations that precipitate anxiety.

Control stimuli as appropriate for patient needs.

Support the use of appropriate defense mechanisms.

Assist patient to articulate a realistic description of an upcoming event.

Determine patient's decision-making ability.

Instruct patient on the use of relaxation techniques.

Administer medications to reduce anxiety as appropriate.

Reprinted with permission from McCloskey, J.C., & Bulechek G.M. (1996). Nursing interventions classification (NIC) (2nd Ed.). St. Louis: Mosby.

TABLE 5-5

Qualifiers for nursing diagnoses

Suggested, But Not Limited to, the Following:

Acute	Severe but of short duration
Altered	A change from baseline
Chronic	Lasting a long time, recurring, habitual, constant
Decreased	Lessened, lesser in size, amount, or degree
Deficient	Inadequate in amount, quality or degree, defective, not sufficient, incomplete
Depleted	Emptied wholly or in part, exhausted of
Disturbed	Agitated, interrupted, interfered with
Dysfunctional	Abnormal, incomplete functioning
Excessive	Characterized by an amount or quantity that is greater than necessary, desirable, or useful
Increased	Greater in size, amount, or degree
Impaired	Made worse, weakened, damaged, reduced, deteriorated
Ineffective	Not producing the desired effect
Intermittent	Stopping or starting again at intervals, periodic, cyclic
Potential for	For use with wellness diagnoses
Enhanced	Made greater, to increase in quality or more desired

From North American Nursing Diagnosis Association. (1994). NANDA nursing diagnoses: Definitions & classifications, 1995-1996. Philadelphia: Author.

judgment for the collected data because the critical defining characteristics of inability to ask for help and inability to problem solve were part of the nursing assessment data for this client.

As a nurse becomes more skilled in the diagnostic reasoning process, more confidence is developed for choosing the appropriate diagnostic label (see Box 5-5). It is a learning process that takes time and experience. The student should ask the instructor and/or a more experienced nurse for help when needed.

Documenting nursing diagnosis

It is extremely important that nursing diagnoses be initially documented on a comprehensive psychiatric nursing history/health assessment as a summary statement,

including the qualifier, related to factors, and the specific data used for the diagnosis. The nursing diagnosis is a two-part label and related to statement. For example, the nursing care plan on pp. 70-71 is based on the nursing diagnosis moderate anxiety related to threat to or change in role functioning. This information should also be transferred to a nursing care plan, a Kardex care plan, or even imbedded in an interdisciplinary treatment plan or critical pathway.

To illustrate the importance of this point, both the comprehensive psychiatric nursing assessment form in Box 5-2 and the nursing care plan on pp. 70-71 provide space for nursing diagnoses to be documented in this way. Documenting in this manner is evidence of a nurse using diagnostic reasoning to select or cluster data, and to determine that the data was in concert with NANDA criteria for the diagnostic category of anxiety.

Some standardized hard copy or computerized nursing care plans, based on NANDA diagnoses, include the defining characteristics, risk, and related to factors on the form or screen. In this case a nurse who selects a particular nursing diagnosis for a client would be instructed to highlight the data that applies to his or her client. Psychiatric nurses are encouraged to document to meet standards of care and professional performance (ANA 1994).

Outcome Identification and Planning

Standard III is *Outcome Identification* and Standard IV is *Planning*. Once an accurate nursing diagnosis is made, outcomes and a plan of interventions related to the nursing diagnosis are developed. The outcomes should:

- Be individually based
- Be mutually agreed on
- Reflect a change in the client's health status
- Indicate specific timelines for short- and long-term outcomes
- Be documented as measurable goals

The nursing care plan on pp. 70-71 illustrates the above outcome criteria. *Planning* refers to the development of a plan of care that prescribes interventions to attain expected outcomes (ANA, 1994). The specific interventions should be based on theory and research reflecting psychiatric nursing practice. Interventions may include psychoeducation related to the client's mental and physical health problems, treatment, and self-care activities.

Nursing care plan

The nursing care plan on pp. 70-71 documents short- and long-term outcomes (goals) for the identified nursing diagnosis of *moderate anxiety related to a threat to or change in role functioning*. It also lists research- and theory-based interventions, as well as the use of a NIC anxiety reduction protocol found in Box 5-6; all interventions relate to assisting the client in meeting the identified outcomes. After reading the theory and research discussed in Chapter 22, the interventions and rationale will be better understood.

In the clinical setting, nurses do not write out a rationale for each nursing intervention. It is expected that the nurse knows the theory and research to support the chosen interventions and could relate it to the client, significant other, or a colleague if requested.

Research-based practice protocols

Whenever possible, standardized, research-based practice protocols or interventions should be used in nursing care plans (Haber et al., 1994). The NIC intervention for anxiety reduction in the nursing care plan on pp. 70-71 is a research-based protocol with established theory and research-based interventions for anxiety. Used in this manner, the protocol saves the nurse time because it does not have to be written on the care plan. A number of the NIC research-based interventions are specific to psychiatric clients and will be illustrated in care plans throughout the clinical and populations at-risk chapters. (See Parts Five and Six of this text.)

There are also established interdisciplinary research-based protocols for clients with psychiatric disorders, such as the major depression practice guideline of the Agency for Health Care Policy and Research (AHCPR) (U.S. Department of Health and Human Services, 1993). This guideline reflects the synthesis of theory and research from a number of disciplines, including nursing. One of the guidelines clearly states that clients with moderate-to-severe major depressive disorders should be treated with medication, regardless of whether psychotherapy is used. A nursing care plan's outcomes and interventions for this type of client would need to reflect the importance of medication management has in the treatment of a client with a major mood disorder.

Documenting outcomes and plans

There is a movement toward simplifying the documentation process without jeopardizing the quality of the nursing care plan. The NIC taxonomy represents research-based interventions for more than 400 commonly occurring clinical client situations (see the nursing care plan on pp. 70-71). By the care plan referring to the anxiety NIC (see Box 5-6) along with other specific interventions, it (1) individualizes the care plan, (2) supports that research-based interventions are being used, (3) avoids a long list of commonly used interventions being written on a care plan, (4) eliminates the need for the nurse to write out the NIC interventions, and (5) provides for accuracy of the protocol.] The actual NIC protocol can be placed in the client's chart, attached to the nursing care plan, and/or remain in a nursing protocol manual on the unit. Any of these methods enable the nurse, who may not be familiar with a particular proto-

col, to review it. If a health care agency uses NANDA and NIC taxonomies, they may already be computerized or in standardized typed format, which facilitates their use.

Interdisciplinary treatment plan

In some situations the interdisciplinary treatment plan (ITP) indicates the responsibilities of various members of the professional health team for a client's care. The ITP is usually based on the medical or psychiatric diagnosis-related groups (DRG), that is, the medical or DSM-IV diagnosis. This type of ITP may be referred to as a Care Map, critical path, or a managed care plan. Although some are quite lengthy, for example, each page may cover each day of hospitalization, many now are one to two pages in length (Zander, 1994).

The ITP does not preclude the use of a nursing care plan. One way of using the nursing care plan is to include the nursing diagnosis(es) in the nursing intervention section of an ITP. In fact, it is suggested that "see NCP for nursing diagnosis moderate anxiety," be written in this section. The individualized care plan could be included in the client's chart and would serve as documentation that psychiatric-mental health standards of care were met and that nursing played a significant role in helping the client meet expected goals. ITPs for specific disorders are presented in Part Five, and an example is given on p. 72.

Implementation

Implementation is the fifth standard of care. It is a "process" standard and it indicates that the psychiatric nurse implements the interventions identified in the plan of care. The following interventions are used by the nurse functioning at the basic level of psychiatric nursing:

- Counseling
- Milieu therapy
- Self-care activities
- Psychobiological interventions
- Health teaching
- Case management
- Health promotion and health maintenance

Each of these interventions are discussed in Parts Five and Six of this text. The fifth standard of care also indicates that at the advanced level, the certified clinical nurse specialist, in addition to carrying out the basic-level interventions or functions, also may provide consultation, engage in psychotherapy, and prescribes pharmacologic agents where permitted by state statutes or regulations (ANA, 1994).

The basic difference between Standard IV (Planning) and V (Implementation) is that (1) the nurse documents the interventions carried out for the established plan of care and (2) the indicated interventions reflecting

NURSING CARE PLAN

Anxiety Disorders

NURSING ASSESSMENT DATA

Subjective: increased tension; apprehension, "I get so anxious I can't make the presentation." *Objective:* sympathetic simulation (increased perspiration, palpitations, tense facial muscles) *DSM-IV Diagnosis:* Social Phobia.

NANDA Diagnosis: Moderate anxiety related to threat to or change in role functioning

Outcomes	Interventions	Rationale	Evaluation
Short term 1. Will perform homework assignments given at *weekly* therapy sessions 2. Will take prescribed medication 1 hour before next presentations 3. Will perform relaxation techniques before and during next presentations ***Within 2 weeks*** 4. Will report a decrease in somatic complaints (increased perspiration, palpitations, tense facial muscles) after using medication and relaxation techniques **Long term** ***Within 1 month*** 1. Will report experiencing less anxiety and worry before and during each presentation compared with base line 2. Will identify possible sources of anxiety 3. Will conduct a presentation using anxiety-reducing techniques but without use of medication	• Develop nurse-client relationship. • See NIC interventions for: anxiety reduction and coping enhancement, individualize as necessary. • Use contracting for desired behaviors. • Elicit from client current step-by-step coping process and modify as necessary. • Teach client to identify earliest signs and symptoms of anxiety and to rate anxiety level on Graphic Anxiety Scales (GASs). • Teach client muscle relaxation and guided imagery techniques, and encourage use at first signs of anxiety. • Help client identify earlier anxiety provoking situations related to speaking in front of groups. • Discuss with client engaging in the above interventions as homework.	• Presence of the nurse has been shown to decrease anxiety; developing trust and open communication is prerequisite to assisting the client in meeting desired outcomes: • There is consensus and research data to support that the specified NIC interventions reduce anxiety and help individual to cope. • Contracting is a basic principle of cognitive therapy. • It is necessary to determine client's self-schema (cognitive map) so client develops a schema that will work. • GASs are a self-report of trait and state anxiety that will help the client keep a record of signs and symptoms related to various levels of anxiety. They assist in teaching client cognitive therapy principles, which is part of their homework. • These are known techniques for decreasing anxiety (see Chapters 14 and 22). • Knowing the sources of anxiety is the first step toward controlling it.	**Short term** 1, 2, 3. Met in 1 week. 4. Met in 2 weeks **Long term** 1. Partially met *in 1 month.* Experiences *less anxiety* and worry before presentation *but still experiencing some (e.g., increased perspiration and slight palpitations)* compared with initial visit. Review relaxation techniques to be used during presentation. 2. Not met. Continue with NPR and reevaluate expected outcome with interdisciplinary team. 3. Not met. Evaluate plan for this outcome with interdisciplinary team.

NURSING CARE PLAN

Anxiety Disorders—cont'd

Outcomes	Interventions	Rationale	Evaluation
	• Discuss with client desired effect and side effects of beta-adrenergic antagonists such as Atenolol, and the need to report effects.	• Research has demonstrated positive outcomes of Atenolol with phobic clients.	
	• Monitor client response to medication and observe for side-effects.	• Teaching and monitoring medications, as well as communicating with members of the health team, are part of a nurse's case management roles, as is his or her legal/ethical responsibility.	
	• Collaborate with client and multidisciplinary team to assess effectiveness of treatment plan.		

the nurse's designated level of practice. Regardless of setting, the psychiatric-mental health nurse must document that the plan has been implemented. Embedded in this standard and the final standard is that discharge planning was initiated. Various chapters throughout the text address the roles and actions discussed in this standard.

Evaluation

Evaluation is the final standard of care. It is essential that the nurse evaluate the progress the client has made regarding expected outcomes. Evaluation is a formal process that takes place and is documented at designated periods indicated by the timeline of the goal, and before and on discharge.

In addition, outcomes are evaluated on a continual basis during the client's hospitalization or period of community-based treatment program, or any time the nurse is in contact with the client. Through evaluation, new data surfaces, which might indicate that a nursing diagnosis may be resolved; a new diagnosis may emerge; outcomes may be met, partially met, not met, and/or in need of revision; and new plans may be needed. Complete evaluation of the expected outcomes of a nursing care plan requires collaboration with the client.

The nursing care plan at left demonstrates one way to document the evaluation of outcomes. Use of qualifiers such as partially met or not met are recommended. The

examples in the evaluation column of the NCP indicate that in relation to the short-term goals, all were met in the designated timeline. If the outcomes had been met earlier than anticipated, the documentation reflects this information. In each case, data should support the conclusion and a change in plan. The sample NCP indicates that the first long-term goal was only partially met. The stated documentation supported this conclusion and indicated a revised plan.

Evaluation, as a standard or component of nursing process, is ongoing, sophisticated, and a complex critical-thinking process that provides for continuity of care. The documentation of evaluation of care demonstrates nursing's accountability to the consumer of mental health care and to society (ANA, 1994).

KEY POINTS

• Psychiatric nursing is the diagnosis and treatment of human responses to actual or potential mental health problems.
• The nursing process is presented as psychiatric-mental health nursing's six standards of care: assessment, diagnosis, outcome identification, planning, implementation, and evaluation.
• Diagnostic reasoning is defined as a process that enables an observer to assign meaning and to classify phenomena in clinical situations by integrating observations and critical thinking.

∷ INTERDISCIPLINARY TREATMENT PLAN

Critical Pathway: Anxiety 300.0X; Panic 300.0X, PTSD 309-89

Patient Name: _____   Case Manager: _____   Physician: _____   Medical Record # _____
Admit date: _____   Expected LOS: _____   UR days certified: _____   Discharge Date: _____   Actual LOS: _____

Day/Date:	0–8 Hours	8–24 Hours	Day 2	Day 3	Day 4	Day 5
ASSESSMENTS AND EVALUATIONS	Nursing Nutritional screen Admit note Precautions	H & P, Social HX, RT/TA; Dr. Initial TX Plan/Admit Note, AIMS Assess sleep patterns	Precaution Evaluation	Psych Eval done Social Hx on chart Precaution Evaluation Assess for level of care	Assess for readiness for discharge	Assess for goals achieved
PROCEDURES	Lab ordered-Admit profile UA, UDS, UCG, EKG, Other:	Lab done: UA, UDS, UCG, EKG Other:	Lab results checked Abnormals called to Dr.	Follow-up for abnormal lab results		
CONSULTS	IT ordered Y/N FT ordered Y/N GT ordered Y/N Psych Testing Order Y/N	GT started Psych Testing done	Schedule MTP meeting	IT started, FT started Psych Testing Results Home Contract		
TREATMENT PLANNING	NI: Axis III		RT/TA started School started (youth)	Master TX Plan Updated RT/TA entry	MTP reflects psych testing results	Assess client support network
INTERVENTIONS	Assess Suicidal/Aggressive potential	Communicate in calm nonthreatening manner	Low stumli, identification of causative factors	Explore anxiety triggers	Help develop and rehearse problem-solving skills	Encourage independent decision making
MEDICATIONS	Meds ordered, Informed Consent		Drug interaction checked by Pharmacist/Dr. signs informed consent	Antianxiety meds as short term intervention only	Meds evaluated/readjusted	Discharge instructions for medication self-admin
LEVEL TEACHING	Level ordered Patient Rights Orient to Unit	Orient to Program	Reevaluate Medication Teaching Stress Reduction; Goals	Reevaluate for PHP Meds reinforced; Positive coping mechanism	Reevaluate for D/C Decision making; Relaxation techniques	Reevaluate Promote self-reliance and diversional activities
NUTRITION/DIET CONTINUM OF CARE	Diet Ordered: Initial D/C Plans	Chart daily intake Outcome survey	Chart daily intake Evaluate support system	Weight, chart intake D/C Plan update/revise	Chart daily intake After Care Plan written	Diet D/C instruction Outcome survey
PATIENT OUTCOMES	Controls self-harm/aggr.	Patient feels more secure	Anxiety levels decreased	Anxiety cycle interrupted	Uses problem solving skill	Promote cntl/self-worth

NOTE: (Variances included on the second page of the pathway) which is not shown; © 1994 Strategic Clinical Systems, Granbury, Texas.

CRITICAL THINKING QUESTIONS

A student nurse, Amber, is finishing her 7-week clinical rotation in psychiatric-mental health nursing. She overhears a discussion at the nurses' station between two of the nurses. One staff nurse, Ms. R., states that the nursing process is a waste of time and that only the psychiatrists and psychologists use the diagnostic process. The case manager of the unit, Nurse M., states that she disagrees with Nurse R. Nurse M. states that NANDA's taxonomy can be used with interdisciplinary treatment plans and that they are not in conflict with standardized nursing care plans. She ended the discussion noting that NANDA diagnoses help to provide data not only for documenting JCAHO's standards for health care settings treating psychiatric clients but also for psychiatric nursing standards of care (ANA, 1994). Amber relates the discussion to her fellow students during postconference. Her instructor asks the following questions:

1. How would you answer Nurse R.?
    A. Include the similarities and differences between the nursing process and the diagnostic process used in deriving DSM-IV diagnoses.
    B. Discuss the rationale for including a two-part nursing diagnosis statement when documenting your diagnosis for a client experiencing a mental health disorder.
    C. What are the similarities and differences between NANDA's taxonomy of nursing diagnoses and the NIC taxonomy?
2. How would you answer Nurse M.?
    A. Do you agree or disagree with Nurse M. regarding interdisciplinary treatment plans and standardized nursing care plans? Support your answer.
    B. What do you think is the rationale for Nurse M. stating that the use of NANDA's diagnoses meet psychiatric-mental health nursing's standards of care (ANA, 1994) and JCAHO's standards for health care settings treating clients with mental illnesses?

- Assessment refers to the systematic collection of objective and subjective data about a client.
- Subjective data include reports or experiences described by the client; these descriptions are exactly what the person states are his or her thoughts and feelings and are referred to as *symptoms*.

- Objective data are behaviors observed in the client or findings of diagnostic tests; these are considered objective indicators of health or deviations of health or human responses to problems and are referred to as signs.
- A comprehensive nursing assessment provides information regarding a client's spirituality/philosophical, emotional and biological/gender growth and developmental stages, sociocultural background, and psychological aspects of current and/or previous psychiatric history.
- A NANDA nursing diagnosis refers to a clinical judgment about individual, family, or community responses to actual and potential health problems/life processes. Nursing diagnoses provide the basis for selection of nursing interventions to achieve outcomes for which the nurse is accountable.
- NANDA's main "components" of a nursing diagnosis are the label, definition, defining characteristics, related factors, and risk factors.
- NIC interventions are research-based practice guidelines for common clinical problems, which are also approved by ANA for clinical use.
- ITPs indicate the responsibilities of various members of the health team for a client's care. An ITP may be referred to as a Care Map, critical path, clinical pathway, or a managed care plan.
- The implementation standard of care reflects the following interventions that are used by the nurse functioning at the basic level of psychiatric-mental health nursing: counseling, milieu therapy, self-care activities, psychobiological interventions, health teaching, case management, health promotion and health maintenance.
- Evaluation of client outcomes is an ongoing, sophisticated, complex, critical thinking process that provides for continuity of care.

REFERENCES

American Nurses Association. (1995). *Nursing: A social policy statement.* Kansas City, MO: Author.

American Nurses Association. (1994). *A statement on psychiatric-mental health clinical nursing practice and standards of psychiatric-mental health clinical nursing practice.* Washington, DC: American Nurses Publishing.

American Nurses Association. (1991). *Standards of clinical nursing practice.* Kansas City, MO: Author.

American Psychiatric Association. (1994). *Diagnostic and statistical manual of mental disorders DSM-IV* (4th ed.). Washington, DC: Author.

Carnevali, D. L., & Thomas, M. D. (1993). *Diagnostic reasoning and treatment decision making in nursing.* Philadelphia: J. B. Lippincott.

Dunn, J.R. (1993). Medical skills and knowledge: How necessary are they for psychiatric nurses? *Journal of Psychosocial Nursing and Mental Health Service, 31*(12), 25.

Haber, J., Feldman, H.R., Penney, N., Carter, E., Bidwell-Cerone, S.R., & Hott, J.R. (1994). Shaping nursing practice through research-based protocols. *The Journal of the New York State Nurses Association, 25*(3), 4-12.

Joint Commission on Accreditation of Healthcare Organizations (1995). *Mental health manual.* Oakbrook Terrace, IL: Author.

Kaplan, H.I., Sadock, B.J., & Grebb, J.A. (1994). *Kaplan and Sadock's synopsis of psychiatric behavioral sciences clinical psychiatry* (7th ed.). Baltimore: Williams & Wilkins.

Krainovich-Miller, B., Haber, J., Adler-Klein, D., & Parry, M. (1995). *The experience of caring in an AIDS population: Patient, nurse, and physician perspectives.* (Unpublished manuscript).

Levin, R.F., & Crosley, J.M. (1986). Focused data collection for the generation of nursing diagnoses. *Journal of Nursing Staff Development, Spring,* 56-64.

McCloskey, J.C., & Bulachek, G.M. (1996). *Iowa intervention project: Nursing interventions classification (NIC)* (2nd ed.). St. Louis: Mosby.

McCormick, K.A., Lang, N., Zielstorff, R., Milholland, D.K., Saba, V., & Jacox, A. (1994). Toward standard classification schemes for nursing language: Recommendations of the American Nurses Association Steering Committee on databases to support clinical nursing practice. *Journal of the American Medical Informatics Association (JAMIA), 1*(6), 421-427.

Mulhearn, S. (1989). The nursing process: Improving psychiatric admission assessment. *Journal of Advanced Nursing, 14,* 808-814.

North American Nursing Diagnosis Association. (1994). *NANDA nursing diagnoses: Definitions and classification 1995-1996.* Philadelphia: Author.

Peplau, H.E. (1987). List of intellectual and interpersonal basic skills. *Nursing Times, 83*(1).

Potter, P. (1994). *Pocket guide to health assessment* (3rd ed.). St. Louis: Mosby.

U.S. Department of Health and Human Services. Depression Guideline Panel. (1993). *Depression in primary care: Volume 2: Treatment of major depression* (AHCPR Publication No. 93-0551). Rockville, MD: Author.

Chapter 6

Understanding the Influence of Culture

Josepha Campinha-Bacote

LEARNING OUTCOMES

After studying and applying the concepts of this chapter, the learner will be able to:
- Define culture and its characteristics.
- Discuss the relationship between culture, health, and illness.
- Define diagnostic and treatment issues in psychiatric nursing when caring for culturally diverse clients.
- Identify components of cultural competence.
- Discuss culturally specific interventions.

KEY TERMS

Acculturated interacting style
Beliefs
Bicultural interacting style
Color-blind
Covert racism
Cross-cultural diagnosis
Cultural awareness
Cultural blind spot syndrome
Cultural blindness
Cultural competence
Cultural encounter
Cultural ignorance

Cultural imposition
Cultural knowledge
Cultural skill
Culturally immersed
Culturally liberated
Culturally responsive
Culturally sensitive
Culturally specific care
Culturalogical assessment
Culture
Culture-bound syndrome
Customs

Emic
Enculturation
Ethnic pharmacology
Ethnocentrism
Ethnosensitivity
Intra-ethnic variation
Labeling
Overt racism
Personalistic
Stereotype
Traditional interacting style
Values

The relationship between culture and mental illness remains controversial in the field of mental health. Many authors assert that culture is a direct determinant of disease and illness, but others argue that no direct relationship between culture and mental illness exists, because no person lives in a "nonculture" (Kalkman and Davis, 1980). Nonetheless, psychiatric nurses are exposed to individuals, families, and communities experiencing culture-bound illness, in which symptomatology closely mimics psychiatric disorders (Campinha-Bacote, 1989). The only responsible choice for a psychiatric nurse is to explore effective and culturally relevant ways to assess, diagnose, and treat individuals, families, and communities from culturally diverse backgrounds. The purpose of this chapter is to examine important cultural factors that facilitate the effective practice of psychiatric nursing.

CULTURE AND HEALTH

The concept of culture and its relationship to health beliefs and practices is essential to understand when discussing the issue of cultural competence in psychiatric nursing. The literature is saturated with definitions of culture. For the purpose of this chapter, Tylor's definition will be used. Tylor (1871) defined *culture "as that complex whole which includes knowledge, belief, art, morals, law, custom, and any other capabilities and habits acquired by man as a member of society."*

Many factors other than ethnicity constitute a cultural group. Geographical location, gender, religious affiliation, sexual orientation, occupation, a physically challenged state of health (e.g., blindness or deafness), education, and socioeconomic status are only a few variables that draw individuals together to form a distinct cultural group.

There are several characteristics of culture, being that it is learned. Culture is acquired by personal experience. *Enculturation is the process by which culture is transmitted from one generation to another.* Culture is also shared, defining dominant patterns of values, attitudes, beliefs, and behaviors. It can therefore be concluded that culture connotes shared beliefs and patterns of behavior that are learned through socialization (Tripp-Reimer, 1984).

Culture is a combination of values, beliefs, and customs. *Values give an individual a sense of direction, as well as meaning to life.* They guide the individual internally to do what he or she "ought" to do in certain situations (Tripp-Reimer, 1984). Values are responsible for developing a person's perspective by establishing a hierarchy of needs and goals, and by limiting alternative choices. Values are held on an unconscious level and are learned. Health behaviors are generally consistent with personal cultural values.

Beliefs include knowledge, opinions, and faith concerning various aspects of a person's world. An individual's definition of illness is part of his or her belief system and is determined largely by cultural factors. The final component of culture is custom. *Customs are practices or habitual lifeways expressed by a specific cultural group.* Customs are the easiest to assess and describe because they are directly observable. Home remedies are examples of customs that play a vital role in the health practices of individuals. Table 6-1 depicts the basic characteristics of culture.

A direct relationship between culture and health practices exists, and of the many factors that are known to determine health beliefs and behaviors, culture is the most influential variable (Harwood, 1981). Culture has been shown to influence a person's concept of disease and illness. Disease and illness are not interchangeable terms, and a distinction has been made by Rosen, Kleinman, and Katon, 1982:

> Disease may be defined as the malfunctioning of biological and/or psychological processes, whereas illness may be defined as the perception, evaluation, explanation, and labeling of symptoms by the patient and his family and social network.

The cultural aspect of health is an important and influential variable to consider when providing nursing care to individuals, families, and communities from diverse cultural backgrounds, since "culture is tightly interwoven into the life of man and continually pervades his thinking, actions, feelings, and particularly his health state" (Leininger, 1967). The client's world view (beliefs and values) dictates how he or she sees the world. This world view is referred to as the emic view of the client. An *emic view is the native view of the client's presenting problem.* For example, some individuals hold a personalistic view of illness causality. *A personalistic view of illness is when an individual believes that his or her illness is related to an active, purposeful intervention of an agent who may be human, nonhuman (evil spirit), or supernatural.* It is important to understand this emic perspective to provide culturally relevant nursing care.

CULTURAL ISSUES IN PSYCHIATRIC NURSING

Diagnostic and treatment issues are critical to examine when caring for culturally diverse clients. Diagnostic clarity may be confounded by differences in behavioral expressions of mental disorders in various cultures. In addition, the relationship between ethnicity and diagnosis remains a controversial issue in the field of psychiatry. Conflicting research findings appear to group in three categories:

TABLE 6-1

Basic characteristics of culture

CHARACTERISTIC	DESCRIPTION	EXAMPLE
Culture is learned.	Culture is a learned set of values, beliefs, and behaviors that are shared by a group of people who learn them through formal and informal channels. Culture is not genetically inherited—unlike race, which refers to biologically inherited characteristics that are observable in physical traits.	Cuban family members learn that humor is a way of making fun of people, situations, or things known as *chateo*. Humor also includes modifying situations through exaggeration, jokes, and satirical expressions or gestures.
Culture is transmitted.	Culture is passed from one generation to another by a person; this process is known as enculturation.	In the Asian culture the concept of the family extends both backward and forward. The individual is seen as a product of all generations of his or her family from the beginning of time. The transmission of this concept is reinforced by rituals such as ancestor worship and family record books. Personal actions reflect not only on the individual, but also on all generations—past, present, and future.
Culture is shared.	Culture is a shared set of assumptions, values, beliefs, attitudes, and behaviors of a group. Sharing a common culture allows members of a cultural group to predict one another's actions and to react accordingly.	An assumption of traditional Arab culture is that a woman will not make eye contact with a man other than her husband. All decisions are made by her husband. Since a woman may not be touched by another man, health care may be provided only by another woman.
Culture is integrated.	Universal aspects of culture include religion, politics, economics, art, kinship, diet, health, and patterns of communication. It is difficult, if not impossible, to study only one aspect of a culture because all categories are interrelated.	In Ireland and the United States the primary cultural force and national unifier of Irish culture has been the Catholic Church. In fact the parish rather than the neighborhood has traditionally defined the family's social context.
Culture contains ideal and real components.	Ideal cultural patterns are called norms, which prescribe what people ought to do in a particular situation. Norms may be reinforced through legal or social means. Real behavior may diverge from ideal behavior and still be acceptable.	The American mainstream culture condemns the drinking of alcohol on a daily basis. However, those who do so, but "hold their liquor well," are regarded with only minimal disapproval.
Cultures are dynamic entities that are continuously evolving.	Cultural change is an ongoing but slow process. All aspects of culture do not change simultaneously. Cultural habits and superficial behaviors are easier to alter than are deep-rooted values and beliefs that are acquired early in life.	Although Italian Americans have become an integral part of American society, values regarding the family roles of men and women are often more traditional than values regarding roles of men and women in the workplace.

Continued.

TABLE 6-1 — cont'd

Basic characteristics of culture

CHARACTERISTIC	DESCRIPTION	EXAMPLE
Individual behavior is not necessarily representative of the culture.	Although the culture defines the dominant patterns of values, beliefs, and behaviors, it does not determine all the behaviors in any group. Variation from the dominant pattern of behavior encountered in one individual is called eccentric behavior. The meaning of this behavior within the culture will determine whether it is regarded as normal, eccentric, or deviant. A group of people within a society who share values, beliefs, and behaviors that differ from those of the dominant culture are referred to as a subculture.	Male and female roles are strictly defined in traditional Greek culture. Women are secondary to men. The man is the head of the family. Men work and provide for their families; it is a dishonor if the wife works outside the home. Within this cultural context, a Greek woman who is a proponent of the feminist movement might be viewed as eccentric or deviant, depending on how vocal she is or how much her beliefs disrupt the community.

- Those that find a difference in psychiatric diagnosis based on ethnic identity
- Those that find no difference
- Those for which evidence is inconclusive and therefore no judgment can be made about psychiatric diagnosis and ethnicity (Flaskerud and Hu, 1992).

Diagnostic controversy also includes the role of psychiatric nurses and their ability to maintain diagnostic objectivity in cross-cultural situations (Campinha-Bacote, 1995a).

***Cross-cultural diagnosis** is the ability of the nurse from one culture to make an accurate diagnosis for a client from another culture.* There are many variables that may limit the psychiatric nurse's ability to make cross-cultural diagnoses. One variable is ethnic background of the nurse. For example, European American psychodiagnosticians may have a lower threshold of psychiatric evaluation before assigning a diagnosis of schizophrenia to African Americans (Neighbors et al., 1989). Specifically, fewer symptoms are required to be present before diagnosing an African-American client as having schizophrenia as compared with European-American clients having schizophrenia. This misdiagnosis is related to the labeling process.

***Labeling** refers to assigning a particular impression or diagnosis specific to a client.* Different cultures vary greatly in what they consider mentally normal and abnormal, so psychiatric nurses need to be aware of factors that combine to create the phenomenon called labeling process. Box 6-1 contains questions that nurses must ask themselves when assessing and labeling clients.

The *Diagnostic and Statistical Manual of Mental Disorders, Fourth Edition* (DSM-IV) (1994), is one of the major classification systems used in the labeling process of mental illness. Historically, this manual has not been sensitive to cultural aspects affecting the diagnostic process. However, particular effort has been made to enhance the relevance of DSM-IV internationally, as well as to the culturally and ethnically diverse population of the United States (Wilson and Skodol, 1994). The DSM-IV now includes three types of information related to ethnic and cultural issues: (1) a discussion of cultural variations in the presentation of disorders, (2) a description of several culture-bound syndromes in an appendix, and (3) an outline for cultural formulation for assessment of culturally and ethnically diverse clients in an appendix (Wilson and Skodol, 1994). These recent changes in the DSM-IV are an initial step toward increasing diagnostic clarity in cross-cultural situations.

Culturally specific issues in psychiatric nursing also include several treatment issues, especially in the areas of psychopharmacology. Psychiatric nurses must be aware of the field of ethnic pharmacology. ***Ethnic pharmacology** is the growing field of study that investigates variant responses to drugs in ethnic groups.* For example, Askenazic Jewish individuals respond differently to specific neuroleptic agents with regard to side effects. Clozapine (Clozaril), used to treat schizophrenia, was associated with the development of agranulocytosis in 20% of Jewish clients, although it occurs in only 1% of clients with chronic schizophrenia in the general population (Liberman, Yunis, and Egea, 1991). Another example is Hispanics taking tricyclic antidepressants. Hispanics experience side effects at half the dosage observed in European Americans (Marcos and Cancro, 1982).

Most clinical drug trials are conducted on European-American men. More recently, clinical trials have begun

Box 6-1

Nurse's Self-Assessment in Labeling Clients

- How do I define this behavior?
- How is my cultural, religious, or social environment influencing me?
- To what degree am I attempting to understand the client's behavior from a relativistic or an ethnocentric perspective?
- To what degree am I stereotyping the client?
- To what degree am I being influenced by others (such as family or team members) who I hold in high regard?
- What objective data are there to substantiate the label given?
- To what degree am I expressing a professional assessment or a personal opinion?
- Are there underlying political or financial motives for the label given?
- What will be the results to the client if this label is given to this behavior?
- To what degree does this client confront a sensitive issue or perceived weakness in me?

to include European-American women. However, specific ethnic groups, regardless of gender, continue to be an underrepresented group in research studies regarding clinical drug trials.

Another treatment issue for the psychiatric nurse is ethnicity and family therapy. Culture is deeply tied to the family, and increasing evidence shows that ethnic values are retained for many generations (McGoldrick, Pearce, and Giordano, 1996). The major family models, however, have not made explicit reference to these cultural differences. Therefore when conducting family therapy sessions with families from diverse cultural groups the psychiatric nurse must be knowledgeable about cultural variations in treatment issues. McGoldrick, Pearce, and Giordano (1996) stated that the family therapist must be aware of the following:

- Definitions of family differ greatly from culture to culture
- Family life cycle phases vary for different ethnic groups
- Cultural groups vary in the emphasis they place on different life cycle transitions
- Cultural groups differ in what they see as problematic and how they see the solution to the problem
- Cultural groups vary in their attitudes toward seeking help.

The use of folk health systems and folk remedies represent still another treatment challenge for the psychiatric nurse. It is common for individuals to seek care from both professional and folk health care systems. Powers (1982) reported a case study in which a client who believed that someone had "worked roots on her" sought treatment from professional health care providers, as well as from the local "root doctor." Similarly, some Mexican-American clients seek spiritual treatment through a curandero or curandera (male or female folk healer). The psychiatric nurse cannot assume that because clients are receiving care from professional health care providers that they are not also receiving care from folk health care systems. It is the role of the nurse to assess what types of health care systems and folk remedies are being used and to negotiate a treatment plan that reflects, respects, and incorporates both health care systems.

If nurses are not knowledgeable about various cultural home remedies used by clients, they may misdiagnose a behavior as representing a psychiatric problem. An example is the Vietnamese folk medical practice of dermabrasion, a home treatment for such health conditions as fever, chills, and headaches (Tripp-Reimer, 1984). First, oil is massaged into the skin until the skin becomes warm. A coin is then used to firmly stroke the skin to produce petechiae. This folk custom, if misinterpreted, can be misdiagnosed as physical abuse.

The psychiatric nurse must be able to differentiate between psychopathology and a normal cultural expression. Failure to make this distinction may result in diagnostic and treatment errors with culturally diverse clients.

Cultural Competence in Psychiatric Nursing: A Conceptual Model

Cultural competence is defined as a set of congruent behaviors, attitudes, and policies that come together in a system or agency, or among professionals, and enable that system, agency, or professionals to work effectively in cross-cultural situations (Cross et al., 1989). These authors view cultural competence on a continuum, ranging from cultural destructiveness to cultural proficiency. The American Academy of Nursing (AAN) *Expert Panel Report on Culturally Competent Nursing Care* (1992) defined culturally competent nursing care as:

> Care that is sensitive to issues related to culture, race, gender, and sexual orientation. This care is provided by nurses who use cultural nursing theory, models, and research principles in identifying and evaluating the care provided. It is also care that is provided within the cultural context of the clients.

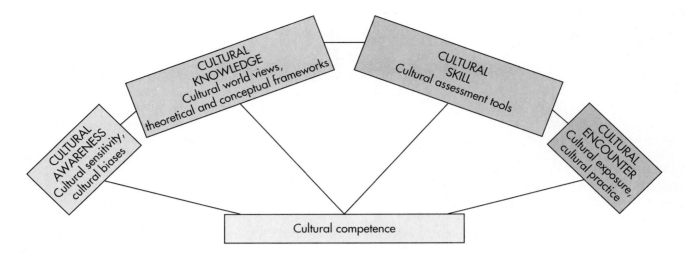

Fig. 6-1   A culturally competent model of care.

Campinha-Bacote (1994a) defined cultural competence in psychiatric nursing as a process, not an endpoint, in which the psychiatric nurse continually strives to achieve the ability to effectively work within the cultural context of an individual, family, or community from a diverse cultural or ethnic background. In this model, Campinha-Bacote identified cultural awareness, cultural knowledge, cultural skill, and cultural encounters as components of cultural competence that is illustrated in Fig. 6-1. This model will provide the framework to develop the skills of cultural competence.

Cultural Awareness

Cultural awareness is the deliberate and cognitive process in which the psychiatric nurse becomes appreciative and sensitive to the values, beliefs, lifeways, practices, and problem-solving strategies of a client's culture. During this process, nurses must examine their biases and prejudices toward other cultures, as well as explore their own cultural background. This task is necessary, since there is a tendency for a person to be ethnocentric regarding his or her own values, beliefs, and practices. *Ethnocentrism is the tendency of an individual (or group) to feel that his or her own lifeways are the most desirable, acceptable, or best, and to behave in a superior manner to another culture's lifeways* (Leininger, 1978).

Ethnocentric tendencies can lead to cultural blindness. *Cultural blindness is the inability of the nurse to recognize not only his or her own lifestyle, values, and modes of behavior but also those of another individual because of strong ethnocentric tendencies* (Leininger, 1978). Without being aware of the influence of personal cultural values, there is a risk for the nurse to engage in cultural imposition. As defined by Leininger

(1978), *cultural imposition is the tendency of an individual to impose their beliefs, values, and patterns of behavior on another culture.* Pedersen (1995) suggested several techniques to stimulate cultural awareness: (1) experiential exercises (role plays, role reversals, simulations); (2) field trips; (3) guided self-study with a reading list; (4) critical incidents; (5) panel discussions; (6) audiovisual presentations; (7) interviews with consultants and experts; and (8) bicultural observations. Pedersen's goal in this "awareness focus" is to assist the health care provider in becoming aware of the contrast and conflict between his or her background and the client's cultural background.

In gaining cultural awareness, psychiatric nurses must become aware of the different interacting styles in which they may engage when interacting with culturally diverse clients. Bell and Evans (1981) described five interacting styles:

1. *Overt racism is when nurses interact with culturally diverse clients out of deep-seated prejudices, which they may have toward that specific cultural group.* The nurse may use the power of his or her attitudes and behavior to dehumanize the client.
2. *Covert racism is an interacting style in which the nurse is aware of his or her fears toward a specific cultural group but knows that open expression of those attitudes is inappropriate.* The nurse attempts to hide his or her true feelings.
3. *Cultural ignorance is when the nurse has little or no prior exposure to the specific cultural group and experiences fear of his or her inability to relate to the client.*
4. The *color-blind nurse denies the reality of cultural differences that are important to effective*

interactions. In this interacting style the nurse has made a decision that he or she is committed to equality for all people and therefore treats all people alike, regardless of cultural background.

5. The **culturally liberated** *nurse does not fear cultural differences and is aware of his or her attitudes toward specific cultural groups.* This nurse encourages the client to express feelings about their ethnicity and uses these feelings as a shared learning experience.

Nurses must be aware of the interacting style in which they are operating and strive toward a culturally liberated interacting style.

Borkan and Neher's (1991) developmental model of ethnosensitivity can be used as a framework to further assist nurses in gaining cultural awareness and sensitivity. They assert that ethnosensitivity can be viewed on a continuum of personal growth, advancing from ethnocentrism to ethnorelativity. This developmental model begins with the ethnocentric position of fear and mistrust toward culturally diverse groups and progresses through phases of denial of a person's biases, negative stereotyping of cultural groups, minimization of cultural differences, acceptance of differences, empathy toward culturally diverse groups, and finally an ethnosensitive attitude of integration. The ultimate goals of this model are fostering **ethnosensitivity,** *the ability to appreciate values and behaviors within the context of specific cultural norms and the application of this ability to clinical practice.*

It is important to understand that the level of cultural sensitivity a nurse exhibits is likely to vary according to the cultural or ethnic group encountered. For example, a nurse may be ethnosensitive toward Asians and ethnocentric when interacting with Native Americans. Therefore the developmental stages of ethnosensitivity should not be considered mutually exclusive (Borkan and Neher, 1991). The process of gaining cultural awareness and sensitivity is an important first step in the journey toward cultural competence. However, a **culturally sensitive** *approach requires only an awareness of the values, beliefs, lifeways, and practices of an individual,* whereas a **culturally responsive** *approach incorporates the individual's values, beliefs, lifeways, and practices into a mutually acceptable treatment plan* (Campinha-Bacote, 1989). Psychiatric nurses must go beyond cultural awareness and cultural sensitivity and develop other needed components of cultural competency.

Cultural Knowledge

Cultural knowledge *is the process by which the nurse seeks and obtains a sound educational foundation concerning the various world views of different cultures.*

The goal of cultural knowledge is to become familiar with a culturally or ethnically diverse group's world view, beliefs, values, practices, lifestyles, and problem-solving strategies. The fields of transcultural nursing, sociology, transcultural psychiatry, anthropology, and medical anthropology can provide nurses with this educational foundation. To acquaint nurses with content relevant to cultural knowledge, this section presents information on etiological explanations of illness causality, interacting styles within cultural groups, culture-bound illnesses, and ethnic psychopharmacology.

Etiological explanations of illness causality

Most professional health care providers ascribe to a biomedical view of an individual's initial health care problem, which assumes that disease is a result of cause-and-effect relations of natural phenomena (Henderson and Primeaux, 1981). Professional medicine gives little credit to supernatural theories of illness causality and refers to this viewpoint as primitive, irrational, superstitious, and/or nonprofessional. However, specific ethnic and cultural groups strongly believe in magic and supernatural forces as etiological factors of disease and illness.

Foster (1976) divided beliefs about illness causality in nonprofessional medical systems into two broad categories: (1) personalistic and (2) naturalistic. The personalistic viewpoint regards illness as a condition related to active, purposeful intervention of an agent who may be human (witch, sorcerer), nonhuman (evil spirit), or supernatural (a deity or powerful force). In the naturalistic view of illness causation, health is conceived to be a state of equilibrium and when imbalance occurs, it triggers illness. The naturalistic view of illness explains ill health as natural forces or conditions such as cold, heat, wind, and dampness. Foster's categorizations of illness causality are not mutually exclusive. In many instances, more than one theory may be recognized by a specific cultural group. Although cultural groups may vary in their commitment to any one theory of illness, most people are committed to either a naturalistic or personalistic view to explain a majority of illnesses (Foster, 1976).

Interacting styles within cultural groups

In obtaining cultural knowledge, it is also important to be knowledgeable of the different interacting styles within culturally diverse groups. Bell and Evans (1981) assert that there are four different types of interacting styles within a specific cultural group: acculturated, culturally immersed, traditional, and bicultural. The **acculturated interacting style** *is when a client from a culturally diverse ethnic group makes a conscious or subconscious decision to reject the values, beliefs, practices, and general behaviors associated with his or her own cultural group.* In contrast the **culturally immersed** *client rejects all values, except those held by his or her culture.*

They are often labeled "militant" or "difficult to work with." This client becomes immersed in his or her own culture as a survival mechanism. In the *traditional interacting styles, the client neither rejects nor accepts his or her ethnic identity.* They do not disclose personal information and therefore are difficult to reach. These individuals have been taught the motto: "Do not air your dirty laundry to anyone." The *bicultural interacting style* demonstrates *the pride that the client has for his or her identity, history, and cultural traditions, while still feeling comfortable in the mainstream world.* The bicultural person values integrated living and ethnic diversity.

It is important to understand these different interacting styles of culturally diverse clients when rendering culturally specific services because the acculturated client may reject the nurse's attempt to provide culturally relevant services, whereas the culturally immersed client will demand culturally specific services. An example is a third-generation Mexican-American client who has been raised in a predominantly European American community. This client does not speak Spanish and selectively does not relate to other Mexican Americans. It is important for the nurse to realize that this client may be acculturated, and it may not be appropriate to design culturally specific interviews based on Mexican-American world view.

Culture-bound illnesses

Obtaining knowledge of culturally diverse populations will prevent possible misdiagnosis of clients. Diagnostic clarity may be confounded by differences in behavioral expressions of mental illness in various cultures. This select expression of an illness within cultures is referred to as a culture-bound syndrome. Leff (1981) defines *culture-bound syndrome as the features of an illness that vary from culture to culture.* Susto, falling-out, voodoo illness, and mal ojo, are a few examples of culture-bound illnesses that the psychiatric nurse may encounter when caring for various cultural groups.

Falling-out and voodoo illness are two culture-bound illnesses that may be seen in some African-American and black Caribbean cultures. Falling-out is manifested by the sudden collapse and paralysis, and the inability to see or speak (Westermeyer, 1985). However, the individual's hearing and understanding are still intact. Voodoo illness is a belief that illness or death may come to an individual through a supernatural force. Voodoo illness is more commonly referred to as *rootwork, hex, fix, witchcraft, a spell, black magic,* or *a trick* (Campinha-Bacote, 1986). The symptoms include gastrointestinal (GI) and behavior disorders such as nausea, vomiting, diarrhea, food that does not taste right, convulsions, muscle weakness, paralysis, and complaints that animals are living in the client's body (Campinha-Bacote, 1986).

Susto and mal ojo are two culture-bound illnesses noted in some Hispanic populations. Susto, or soul loss, is the belief that a frightening experience can cause illness. When this fright occurs, it is believed that the soul of the victim has been captured by spirits. Symptoms include anorexia, listlessness, apathy and withdrawal (Harwood, 1981). Mal ojo, or evil eye, embodies the belief that social relations contain dangers to an individual. It is stated that women and children are more susceptible to this illness because they are considered weaker. The belief is that a "strong" person with "vista fuerte" (strong vision) can exert a negative power over the weaker person causing them to become ill. Symptoms such as fever, rashes, nervousness, and irritability appear abruptly.

Since these culture-bound illnesses imitate psychopathology, there is a serious concern for misdiagnosis in culturally diverse ethnic groups. Adebimpe (1981) reports that over the years, a major diagnostic issue has been the high frequencies of the diagnosis of psychosis and the low frequency of depression in African-American clients. Mukherjee et al. (1983) also confirm the incidence of overdiagnosis and misdiagnosis of schizophrenia among African-American and other ethnic groups.

Worthington (1992) conducted an in-depth review to critically examine the professional literature on racial and ethnic factors pertaining to misdiagnosis of the African-American client. She found that most researchers related diagnostic and treatment issues to race. As a result of the great potential of misdiagnosis of mental illness among culturally diverse groups, a cultural assessment is one obvious solution to this problem. Unfortunately, most clients do not receive culturally based assessments, and misdiagnosis continues to present a problem for most culturally or ethnically diverse populations.

Ethnic pharmacology   Most of the literature on cultural competence focuses on therapeutic barriers formed by ethnic difference and the interpersonal process of interacting with an ethnically diverse cultural group. One area of cultural competence that is neglected in providing culturally relevant services to ethnic populations is ethnic and racial differences in response to drugs (Campinha-Bacote, 1994b). In obtaining cultural knowledge, it is important to acquire knowledge regarding the culturally diverse group's response to medications.

Pharmacogenetic research in the last 15 years has uncovered significant differences among racial and ethnic populations with regard to metabolism rates, clinical drug responses, and side effects. These findings gave rise to the field of study called ethnic pharmacology. Ethnic pharmacology (also referred to as pharmacoanthropology) is the field of study that investigates variant responses to drugs in ethnic or racially distinct groups (Kudzma, 1992).

Several factors are involved in determining responses to a specific drug in ethnic groups. These factors include environmental, genetic, cultural, and structural variations in ethnic groups. For example, among African Americans and European Americans, only 9% are considered to be slow metabolizers, whereas as high as 32% of Asians are considered to be slow metabolizers. This difference is important, because if a drug is metabolized more quickly than usual, drug effects may be below optimal response or even ineffective. Lin, Poland, and Lesser (1986) stated that ethnic groups such as Asians, who metabolize drugs more slowly, will experience a greater risk of side effects with neuroleptic medication. Specifically, 95% of Asians will experience extrapyramidal symptoms (EPS), whereas only 67% of European Americans and African Americans will experience this side effect. In addition, Campinha-Bacote (1991a) reported that African-American psychiatric clients experience a higher incidence of EPS with haloperidol decanoate (Haldol) than European Americans.

The process of attaining cultural knowledge is intended to provide the psychiatric nurse with a general overview of different cultures and their world views. Physiological, as well as psychological, social, spiritual, and environmental dimensions are valuable in understanding culturally diverse groups. The nurse can use this basic knowledge as a foundation when interacting with specific cultural groups. However, nurses cannot rely solely on textbooks for culturally specific knowledge. They must also develop the skill necessary to obtain knowledge directly from the client. This skill will prevent possible stereotyping of specific cultural groups.

Cultural Skill

Cultural skill involves the process of learning how to conduct a cultural assessment. This skill allows the nurse to individually access the client's cultural values, beliefs, and practices without depending solely on written facts about that specific cultural group. The nurse learns about the client's perception regarding health and illness, as well as the client's perception of what treatment should be rendered.

Although it is essential to conduct an assessment with culturally diverse groups, it is also necessary to ensure that every client receives a cultural assessment. Every client has values, beliefs, and practices that must be considered when rendering health care services. Therefore cultural assessments are not limited to specific ethnic groups but rather should be conducted with each individual. Conducting a cultural assessment with each client will prevent the "cultural blind spot syndrome." Buchwald, et al. (1994) defines the *cultural blind spot syndrome* as follows: *"Just because the client looks and behaves much the way you do, you assume there is no cultural differences or potential barriers to care."*

Cultural assessment tools
Culturological assessment is a systematic appraisal or examination of individuals, groups, and communities, regarding their cultural beliefs, values, and practices to determine explicit needs and intervention practices within the cultural context of the people being evaluated (Leininger, 1978). Psychiatric nurses should be aware of the available cultural assessments within a variety of disciplines.

Kluckhohn and Strodtbeck's (1961) Model of Variation in Value Orientation provides a conceptual framework for assessing cultural groups in five dimensions:

- Human nature
- Person-nature
- Time sense
- Activity
- Social relations

The component of human nature assesses whether a client views people as both good and bad, mostly good, or "cannot be trusted." The person-nature component assesses whether the client experiences relationships that reflect the perspective that life is largely determined by external forces such as fate, God, or genetics; or those that reflect experiences and relationships that people should conquer to control life. Time sense assesses if people value history (past), the moment (present), or value planning and goal setting (future). The activity component assesses whether the culture is "doing" oriented (oriented toward achievement) or "being" oriented. The final dimension is social relations. The nurse must assess whether the client views that some people are born to lead or whether the client believes that some people are born to follow.

Table 6-2 illustrates the diversity of traditional tendencies in value orientation among some American ethnic groups. Such understanding provides an explanation for client behavior, highlights potential barriers to participating in psychiatric treatment, and signals potential value conflicts between the nurse and the client. Kleinman, Eisenburg, and Good (1978) have suggested eight open-ended questions conducting a cultural assessment (Box 6-2).

The cultural assessment tool of Leininger (1978), can be used across all subspecialties of nursing. Leininger (1978) identified the following nine major domains to consider when conducting a cultural assessment:

- Patterns of lifestyle
- Specific cultural values and norms
- Cultural taboos and myths
- World view and ethnocentric tendencies

TABLE 6-2

Tendencies in value orientation of selected American ethnic groups

				ORIENTATION	
ETHNIC GROUP	TEMPORAL	ACTIVITY	RELATIONAL	PEOPLE TO NATURE AND THE SUPERNATURAL	INNATE NATURE OF HUMAN BEINGS*
Northern European Americans	Future over present	Doing	Individualistic	1. Dominant 2. Harmony with nature 3. Subjugated	1. Mixed 2. Evil 3. Good
African Americans	Present over future	Being	Collateral-lineal	1. Subjugated 2. Dominant 3. Harmony with nature	1. Mixed 2. Evil 3. Good
Mexican Americans	Present	Being	Lineal-collateral	Subjugated	1. Mixed 2. Evil 3. Good
Puerto Rican Americans	Present over future	Being	Lineal-collateral	Subjugated	1. Mixed 2. Evil 3. Good
Native Americans	Present	Being	Collateral-individual	Harmony with nature	1. Good 2. Mixed 3. Evil
Chinese Americans	Past-present	Being	Lineal	Harmony with nature	1. Good 2. Mixed 3. Evil

Numbers 1, 2, and 3 indicate rank order dominance of the innate human nature value orientation in that culture.

• General features that the client perceives as different or similar to other cultures
• Health and life care rituals and rites of passage to maintain health
• Degree of cultural change
• Caring behaviors
• Folk and professional health-illness system used

According to Leininger (1978), the two guiding principles that can help the nurse make an accurate culturological assessment are to (1) maintain a broad, objective, and open attitude of individuals and their culture; and (2) avoid seeing all individuals alike.

Communication style involves obtaining information on the client's language and dialect preference, as well as nonverbal social and ethnic customs. Orientation refers to the client's ethnic identity. Asking the client the ethnic or cultural group with which he or she identifies allows the client to choose his or her orientation without being labeled by the nurse. Orientation also refers to how closely the client adheres to traditional habits and values of his or her cultural group. Nutritional information can be obtained by asking such questions as:

• Are there ethnic foods that the client prefers?
• Are there foods the client is encouraged to eat when sick?
• Are there foods to be avoided because of ethnic origin, health status, or illness?

Family relationship data involve such questions as asking the client his or her definition of family and how decisions are made in the family. Some examples of questions for gaining information regarding the client's health beliefs are as follows:

• Does the client rely on any self care or traditional folk medicine practices?
• How does the client explain illness?
• How does the client respond to hospitalization?

Educational and religious information can be obtained by asking the following questions:

Box 6-2

Cultural Assessment Tool

What do you think has caused your problem?

Why do you think it started when it did?

What do you think your sickness does to you?

How severe is your sickness?

What kind of treatment do you think you should receive?

What are the most important results you hope to achieve from these treatments?

What are the chief problems your sickness has caused?

What do you fear the most about your sickness?

From Kleinman, A., Eisenburg, L., & Good, B. (1978). Culture, illness, and care. Annals of Internal Medicine, 88, 251.

- Does the client prefer printed literature or audiovisual learning tools?
- Does the client learn by trial and error or by didactic methods?
- Does the client have a religious or spiritual preference?
- To what religious beliefs, sacred rites, religious sanctions, or restrictions does the client adhere?
- What religious persons will be involved in the client's health care?

Conducting a cultural assessment in a culturally sensitive manner

Cultural skill involves the process of developing a personal style in asking questions in a culturally sensitive manner. The nurse's approach to interviewing the client must be done in a culturally sensitive manner. For example, if the nurse uses Leininger's (1978) culturological assessment tool, how does the nurse ask questions regarding the clients cultural taboos? Does the nurse directly ask, "What are your cultural taboos?" An alternative way of asking this question in a culturally sensitive manner is, "Are there any treatments or types of care that may be offensive to you?"

Cultural skill acquisition

Buchwald et al. (1994) suggested the following techniques for eliciting cultural content from the client in a sensitive manner:

- Listen with interest and remain nonjudgmental about what is said.
- Develop alternative styles of questioning by adopting a less direct and more conversational approach to assessing the client's cultural background.
- Frame questions in the context of other clients or the client's family members.

Using the approach of Buchwald et al. to frame a question in the context of other clients or the client's family member, the nurse might say, "I know another client who had (give example of) an idea of what was wrong. Do you think that?" or, "What does your mother think is causing your problem?" Attributing the explanation to another person can help clients disclose health beliefs and practices that they feel uncomfortable expressing directly (Buchwald et al., 1994).

Another approach to conducting a cultural assessment in a sensitive manner, is to integrate cultural questions into the initial assessment. In contrast to having a separate cultural assessment form or tool, nurses may find it more useful to revise their existing general assessment form or admission form to reflect culturally relevant questions. This integrated approach results in having culturally relevant questions embedded into the nurse's existing assessment form. Culture is not "singled out" but rather appropriately integrated into the client's initial nursing history (Campinha-Bacote, 1995b).

Cultural Encounters

*A **cultural encounter** is a process that allows the nurse to directly engage in cross-cultural interactions with clients from culturally diverse backgrounds.* At times, we may believe that because we have studied a specific cultural group or interacted with three or four members from a specific cultural group, we are knowledgeable about the cultural group. In fact, these three or four individuals' values, beliefs, and practices may or may not represent the stated values, beliefs, and practices of that specific cultural group about which the nurse has read. This is because of intra-ethnic variation. ***Intra-ethnic variation** asserts that there is more variation within a cultural group than across cultural groups* (Campinha-Bacote, 1991b). It is extremely important to directly interact with clients from diverse cultural groups to refine or remodify one's existing knowledge about a specific cultural group. Face-to-face experiential encounters will at times negate and contradict the academic knowledge one has learned about that cultural group. The failure to directly interact with another cultural group will only stereotype that culture. A ***stereotype** is an oversimplified mental picture of a cultural group.* The nurse must continuously make it a priority to have cultural encounters to prevent such possible stereotyping that may occur when knowledge is being obtained. This experimental knowledge will serve as a sound framework in developing culturally relevant nursing interventions.

CULTURALLY RESPONSIVE INTERVENTIONS

***Culturally specific care** refers to the particularistic values, beliefs, and patterns of behavior that tend to be* *special, local, or unique to a designated culture and which do not tend to be shared with members of other cultures* (Leininger, 1978). The AAN of Expert Panel Report (1992) stated that nurses are central to the potential of developing and maintaining programs that deliver culturally competent health care. Leininger's (1991) Theory of Culture Care Diversity and Universality serves as a framework for nurses in providing culturally specific care. The three major modalities of Leininger's (1991) framework that guide culturally specific care include (1) cultural care accommodation (negotiation); (2) cultural care preservation (maintenance); and (3) cultural care repatterning (restructuring). Ethnomusic therapy is one example of a culturally specific intervention.

Ethnomusic therapy uses ethnic music as an intervention with ethnically diverse clients. Enthomusic therapy has the potential to (1) enhance interpersonal communication for clients of a specific ethnic group, and (2) moti-vate clients unresponsive to mainstream music therapy by using culturally relevant musical experiences (Morena, 1988). For example, in the African-American culture, a majority of "blues" music deals with situations and problems about which African Americans feel a sense of helplessness and confusion (Goines, 1973). Blues music is about something real, and the singing of or listening to blues lyrics has the potential to effectively release emotions for some African-American clients with a psychiatric disorder. In fact, Goines argued that blues music developed as a simple and inexpensive form of psychotherapy for African Americans.

Campinha-Bacote (1991a) developed a culturally specific program for African-American clients with a dual diagnosis of substance abuse and mental illness (SAMI). She described several culturally specific interventions to consider when delivering mental health services to African-American clients. She compared these culturally

TABLE 6-3

Similarities and differences between a traditional SAMI program and a culturally specific SAMI program

TRADITIONAL	CULTURAL SPECIFIC
Uses Bennett et al. (1983) conceptual model of the dual problem client	Uses a modified version of Bennett et al. (1983) conceptual model in addition to the culturally specific models of Phillips (1988), and Bell and Evans (1981)
Uses group and individual therapy with a professional orientation (e.g., psychoanalytical)	Uses group and individual therapy from an African-American perspective (e.g., ethnomusic therapy, humor therapy)
Treatment focuses exclusively on the dual diagnosis (e.g., SAMI)	Treatment focuses not only on the dual diagnosis problem, but also considers the total health needs of the client, (e.g., morbidity or mortality issues of African Americans)
Physical environment does not play a critical factor in treatment	Physical environment plays an important factor in treatment to reflect the client's cultural background (e.g., African-American pictures and symbols present)
Therapist accepts the client's presenting diagnosis (no need for rediagnosis or conducting a culturological assessment)	As a result of misdiagnosis of minorities, there is an essential need to rediagnose the client by completing a culturological assessment
Biological and genetic responses to medication are not an issue	Need to consider biological and genetic responses to medication (e.g., higher incidence of EPS in young black men on haloperidol [Haldol]; need to consider ethnicity and psychopharmacology)
Referrals are obtained through telephone contact and appointments that are set up by inpatient programs at hospital discharge	Referrals are obtained by focusing on the establishment of a personal contact and a close relationship with the client while he or she is in an inpatient setting (e.g., client attends an inpatient treatment program while also attending the outpatient culturally specific SAMI program)

From Campinha-Bacote (1991a). Community mental health services for the underserved: A culturally specific model. Archives of Psychi-atric Nursing, 5(14), 229-235.

specific interventions to a traditional program treating European American clients with a diagnosis of substance abuse and mental illness. These similarities and differences are displayed in Table 6-3.

Community Services for Underserved and Culturally Diverse Populations

Underutilization of mental health services by ethnic groups continues to pose a problem for community mental health centers. In 1981 the National Institute of Mental Health sponsored a review of the community support programs for mental health services with a special focus on ethnic groups. The results of this review demonstrated the need to develop model programs and clinical treatment standards that were culturally and ethnically appropriate (Martin, 1988). Campinha-Bacote (1991b) stated that culturally appropriate services must be available, accessible, appropriate, acceptable, and adoptable.

There has been an increase in the number of programs and services that are available to culturally diverse populations. However, these programs have not been easily accessible or affordable for individuals, families, and communities who need them the most. Availability is only one criterion in the provision of culturally relevant services. Culturally responsive programs must not only be available, but also must be accessible and affordable to culturally diverse and underserved populations. Several factors, such as geographical location and socioeconomic status make culturally relevant programs a myth to many underserved and ethnically or culturally diverse populations.

Culturally relevant services may be available, accessible, and affordable, but not acceptable to culturally diverse populations. To render services that are culturally acceptable involves a partnership with the client, family, or community. Such strategies as focus groups can provide nurses and other health care professionals with insight into what is acceptable for a particular cultural group.

Although a nurse may possess cultural awareness, cultural knowledge, and cultural skill, and may have had several cultural encounters, he or she must also possess the desire to work with culturally different clients. As defined by Covey (1989), desire is the motivation and the "want to do." This genuine desire paves the way for the development of culturally responsive programs that are available, accessible, affordable, acceptable, appropriate, and adoptable (Fig. 6-2).

Clients must also find services culturally appropriate and be willing to adopt them as their own. Culturally relevant programs that are adaptable lend themselves for adoption. Therefore if services to culturally diverse and underserved clients are intended to be culturally responsive, they must meet the criteria of being available, accessible, appropriate, acceptable, and adoptable. The Community Resources box on p. 88 lists several organizations that offer and promote multicultural services.

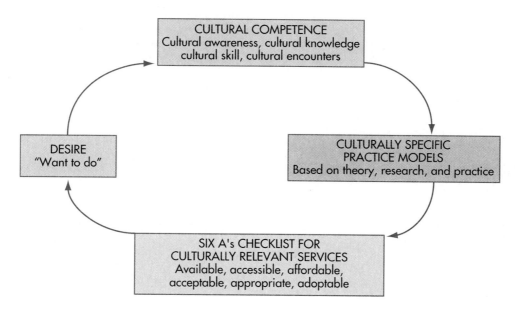

Fig. 6-2 A model of health care service delivery for underserved and ethnically/culturally diverse populations.

COMMUNITY RESOURCES

National Alliance for the Mentally Ill (NAMI)
Minority Group Community Resources
(800) 750-6264

Association of Multiethnic Americans
1060 Tennessee Street
San Francisco, CA 94107

Holt International Children's Services
P.O. Box 2880
Eugene, OR 98402
(541) 687-2202

Council of International Books for Children, Inc.
1841 Broadway
New York, NY 10023
(212) 966-1990

Multiethnic Unity Effort (MUE)
c/o Cheryl Paxson
P.O. Box 522
Waukegan, IL 60079
(708) 367-1782

National Coalition to End Racism in American Child Care System, Inc.
(Support group for transracial adoptions)
22075 Koths
Taylor, MI 48180
(313) 295-0257

Interrace Magazine
P.O. Box 1001
Schenectady, NY 12301-1001

National PTA Prejudice Club
700 N. Rush Street
Chicago, IL 60611

Blacks Educating Blacks About Sexual Health Issues
(BEBASHI)
1319 Locust Street
Philadelphia, PA 19107
(215) 546-4140

Coalition of Hispanic Health and Human Service Organizations
(COSSMHO)
1030 15th Street NW
Washington, D.C. 20005
(202) 371-2100

Multicultural Prevention Resource Center (MPRC)
1540 Market Street, Suite 320
San Francisco, CA 94102
(415) 861-2142

Office of Minority Health Resource Center
P.O. Box 37337
Washington, D.C. 20013-7337
(213) 385-1474

Outreach to African American and Hispanic Families
A Manual for NAMI Affiliates
Thresholds National Research and Training Center
2001 N. Clybrian Avenue
Suite 302
Chicago, IL 60614
(312) 348-5522

Culturgram
Information regarding different cultures
Bringham Young University
David Kennedy Center for International Studies
Publication Services
280 HRCB
Provo, Utah 84602
(801) 378-6528

AT&T Language Line Services
Offers translations in more than 140 languages
(800) 752-6096

KEY POINTS

- Culture-bound illness mimics psychopathology.
- Many factors other than ethnicity constitute a cultural group. Geographical location, gender, religious affiliation, occupation, education, socioeconomic status, sexual orientation, and a physically challenged state of health (blindness, deafness) are but a few variables that draw individuals together to form a distinct cultural group.
- Culture is a combination of beliefs, values, and customs.
- Diagnostic clarity in psychiatric nursing may be confounded by differences in behavioral expressions of mental illness in cultural and ethnic groups.
- Treatment issues in caring for culturally diverse clients include pharmacological considerations (ethnopharmacology), ethnicity and individual/family therapy approaches, and the use of folk health care systems (folk healers, curanderos).
- The four components of cultural competence are (1) cultural awareness, (2) cultural skill, (3) cultural knowledge, and (4) cultural encounters.

- There is a tendency to be ethnocentric regarding one's own values, beliefs, and practices.
- It is important to conduct a cultural assessment on *all clients,* not just clients who represent a specific ethnic group. Every client has values, beliefs, and practices that must be considered when rendering nursing care.
- The basic premise of the cultural assessment is that clients have a right to their cultural beliefs, values, and practices, and these factors should be understood, respected, and considered when rendering culturally competent care.
- Culturally responsive services to culturally diverse clients must be available, accessible, affordable, acceptable, appropriate, and adoptable.

CRITICAL THINKING QUESTIONS

On July 16, 1997, Mr. Gomez, a 47-year-old Mexican-American man is brought into your hospital with the presenting problem that he is going to die within the next 3 days. You discover that he is in excellent health and has no major health problems. He tells you that he has been cursed by his ex-wife, who now lives in Mexico. He further adds that when they ended their marriage 3 months ago, his ex-wife consulted a briuja (witch) who put a spell on him. He believes that this spell will cause him to die on July 19, 1997 at midnight. You try to comfort him, but he states, "You have to believe me! I'm going to die! Please help me!"

1. What is your initial assessment of Mr. Gomez?
2. Describe two culturally sensitive responses to Mr. Gomez's plea for help with the spell? Give a rationale for each response.
3. What are some of the diagnostic and treatment issues in caring for Mr. Gomez? Identify at least three issues.
4. Describe a culturally specific intervention for Mr. Gomez.
5. How would you interpret Mr. Gomez's presenting problem from an emic perspective?
6. What are other pieces of information that are critical to know about Mr. Gomez's case? Why?

REFERENCES

Adebimpe, V. (1981). Overview: White norms in psychiatric diagnosis of black American patients. *Journal of Psychiatry, 138*(3), 279-285.

American Academy of Nursing Expert Panel Report. (1992). Culturally competent health care. *Nursing Outlook, 40*(6), 277-283.

American Psychiatric Association. (1994). *Diagnostic and statistical manual of mental disorders, fourth edition,* Washington, DC: Author.

Bell, P., & Evans, J. (1981). *Counseling the black client.* Center City, MN: Haxelden Education Materials.

Borkan, J., & Neher, J. (1991). A development model of ethnosensitivity in family practice training. *Family Medicine, 23*(3), 212.

Buchwald, D., et al. (1994). Caring for patients in a multicultural society, *Patient Care, 28*(11), 105-123.

Campinha-Bacote, J. (1986). *Consideration of the cultural belief systems of individuals experiencing conjure illness by public health nurses and emergency room nurses: An exploratory study.* Dissertation, University of Virginia, Charlottesville.

Campinha-Bacote, J. (1989). Beyond cultural sensitivity. *Pacesetter, 16*(3), 3.

Campinha-Bacote, J. (1991a). Community mental health services for the underserved: A culturally specific model. *Archives of Psychiatric Nursing, 5*(14), 229-235.

Campinha-Bacote, J. (1991b). *The Process of Cultural Competence In Health Care: A Culturally Competent Model of Care.* Wyoming, OH: Perfect Printing Press.

Campinha-Bacote, J. (1994a). Cultural competence in psychiatric mental health nursing: A conceptual model. *Nursing Clinics of North America, 29*(1), 1-8.

Campinha-Bacote, J. (1994b). Ethnic pharmacology: A neglected area of cultural competence. *Ohio Nurse Review, 69*(6), 9-10.

Campinha-Bacote, J. (1995a). Transcultural psychiatric nursing: Diagnostic & treatment issues. *Journal of Psychosocial Nursing, 32*(8), 41-46.

Campinha-Bacote, J. (1995b). The quest for cultural competence in nursing care. *Nursing Forum, 30*(4), 19-25.

Covey, S. (1989). *The seven habits of highly effective people.* New York: Simon & Schuster.

Cross, T.L., Bazron, B., Dennis, K.W., & Isaac, M.R. (1989). *Towards a culturally competent system of care.* Monograph produced by the CASSP Technical Assistance Center, Georgetown University Child Development Center, Washington, DC.

Flaskerud, J., & Hu, L. (1992). Relationship of ethnicity to psychiatric diagnosis. *The Journal of Nervous and Mental Disorders, 180*(5), 296-302.

Foster, G. (1976). Disease, etiologies, in non-western medical systems. *American Anthropologist, 78,* 777.

Goines, L. (1973). The blues as black therapy. *Black World, 23,* 28-40.

Harwood, A. (1981). *Ethnicity and medical care.* Cambridge, MA: Harvard University Press.

Henderson, G., & Primeaux, M. (1981). *Transcultural healthcare.* Redwood City, CA: Addison-Wesley.

Kalkman, M., & Davis, A. (1980). *New dimensions in mental health-psychiatric nursing.* New York: McGraw-Hill.

Kleinman, A., Eisenburg, L., & Good, B. (1978). Culture, illness and care. *Annals of Internal Medicine, 88,* 251.

Kluckhohn, F.R., & Strodbeck, F.L. (1961). *Variations in value orientations.* New York: Row Peterson & Company.

Kudzma, E. (1992). Drug response: All bodies are not created equal. *American Journal of Nursing, 12,* 48-51.

Leff, J. (1981). *Psychiatry around the globe.* New York: Marcel Dekker.

Leininger, M. (1967). The culture concept and its relevance to nursing. *Journal of Nursing Education, 6*(2), 27.

Leininger, M. (1978). *Transcultural nursing: Theories, concepts and practices.* New York: John Wiley & Sons.

Leininger, M. (1991). *Culture care diversity and university: A theory of nursing* (Publication No. 15-2402). New York: National League for Nursing Press.

Liberman, J., Yunis, J., & Egea, E. (1991). HLA-B38, DR4, DQW3 and clozapine induced agranulocytosis in Jewish patients with schizophrenia. *Archives of Psychiatry, 47,* 945-948.

Lin, K., Poland, R., & Lesser, I. (1986). Ethnicity and psychopharmacology. *Culture, Medicine and Psychiatry, 10,* 152-265.

Marcos, L., & Cancro, R. (1982). Pharmacology of Hispanic depressed patients: Clinical observations. *American Journal of Psychotherapy, 36,* 508-512.

Martin, M. (1988). Differences from the basis for inclusion. *Community Support Network News, 4*(4), 1-2.

McGoldrick, M., Pearce, J., & Giordano, J. (1996). *Ethnicity and family theray* (2nd ed.). New York: Guilford Press.

Morena, J. (1988). Multicultural music therapy. *Journal of Music Therapy, 25,* 17-27.

Mukherjee, S., Skukla, S., Woodle, J., Rose, A., & Olarte, S. (1983). Misdiagnosis of schizophrenia in bipolar patients: A multiethnic comparison. *American Journal of Psychiatry, 40*(12), 1571-1574.

Neighbors, H., Jackson, J., Campbell, L., & Williams, L. (1989). The influence of racial factors on psychiatric diagnosis: A review and suggestions for research. *Community Mental Health Journal, 25,* 301-311.

Pedersen, P. (1995). *A handbook for multicultural awareness* (2nd ed.). Richmond, VA: American Association for Counseling and Development.

Powers, B. (1982). The use of orthodox and black American folk medicine. *Advances in Nursing Science, 4*(3), 37-47.

Rosen, G., Kleinman, A., & Katon, W. (1982). Somatization in family practice: a biopsychocial approach. *The Journal of Family Practice, 14*(3), 493.

Tripp-Reimer, T. (1984). Cultural assessment. In J. Bellack & P. Bamford (Eds.), *Nursing assessment.* Long Beach, CA: Wadsworth Health Sciences Division.

Tylor, E. (1871). *Primitive culture.* Vol. I. London: Bradbury, Evans.

Westermyer, J. (1985). Psychiatric diagnosis across cultural boundaries. *American Journal of Psychiatry, 142*(7), 798-805.

Wilson, H., & Skodol, A. (1994). Special report DSM-IV: Overview and examination of major changes. *Archives of Psychiatric Nursing, 8*(6), 340-347.

Worthington, C. (1992). An examination of factors influencing the diagnosis and treatment of black patients in the mental health system. *Archives of Psychiatric Nursing, 6*(3), 195-204.

VIDEO RESOURCES

Mosby's Community Health Nursing Video Series: *Culture in the Community.*

Mosby's Communication in Nursing Series: *Communicating with Clients from Different Cultures.*

Chapter 7

Understanding People Across the Life Cycle

Judith Haber

LEARNING OUTCOMES

After studying and applying the concepts of this chapter, the learner will be able to:

- Discuss the system's properties of wholeness and interrelatedness as they relate to developmental processes across the life cycle.
- Discuss the relative nature of developmental norms.
- Compare and contrast the major developmental theories presented in this chapter.
- Describe the relevance of developmental theory to nursing practice.
- Identify the stages of the life cycle.
- Analyze physical, cognitive, and psychosocial development at each life cycle stage.
- Evaluate educational needs of individuals or families at specific life cycle stages.

KEY TERMS

Activity theory	Disengagement theory	Object constancy
Anxiety	Emergent self	Separation
Continuity theory	Gender identity	Subjective self
Core self	Individuation	Verbal self

Integral with the practice of psychiatric mental health nursing is understanding the processes of human development across the life cycle. Nurses need to understand the complex physical, cognitive, and psychosocial factors associated with growth and change at each stage of the life cycle. This knowledge base provides a context for the following:

1. Understanding predictable changes in people during key developmental transitions
2. Understanding variations in developmental processes that set the stage for vulnerability or risk for specific age groups across the life cycle
3. Understanding the behavior of the client with mental illness in the context of developmental life cycle experiences
4. Providing a framework for the application of the nursing process with clients whose problems may reflect dysfunctional developmental processes

When nurses understand life cycle developmental changes, they are able to appreciate the uniqueness of each person as he or she progresses through the life cycle. They are also able to assess whether people are progressing within anticipated parameters and determine whether variations in identified areas is indicative of actual or potential health problems. Assessment facilitates health promotion, illness prevention, early case finding, intervention, and health maintenance activities.

The purpose of this chapter is to (1) acquaint students with selected developmental theories, (2) highlight key physical, cognitive, and psychosocial experiences associated with each developmental stage across the life cycle, and (3) apply the nursing process to selected developmental issues experienced by clients during important developmental transitions.

ORGANIZING THEORIES

Professional nursing practice is derived from a theory base from which the nurse selects concepts that are used to understand client behavior and guide the application of the nursing process. Developmental theories provide a framework for examining the life cycle. The theories of Freud (1972), Sullivan (1953), Erikson (1963), Mahler (1975, 1980), Stern (1985a, 1990), Piaget (1962, 1963), Kohlberg (1969), and Gilligan (1982, 1990), among others, have contributed to the understanding of human development. Other theorists such as Lidz (1968), Levinson et al. (1978), and Sheehy (1995) have focused on developmental processes from youth through middle adulthood. Havighurst and Albrecht (1953) and Neugarten (1968) described the developmental process of late adulthood. All theories are discussed in the appropriate developmental sections of this chapter.

PERSONALITY DEVELOPMENT
Freud: Psychosexual Development

Freud (1972), founder of the psychoanalytical school, described stages of psychosexual development from birth through adolescence (Table 7-1). He also focused on aspects of consciousness (i.e., conscious, preconscious, and unconscious) and personality (i.e., id, ego, and superego).

The major assumption of Freud's theoretical model is that all behavior is meaningful. Freud, a psychoanalyst, considered every thought, feeling, action, and dream to be an expression of a unique and important aspect of the person. He considered the primary motivation of behavior to be ***anxiety, which is an unconsciously motivated experience of tension or dread related to loss of self-image.***

TABLE 7-1

Freud's stages of psychosexual development

STAGE	AGE	CENTRAL TASK
Oral	Birth to 18 months	Learning to deal with anxiety-producing experiences by using the mouth and tongue
Anal	18 months to 3 years	Learning muscle control, especially that involved with urination and defecation
Phallic	3 to 6 years	Learning sexual identity and developing awareness of the genital area
Latency	6 to 12 years	Quiet stage during which sexual energy is repressed and sexual development lies dormant
Genital	12 years to adulthood	Developing sexual maturity and learning to form satisfactory relationships with the opposite gender

TABLE 7-2

Erikson's stages of psychosocial development

STAGE	AGE	CENTRAL TASK
Infancy	Birth to 18 months	Trust versus mistrust **Positive resolution:** Learning to trust others; developing a sense of trust in self **Negative resolution:** Mistrust, withdrawal, and estrangement
Early childhood	18 months to 3 years	Autonomy versus shame and doubt **Positive resolution:** Learning self-control and the extent to which the environment can be influenced by direct manipulation **Negative resolution:** Compulsive self-restraint or compliance; willfulness and defiance
Late childhood	3 to 5 years	Initiative versus guilt **Positive resolution:** Learning the extent to which assertiveness and purpose will influence the environment; beginning ability to evaluate one's own behavior **Negative resolution:** Lack of self-confidence, pessimism, fear of wrongdoing, and overcontrol and overrestriction of own activities
School age	6 to 12 years	Industry versus inferiority **Positive resolution:** Learning to use energies to create, develop, and manipulate; development of a sense of competence **Negative resolution:** Disappointment in own abilities, loss of hope, sense of being mediocre, and sense of inadequacy
Adolescence	12 to 20 years	Identity versus role diffusion **Positive resolution:** Integration of life experiences into a coherent sense of self; plans for actualizing one's abilities **Negative resolution:** Doubt about sexual identity; inability to find an occupational identity; personality confusion
Young adulthood	18 to 25 years	Intimacy versus isolation **Positive resolution:** Development of an intimate relationship with another person; commitment to work **Negative resolution:** Avoidance of intimacy; avoidance of relationship, career, and lifestyle commitments
Adulthood	21 to 45 years	Generativity versus stagnation **Positive resolution:** Establishing a family and guiding the next generation; expansion of creativity, productivity, and concern for others **Negative resolution:** Self-concern, self-indulgence, pseudointimacy, and lack of interest and commitments

Continued.

TABLE 7-2—cont'd

Erikson's stages of psychosocial development

STAGE	AGE	CENTRAL TASK
Maturity	45 years to death	Integrity versus despair **Positive resolution:** Acceptance of one's life as having been meaningful, fulfilling, and worth-while; extension of interests and relationships; providing a legacy for the next generation **Negative resolution:** Fear of death, sense of loss, and lack of perceived meaning in one's life

Freud's notion of sequential stages of psychosexual development has been challenged in recent years by psychoanalytical theorists who propose that there are no critical stages in a child's life but rather a long continuum of important everyday interactions with parents and significant others (Stern, 1985a). Another theoretical challenge is posed by neurobiologists who hypothesize that maturation is a vast array of carefully timed neurodevelopmental processes (Schore, 1994).

Erikson: Psychosocial Development

Erik H. Erikson (1963) was a psychoanalyst who added another dimension to Freud's theories—society. He hypothesized that every person is a product not only of heredity and experience but also of society. Thus all personal anxiety, for example, reflects social concerns. Erikson emphasized the ego and its development. He thought that the gradual stage-by-stage growth of ego identity (Table 7-2), based on experiences of social health and cultural solidarity, culminates in a sense of humanity.

Erikson's theory, like Freud's, remains empirically unvalidated. Moreover, the basis of Erikson's theoretical perspective is derived largely from male norms with which women are compared. As such, lack of empirical support and possible gender bias should make nurses cautious about the generalizability of Erikson's work.

Sullivan: Interpersonal Development

Harry Stack Sullivan (1953) formulated a theory that major life events and sources of serious difficulty are the result of interpersonal relationships within a societal context. Sullivan saw human beings as gifted animals who must be socialized before they become able to live in a social organization. Sullivan's (1953) theory implies that anxiety is, in a sense, intolerable; he thought that learned ways of coping with anxiety can limit the capacity to have meaningful experiences later in life. The motivation for behavior, in Sullivan's view, is avoidance of anxiety

and the satisfaction of needs. Sullivan's behavioral theories centered on interpersonal growth and development (in contrast with Freud's emphasis on psychosexual development and Erikson's focus on social growth and development) (Table 7-3). Nurses need to remember that Sullivan's interpersonal theory remains empirically unverified, and as such, they should generalize from the theory to clients with caution.

Stern: Development of Self

Daniel Stern (1985a, 1990), a psychoanalyst, has combined psychoanalytical theory with concepts of developmental psychology to propose a theory about how the self emerges during infancy. Stern believes that infants differentiate themselves from birth and progress through increasingly complex modes of relatedness.

Stern's research about infants has been based on his observations of infants, the observed infant, and reconstructions about infants as related by adults in later life, that is, the clinical infant. The entities are not the same, but there is overlap, or an area in which they interface. In Stern's (1985a) view the information provided by the clinical infant provides subjective validity about the observed infant.

Findings of the studies about the observed infant have led to Stern's theory about the development of self. He proposes that four domains of self emerge in the first 2 years of life: the ***emergent self,*** *which occurs from birth to 2 months,* the ***core self*** *from 2 to 6 months,* the ***subjective self*** *from 9 to 18 months,* and the ***verbal self,*** *which emerges some time after that.* Each domain does not end abruptly as another begins but rather becomes integrated within the person throughout the life cycle.

Stern's (1985a) theory is new and in the early stages of empirical testing. His integration of many theories with a research model has generated much discussion in self-psychology and psychoanalytical circles. However, generalizability of the findings of Stern's work awaits further validation.

TABLE 7-3

Sullivan's interpersonal developmental schema

STAGE	AGE	CENTRAL TASK
Infancy	Birth to 18 months	Learning to count on others to gratify wishes and needs
Childhood	18 months to 6 years	Learning to accept interference with one's wishes in relative comfort, to delay gratification
Juvenile	6 to 9 years	Learning to form satisfactory relationships with peers
Preadolescence	9 to 12 years	Learning to relate to a friend of the same gender
Early adolescence	12 to 14 years	Learning to master independence and to establish satisfactory relationships with members of the opposite gender
Late adolescence	14 to 21 years	Developing an enduring, intimate relationship with a member of the opposite gender

TABLE 7-4

Mahler's separation-individuation process

STAGE	AGE	PROCESS
Symbiosis	Birth to 4 to 5 months	Development of a symbiotic bond with the nurturing figure
Separation-individuation		
Phase 1: Differentiation	Phase 1: 4 to 5 months, to 7 to 10 months	Increasing awareness of self as a separate person; beginning imitative use of autonomous ego functions
Phase 2: Practicing	Phase 2: 7 to 10 months, to 16 to 18 months	Development of an acute awareness of self as a separate person; resolution of separation anxiety; expanded use of autonomous ego functions such as memory, perception, and reality testing leads to internalization of mental images that results in object constancy
Phase 3: Rapprochement	Phase 3: 16 to 18 months to 25 months	
Phase 4: Object constancy	Phase 4: 25 to 36 months	

Mahler: Development of Separation-Individuation

Mahler's (1975, 1980) research has provided a detailed theory about the separation-individuation process, which takes place during the first 3 years of life and is summarized in Table 7-4. *Separation involves the development of a mental picture of self as distinctly separate from other people. Individuation involves the development of autonomous ego functions that produce intrapsychic autonomy such as cognition, perception, memory, and reality testing.* Both processes culminate in *object constancy—the development of a whole, internalized image of the object that can be maintained, irrespective of either satisfying or unsatisfying experiences.* An example of object constancy would be a 30-month-old child who is able to leave his or her mother for a time, become involved in current activities, later ask where mommy is, and become reabsorbed in the activity when mommy does not appear. This child is sustained by an internalized representation of mommy that exists whether she is present or absent.

However, nurses need to remember that Mahler's separation-individuation theory is in contradiction to Daniel Stern's self-development theory. Although there is some research evidence to support her findings, there

TABLE 7-5

Piaget's theory of cognitive development

STAGE	AGE	COGNITIVE PROCESS
Sensorimotor	Birth to 18 months	Learning about self and the environment through sensorimotor exploration of objects and events and imitation
Preoperational		
Preconceptual phase	2 to 4 years	Learning to think in terms of mental images; development of expressive language and symbolic play
Intuitive phase	4 to 7 years	Learning to separate disparate objects and events into a rudimentary classification system; egocentric thought is reflected in persistent thought and animism; expansion of expressive language
Concrete operations	6 to 8 years, to 12 years	Learning to reason in a systematic way and apply rules to things that are seen and heard; beginning of abstract thought and reversible operations
Formal operations	12 years through adulthood	Learning to think using abstract, conceptual operations; refinement of reasoning abilities leads to the capacity to visualize multiple logical relationships between classes or between and among several different properties

are also data supporting Stern's work. Mahler may eventually be regarded as a classical theorist in relation to the development of self as more data emerge to definitively support the more contemporary ideas of Stern (1985a, 1990) and others.

Piaget: Cognitive Development

Piaget's (1962, 1963) theory is primarily concerned with cognition, the process of knowing and understanding. He was concerned with how we come to know what we know—with explaining how different methods of thinking develop in children and adolescents. The theory stresses both biological changes and maturation as determinants of cognitive development. The stages of cognitive development are summarized in Table 7-5.

Piaget's theory of cognitive development has been widely accepted by educators and health professionals. However, contemporary cognitive-developmental theorists critique Piaget's work by pointing out that his theory was developed through observation of a small sample of children, largely his own four children, all male. Moreover, current observations of children's cognitive development highlight the idea that cognitive development is not a rigid stage-by-stage process. Rather, it is much more of an individual progression.

Kohlberg and Gilligan: Moral Development

A six-stage theory of moral development, summarized in Table 7-6, was proposed by Kohlberg (1969, 1973). He emphasized cognitive development and social experience as requirements for sequentially moving to more advanced moral stages.

Kohlberg's theory is empirically based on a study of 84 boys whose development Kohlberg has followed for over 20 years. Although Kohlberg claims universality for his stage sequence, other subject populations not included in his original sample rarely reach stages 5 or 6. Prominent among those who thus appear to be deficient in moral development (when measured by Kohlberg's scale) are women, whose judgments seem to exemplify the third stage of his six-stage sequence. Their morality is conceived in interpersonal terms, and goodness is equated with helping and pleasing others.

Much controversy has been generated by Gilligan (1982, 1988, 1990), who proposes that the very traits that have traditionally defined the "goodness" of women (their care for and sensitivity to the needs of others) paradoxically are those that mark them as deficient in moral development. Rather than trying to "fit" women into the male developmental paradigm, another perspective is needed. A study of women's lives reveals developmental concepts that outline moral development in a different manner, one in which moral problems arise from conflicting responsibilities and relationships rather than from competing rights. For its resolution, this perspective requires a mode of thinking that is contextual and narrative rather than formal and related to abstract rights and rules (Gilligan, 1982).

This difference in how men and women understand and think about a moral problem may be seen as the crit-

TABLE 7-6

Kohlberg's stages of moral development

STAGE	CHARACTERISTICS
Premoral Levels	
1. Obedience and punishment orientation	Wrongdoing viewed in terms of damage done; emphasis on submission to authority
2. Instrumental relativist orientation	Acts satisfying to self and sometimes to others defined as right
Conventional Morality	
3. Interpersonal concordance orientation	Morality of maintaining good relations and approval of others
4. Orientation toward authority, law, duty	Respect for authority and maintaining social order for social order's sake
Levels of Principled Moral Reasoning	
5. Social contract orientation	Morality of accepting democratically contracted laws
6. Universal ethical principles orientation	Morality of individual principles of conscience; do what seems right, regardless of reactions of others

ical reason for womens' "failure" to develop to the highest level according to Kohlberg's system. In Kohlberg's model the highest stage of moral development is derived from a reflective understanding of human rights (Kohlberg and Gilligan, 1971). Consider the primary distinctions: the morality of rights differs from the morality of responsibility in its emphasis on separation (male) rather than connection (female) and in its perspective about the individual rather than the relationship. Traditional moral development paradigms are under intense scrutiny at this time, as is reflected by the above feminist perspective.

Fowler: Spiritual Development

Spiritual beliefs are closely related to moral and ethical concepts and judgment. Spiritual beliefs provide children and adults with meaning, purpose, and hope in their lives. The quest for spiritual understanding and forgiveness is present, even in very young children. Research in spiritual development is limited and subject to criticism, particularly in relation to life stage models proposed by theorists such as Kohlberg, Piaget, Erickson, and others. In understanding that a unique developmental timetable for each person exists, a stage framework for spiritual development also provides a useful approach to assessing the approximate level of development for each child.

Extending beyond religion, which is an organized set of beliefs and practices, spirituality affects the whole person—mind, body, and spirit. As illustrated in Box 7-1, Fowler (1974) has identified seven stages in the development of faith, five of which parallel and are closely as-

sociated with cognitive, moral, and psychosocial development through adolescence.

THE LIFE CYCLE

Nine life cycle stages are presented in the following sections, which highlight important physical, cognitive, and psychosocial patterns that are *generally* characteristic of particular life cycle stages. However, each person's developmental process should be regarded as proceeding on an individual timetable that allows for personal uniqueness. Table 7-7 highlights mental health needs across the life cycle. The Community Resources box on p. 100 lists organizations related to developmental needs at different life-cycle stages.

Infancy (Birth to 18 Months)

Physical development in infancy

During infancy, the most important physical functions are the rhythmic integration of body processes such as sleeping, eating, elimination, sensory perceptions, and movement. Rhythmic body processes are initially erratic; stable, predictable patterns need to be developed through both internal regulatory mechanisms and interpersonal interactions. Internal regulatory mechanisms are the rhythms with which the infant experiences body needs. Initially, the needs do not necessarily occur in regular patterns; only gradually do they take on a predictable rhythm. As needs arise, tension is felt. The way the nurturing figure deals with these needs will either reduce tension or allow it to continue (Sullivan, 1953; Mahler, 1975; Stern, 1985a, Schore, 1994).

TABLE 7-7

Mental health needs across the life cycle

FAMILY LIFE CYCLE STAGE	MENTAL HEALTH NEEDS
Single young adults	Relationship effectiveness Sexually transmitted diseases Safe sex Violence prevention Drug and alcohol prevention Assertiveness training Depression screenings Suicide prevention
Joining of families	Premarital counseling Family planning Genetic counseling Enhancing marital effectiveness Stress management
Families with young and school-age children	Preparation for childbirth Parenting effectiveness Child-abuse prevention Parent-child interaction training Tactile/kinesthetic stimulation programs Enhancing marital effectiveness ADD/ADHD/LD parent and child support groups Violence prevention Stress management Adjustment to situational crises: pregnancy loss, congenital deformities, mental retardation, prematurity, infertility, divorce, death
Families with adolescents	Drug and alcohol prevention Violence prevention Sexually transmitted diseases Safe sex Assertiveness training Values clarification Depression screening Suicide prevention Parenting effectiveness Dealing with divorce
Middle adulthood	Redefining life goals Dealing with the empty nest Parenting effectiveness for midlife parents Coping with adult children who return home Parenting grandchildren Renegotiating the marital relationship Coping with disabilities and death of parents and grandparents Caregiver support Developing lifestyle changes Coping with unemployment Coping with onset of physical health problems Developing new sources of meaning Stress management

TABLE 7-7—cont'd

Mental health needs across the life cycle

FAMILY LIFE CYCLE STAGE	MENTAL HEALTH NEEDS
Late adulthood	Facilitating functional capacity
	Retirement planning
	Dealing with loss while remaining optimistic
	Maximizing support systems
	Maximizing involvement
	Promoting intergenerational connectedness
	Caregiver support groups
	Reminiscence
	Suicide assessment
	Maintaining independence

Box 7-1

Development of Faith

STAGE 0: UNDIFFERENTIATED

This stage of development encompasses the period of infancy when children have no concept of right or wrong, no beliefs, and no convictions to guide their behavior. However, the beginnings of faith are established with the development of basic trust through their relationships with the primary caregiver.

STAGE 1: INTUITIVE-PROJECTIVE

Toddlerhood is primarily a time of imititating the behavior of others. Children imitate the religious gestures and behaviors of others without comprehending the meaning or significance in these activities. During the preschool years, children assimilate some of the values and beliefs of their parents. Parental attitudes toward moral codes and religious beliefs convey to children what they consider good and bad. Children follow parental beliefs as part of their daily lives rather than through understanding of their underlying concepts.

STAGE 2: MYTHICAL-LITERAL

Through the school-age years, spiritual development parallels cognitive development and is closely related to children's experiences and social interaction. Most children have a strong interest in religion during the elementary school years. The existence of a deity is accepted and requests to an omnipotent being are important and expected to be answered. Good behavior is rewarded and bad behavior is punished. Children's developing conscience bothers them when they disobey. They are able to articulate their faith and may even begin to question its validity.

STAGE 3: SYNTHETIC-CONVENTION

As children approach adolescence, they become increasingly aware of spiritual disappointments. They recognize that prayers are not always answered. They begin to reason, to question some of the established parental religious standards, and to drop or modify religious practices.

STAGE 4: INDIVIDUATING-REFLEXIVE

Adolescents become more skeptical and begin to compare the religious standards of their parents with the standards of others. They attempt to determine which to adopt and incorporate into their own set of values. They also begin to compare religious standards with scientific viewpoints. It is a time of searching rather than reaching. Adolescents are uncertain about many religious ideas but will not achieve profound insights until late adolescence or early adulthood.

COMMUNITY RESOURCES

Raising Our Children's Kids: an Intergenerational Network of Grandparenting
ROCKING
P.O. Box 96
Niles, MI 49120

National Coalition of Grandparents
137 Larkin Street
Madison, WI 53705

American Association of Retired People
AARP
601 E Street NW
Washington, DC 20049

Gray Panthers
311 South Juniper Street
Suite 601
Philadelphia, PA 19107

Alzheimer's Disease Association
919 North Michigan Avenue
Chicago, IL 60611-1676
(800) 272-3900

American Fertility Society
2140 11th Avenue, South
Suite 200
Birmingham, AL 35205

Planned Parenthood of America
810 Seventh Avenue
New York, NY 10019

National Mental Health Association
1021 Prince Street
Alexandria, VA 22314

Menopause News (newsletter)
2074 Union Street
San Francisco, CA 94123
(415) 567-2368

Midlife Woman (newsletter)
5129 Logan Avenue South
Minneapolis, MN 55419-1019
(612) 925-0020

National Committee to Prevent Child Abuse
332 South Michigan Avenue
Suite 1600
Chicago, IL 60604
(312) 663-3520

National Resource Center on Worksite Health Promotion
777 North Capitol Street NE
Suite 800
Washington, DC 20002
(202) 408-9320

Resource Center on Substance Abuse Prevention and Disability
1331 F Street NW
Suite 800
Washington, DC 20077-1514
(202) 783-2900

National Association for the Education of Young Children
1834 Connecticut Avenue NW
Washington, DC 20009
(800) 424-2460

For example, infants experience hunger-satiation cycles about every 3 to 4 hours but not necessarily on a predictable schedule. How the nurturing figure meets this need establishes associations that will be connected with the feeding process in the future. The parenting figure must be sensitive to cues that the infant is experiencing hunger and be flexible and available to provide both food and emotional warmth. The infant learns to correlate being hungry with the need to eat and the relief of hunger with ingesting food. The rhythm of this cycle becomes predictable to both mother and infant.

They develop a set of cues for indicating need and responding to it.

Sleep-wake rhythms also vary greatly during the first year of life. Immediately after birth, infants spend most of their time sleeping. Their sleep-wake cycles, however, are short and unpredictable. Parents must be willing to modify their own cycles until the infant's cycle lengthens. From the beginning, infants may demonstrate distinct preferences with regard to sleeping and waking. Most infants move toward longer sleep-wake periods and sleep through the night by 4 to 7 months. Others prefer to sleep during the day and remain wakeful at night. Parents who are used to sleeping uninterruptedly at night may discover a mismatch between their rhythm and their infant's. This lack of synchrony can make it difficult for the parents to remain emotionally available to their child; they may find themselves increasingly fatigued and irritable. Over time, infants usually settle into a morning and afternoon nap and a full night of sleep. However, variations do exist; families have to develop a match that accommodates both children's and parents' sleep-wake rhythms.

Cognitive development in infancy

Infants have the potential for cognitive development and demonstrate increasing maturation of cognitive abilities throughout infancy. Nelson and Collins (1991) and Baillargeon (1991) have demonstrated that the cognitive abilities of infants were underestimated by Piaget. Such researchers propose that as early as 2-1/2 months of age, infants know that objects are solid and continue to exist even when they are out of view. However, it is only after 6 months that an infant will begin to understand that an object's motion is subject to the laws of gravity and inertia. It has been demonstrated that infants of less than a year have a wide range of perceptual abilities: they can visualize separate objects from a background, and they know that objects cannot move through one another and that they continue to exist when hidden. In other studies (Nelson, 1991), 1-month-old infants have recognized images of objects they have only felt in their mouths (see Teaching Points below). By 6 months, infants can distinguish between pictures they have never seen, those with which they are familiar, and those that they have seen infrequently. Infants can develop mental representations, formerly thought to develop around the age of 18 months to 2 years, and call on them to compare old and new information. During a research study, for example, an 8-month-old infant had a dramatic electrical response to a ball (known only by touch) when shown pictures of the ball, in contrast to pictures of other objects.

Psychosocial development in infancy

Development of a sense of self The psychosocial tasks of the first 18 months of life have been described differently by major theorists. Freud (1972) proposed that this, the oral period of development, centers around learning to deal with anxiety-producing experiences by using the mouth and tongue. Erikson (1963) and Sullivan (1953) proposed that the development of trust is the central psychosocial task of infancy. Mahler (1975) stated that infancy is characterized by the symbiotic relationship between mother and infant that progresses in the direction of the infant's increasing awareness of self as a separate person. Stern (1985a, 1990), Schore (1994), and Kohut (1984) propose that the infant's sense of self and social experience begin in a differentiated way from birth.

The helplessness of infants forces them to trust that the nurturing figure will gratify basic physical and emotional needs. Predictability and continuity are internalized through the developing olfactory, visual, auditory, and tactile senses. During this life-cycle stage, visual stimulation, embedded in mutual gaze interactions between caregiver and infant, is an essential component of a growth-promoting environment. The caregiver's face is the most important source of affective information and face-to-face interaction serves as a visual imprinting stimulus for the infant's developing nervous system (Schore, 1994).

The relationship with the mother or other nurturing figure is the foundation for the self-concept. The infant whose needs are met in a positive way will experience both the mother and the self as good. This is a basis for trust in self and others. As a result of varied interchanges between the nurturing person and the child, confidence is developed.

In infancy the mouth is the primary vehicle for communication and gratification. Consequently, feeding becomes an important activity. Prompt feedings accompanied by ample tactile stimulation increase the infant's confidence that needs will be met and that the environ-

TEACHING POINTS

Parents of Infants

Nurses should teach parents of infants the importance of mutual gaze interactions in which the caregiver's smiling facial expression stimulates positive affect in the infant. In response the child's internally pleasurable state is communicated back to the caregiver.

Nurses need to explain that the reciprocal caregiver-infant stimulation generates a mutual state of heightened affect, which is essential to learning about communication. These interactions imprint events in the child's right hemisphere, thereby facilitating maturation of the limbic system, which is involved in socio-emotional functions.

ment can be trusted. Sporadic feedings and inconsistent feelings communicated by the mother will lead to uncertainty, anxiety, and mistrust. Then the infant's anxiety will be manifested in behavior that may generate further inadequate or inconsistent nurturing patterns—thus a cycle of anxiety and mistrust of others and the environment is developed. Maladaptive behavior patterns emerge quickly in an infant. A sequence of protest, crying, withdrawal, despair, and death can appear within 4 to 6 weeks of inadequate nurturing and stimulation.

During infancy, three different senses of the self, each related to a different domain of self-experience and social relatedness, are observable. The sense of **emergent self,** *which forms from birth to age 2 months is characterized by a beginning awareness of self-organizing processes that are precognitive and presocial.* However, data indicate that infants are able to differentiate self from others and selectively respond to external social events. For example, 3-day-old infants were placed on their backs and breast pads taken from their nursing mothers were placed at one side of their heads. Breast pads from other nursing women were placed on the other side of the infant head. The newborns reliably turned their heads toward their own mother's pads, regardless of which side the pads were placed, indicating they could discriminate the smell of their own mother's milk. (Stern, 1985a).

During the period from 2 to 6 months, infants consolidate the sense of a **core self** *as a separate cohesive bounded physical unit with a sense of their own purpose, feelings, and continuity in time.* Infants are fascinated by and become proficient at purposefully manipulating objects and at interacting with people. They respond to the islands of consistency in significant others. For example, they will turn their head and begin to laugh at familiar adult baby talk even before it is in their direct visual gaze. Infants will also, for example, regulate the level of excitation by averting their gaze to cut out stimulation that has risen above the optimal range.

From *7 to 18 months,* the **subjective self** *emerges. This period of life is equally devoted to developmental tasks of independence and seeking and creating a union with significant others, that is, learning that one's thoughts and feelings can be shared with another.* For example, if a mother points to the mirror, the 9-month-old infant follows past her finger to the mirror and then turns around, looks at her and appears to use the feedback from her face to confirm, in a sharing way, that they have arrived at the intended target. Similarly, when infants encounter uncertain situations, they are observed to look back at the mother for cues from her facial expression and other affective signs to help resolve their uncertainty. Attunement of feeling states, that is, tuning in to the other's feelings—whether the other is parent or infant—is also characteristic of this period of

life (Stern, 1985b; Oatley and Jenkins, 1992).

In midinfancy, children also demonstrate a high level of emotional arousal and elevated activity level that is often described as boundless energy. This is associated with heightened activity of the sympathetic component of the autonomic nervous system. This reflects unmodulated excitatory activity of early maturing, reticular formation of brain stem systems responsible for arousal (Thompson, 1990). In late infancy, this excitatory activity is decreased as a result of the later neural maturation of the inhibitory parasympathetic processes in the frontal lobes.

Parents' attitudes and understanding of development will, in part, determine the extent to which the child engages in exploratory behavior. Parents who understand that exploratory behavior is a vehicle for learning will encourage and facilitate it and will be less concerned about the domestic disarray that often results. For example, parents can provide age-appropriate toys that will facilitate this process and not forbid a child to play with more than one toy at a time. However, realistic limits and boundaries (based on safety, consideration for others, and the family's own needs) should begin to be established and consistently enforced. Children who feel free to explore within safe, secure boundaries and whose efforts are rewarded will develop self-confidence and enthusiasm about themselves and their environment.

If children leave this stage without having developed a strong sense of self and trust in others, they may encounter problems in later life: mistrust, superficial relationships, lack of self-confidence, dependency, boundary problems, and depression.

Early Childhood (18 Months to 3 Years)

Physical development in early childhood

Neuromuscular coordination improves as the nervous system matures and as muscles grow larger and increase in strength. Practice refines neuromuscular skills and improves the efficiency with which such skills are used. For example, by age 2, children walk upstairs, holding on to someone's hand, a rail, or a wall and placing both feet on each step before proceeding to the next. By age 3, they alternate feet (one to a step) and do not hold on to anything. Neuromuscular coordination leads to gross and fine motor accomplishments. Gross motor accomplishments involve use of the large muscle groups such as the arms and legs. The 2-to-3 year old is usually able to throw a ball overhand, pedal a tricycle, and jump in place. Fine motor accomplishments involve the use and coordination of small muscle groups such as the fingers. The 2-to-3 year old is usually able to build an eight-block tower, copy a circle, imitate a vertical line, and string large beads. Parents need to encourage physical activity that enhances the development of gross and fine motor skills.

Cognitive development in early childhood

Cognitive development expands as the child enters toddlerhood. Piaget called this the stage of preoperational thought, which lasts from ages 2 to 7 years. Children are increasingly able to form mental images rather than assimilate them only through exploration and manipulation. The outcome is that children are no longer limited to present physical experiences but can transcend time and space by remembering and by thinking about things that are out of sight. For example, current research findings (Bauer and Mandler, 1989) indicate that 20-month-old infants can imitate sequences they saw as long ago as 6 weeks earlier. At age 3 years, a verbal or visual cue given 6 months to 1 year earlier can trigger a long-term memory for a sequence of events that can now be repeated.

Play becomes more symbolic. Children coordinate mental and action images that provide the basis for thinking about and imagining events and their interpersonal life. Acquisition of expressive (verbal) language in the form of words, phrases, and then sentences provides a way to share meanings that are mutually agreed on. However, children are still often unable to phrase questions that help clarify their thoughts.

The ability to use mental images, although it is established in early childhood, will not be refined for several more years. For example, young children often have difficulty differentiating between the real and the unreal—for instance, between actual events and fantasies. Thus witches, goblins, ghosts, and dreams seem real. The concept of time also remains nebulous for young children, who have difficulty understanding the difference between yesterday, today, and tomorrow.

Psychosocial development in early childhood

The psychosocial tasks of the second and third years of life revolve around the development of autonomy and the emergence of the verbal self (Stern, 1985a).

Development of self Stern (1985a, 1990) describes the emergence of the *verbal self (after 18 months)*. Unlike Mahler (1975), he proposes that *the child's core self, now solidified, enables the youngster to seek sharing experiences with others more than ever before.* Evidence about the objectification of self is demonstrated when rouge is put on a child's cheek and a mirror is pointed to by an adult. The child, instead of just pointing past the parent's finger to the image in the mirror, as might have been the case at a younger age, will touch the rouge on his or her cheek visible in the mirror. In other words, the child now knows that it is he or she, a separate self, whose cheek has the rouge. Because children now have verbal language, they use pronouns such as *I, me*, and *mine* to refer to self and have the tools to narrate a story about self.

Gender identity It is also about this time that *gender identity* becomes stable and *the child recognizes that the self, as an entity, can be categorized as either boy or girl* (Gilligan, 1982). The gender label is internalized early and subtly through imitation of parents' expressions as they refer to children's gender (e.g., "That's a good girl" or "That's a good boy").

By the time children are 3 years old, they have acquired considerable knowledge of and a preference for gender-appropriate behaviors. Gender-appropriate behaviors are learned within the family system. Each family has its own concept of what constitutes male or female attributes and the types of gender-linked behavior they wish to cultivate in their children. These beliefs are conveyed to the children by a variety of means (e.g., toys elected for them and activities in which they are encouraged to participate) and parents exert special efforts to gain cooperation with their expectations.

However, with the increasing number of flexible gender roles being enacted in families and on prime-time television, children's stereotypical perceptions of men and women may be changing. Children who are familiar with shows that depict men performing traditionally feminine tasks such as cooking, cleaning, child care, and women employed outside the home have a more contemporary view of gender-related roles (Rosenwasser, Lingenfeller, and Harrington, 1989).

Socialization Children begin to learn socially acceptable behavior when they can forgo self-gratification to some extent and incorporate their parents' demands, which are representative of the larger society. At this period, sexuality and gratification center on the anal zone of the body. Issues of control—which can develop into a power struggle—have to do primarily with the child's need to coordinate "holding on" and "letting go."

Neurobiologically, studies have shown that the right hemisphere orbitofrontal region of the brain is involved in regulation of bladder capacity and that individual orbital neurons respond to the odors of urine and feces. The right hemisphere is known to be dominant for the analysis of information received by the individual from his own body and for the generation of internal images of (disgust, shame) faces. The orbitofrontal area matures during the second year of life, functioning to balance internal desires (pleasures of holding onto or handling urine or feces) with external reality (accepting parental expectations to let go and become toilet-trained) (Schore, 1994).

Toilet training is probably the most important example of this neurobiological maturation coupled with development of socialization. It is accomplished only when the child achieves neurobiological maturation and complies with the parents' wishes to retain their approval and love and reduce anxiety to a minimum. Children who are not expected to exercise control beyond their physical capacities will experience satisfaction over this achievement.

Children of this age also demonstrate other evidence of self-regulation that illustrates the interplay of neurobiological excitators and inhibitory forces that influence affect and socialization. They begin to learn rules of social behavior (how to act at the table, not to kick or bite) and guidelines for safety (not to touch dangerous objects). Realistic, consistent limits set by parents will support children's own efforts at self-control. If their developing autonomy is respected, children will come to feel that they can cope with difficulties and feel confident. Basic concepts that help establish a balance between love and hate, cooperation and willingness, and self-expression and suppression are developed.

Failure to negotiate the tasks of this stage is manifested in feelings of shame and doubt, fear of self-disclosure, and ritualistic behavior. In adulthood, lack of autonomy and other relatedness may persist and express itself as defiance, oppositional behavior, excessive need for control, order, and approval, overconforming behavior, and irrational rituals.

Middle Childhood (3 to 6 years)

Physical development in middle childhood
Physical development continues at the slow, even rate of early childhood. Refinement of gross and fine motor skills continues as the nervous system matures and as physical activity provides opportunities for practice. Children in this age group can usually run with ease, hop on one foot, catch a bounced ball, and walk backward. They can draw crude figures, copy a square, and begin to write letters and numbers. Parents need to provide age-appropriate activities that will enhance development. (Whaley and Wong, 1995).

Cognitive development in middle childhood
According to Piaget (1962, 1963), at this age, cognitive development continues in the preoperational stage; children make the transition to the intuitive phase of preoperational thinking, which refers to the emerging ability of young children to separate dissimilar objects and events into some basic classification pattern. By adult standards, however, their classifications often remain unsystematic. For example, a boy of 4 was given 12 pieces of red paper shaped in circles, squares, and rectangles and was asked to put them into groups that looked alike. The child returned 5 minutes later with all the shapes in one bag. When asked why he had not separated them into groups, he replied, "Oh, I did. They're all the same color, so I have one group." This made perfect sense to the child. The adult, thinking in a more sophisticated way, had expected the child to classify the objects by shape.

Thought is egocentric during this phase; that is, children view everything in relation to themselves. This orientation makes it difficult for them to shift attention from one need, desire, or aspect of a problem to another and can make them appear single-minded, persistent, and stubborn. For example, a 5 year old, struggling with the abstract concept of death, persists in asking questions about what happened to grandpa after he died. Egocentric thought is also exhibited in animism—attribution of life, consciousness, and will to physical objects. Pincushions feel the prick of a pin. Weeds hurt when they are pulled out of the ground. Clouds feel heavy when they are full of rain. The nature of the child's thinking also gives lifelike qualities to dreams, names, and events (Piaget, 1963).

Expressive language becomes increasingly sophisticated as sentences grow in complexity. Several ideas may be grouped in a sentence. Use of pronouns increases, and vocabulary multiplies rapidly. Pronunciation of words improves, so the child's speech is better understood by others.

Psychosocial development in middle childhood
The psychosocial tasks of the third to sixth years of life revolve around the development of identity and initiative (Erikson, 1963).

Development of relationships   The emergent self, core self, subjective self, and verbal self all remain fully functional and will be active, and continue to develop and coexist throughout life. As a result, the child's simultaneous sense of separateness and connectedness provides a sense of identity and expands the child's world (Stern, 1985a). The focus shifts from a preoccupation with self and parenting figures to a wider circle of significant people, including siblings, relatives, friends, and peers. Children see themselves in an adult-dominated world and form attitudes toward authority. Issues of initiative, compliance, and defiance are dealt with by role modeling and setting limits.

At the younger end of this age group, relationships with peers take the form of "parallel play"; children play together in a group, but each child usually focuses on a separate project. They come together only occasionally for cooperative activity. While children are playing separately, however, they are gaining the positive benefits from the presence of others for example, empathy and stimulation. Children may turn from exclusive consideration of their own needs to consideration of the needs of others. They begin to appreciate the rights and feelings of other people. Social abilities develop as relationships expand and feedback is received about behavior from significant others. These abilities include leading, following, sharing, and competing. However, as they approach ages 5 and 6, they begin to play more cooperatively, creating elaborate games of make-believe or complex buildings of blocks (Erikson, 1963).

Having discovered the self as a separate person, children develop a sense of initiative and become curious about how much they can do, what they can become, and who else they can be. The child finds answers to these questions through observation, investigation, and play. Observation of diverse phenomena leads to many questions from the curious preschooler. "Why?" is the standard question as the child attempts to satisfy curiosity and deal with an expanding world. Exploration of self and the environment is vigorous and involves discovery of ways to undertake, plan, and carry out a task. Rivalry is everpresent because the child wants to succeed, win, and demonstrate superior ability. From this kind of successful exploratory activity the child begins to develop a feeling of being, to some extent, the master of his or her own fate. Play offers an opportunity for imagination and fantasy and for experiments with roles and interpersonal styles. (The child often plays "house" or dresses up and pretends to be another person.) Through play, a child gets a sense of what life is like for other people.

Sexual identity   During this period, sexuality and gratification center on the genital area. Sexual identity and rivalry with the parent of the same gender for attention of the parent of the opposite gender become important. (The child may even express a desire to marry the parent of the opposite gender.) Children are preoccupied with sexual topics and body parts. They often react with surprise and shock to observation of genital differences between men and women. Girls often wonder why they do not have a penis and may begin to feel inferior because they are missing this body part. Fantasies about reproduction abound (children commonly think that a person can become pregnant by swallowing a seed).

Sexual identity is developed through identification with the parent of the same gender as infantile sexual striving toward the parent of the opposite gender is renounced. Children recognize that they cannot have the same kind of relationship with the parent of the opposite gender that Mommy or Daddy does. Fantasy, imagination, and preoccupation with the body result in normal guilt about dreams, wishes, and thoughts relating to self and parents.

Gender role standards are increasingly differentiated and continue to be developed throughout childhood. Gender role behaviors, an important part of sexual identity formation, are consolidated through play activities such as "dress-up," "playing house," and "going to work." Since the women's movement, more liberal views regarding gender role stereotyping are more apparent.

Development of internal controls   During this period a rudimentary sense of superego or conscience develops as external prohibitions are internalized and incorporated as part of the self. Parents or other significant caregivers, through external responses and feedback, influence the child's developing moral capacities by shaping the neurobiological structures in the right hemisphere and the orbitofrontal cortex that are involved in empathetic and moral behaviors.

Children begin to establish an internal value scale of right and wrong and develop capacity for empathy and signal anxiety, which is anticipation of wrongdoing by connecting a wish with its consequence. The development of conscience also serves to self-regulate their initiative. Children not only fear the consequences of being caught in wrongdoing by their parents but also fear being tormented by their own self-accusations and prohibitions. The development of conscience is necessary for the formation of moral values. However, the child's conscience can be punitive and cruel. If children experience excessive shame or guilt about their feelings, thoughts, or actions, they will deny their own wishes and curtail their activities. Children need to develop internal coping mechanisms that will regulate impulsive and aggressive behavior without becoming burdened by unrealistic self-restrictions that limit expansion of skill and energies. Ideally, superego development will be constructive, and this will be demonstrated by evidence of a beginning value system. Ideal traits, behaviors, and role models are internalized by children so that they become inner standards and goals that provide direction for behavior and thus contribute to self-assurance and independence (Erikson, 1963; Schore, 1994).

Children who are adjusting well will talk about the future and their possible roles in it. On the other hand, children may feel that they have no right to dream. The secure child feels worthy and competent even though small. Failure to successfully negotiate the issues of this developmental stage leads to psychosexual confusion, rigidity, and guilt, loss of initiative, and reluctance to explore new skills.

Late Childhood (6 to 12 Years)

Physical development in late childhood

There is a distinct change in body image as children move from the toothless, babyish look of the 6 year old to the lean, muscular preadolescent look of the 11 or 12 year old. Children may approach puberty during this period, have a growth spurt, and begin to develop secondary sex characteristics, and girls may begin menstruating.

Fat deposits are burned off and muscles grow stronger as children engage in physical activity. Gross motor coordination becomes increasingly refined as children ride bicycles and skateboards, swim, play baseball, run, climb, and jump. Fine motor coordination develops as children write, paint, model clay, weave, collect stamps, sew, take photographs, build models, and so on. Parents often describe their child as becoming physically competent during this period—youngsters who can really be a help in many situations (Whaley and Wong, 1995).

Cognitive development in late childhood

According to Piaget (1963), during this stage, cognitive development makes a transition from preoperational thought to concrete operations. This period begins somewhere between ages 6 and 8, depending on the child. Concrete operations involve the ability to reason in a systematic way and to apply previously learned rules to new tasks and situations. That is, rules now help children understand and classify new phenomena. The rules constantly undergo revision. For example, a school-age child who sees an infant alone in a room will reason that a mother must be nearby because infants cannot take care of themselves. When a group of adults enters the room, the child will search out the person most likely to be the mother. If the mother does not go over to the infant and if the father attends the infant instead, the child will have to revise the rule to include the fact that adults other than mothers also take care of infants.

Children who perform concrete operations can mentally reverse the operations—they can imagine how things were before the operations took place. This ability depends on a skill called conservation. Conservation is the ability to understand that a quantity does not change simply because the form it takes varies. For example, a child who can "conserve substance" realizes that a given amount of water does not change when it is poured from a short glass to a tall glass. This skill enables the child to view the same situation in a variety of ways. A child at this age is also able to classify phenomena according to similar attributes and order them serially by height, size, shape, and so on. The ability to synthesize diverse phenomena, formulate relationships, and speculate about causality provides a foundation for objectivity and problem solving, and these in turn lead to the development and/or refinement of abstract rather than rote learning—a capacity fundamental for the development of academic skills.

Psychosocial development in late childhood

The psychosocial tasks of the 6-to-12 year old revolve around industry and learning.

Self-concept The child believes the aphorism, "I am what I learn." Self-esteem is derived from accomplishment, and the child learns to win recognition by producing things. Children take pride in mastering tasks and feeling useful. Both boys and girls feel good about themselves when their diligence produces a completed task. Positive appraisal from significant people such as parents, teachers, and friends reinforces their good feelings. Although some feelings of inadequacy are bound to occur during late childhood, a sense of industry can be fostered by sensitive adults who counterbalance negative feedback with constructive criticism, suggestions, and praise.

Sexuality Theorists such as Freud (1972) and Erikson (1963) have stated that the school-age period is one of sexual latency, that is, sexual energy is sublimated into industry, sports, and learning. However, current research indicates that for many children sexual curiosity actually increases. They tell each other the "facts of life" and share "dirty jokes," and many read anything related to sex that they can get their hands on. Toward the end of late childhood, sexual desires intensify, and there may be a reappearance of masturbation and sexual fantasy. Much of this sexual feeling is mixed with aggression and is sublimated into physical activity. However, changes in body image lead to intense preoccupation with appearance, especially if physical changes occur at this point. At this stage, sexuality is also a consolidation of "feeling male" or "feeling female" and thus sets the stage for puberty.

Peer relationships For children of school age, the peer group and the school become major influences on socialization, along with the family. As friends and "ego ideals" such as teachers become the center of the child's universe, parents' influence decreases. Through cooperation, compromise, and collaboration, children take their place in their peer group, which is the core of their social life. Friends are used as sounding boards, and the group becomes a testing ground for values and attitudes learned at home. In many cases the peer group can be more democratic than the home. Rules are not laid down by authority figures but are debated, with some or all of the group having a say in what they should be. Home values and attitudes may be strengthened or watered down.

During late childhood, friendships become more stable. Friends of the same gender are sought out, and "best friends" develop. Individual friendships provide opportunities for intimacy, sharing, and self-disclosure that may not have been experienced previously outside the family. Female rather than male friendships are characterized by connectedness and sharing; male friendships remain more competitive (Gilligan, 1981). Group relationships usually involve organized activities, such as scouting, sports, and community group projects, which provide a sense of belonging, teamwork, and cohesiveness. Other group activities such as secret societies, gangs, and team sports offer opportunities for playful aggression and acceptable sublimation of hostility (Freud, 1972; Erikson, 1963).

One of the crucial tasks of school-age children is moral development, which in this stage depends less on children's automatic obedience to parents and more on their internal judgments. This is equivalent to Kohlberg's (1969) stages 3 and 4, conventional morality, discussed earlier in this chapter. As the superego or conscience matures, children begin to discriminate between their own motives and motives derived from parents' demands. By late childhood, children can be expected to understand most of the things that family and society define as unacceptable, but they cannot always be expected to have control over their unacceptable urges. Nor can they always be expected to consider the rights and needs of others. To reach other levels of moral judgment, children need experience in choosing what is right and wrong, and in reasoning the whys and wherefores of their choices. Ultimately, they will be able to distinguish between right and wrong without external reminders.

Failure to develop self-esteem and a sense of mastery at this stage may lead to feelings of inadequacy and inferiority that persist in later life. A child who has not developed a sense of initiative may be unprepared for school, or the school itself may fail to help the child develop necessary skills. The child may conclude, "I'll never be good at anything," and may increasingly display reluctance to explore the environment and human relationships.

Adolescence (12 to 18 Years)

Physical development in adolescence

The onset of puberty (changes accompanying the arrival of sexual maturity) varies from person to person. Puberty usually encompasses 1 to 2 years of rapid growth and development before a girl or boy becomes capable of reproducing children. Sexual maturity is preceded by the development of secondary sex characteristics. In girls, as hormonal changes occur and estrogen is secreted, the breasts begin to enlarge, pubic and axillary hair appears, the hips widen, and menstruation begins. This process begins at about age 11, but time of onset can vary widely from age 9 to age 15. In boys, as behavioral changes occur and androgens are secreted, the penis, testes, and scrotum increase in size, pubic hair appears, the voice deepens as the shape of the larynx changes, the hips become slimmer, the body becomes more muscular, and the production and emission of sperm begin. Facial, body, and axillary hair appears with later physical changes. Puberty begins about 2 years later in boys than in girls, around age 13. As with girls the time of onset of this process can vary widely. In both genders, endocrine changes also include activation of the sweat and facial oil glands. The increased activity of these glands predisposes the adolescent to have body odor, pimples, and blackheads, which constitute a disturbing alteration in body image.

Height and weight increase dramatically; full adult height and weight are attained during adolescence. Girls are initially taller than boys, but boys generally become taller in middle to late adolescence. The sudden and dramatic changes in body proportions often contribute to feelings of awkwardness, clumsiness, and self-consciousness.

Cognitive development in adolescence

The last stage of cognitive development, formal operations, occurs during adolescence, although recent research indicates evidence of abstract thinking in earlier stages of childhood. This stage provides the foundation for cognitive operations throughout adulthood. Formal operations involve abstract conceptual thought. The ability to reason becomes increasingly complex as the adolescent is able to see multiple logical relationships between classes or between and among several different properties (such as height, weight, and density).

Research indicates that the development of formal-operations skills to some extent may be a function of culture and education. In areas where children begin school early and are given extensive instruction in written language, formal operations emerge before the teenage years. Written language helps children go beyond concrete here-and-now thinking. Children who read are helped to think about abstract as well as concrete possibilities. Nonreaders, poor readers, and people in cultures that do not use written language extensively may not reach the formal-operations stage at all.

Psychosocial development in adolescence

Consolidation of self-concept Psychologically, a sense of personal identity is being forged in adolescence. The adolescent asks, "Who am I?", "Where have I been?", "Where am I going", "What will I become?" Adolescence provides the opportunity to ask those questions and emerge with answers.

Classical developmental theory (Freud, 1972; Erikson, 1963) proposes that the major psychosocial task of adolescence is the development of autonomy and the renunciation of one's childhood relationships. Indeed, in Western cultures, autonomy becomes the distinguishing feature of the mature adult. However, findings of studies about self-development in women and girls seem to contradict classical theories that consider separation and individuation to be universal adolescent issues (Gilligan, 1982; Belenky, 1986; Lyons, 1988; Stern, L., 1990; Goodrich, 1991). Although for men the movement is toward independence and autonomy, for women, it is toward both independence (self-care) and connectedness. For women, both are compatible, not contradictory, and function in the service of each other. Independence comes within attachment to others and transforms both, leading to a new way of being and a new way of interacting with others. For boys the development of autonomy and for girls the development of autonomy and connectedness take place over approximately 6 or more years.

It is difficult for parents to know how to react to young people who are adults 1 minute and children the next. Parents need to strike a balance between freedom and realistic expectations. The process of separating from parents brings feelings of loss and emptiness that, although normal, are difficult for the adolescent to express and resolve.

Adolescents begin to blend "wants" and "shoulds" of significant others with their own, but judgments by significant others still largely determine their sense of self-worth. Sexuality must be dealt with and expressed in acceptable ways. This is a problem for the adolescent who is often overwhelmed by sexual feelings and has no outlet for them other than self-stimulation. The adolescent needs to know that these feelings are completely normal.

Moral development   Moral development in adolescence coordinates with the establishment of abstract thinking. Gender differences in moral reasoning become apparent (Gilligan, 1982, 1988, 1990). Male subjects, who were the focus of Kohlberg's (1969) research and theory building, demonstrate evidence of his stage 5 and 6 model, that of morality of justice and rights. The moral dilemmas of this perspective center around conflicts of fairness, impartiality, and objective measures of choice that ensure fairness in arriving at a decision. However, female subjects focus on the morality of care that rests on an understanding of relationships as reciprocal. In a morality of care, resolution of moral conflicts are sought by restoring relationships or connections between people and in carrying through activities of care, ensuring that good will come to others or that hurt/suffering will be stopped for others or oneself (Gilligan, 1982; Belenky, 1986; Lyons, 1990). These differences in moral perspective closely parallel gender differences in relation to self-concept development. Once again, men focus more than women on individual or societal issues as they affect one's own values and principles as judged by an impartial, objective measure that ensures fairness in arriving at a decision. Women focus more than men on issues of self in relation to others—issues surrounding potential fractures between people and how to care for self, especially in considering care of others. Evaluation of resolution is not necessarily judged by objective measures.

As adolescents strive to understand the meaning and purpose of life, they examine, clarify, and perhaps modify childhood and parental values and develop a foundation for their own adult values. They will naturally be confused and disappointed when role models or mentors make mistakes or demonstrate inconsistent or immoral behavior—for example, when an athletic coach preaches fairness on the playing field but then urges the team to win in any way it can.

Many health-related societal issues provide fertile territory for ethical issues considered by adolescents. Societal problems related to violence, gun control, alcohol and drug abuse, smoking, acquired immunodeficiency syndrome (AIDS) and other sexually transmitted diseases, safe sex, teenage pregnancy, divorce, and domestic violence are of concern to teenagers of this decade. A nationwide poll of teenagers suggests that many lead lives shadowed by adult concerns such as those listed above (Chira, 1994). Simultaneously, teenagers feel that their parents are sometimes or often unavailable to them, a result that did not appear to depend on whether their mothers worked outside the home. Adolescents also said their parents were not spending much time with them or communicating well with them.

If teenagers see in one another their greatest comfort and source of support, they also see their peers as the greatest menace. Most teenagers polled said other teenagers were far more likely than adults to commit crimes against them, describing them as less mature, more impulsive, and susceptible to group pressure (Chira, 1994). Consider the fact that although violent crimes have decreased nationwide in the past 10 years, arrest rates for violent crimes committed by youngsters ages 10 to 17 doubled between 1983 and 1992. The majority of these crimes are committed between 3 PM and 6 PM. What is the relationship between this statistic and the fact that 3 million "latchkey" children go home to no daytime caregiver supervision? What action can teenagers take to address this ethical issue?

Adolescents will challenge, test, and perhaps even reject social, moral, and religious norms under which they have been raised. Attendance at a place of worship may diminish; interfaith dating may occur. Parents' commitment or lack of commitment to a religion may be questioned; religious practices may be seen as hypocrisy. At this time, beliefs of a peer group are often respected more than those of the family. However, the belief system that people ultimately adopt as adults is usually more similar to than different from their parents' even if they have protested and rebelled during adolescence.

Social relationships   Socially adolescents are in role transition; they must form a concept of acceptable social roles through experimentation. Their inner lack of trust in themselves is manifested in conformity to a group. Cliques and gangs are often intolerant of those who do not belong. Rigid clothing styles, mannerisms, fetishes, and codes of behavior reflect a need to be accepted, wanted, and loved. Even when the group's purpose or code of conduct is destructive, as is true for many teenage gangs or cults, the need for belonging and self-affirmation overrides cognitive, emotional, or moral doubt. If the adolescent experiences acceptance in a group, then individual intimate relationships will probably be sought. On the basis of these, a more or less enduring relationship with a significant other may develop, and first love may be experienced (Sullivan, 1953).

Educational and career concerns   Contemplation of the future—"who I want to be and what I want to do"—

begins in adolescence, and finding a career becomes a concern. The adolescent is continuously bombarded by questions about career plans. Uncertainty is compounded, since people of this age have not participated extensively in the world of work and have observed only fragments of work situations and job roles. Consequently, they may find it difficult to commit themselves to a full-time job or to identify career choices (Nemiroff and Colarusso, 1990).

Other problems like teen-age pregnancy (and everyday in the United States 1,340 teenagers give birth) decrease educational and career opportunities for both teen-age mothers and fathers who prematurely must assume financial and parenting responsibilities (Alan Guttmacher Institute, 1995).

Incomplete resolution of the tasks of this stage may result in failure to consolidate an idea of "who I am," which leads to role confusion, deficits in assuming responsibility, a sense of inadequacy in controlling the self, and an inability to compete successfully.

Young Adulthood (20 to 29 Years)

Young adulthood is a time when men and women struggle with the urge to remain dependent and sheltered by others as opposed to the urge to prepare for and master the future. Today, young adulthood often stretches through the twenties in a "provisional" kind of adulthood until an individual is close to age 30, moving all the other adult stages back by up to 10 years.

The last 10 years have seen a 20% decrease in the average real income and a corresponding 46% drop in under-25 year olds who own their housing units, as well as a 21% decline in those who are renting (U.S. Bureau of the Census, 1990). Those who do move back home seldom do so because they are lazy or unmotivated. They are making an economically sound and usually painful decision. Few young adults want to share a sink with Dad and many feel inhibited about entertaining friends in Mom's living room. Table 7-8 illustrates the major developmental theories and tasks of young adulthood.

Physical and cognitive development in young adulthood

Young adulthood is essentially a period of psychosocial development. Physical development has been completed, except that men (more often than women) may continue to grow. Cognitive development of high-order cognitive operations has been completed. The young adult continues to refine and expand use of such operations.

Psychosocial development in young adulthood

Equipped with only a provisional sense of identity, the young adult is usually caught between wanting to prolong the irresponsibility of adolescence and wanting to assume adult commitments. However, a central task of this period is differentiation of self from the nuclear family in which one grew up (Aylmer, 1989). Irresponsibility is more easily continued by those who do not begin to work, either because they remain in school or for other reasons. Some young adults want to make intelligent adult commitments, but they worry about making irre-

TABLE 7-8

Developmental theories of adulthood: Lidz, Sheehy, Levinson, Neugarten		
STAGE	**AGE**	**TASK**
Young Adulthood	20 to 29 years	Development of a life dream; development of an occupational choice that represents the selection of a way of life Decision making about marital, parenting, or relationship choices and options Differentiation of self from the nuclear family
Adulthood	30 to 45 years	Extension or revision of work and relationship commitments Childbearing and childrearing Consolidation of self-identity Commitment to the marital system Redefining the marital relationship to allow for the transition to parenthood
Middle Adulthood	45 years, to 65 to 70 years	Reintegration of self-identity Acceptance of aloneness and individuality; extension of relationships Renewal and extension of secondary interests Launching of children and grandparenting Acceptance of physical manifestations of aging Redefined attitudes about money, religion, and death

vocable decisions that will lock them into a permanent structure. This is particularly true for those confused by a seemingly bewildering array of career and lifestyle options. Others want to forge new creative paths that will involve them in pursuits that are not accepted norms for adulthood. For example, some young people may join a commune or a religious cult, and some may pursue scholarly, political, artistic, or other nonmaterialistic interests. Others may choose more traditional paths, such as career, marriage, and parenthood at this time.

Some young men and women at this time are likely to embark on careers that will enable them to realize the occupational dreams of childhood (Nemiroff and Colarusso, 1990). They may also formulate short- and long-term goals in traditional or nontraditional careers. In the past, women making the transition into adulthood usually focused on getting married and having a family. The expected role for women was primarily that of wife, mother, and homemaker. However, this traditional role has changed, and many new options now exist for women, half of whom continue to work outside the home after having children. Today, young women formulate the same kinds of occupational goals as men. Thus they too have short- and long-term career goals in traditional and nontraditional careers.

Contributing to this trend is that the current generation of young adults has experienced a sharp decline in spending power. Most young Americans will be unable even to match their parents' single paycheck, middle-class lifestyles (Bartlett and Steele, 1992; Estess, 1994).

Although choosing a marriage partner and starting a family are major tasks of young adults, there is an increasing acceptance of diverse lifestyles that support a wide range of commitment and intimacy. Many young adults choose alternative options. Childless marriages, postponement of parenthood, cohabitation (living together), and remaining single or not marrying until the late twenties or thirties are increasingly acceptable. For those who elect to marry, the motivation must be seriously examined. The marital relationship at its best represents true integration and leads to interdependence rather than dependence. Such "closeness without fusion" must be managed so that intimacy is possible but neither partner merges, loses, or gains self-identity at the expense of the other. Commitment to a new family system becomes a major focus (McGoldrick, 1989; Bartlett and Steele, 1992).

To some people, young adulthood may appear to have been wasted if traditional or acceptable paths are not followed. One commonly hears family members say, when talking about a young adult, "When is he (or she) going to stop fooling around and get busy being a grown-up?" It is important to remember, however, that experimentation at this stage may be necessary. Some people need

time to integrate identity, role, and separation issues to achieve a workable balance (Walters et al, 1988).

Young adults continue to sort through the values and beliefs they learned as children and strive to arrive at a belief system of their own. Essentially they ask, "What do I believe in?" and "What do I see as the fundamental purpose of life?" Parents' values are discarded, modified, or adopted according to how well they integrate with the young adult's own emerging beliefs. Spirituality is usually not a primary concern for young adults; there is too much else going on in their lives as they establish themselves in the adult world. However, societal or personal crises (such as war, natural disasters, traumatic accidents, or death of a significant other, [e.g., a parent or friend]) may intensify the search for meaning. Young adults who marry and begin to raise a family during this period are likely to develop an identity that includes religious and moral values that they will pass on to their children.

Young adults who fail to achieve personal integration during this stage may have their options cut off too early. They may make decisions about work, marriage, and parenthood on the basis of values and wishes of others rather than their own. People who fail to develop some form of intimate relationship at this stage risk isolation later in life—avoidance of close relationships or participation only in relationships that are short-lived, superficial, and stereotyped.

Adulthood (30 to 45 Years)

Adulthood is a time when men and women have a sense of personal integration and work toward taking their place in the world. Table 7-8 illustrates the major developmental theories and tasks of adulthood.

Physical and cognitive development in adulthood

The physical changes that occur in adulthood vary widely from person to person. Physical growth has ceased, and body integrity depends greatly on diet, exercise, rest, stress, genetic factors, and whether health problems or disabilities develop. The first physical signs of aging may appear in the late twenties and throughout the thirties. Skin begins to lose its resilience and elasticity, and wrinkles appear. This may be upsetting to men and women unless they feel that wrinkles add character to their appearance. Hair may grow more slowly, be lost, or turn gray. Genetic predisposition to baldness or early graying, nutritional factors, disease, drugs, and hormones may contribute to these changes.

Cognitively, adulthood is a productive stage. Brain weight and maturation of brain cells peak in the late 20s. Although a gradual shrinking process begins after that, cognitive functioning remains high throughout this period. Abstract thought is applied to a wide range of phenomena; inductive and deductive logic are used to solve problems and deal with human relationships.

Psychosocial development in adulthood

In adulthood, multiple role changes occur. Adults in their thirties assume new roles as workers, lovers, spouses, parents, and participants in the community.

In the world of work, adults in their thirties are busy setting goals, trying to bring about significant change, and seeking mentors who can guide them in their careers. Hope and energy abound, and demonstrating competence is of great importance. Some adults continue to explore and experiment with career options into their thirties. At this time, people begin to build a foundation for a safe future, but decisions are still not viewed as irrevocable (Sheehy, 1995).

Other major choices are made at this time if they have not been made before. Options for marriage and parenthood may be considered and implemented. These options include considerations of committing to the marital system, as well as redefining the marital relationship to allow for the transition to parenthood (Carter and McGoldrick, 1989).

Selection of a lover or spouse creates an opportunity for intimacy and consolidation of sexuality without loss of differentiation. Some people elect to remain unmarried. Others may enter into a significant lasting relationship with another person without formal marriage.

Those who choose to marry are confronted with a variety of relationship issues. For women, the question of combining marriage and career arises. Questions about having a family emerge. Some couples decide to have children immediately or shortly after marriage. When this decision is made, some women opt to interrupt their career for a number of years, whereas other women choose to return to work or to start working shortly after an infant is born. Some couples decide to postpone parenthood indefinitely. The decision the couple makes will result in role and identity shifts. A decision to postpone parenthood may imply that an occupational role or identity is paramount; a decision to have children or to stay home and nurture them may bring the parenting role and identity to the forefront. Conflict can occur when both marriage and career are desired. This dual objective requires role modification for both partners so that marriage, family, and careers can be successfully combined (Bradt, 1989). The thirties and early forties always present maximum role demands.

Women often continue to work during the childrearing years. More than 50% of women with children work. The number of married mothers working full time who have one or more preschool children at home tripled between 1961 and 1991, jumping to 60%. That revolutionary trend will only continue (Sheehy, 1995). Projections

suggest that new mothers will be lucky to take off 10 or 15 weeks to stay home with newborn children over their worklife.

The dual career or worker family has become not just a luxury but an economic necessity. Consider that over the past 20 years, a married couple in which the wife was in the paid labor force had a 14% increase in real income. When the wife was not in the labor force, such a family took a 9% decrease in real income. This sobering difference explains a great deal about the explosion of women working outside the home. Women now in their thirties and forties, are expected to spend nearly three quarters of their adult lifetimes working outside the home (Sheehy, 1995).

Moreover, many women, as single head-of-households, continue to work because they represent 26% of households with children under 18 who have only a mother at home. Another 4% have only a father. Since 1970 the number of single parents has tripled, from about 4 million to about 12 million (US Bureau of the Census, 1990).

Women struggle with the eternal problem of how to balance it all. They work hard at juggling the roles of wife, mother, and worker. They often find themselves overwhelmed by the enormity of having not one career, but three. This contributes to the superwoman phenomenon of women feeling they have to do it all perfectly without ever dropping the ball. This is a potential source of stress to adult working women.

Men in their 30s and 40s are much more aware of their parental and household responsibilities than previous generations. This trend is demonstrated by fathers who take family leaves to share in the care of newborn or sick children, the record number of fathers seeking and receiving joint custody, and fathers equally involved with concerns about child care resources (Hoffman, 1995).

Single men and women in their 30s may question earlier decisions about postponement of marriage and parenthood. They may have achieved their career goals and may now be ready to forgo a career or combine it with marriage and/or parenthood. Relationships and parenthood may now seem more important than achievements. Single people may be ready for a change.

Many couples and single persons do opt to postpone parenthood until the mid-to-late thirties or early-to-mid forties, when the biological clock ticks ever more loudly. Although the average age of first-time mothers is 23.7, only 2 years higher than in 1960, there is a record number of first-time babies being born to couples and single people who choose to become parents after age 35.

Middle Adulthood (45 to 65 or 70 Years)

Adults currently entering midlife are set to become the longest living humans in American history. At least half of this cohort can expect to live into their eighties and nineties. The fastest growing segment of the population is women between 45 and 54. As such, midlife represents the beginning of the second half of life (see Table 7-8).

Many adults in their forties and fifties feel that they are at the height of their professional, emotional, and spiritual fitness. They have a sense of physical well-being not noted in previous generations of midlifers. In fact, many people in middle adulthood perceive themselves to be a full 10 years younger than their chronological age.

Men and women in their fifties and sixties often find their identity and commitments restabilized. They can enjoy the privileges of the middle years without envying others.

Physical and cognitive development in middle adulthood

During middle adulthood, there is a gradual slowing of all physiological functions, and tissues have less capacity to regenerate. Degenerative changes such as arthritic joint disease may begin at this time. Other changes occur, such as wrinkling and sagging caused by loss of tissue elasticity; balding and graying continue. Varying amounts of distress are experienced because of these changes.

The outstanding physical changes during this period, in both men and women, have to do with the reproductive system. The reproductive organs begin to atrophy with advancing age. The end of the female reproductive cycle is relatively clearly marked by menopause, which occurs between the ages of 40 and 55. The male climacteric is gradual, and the point at which it is concluded is less obvious; whether it is a purely physical syndrome is uncertain. Neither menopause nor the male climacteric need appreciably alter the sex drive. It may remain powerful throughout the life span.

Cognitive development does not advance. In fact, nerve impulses in the brain travel more slowly across neurons, causing a decrease in reaction time. However, in spite of these degenerative changes, most people retain full use of their intellectual abilities throughout the middle years. They continue to add new words to their vocabulary and organize and process new information. The degree to which intellectual functioning is maintained in the middle years appears to be a function of ongoing mental stimulation and variation in life experience.

Psychosocial development in middle adulthood

The midlife crisis is a period of acute psychosocial discomfort experienced by many as men and women face the discrepancy between their youthful ambitions and their actual achievement. They may feel bored and dissatisfied with the way their life has developed; they may feel ambivalence and uncertainty about the future. The loss of youth and all it entails must be mourned for men and women to move on with renewed vigor.

Multiple role changes occur. Children leave the home, and active parenting is completed, unless parenthood has been postponed until the late thirties or forties. Then parenting is only beginning at midlife. Where active parenting is completed, some former meaningful roles are gone. Women in their forties whose lives have been bound up in motherhood and managing the household may feel that they have lost their purpose in life as their children become increasingly independent. Even women who have had careers and whose identities have not been as wrapped up in parenting experience a loss when their children leave home. Many men have a similar sense of loss. The "empty nest" syndrome stems from the temporary sense of loss and purposelessness both men and women experience at this time. As children leave to lead their own lives, new sources of meaning and purpose must be developed by parents.

Men in midlife may feel that their career paths have never been more vital. Others feel that opportunities for advancement are limited and that younger people with better knowledge and skills are crowding them out. Still others are dealing with the crisis of unemployment or forced early retirement related to workplace restructuring (Friedmann and Webb, 1995). They may have to give up the idealized self of the twenties and thirties for a more realistic one. Men also question what the purpose will be for the rest of their lives. They may have to give up early hopes and dreams and find value in what they have actually accomplished and still can accomplish. Many men and women must confront the necessity of finding a new career, or the fact that they have become unemployable. Even people who have attained their goals need new ideas to renew their zeal (McCullough and Rutenberg, 1989).

A generation ago, adults had only one career. Today, with fierce workplace competitiveness, restructuring, economic constraints, increased life expectancy, and shrinking retirement entitlements, the traditional work or career ladder no longer exists. Both men and women in their forties and beyond can be expected to work into their seventies having multiple career paths that capitalize on basic skills and talents developed in earlier years. Sometimes educational or vocational retooling is a necessity.

The marital relationship also changes. Husbands and wives are alone together as they have not been in years, unless parenthood is a midlife event or children begin returning home to live as the last child is launched (Estess, 1994). In fact many persons who have children in their late thirties and forties will spend their midlife years attending children's athletic events, and chaperoning school trips, and proms.

Empty nesters may find that they no longer share interests or values or that they have gotten into the habit of communicating through their children. They may find that they need to renew their relationship and develop new interests that will enrich their lives. Role reversals occur. Adults become parents to their own parents as the parents age and become infirm. Caregiver burden and strain is a common cause of stress as midlife children assume responsibility for aging parents as they become increasingly frail. Stress on family systems resources creates strain that challenges the well-being of family members (Fink, 1995). The last shreds of childhood are severed. The adult realizes that "I am alone." This moment of self-confrontation is often terrifying (Walters et al., 1988; Thomas, 1995).

In their middle years, men and particularly women who earlier elected not to marry and or become parents often have to confront the fact that they will not bear children. This awareness can lead to feelings of depression.

Physical changes occur that reflect changes in body image. There is a growing difference between the sexual capacity of men and women. Men find that they are unable to perform as frequently as in previous years. Women, on the other hand, experience no loss of sexual ability and may actually feel increased desire, owing to freedom from fear of pregnancy, freedom from the responsibilities of earlier years, and a positive redefinition of self, particularly if they have multiple sources of meaning in their lives. However, menopause and the accompanying physiological changes may contribute to temporary emotional disequilibrium and add to a woman's sense of loss and depression. However, this sense of disequilibrium is usually just a pause in the menopause experience (Sheehy, 1991; Barbach, 1993). Once over 50, women, more than men, exhibit renewed self-confidence and what Sheehy (1995) calls "postmenopausal zest."

The capacity for love and intimacy is not decreased for men or women, and sexuality in the middle years can be most fulfilling if creative approaches are taken to sexual activity. The general physical process of aging, however, confronts people with their own mortality. Illness and death among friends and relatives makes it difficult to deny that endurance and physical capacity are decreasing. But in a youth-oriented culture, many people do try to hold on to a youthful self-concept. They look back at the past to evaluate whether they want to pursue such youthful pleasures now. They may seek the exclusive company of people younger than themselves, have extramarital affairs with younger people, or maintain a frantic pace of life. They may dye their hair, have cosmetic surgery, or dress in a youthful way. All these activities may be attempts to deny the aging process and to maintain a sense of vigor and self-esteem (Sheehy, 1995; Levinson, 1978; Julian, McKenry, and McKelvey, 1992).

If the tasks of midlife—self-confrontation and change—have been accomplished, men and women may find their fifties and sixties to be the most personally rewarding period of their lives. People come to terms with mortality and reconcile what is with what might have been. The fifties and sixties become a stable psychological state of mastery (Sheehy, 1995). Reaching this state of mastery is one of the best predictors of good physical, mental, and psychological functioning in old age (Goleman, 1994; Thomas, 1995).

Marriage, if it survives to midlife, can provide opportunities for renewed intimacy, once children no longer occupy so much of the partners' time. Adults in the later middle years become concerned with generativity—establishing and guiding the next generation. Parents recognize their children as separate adults, not merely extensions of themselves. They enjoy family events such as marriage of children and birth and growing up of grandchildren. People who have not married or had children of their own may expand and deepen relationships with nieces and nephews, younger colleagues, or students.

Involvement in community activities can provide an expanded network of social relationships at a time when friendship networks tend to contract because of geographic moves and death. Interests left dormant during earlier preoccupation with establishing a family, a career, or both, can be redeveloped. Previous hobbies or interests can blossom and become involving. For example, a builder concentrated his interest and skill on building a sailboat, a hobby left untouched from his teenage years. A woman turned a lifetime love of cooking into a money-making venture when she started a catering business.

The basic crisis of the middle years is one of introspection, self-confrontation, a search for meaning, and renewal. The process of peeling away the layers is often painful because feelings that have been buried for years may emerge. People are not sure they like what they see. However, this is a unique opportunity to put things together and come to accept oneself with renewed vitality.

As a result of their own reassessment middle-age people are often more flexible about accepting philosophical, moral, ethical, spiritual, and religious differences among people; they accept the right of each person to choose a belief system. Within individual contexts, people may be able to renew their commitments to religious doctrines. Participation in church-affiliated activities often increases during the middle years. However, spiritual beliefs often extend beyond the confines of one's own religion. A sense of philanthropy may create a deep commitment to ecumenical religious and secular interests, and to the community (Kohlberg, 1973; Sheehy, 1995).

Accepting their own mortality leads midlife people to grapple with the need for transcendence—when they accept the inevitability of death, there may be a concurrent need to believe in some form of immortality. However, immortality need not be envisioned as personal survival. For some people, it can take the form of accomplishments that will live on; and for some it is seen in links with other generations—children, grandchildren, nieces, nephews, and other significant youngsters. People place more and more importance on immortality as their own sense of vulnerability becomes acute and as their parents and peers grow infirm and die (Erikson, 1963).

If these issues are not confronted in middle adulthood, they crop up again in later years. Failure to negotiate these tasks and accept one's own finiteness results in denial, depression, stress-related health problems, boredom, and stagnation.

Late Adulthood (65 or 70 Years to Death)

In general, people reach their sixties and seventies in better health and with a longer life expectancy than ever before. People in their sixties need to develop a life plan for making the next 20 or 30 years they are likely to live, a quality phase of the life cycle. The way in which people experience late adulthood appears to be a function of a complex interrelationship of physical, cognitive, and psychosocial factors. Table 7-9 illustrates major theories and tasks of late adulthood.

Physical and cognitive development in late adulthood

The physical appearance and cognitive functioning of people over 65 vary as much as those of people of earlier developmental stages. Chronological age cannot be used as a predictor of physical and cognitive decline. The physical and cognitive aspects of aging are, to some degree, a result of changes in the ability of individual cells to perform specialized, integrated functions. Brain cells do not die off in annual batches. Rather, they shrink or grow dormant in old age, particularly from lack of stimulation and challenge (Sheehy, 1995). Even in an older developed brain, "sprouting" can take place in which new neural processes form additional synapses. Nearly one third of individuals enjoy full mental alertness throughout late age (Powell, 1994). Although change is inevitable, most researchers agree that no functional mental decline begins before age 60 or 65, although short-term memory can become somewhat less reliable. The rapidity and extent of change are highly correlated with the individual's investment or lack of investment in living, acquired cognitive mastery techniques, accumulated wisdom, and focus.

Physical changes   During the gradual onset of aging, the body experiences degeneration in structure and functioning. Loss of bone density and mass (osteoporosis) causes a compression of bones, especially in the vertebral area, so that there is a slight decrease in height. All bones break more easily and heal more slowly. A loss of cartilage makes painful joint complaints more prevalent and decreases range of movement and mobility. A curved posture becomes increasingly common with age.

Visual acuity decreases beyond the sixties. Because of changes in the eye, older people accommodate more slowly to light and dark, color, and depth. Night driving may be more hazardous for this reason. Color and depth perception are also less accurate.

Hearing acuity decreases with age as the mean pure

TABLE 7-9

Developmental theories of late adulthood: Havighurst, Lemon, Neugarten, Erikson, Sheehy		
STAGE	**AGE**	**TASK**
Late Adulthood	65 to 70 years to death	Capacity to feel whole, worthwhile, and happy because of one's social and mental powers, whether or not health is perfect; lack of preoccupation with health, physique, and body comfort
		Adjusting to decreased physical strength and health, to retirement and reduced income, and to death of a spouse
		Capacity to accept the death of the body as less important than knowing that a future has been built through children, other relationships, and community, contributions—a feeling of enduring significance—capacity to adjust to current life situations
		Adjusting and adopting social roles in a flexible way
		Establishing supportive living arrangements that maintain maximum independence

tone threshold at all sound frequencies increases in both genders. Many older people, either unaware of or hesitant to admit a hearing loss, may pretend to understand messages that they do not hear completely. They may try to piece together what they did hear and fill in the blanks. As a result, they may receive the wrong message.

Taste buds and the sense of smell decrease with age; this contributes to a loss of appetite—and loss of appetite, in turn, may lead to an unbalanced diet and inadequate nutritional intake, especially if finances are limited or preparing food becomes difficult. The integrity of teeth depends on regular dental maintenance. Many people retain their own teeth, but others wear partial or full dentures.

Changes in skin and tissue are common. Pigment deposits in the skin may produce "age spots"; loss of elasticity produces wrinkles and jowls. The sebaceous glands slow down, and the skin may become dry and scaly. There is also a decrease in body hair and an increase in facial hair, owing to a decrease in hormone secretion.

Sexual activity usually diminishes during this stage, more so in men than in women. In men the erectile capacity decreases, and ejaculation may or may not occur even if an erection is attained. In women, vaginal lubrication diminishes because of estrogen depletion, so artificial lubricants may be necessary during intercourse, if the woman does not take hormone replacement therapy. However, the capacity for sexual functioning does not disappear. Ongoing sexual behavior will depend on attitudes about sexual activity for this age group, interest, availability of a partner, and health status. Sex becomes a recreative rather than procreative activity. Although arousal and orgasm diminish in intensity and frequency, sexual activity can continue to provide a physical and emotional bond that creates and expresses intimacy, affection, and tenderness.

Health problems become an increasing concern. Cardiovascular, pulmonary, and renal problems can be treated medically but may eventually take their toll. Cancer is prevalent in this age group (Ebersole and Hess, 1994).

Research findings indicate that courage in dealing with chronic illness, so common in this age cohort, can transform a struggle into a challenge (Finfgeld, 1995). Persons with courage have (1) a strong commitment to cognitively convert a struggle into a challenge, (2) long-term determination that will sustain the transformation process over the course of the chronic illness, and (3) perceived control over the situation based on their remaining physical stamina, knowledge base, or psychic strength.

Cognitive changes   Cognitive changes occur in late adulthood. However, their extent is variable. Some of what is considered cognitive impairment results from at-

titudes toward older people. Society expects people to become mentally deteriorated, or "senile," as they age. If this attitude is incorporated by older people, they begin to perceive themselves as cognitively inept, become less willing to use the cognitive skills they do have, and become apprehensive about intellectual activities. Thus cognitive deterioration becomes a self-fulfilling prophecy. In fact, however, older people can maintain cognitive integrity if extra time is allowed for assimilation and mastery, if adequate social stimulation is provided, and if they are valued by themselves and others as meaningful participants and contributors.

Psychosocial development in late adulthood

Much has become known about the older adult psychosocially. There are several theories about certain aspects of psychosocial aging, but inadequate evidence exists to formulate a single theory. According to the *disengagement theory proposed by Cummings and Henry (1961) aging people and society inevitably withdraw from each other physically, emotionally, and socially. In this process both society and the individual prepare for death.*

The **activity theory** *formulated by Lemon et al. (1972) is opposed to the disengagement theory and is currently more popular. According to this theory, the majority of older people maintain a fairly high level of activity and engagement. The degree of engagement or disengagement is influenced more by past lifestyles and social and economic forces than by aging itself.*

The **continuity theory** *proposed by Havighurst et al. (1953) focused on the relationship between life satisfaction and activity as an expression of enduring personality traits.* This theory makes the following three important assumptions:

1. In normal aging, personality remains consistent in men and women.
2. Personality influences role activity and investment in activities.
3. Personality influences life satisfaction regardless of role activity.

These theories can be seen as representing different points on a continuum. It is likely that most people fall somewhere in between. Although older people reduce activities in some areas, such as work, they may increase activities in other areas, such as hobbies. Reduction of activity occurs as energy decreases. However, selective meaningful involvement may continue. Neugarten et al. (1968) state that level of activity will be influenced by patterns established in younger years. Disengagement may occur involuntarily owing to death of spouse and peers and concomitant lack of social support, lack of finances or transportation, or poor health.

The central psychosocial tasks of late adulthood involve loss and change. Changes in roles, activity, social relationships, finances, and living arrangements frequently occur. Loss is experienced with death of a spouse and friends and decreased independence. The changes noted above can also be perceived as losses if they are extensive or occur in areas of great importance. Redefining a lifestyle includes dealing with retirement, death of a spouse, rearrangement of social relationships, loss of independence, and altered living arrangements.

Retirement   Retirement is often a crisis because it threatens identity, integrity, and self-esteem. In a production-oriented society, where (especially for men) one's major social role is occupational, retirement, whether voluntary or forced, may mean loss or reduction of income, influence, responsibility, authority, status, social relationships, creativity, activity, and control over the environment.

Retirement may be less of a crisis for women who have primarily been homemakers. They have already had to adjust to a form of retirement when child rearing was completed in their late forties or fifties. However, a husband's retirement may result in loss of privacy and increased demands on a woman's personal time. Women who have combined homemaking and a career, which is rapidly becoming the norm, not the exception, may also find retirement less of a crisis, since they have undergone many changes in and modifications of roles.

Retirement does not affect everyone in the same way. Several factors contribute to the way it is experienced:

1. Degree to which leisure-time activities have been developed and are seen as meaningful and ego-enhancing
2. Degree to which attitudes and perceptions of self-worth are determined by one's work
3. Degree to which friendships and social involvement have been developed and can be maintained
4. Degree to which changes in income will inhibit retirement activity and determine lifestyle
5. Degree to which the spouses look forward to increased opportunities for time together and whether these expectations are met

Death of spouse   Women outlive men by an average of 8 years and are much more likely to experience loss of a spouse than are men (Gale, 1993). The loss is significant, because it not only involves the death of a lifelong companion but is also an undeniable reminder of one's own mortality. Reaction to the loss of a spouse will depend on the quality of the relationship, the amount of warning there was of the approaching death, the survivor's degree of independence, sources of inner strength, the supportiveness of family and friends, and any financial burdens that may exist (Moloney, 1995).

For a woman the loss of a spouse deprives her not only of a significant other but also of any identity that she may have achieved through her husband's social and economic position. If a woman has not developed an individual identity, she must now redefine herself socially and economically. For example, a woman who has never learned to balance a checkbook may suddenly have to handle financial matters for herself, or a woman who was married for 40 years may choose to enter the dating world in search of companionship.

However, men are more apt to suffer acute loneliness after the death of their wives. The wife is often the husband's only confidant and friend. Men may feel that they must be courageous and unemotional in their bereavement, and they may have nobody with whom to share their grief. Also, some men are less independent. Living alone and taking care of themselves may be difficult: laundry, housecleaning, shopping, and cooking may be unfamiliar tasks. Twice as many widowers remarry as widows—possibly for these reasons, and possibly because women have more opportunities for companionship without remarrying than men do. The suicide rate is highest among single white men above the age of 65.

One's own death   Life, of course, does not continue indefinitely. Some people deal with the prospect of death by denying it; others seem to accept it, saying that they have lived full lives and have no fear of personal extinction. Some cultures—U.S. society included—avoid the subject of death and thus make it difficult for people to verbalize their positive or negative feelings about it. This often leads to suppression of fear, increased anxiety, and maladaptive behavior.

Social relationships   Peer groups of old close friends grow smaller as friends die and move away; and three fourths of older people live apart from their families. Opportunities for social contacts shrink unless people reach out and form new relationships. It is easy for the elderly to sink into isolation, loneliness, boredom, and despair. At a time when they feel that social connectedness is vanishing and that their worth as social beings is gone, they must repattern their social world so that they do not become isolated. Senior citizens' centers, church groups, "volunteer grandparent" groups, and residential complexes are examples of support systems for the elderly that are vehicles for expanding social relationships (see Chapter 35).

Intergenerational connectedness with family, particularly children and grandchildren, can be satisfying if the older adult is not perceived in a negative way by family members, made a scapegoat for family problems, or excluded from an active role in the family. The desire to leave a legacy, to pass something personal along to others in the next generation, can often be accomplished in grandparent-grandchild relationships; grandparents pass on skills, family history, and the wisdom gained through experience to their grandchildren. This enables them to feel a sense of immortality and a link with the future. Such a legacy can also be transmitted through mentoring relationships with other young people or the community (Erikson et al., 1986; Kaufman, 1987).

Maintaining independence Ongoing health problems and disability may result in dependence on others for care, support, and security. The older adult has fewer support systems. For example, an older adult may live far from family and be widowed, without friends, and unaware of community resources. Lack of financial resources also may inhibit the seeking of needed services. Meals-on-Wheels, homemaker services, community health nurses, senior citizen clinics, Dial-a-Ride, and state aid to the elderly are all community services available to help people care for themselves and remain as independent as possible.

Altered living arrangements A need to alter living arrangements can come about because of physical limitations, changes in financial status or family configurations, changed relationships, and deteriorating neighborhood conditions.

Physical limitations can lead to a loss of the ability to live independently. Sometimes only a relatively minor change will solve a problem; for example, a woman who had had a severe heart attack moved from a third-floor walk-up apartment to a lobby-level apartment. Physical disability may also necessitate supervision. The degree of supervision required can vary from a spouse or adult child who becomes caregiver, to a nighttime sitter, to a full-time homemaker, to a respite care facility, to a skilled nursing facility. Only 5% of the elderly live in institutions; most maintain themselves in community settings.

Changing family configurations most commonly result from loss of a spouse and geographic separation from children. Loss of a spouse through death leaves the survivor alone and faced with a decision to live alone, find a companion, or move in with other family members. In most cases, family members are unwilling or unable to have a parent move in even if they assume role of caregiver. They may feel that this would set the stage for multigenerational conflict between grandparents, parents, and children; or they may not have space for an extra person. Older people themselves may not want to live under someone else's roof, even if invited. They often feel like a "fifth wheel," with no authority, role, or corner to call their own. Older adults must thus come to terms with the decision to remain alone or find a place where they will belong (Walsh, 1989).

Options for altered living arrangements are available to individuals or couples in late adulthood. Many older people leave established neighborhoods and head south to the warmth of Florida, Arizona, and California; others move to senior housing in their own communities. Retirement communities provide transportation, an age-appropriate social network, and sense of community that may be missing for the older adult who remains in a heterogeneous community.

Changes in finances may necessitate a move to more modest surroundings. This may be accompanied by loss of status, prestige, and self-worth, and it may mean separation from any social network that is not accessible with available transportation. Many older adults exist on fixed incomes; when income does not increase with inflation, the older person may become impoverished. This often results in the entrapment of older people in deteriorating neighborhoods, the only ones they can afford. Their living arrangements are substandard; they are often terrorized by neighborhood crime. They huddle in isolation, powerless to help themselves. Community resources can help such people locate more adequate, safer housing that is government-subsidized or privately owned.

Spiritual issues

Despite losses, potential crises, and undercurrents of grief running through their lives, members of this older age group are courageous; they are concerned with actualizing their remaining possibilities and maintaining integrity and dignity (Finfgeld, 1995).

Moral issues reemerge as a priority in late adulthood. Although death looms, people still have time to contemplate moral issues, especially mortality, immortality, and transcendence.

For men there is a shift in moral judgments from those related to logical justification to a dialectic resolution between justice and personal caring that has been more characteristic of adult women (Rybash, Roadin, and Hyes, 1983). This reflects the older person's shifting concerns (irrespective of gender) from social, legalistic matters to interpersonal concerns (Kohlberg, 1973; Rybash, Roadin, and Hyes, 1983).

Religion is a significant factor in happiness, usefulness, and personal adjustment in older people, especially men and those over 70. Research indicates that people who have grown up with a religious affiliation continue it for as long as possible. Activities related to a church or synagogue often became the focus of the social world and decrease only when a person becomes ill or transportation is not available. Religious activities within the home may increase as well.

Older people who do not have a religion or an abiding sense of the spiritual may feel purposeless, worthless, unloved, and perhaps abandoned by God, and they may fear death. They may struggle frantically to find some belief that will help them deal with the inevitable end of

CRITICAL THINKING QUESTIONS

Lois and David L., age 50 and 53, are the parents of three children. Their oldest daughter Joan, age 29, and her husband Alex, age 32, have been married for 1 year and are the parents of a 2-month-old girl, Alexa, who is also the first grandchild and great-grandchild. Although Lois and David like Alex, they are concerned about his stability; he has held four jobs in the 2 years that Joan and Alex dated and were married. Currently, he is not working. Joan, who had hoped to stay home with Alexa for at least 3 months, returned to work 2 weeks after the infant's birth to preserve her job as a bank assistant manager because this is their only source of income until Alex "finds himself." She is feeling exhausted and resentful that Alex gets to stay home and take care of Alexa while she has to go to work. Alex, on the other hand, feels bored and restless at home.

Lois, an only child, was a midlife surprise to parents who had long given up hope of having a child. Her mom, a widow for 10 years, died last year at 87 after a 3-year bout with cancer. Lois was her mom's major caregiver and David's parents, who live in Florida and are increasingly frail, are a constant concern. David's father has failing eyesight, but insists on driving although he has had numerous "fender-benders." Last night, his father called to say that his mother slipped getting out of the shower, fractured her hip, and is in the hospital.

David, an aviation mechanic, works for an aircraft company scheduled for closure in the near future because of defense budget cutbacks. Lois, who works as a secretary for the Board of Education, wonders whether all families are like theirs and how they will cope with the latest family crisis.

1. What would be the most important assessment variables to consider when assessing the mental health needs of this family?
2. What are the most appropriate intervention activities for the nurse to use in helping this family cope effectively with their life cycle issues?
3. What are the mental health needs of Lois and David? Of Joan and Alex?
4. What kinds of community resources would provide a support system for this family?
5. What kinds of intergenerational issues are evident?
6. What are the major life cycle issues for the members of this intergenerational family?

life. Most people with strong religious beliefs do not fear death; rather, they accept it as an inherent part of life. If they are anxious, it is about the process of dying, not death itself. They fear losing control as death approaches, being unable to obtain help when they need it, and being abandoned (Erikson, 1963).

Those who do not cope effectively, who do not reach out, become bored and stagnant. Many also become bitter and withdrawn, feeling themselves to be victims of their age. Because processes of decline and growth occur concomitantly but not in equal balance, it is of utmost importance for caregivers to examine the symptoms before making judgments about any client. More than with any other age group, it is necessary to be aware of stereotyped attitudes toward the aging process, the wide variety of individual differences that do exist, and the effectiveness of intervention.

KEY POINTS

- Development is a continuous evolutionary process that becomes increasingly complex and diverse.
- Developmental processes are unique for each person and emerge from continuous interaction with the environment with relative (not absolute) developmental norms.
- Organizing developmental theories of Freud, Erikson, Sullivan, Stern, Mahler, Piaget, Kohlberg, Gilligan, Fowler, Levinson, Sheehy, Neugarten, and Havighurst contribute to the understanding of developmental processes.
- The life cycle can be viewed in terms of physical, cognitive, and psychosocial forces that provide a holistic perspective for assessing developmental processes at each life cycle stage.
- The life cycle is divided into nine stages: infancy, early childhood, middle childhood, late childhood, adolescence, young adulthood, adulthood, middle adulthood, and late adulthood.
- Nurses need a thorough understanding of developmental processes to understand people's feelings, thoughts, and actions to differentiate functional from dysfunctional developmental processes.

REFERENCES

Alan Guttmacher Institute. (1995). Personal communication.

Aylmer, R.C. (1989). Launching the single young adult. In B. Carter & M. McGoldrick (Eds.), *The changing family life cycle* (2nd ed.). Boston: Allyn & Bacon.

Baillargeon, R. (1991). The object concept revisisted: New directions in the investigation of infants physical knowledge. In C.E. Granrud (Ed.), *Visual Perception and Cognition in Infancy.* Carnegie-Mellon symposia on cognition (Vol. 23.). Hillsdale, NJ: Erlbaum.

Barbach, L. (1993). *The pause: Positive approaches to menopause.* New York: Signet.

Bartlett, D.L., & Steele, J.B. (1992). *America: What went wrong?.* Kansas City, MO: Andrews and McMeel.

Belenky, M. et al. (1986). *Women's ways of knowing.* New York: Basic Books.

Bradt, J. (1989). Becoming parents: Families with young children. In B. Carter & M. McGoldrick (Eds.). *The changing family life cycle* (2nd ed.). Boston: Allyn & Bacon.

Carter, B., & McGoldrick, M. (1989). Overview: The changing family life cycle: A framework for family therapy. In B. Carter & M. McGoldrick (Eds.), *The changing family life cycle* (2nd ed.). Boston: Allyn & Bacon.

Chira, S. (1994, July 10). Teenagers, in a poll, report worry and distrust of adults. *The New York Times.*

Cummings, E., & Henry, W.E. (1961). *Growing old: The process of disengagement.* New York: Basic Books.

Ebersole, R., & Hess R. (1994). *Toward healthy aging: Human needs and nursing response* (4th ed.). St. Louis: Mosby.

Erikson, E.H. (1963). *Childhood and society.* New York: W.W. Norton.

Erikson, E., Erikson, J., & Kivnick, H. (1986). *Vital involvement in old age: The experience of old age in our time.* New York: W.W. Norton.

Estess, P.S. (1994). When kids don't leave. *Modern Maturity, 37,* 6, 56, 57, 90.

Finfgeld, D.L. (1995). Becoming and being courageous in the chronically ill elderly. *Issues in Mental Health Nursing, 16,* 1, 1-11.

Fink, S.V. (1995). The influence of family resources and family demands on the strains and well-being of caregiving families. *Nursing Research, 44,* 3, 139-146.

Fowler, J.W. (1974). Toward a developmental perspective on faith, *Religious Education, 69,* 207-219.

Freud, S. (1972). *A general introduction to psychoanalysis.* New York: Pocket Books.

Friedemann, M.L., & Webb, A.A. (1995). Family health and mental health six years after economic stress and unemployment. *Issues in Mental Health Nursing, 16,* 1, 51-66.

Gale, B.J. (1993). Psychosocial health needs of older women: Urban versus rural comparisons. *Archives of Psychiatric Nursing, 7,* 2, 99-105.

Gilbert, P. (1992). *Depression: The evolution of powerlessness.* New York: Guilford Press.

Gilligan, C. (1982). *In a different voice.* Cambridge, MA: Harvard University Press.

Gilligan, C. (1988). Exit-voice dilemmas in adolescent development. In C. Gilligan, J.V. Ward, & J.M. Taylor (Eds.), *Mapping the moral domain.* Cambridge, MA: Harvard University Press.

Gilligan, C. (1990). Listening to voices we have not heard. In. C. Gilligan, N. Lyons, & T. Hammer. (Eds.), *Making connections.* Cambridge, MA: Harvard University Press.

Goleman, D. (1994, April 26). Mental decline in aging need not be inevitable. *The New York Times.*

Grotstein, J.S. (1990). Invariants in primitive emotional disorders. In L.B. Boyer & P.L. Giovacchini (Eds.), *Master clinicians on treating the regressed patient.* Northvale, NJ: Jason Aronson.

Havighurst, R.J., & Albrecht, R. (1953). *Older people.* New York: Longmans.

Hoffman, J. (1995, April 26). Divorced fathers make gains in battles to increase rights. *The New York Times.*

Julian, T., McKenry, P.C., & McKelvey, M.W. (1992). Components of men's well-being at mid-life. *Issues in Mental Health Nursing, 13,* 4, 285-299.

Kaufman, S. (1987). *The ageless self: Sources of meaning in late life.* Madison, WI: University of Wisconsin Press.

Kohlberg, L. (1969). The cognitive-developmental approach to socialization. In D. Goslin (Ed.), *Handbook of socialization.* Chicago: Rand McNally.

Kohlberg, L. (1973). Continuities in childhood and adult moral development revisited. In P. Boltes & K.W. Shaire (Eds.), *Life span developmental psychology.* New York: Academic Press.

Kohlberg, L., & Gilligan, C. (1971). The adolescent as a philosopher: The discovery of self in a post conventional world. *Daedalus,* 100.

Kohut, H. (1984). *How does analysis care?* Chicago: University of Chicago Press.

Lemon, B., Bengtson, V., & Peterson, J. (1972). An exploration of the activity theory of aging. Activity types and life satisfaction among in-movers to a retirement community. *Journal of Gerontology,* (27), 511.

Levinson, D.J. et al. (1978). *The seasons of man's life.* New York: Ballantine.

Lidz, T. (1968). *The person: His development throughout the life cycle.* New York: Basic Books.

Lyons, N.P. (1988). Two perspectives: On self, relationships and morality. In C. Gilligan, J.V. Ward, & J.M. Taylor (Eds.), *Mapping the moral domain.* Cambridge, MA: Harvard University Press.

Mahler, M. (1975). *The psychological birth of the human infant: Symbiosis and individuation.* New York: Basic Books.

Mahler, M. (1980). *The rapprochement subphase of the separation-individuation process.* In R.F. Lax, S. Bach, & J.A. Burland (Eds.), *Rapprochement: The critical subphase separation-individuation.* New York: Arronson.

McGoldrick, M. (1989). The joining of families through marriage: The new couple. In B. Carter & M. McGoldrick (Eds.), *The changing family life cycle.* Boston: Allyn & Bacon.

Moloney, M.F. (1995). A Heideggerian hermeneutical analysis of older women's stories of being strong. *Image, 27:2,* 104-109.

Nelson, C.A. (1991). Neural correlates of recognition memory in the first post natal year of life. In G. Dawson & K. Fischer (Eds.), *Human Behavior and Braun Development.* New York: Guilford Press.

Nelson, C.A., & Callius, P.F. (1991). Event-related potential and looking-time analysis of infants' responses to familiar and novel events: Implications for visual recognition and memory. *Developmental Psychology, 27,* 1, 50-58.

Nemiroff, R., & Colarusso, C.A. (1990). *New dimensions in adult development.* New York: Basic Books.

Neugarten, B. et al. (1968). *Middle age and aging.* Chicago: University of Chicago Press.

Oatley, K., & Jenkins, J.M. (1992). Human emotions: Functions and dysfunction. *Annual Review of Psychology, 43,* 55-85.

Piaget, J. (1932). *The moral judgment of the child.* London: Routledge.

Piaget, J. (1962). The stages of the intellectual development of the child. *Bulletin of the Menninger Clinic, 26,* (4103), 120-132.

Piaget, J. (1963). *The child's conception of the world.* New York: Littlefield, Adams.

Powell, D. (1994). *Profiles in cognitive aging.* Cambridge, MA: Harvard University Press.

Preto, N.G. (1989). Transformation of the family system in adolescence. In B. Carter and M. McGoldrick (Eds.), *The changing family life cycle.* Boston: Allyn & Bacon.

Rogers, M. (1988). Nursing science and art: A prospective. *Nursing Science Quarterly,* 1(3), 99-102.

Rosenwasser, S.M., Lingenfelter, A.F., & Harrington, A.F. (1989). Nontraditional gender role portrayals on television and children's gender role perceptions. *Journal of Applied Developmental Psychology, 10,* 97-105.

Rybash, J., Roadin, P., & Hyes, W. (1983). Expressions of moral thought in late adulthood. *Gerontologist, 23,* 254-263.

Satinover, J.B., & Bentz, L.T. (1992). Aching in places where we used to play. *Quadrant: The Journal of Contemporary Jungian Thought, 25,* 1, 21-57.

Schore, A.N. (1994). *Affect and regulation and the origin of self: The neurobiology of emotional development.* Hillsdale, NJ: Lawrence Erlbaum Associates.

Sheehy, G. (1991). *The silent passage: Menopause.* New York: Pocket Books.

Spiegel, S. (1987). The interpersonal world of the infant symposium. *Contemporary Psychoanalysis, 23* (1), 6-16.

Stern, D. (1985a). *The interpersonal world of the infant.* New York: Basic Books.

Stern, D. (1985b). Affect attunement. In J.D. Call, E. Galenson, & R.L. Tyson (Eds.), *Frontiers of infant psychiatry* (Vol. 2.). New York: Basic Books.

Stern, D. (1990). *Diary of a baby.* New York: Basic Books.

Stern, L. (1990). Conceptions of separation and connectedness. In C. Gilligan, N. Lyons, & T. Hammer (Eds.), *Making connections.* Cambridge, MA: Harvard University Press.

Sullivan, H.S. (1953). In H.S. Perry (Ed.), *Interpersonal theory of psychiatry,* New York: W.W. Norton.

Thomas, S.P. (1995). Psychosocial correlates of women's health in middle adulthood. *Issues in Mental Health Nursing, 16:*4, 285-314.

Thompson, R.A. (1990). Emotion and self-regulation. *Nebraska symposium on motivation,* Lincoln, NE: University of Nebraska Press.

U.S. Bureau of the Census. (1990). *United States census of population and housing summary (Tape file 3-C).* Washington, DC: Author.

Von Bertalanffy, L. (1968). *General systems theory.* New York: Braziller.

Walsh, F. (1989). The family in later life. In B. Carter & M. McGoldrick (Eds.), *The changing family life cycle.* Boston: Allyn & Bacon.

Walters, M. et al. (1988). *The invisible web: Gender patterns in family relationships.* New York: Guillford Press.

Whaley, L., & Wong, D. (1995). *Nursing care of infants and children* (5th ed.). St. Louis: Mosby.

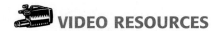 **VIDEO RESOURCES**

Mosby's Communication in Nursing Video Series: *Communicating Across the Lifespan.*

Chapter 8

Therapeutic Communication

Judith Haber

LEARNING OUTCOMES

After studying and applying the concepts of this chapter, the learner will be able to:
- Describe communication as a circular process.
- Discuss the components of verbal and nonverbal communication.
- Discuss cultural factors that influence communication.
- Apply the principles of therapeutic communication to nurse-client interactions.
- Discuss physical and psychosocial attending skills that facilitate nurse-client interactions.
- Discuss how specific therapeutic responding strategies facilitate nurse-client interactions.
- Discuss barriers to therapeutic communication and their consequences in nurse-client interactions.

KEY TERMS

Appearance	Facilitative questions and statements	Proxemics
Attending	Feedback	Reflection
Attending skills	Focusing	Restatement
Clarifying	Kinesics	Silence
Communication	Nonverbal communication	Stating observations
Confrontation	Paralanguage	Summarizing
Conveying information	Perception	Verbal communication
Empathy	Presence	

ommunication is a dynamic information-sharing process that occurs between people and their environment. Communication occurs between and among all people in all situations and circumstances of life. It occurs between family members, friends, and colleagues, as well as between nurses and clients. Since communication is an essential tool of psychiatric nurses, understanding therapeutic communication is crucial (Peplau, 1963).

Communicating therapeutically with clients is a skill that must be learned and mastered by all nurses, but especially by psychiatric nurses for whom the therapeutic use of self is the primary tool for working effectively with clients. This enables psychiatric nurses to meet standards of care and implement psychiatric nursing role functions.

Communication may appear simple at first. Surely we communicate with others every day of our lives. In fact, though, communication is a complex process. Nurses may assume that they know how to listen and respond to clients and fail to develop the skills of therapeutic communication, a major intervention modality of psychiatric nursing. The purpose of this chapter is to provide a framework for understanding therapeutic communication and its relevance to psychiatric nursing by presenting the principles and techniques of therapeutic communication, discussing barriers to therapeutic communication, and applying these principles to the nursing process.

DEFINITION OF COMMUNICATION

Communication is a continuous circular process by which information, such as ideas and feelings, is transmitted between people and their environment. Communication involves symbols, such as written words, and spoken language. Words in spoken language are also symbols. The ultimate goal of communication is to understand and be understood.

Communication is both verbal and nonverbal and occurs within an environmental context of cultural, family, and individual life experiences. Verbal and nonverbal communication provide essential client assessment data.

Verbal Communication

Verbal communication refers to spoken or written words that comprise the symbols of language. In verbal communication the meanings of the words are derived not only from the words themselves but also from their order in phrases, sentences, and paragraphs. Some groups of words convey special meanings: these groups include figures of speech, jokes, proverbs, clichés, and mottos. Such messages may have both an abstract and concrete interpretation. For example, the proverb "A

stitch in time saves nine" can be interpreted abstractly to mean that preventive health measures may forestall bigger health problems in the future. Sentences and phrases like this have acquired special meaning over time and can succinctly convey a great deal. However, nurses should remember that expressions such as proverbs may be culturally relevant. Thus clients from diverse cultures may lack familiarity with them and how to interpret them from a mainstream western culture perspective.

Certain clients have difficulty expressing verbal language. Clients with schizophrenia have problems abstracting and using words to convey meaning that is reality-oriented. When asked what the proverb "People who live in glass houses shouldn't throw stones" means, the client with schizophrenia is likely to answer, "When you live in a glass house, you'll break your house if you throw stones at it." Nurses must assess whether the client's inability to abstractly interpret a proverb is related to cognitive dysfunction, such as loss of abstract thinking, or represents a cultural phenomenon. Clients with depression often have difficulty thinking of and verbally stating the words that convey what they feel. When asked to describe how she was feeling, a client with depression softly stated, "Gray," and could not expand this one-word verbalization. However, this single word conveys a lot of emotion to the client with depression.

Nonverbal Communication

Nonverbal communication is communication without words. It includes messages created through body motion and the use of space, sound, and touch (Northouse and Northouse, 1992). Nonverbal communication includes nonverbal behaviors that contribute meaning to verbal messages or convey their own message. Body movement, gestures, eye contact, appearance, posture, manner of dress, and makeup are nonverbal messages to which nurses must be attentive.

Nonverbal communication does not encompass language but can be vocal or nonvocal. This statement may sound contradictory because nonverbal communication is usually thought of as silent. However, vocal sounds that are not words fall within the category of nonverbal communication. The groan or scream of a client about to engage in aggressive behavior would be vocal nonverbal communication, whereas the smile or frown of a withdrawn client would be nonvocal nonverbal communication (Box 8-1).

Nonverbal messages are recognized through observation. Four ways in which they are expressed are as follows:

1. *Kinesics—body motion*
2. *Paralanguage—voice quality and use of sounds in nonlanguage vocalizations*

3. *Proxemics*—*use of space*
4. *Appearance*—*use of clothing and other objects to communicate a personal image*

Table 8-1 illustrates the ways in which nonverbal messages are expressed.

FACTORS THAT INFLUENCE COMMUNICATION

Many factors influence the communication process. Culture, perceptions, values, social class, relationships, content of the message, and context of the message all contribute to the outcome of the communication process.

Culture

"Culture is communication and communication is culture" (King, Novik, and Citrenbaum, 1983). Culture influences all aspects of communication. People are taught by their culture how to communicate through verbal and nonverbal symbols such as language, gestures, facial expressions, clothing, and rituals. Cultural attitudes—including generalizations and stereotypes—influence how people see each other and relate to each other within and across cultural boundaries.

Psychiatric nurses continually meet clients from cultures different from their own. They are challenged to effectively communicate with clients who may speak a different language or for whom gestures, eye contact, clothing, or rituals have a far different meaning. For example, Asian clients often seek mental health treatment only as a final alternative. During initial meetings with mental health professionals, they do not maintain eye contact, engaging in polite small talk and taking care not to reveal personal information that would further expose their secret about a family member having a psychiatric problem. If the psychiatric nurse does not understand this cultural influence on communication, she or he may conclude that the client and/or family may be avoiding involvement in the treatment process. A conclusion like this can inhibit the development of effective communication. Rather, the nurse who understands the meaning of this cultural pattern respects the family and significant others, is patient, and engages in superficial conversation until the family feels enough trust to share more-personal thoughts and feelings (see Chapter 6).

Perceptions and Values

A *perception* *is a personal internal experience of the environment that influences how the communication is interpreted and understood.* Values are individualized rules by which persons live. Both perceptions and values are influenced by cultural and family socialization

Box 8-1

Implications of Nonverbal Communication for Nursing Practice

- Respond to nonverbal behavior by confirming and clarifying its meaning and significance to client through use of the following:
  - Facilitative questions that clarify and increase client awareness
  - Content and feeling reflection that attempts to validate client feelings, show acceptance, and request elaboration by the client
- Assess level of clients spatial tolerance by observing the distance the patient maintains with other people.
- Allow hospitalized clients, whenever possible, to control and enjoy personal possessions and private living space no matter how small or seemingly insignificant.
  - Encourage clients to wear personal clothing and keep personal items.
  - Allow clients free access to their personal living quarters.
  - Allow clients to have free access out of doors as soon as possible.
- Minimize control issues by having communication take place in a neutral area that belongs to neither person.
- Make communication easier by having both participants at similar levels when seated or standing.
- Use touch judiciously. Clients who are suspicious or sensitive to issues of closeness may perceive a casual touch as an invasion or invitation to intimacy that may even be more frightening.
- Clearly communicate explanations before and during procedures requiring physical contact.
- Recognize the potential for touch to be interpreted in a sexual way, thus creating problems related to the sexual conduct of the nurse within the nurse-client relationship.
- Recognize your own nonverbal cues that communicate interest, respect, and genuineness. Equally important is recognizing negative nonverbal cues that communicate boredom, judgmentalness, anger, or anxiety.
- Identify cultural differences in nonverbal communication through interventions that respect cultural variations.

processes and, in turn, influence the communication process. For example, in a culture where the open expression of feelings is positively valued, families may socialize their children to express both positive and negative feelings freely, even if uncontrolled outbursts of temper are the result. As an adult, a member of such a family may enter the mental health system through the emergency room after arrest for assault. The client and family may perceive this behavior as "letting off steam." However, both the legal and mental health systems would perceive this behavior as dysfunctional. The com-

TABLE 8-1

Ways in which nonverbal messages are expressed

EXPRESSION OF NONVERBAL MESSAGE	DEFINITION	IMPLICATIONS	EXAMPLES
Kinesics	Study of body motion:		
	• Facial expression	Single most important source of nonverbal messages.	Joe B. states, "I'm looking forward to being discharged from the hospital." However, the facial expression is frowning.
	• Posture	Reveals self-concept and mood state. Posture that is stooped or slumped versus erect and attentive often communicates a message of withdrawal and low self-esteem. Gait also relates to posture.	Amy R., a client with depression is observed sitting in a corner chair. Her posture indicates that her legs are tucked up, her arms crossed, and her head down buried in her arms.
	• Gestures	Body movements and gestures carry emotional messages that provide clues about how people feel about themselves and others. • Hand gestures convey indifference, relaxation, agitation, excitement • Fidgeting suggests unease, impatience, anxiety, or escalating aggressiveness	Ralph M. had been sitting quietly in the day treatment lounge. He began to fidget, run his hands through his hair, wordlessly shaking his head back and forth and shaking his leg. The nurse, knowing Ralph's history of aggressive episodes, assessed this nonverbal behavior as an indication of a potential explosive episode. She and two aides escorted Ralph to a quiet room before his agitation increased further.
	• Eye contact	Communicates level of interest or involvement with current interaction. Communicates feelings associated with the issue being discussed. Eye contact may be culturally related.	Ann P. felt a great deal of shame about her recent rape experience. She averted her eyes while haltingly discussing this traumatic event. People from Asian cultures regard direct eye contact as impolite; lack of direct eye contact from such clients is normal, not an expression of avoidance.
	• Touch	Conveys feelings that accentuate the way in which emotions are communicated. Touch communicates feelings that range from tenderness and warmth to anger and resentment.	Frances R., a withdrawn silent client, had been sitting with the nurse for 15 minutes a day for the past 4 days. Yesterday morning the nurse noticed Frances' hands resting on the arms of her chair. Today her fingers were making tentative movements toward the nurse's hand. As the nurse saw this happening, she reached out to be available to Frances if she indicated interest in this contact.

TABLE 8-1—cont'd

Ways in which nonverbal messages are expressed

EXPRESSION OF NONVERBAL MESSAGE	DEFINITION	IMPLICATIONS	EXAMPLES
			Frances moved her hand onto the nurse's open palm, rested it there, then curled her fingers around it. She sat back with a sigh, closed her eyes, and sat back quietly in her chair.
		It is important to be sensitive to cultural and personal norms and boundaries so that they are not violated (Tommasini, 1990).	Glenda B. had been sexually molested as a child. As an adult, she continued to feel dirty and thought that the touch of others would contaminate her. She even avoided introductory handshakes intended to convey friendliness.
Paralanguage	Paralinguistic behavior refers to the way in which the voice is used: • Tone of voice • Inflection • Spacing of words • Emphasis • Pauses • Nonlanguage vocalizations (e.g., grunting, laughing, and sobbing	Paralinguistic behavior is recognized by listening to nonword vocalizations, as well as tone of voice that either confirm, emphasize, or contradict verbal messages.	Bob F., a manic client, spoke rapidly in a loud voice, punctuated by bouts of hysterical laughter. In contrast, Paul B., a client with depression spoke softly, hesitantly, and without expression in his voice other than periodic sighs.
Appearance	Appearance refers to the way in which people use clothing and other objects to convey a message	Clothing, jewelry, hairstyle, beards, makeup, and eyeglasses are some of the articles that people put together in characteristic and unique ways. A change in a person's appearance can indicate developing problems.	When Nina K. was moving toward a manic state, her makeup became very bright and was applied too heavily. She dyed her hair with purple streaks and wore many pieces of jewelry and clothes in loud colors that did not match.
			In contrast, Ralph V., a retired man, 75 years of age, was always immaculately groomed and wore coordinated sports outfits. After the death of his wife, he was often observed in the street unshaven, wearing ragged, mismatched clothing and having strong body odor. Shortly thereafter he was hospitalized for severe depression.

Continued.

TABLE 8-1—cont'd

Ways in which nonverbal messages are expressed

EXPRESSION OF NONVERBAL MESSAGE	DEFINITION	IMPLICATIONS	EXAMPLES
Proxemics	Study of space and territory as it is used during personal transactions.	The amount of space (physical area) persons need, prefer, or desire defines their spatial requirements, as follows: • Territory is a specific limited space belonging to someone who defines its boundaries and controls it. People define homes, rooms, areas, pieces of furniture as their territories. They experience a sense of security when their territory is clearly demarcated and respected by others. Behavior that violates or intrudes on other's territory may elicit tension, defensiveness and aggression. • Distance zones are space requirements in relation to others. Four distance zones in North America are as follows: - Intimate space (up to 18 inches) allows for maximum sensory stimulation. - Personal space (18 inches to 4 feet) used for close relationships and touching distances. Visual sensation is improved over the intimate range. Voice level moderate. - Social-consultative space (9 to 12 feet) for less personal, business, and social relationships. Speech must be louder. - Public space (12 or more feet) used in issuing speeches and for other public occasions. Culture and geographic location influences the use of territory and distance by prescribing how, when, and who may use them without causing discomfort.	When Sandy B. came to the nurse's office, she always sat in the chair across from the nurse. If the nurse invited her to move her chair closer, she would say, "No, this is my zone. I don't ever come any closer and don't you either." Psychiatric clients define specific areas such as their room, dresser, or closet as belonging to them. They may also define an area of the hall, day room, or lounge, as well as a particular chair or couch as theirs, reacting possessively if someone intrudes on their territory.

munication process between family and nurse can become stalled if each party is unwilling to move beyond communicating its individual perception.

Social Class

Social class has a significant influence on communication. Verbal and nonverbal communication may differ between social classes in relation to slang, cliches, gestures, and appearance. Such differences may create communication barriers between people of different social classes. When nurses and clients are from different social classes, each may feel misunderstood and withdraw without trying to develop an effective nurse-client relationship. Nurses must be careful to communicate with clients in a way that is meaningful to the clients, explaining treatments in understandable language and inviting them to be collaborative partners in the treatment plan, even if they do not have all of the psychiatric terminology at their fingertips. Moreover, nurses must understand the environmental constraints with which clients from cultures of poverty must cope. Otherwise, such clients tend to withdraw from the health care system because they feel "put down" or misunderstood, as in the following example:

Rachel G., a single mother with six young children, is assigned to the mental health clinic for treatment of her depressive disorder. She arrives late for her therapy appointment with five of her six children trailing behind her. The nurse had planned to discuss depression and medication therapy with her. Because the nurse is running on a tight schedule and Rachel is late, she is annoyed and impatient. Tempted to lecture Rachel about lateness and then proceed to describe depression and her antidepressant medication in technical terms, she says, "No, I won't do that. It will be too overwhelming. That would be meeting my needs and would just turn Rachel off." Instead, in the 30 minutes of the session that remained, she invited Rachel and the children into her office, gave the children fruit rolls to eat and toys to play with, and encouraged Rachel to talk about her problems, her lack of social and financial supports, her transportation difficulties (three buses to get to the clinic), and her feelings of incompetence in managing her life. Rachel left the session feeling that the nurse was interested in her as a person and said she would be back next week with questions about her medication. The nurse thought about how she would deal with the "lateness" issue if it became a recurring incident.

Relationships

Another factor that influences communication is relationships between people. One aspect of relationships is known as level of relatedness, which is a function of both intimacy and perceived role status and authority.

Husband and wife, child and parent, or best friends will relate differently than will two people who are strangers or two other people, one of whom is the nurse, the other the client. Nurses will relate to their family members in a different way than they will relate to clients. Family relationships are much more intimate and close than the more professional, objective, and therapeutic nurse-client relationship. Clients may communicate with physicians in a way that differs greatly from the way they interact with nurses.

A second aspect of relationships is emotional climate. Whether the emotional climate is relaxed or tense will affect both *what* is communicated and *how* it is communicated, as in the following example:

The emotional climate on the psychiatric unit was uncharacteristically tense after the suicide of a client. However, it was not until the weekly community meeting 2 days later that the higher anxiety level was expressed by clients who angrily blamed the staff for not preventing the suicide of their peer. The clients chose the safety of a large group setting and anger to express fear about their own safety.

Content of the Message

The content of a message can either change or defuse the atmosphere of an interaction. When a client talks

TABLE 8-2

Words potentially toxic to clients and alternative words

TOXIC WORD	ALTERNATIVE WORD
Anxious	Nervous
	Upset
Guilty	At fault
	Responsible
	In error
Angry	Uptight
	Annoyed
	Irritated
	Dismayed
Blame	Responsibility
Masturbate	Self-pleasure
Forsaken	Distant
Abandoned	Left out
Humiliated	Belittled
	Minimized
	Unappreciated
Disgraced	Put down
Shame	Embarrassment
	Remorse
	Regret

about feeling worthless or enraged about a rape or incest experience, certain feelings are aroused that can affect how the message is sent and received. For example, Joan B. hinted that she had had a traumatic sexual experience. The nurse, depending on the feelings aroused by the potential emotional charge of the data, could either change the subject, ask questions that would yield a yes-or-no answer, or convey interest in hearing more about the traumatic experience. Many times nurses can defuse the intense, toxic, or charged nature of a message by being sensitive to emotionally charged words and using language skillfully.

Table 8-2 lists words that can be toxic to clients and the alternative word choices that will facilitate rather than inhibit communication.

Context of the Message

The context, or place, where the interaction takes place will influence the communication process. Nurses who expect clients to share personal thoughts and feelings must provide a private environment in which that self-disclosure can comfortably take place. The lounge, dayroom, or home are not private places; a private conference room, office, or separate room in the home is more appropriate.

PRINCIPLES OF THERAPEUTIC COMMUNICATION

Therapeutic communication is the hallmark of a therapeutic nurse-client relationship (Peplau, 1963). It is the art and process of reaching a person by means of verbal and nonverbal messages designed to facilitate health. Each message is deliberately chosen and considered in relation to each client's need for growth.

Therapeutic communication in nursing has the following five goals:

1. Exploration of the client's feelings, thoughts, behaviors, and experiences.
2. Distinguishing those thoughts, feelings, and behaviors that are functional from those that are not.
3. Assisting clients to make this distinction.
4. Understanding of the roles played by the client and other significant people that contribute to identified problems.
5. Action directed at resolving problematic areas of the client's life through the identification and implementation of alternative options.

THERAPEUTIC COMMUNICATION SKILLS

It is common for a beginning nurse not to know how to respond to a client or what to say next. Relying on social skills like those used for developing friendships has proven to be unsuccessful in establishing a therapeutic relationship with a client. Therefore nurses and other health professionals have developed a set of attending and responding strategies, called therapeutic communication skills, for developing effective relationships with clients (Egan, 1975; Egan, 1977). The following sections present attending and responding skills that can be used as guidelines for facilitating communication. It is important for the reader to understand that these are not intended as a set of rules. Communication and people are too complex for rules to be rigidly applied. Each nurse must modify the skills so that they fit his or her style—the stage of the nurse-client relationship—and adapt them so that they are relevant to each interaction.

Attending Skills

Therapeutic interactions require something that can be called presence. ***Presence involves being with a person both physically and psychologically and with a certain degree of intensity. Attending is using the self so as to communicate to another person that one is paying attention***—for example, that one is listening to what is being said. ***Attending skills involve physical skills (making the body attentive) and psychosocial skills (making the mind attentive).***

Physical attending skills

The body plays a large part in interpersonal communication. What is done with the body can emphasize, or on the other hand, confuse or contradict, a message that is being communicated in words.

For example, Marshall sat in a chair turned toward the wall in a corner of the dayroom. His knees were drawn up to his chest, his head rested on his knees, and his arms hugged his lap. Jana, his nurse, approached and said:

> "Hello, Marshall, I'd like to sit down and spend some time with you." Marshall did not move or respond verbally. Jana said, "I'm going to sit quietly with you for a few minutes." The lack of verbal response from Marshall confirmed the closed nature of his body posture and location in the dayroom.

It is impossible not to communicate with the body. What is done with the body and how it is done will either facilitate or inhibit the interactive process.

Six basic physical attending skills are as follows:

1. Facing the other person squarely. This is the basic posture of involvement. Facing another person squarely, or at a slight angle, says "I'm available to you; I choose to be with you." Turning the body away from another person while talking lowers the level of involvement with that person.

2. Adopting an open posture. Crossed arms and crossed legs can be signs of defensiveness or lessened involvement with others. An open posture, especially open arms, is a sign that the listener is open to the other person and to what he or she has to say. It is also considered a nondefensive position.

3. Leaning toward the other person. This is another sign of presence, availability, and involvement. It indicates that the listener is making a consistent effort to take in what the other person is communicating.

4. Maintaining direct eye contact. The listener should spend much of the time looking directly at the other person. Some people object to this idea; they say that this can be frightening or can make the other person uncomfortable. However, there is a difference between staring another person down (which may be an attack) and maintaining the direct eye contact indicative of interested involvement.

5. Creating a relaxed environment. The listener should sit or stand quietly without excessive movement and fidgeting. This does not imply that one should sit rigidly in a fixed position, which would communicate negative tension and discomfort. Relaxed posture communicates a natural readiness and ease in listening to what is being said. It says "I feel comfortable with you." Comfort relates to factors such as seating, lighting, noise level, and space. Seating should be comfortable, but not so relaxing that people want to go to sleep. Lighting should be soft, but bright; dim or glaring light is harsh and can be distracting. The noise level should be low so that it is not distracting. Space should meet the territorial needs of the people involved. Placement of persons and furniture should reflect boundary needs.

   It is important to observe how people use interpersonal space. Space can be used to increase or decrease interpersonal distance, and it is often an indicator of intimacy and involvement.

6. Creating privacy. It involves providing for privacy and comfort. Privacy is the degree to which people can interact without interference, distraction, and loss of confidentiality. Privacy is usually ensured by setting apart an area or room for the people who are interacting.

Psychosocial attending skills

Active listening is a psychosocial attending skill that involves listening to all the messages the other person is sending. It involves paying attention to two sources of messages, spoken words and nonverbal behavior. This type of listening is an active rather than a passive process; it conveys respect for the other person and thus will facilitate the development of relationships (Kemper, 1992; Sundeen et al., 1994).

The spoken word   The effective listener tries to hear both content and feelings that are being verbally communicated. The listener wants to know about the experiences, behavior, and underlying feelings of the speaker. This material enables the listener to identify patterns and themes that become important keys to understanding the person within his or her own frame of reference. Table 8-3 presents psychosocial listening skills and examples that relate to verbal messages (Egan, 1975).

Nonverbal behavior   Much of the meaning of a message—65% or more—is conveyed by nonverbal behavior, although many nonverbal behaviors are interpreted by verbal symbols. Verbal and nonverbal behaviors complement each other and consequently cannot be examined independently. The four major forms of nonverbal messages discussed earlier in the chapter—kinesics, paralanguage, proxemics, and appearance—can be seen as ways of:

1. Confirming what is being said
2. Strengthening and emphasizing what is being said
3. Adding emotional color to what is being said
4. Confusing or contradicting what is being said

Hence, verbal and nonverbal behavior fit together and function to confirm, complement, or contradict each other. The listener puts this information into context so that the communication can be understood and responded to appropriately.

Therapeutic Responding Strategies

Therapeutic responding strategies are ways of talking with clients that encourage them to communicate in a manner that facilitates their growth.

   Responding strategies should be direct and pertinent and contain words that are understood by the client. They should convey a clear meaning, allow for a response from the client, and be repeated as required by the client.

   Thirteen common therapeutic responding strategies are listed in Box 8-2. They can be used by nurses within the context of the nurse-client relationship and are discussed on the following pages.

Facilitative questions and statements

Facilitative questions and statements are sometimes referred to as broad openings and open-ended questions. Nurses use these strategies to encourage clients to discuss their problems in a descriptive manner in which various answers will be possible. Questions and statements of this kind encourage clients to express ideas and feelings in their own words. When facilitative ques-

TABLE 8-3

Psychosocial listening skills that relate to verbal messages

SKILL	EXAMPLE
1. Focus your complete attention on the speaker. Do not be preoccupied with yourself. Suspend thinking about your own experiences and problems and suspend personal judgments about the client.	Nurse: I told you that I would be back in a half hour, when I would be able to give you my complete attention. So [facing the client with direct eye contact], tell me how your job interview went.
2. Listen to everything that is being said. It is important to get a total picture of the person's verbal communication. Selective listening, which is often used to keep the anxiety of the listener in check, is ineffective because it may keep the listener from hearing important information. Examples of selective listening are hearing superficial instead of intimate things, praise instead of criticism, and positive parts of sentences instead of disturbing parts—or vice versa.	Client: I feel so worthless. I don't know how I get up in the morning. Nurse: Tell me more about that feeling of worthlessness. It sounds like it's draining you, and I'd like to get a more complete picture of it.
3. Analyze the verbal message that is being communicated. A speaker may relate both relevant and irrelevant information. The listener needs to sort it out and come up with the essence of the message so that he or she can begin to make sense of what is being heard.	Client: I left the house, I wandered around, I visited a couple of people, I don't know, I just don't know . . . Nurse: It sounds like you were feeling lost or directionless at that point . . . Client: Yes, yes, that's it!
4. Identify themes and patterns in the verbal communication. After the sorting process has taken place, the listener will realize that there is a structure to what is being expressed. Themes and patterns relate to this structure and convey underlying meanings. Examples of themes and patterns are feelings of powerlessness at work, excessive reliance on others for positive feelings about self, talking only in a positive way, and avoiding talking about personal strengths. Identification of themes and patterns enables the listener to respond with understanding.	Client: I go out socially and feel like I'm going to panic. I sit home and think about it and that happens. I feel like something awful will happen if I let them [people] get too close. Nurse: From what you've told me on several occasions, closeness makes you feel uneasy, and you aren't sure about your ability to control how close people get to you.
5. Summarizing the content and feelings that have been expressed. It is important to summarize not only content but also feelings.	Nurse: If I had to summarize what I've heard you say, it seems like feeling that you can be in charge of yourself is a major concern.

tions and statements are used, clients improve their ability to observe, describe, and analyze their thoughts, feelings, and experiences. Steps 1, 2, and 3 in Table 8-4 illustrate examples of this process.

In contrast, strictly structured questions that limit response options are inappropriate except for obtaining narrowly factual answers. For example, the question "Who was with you?" has a limited range of possible answers: family, friends, strangers, and their names. However, if you want only the names of the people, then a structured question of this kind *is* appropriate. An open-ended, facilitative phrasing of the question would be, "Tell me about the people you were with." Such phrasing would tend to uncover not only who the other people were but also something about each of them.

Reflection

Reflection *involves two dimensions of communication: content and feeling.* Reflecting the content of a message means repeating a client's basic statement. This provides the client with an opportunity to hear and think about what he or she has said. The danger inherent in content reflection is that it can become simply hollow repetition, and the nurse can end up sounding like a parrot. If content reflection is misused or overused, it will not be therapeutically effective. Here is an example of content reflection:

Client: I'm so discouraged. I thought I'd be home from the hospital today.
Nurse: You sound upset that you're not going home.

Box 8-2

Therapeutic Responding Strategies

1. Facilitative questions and statements
2. Reflection
3. Restatement
4. Focusing
5. Clarifying
6. Conveying information
7. Providing feedback
8. Stating observations
9. Connecting islands of information
10. Confrontation
11. Summarizing
12. Silence
13. Humor

Reflection of feelings means verbalizing what is implied or hinted at by a client. In reflecting feelings the nurse seeks to identify the underlying meaning of content. Themes, patterns, and indirect expressions of thoughts and feelings emerge as the nurse considers what the client is really expressing. The nurse goes beyond what the client has explicitly stated and provides additional material for the client to consider. Verbalizing the implied is useful because it helps provide an objective picture of the situation and helps the client view problems in greater depth and with increased accuracy. It also encourages the client to make additional clarifying comments. Here is an example of reflection of feelings:

Client: I'm so discouraged. I thought I'd be home from the hospital today.

Nurse: It sounds as though you feel discouraged because you're still in the hospital and you expected more of yourself than has happened. Tell me more about what you are thinking.

Client: Yes, I thought I would feel less depressed by now. I always expect a lot of myself; my family does too.

Nurse: Your progress is slower than you anticipated. Perhaps you feel disappointed in yourself?

Client: Yes, in the past I've always looked forward to going home and picking up my responsibilities, but this time . . .

Nurse: It sounds as if this time you're not sure you can do it.

Client: I don't think I can do it in the same way. Maybe that's better; I should think of how I can change what I expect of myself.

Lead-in words or statements such as "It seems as if," "It appears to me," "I am hearing a lot of," or "Perhaps you"

are good openers to reflective interventions. This responding strategy is also illustrated in Steps 3 and 4 of Table 8-4.

Restatement

A nurse can convey understanding of what a client has just said by **restatement.** *This means that the nurse paraphrases the main content and feeling of the client's message, using new (and probably fewer) words.* Paraphrasing also helps to highlight important parts of the client's message that might otherwise be lost or obscured by details. Restatement indicates that the nurse is listening to the client and trying to enter and understand the client's frame of reference. This *identification with the client is called* **empathy** and is therapeutic because it makes clients feel understood, and encouraged to continue sharing inner thoughts and feelings with their understanding listener (Alligood, 1992). The following dialogue illustrates the use of restatement as a form of empathy.

Client: I don't know what's going on. I study hard, but I just don't get good marks. I think I study as hard as anyone else, but all my efforts seem to go down the tube. I don't know what else to do.

Nurse: It sounds as if you feel frustrated because even when you think you try hard, you don't get the result you want. Perhaps you also feel a little sorry for yourself.

Client: That's exactly it. I think the feeling sorry part is even worse than the frustration.

The lead-ins suggested for reflection can also be used appropriately with restatement. Steps 4 and 5 of Table 8-4 also illustrate this type of responding strategy.

The use of empathy by a nurse is an important aspect of therapeutic communication. Furthermore, it is the client's perception of being understood in an empathic way that is associated with a reduction of tension, stress, and anxiety. The Perception of Empathy Inventory (PEI) developed by Wheeler (1990) measures the client's perception of the nurse's empathy.

Focusing

Focusing is a responding strategy that creates order, guidelines, and priorities. The nurse assists the client in identifying problems and establishing their relative importance, which helps establish an order for dealing with them. Such structuring can help clients who present a wide array of problems, have no idea of which problems are most important, and do not know where to begin working on them. Focusing can also take the form of establishing contract guidelines (time, place, length of treatment, fee, and so forth) for nurse-client interactions. An example of a focusing statement follows:

TABLE 8-4

Facilitative questions and statements that improve client's ability to process ideas, feelings, and experiences

STEP	EXAMPLE
1. Observe—to notice what went on or what goes on	Tell me about yourself. Could I share that thought with you? Tell me, what did you notice? Tell me every detail from the beginning. To what degree do you feel that way? Then what? Go on. . . .
2. Describe—to be able to recall and tell the details and circumstances of a particular event or experience	Tell me more. Give me an example. Describe that further. If you remain the same, how would you envision yourself 10 years from now? What did you feel at the time? What happened just before? How did she respond to your comment? What did you feel at the time?
3. Analyze—to be able to review and work over the data with another person to gain greater understanding	Please explain. Help me to understand that. What do you mean? What was the importance of that event? What do you see as the reason? How do you think that happens to you over and over again? What was your part in it?
4. Formulate—to be able to restate in a clear, direct way the relationship between thoughts, feelings, and experiences	What would you say was the problem? Tell me again. Can you tell me the essence of the problem?
5. Validate—to be able to confirm with an-other person one's thoughts, feelings, and perceptions	Is this what you meant? Let me restate. Is this what you were saying? Tell me again how you see it. Am I correct in concluding that? If I hear you correctly, you are telling me . . . Are you saying that . . . ?
6. Test—the ability to try out new thoughts, feelings, or behaviors	What would you do if a situation like this came up again? In what way can you use this conclusion to prevent playing a passive role again? What difference will it make now that you know this? In what way will this understanding help you in the future?

Adapted from Peplau, H. (1963). Process and concept of learning. In S. Burd & M. Marshall (Eds.), Some clinical approaches to psychiatric nursing. *New York: MacMillan.*

Nurse: You've described several problems to me. As I hear them, they would be loneliness, dissatisfaction with your schoolwork, obesity, emotional distance from your father, and inability to be assertive. Which one would you say is most important, and which would you want to begin work on first?

Focusing also involves keeping the flow of communication goal directed, specific, and concrete. It helps clients to be clear rather than vague, specific rather than general, oriented to reality rather than oriented to fantasy, and purposeful rather than rambling. This focusing keeps discussions concentrated on central issues related to important problems. Related techniques such as encouraging description, placing events in time sequence, and encouraging comparisons can be used to promote specificity and analysis of problems. An example of focusing follows:

Client: I feel so down today . . .
Nurse: Tell me more about what you are thinking and feeling . . .
Client: I'm so tired. I feel like lead. I feel sad too. I could cry at the drop of a hat . . .
Nurse: How long have you been feeling that way?

This responding strategy is illustrated in step 3 of Table 8-4.

Clarifying

Clarifying demonstrates the nurse's desire to understand the client's communication (Sundeen, et al., 1994). Clarification is often necessary because client's communications are not always direct and straightforward when clients are out of touch with reality, intoxicated, or reluctant to share feelings with another person. The nurse should not hesitate to let a client know (tactfully) that something is not understood. A client's communication may be confused, fragmented, disorganized, symbolic, hesitant, or incomplete. If the nurse allows communication to continue in this way without seeking clarification, the client will not know that he or she is not understood. Valuable time will be wasted, opportunities for feedback and correction will be missed, and a serious problem may remain undiscovered. In addition, the client may develop doubts about the nurse's ability to understand. Clients are perceptive; they soon come to recognize nurses who pretend to understand but do not.

Clarifications are often tentative, phrased as general questions or statements: "I'm not sure I'm following what you're saying. Are you saying that . . . ?" or "Could you go over that again, please?" At other times clarification can take the form of a specific question such as asking a client to clarify a particular idea or feeling that is confusing to either the client or the nurse. Consider, for ex-

ample, an interaction in which a depressed client is attempting to differentiate between what she *wants* to do for herself and what she feels she *should* do for herself:

Client: I just want to break free and do things that I want to do. But I shouldn't want that, because I should be acting like a responsible person . . . Oh, it's so confusing . . .
Nurse: Let's take a moment to clarify what you're thinking. Are you saying that there is an irresponsible child part of you and a responsible adult part of you, and that you can't fit the two together into a whole person that functions smoothly.
Client: Yes, that's it, it's very confusing. I feel as if I'm going to be either one or the other, either totally irresponsible or entirely responsible. Either extreme is exhausting.
Nurse: Well, what other alternative can you come up with?

Clarification allows the nurse to confirm or verify her perception of the client's message or behavior. This process is also illustrated in steps 5 and 6 of Table 8-4.

Conveying information

Information is conveyed to a client by making statements that supply data. New input encourages further clarification. Withholding useful information may prevent the client from making informed choices or decisions. When a client is seeking direct information, the nurse should not ask the client what he or she thinks is the answer. In most cases, if the client knew the answer, the information would not have been requested. When *conveying information,* nurses need to avoid giving advice or providing interpretations, as in the following example:

Client: I feel nauseous and have diarrhea. Why do I feel so sick?
Nurse: You may be having side effects from the lithium you're taking. Let me check your latest lithium level.

Providing feedback

Feedback involves giving constructive information to clients about how the nurse perceives and hears them. The nurse describes his or her perceptions about clients' thoughts, feelings, and behaviors in interactions. This feedback offers the clients an opportunity to verify, modify, or correct the nurse's perceptions. It also provides an opportunity for clients to see how others perceive them. Feedback of this kind serves as a validation system ensuring that the nurse accurately understands the client.

Feedback also provides clients with an opportunity to examine and integrate their own conflicting or scattered thoughts and feelings, as in the following example:

Client: I don't know what I believe about myself any more. I still hear my dad telling me that I'm destined to be a great achiever. But I also hear him telling me that I'm too weak to stand up under pressure.

Nurse: What I'm hearing you say is that you live with two opposing scripts: a "you will be great" script and a "you will be a failure" script. Those scripts sound contradictory. It's not surprising to me that you feel confused.

Client: That's right. Which script do I believe? Which is the real me? How do I sort that out?

Step 5 of Table 8-4 also illustrates the strategy of providing feedback.

Stating observations

Stating observations involves descriptions by the nurse of interpersonal dynamics in the nurse-client relationship. These dynamics explain connections between overt behavior and underlying thoughts and feelings in nurse and client. They enable feelings having to do with transference and countertransference to surface for examination, clarification, and resolution. Stating observations is most appropriately used when trust has been established in the nurse-client relationship. Following is an example of stating observations:

Nurse: You were telling me about fighting with your mom this weekend, and suddenly you began fidgeting and looked away, and then you got up to take a walk. When I called to you, you told me to go to hell.

Client: That's right—shove it.

Nurse: I wonder how you feel when I encourage you to talk about something that makes you uncomfortable.

Steps 2 and 3 of Table 8-4 illustrate how stating observations encourages the client to describe and analyze thoughts, feelings, and behavior.

Making connections

Nurses assist clients in **making connections** between *feelings, thoughts, experiences, and behavior. This process helps the client connect seemingly isolated phenomena by filling in blanks and establishing relationships.*

The nurse must strive for accuracy in making such connections and present them collaboratively to the client as theories for consideration, not as statements of fact. It may take considerable discussion between nurse and client for an accurate picture to be established. For example, a nurse and client were working toward identifying factors contributing to the client's social withdrawal, particularly her reluctance to engage in relationships with men. The following interaction took place:

Client: I'm uncomfortable, really anxious, in a social situation. Not so much with adults, people older than myself, but more with my peers.

Nurse: Have you thought about what it is about relating with young men and women, as opposed to older adults, that makes you tense and want to withdraw?

Client: With older people, I feel that I know what to say and how to act. I know the "good little girl" role very well. But with friends . . .

Nurse: Are you saying that a parent-child or adult-child interaction is a known, comfortable situation that you don't feel the same urge to run from?

Client: Yes. It's as if I know they'll take care of me; I may not like it, but it will be basically okay.

Nurse: What do you suppose the connection is between relating with peers, feeling anxious, and needing to withdraw socially?

Client: I have to be adult in that kind of relationship, you know, be responsible for myself. I don't think I can do that. I'm petrified of being an adult with another adult.

This example provides an abbreviated version of the kind of interaction needed to connect islands of information and find a pattern; an actual interaction might take much more time. The nurse and client in the above example might have had to connect many more pieces of data before a complete picture was formulated. Steps 3 to 6 of Table 8-4 illustrate the process of making connections.

Confrontation

Confrontation is a responding strategy that encourages congruence between verbal and nonverbal communication. Confrontation calls attention to discrepancies between what the client says (verbal communication) and what the client does (nonverbal communication). This process involves describing the message you are perceiving, describing the perceived contradiction, smoke screen, distortion, or evasion in the words the client has used, and waiting for a client response (Egan, 1975).

Contradiction: I hear you tell me that your husband doesn't care about you because he hasn't visited you, but you told me you sent him a letter asking him not to visit you. I'm confused.

Distortion: I understand what makes you mistrust your brother, but what is it that makes you think that all other people will also betray you?

Games, smoke screens: I appreciate your wanting to discuss in private what happened in the group tonight, but I'm a little uncomfortable being singled out like this. I think that all of us should look at the level of trust in the group.

Evasions: I have a sense of vagueness when you tell me you're angry with your husband. I don't

Box 8-3

Assessment Factors Related to Confrontation

- The client's stress level
- The client's level of anger and volatility and tolerance for hearing another perception
- The stage and related level of trust in the nurse-client relationship
- The client's need for personal space or closeness
- The strength of the client's defense mechanisms
- The nurse's comfort level and available support systems

hear what it is he does that makes you feel unappreciated.

Steps 1 to 5 of Table 8-4 illustrate therapeutic questions and statements that can be used effectively with confrontation. Box 8-3 lists assessment factors to be considered before using confrontation with clients.

Confrontation must be timed appropriately to be effective. In the initial stages of the nurse-client relationship, confrontation is used infrequently. In this situation, the nurse states his or her observations about contradictory behavior. In the working phase of the relationship, confrontation is used more frequently and directly by focusing on discrepancies between words and actions, distortions, evasions, and smoke screens such as when the client demonstrates insight about the effect of drinking behavior on his marriage but continues to exhibit daily drinking behavior. Inexperienced nurses often avoid confrontation, fearing it will be hurtful or destructive to the client. Indeed it can be nontherapeutic if it is used to vent the nurse's feelings of anger, frustration, or futility. However, research indicates that effective helpers use confrontation often, confronting clients with their assets more often in earlier interviews and with their limitations in later sessions. Whenever confrontation is used, it should be communicated in a nonjudgmental manner that conveys caring and encourages the client to expand their awareness and grow (Balzer-Riley, 1996).

Summarizing

Giving feedback to a client about the general substance of an interview or a portion of the interview, as seen by the nurse, is called **summarizing.** This technique unifies a number of pieces of information into main themes of content and feeling. By highlighting the most significant data, the nurse can determine with the client the progress they have made and whether the information obtained is accurate. They can also use these data for making future plans. This cooperative nurse-client interaction gives clients a sense of contributing to the resolution of their problems and thus reaffirms their sense of self-worth and feelings of being understood. An example of a summary statement follows (the client is a middle-age man fighting alcohol abuse):

Client: I know drinking doesn't really help me in the long run. And it sure doesn't help my family. My wife keeps threatening to leave. I know all this. But it's hard to stay away from the booze. Having a drink makes me feel relieved.

Nurse: You're aware of some of the ways that drinking is not very helpful to you [summarization of content], yet you feel better, less overwhelmed, after a drink [summarization of affect].

Steps 4 and 5 of Table 8-4 provide other examples of questions and statements that help nurses to effectively summarize client communication.

Humor

Constructive humor is a responding strategy that helps communication by breaking down barriers, by making people feel good, and by bringing people closer together (Buxman, 1988; Davidhizer, 1992; Balzer-Riley, 1996). It can also neutralize emotionally charged interpersonal events. To be able to laugh at a tough situation provides temporary relief from stress, fear, or worry (Balzer-Riley, 1996). Through the use of humor, clients may be able to "jokingly" express feelings of fear or embarrassment. Clients may "test the water" by bringing up a secretly serious subject through the use of light banter to see how it is received by the nurse.

Client: I'm going to go to the dance at church Friday night, but who do you think would want to dance with an "ugly devil" like me?

Nurse: It sounds like you are making light of a real concern. Would you like to tell me what really worries you about this? I'd be glad to listen.

Genuine interest on the part of the nurse provides an accepting environment for the client to express his or her deeper concerns. In contrast, humor also provides a vehicle for the nurse and client to share their humanness. For example, a client tensely tells the nurse about how he missed the bus to work, arrived late, and discovered that he had put his shirt on inside out. The nurse smiles and tells him she can empathize because just yesterday she arrived at work and noticed that she was wearing two different shoes. The client chuckled and said, he thought he was the only one to whom these embarrassing things happened. This interaction provided some comic relief at a time when the client felt overwhelmed by his own inadequacies. He was able to verbalize that everyone is human.

Nurses must exercise judgment about deciding with which clients it is appropriate to use humor. For exam-

Text continued on p. 140.

TABLE 8-5

Barriers to therapeutic communication

BARRIERS	DYNAMICS	NONTHERAPEUTIC EXAMPLES	THERAPEUTIC EXAMPLES
Giving advice	The nurse offers solutions and advises the client about what course of action to take. This approach denies the client's ability to formulate solutions to problems and assume responsibility for the direction of his or her life, devalues the client, and keeps the nurse in a position of control.	"Why don't you _____" "If I were you _____" "It would be best if _____" "Let me suggest _____"	"I hear what you are saying." "What would you suggest?" "What other alternatives have you come up with?"
Giving false reassurance	The nurse offers information to the client that is not based on fact and truth, and differs from conveying information or giving realistic feedback. Reassurance denies the client's right to the feelings being experienced and closes off communication about them. All the client's real feelings remain undiscussed and unexplored. This action shows the client that his or her feelings are not being taken seriously. It is also a self-protective action of the nurse who cannot listen to the client's painful feelings.	"Don't worry." "You'll feel better tomorrow." "Everybody feels that way." "It's not that bad." "Things always look worse before they get better."	"What worries you about that?" "This is a difficult time for you _____" "Tell me what you are thinking." "What's the worst thing about this for you?"
Changing the subject	The nurse diverts the focus of the interaction at crucial times to something less threatening. Changing the subject usually occurs when the nurse is unwilling or unable to listen to painful feelings being expressed by the client. This communicates to the client that the nurse cannot stand to hear what the client has to say and is not able to talk about what is important to the client. Communication may remain superficial.	"Let's discuss that later _____" "Let's leave that and talk about _____" "I forgot that I wanted to ask you about _____"	"That sounds important, so go on and tell me more." "I know that's painful for you to talk about, but try to tell me how you're feeling." "Let's look at that further."

TABLE 8-5—cont'd

Barriers to therapeutic communication

BARRIERS	DYNAMICS	NONTHERAPEUTIC EXAMPLES	THERAPEUTIC EXAMPLES
Being judgmental	The nurse responds to the client with value-laden judgments that come from the nurse's value system. Those are critical evaluative statements that label the client and do not convey acceptance of him or her as a unique person. Being judgmental conveys stereotyped attitudes toward others and lack of acceptance of individual differences. The client is only approved and accepted if he or she conforms to the nurse's values.	"You're wrong." "I should have known—all you men are alike." "You're just another lazy teenager—you have it too good at home." "What right do you have to consider an abortion? You're married."	"Your interpretation is different. I'd like to hear more about how you see the situation." "I've heard other men express that point of view. I'd like to understand where you're coming from when you say that." "How difficult is it for you to be moving toward independence?" "I may not agree with your decision, but I can understand your reasons for arriving at that choice."
Giving directions	The nurse approaches the client with specific directions to be followed and often lectures the client about the advisability of following this course of action. This approach denies the client's ability to think through and arrive at solutions to problems. It reinforces and maintains the dependent-child position of the client. It is a protective maneuver for the nurse who has difficulty sharing control and power.	"That's not the way _____." "These are the facts—this is the way it should be done." "You must follow these directions." "Listen to me _____"	"Which do you think would be best?" "Let's look at your options." "Can you come up with another way to accomplish this?" "How would you approach this situation?"
Excessive questioning	Excessive questioning on the part of the nurse controls the nature and range of the client's responses. The nurse can be perceived by the client as an interrogator who is demanding information without respect for the client's ability or readiness to respond. Strictly structured questions limit the client's responses to yes, no, and naming of facts. Questions that ask why tend to make the client feel defensive: often he or she does not	"Why do you feel that way?" "What's the real reason?" "Where have you been?" "Do you feel angry?"	"What was happening when you began to feel that way?" "Tell me more about that." "I've missed you. Can you tell me what's been happening with you?" "Can you describe in words how you're feeling right now?"

Continued.

TABLE 8-5—cont'd

Barriers to therapeutic communication

BARRIERS	DYNAMICS	NONTHERAPEUTIC EXAMPLES	THERAPEUTIC EXAMPLES
	know why. Thus a stressful rather than a helpful situation is created. Excessive questioning by the nurse is self-protective. It initially reduces the nurse's anxiety by filling in gaps in an interaction. However, the client may feel overwhelmed and may ultimately withdraw.		
Using emotionally charged words	The nurse uses emotionally charged words with the client who cannot tolerate or accept such feelings. The client may withdraw physically or emotionally. Clients often have much shame and embarrassment about their feelings, especially those they perceive as negative, and they have difficulty communicating them to another person. The nurse who uses words like *angry, guilty,* and *hostile* before the client is ready to hear or speak them is misjudging the client's pace and risks losing the client's involvement. When more comfortable with feelings, the client will choose comfortable words to illustrate an experience. The nurse should use low-key words that the client uses and is comfortable with (see Table 8-3).	"Your mother makes you feel pretty angry." "You feel guilty about what happened." "You describe your wife as acting crazy."	"How do you feel about what she did?" "I wonder whether you feel at all responsible for what happened?" "You describe your wife's behavior as having changed in the past week."
Challenging	The nurse sometimes feels that if the client is challenged to prove unrealistic ideas or perceptions, the client will realize that there is no proof to support such ideas and will be forced to acknowledge what is true. The nurse forgets that unrealistic thoughts, perceptions, and feelings serve a purpose	"You can't be the president of that company!" "You can't really hear the devil saying that you're wicked."	"It sounds as though you'd like to be able to think of yourself as an important person." "The voices you say you hear seem to make you feel that you haven't lived up to your beliefs and values."

TABLE 8-5—cont'd

Barriers to therapeutic communication

BARRIERS	DYNAMICS	NONTHERAPEUTIC EXAMPLES	THERAPEUTIC EXAMPLES
	for the client and will not be given up until that purpose can be fulfilled in healthier ways. When challenged, the client feels threatened and tends to cling to and expand such misinterpretations because they provide support for his or her point of view.		
Making stereotypical comments	Offering trite expressions and meaningless cliches as responses diminishes the value of the nurse-client interaction. Such comments by the nurse imply lack of understanding of a client's uniqueness. Nothing about either the client or the nurse is really communicated by such statements, which create or maintain distance because the nurse is acting in a mechanical way as a substitute for giving a more personal, considered response. The nurse communicates an unwillingness to delve further into the client's feelings. Behind a nurse's automatic responses may be equally stereotyped attitudes.	"You're looking chipper today, Tom." "Keep your chin up, Mary; it won't be much longer now."	"I've noticed you smiling a few times this morning. Is that an indication of how you're feeling?" "How difficult is it for you to keep your motivation at a high level?"
Self-focusing behavior	Self-focusing behavior is characterized by the nurse's excessive interest in or preoccupation with his/her own thoughts, feelings, or actions. When thoughts or feelings involve total self-absorption, they detract from or interfere with effective interaction with the client and fulfillment of the interview goals. In cognitive self-focusing, the nurse devotes less attention to what the client is saying and more attention to answering the	Nurse (thinking to himself or herself: Now what? What do I say? What if he doesn't answer? What did he say he was thinking before? Then aloud): "Oh, excuse me; could you repeat that? I didn't hear what you said."	The nurse caught her attention wandering as she worried about her ability to communicate therapeutically. She noticed that she was not listening as attentively as she should and knew she should validate whether she had heard the client's message accurately. "If I understand you correctly, Mr. Brown, you said that . . ."

Continued.

TABLE 8-7—cont'd

Barriers to therapeutic communication

BARRIERS	DYNAMICS	NONTHERAPEUTIC EXAMPLES	THERAPEUTIC EXAMPLES
	client correctly, asking the right follow-up question, or having another question to ask if the first does not work. Self-focusing occurs when the nurse verbalizes his or her own feelings during an interview and does not focus on those of the client.		
Double-bind messages	The nurse delivers two conflicting messages, one verbal, the other nonverbal. The nonverbal message contradicts the verbal message. It is unclear which message is to be obeyed. There is also an injunction against noticing that the contradiction exists. As a result, the client is unable to confront the inconsistency to determine which is the real message. The client may feel paralyzed about selecting a course of action and feel that there is no escape from the situation.	Client: "I get these sudden bursts of temper. I don't know what comes over me. It's like I'm going to explode. Am I scaring you? [notices nurses's fidgeting] . . ." Nurse: "No, not at all. I'm interested in what you have to say [picks her nails, no eye contact, fidgets in chair] . . . Tell me more [continues to fidget, runs hands through hair, skin color pales] . . ." Client [thinking to herself]: Is she scared or not? I don't know whether she really wants me to continue.	Client: "I get these sudden bursts of temper. I don't know what comes over me. It's like I'm going to explode. Am I scaring you? [notices nurse's fidgeting] . . ." Nurse: "It sounds scary to have such intense feelings that you seem not to be able to control. I think it does make me uncomfortable more than secure to hear such intensity. But I'm not scared of you." Client: I was confused by your fidgeting. I didn't know if I should go on." Nurse: "I'm glad you told me that so I could clarify the matter for you. Please go on . . ."

ple, clients who are suspicious and paranoid may misinterpret humor as a personal attack.

Silence

Silence is a responding strategy that gives the nurse and the client a way to interact without words. It is a period during which the nurse waits without interruption for the client to begin or resume thinking. Silence gives clients an opportunity to collect and organize their thoughts and thereby increase their awareness of their problems. Silence can also convey acceptance, concern, support, and the message that talking is not always necessary in a therapeutic relationship. A comfortable silence lets clients see the nurse as a person who is willing to let them give cues as to when the conversation will begin again, as in the following example:

Gary W., a client, had been discussing his father's death at age 35 and his own panic attacks, including chest pain and choking sensations, that began following his thirty-fourth birthday. He describes walking into his father's bedroom and being unable to wake him up from his nap. Gary's voice tapers off, and he becomes silent, looking down at his hands in his lap. The nurse uses the silence as an opportunity to observe Gary, assess his level of anxiety, allow him to collect his thoughts and feelings, and wait for him to respond. Approximately 5 minutes elapse, during which the nurse sits quietly, maintaining eye contact and an interested, open posture. Gary raises his head and says, "I can't believe the rush of memories that just went through my head. I needed those few minutes to just let them wash over me. Thank you for being patient with me."

Although silence is an effective communication skill, competence is needed to employ it correctly. Socially, most people do not feel comfortable with silence. If there are lulls in a conversation, people feel that something is wrong. Therefore it is not unusual for a nurse to feel this way about silence during a nurse-client interaction. Nurses may feel compelled to break silences because they are self-conscious and uncomfortable. Nurses may need to practice this skill often before they can use it with confidence.

Therapeutic communication skills are used throughout the nurse-client relationship—when it is initiated, as it progresses, and when it is terminated. The use of communication skills in this context will be explored in detail in Chapter 9. The skills are also used during the assessment process, when data about client, family, and community are being collected. While working with clients and colleagues, nurses will find that therapeutic communication skills are invaluable in establishing and conducting effective interpersonal relationships.

BARRIERS TO THERAPEUTIC COMMUNICATION

In the previous section, skills for therapeutic communication were presented. It is important for the nurse to realize that there are also barriers to therapeutic communication. Barriers are an inevitable part of the communication process: they are protective behaviors that arise when clients perceive interactions as threatening and likely to increase self-exposure, insecurity, and helplessness. If barriers are unchecked, they will prevent the nurse and client from continuing the work of the interaction by interfering with each person's ability to attend and respond to the messages the other sends. When barriers to therapeutic communication occur, the primary goals for the nurse are to (1) recognize that a barrier exists, (2) identify the purpose or need served by such a behavior, (3) identify appropriate alternative therapeutic behavior, and (4) implement the alternative therapeutic behavior in the interaction so that therapeutic communication can be resumed. Table 8-5 summarizes barriers to therapeutic communications that are commonly experienced by nurses.

KEY POINTS

- Communication is a continuous circular process by which information is transmitted between people and their environment.

- Communication consists of verbal and nonverbal messages. Verbal messages are communicated through language. Nonverbal messages are expressed through kinesics, paralanguage, proxemics, and appearance.
- Factors that influence communication include culture, perceptions, values, social class, relationships, content of the message, and context of the message.
- Therapeutic attending skills are listening skills and include physical and psychosocial attending skills.
- Therapeutic responding strategies are ways of talking with clients that encourage them to communicate in a manner that facilitates their growth. These strategies are ways of helping clients engage in a process of self-explanation, self-understanding, and change.
- Barriers to therapeutic communication are protective behaviors that arise when interactions are threatening and likely to increase self-exposure, insecurity, and helplessness. If barriers are unchecked, they will prevent the nurse-client relationship from developing in an effective manner.

 CRITICAL THINKING QUESTIONS

Ginny is an attractive, articulate 25-year-old woman with a diagnosis of depression who is stylishly dressed at all times. She is often sought out by other clients in the day treatment program who want to talk to her or do activities with her. However, Ginny repeatedly talks about her feelings of low self-esteem. She feels unattractive and states that she is unpopular because she is ugly and unappealing.

Based on the data:

1. Which responding strategy would you select to deal with Ginny's communication?
2. What is your rationale for this choice?
3. Differentiate between constructive and destructive confrontation.
4. Explain the relationship between use of confrontation and stages of the nurse-client relationship.
5. What self-assessment factors must nurses consider when using confrontation as a responding strategy?

REFERENCES

Alligood, M.R. (1992). Empathy: The importance of recognizing two types. *Journal of Psychosocial Nursing, 30,* 3, 14-17.

Balzer-Riley, J. (1996). *Communications in nursing: Communicating assertively & responsibly in nursing: A guidebook.* St. Louis: Mosby.

Buxman, K. (1991). Humor in therapy for the mentally ill. *Journal of Psychosocial Nursing, 29,* 6, 31-35.

Davidhizar, R. & Bowen, M. (1992). The dynamics of laughter. *Archives of Psychiatric Nursing, 6,* 132-136.

Egan, G. (1975). *The skilled helper.* Belmont, CA: Wadsworth.

Egan, G. (1977). *You and me.* Monterey, CA: Brooks/Cole.

Kemper, B.J. (1992). Therapeutic listening: Developing the concept. *Journal of Psychosocial Nursing, 30,* 7, 21-26.

King, M., Novik, L., & Citrenbaum, C. (1983). *Irresistible communication: Creative skills for the health professional.* Philadelphia: W.B. Saunders.

Northouse, P.G., & Northouse, L. (1992). *Health communication strategies for health professionals* (2nd ed.). Englewood Cliffs, NJ: Prentice-Hall.

Peplau, H. (1963). Process and concept of learning. In S. Burd & M. Marshall (Eds.). *Some clinical approaches to psychiatric nursing.* New York: Macmillan.

Ruesch, J. (1968). *Therapeutic communication.* New York: W.W. Norton.

Sundeen, S.J., Stuart, G.W., Rankin, E.A.D., & Cohen, S.A. (1994). *Nurse-client interaction: Implementing the nursing process* (5th ed.). St. Louis: Mosby.

Tommasini, N.R. (1990). The use of touch with the hospitalized psychiatric patient. *Archives of Psychiatric Nursing, 4,* 213-220.

Wheeler, K. (1990). Perception of empathy inventory. In O. Strickland & C. Waltz (Eds.). *Measurement of nursing outcomes* (Vol. 4). New York: Springer.

VIDEO RESOURCES

Mosby's Communication in Nursing Video Series:

Basic Principles for Communicating Effectively in Nursing

Communicating with Clients and Colleagues: Effectiveness in the Caring Environment

Communicating with Clients and Colleagues from Different Cultures

Communicating with Difficult Clients and Colleagues

Communicating with Clients with Mental Disorders or Emotional Problems

Communicating Across the Life Span: Children, Families, and the Elderly

Chapter 9

The Nurse-Client Relationship

Anita Leach McMahon

LEARNING OUTCOMES

After studying and applying the concepts of this chapter, the learner will be able to:
- Analyze the components of the self system.
- Apply the process of self-awareness and principles of therapeutic use of self to therapeutic nurse-client relationships.
- Discuss the nature of therapeutic relationships as they exist in today's health care environment.
- List the components of the counseling role of nurses.
- Trace the historical evolution of counseling strategies used by psychiatric-mental health nurses.
- Implement brief relationship interventions with clients in the mental health system.
- Discuss the dynamics and roles of the nurse inherent in each of the phases of a therapeutic relationship.
- Design a relationship contract for use with mental health clients in brief relationships.

KEY TERMS

Autodiagnosis	Genuineness	Self-concept
Brief relationships	Identity	Self-esteem
Concreteness	Immediacy	Self-intervention
Confrontation	Reactivity	Testing behaviors
Contracting	Resistance	Therapeutic relationship
Counseling	Respect	Therapeutic use of self
Countertransference	Self	Transference
Empathy	Self-awareness	

The work of nursing takes place within the context of a therapeutic relationship. A therapeutic relationship is a unique, complex, dynamic, interactive alliance that evolves between two persons. It involves a two-way interactive process during which nurse and client communicate needs and feelings to each other. Both bring to the encounter their unique selves and individual means of reacting emotionally; each communicates in ways that affect the other. The client's needs, feelings, and expectations affect the nurse, and the nurse's responsiveness influences the client.

Dramatic changes in the delivery of mental health care have had significant effects on the nature of nurse-client relationships. The transformed health care environment has led to a shift in the context of the therapeutic relationship from having the luxury of time to having brief time with clients. Furthermore, the work with clients has shifted from intense exploration of interpersonal issues to strategies that encourage action. Nurses in primary care settings provide integrated services to clients with mental illness and must establish sustained interactive partnerships with them, their families, and communities.

The purpose of this chapter is to acquaint the student with the components of the therapeutic relationship and the counseling role of psychiatric nurses. The therapeutic process, brief counseling strategies, and the dynamics that occur during the phases of therapeutic relationships are discussed.

THE NURSE AS THERAPEUTIC PERSON

Understanding of another begins with understanding of self. Nursing takes place in an interpersonal setting and deals with relationships and interactions concerning the self, and self interacting with others. Feelings, thoughts and behaviors continually emerge and change as a result of the dynamic, reciprocal interaction between nurses and clients.

Competency in nurse-client relationships implies that nurses possess the following personal and professional characteristics:

- Acceptance of clients as unique individuals with legal rights to ethical treatment.
- Conviction that clients are capable of change.
- Commitment to an increased understanding of self and the client.
- Willingness to risk becoming involved in the interpersonal process.
- Willingness to be an advocate for clients.
- Commitment to know and understand themselves, their skills, and their limitations.
- Knowledge of the nursing process, therapeutic relationship skills, communication theory, communication techniques, available community resources, and dysfunctional behaviors of clients.
- Respect for the client's right to confidentiality

Nurses, like clients, experience varying degrees of anger, guilt, frustration, helplessness, hope, self-control, love, joy, or other feelings. When nurses react to clients spontaneously, without conscious exploration of self or without therapeutic purposes, the interactions may not be therapeutic.

This section addresses the components of the self, self-awareness, therapeutic use of self, and self-intervention strategies for nurses and clients.

The Self

Self describes one's own person as distinguished from others in the environment. It is who one is as a separate and whole person. It consists of physical, cognitive, affective, behavioral, and social dimensions.

The self is never constant. It is forever changing and emerging in new ways. The emergence of self is influenced by interactions with others as well as by interaction with one's environment. It incorporates self appraisals as well as appraisals made by others. The Johari window diagrammatically depicts four dimensions of self and how these relate to self-awareness in interpersonal relationships (Fig. 9-1). These include the following:

- *The public self,* the self that is presented to and observed by others.
- *The semipublic self,* the self as others perceive it and of which one may not be aware. It is an area of the self that can be enhanced through feedback from others.
- *The private self,* the self that is known but not revealed to others. There will always be some knowledge about self that is not disclosed to others and some that is shared only with persons with whom one has an intimate relationship. When persons have a great reluctance to share information about themselves, they are experienced as closed and distant by others and have an increased risk of loneliness and social isolation. Reluctance to share self-knowledge increases the risk of inaccurate information about self, misperceptions derived from unverified information, and behavior that interferes with effective functioning.
- *The inner self,* the self that is unconscious and unknown even to the individual because its content is too anxiety-provoking to be consciously acknowledged. Knowledge about self that is stored in the unconscious continues to influence perception, thinking, feeling, and behavior, an influence that is not always recognized by the person. The influence

	Known to self	Not known to self
Known to others	I Public self	II Semipublic self (blind area)
Not known to others	III Private self	IV Inner self (area of unknown)

Fig. 9-1 The Johari Window. Each quadrant (or window pane) describes one dimension of the self.

may impose limits on functioning; generate impulsiveness, inappropriate behavior, or unpleasant feelings; or interfere with the development and maintenance of relationships. The inner self, when explored with a supervisor, counselor or other guide, facilitates insight into behaviors and feelings that stem from the unconscious.

A person's sense of self, one that is differentiated from the rest of the world, does not develop all at once. Nor does it ever develop in a final way. The self represents each person's unique pattern of values, attitudes, feelings, ideas, and needs. This pattern results from biological heredity, beliefs, and values developed within the family and culture, formal learning experiences, and interpersonal relationships. Together, these factors contribute to the emergence of a unique self-concept.

Self-Concept

The ***self-concept is the sum total of perceptions, feelings, and beliefs about oneself. It includes characteristics and personality traits and an evaluation of the worth or desirability of these traits.*** It is a totality of a person's attitudes, beliefs, judgments, and values held in relation to one's behavior, abilities, and qualities. Self-concept is the way the person perceives his or her abilities and worth. The self-concept reflects the individual's integration of self—body, mind, and spirit.

Self-concept is influenced by the responses of significant others, how those responses are perceived and internalized, and how they influence behavior. How nurses perceive themselves influences their ability to engage in therapeutic interactions.

Self-Esteem

Self-esteem is the evaluative internal image of oneself formed by the interaction of one's bodily experiences with influential variables in the environment. Self-

esteem ***is an evaluative dimension of self-concept as it can be either positive or negative. It reflects self-acceptance.*** Positive self-esteem requires self-acceptance and a healthy attitude toward one's own worth and limitations.

Interactions with others influence self-esteem. Such interactions may generate feelings toward the self such as pride, joy, shame, respect, love, or hate. Self-esteem is also influenced by one's own and others recognition of personal achievements. Accomplishment of goals, being valued and cared about by others, and acting in ways that are consistent with one's personal values and belief system are other factors that contribute to self-esteem.

Nurses engaged in therapeutic relationships with clients need positive self-esteem. They need to feel that they are worthy, competent, and loved. Positive feelings about oneself facilitates involvement in therapeutic relationships with clients. Self-esteem contributes to the nurses motivation, achievement, and sense of personal worth and power.

Identity

A sense of ***identity,*** which is a part of the self, *is the awareness of being a person separate and distinct from all others.* The phenomenological aspects of identity include a realistic body image, subjective self-awareness, consistent attitudes and behaviors, personal continuity over time, authenticity, and one's gender, ethnicity and conscience (Akhtar and Samuel, 1996). Each of these societal identity characteristics has an evaluative dimension.

Insight into a person's identity is provided by the answers given to the question, "Who am I?" It is based on the integration of the body image and self-concept. One's identity is not static. It is a product of continually changing psychological, social, physical, and developmental processes. Nurses involved in therapeutic relationships with clients bring to these encounters their unique identity. The nurse's identity as a person and as a professional, as well as the client's identity, influences the therapeutic process.

Self-Awareness

Self-awareness is the recognition of one's own uniqueness. It encompasses self-knowledge about one's behavior and its impact on self and others, feelings toward self and others, one's needs and wishes, and one's sense of life purpose. Self-awareness is a keystone in therapeutic relationships. It is influenced by the degree to which one has an accurate view of the different dimensions of self (see Fig. 9-1).

Part of the self exists in conscious awareness, other parts of the self are better known by others, and other parts are private and known only by the self. Still other

Box 9-1

Self-Assessment Questions That Promote Self-Awareness in the Nurse

Who am I?

What is my purpose in life?

What are my talents and strengths?

How do I interact with men? With women?

What are my most common interactive patterns with authority figures? With those I perceive as inferiors?

Do I behave in a particular way with people I like? Dislike?

How do I express anxiety?

What types of clients frighten me? Generate anger within me? Make me sad?

What emotions are stirred in me when I interact with this client?

Are there certain types of clients I consistently avoid?

How do I behave with this client?

Does this client remind me of someone I know?

What kinds of clients generate the greatest reaction in me?

How have I grown in the last week, month, or year?

In what ways have I identified with nursing?

What are the high points of my professional practice? What are the low points?

How do my experiences, family belief system, values, and attitudes influence the way I see this client?

What events in my life have had an important influence on my thinking, feeling, or behavior?

---

parts are largely undiscovered. Each person has the potential for expanding individual self-awareness as he or she becomes more fully acquainted with each dimension. Questions that will promote greater self-awareness in the nurse are found in Box 9-1.

Self-Assessment

The process of using self therapeutically requires that nurses identify their own feelings, thoughts, and behaviors that emerge in response to clients' behaviors or external factors. The process of self-assessment leads to *autodiagnosis,* that is, *to knowledge about the self.* Specific suggestions for facilitating the self-assessment process are found in Box 9-2. Self-awareness involves recognition of the freedom and responsibility individuals have to make choices and changes congruent with their self-image. Self-assessment facilitates the formulation of a personal philosophy that, for nurses, would include nursing as their vocation and an integral part of their life purpose. Self-assessment contributes to nurses' quest for wholeness as people and as members of a profession.

Self-assessment is an essential ingredient of therapeutic use of self and an integral part of therapeutic relationships. The process of self-assessment enables nurses to learn about themselves in the context of the therapeutic relationship. The process uncovers how the person (nurse) interacts with the other person (client). It reveals to nurses how they use their strengths and modify their weaknesses to enable clients to move toward wholeness and develop functional ways of coping, problem solving, and interacting effectively.

Self-Intervention

Self-intervention is *a process of understanding and modifying forces within the self that provoke anxiety*

and interfere with the nurse-client relationship. If nurses ask clients to examine their inner selves and modify dysfunctional patterns in their lives, they too must engage in a similar process. Reaching self-awareness increases self-understanding, self-acceptance, and options for action. A person's *reactivity* is *the spontaneous response he or she has to the interpersonal situation. It is the input from another that triggers or sets off affective, cognitive, social, or behavioral responses within oneself.* Intervening with self enables nurses to deal with their own reactivity and "triggers" and thus help clients with all kinds and degrees of problems.

Striving for self-awareness involves a dynamic, ongoing process of discovery and change. Nurses attempt to discover the forces within themselves that influence the nurse-client relationship. Once these thoughts, feelings, values, and behaviors have been discovered, specific ways in which they positively or negatively affect relationships with clients are examined. In addition, ways to modify negative forces so that they can increase nurses' effectiveness as caregivers are identified. Nurses engage in the self-intervention process in several ways.

- *Individual introspection to design change.* The perceptual field often has blind spots that limit the ability to see oneself and others clearly. Consequently, introspection has limitations, at least for beginners who may not have extensive self-understanding or experience with the self-awareness process.
- *Supervisory relationship with a liaison nurse, clinical specialist, or instructor.* Supervisory relationships are designed to monitor the nurse-client relationship, provide objective feedback regarding the process and content of the relationship, and provide an arena for identifying strategies for implementing and evaluating change.

Box 9-2

Suggestions for Facilitating the Autodiagnosis Process

- Use active listening skills to identify positive and negative patterns in interpersonal style.
- Reflect on past life influences that have been instrumental in creating the person that exists today.
- Identify how various past experiences and learning are influencing the current relationship.
- Explore any conflict between feelings, thoughts, values, and behavior and the way in which conflict is manifested in the nurse-client relationship.
- Analyze clients' behavior that you perceive has precipitated problematic feelings or conflict.
- Accept feelings, thoughts, and values for what they are.
- Recognize cognitive, affective, behavioral, and physical stress in your own personal and professional life.

- *Professional counseling.* Self-awareness and personal growth are facilitated by the counseling process.
- *Supervision by a peer group.* Groups provide a forum for case presentations. Objective feedback about problems experienced in the nurse-client relationship, as well as suggestions for change are given. Supervision can be viewed as an opportunity for collaborative exchange, which becomes a learning experience for everyone involved.
- *Nursing or interdisciplinary team conferences.* Team meetings offer another opportunity to participate in a collaborative learning experience. Different team members working with the same client, or group of clients, take the opportunity to present their views of the client, their work with the client, and problems encountered. They provide a forum for the exchange of thoughts, feelings, and potential strategies.
- *Ongoing use of stress management.* Stress management techniques enhance the effectiveness of nurses engaged in therapeutic relationships with clients. Regular use of stress-alleviating strategies helps nurses maintain mind-body-spirit balance in their lives (see Chapter 14).

THE THERAPEUTIC RELATIONSHIP

A *therapeutic relationship is a dynamic interactive process convened to help one of the participants, the client, achieve a planned goal. It is a pivotal therapeutic process that involves nurses' therapeutic use of themselves in specific, time-limited, goal-directed interactions with clients who are experiencing health-related difficulties.* It is a client-centered relationship that seeks to promote mental health, productivity, and improved quality of life for clients. It is the medium for the exchange of all forms of information, feelings, and concerns, a factor in successful therapeutic regimens, and an essential ingredient in the satisfaction of both nurse and client.

The therapeutic relationship in a transformed health care environment takes the form of a partnership or therapeutic alliance in which nurse and client work together to pursue common goals and interests (Wilson and Hobbs, 1995). It assumes that clients are capable of participating in their own care and have the capability to access care when it is needed. Therapeutic relationships require the art of caring and focus on effecting change, promoting growth, and healing the emotional pain of clients. Although every relationship is unique, each has several components that can be observed and studied (Forchuk, 1995).

Therapeutic Interaction Models

Multiple models exist that determine how therapeutic relationships should evolve. In the section that follows, models most commonly used by nurses are discussed.

Interpersonal model

Hildegarde Peplau (1952), a nurse theorist, draws her theory about therapeutic interaction from the interpersonal work of Sullivan and in part from learning theory. Her work provides a systematic framework for examining current nurse-client interpersonal experiences. Nurses help clients *observe* their behavior and describe it in detail. Nurses help clients *analyze* this information and *formulate* connections that the nurse *validates*. Finally, clients are taught to *integrate* the learning into new behaviors (see Chapter 8).

Peplau described the importance of self-assessment by nurses. By examining their own interpersonal behaviors as they affect the nurse-client relationship, nurses are able to use themselves therapeutically. The concept of therapeutic use of self is pivotal to Peplau's framework.

Therapeutic use of self The concept of ***therapeutic use of self*** *implies that nurses use their personal identity to promote self-actualization and healing in their clients.* They bring to the interaction their perceptions, values, expectations, emotions, and expertise to assess the interaction, explore resulting feelings, thoughts, and behaviors, and to identify the meaning and impact of these on themselves, their clients, and the relationship. Therapeutic use of self means that nurses, not just procedures or techniques, facilitate healing. Like all people, nurses have unique personalities, are at specific developmental levels, and have needs, coping strategies, and unique histories that influence their interactions. They have distinctive, idiosyncratic ways of experiencing and responding to the interactive process.

Interpersonal roles of the nurse Peplau (1952) suggests that the interactive roles in which the nurses engage in the therapeutic nurse-client relationship include the following:

- *Stranger*—Assumed by both nurse and client at the outset of the relationship

When clients and nurses first meet, they are strangers. They are subject to many doubts, concerns, and fears as they consider a commitment to the therapeutic process. Although many new nurses experience fear, most can recognize it as a natural result of the therapeutic encounter, a situation that entails taking risks. The nurse-client relationship requires courage, which comes more easily when fear is accepted as appropriate.

Failure to come to grips with ever-present fears poses a serious barrier to the development of the nurse-client relationship, since clients who elicit fear sense the effect of their behavior. Fears borne in secret are intensified and generalized. Fear brought out into the open—shared with an instructor, classmate, peer, or supervisor—can be named and understood.

Some common fears and concerns of nurses at the outset of a therapeutic relationship include the following:

- Fear of rejection by clients
- Fear of exploiting clients
- Feelings of helplessness
- Fear of physical aggression by clients
- Fear of "catching" a psychiatric disorder

Similarly, clients experience concerns about engaging in therapeutic relationships. They may not understand the nature of the process, may be overwhelmed by it, or may have had previous negative experiences or outcomes. Accepting help takes on different meanings for each client. For some, expectations are that nurses will "rescue" them, whereas others may think that they need to give up all power of the nurse. Acknowledging the concerns of nurses and clients as "normal" facilitates rapport building in the relationship.

- *Teacher*—Assumed by nurses to facilitate learning by clients. Today, nurses assume key roles in psychoeducation. Chapter 16 discusses the educative role of the nurse.
- *Resource Person*—Assumed by nurses in their case management activities. Nurses are expected to provide health information and support to client consumers. Chapter 17 delineates case management functions of psychiatric nurses.

- *Surrogate*—Assumed by nurses and assigned by clients who view the nurse in roles of the clients' past significant others (similar to transference). The nurse enables clients to delay gratification and invest emotional energy in goal achievement.
- *Leader*—Assumed by nurses as they engage in the nursing process (see Chapter 5).
- *Counselor*—Assumed by nurses to help clients integrate facts and feelings associated with their symptoms into the total life experience.

Nurses practice problem-solving approaches and teach them to clients. The ANA, in its psychiatric-mental health nursing's *Standards* (ANA, 1994), highlighted the **counseling** role and defined it as the following:

A specific time-limited interaction of a nurse with a client, family, or group experiencing immediate or ongoing difficulties related to their health or well-being. The difficulty is investigated using a problem-solving approach for the purpose of understanding the experience and integrating it with other life experiences.

Core dimensions of the therapeutic relationship
A number of facilitative interpersonal processes have been conceptualized by investigators attempting to identify and operationally define helper behaviors during the therapeutic relationship process. Carkhoff's core dimensions (Carkhoff, 1968) describe a way of "being with" a client so that goal achievement takes place. Genuineness, empathy, respect, and concreteness are the responsive dimensions of therapeutic relationships, whereas confrontation and immediacy are thought to be the action components. Table 9-1 defines the core components and illustrates each with an example.

Brief relationships
Brief relationships involve a time-limited, dynamic, outcome-oriented process. They are the hallmark of managed care environments because traditional (long-term) approaches to the therapeutic process fail to meet the demand for accessible and cost-effective care. Consequently use of non-traditional models for building therapeutic alliances has evolved. Emphasis has shifted from "fixing" clients to mobilizing their own strengths and resources to deal with problems. Clients entering into the therapeutic process expect a structured, problem solving, resolution style of interaction. Box 9-3 lists and describes characteristics of brief therapeutic relationships (Hoyt, 1994).

Time is the central organizing concept in brief relationships (Mann, 1995), that is, the duration of the therapeutic relationship is implicitly and explicitly limited. The key to time-limited intervention is identification of

TABLE 9-1

Core dimensions of therapeutic relationships

CORE DIMENSION/DEFINITION	EXAMPLE
Empathy The temporary experiencing of another individual's feelings; expressions that convey the nurse's accurate recognition of the feelings, motives, and meanings underlying a client's communications. It is the ability "to get inside another's skin" and subjectively feel with a client while objectively observing behavior.	*Client:* (Crying and obviously upset) "We've only been married for a year and now I have breast cancer." *Empathetic response:* "Putting your feelings about having cancer together with your feelings for your husband must be overwhelming."
Respect Communication of acceptance of the client's ideas, feelings, and experiences; recognition of a client's potential for self-actualization.	*Client:* Mrs. B. is a Christian Scientist. She is incontinent because of bladder and bowel cancer. She has an order for an indwelling catheter and pain medication. She tells you, "I really don't want any scientific treatment. I just want to make things easier for my husband." *Respectful response:* "I really understand. Perhaps you want to discuss the catheter with your husband before you decide if I should put it in."
Genuineness Spontaneous expressions conveying an individual's inner experience.	*Client:* "I know tomorrow is your last day working with me. I'm really angry you're leaving." *Genuine response:* "I will miss you too. I have appreciated the time we have spent sorting out your problems. It's hard to break away from people we care about."
Concreteness The clear, direct expression of personally relevant perceptions, values, and feelings as they exist in the present relationship. It is used to help clients focus on specific problems and significant details.	*Client:* "Everything about this place is exasperating. I'm getting no where." *Concrete response:* "Tell me one specific thing that has upset you. Perhaps we can solve the issue together."
Immediacy A dimension of communication that deals with the relationship-building element of the helping process; expressions emphasizing immediacy draw relationships between clients overt communications and their underlying impressions of what is going on between client and nurse into the here and now.	*Client:* (An outpatient who has been putting off the decision to leave her abusive husband.) "I'll get all the paperwork together soon." *Immediate action response:* "I'm sure this is not easy for you. Let's select one part of the paperwork and decide when you will file it."
Confrontation Communications that call attention to significant discrepancies in the client's experience; verbal messages that are intended to help a client recognize information that is not consistent with his or her self image.	*Client:* (Michael is an adolescent who consistently disrupts group meetings with angry outbursts.) "I really don't care about this stuff. I'm leaving now." *Confrontation:* "Michael will you stay here now. Everytime we begin to talk about families you seem to become angry and make excuses to leave the group. You say you don't care, but your actions say you care very much."

Box 9-3

Characteristics of Brief Therapeutic Relationships

- Contacts are aimed at solving immediate and specific problems.
- Response is rapid and involves early engagement of the client.
- There are clear definitions of client and counselor responsibilities.
- Emphasis is placed on the client's competencies, resources, and involvement.
- Goals are behavioral and measurable and have specific time boundaries.
- Time boundaries are flexible and creative. The length, frequency, and timing of contracts vary according to client needs.
- Interdisciplinary cooperation and case management strategies facilitate a more holistic view of clients.
- Multiple formats and modalities of treatment are encouraged and are used sequentially or simultaneously to meet client-determined goals.
- Intermittent long-term relationships with clients are encouraged. A "cure" philosophy is replaced by ongoing caring.
- Therapeutic sessions are results-oriented. Symptom relief is the goal of the brief encounters that occur in the context of ongoing therapeutic relationships.

the central issue. An example of the identification process follows:

> Sheila, a 45-year-old successful career woman, seeks help from the nurse practitioner in the primary care clinic because of anxiety and ambivalence related to a recent decision to change careers. She has been a widely recognized scientist for several years. After two assessment meetings, her history revealed a chaotic childhood and two failed marriages. The nurse identifies Sheila's central issue as follows:
>
> Sheila has been highly successful despite numerous difficulties. The anxiety and ambivalence she feels now is a result of the dichotomy between her public image and the private feelings of insecurity she has about herself.

The central issues in this example involved time (history), affect (feelings of anxiety and ambivalence), and Sheila's image of herself. Symptom relief becomes a byproduct of the time-oriented process, not its goal. The number of sessions needed to resolve the issues is mutually determined by nurse and client and the date for the final meeting is agreed on once the central issue is identified (Delaney et al, 1995).

The management of the therapeutic relationship and reframing it as a therapeutic, "working" alliance sets the stage for a holistic system approach to clients' issues. Interpretations, statements by the nurse about central issues and solutions, are common in brief relationships. They focus on the present and must make sense to the client, and, as in more traditional therapeutic processes, the timing of them is key to behavioral change.

Flexibility and creativity are other essentials of the brief relationship process. Techniques such as prescribing homework or requiring clients to keep diaries are used but do not substitute for the personal connectedness between the client and the therapist.

Brief relationships may take the form of single client-nurse encounters. Single sessions with clients may encompass the whole relationship process. This occurs when client and nurse mutually agree to one meeting. Generally such meetings are longer than the usual "50-minute hour," but they encompass all the phases of any therapeutic relationship. Single sessions also serve as periodic "checkups" for a client who may need to become "unstuck" or get "back on track" (Schneider and Ross, 1996). Nurses in general hospital settings often use single sessions to enhance the psychosocial outcomes of their clients.

Brief nurse-client relationships are not for everyone. Those who are most likely to benefit from brief therapeutic intervention include the following:

- Clients with specific, well-defined problems
- Clients needing only reassurance for their reactions to an issue
- Clients with family members who are supportive and can serve as "co-therapists"
- Clients needing evaluation and referral
- Clients who are spontaneous improvers

Clients less likely to benefit from brief therapeutic relationships are those who are homicidal or suicidal and require inpatient care; those whose symptoms have strong biological or chemical origins (e.g., clients with schizophrenia, bipolar disorder, panic disorder, or alcohol or drug disorders; those requesting long-term self-exploration; and those needing ongoing support to resolve childhood or adult abuse).

PHASES OF THERAPEUTIC RELATIONSHIPS

Therapeutic relationships are dynamic. They involve an ongoing, ever-changing process that has a beginning, midpoint, and end. The therapeutic process is a historical or temporal process, interweaving expectations and concerns of nurses and clients. Every contact (session) has within it definable characteristics. Furthermore, as the relationship evolves within a session or over time, distinctive, yet interrelated phases of the process may be identified. Commonly, these phases are not distinct but flow into one another. The time when each phase occurs, and its duration, can vary widely and depends on the specific context of care. For example, the tasks of all the phases may be accomplished in 3 to 4 days by clients in a short-term inpatient crisis unit, 3 to 4 weeks in a diagnostic unit, or one session in an emergency room setting. On the other hand, clients in longer-term treatment, or those engaged in ongoing outpatient therapy, may experience the phases more slowly.

In her work, *Interpersonal Relations in Nursing,* Peplau (1952) identified for the first time four phases of the nurse-client relationship: orientation, identification, exploitation, and resolution.

During the *orientation* phase (preinteractive, beginning), the client seeks assistance, conveys needs, and shares preconceptions and expectations regarding the process with the nurse. The nurse responds to the client, defines the boundaries of the relationship, gathers data, listens attentively, and clarifies the goals and purposes of the relationship. Nurses explore and clarify their own preconceptions and expectations and begin the self-assessment process.

The identification and exploitation phases pull together what may be thought of as the working stage of the relationship. In the *identification* stage, clients respond to the help offered by the nurse, begin to explore feelings, identify with the nurse, and fluctuate between independence and dependence in the relationship. Nurses provide structure, focus on clients, and facilitate the expression of problems and feelings.

The *exploitation* stage as defined by Peplau is the time when clients exploit or use the help offered by nurses. Clients change behaviors and access services. Nurses continue to explore clients' feelings and behaviors, deal with resistances (stalls) in the relationship, and facilitate clients' achievement of goals.

Peplau described the *resolution* stage as the point in time when clients abandon their old behaviors, engage in new problem-solving skills, and exhibit the ability to view themselves positively. Nurses encourage self-care and begin work with the clients to negotiate termination of the nurse-client relationship.

In the present managed care climate brief relationship models that modify the traditional phasing of therapeutic relationships are being used. Table 9-2 suggests a framework that incorporates traditional phases and the brief models for therapeutic relationships. The mnemonic, DWARF, is used to suggest each of the phases: **D**esigning, **W**arm-up, **A**greement, **R**ehabilitation, and **F**inishing.

Designing the Therapeutic Relationship

To be successful, therapeutic relationships need planning. Preparation by the nurse, before the actual beginning of a therapeutic relationship, occurs a number of ways. Nurses first prepare themselves by acquiring a knowledge base that includes understanding the growth and development of individuals and by appreciating how family dynamics and environmental, cultural, and gender diversity affect a person. An understanding of the biopsychosocial theoretical correlates of each of the DSM-IV clinical disorders facilitates competency. Comprehending the communication process (see Chapter 8) and appreciating the importance of self-awareness promote relationship growth. Recognition of the differences between social and therapeutic relationships is also helpful to the beginning nurse (Table 9-3).

Practical details

Structuring practical skills can facilitate the beginning of a therapeutic relationship. The first interview is struc-

TABLE 9-2

Phases of the therapeutic relationship (DWARF)	
PHASE	**DEFINITION**
Designing	Establishing the practical details of the therapeutic encounter
Warm-up	Beginning the therapeutic relationship, building rapport, and engaging each other in the therapeutic process
Agreement	Mutually negotiating a contract that states outcomes of the therapeutic relationship
Rehabilitation	Working to facilitate movement toward mutually set goals through negotiation of defenses, transference, and countertransference
Finishing	Terminating and evaluating the therapeutic relationship at a mutually negotiated end time while maintaining openness to future therapeutic contracts to allow clients "time up" to reconsider the direction of their life goals

Courtesy Anita Leach McMahon. Used with permission.

TABLE 9-3

Differences between social and therapeutic relationships

THERAPEUTIC RELATIONSHIP	SOCIAL RELATIONSHIP
Client's expression of feelings, ideas, and actions is not limited to socially acceptable behavior. Clients may express their thoughts, feelings, and actions as long as they are not destructive to themselves or others.	Each person expects to be respected and liked by the other. Freedom to express feelings, ideas, and behavior is limited by socially acceptable protocols. Social codes of conduct that govern expression vary with age, gender, nationality, social class setting of interaction, and other factors.
The expectation is that nurses will accept clients as they are and will begin work with them at the *client's* level of functioning. Nurses are expected to use therapeutic procedures in the problem-solving process, these may include the offer of help but only as clients need it and are ready to use it.	Individuals differ widely in their tolerance for socially inappropriate behavior. Although there is a wide margin of intolerance, there is no obligation to understand or tolerate behavior that strains the relationship.
Integrity is present at all times. Promises and appointments are only made when they can be kept. The nurse refrains from insincere praise, false reassurance, superficial comments, and social cliches. Clients are expected to discuss their problems and formulate strategies to solve them.	No obligation regarding honesty. People may give each other advice without even considering the unique facets of a problem or may urge solutions for people who are capable of making their own choices. Individuals have the option of avoiding any discussion of problems.
The expectation is that the content of the interaction will be professional and confidential.	No such agreement, except when an individual specifically requests it.
Nurses are expected to examine their own behaviors, study their effects on clients, and attempt to become more aware of their responses to interpersonal situations.	Individuals depend largely on intuitive responses for cues in each other's behavior to keep the relationship on a mutually satisfying basis.
Nurses assume responsibility for conscious direction of their behavior to provide a therapeutic experience for the client. Ongoing study and supervision broadens nurses' knowledge of the theoretical basis for therapeutic interventions and assists in the development of clinical skills.	There is no obligation to consciously examine social interactions or to work toward greater self-awareness.

tured so that data can be collected by the nurse and the client can feel at ease. Arrangements are made to meet in a relaxing physical environment that includes comfortable seating, a low noise level, soft nonglare light, and a private area free of interruptions and distractions.

Warm-Up

The warm-up phase of a therapeutic relationship has been referred to as the orientation phase, the establishing phase, and the downward or inward phase. It is simply the early stage of any therapeutic relationship. During the warm-up phase the critical tasks to be accomplished are establishment of a working alliance or rapport between the nurse and client and identification of the client's chief problem or area of concern. During this phase, nurse and client, who are strangers to one another, meet. Neither can predict much about how the relationship will de-

velop. The things that will happen throughout the relationship can, at best, only be anticipated. Some practical do's and don'ts useful to the nurse during the warm-up phase of a therapeutic relationship are listed in Table 9-4.

Building rapport

The initial interview is usually completed within a short time; but whether it is short or long, rapport must be established. One might refer to establishing rapport as the process of engaging the client. Spontaneity, freedom to be oneself, clarity, openness, physical and psychological closeness, and intimacy are the signs of rapport. Both nurses and clients feel peaceful, comfortable, and even joyous when rapport has been established. Initial support is, in a sense, the foundation on which the reminder of the relationship rests. The initial contact influences the success or failure of future therapeutic interventions.

TABLE 9-4

Do's and don'ts for the warm-up phase

DO	DON'T
Have a conscious objective and state the purpose of the interview.	Don't assume the person will accept you because of your role—you are a stranger.
Give the person your undivided attention. Be unhurried.	Don't deprive the person of their individuality—do not categorize them.
Be aware of, sensitive, and responsive to nonverbal communications.	Don't be overly pessimistic regarding a person's ability to change.
Listen. Secure sufficient information to make a realistic evaluation.	Don't minimize the seriousness of the situation by giving premature and/or false reassurance.
Be professional but warm, accepting, supportive, and objective.	Don't express moral or ethical judgment or disapproval of attitudes and ideas.
Recognize and respect culturally influenced values and behaviors.	Don't try to impress the person with your superior knowledge.
Use a language the person understands and can accept.	Don't be defensive.
Recognize your own feelings and how they affect your behaviors.	Don't monopolize or dominate the interview or let the person being interviewed control it.
Make clear that the final responsibility for action rests with the client.	Don't get information to satisfy your own curiosity.
Help him or her develop an awareness of consequences and possible alternatives.	Don't divulge confidential information.

Agreement

As the early phasing of a therapeutic relationship evolves, client and nurse mutually negotiate a contract or agreement that states the specific therapeutic goals and outcomes of their time together. Therapeutic relationships focus on helping clients deal with problems that take place during contracted time, when rules for a therapeutic relationship are operative. It is similar to Peplau's identification phase.

Contracting

Contracting usually takes place during the initial interview between nurse and client and *is the negotiation of an agreement that stipulates the means of achieving specific behavioral change in the client.* The expectations of both nurse and client are explicitly stated. Many clients have misconceptions about the helping relationship; nurses therefore assume an educative role during the process of making the contract. Contracts usually contain the following components:

- Purpose of sessions
- Mutual expectations
- Goals and means of achieving them

- Boundaries
- Confidentiality statement

Setting boundaries

Issues related to the boundaries of therapeutic relationships may occur at any time in the course of treatment but are best dealt with at the outset of therapeutic encounters and may be included in the therapeutic contract. *Boundaries may be thought of as the rules or expected behaviors that govern meetings between clients and nurses.* Establishing boundaries takes on added significance in the mental health system because the symptoms experienced by some clients put them at risk to violate them. It is the responsibility of the nurse to set clear boundaries for the therapeutic relationships. Tangible boundaries that are set and negotiated at the onset include the following:

- Time, place, frequency, and duration of meetings
- Compensation for professional services
- Guidelines that prohibit the exchange of gifts
- Guidelines restricting physical contact between client and nurse; sexual contact never permitted

Boundaries that are less tangible but are nonetheless important to the professional role of psychiatric nurses involved in therapeutic relationships include:

- Setting firm therapeutic limits with clients.
- Dressing professionally. Suggestive, flamboyant, or seductive clothing is unacceptable. Nurses who expect to be treated professionally should dress accordingly.
- Using language that conveys caring and respect. Sexually explicit or vulgar language violates boundaries. Use of first or full names should be mutually negotiated by client and nurse and reflect the custom of the place where treatment takes place.
- Using self-disclosure discriminately. Self-disclosure is appropriate when its purpose is to model or educate, foster the therapeutic alliance, or validate a client's reality.

Negotiating outcomes

Identifying clients' goals is an important part of the agreement phase of a therapeutic relationship. The term *goal* and *objective* does not suggest that the future is predetermined; a goal or an objective is, rather, an image of the future that suggests approaches and legitimizes the helping relationship. Outcome negotiation follows a comprehensive assessment for the client (see Chapter 5) and determines the focus of the therapeutic relationship.

Goals or outcomes established for any therapeutic relationship are intended to facilitate the client's self-understanding, self-acceptance, and self-respect; to help the client achieve a clear personal identity; to increase the client's ability to form intimate, interdependent relationships; and to enable clients to give and receive love. For each client, unique goals are established to facilitate improvement in function. Goals may be established and be achieved within a short time period or may be ongoing and long-term (see Chapter 5).

Rehabilitation

The process of behavioral change occurs during the working or rehabilitation phase of a therapeutic relationship. This time is also called the middle phase and corresponds to Peplau's exploitation phase. It follows data gathering and implies that rapport and trust are established between client and nurse.

The transition to the rehabilitation phase of a therapeutic relationship may be rapid or gradual. It is signaled by the client's willingness to assume a more active role in self-exploration. Taking into account the accomplishments during the warm-up and agreement time, nurses and clients can pursue activities aimed at enabling clients to cope with, or profit from, exploration of the stated problem.

The rehabilitation phase is the point in the interview when nurses guide clients to explore "the heart of the matter." It is the time of growth and change. It is a time when clients learn, continue to test, and integrate new behaviors. It requires hard work and painful uncovering of the past so as to link it to the present. Clients are encouraged to take risks—since risk is inherent in change—and persevere through to the therapeutic end.

Several unconscious phenomena occur during this time. Testing behaviors, resistance, transference, and countertransference may become operative and must be worked through to achieve expected outcomes. Ongoing evaluation of these phenomena and renegotiation of therapeutic goals are the work of the rehabilitation phase of relationships.

Maximizing the client's self-awareness of the growth accomplished becomes the desired outcome. During the middle phase of the relationship, plans for termination are made more specific, and clients are encouraged to begin the transition to another phase of treatment.

Testing behaviors

Not all therapeutic relationships run smoothly. Clients, like nurses, live through moments of fear and uncertainty. Clients may not recognize, understand, or claim their misgivings. They need to grapple with a number of threats to their self-image as they invest in a relationship that involves receiving help. Some of the behaviors displayed by clients at this juncture are labeled *testing behaviors. Clients act in ways that challenge nurses to see if they can be trusted. Clients may try to shock or surprise the nurse to control the relationship or elicit an emotional response.*

Sometimes clients attempt to convert a therapeutic relationship to a social one, thereby testing the limits of the therapeutic encounter. There are times in a therapeutic relationship when social exchanges are appropriate, for example, during recreational games with clients. In these instances the nurse uses the interaction to acquire information about clients' behaviors, their perception of self, and their ability to sustain a social relationship. The game playing can be a therapeutic strategy for developing trust, a time for nurse and client to get to know each other. Other examples of testing behaviors used by clients are found in Box 9-4.

Underlying testing behavior is the issue of trust. The client is making judgments about the trustworthiness of the nurse. The role of the nurse focuses on the purpose and structure of the therapeutic relationship. In turn the client's involvement in the relationship becomes less anxiety-producing.

It is important to recognize that testing is inevitable and a part of normal human reluctance to expose painful emotional information about the self, significant others, and one's family. This reluctance is a defense that protects the self from threats to psychological integrity

Box 9-4

Testing Behaviors of Clients

Attempting a social relationship
Casting nurse into parental role
Judging whether the nurse trusts them
Attempting to take care of nurse
Avoiding discussion of problems
Asking for personal data about the nurse
Violating personal space of nurse and others
Seeking attention from the nurse
Challenging the nurse's commitment to the process
Revealing information that shocks the nurse
Touching the nurse inappropriately

and from becoming overwhelmed. Sustaining the therapeutic relationship patiently to help clients increase self-awareness and feel safe while simultaneously addressing central issues facilitates the clients movement toward goals.

Other common concerns are disclosure requests made by clients for personal data about the nurse. These requests test the therapeutic relationship by attempting to convert it to a social one. Nurses appropriately provide clients with information about their professional credentials but limit discussion about other aspects of their lives. Personal information is not shared, since it has the potential to be used later to "put down" staff. Self-disclosure of a personal nature may also burden clients or become a source of fantasy or distortion.

Inappropriate touching by clients is another troublesome testing behavior. Clients may act out nonverbally what they are unable to express in words. As a general rule anything that is acted out will not be talked about. Therapeutic relationships are verbal processes, and since certain nonverbal behaviors block this process, it is important that the nurses discuss such behaviors with clients. As a relationship evolves, clients may engage in attention-seeking behavior, test the nurse's commitment to them, use statements intended to shock, or even devalue the nurse.

Other clients may avoid discussion of painful issues by talking about social happenings, as in the following example:

Tom tells Olive about a movie he saw recently. Olive focuses the relationship process in the here and now. She likens the topic to the client's problem. "This movie seems important to you. Tell me what meaning the movie has in your life?"

Clients may also attempt to shock nurses or throw them off guard. They are testing whether or not the

nurse is able to handle "real" problems. At such times nurses need to remain calm, maintain a neutral stance, show interest, and explore what the statements mean to the client.

The statements made by the client may be true. If such disclosure occurs when the relationship is well-established, it may be a sign that the client is ready to work on resolutions of problematic feelings and behavior. However, if the disclosure is early in the relationship, clients may be attempting to evoke shame, to embarrass, or to disgust the nurse.

Testing behavior challenges the nurse to remain focused and goal-oriented. Careful self-assessment in such situations enables nurses to use what clients are saying or doing to intervene therapeutically with them. When the relationship proceeds therapeutically, client and nurse will come to expect outcomes such as independence, spontaneity, mutual trust, self-awareness, honesty, responsibility, and acceptance of reality.

Negotiating resistance

Resistance is a term that was originally introduced by Freud and *has come to mean all the phenomena that interfere with and disrupt the smooth interactional flow of feelings, memories, and thoughts. It is an individual's attempt to remain unaware of anxiety-producing aspects of the self.* People fear being blamed, being shamed, or being found incompetent. Sometimes their feelings of guilt are so painful that they cannot be shared. When such feelings and fears exist, resistance may occur. Resistance generally results in avoidance behavior by both nurse and client thus slowing the work of a therapeutic relationship.

Several forms of resistance or avoidance behavior have been identified. Clients may suppress or repress important information. Others may "recover" quickly with a flight into health so as not to continue the therapeutic process. Other forms of resistance include having a hopeless outlook, acting out, or engaging in irrational behavior. Keeping interactions superficial and social also contributes to resistance. For some clients, recovery is so frightening that despite intellectual insight into their issues, behaviors remain unchanged and movement toward established outcomes becomes stalled.

Nurses may contribute to the resistance that occurs in therapeutic relationships. Feelings that have been generated in client and nurse about each other, or misperceptions of the client's progress, may be at the root of the failure to move the process in a therapeutic direction. Self-assessment facilitates nurses' awareness of feelings and behaviors that contribute to stalling the therapeutic process. Table 9-5 lists common behaviors and feelings that may stall the therapeutic relationship process and suggests solutions that derive from the nurse's self-assessment.

TABLE 9-5

Behaviors and feelings in therapeutic relationships that contribute to resistance

BEHAVIORS/FEELINGS	SOLUTION DERIVED FROM SELF-ASSESSMENT
Ambivalent feelings	Recognize that ambivalence is happening Accept and understand self and others
Pessimistic feelings	Look for a client's assets, not just his or her problems Set realistic goals Develop optimism about goals of the relationship
Feeling superior	Give supportive encouragement Realize human limitations Develop respect for self and for the client Be supportive rather than reassuring
Misuse of confrontation	Stay with here-and-now issues Use immediacy and empathetic understanding Be aware of "timing" when making alterations
Misjudging independence	Acknowledge the misjudgment Ask what clients can do for themselves Reassess client and family capabilities Do not infantilize client
Labeling	Acknowledge feelings and reasons for label Describe rather than label
Overidentification	Acknowledge the existence of overidentification Look at the client's problem from all perspectives Discuss countertransference with a supervisor
Overinvolvement	Do not allow client to deny reality of illness Avoid social invitations from the client Avoid calling the client at home Avoid any secondary financial gains
Painful feelings	Explore the possible sources of painful feelings Avoid isolation and withdrawal from client Use autodiagnosis
Misuse of honesty	Fulfill promises in a timely manner Answer questions directly and honestly Avoid omissions in conversations with the client Avoid hedging when asked direct questions

Listening pitfalls (see Chapter 8)
  Listening poorly
  Selective listening
  Listening only to the content
  Listening only to the affect
	Avoid excessive verbalization
	Avoid giving advice and making decisions for the client
	Avoid faking attention, interrupting, and asking clients to repeat what they have said
	Maintain eye contact
	Avoid changing the subject
	Keep the interaction client-focused

Negotiating transference

Two unconscious phenomena, transference and counter-transference, occur in all relationships. In psychoanalytic theory the term *transference refers to an interpersonal experience (not recognized by the person) in which the feelings, attitudes, and wishes originally linked with significant figures in one's early life are attributed to others who represent these people in the current situation.* Transference is generally expected in therapeutic relationships. The following example is used to illustrate transference phenomena.

Charlie is a 57-year-old man admitted for evaluation. During his first meeting with Amelia, the nurse, he is critical, demanding, and generally unpleasant. Amelia initially responded to Charlie with silence and by distancing from him. She felt frustrated by his failure to share feelings.

Amelia speaks with the team and makes use of self-assessment. She recognized that Charlie reminds her of her father, who tends to be a "critical expert" with her. Once freed of her negative reactions to Charlie she is able to explore his behaviors. She asks, "How do you think things are going between us?" Charlie responds by saying he is angry with her. "Perhaps I remind you of someone else." Charlie blurts out, "You are just like my mother. You are always analyzing me. You make me very angry." Amelia continues to explore the anger. "What is it about me that provokes your angry feelings?" Charlie responds, "You seem to be judging me. I like you, but you are so much like my mother."

Clients' transference interferes with their ability to accurately possess the here and now. Clients may repeat interaction patterns that were characteristic of earlier relationships. They may begin to project onto nurses their past or present attitudes toward family members or people in authority. Thus they may experience nurses as they might have experienced other people who have played significant roles in their lives. Clients may form a single image, or multiple images of nurses, some of which are distorted by past events. Transference alters a client's reality-based perception of the nurse. In the previous example, Charlie, the client, saw the nurse as parent and himself as child, thus creating dependency. Charlie's expectation was that he would be told what to do but when Amelia did not respond to the expectation he became angry with her. The therapeutic process recreated Charlie's past experience with his mother in the person of the nurse.

Negotiating countertransference

The term *countertransference is used to describe all the feelings that nurses experience toward clients. It is the conscious or unconscious response occurring in nurses as they interact with clients. Wishes and conflicts originating in the helper's own relationships with significant others are transferred onto the client.* Countertransference may result in resistance and certainly impedes the rehabilitative work of the relationship.

Attraction, warmth, and concern are common positive countertransference reactions; but negative responses to the client, such as discouragement, resentment, boredom, guilt, and anger, are equally typical. Changes in the nurse's behavior toward clients occur when countertransference is unrecognized or when it evokes anxiety. When it occurs, the overt communication of nurses may be unrelated to their inner feelings. Thus while nurses may appear to be attending to the client's concerns, their energies are in fact being diverted toward efforts to recapture a feeling of personal security. They react the way they think they should, in a rehearsed, "professional" fashion. Clients can often sense the discrepancy between the nurse's outward appearances and their inner selves:

In the previous example Amelia was experiencing countertransference. She unconsciously reacted toward Charlie as if he were her father. Charlie may have been responding to Amelia's discomfort. Although Amelia did not verbally express her discomfort, she initially withdrew and was silent with him. Charlie "tuned in" to Amelia's inner discomfort and began to react to her as if she were his mother.

Nurses may suspect that countertransference is occurring if they are ignoring selected data about clients, blaming them, being smug about their own opinions, or being rigid about the structure of a relationship.

Finishing

The completion of the finishing phase of a therapeutic relationship has been called the termination stage, the closing or ending phase, and the resolution stage. It is the time in a relationship when client and nurse mutually decide to interrupt a scheduled contract because previously contracted outcomes have been achieved.

Termination may occur at the end of a single interview, following a brief inpatient therapeutic relationship, or after months of outpatient therapy. Clients' reactions to ending a particular segment of a therapeutic encounter are affected by the meaning they ascribe to it, the duration of the relationship, and the extent to which goals have been achieved. The finishing process begins in the early stages of the relationship when goals are set and is completed when both nurse and client think that their goals have been achieved.

Finishing or ending a particular aspect of an ongoing relationship is much like the process that occurs when a primary care physician tells a client that he or she does not have to come again unless the problem "flares up." It is separation for a time. This slant on termination of a therapeutic relationship deviates from traditional wisdom but does reflect Peplau's idea of *resolution* of a focused issue. In a sense the therapeutic relationship does not end but the clients transfer their new skills and behaviors back to their everyday environment. It is a time to summarize all the data about central issues and to reiterate learned strategies to cope with problems. It is the hallmark of seamless, integrated care.

Ideally the timing of the endpoint in a therapeutic relationship is agreed on by the treatment team, client, and nurse. Criteria that can be used to determine when termination is appropriate may include the following:

- Experience of relief from the problem or central issue that initiated the relationship
- Observation of increased social functioning and decreased social isolation on the part of the client
- A strong sense of self-integration
- Achievement of specific predetermined goals

Anxiety about anticipated change occurs in clients when they realize they will not have the security of scheduled support. Anticipating the endpoint of the relationship activates a grieving process. The purpose of the grieving process is effective separation. The process is complete when client and nurse internalize the loss of the therapeutic relationship in its present form, knowing that future encounters may be needed and are possible.

It is not unusual in the finishing stages of a therapeutic relationship, particularly one that has been of long duration, for clients to begin to experience a variety of somatic symptoms. They may become depressed and preoccupied with guilt. They may wonder whether it was something they did that caused the relationship to end. A stiff manner, designed to hide anger, often develops. For awhile, the client may decompensate, that is, lose the capacity for initiating or maintaining healthy patterns of behavior. To reduce their anxiety, clients may use defense mechanisms such as acting out, dependency, resignation, denial, and reaction formation (see Chapter 22).

In a single session or other brief encounter, clients may save important information until the last few minutes of the therapeutic time. At this time it is important to remain focused on goal fulfillment and achievements.

Hospitalized clients about to be discharged may leave the hospital precipitously, "against medical advice." Some clients abruptly end the relationship by refusing to keep appointments with the nurse. When clients run away from the hospital or sign out early, the ending process does not occur and nurses and client may both experience a sense of incompleteness.

Termination or ending strategies begin with the nurse's comfort with the impending separation. The single most important nursing intervention during the finishing phase of a therapeutic relationship is alerting the client to the endpoint. The nurse conveys that leaving is not something he or she does to the client but rather something done *with* the client. Summarizing situations that occurred throughout the relationship, exchanging memories, and evaluating goals are experiences that nurses share with clients.

Clients are reassured that they can reestablish a therapeutic relationship at a future point if new problems need resolution. For some clients with chronic illness regular checkups may be scheduled.

KEY POINTS

- Understanding of another begins with understanding oneself.
- The process of using self therapeutically requires that nurses identify their own the feelings, thoughts, and behaviors that emerge in response to a client. Self-assessment facilitates this self-awareness.
- The self may be public, semipublic, private, or unknown.
- A sense of identity is the awareness of being a person separate and distinct from all others.
- Peplau's model emphasizes therapeutic use of self and the psychiatric nursing roles of stranger, teacher, resource person, surrogate, leader, and counselor.
- Core dimensions used throughout a therapeutic relationship include empathetic understanding, genuineness, respect, concreteness, confrontation, and immediacy.
- Brief relationship or short-term psychotherapy is a time-limited, dynamic, outcome-oriented process that is appropriate when clients experience acute problems, have a history of rapid adjustment, and have a healthy relationship style and an existing support system.
- Peplau identified orientation, exploration, identification, and resolution as the stages of therapeutic nurse-client encounters.
- The mnemonic DWARF is used as a guide to the phases of brief therapeutic relationships. The phases include **D**esigning, **W**armup, **A**greement, **R**ehabilitation, and **F**inishing.
- The designing or preinteractive phase of a therapeutic relationship includes self-preparation by the nurse and attention to the practical details necessary for interacting with clients.
- The beginning or warm-up stage of a therapeutic relationship is the time when rapport is built, the boundaries and goals for the relationship are established, and contacts are formalized.
- The middle stage of a therapeutic relationship is referred to as the working or rehabilitative phase. Under the guidance of the nurse, clients explore their feelings and behaviors and test new ways of relating. Resistance, transference, and countertransference phenomena are worked through to achieve behavioral change.
- The time just preceding a separation between nurse and client is referred to as the termination or finishing phase of a helping relationship. It is a time when clients "separate" from the nurse, summaries are exchanged, memories are shared, and goals are evaluated.

CRITICAL THINKING QUESTIONS

Sally is a nursing student who is beginning her psychiatric rotation at the local Veteran's Administration hospital. She is shy and was somewhat timid during orientation to the unit, often looking at the locked door. She feels relieved that her assigned client, Marcella, is a 22-year-old college student like herself and feels confident that she will be able to establish a therapeutic relationship with her.

Marcella was brought to the hospital 2 days ago by her father after a suicide attempt. At the team meeting the staff reported that Marcella had been hospitalized here before and at that time had accused her father of raping her. Her father is a high-ranking military officer stationed at the local military base. Marcella's mother died when she was 8 years old. During the last hospitalization, Marcella subsequently denied her original story and was discharged to her father's care. She returned to college and seemed to be doing well until the Christmas break.

Over the weekend, Marcella was often found standing in the middle of the room looking as if she were lost. She repeated over and over that "he did it again." Liquid Haldol was prescribed for Marcella, even though she personally was unable to sign a consent for treatment. Her father had health care power of attorney.

Sally attempts a therapeutic interaction, but Marcella is vague and nonresponsive. She appears to be actively hallucinating. Sally has an interaction study assignment to complete, so she attempts to elicit a verbal response while sitting with Marcella in the day room. Sally realizes that she will probably not be suc-

cessful because of Marcella's symptoms but continues anyway. Sally is feeling very inadequate and can sense that her anxiety is increasing.

After about 5 minutes of receiving only stares for responses, Sally asks if what the staff is saying is true—that she was raped by her father? Marcella does not verbally respond at first but is incontinent of urine while sitting in the chair. When Sally is assisting to clean and redress her, Marcella begins speaking. She tells Sally, "The only one that can help me is my mother. This all started when she died. My father smothered me. He killed me."

1. What self-assessment questions would be appropriate for Sally to ask herself about her initial feelings toward Marcella?
2. What reactions are *you* experiencing about this client?
3. What potential legal and ethical issues are revealed in the case study?
4. How would you interpret Marcella's incontinence and disclosure about her father?
5. Would you discuss the information you gained from Marcella with her father? Why or why not?
6. What are Marcella's strengths?
7. How can these be used as part of the team plan for Marcella?
8. Is Marcella a candidate for short-term rehabilitation? Why? Why not?
9. What therapeutic strategies would you use during an initial encounter with Marcella?
10. What short-term outcomes could you negotiate with Marcella?

REFERENCES

Akhtar, S., & Samuel, S. (1996). The concept of identity: Developmental origins, phenomenology, clinical relevance, and measurement. *Harvard Review of Psychiatry, 3*(5), 254-267.

American Nurses Association. (1994). *A statement on psychiatric-mental health clinical nursing practice and standards of psychiatric-mental health nursing practice.* Washington, DC: American Nurses Publishing.

Carkhoff, R. (1968). *Helping and human relations.* New York: Holt.

Delaney, K., Ulsafer-VanLanen, J., Pitula, C.R., & Johnson, M.E. (1995). Seven days and counting: How inpatient nurses might adjust their practice to brief hospitalization. *Journal of Psychosocial Nursing, 33*(8), 36-40.

Forchuk, C. (1995). Uniqueness within the nurse client relationship. *Archives of Psychiatric Nursing, 9*(1), 34-30.

Hoyt, M.F. (1995). Characteristics of psychotherapy under managed care. *Behavioral Healthcare Tomorrow, 3*(5), 59-62.

Mann, J. (1981). The core of time-limited psychotherapy: Time and the central issue. In S. Budman (Ed.). *Forms of Brief Therapy.* New York, NY: Gilford Press, 25-43.

McCloskey, J.C., & Bulechek, G.M. (1995). *Nursing interventions classification (NIC).* (2nd ed.). St. Louis: Mosby.

Peplau, H. (1952). *Interpersonal relations in nursing.* New York: Putnam.

Schneider, S.E., & Ross, I. (1996). Ultra-short hospitalization for severely mentally ill clients. *Psychiatric Services, 47*(2), 137-138.

Wilson, J.H., & Hobbs, H. (1995). Therapeutic partnership: A model for clinical practice. *Journal of Psychosocial Nursing, 33*(2), 27-30.

Part Three

Nursing Interventions

Chapter 10

Crisis Intervention

Mary Rosedale

LEARNING OUTCOMES

After studying and applying the concepts of this chapter, the learner will be able to:
- Define crisis.
- Identify characteristics of the crisis state.
- Examine the neurobiological basis of the crisis response.
- Differentiate among maturational, situational, and social crises.
- Complete a crisis assessment.
- Develop a crisis intervention plan that includes potential solutions and methods for accomplishing them.
- Implement a crisis intervention plan.
- Evaluate the effectiveness of the crisis intervention plan.

KEY TERMS

Balancing factors	Crisis prevention	Situational crisis
Crisis	Maturational crisis	Social crisis
Crisis intervention		

crisis is a part of life in American society and many other Western societies. People have become accustomed to thinking about a crisis, concluding that exposure to certain events such as terrorism, natural disaster, or personal tragedy precipitate a crisis. The notion of a crisis has been expanded to incorporate situations that connote a sense of loss, threat, or critical change such as unemployment, divorce, or retirement. Yet many people respond to these challenges with a remarkable degree of courage and creativity, a striving toward life and growth that is inspirational. It is not the event itself that constitutes a crisis. Instead, it is the individual's perception of the event as threatening, overwhelming, or harmful and the resulting sense of distress that mounts as the person is temporarily unable to modify this inner and outer reality that characterize a crisis. *Crisis intervention refers to the timely and skillful use of the nursing process toward alleviating the environmental, emotional, perceptual and cognitive impact of the crisis while enhancing the capacity for growth, development, and change.*

The purpose of this chapter is to discuss the concept of crisis and the types of crises and to examine a crisis intervention model that enables students to analyze and intervene in individual and family crises.

DEFINITION OF A CRISIS

A *crisis is a turning point, resulting from a stressful event or threat to one's well-being. It occurs where a conflict, problem, or situation of importance is perceived as threatening and not readily solvable by past methods.* Anxiety increases, effective cognitive functioning decreases, and behavior becomes disorganized. The person urgently seeks help because old problem-solving methods do not work. Crises share identifiable characteristics. Table 10-1 identifies the characteristics of a crisis.

DEVELOPMENT OF A CRISIS

Identifiable phases of crisis, which are psychosocial in character, lead to an active crisis state. Parad and Parad (1990) describe a four-phase sequence in the development of crisis that will be illustrated in the following clinical example.

Eleanor is a 76-year-old, widowed Holocaust survivor and mother of two daughters. Estranged from her eldest daughter, Laura, she resides with her other daughter, Karen, age 38. When asked about the separation from her eldest daughter, Eleanor offhandedly reports, "She says I'm totally consumed with Karen." The choice of metaphor is illuminating, since Karen has just been hospitalized for treatment of recurrent anorexia nervosa.

Phase 1

A specific and identifiable stressful precipitating event occurs. People commonly experience feelings of discomfort and bewilderment.

Her daughter's hospitalization was a stressful and disturbing event. Attempting to recap and make sense of the situation, Eleanor described averting her eyes from her daughter's dinner plate and clearing the dishes as Karen inevitably headed upstairs to the bathroom. Confronted with the reality that her daughter was vomiting and was in a life-threatening situation, Eleanor conveyed a sense of bewilderment and implored the nurse to understand: "I wanted to give her space; I had no idea that it had gotten so bad."

Phase 2

The event is perceived as a threat and produces an increase in anxiety. Attempts are made to cope with and to resolve the crisis through characteristic problem-solving methods and defense mechanisms such as analyzing the event, talking it over with friends, or denying the reality of the situation. Feelings of danger and confusion are often experienced. If efforts at this stage are ineffective, the person feels he or she is at an impasse and moves on to the next phase.

For Eleanor, hospitalization and the unanticipated reality that her daughter was dangerously ill represented the external threat. Before the event, she had thought herself a good mother and keen observer of events and people. Her sense of self was shaken and this constituted the internal threat. Looking back on her life, she felt that she had achieved nothing and that she had failed in the very areas she valued most. Customary problem-solving techniques of analyzing and reconstructing the event only led to anxiety and guilt. Whereas she could usually talk problems over with Karen, she now felt alone and unable to deny the problem.

Phase 3

Increased anxiety and disorganization occur and may be manifested cognitively, physically, behaviorally, or socially (see Table 10-1). At this phase, common feelings include desperation and apathy.

Eleanor described feeling as though she was in a cloud. She appeared dazed and asked the nurse to repeat questions. Perceiving the external experience as hopeless and neverending, she portrayed Karen as incurable. Recounting a personal sense of courage and fortitude associated with tragedy and noting her changed self-perception, she said: "I used to be like Jacqueline Kennedy but now I'm like John Kennedy; I feel that I've been assassinated." She experienced intermittent headaches and episodes of exhaustion and insomnia and

TABLE 10-1

Characteristics of crisis

CHARACTERISTIC	EXPERIENCE	EXAMPLE
Identifiable precipitant	Loss	Death of loved one Divorce Job termination Destruction of home or property
	Transition	Moving to another community Graduation from school, entry into work Marriage Birth of a child
	Challenge	Job promotion Career change
	Cluster stress events	Combined stress of several events occurring simultaneously such as divorce, transition to being single, challenges of single parenting and financial independence
Perception of threat	The magnitude of danger experienced is based on the perceived degree of external alarm and internal alarm	*External alarm:* environmental risk to safety and security such as loss of relationship, role, income, or property; *internal alarm:* belief that important values, life goals, or views about oneself and about the world are in jeopardy
Mounting tension	Stress not alleviated by usual methods; intensity and duration surpass manageable levels	Usual coping methods such as talking matters over with friends, "waiting it out," exercising, throwing oneself into work and engaging in diversional activities do not work; the level of stress continues to escalate
Outbursts of anxiety	Cognitively	Racing thoughts, inability to think clearly, difficulty concentrating, indecisiveness; exaggerated view of the situation as unsolvable, inescapable, neverending, and magnified view of threat to the self structure as "falling apart"
	Physically	Development of somatic symptoms such as headaches, back pain, abdominal pain, loss of appetite, vomiting, and diarrhea
	Behaviorally	Impulsive, disorganized, erratic action, "hit-or-miss" attempts to modify experience rather than customary problem-solving, disturbance in usual patterns of eating, sleeping, dreaming, lovemaking, working
	Socially	Disruptions in usual relationships, withdrawal from or conflict with others

TABLE 10-1—cont'd

Characteristics of crisis

CHARACTERISTIC	EXPERIENCE	EXAMPLE
Time-limitation	By its nature the experience of crisis is felt to be interminable; however, the intensity cannot be sustained over an extended period of time. Crises are generally resolved positively or negatively in 4 to 6 weeks	After a crime such as a mugging the victim tends to feel unsafe, to become hypervigilant with an exaggerated startle reflex. Over time, the person may view the experience promoting a positive change such as a change in lifestyle or perspective. The person may learn personal self-defense skills, feel in control of self, and resume usual functioning. In contrast the person may conclude that the world is an unsafe place and never return to the previous trusting state.
Help-seeking	An enhanced willingness to pursue and accept outside assistance	*Feelings of helplessness:* "I can't manage this myself"; *urgency:* "I need help now" are common self-descriptions.

described pacing back and forth in her empty home. She stopped going to the synagogue and refused phone calls from friends. In a powerful statement that depicts how the meaning of an event is shaped by experience, background, and culture, she asserted: "You can never comprehend the shame of a Holocaust survivor whose own child starves herself. I can't face people."

Phase 4

The person mobilizes internal and external resources and tries out new problem-solving methods or redefines the threat so that old methods can work. This is a prime time for intervention as feelings of helplessness and urgency lead people to seek and accept assistance. Resolution can occur in this phase if new or old problem-solving methods are put into action and are effective.

Resolution of the crisis can lead to a return to a pre-crisis level of functioning or to an increase or decrease in the person's functional level. This sequence is illustrated in Fig. 10-1.

With crisis intervention, Eleanor redefined her problem as one of excessive reliance on Karen. She recognized that for the past 5 years, she had neglected her eldest daughter and had increasingly isolated herself from friends and community supports. Now that Karen was hospitalized, it was not surprising that she felt unbearably alone with no situational supports to help her cope with the stress. The nurse assisted Eleanor in expanding support systems, decreasing her anxiety, and expressing feelings about past and present losses to support progression through grief stages.

Eleanor recontacted her eldest daughter Laura, who was receptive to reconnecting with her mother. She planned activities with Laura and with friends, volunteered to organize a Holocaust memorial exhibition at the local library, and was introduced to a multiple family group—a treatment method that merges theoretical concepts of crisis groups and family crisis therapy.

As family relationship patterns began to shift, Eleanor was able to more realistically view her position as support for her daughter's recovery and the crisis was resolved.

THE NEUROBIOLOGICAL BASIS OF THE CRISIS RESPONSE

Much as the perception of stress prompts one to use psychological capacities for coping, physiological resources are tapped so that the body is geared to combat or defend against threat. If the stress is not decreased, the sustained neurobiological responses produce a kind of circuit overload—capacities are overtaxed, and the prolonged use of physiological mechanisms produce negative consequences. Robinson (1990) describes the components of the crisis response as follows:

Phase 1: Immediate Physiological Processes

The autonomic nervous system is activated when an individual perceives a threat or demand from the environment. The hypothalamus stimulates the sympathetic fibers as the body prepares for "fight or flight." Within 2 to 3 minutes, sympathetic nerve fibers release the catecholamines of epinephrine and norepinephrine, which

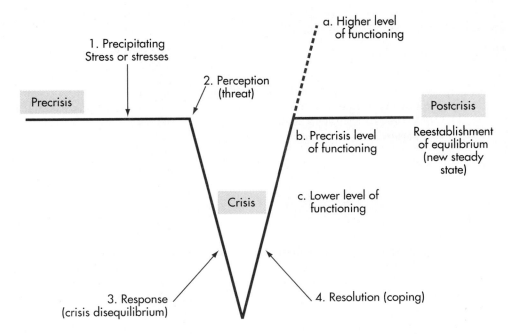

Fig. 10-1 The crisis intervention "roller coaster."

last between 5 and 10 minutes. Anxiety is experienced and can be observed both through a person's verbal report, as well as clinical signs, including perspiration, tremulousness, and rapid pulse and breathing.

Phase 2: Intermediate Response

Following the secretion of epinephrine and norepinephrine, these neurotransmitters travel to the end organs where they maintain the processes already initiated. These sympathetic effects are maintained for 1 to 2 hours. The adrenal medulla does not continue its response but is reactivated only after the central nervous system triggers the sympathetic nervous system again. The catecholamines also stimulate gluconeogenesis, which provides the body with additional energy.

Phase 3: Long-Term Response

Three pathways of the endocrine system perpetuate the long-term effects of stress: the adrenocorticotropic, the thyroxine, and the vasopressin pathways. The adrenal cortex secretes two types of corticoids: the mineralocorticoids and glucocorticoids. Aldosterone, a mineralocorticoid, raises the systemic blood pressure. Cortisol, which is a representative of the three glucocorticoids, is pivotal to the breakdown of fats and proteins for energy. Their prolonged secretion, however, has negative effects such

as overtaxing the liver, sustained skeletal muscle breakdown, and continued salt and water retention. The effects of thyroxine are not observed until it peaks at about the tenth day following the stressful event, and the effect may last 6 to 8 weeks. Thyroxine increases the body's metabolism as much as 60% to 100%. This is why people may have weight loss. Vasopressin is released from the posterior pituitary gland and elevates blood pressure. The concept of crisis response can be understood on a time continuum characterized by initial neurobiological reactions and subsequent response phases.

CRISIS THEORY PARADIGM

Aguilera (1994) developed a crisis paradigm that provides a framework for examining the presence or absence of balancing factors in a crisis. *Balancing factors include the person's perception of the event, situational supports, and coping mechanisms.* Strengths or weaknesses in any one of these factors can be directly related to the onset of crisis or to its resolution. This paradigm helps to explain how two people faced with the same objective event may respond very differently. In the realm of human experience, there are additional dimensions through which an event is processed. One person may view an episode as devastating and intractable, whereas for another person it may enact the striving to overcome and transcend handicap.

Effective resolution of crisis is more likely to occur if:

1. *The perception of the precipitating event is realistic rather than distorted.* If the event is perceived realistically, there will be recognition of the relationship between the event and feelings of stress. Problem-solving can then be appropriately directed toward reduction of tension and resolution of the stressful situation. If the perception of the event is distorted, there may be no recognition of the relationship between the event and feelings of stress. The clinical example below illustrates the importance of assessing the perception of an event.

Catherine, a 67-year-old widow of 1 year came to the mental health clinic at the suggestion of the police. Eight months ago she was the victim of a burglary. Since that time she has repeatedly called the police department with the complaint of menacing sounds in her home, creaks and thumps that could never be explained. Now she lays awake at night, listening for danger in the stillness. The safety and security of her home is gone, all she sees is remote hiding places, locks, and burglar alarms. Tearfully she notes, "Even the police have deserted me." As the nurse explored Catherine's perception of the problem and her sense of being "deserted," it became clear that Catherine had always felt protected by her husband. The crime event quite literally "drove home" the fact that he was no longer there to protect her. Catherine revised her perception of the problem to include grieving for her husband's loss.

2. *Situational supports are available to the person; people in the environment can be depended on to help solve the problem.* When situational supports such as family, friends, teachers, counselors, or religious advisors are not available, the person may feel overwhelmed, alone, vulnerable, and without anchor. Part of the crisis-intervention plan includes helping clients to mobilize and/or develop support systems that become interpersonal resources, as depicted in the following clinical example:

Ralph, a 44-year-old midwestern farmer came to the crisis clinic saying he was on the verge of emotional and physical collapse. Three months earlier, his farm was threatened by a series of storms that ultimately destroyed the bulk of his crop. Facing an economic crisis, his wife Gwen found employment at the local mercantile. Ralph helped out with the child and home care responsibilities but now experienced his wife as increasingly demanding and unsatisfied with his every effort. Angrily he asserted "maybe I wasn't cut out to be a housewife." As the nurse explored available situational supports, Ralph reported that there was no one to whom he could turn. Although he knew everyone in the town, his wife's employment prompted him to feel glaringly exposed

in his failure to support the family. When Gwen asked him to run town errands, he refused because he was afraid he would come into contact with contemptuous neighbors. The nurse gave him the assignment of contacting one person who shared the potential loss of livelihood prompted by the storms. The following week, Ralph reported that he and Gwen had dinner at a neighbor's house. They agreed that the economic crisis although disastrous, was season-limited and that the community had to pull together just as they had in the days of his father and grandfather. His physical complaint disappeared.

3. *Coping mechanisms that alleviate anxiety are available.* Over a lifetime, persons develop coping mechanisms, which can be cognitive, emotional, or spiritual. Available coping mechanisms are behaviors in which a person usually engages when he or she has a problem (e.g., sitting down and trying to think it out with a friend). Some cry it out or try to get rid of their feelings by yelling or swearing, kicking a chair, or slamming a door. Others go jogging or walking to engage in other types of physical activity. Such coping mechanisms have been found effective in maintaining emotional stability and have become a part of the person's lifestyle in dealing with the stresses of daily life. When a new stress-producing situation arises and learned coping mechanisms are not effective, anxiety is experienced. The person engages in efforts to "do something" to relieve the discomfort of anxiety. The following clinical example illustrates both the failure of previous coping mechanisms to moderate a stressful event and the role of the interdisciplinary team in crisis intervention:

Jennifer, a 26-year-old housewife came to the emergency room with the hand of her trembling 8-year-old son, Billy, clutched in her own. She told the triage nurse that although her husband Jim had been violent toward her in the past, he had never struck Billy. Tonight, "after a few beers with his friends," Jim came home and demanded to know who she had been talking with on the phone. He accused her of having an affair and threw her against the wall. Billy ran to protect his mother but was cast to the floor with Jim's fisted blow to his chest. Later that night, she secretively gathered her son and slipped out of the house.

Jennifer said she had tried everything she could think of to be a good wife. She listened to Jim's difficulties at work, tried to help with his problems, kept her own difficulties to herself, encouraged him to spend time with his friends, asked him to join Alcoholics Anonymous, stopped calling and seeing friends for fear of Jim's jealousy, prayed, and pretended that things were getting better. There were no relatives to whom she could turn. Faced with the crisis event of her son's abuse, Jennifer no longer believed that her previous coping methods would help.

The nurse notified the surgical resident, the child welfare authority, and the social worker. After physical examination, the resident ordered a series of x-rays for mother and son and consulted adult and pediatric orthopedists. For Jennifer, x-rays revealed past healing fractures of her wrists and right arm. Billy's x-rays showed two acute rib fractures requiring his admission to the hospital. The pediatric unit nurses were notified of the admitting situation and immediately restricted Jim's visitation. The social worker advised Jennifer about shelters for battered women and children, and support groups for abuse victims. Jennifer accepted the referrals and was ushered to a shelter by a crisis volunteer. Through her continued relationship with a caseworker from the child welfare authority, she obtained legal assistance in pressing charges and ultimately divorced Jim.

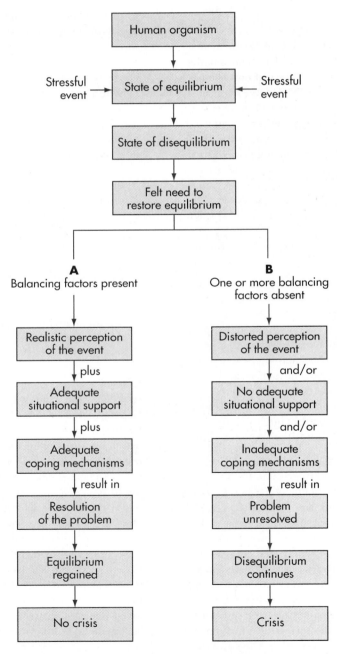

Fig. 10-2   Aguilera's crisis theory paradigm. (From Aguilera, D.C. (1994). *Crisis intervention: Theory and methodology* (7th ed.). St. Louis: Mosby.)

The balancing factors described on p. 167 are presented in Fig. 10-2 in the crisis theory paradigm developed by Aguilera (1994).

TYPES OF CRISES

Three types of crises can be identified: anticipated maturational crises of the life cycle, unanticipated situational crises, and unanticipated social crises (Hoff, 1989). It is common for a person to experience more than one type of crisis at the same time.

Maturational Crises

Maturational crises, sometimes called developmental crises, are predictable life events that occur gradually in the course of the life cycle. The nature and extent of the maturational crisis is influenced by the four factors listed below. An example of such a crisis follows:

1. *The success with which previous life transitions have been mastered.*
2. *Role models provide the person with examples of how to act in a new role and give the person heroes (i.e., persons to emulate, by which to be inspired and supported).*
3. *Interpersonal resources such as relationships that influence a person's ability to grow and change.* Persons who experience extreme anxiety not moderated by situational supports may require professional assistance to cope with and resolve problematic situations.
4. *The degree to which others accept or resist the new role.* The greater the resistance, the more difficulty in making a change (see Chapter 7).

Gina, a 17-year-old single mother, stated that she had a baby so that someone would love her unconditionally. She described neglect by her own mother and expressed an ardent desire to be different, to be a good mother, and to "do it on my own." She had no contact with the baby's father and although they lived in the same house, she and her own mother barely spoke. Easily frustrated with the baby's crying, she felt rejected when the infant was not soothed by her cooing and rocking. Thinking that each cry was an indictment of her failure as a mother, she felt driven to scream at and shake the infant. She thought herself "a terrible person" and described nightmares, tremulousness, and a "pounding" heart rate. She came to the crisis clinic saying: "I'm afraid I might hurt my baby."

The unresolved dependency issues that kept Gina focused on the unmet need for love, inhibited movement to adolescence. Gina's struggle with developmental tasks of self-definition and independence without having resolved earlier issues led to the maturational crisis of adolescence (Slaikeu, 1990a).

Seeking to resolve the crisis by meeting both dependency needs for "unconditional love" and adolescent needs for self-definition through identification of self as a "good mother," Gina had a baby. This precipitated the compounding maturational crisis of motherhood.

Situational Crises

Situational crises occur when unanticipated events threaten a person's biological, social, or psychologic integrity. Examples include loss of a loved one, loss or change of job, financial changes, geographical move, unwanted pregnancy, birth of a premature or disabled child, and illness in self or significant other (Slaikeu, 1990b).

Parad and Parad (1990) state that the unpredictable nature of these events introduces an element of hazard that does not exist in the anticipated maturational crises. The element of unpreparedness increases the potential for disruption of lifestyle. Parad and Parad (1992) describe the dynamic interactions among participants in the crisis drama, as illustrated in the following example:

John B., age 45, was offered a vice presidency in a California engineering firm that had just secured a large government contract. The offer was too good to refuse. His family, consisting of his wife and three children, ages 12, 15, and 17, reluctantly moved from their lifelong Connecticut home to Los Angeles. After 6 months of work, the contract fell through. John's firm went bankrupt, and he was out of a job. At the same time, John's wife was depressed and lonely, 3,000 miles from family and friends. Now she was faced with financial insecurity as well. The children were having difficulty adjusting to a different academic program and making new friends. The financial crisis led John to begin drinking heavily; he was embarrassed to call his old firm in Connecticut, had few business contacts in the area, and was not making any new job connections. The family's savings were being depleted rapidly.

The job change and geographical move initiated a sequence of events that involved all family members. The hazardous situation became a family crisis when John lost his job. Financial stress and loss of self worth, followed by heavy drinking, school problems, and loss of extended family connections combined to create a network of situational crises that would have to be confronted before resolution could take place.

Social Crises

Social crises are accidental, uncommon, and unanticipated crises that involve multiple losses or extensive environmental change (Aguilera, 1994). Examples might include natural disasters such as fires, floods, hurricanes, and earthquakes; national disasters such as wars, riots, or genocide; and violent crimes such as serial rape or murder (Barash, 1990; Caurtois, 1990).

Box 10-1

The Oklahoma City Bombing

- A truck bomb carrying 4,800 pounds of explosives detonated at 9:02 AM on April 19, 1995 outside of the Alfred R. Murrah Federal Building in Oklahoma City, where offices and a day-care center were housed
- Highest death toll of any terrorist act on U.S. soil
- A wave of bomb threats followed the attack, including a fatal attack by an ecoterrorist known as the Unabomber
- Awareness and reaction increased through mass media and Internet
- The bomb was found to be made of commonly available ingredients and the chief suspect was identified as an American citizen, causing anxiety about another attack
- 5,862 crisis workers from the Red Cross, opening more than 600 cases, were part of the relief effort
- A nurse who was injured by falling debris in the rescue effort became one of the casualties
- A total of 169 lives were lost, including many children

The shock value of these events make social crises among the most challenging in terms of individual coping, as illustrated in the example of the 1995 Oklahoma City bombing (Box 10-1).

The most common headline referring to the Oklahoma City bombing disaster read "Terror in the Heartland." The imagery is accurate, since the shock from this event struck at the epicenter of America and at the heart of the fears and insecurities of its citizens. Far away from the "hot spots" of the world, Oklahoma seemed to be an unlikely target for terrorist violence. The incongruity of the event deepened its impact as a social crisis.

Tynhurst (1951) describes three overlapping phases of individual response to community disasters: impact, recoil, and posttraumatic. The impact phase, lasting from a few minutes to 1 or 2 hours, is characterized by both effective action and by some degree of panic or hysteria. Both were in evidence shortly after the blast in Oklahoma. Rescue workers from around the nation were mobilized within a matter of hours, and the President and Attorney General were on television before the end of the working day. At the same time, workers in other federal office buildings panicked, leaving their offices in droves.

In the recoil phase, there is a desire in the community to express an outpouring of emotion regarding the traumatic event. One interesting contemporary example of this was the creation of an electronic sympathy card on the Internet with hundreds of messages from as far away as England and Australia. An electronic resource named HealingNet was established by the National Performance Review to give Federal employees and other concerned citizens a place to vent their feelings and concerns, discuss issues, and begin the healing process. This shows how the concept of community has broadened in the electronic age, but established principles governing community response prevail. The recoil phase was lengthy, partly because the rescue effort dragged on for 16 days after the attack. Impact overlapped with recoil as bomb threats and attacks continued during this time.

The posttraumatic phase continues to this day. Survivors of the blast may be plagued by guilt, anger, nightmares, anxiety reactions, reactive depressions, or even psychotic episodes as a result of the dislocation caused by the assault on their lives. Certainly, the effects of the Oklahoma bombing as a social crisis are still perceptible and will likely not fade from the national consciousness for some time (see Chapter 24).

ROLE OF THE NURSE IN CRISIS INTERVENTION

According to the American Nurses Association (ANA) psychiatric-mental health nursing's *Standards* (1994), psychiatric-mental health nurses provide direct crisis intervention services to people in crisis and serve as members of crisis teams. Crisis intervention is a short-term therapeutic process that focuses on the resolution of an immediate crisis or emergency through the use of available professional personnel, family, and/or environmental resources.

Nurses practice in a variety of traditional settings where crisis intervention is the therapy of choice. Nurses who work on general hospital units deal with crisis resulting from the stresses of hospitalization, illness, and death on a daily basis. Nurses who work in obstetric, pediatric, adolescent, or geriatric settings deal with families undergoing maturational and situational crises. Emergency rooms are deluged 24 hours a day with clients in crisis. Nurses who work on psychiatric units deal with the crisis of first-time mental illness and the crisis of relapse. Within the context of short-term hospitalization, rapid stabilization is the goal. As such, crisis intervention is the form of brief therapy that clients and families receive before discharge and seamless transition to the next phase of treatment.

Likewise, crisis intervention has become a vital component in community settings. Economic pressure to curtail health care costs has resulted in shortened hospital stays, alternatives to hospitalization, and deinstitutionalization of the mentally ill. Increases in the population of older adults with chronic health problems, the prevalence of AIDS, and heightened awareness of substance abuse; sexual molestation; teenage suicide; and child, spousal, and elder abuse has created further demand for emergency and preventive crisis services in the community.

CULTURAL HIGHLIGHTS

Crisis Intervention for Filipino Americans

Assessment

1. Filipino Americans show an increased prevalence of clinical depression compared with the general population and male Filipino-American elderly are especially prone to alcoholism.
2. Among Asian groups in San Francisco, Filipino Americans have the highest percentage of AIDS cases and middle school students have the highest rate of suicide attempts and teenage pregnancy.
3. Most Filipino Americans are first-generation immigrants with potential stressors including unemployment or underemployment, legal and immigration problems, separation from social supports, cultural adjustment, and generational conflict problems that can lead to crisis.
4. Anger and irritability may be expressed literally as "my head is always hot" and anxiety may be translated literally to mean "I feel cold." The expression of symptoms in somatic terms coupled with the use of medical versus mental health resources leads to failure in recognizing symptoms and providing appropriate crisis referral.
5. Filipino Americans may smile when expressing serious problems or oscillate between smiling and crying in a short time. This may lead to minimized assessment of depressive symptoms or to labeling of "inappropriate affect."
6. Shyness, little eye contact, and hesitancy to share "shameful" information and to question the clinician's suggestions when the client does not agree may lead to the clinician's frustration and misinterpretation of cultural characteristics as evidence of passivity or paranoia.
7. Since divorce is not allowed by the Catholic Church (the home country's predominant religion) and is illegal in the Philippines, marital conflict may be endured, and in the case of divorce the event may be perceived as a catastrophic stressor. Aside from the associated cluster stress events such as financial instability and child-rearing difficulties, there is a feeling of *hiya*—the guilt and stigma associated with being divorced among Filipino Americans and back in the Philippines when news of the divorce reaches home (Cabezas, 1982; Munoz, 1987; Tompar-Tiu and Sustento-Seneriches, 1995).

Intervention

1. Encourage development of support systems. Actively involve people who are influential in encouraging the client to seek help and the most influential "elder" in the family structure as a means of eliciting cooperation in treatment. Participation in church-affiliated community centers, particularly in areas with a high concentration of Filipino Americans should be maximized in referrals (Tompar-Tiu and Sustento-Seneriches, 1995).
2. "What has bothered you most? What kind of problems have you experienced?" are more meaningful than, "Are you feeling sad or depressed?" because symptoms are not usually expressed effectively.
3. Monitoring side effects of medications is especially important with Filipino Americans who appear to develop side effects at lower doses of antipsychotics, antidepressants, antianxiety medications, and lithium (Chien, 1989; Lin and Poland, 1989).
4. Selective preventive intervention for adolescent suicide, teen-age pregnancy, AIDS, and alcohol abuse are urgently needed in the Filipino community.

In these, as in all settings, nurses work in collaboration with families, interdisciplinary, and community personnel. The future of crisis intervention will require innovative interactional and network approaches such as the dissemination of information and coordination of services over computer networks. The use of electronic media and networks as resources for crisis intervention and prevention is the wave of the future.

Efforts at delivering quality services while managing their cost will reinforce the importance of brief crisis therapy, approximately two to eight sessions in length. Tools such as critical pathways, a map of the intervention time frame with specific, measurable outcomes for each session and the means toward achieving short- and long-term goals will increasingly be required by insurance companies and managed care organizations.

As cost-effective providers, nurses will be used more often in the roles of primary therapist, case manager, teacher, and researcher. They will directly provide brief crisis therapy, access and coordinate resources, instruct others in time-limited crisis intervention, and generate outcome-based research demonstrating the clinical efficacy and cost-savings of effective crisis management.

Nurses working in crisis intervention work with clients from various cultures. They must be sensitive to the cultural aspects that influence a client's behavior and treatment. The Cultural Highlights box on p. 171 specifies cultural considerations for Filipino Americans.

Legal and Ethical Issues in Crisis Intervention

In crisis intervention, the ethical principle of beneficence (literally "to do good") refers to the calculation of the potential risks and benefits of giving or withholding treatment. The ethical principle of beneficence, the psychiatric-mental health clinical nursing's *Standards* (1994) and legal requirements overlap in supporting appropriate crisis intervention. For example, leaving a suicidal client in a crisis would not only violate professional ethics and standards of practice but could lead to legal liability. Although we live in an age characterized by rampant litigation, the danger of exposure to lawsuit should never paralyze a nurse. In most cases, establishing good communication with clients and families, and acting in a professionally responsible manner will minimize or nullify potential liability risks (see Chapter 3).

OTHER METHODS OF CRISIS INTERVENTION

Crisis intervention uses a variety of strategies in formulating a comprehensive but short-term treatment plan. The methods of crisis intervention presented below represent initial, additional, or alternative intervention strategies.

Telephone Crisis Hotlines

Crisis intervention centers rely heavily on trained volunteers who "staff the telephones." These counselors are often the first to initiate contact with persons in crisis, to identify appropriate community resources, and to refer the client to an appropriate agency without delay. If the situation is assessed as highly dangerous, the counselor assumes directive action such as eliciting the person's whereabouts and dispatching a multidisciplinary crisis team to the home. Telephone crisis counseling is unique in terms of accessibility and availability. Most people have a telephone or ready access to one and the cost for its use is low. Accessibility is critical for crisis clients, especially those who are suicidal or homicidal, and for those unable to leave their homes (elderly, physically disabled). Most hotlines are available day or night, 365 days of the year. (Slaikeu and Simon, 1990).

Emergency Department Crisis Counseling

The nurse working in the emergency department continually encounters people in crisis. On a daily basis, the nurse observes attempted suicides, rape, and assault victims and their families, people with sudden onset illness such as a heart attack, and people with chronic anxiety who present with a myriad of symptoms. All these people are candidates for crisis intervention. The role of the nurse in the emergency department is to assess and define the problem, initiate brief intervention measures such as approaches to reduce anxiety, and provide appropriate referral.

Mobile Crisis Units

In many metropolitan areas the emergency department of major medical centers have a mobile crisis team that goes out into the community or home to assess and triage problems, provide brief crisis therapy, and facilitate appropriate referrals and necessary hospitalization. Mobile crisis intervention has several features:

1. Mobile crisis team can be dispatched immediately.
2. Underserved populations such as the homeless, chronic mentally ill, and elderly can be accessed through the service's mobility.
3. Clients are served in the communities where they live. This provides a clearer picture of the actual crisis situation and facilitates the involvement of situational supports without resorting to costly and unnecessary hospitalization.

Home Care

Home care nurses often encounter clients in crisis—persons who are temporarily unable to negotiate the demands of family life, those who feel unable to cope with the physical limitations they experience, and people who have so long been institutionalized that the realities of basic home functioning feel alien and unknown. The nurse usually has an ongoing relationship with the family and is in a unique position to intervene effectively during crisis. In the home environment, clients can be observed interacting with others, problems can be identified, client and family resources can be identified and mobilized, and brief crisis therapy can be initiated or referred to appropriate crisis intervention resources (see Chapter 21).

Crisis Groups

Crisis groups are short-term groups that also use the problem-solving method of crisis intervention. Persons are referred to crisis groups after severe and panic-level anxiety has been reduced by means of other crisis intervention methods. Leader and group members have interdependent tasks as described in Chapter 11.

As illustrated in the following clinical example, there will often be striking parallels between the way the client acts and his or her problematic behavior patterns in daily life:

> After two group sessions, it became obvious that Mitch would challenge and argue any point made by another group member. The major reason for Mitch's crisis was that at age 50, he was extremely lonely and had no lasting relationships. The members commented on his behavior in the group and questioned him about a relationship between his argumentativeness and his inability to sustain lasting relationships. Betty, another group member, struggling with her own crisis of newly diagnosed cancer, withdrew from the group interaction. Identifying with Mitch's sense of loneliness, she reflected on her social withdrawal since the diagnosis. In an uncharacteristic move, she told the group that as a result of her cancer, she feared that people would think her less human and treat her as an outcast. This thought was so unbearable that she retreated from human contact and felt utterly isolated. Contrary to her fears, no one shrank away. Mitch was stunned that his experience helped someone else. Noting his appreciation of such openness and honesty, he was the most vocal group member in offering support. It was the first time that Mitch empathically related to another group member.

Family Crisis Therapy

Family crisis therapy uses a family therapy model that is problem-focused. It does not delve into general family issues and problems but it focuses on a specific problem that a family has (Koontz, 1991).

Family crisis therapy involves the entire family unit. The family is viewed as a system, with family members involved in an interactive process. A crisis affecting a family member affects all members, producing shifts in the family balance. Since the crisis is viewed as emerging from within the complex web of family interactional patterns, all members are involved in identifying and changing patterns that support the problem and in developing strategies toward resolution (see Chapter 12).

APPLICATION OF THE PHASES OF CRISIS INTERVENTION

During the 4-to-6-week crisis period, a person lowers psychological defenses, seeks new ways of looking at the problem, and struggles to refine or develop ways of coping. The basic human striving for mastery and growth, coupled with the need for others to affirm, support, and enhance the person's capacity for change, make crisis an optimum time for clinical intervention.

The goal of crisis intervention is to reestablish a level of functioning equal to or better than the pre-crisis level. This includes restoration of order, purpose, and meaning in one's life.

Aguilera (1994) identified four phases of crisis intervention: assessment, planning, intervention, and anticipatory planning (evaluation). These phases closely parallel the steps of the nursing process. A crisis intervention protocol developed by McCloskey and Bulechek (1996) is presented in Box 10-2. Using the interventions cited in this protocol, specific actions are referred to as each phase of crisis intervention is discussed in the following section.

Assessment

Assessment is the first phase of crisis intervention. It involves collection of data about the perception of the problem, coping skills, and situational supports. Furthermore, it is used to establish rapport and a collaborative relationship with the client that is conducive to mutual problem-solving efforts. Assessment focuses on the immediate problem rather than the myriad of other problems that may exist.

Nursing task: See Box 10-2, steps 1-7.

Time frame: The precipitating event has usually occurred within 10 to 14 days before the person seeks help. It is not unusual for something to have happened the day or night before, such as threat of divorce, discovery of a child's drug abuse, loss of a job, or unwanted pregnancy. Symptoms usually appear after the stressful event. As the client connects life events with symptom formation, understanding of the precipitating event can occur.

Sample questions: assessing perception of the problem

1. What brought you for help today? How does this problem affect your life right now?
2. What happened in your life that is different?
3. When did it happen?
4. What do you feel right now?
5. When did you begin to feel this way?
6. What is the connection between how you are feeling and the events you described?
7. How do you see this problem affecting your future?
8. What effect is this problem having on others around you?
9. What other factors could be influencing the way you are seeing this problem?

Sample questions: assessing coping skills

1. Has anything like this ever happened to you before?
2. How have you handled other crises in your life?
3. How do you usually decrease tension and anxiety?
4. Have you tried the same methods this time? If not, why not, if it usually works?

Box 10-2

Crisis Intervention Protocol

DEFINITION

Use of short-term counseling to help the client cope with a crisis and resume a state of functioning comparable to or better than the pre-crisis state

ACTIVITIES

Provide atmosphere of support
Determine whether patient presents safety risk to self or others
Initiate necessary precautions to safeguard the patient or others at risk for physical harm
Encourage expression of feelings in a nondestructive manner
Assist in identification of the precipitants and dynamics of the crisis
Assist in identification of past/present coping skills and their effectiveness
Assist in identification of personal strengths and abilities that can be used in resolving the crisis
Assist in development of new coping and problem-solving skills, as needed
Assist in identification of available support systems
Provide guidance about how to develop and maintain support system(s)
Introduce patient to persons (or groups) who have successfully undergone the same experience
Assist in identification of alternative courses of action to resolve the crisis
Assist in evaluation of the possible consequences of the various courses of action
Assist patient to decide on a particular course of action
Assist in formulating a time frame for implementation of chosen course of action
Evaluate with patient whether crisis has been resolved by chosen course of action
Plan with patient how adaptive coping skills can be used to deal with crises in the future

Reprinted with permission from McCloskey J.C., & Bulechek G.M. (Eds.). (1996). Nursing interventions classifications (NIC) *(2nd ed.). St. Louis: Mosby.*

5. If it was tried and did not work, what kept it from working?
6. What else do you think might work?

Sample questions: assessing situational supports
1. With whom do you live?
2. Is there someone with whom you are particularly close?
3. Do you have friends? A best friend?
4. Who is available to help you?
5. Who understands you? Whom do you trust?
6. Are you involved in community activities?

Planning

Planning is the second phase of crisis intervention. Data from all available resources are organized and examined so that specific interventions can be proposed. The nurse decides on the usable situational and environmental supports and the coping skills needing to be developed or enhanced. Interdisciplinary collaboration facilitates improved treatment, referral, and the coordination of diverse services. The clinical example on p. 167 describes the comprehensive crisis intervention plan for Jennifer, a battered woman and her abused child, Billy. In this example, the plan of care is coordinated among emergency room triage nurse, surgical resident, social worker, adult and pediatric orthopedists, pediatric unit staff nurses, crisis volunteer, and caseworker from the child welfare authority. With seamless transition, health care delivery is coordinated between emergency room, pediatric unit, battered women/children's shelter, and victim support services.
Nurse's Task: See Box 10-2, steps 8-10.

Intervention

Intervention is the third phase of crisis intervention. It is goal-directed and focuses on the implementation of measures addressing the specific problem. The nurse is directive, giving the client concrete instruction as to what should be tried as tentative solutions. Throughout the process, the nurse acts as a role model for open, direct communication, innovative thinking, flexibility, and self-awareness.
Nurse's Task: See Box 10-2, steps 10-15.
Time Frame: Depending on the circumstances, interventions may last as little as 2 to 3 days, or they may be conducted in as many as six or eight weekly structured interviews.

Evaluation

Evaluation is the fourth and final stage of crisis intervention. It involves the examination of behavioral outcomes and the interventions toward achieving them. For example, a client returns to work and resumes a usual family role after the situational crisis of a heart attack. Having developed capacities to process stress (i.e., appropriating time to talk with wife and friends, joining a health club) and having learned about healthful practices (i.e., routine checkups, regular exercise, and low cholesterol diet), the client feels increasingly able to cope with life demands. In fact the client may achieve a level of functioning that surpasses pre-crisis conditions. Anticipatory planning refers to instructing the client in how to deal with potential "trouble spots" in future events, based on an evaluation of effective and ineffective crisis intervention strategies.

Nurse's Task: See Box 10-2, steps 16 and 17.

CRISIS PREVENTION: PREVENTIVE INTERVENTION PROGRAMS

Crisis prevention, also referred to as selective preventive intervention, consists of planned activities designed to address the crisis before it occurs. Goals of selective preventive intervention are to eliminate or modify risk, reduce exposure to risk, and reduce vulnerability by reinforcing coping skills. Steps in this process include identification of the problem; identification of the population at risk; and the design of tools, activities, or strategies that are relevant from the perspective of age, gender, culture, and socioeconomic status. Examples include selective preventive intervention for the following:

- Teen-age pregnancy—Educating adolescents about the difficulties including economic difficulties and loss of personal freedom

 COMMUNITY RESOURCES

Crisis Intervention

Al-Anon
For families of alcoholics
Consult local listing

Alcoholics Anonymous World Services*
(212) 870-3400

American Red Cross
Natural and man-made disasters
Consult local listing

Centers for Disease Control National HIV/AIDS Hotline
(800) 342-2437

Child Welfare League of America
(800) 275-2952

Covenant House
Addictions treatment
(800) 999-9999

Crime Victims Advocacy and Support
(800) 671-7837

Divorce Helpline*
(800) 359-7004

Federal Emergency Management Association
Natural disaters
(800) 462-9029

Legal Aid Services of America
(800) 426-3406

Narcotics Anonymous*
(800) 229-7244

National Alliance for the Mentally Ill
(800) 9501-6264

National Clearinghouse for Alcohol and Drug Information
1-800-SAYNOTO

National Council on the Aging
(202) 479-1200

National Mental Health Consumers Self-Help Clearinghouse
(800) 553-4537

Rape, Abuse and Incest National Network
(800) 656-HOPE

Rape Crisis Center
(202) 333-7273

Suicide Prevention and Hotlines*
Check local listing

Women's Crisis Center
(800) 974-3359

*The number cannot be reached from all calling areas, so local directories or operator assistance should be consulted.

- Serious physical injury—Education in defensive driving
- Human innumodeficiency virus (HIV) and acquired immunodeficiency syndrome (AIDS)—Education about what constitutes risky behaviors, how HIV is transmitted and the practice of safe sex
- Teen-age suicide—Bringing together families, teachers, guidance counselors, school officials, and community mental health professionals for education about signs and symptoms of depression and available community resources

Community Resources related to crisis intervention are presented on p. 175.

KEY POINTS

- A crisis is an internal imbalance that occurs in the normal balance of an individual's life that results from a stressful event or perceived threat to one's well-being.
- Perception of an event varies with experience, background and culture.
- Crises occur in a four-phase sequence that begins with the perception of a threat and moves toward crisis if problem-solving strategies are not effective.

 CRITICAL THINKING QUESTIONS

Gary T., age 65, comes into the crisis center looking despondent and disheveled. He has recently been forced to retire from his job of 35 years at the dairy department of a local supermarket. He tearfully relates that all of his friends were at his old job and he does not know what to do with himself. He has a history of alcohol abuse, which has worsened lately and led to conflicts with his wife. He is angry about the insufficient size of his pension check and feels as if his loyalty to the store has been betrayed. He tells the crisis nurse "I feel as if the rug has been pulled out from under me, and there's nothing left."

1. What are your first impressions of Gary? Your thoughts, your feelings, and initial actions?
2. Does Gary present a safety risk to himself? To others? Why or why not? How does this affect your interventions?
3. How might situational supports help Gary resolve his crisis?
4. What successful or unsuccessful coping strategies can you identify from Gary's history?
5. Describe three types of community or support groups that could help Gary through his maturational and situational crises.

- Whether or not a stressful event or threat is defined as a crisis depends on the person's perception of the problem, situational supports, and coping skills.
- Crises are often precipitated by loss, transition, or challenge.
- Maturational crises are the anticipated transition points of the life cycle such as marriage, parenthood, and retirement. Situational crises are unanticipated events such as illness, divorce, and untimely death. Social crises are uncommon, unanticipated events such as floods, fire, or terrorist attacks.
- Crisis intervention is a community-based form of brief therapy that uses a four-step process: assessment, planning, intervention, and evaluation.
- Specific methods of crisis intervention include: individual therapy, crisis groups, telephone counseling, emergency department counseling, and home visits.
- Nurses intervene with clients in crisis in a variety of inpatient and outpatient settings in collaboration with interdisciplinary and community-based personnel.

REFERENCES

Aguilera, D.C. (1994). *Crisis intervention: Theory and methodology* (7th ed.). St. Louis: Mosby.

American Nurses Association (1994). *A statement on psychiatric-mental health clinical nursing practice and standards of psychiatric-mental health clinical nursing practice.* Washington, DC: 1994.

Barash, D. (1990). The San Francisco earthquake: Then and now. *Perspectives in Psychiatric Care, 26*(1), 32-36.

Bell, L. (1977). *Community mental health: a black perspective.* Unpublished manuscript.

Cabezas, Y. (1982). *In pursuit of wellness.* San Francisco: Department of Mental Health.

Caurtois, C. (1990). Adult survivors of incest and molestation. In H. J. Parad & L. Parad (Eds.), *Crisis intervention.* (Book 2, pp. 139-160). Milwaukee: Family Service America.

Chien, C. (1989, May). Culture, ethnicity and psychopharmacology. Paper presented at the annual meeting of the American Psychiatric Association. San Francisco.

Hoff, L.E. (1989). *People in crisis: Understanding and healing* (3rd ed.). Reading, MA: Addison-Wesley.

Kalichman, S.C. (1994). Magic Johnson and public attitudes towards AIDS: A review of empirical findings. *AIDS education and prevention, 6*(6), 542-557.

Koontz, E., Cox, D., & Hastings, S. (1991). Implementing a short-term family support group. *Journal of Psychosocial Nursing, 29,*(5), 5-10.

Lin, K., & Poland, R. (1989). Pharmacology of Asian psychiatric patients, *Psychiatric Annals, 19*(12), 659-663.

McCloskey, J.C. et al. (1996). Crisis intervention. In J.C. McCloskey & G. Bulechek (Eds.), *Nursing interventions classification (NIC)* (2nd ed.). St. Louis: Mosby.

Munoz, F.M. (1987). Depression-prevention research: Conceptual and practical considerations. In R.F. Munoz (Ed.), *Depression prevention.* Washington, DC: Hemisphere Publishing Company.

Parad, H.J., & Parad, L. (1992). Crisis intervention: Yesterday, today and tomorrow. In R. Punukollu (Ed.), *Recent advances in crisis intervention.* (Vol. 1, pp. 3-23). Huddersfield: International Institute of Crisis Intervention and Community Psychiatry Publications.

Parad, H.J., & Parad, L. (1990). Crisis intervention: An introductory overview. In H.J. Parad & L. Parad (Eds.), *Crisis intervention.* (Book 2, pp. 3-68). Milwaukee: Family Services America.

Punukollu, N.R. (1992). *Recent advances in crisis intervention.* Huddersfield, England: International Institute of Crisis Intervention and Community Psychiatry Publications.

Robinson, L. (1990). *Stress and anxiety. Nursing Clinics of North America, 25*(1), 935-943.

Slaikeu, K. (1990a). Developmental life crises. In K. Slaikeu (Ed.), *Crisis intervention: A handbook for practice and research.* (2nd ed.). Boston: Allyn and Bacon.

Slaikeu, K. (1990b). Situational life crises. In K. Slaikeu (Ed.), *Crisis intervention: A handbook for practice and research.* (2nd ed.). Boston: Allyn and Bacon.

Slaikeu, K., & Simon, S. (1990). Crisis intervention by telephone. In K. Slaikeu (Ed.), *Crisis intervention: A handbook for practice and research.* (2nd ed., pp. 319-328). Boston: Allyn and Bacon.

Tompar-Tiu, A. & Sustento-Seneriches, J. (1995). *Depression and other mental health issues: The Filipino-American experience.* San Francisco: Jossey-Bass.

Tynhurst, J.S. (1951). Individual reactions to community disaster. *American Journal of Psychiatry, 107,* 764-769.

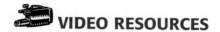 **VIDEO RESOURCES**

Psychiatric Emergencies Video Series Module 1: *Crisis Intervention*

Chapter 11

Working With Groups

Anita Leach McMahon
Joyce Larson Presswalla

LEARNING OUTCOMES

After studying and applying the concepts of this chapter, the learner will be able to:
- Discuss the dynamics of a group.
- Describe the purpose of various kinds of groups.
- Identify growth-producing and growth-inhibiting roles of group members.
- Discuss the impact of various leadership styles on group outcomes.
- Differentiate the phases that occur throughout the life of a group.
- Facilitate healthy group interaction.
- Record a client's participation in groups.

KEY TERMS

Absenteeism	Group content	Rank
Acting out	Group leader	Resistance
Closed group	Group process	Roles
Cohesiveness	Group therapy	Rules
Competition	Groupthink	Status
Countertransference	Heterogeneous group	Subgrouping
Dependency	Homogeneous group	Task group
Fight-or-flight	Norms	Therapeutic group
Group	Open group	Transference

Groups are everywhere. Early socialization takes place within the family group and in groups such as those at school, in day care centers, sports teams, or clubs. Work is accomplished by groups in staff meetings, planning boards, and community councils. Groups also provide social support and are a primary means of adult learning. Groups used therapeutically are an effective method of facilitating personal change and growth.

Clients in the mental health system participate in numerous treatment and rehabilitative groups. Increasingly, groups are used to provide quality services in today's changing health care environment. Numerous social and economic factors have brought about shorter hospitalizations and increasing client acuity. Treatment requires rapid progression through three continuous overlapping phases: assessment, stabilization, and discharge or transitional planning (Crosby and Sabin, 1996).

Both stabilization and transition planning can be accomplished in a group setting. As clients return to their communities, they may participate in numerous groups where they learn, for example, about self-dynamics, how to manage job stress, how to manage their illness and their medications, or how to socialize. Groups differ with respect to goals, the role of the leader, the kind of people in the group, and whether the emphasis is given to prevention, remediation, treatment, or development.

The purpose of this chapter is to equip the learner to facilitate health/group functioning. The learner will be introduced to basic group theory, dynamics present in groups, and the role characteristics of group members. A description of the various groups in which nurses participate is included in the chapter.

DEFINITION OF GROUP

Groups are interdependent associations of two or more persons interacting in such a way that each person influences and is influenced by other group members. A *group comprises a number of persons in a face-to-face setting, accomplishing a task that requires working together.* Group members may:

- Engage in frequent interactions within the group setting
- Define themselves as members of the group
- Be defined by others as belonging to the group
- Share norms with other group members
- Implement a set of interlocking group-determined rules
- Identify with one another through role models or ideals held in common
- Find rewards within the group
- Pursue interdependent goals
- Verbalize a sense of group unity

- Act in similar ways toward the environment outside the group

The life of any group occurs simultaneously at two levels. *Group content refers to what is said in a group and includes the specific information shared by group members.* This information, or content, serves as a focus for discussion. *Group process refers to what is done in a group, that is, what is implied by actions.* Process includes interactions among members, seating arrangements, tone of voice of members, who speaks to whom, and other nonverbal behaviors. One might say that group content refers to what is *said,* and group process to what is *happening.* Content and process constantly occur in groups and provide structure for them, as in the following example:

> Sara is the head nurse on an inpatient crisis stabilization unit. In a monotone voice, she relates recent changes in managed care to her staff. While Sara is speaking, Peter folds his arms and appears uninterested. Eileen yawns, and Susan closes her eyes.

The content in this example is what Sara is telling the group—the factual information about changes in the managed care system. The process is what was happening. Sara speaks in a monotone voice, and Peter, Eileen, and Susan indicate by their behaviors that they are bored. The process in this example indicates that "the group" is probably uninterested in the content.

The duration or "life of a group" is usually determined before the group is formed. Groups may be open or closed. In an *open group the membership changes. As one group member leaves or is discharged, a new member may join the group.* One advantage of an open group is that new members generate different interactions and insights among members. A group formed for the purpose of introducing clients to the milieu on a crisis stabilization unit is an example of an open group. Members come to and leave the group on an ongoing basis.

On the other hand a *closed group is one in which membership is stable and limited. Only those individuals who are present at the start of the group's life attend the sessions.* Although this type of group may be long-term, it often is time-limited. A closed group generally has specific focuses or therapeutic tasks. Two examples are (1) bereavement groups that end when the members resolve the grief process and (2) committees formed to accomplish a specific task.

Groups may be task-oriented or therapeutically oriented, or they may combine these functions. *A task group has direction and is one whose primary purpose is the completion of a predetermined specific goal. It is content-oriented and aims to accomplish tasks, solve problems, or make decisions. A*

TABLE 11-1

Theoretical models

MODEL	GOALS	TECHNIQUES
Person-centered	• Permits clients to explore their feelings • Helps members become increasingly open to new experiences and develop confidence in themselves and their own judgments • Encourages clients to live in the present • Develops openness, honesty, and spontaneity • Makes it possible for clients to encounter others in the here and now and to use the group as a place to overcome feelings of alienation	• Active listening • Reflection of feelings • Clarification • Support, "being there" • Genuineness • Caring • Respect • Understanding
Existential	• Provides conditions that maximize self-awareness and reduce blocks to growth • Helps clients discover and use freedom of choice and assume responsibility for their own choices	• Stresses understanding first and techniques second • No specific set of methods is prescribed
Psychoanalytic	• Provides a climate that helps clients to reexperience early family relationships and uncover buried feelings associated with past events that carry over into current behaviors	• Interpretation • Dream analysis • Free association • Analysis of resistance • Analysis of transference
Adlerian	• Creates therapeutic relationships that encourage participants to explore their basic life assumptions and to achieve a broader understanding of lifestyles • Focuses on clients' strengths and their powers to change	• Analysis and assessment • Exploration of family constellations • Reporting of earliest recollections • Confrontation • Interpretation • Cognitive restructuring • Challenging belief systems • Exploration of social dynamics
Behavioral	• Helps group members eliminate maladaptive behaviors and learn new and more effective behavioral patterns (Broad goals are broken down into precise subgoals)	• Cognitive restructuring • Systematic desensitization • Implosive therapy • Assertion training • Aversive techniques • Operant-conditioning methods • Self-help techniques • Reinforcement • Supportive measures • Coaching • Modeling • Feedback
Rational emotive therapy (RET)	• Teaches group members that they are responsible for their own disturbances • Helps them identify and abandon the process of self-indoctrination by which they keep their disturbances alive • Eliminates clients' irrational and self-defeating outlooks on life and replaces it with more tolerant and rational ones	• Active teaching • Explanation • Persuasion • Lecture • Deconditioning • Role playing • Homework assignments • Assertiveness training

therapeutic group is one with the purpose of personal and emotional growth of members. It is process-oriented.

Many task-oriented groups have therapeutic goals. For example, an activity-oriented task group may have socialization as a therapeutic goal, or a nursing team whose task is the planning of client care may also provide the means for self-learning for the nurse.

Membership in therapy groups may be heterogeneous or homogeneous. *Heterogeneous groups have diverse membership* whereas *homogeneous groups have some characteristics (such as gender or age) or issue (such as divorce, parenting, or a specific diagnosis) in common.*

In a homogeneous group, members tend to discuss common problems. Problems may arise in the therapeutic process of a homogeneous group if the members support one another's defenses; for example, if the members of an AA group support the denial that is prevalent in alcoholism, little growth will occur. On the other hand, sharing common problems can be the primary feeling component in a homogenous group.

The advantage of a heterogeneous group is that members have a variety of stimuli, which facilitates interaction on a deeply emotional level. Ideally, in heterogeneous groups, characteristics of members should be balanced so that clients are not singled out as "different" because of the membership mix. An example of an unbalanced group would be one that is composed of several women and one man.

THEORETICAL FRAMEWORKS

Some group leaders follow specific theoretical orientations that influence the way in which they conduct a group. Generally, they hold the belief that adherence to one theoretical orientation facilitates the success of group work and that a theoretical orientation helps to reach group goals more effectively. Other group leaders however employ an *eclectic* approach. They believe that it is not necessary to use a specific theoretical approach because no one theory can be inadequate in describing group phenomena.

Table 11-1 lists several theoretical models used by group leaders. Goals and techniques employed for each model are listed.

TYPES OF GROUPS

Nurses participate in numerous groups, each of which has specific therapeutic purposes and activities. This section discusses goals and the nurse's role in milieu groups, social skill groups, age-related groups, and support groups, as well as gender-specific, health education, and multicultural groups.

Milieu Groups

Among the types of groups led by nurses in a therapeutic milieu are multifamily groups, community meetings, and transition groups.

Multifamily groups

Multifamily groups, particularly those in inpatient settings, are usually groups with large membership that includes all clients and their families. The multifamily group may be led by a nurse with another team member as a co-leader. Meetings generally occur weekly. The purpose of these meetings is to give family members an opportunity to ask questions, have misinformation corrected, learn how to help the client, acknowledge the difficulty of having a family member with psychiatric symptoms, and share both practical and emotional solutions with one another.

The leaders of the multifamily group start the group discussion and maintain its focus. They are active and directive and know each client, the family issues involved, and the agency's policies and procedures. Recognizing the validity of feelings experienced by families helps to decrease the anxiety of family members. It also helps families to feel that they are a part of the treatment team.

Community meeting

Another large group meeting that may take place in a treatment facility is the community meeting. Most commonly the community meeting occurs in inpatient, day treatment, and halfway house programs. *Community meeting* is a large group gathering for all members of the milieu: clients, doctors, nurses, therapy aides, nursing assistants, house parents, and others. This meeting occurs two or three times weekly, and is generally the only time all staff and clients are together at one time. The goal of the community group meeting is to explore common concerns, complaints, limitations, rules, privileges, and requests. Topics for discussion are broad, although they often focus on problems of daily living, information about medications, treatments, therapies, concerns about jobs and visitors, and questions about discharge or transition to another level of care.

Transition groups

Transition groups are conducted for clients who are admitted or expect to be discharged from their current treatment setting. In some agencies the clients' families are also included in the group. The goal of this group is to provide clients and their families with seamless integrated care, specifically, to facilitate the client's smooth transition to the next level of care. Exchange of feelings among clients and families about the impending transition is facilitated. Often, clients and their families are apprehensive, uncertain, and anxious about how the client will fare in another treatment setting or with a different treatment plan. The normality of these feelings is pointed out to group members in order to decrease some of the stress associated with change. The nurse who leads the group clarifies information about the client's transition date, follow-up treatment, medications, diet, and any restrictions to activity. These groups are also helpful to clients making a transition to a less restrictive treatment environment.

Social Skill Groups

Social skill groups provide clients with the choices they have for learning new skills and spending their leisure time. Occupational and therapeutic recreation specialists often conduct these groups, but nurses help in the planning and selection of clients and often serve as co-leaders.

The leader of a social skill group provides the structure and means for carrying out the specific activity and facilitates communication among members about the group's specific task. Goals of social skill groups include the following:

- Encourage communication
- Learn and practice new skills
- Increase the client's attention span
- Provide outlets for expression of feelings
- Encourage cooperation, healthy competition, and sharing
- Enhance decision-making skills

Some examples of social skill groups include cooking, literature, and exercise groups (Fig. 11-1). In addition to the examples discussed here, other groups may be formed to deal with social skills such as job interviewing, dating, or parenting.

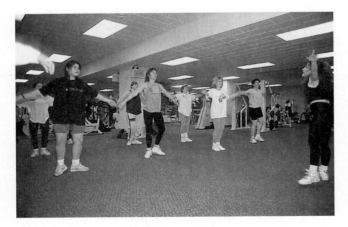

Fig. 11-1 An exercise class for clients at an inpatient psychiatric unit. Exercise classes are one example of a social skills group.

Age-Related Groups

Age-related groups are formed to focus on the issues of a specific developmental age group. The goal of these groups is to facilitate interaction with peers who have similar issues related to age. Age-related groups may be educative or supportive in nature. Examples of age-related groups include play therapy groups for children, adolescent groups, and life-review and reminiscing groups for elderly persons (see Chapters 33, 34, and 35).

Support Groups

Support groups are formed to provide support and problem-solving opportunities for clients who share a common problem or who are distressed about a particular issue. Support groups provide participants with opportunities to:

- Increase their social network
- Share solutions to common problems
- Reshape perceptions of self and the environment

Clients in the mental health system are encouraged to be members of many support groups. Support groups include those formed for divorced and separated individuals, widows and widowers, incest survivors, rape victims, caregivers of the elderly, recovering alcohol and drug abusers, and clients with eating disorders. Clients generally feel more comfortable expressing themselves in a group of individuals "who have been there." Clients garner support from knowing they are not alone with their experiences and can share solutions to their common problems. As a result of the supportive process, clients begin to perceive themselves and their problems in new ways. Leaders of support groups are generally professionals but may be peers or volunteers who have background in group management. Examples of support groups discussed here are quality-of-life, caregiver, and bereavement support groups.

Quality-of-life support groups

Groups may be formed to support the quality of life of clients who have experienced acute psychiatric symptoms, and as a result, have become a part of the mental health system. Clients bring with them to their treatment their quest for inner understanding. Their struggle is for context, interpretation, and absorption of the illness experience.

The illness experience may change, deepen, and challenge the inner life of the clients' spirit. Some clients may want to discuss these inner struggles and changes with others. Support groups with a focus that is spiritual provide for this sharing. Spirituality is defined as the pursuit of that which gives meaning and value to life.

The "what" questions (what is this medicine for?) are understood; but clients often ask "why" questions (why is this happening to me?). Nurses as group leaders of quality-of-life groups can tap the unseen world of the spirit that is crucial to healing, recovery, and health. Such groups can be structured to provide a safe environment to "enspirit" or inspire clients by encouraging them to address their "why" questions (Copp and Copp, 1993).

Caregiver support group

Caregiver support groups are generally professionally led groups formed to support the family members of acutely ill and chronically ill children, adults, and the elderly. Family members are most often parents, adult children, or spouses. Examples of the membership in these groups include the parents of children with leukemia, adult child caregivers for the elderly, family members of those with mental illness, individuals with a family member who has a chronic illness, and spouses of individuals with Alzheimer's. The goals of caregiver support groups include the promotion and maintenance of the caregiver's health, enhancement of their coping skills, acquisition of knowledge about available community resources, and socialization with others having similar responsibilities. Several types of support groups are discussed throughout this text.

Bereavement support groups

Bereavement groups are formed to support those clients who are grieving the loss of a significant other. Members of bereavement groups might be considered "survivors." These goals of bereavement groups include the following:

- Providing an acceptable outlet for the expression of grief and loss
- Providing strategies for coping with the changes created by the death of a loved one
- Promoting socialization

Nurses who lead bereavement groups facilitate the interaction of members but generally maintain a supportive, nondirective role. In some groups the nursing role may be educative. Themes in bereavement groups revolve around the client's ability to manage loneliness. For widows and widowers, socialization as a single person, adapting a new lifestyle, and assuming the responsibilities and tasks of the deceased spouse are common themes.

Self-Help Groups

Self-help groups are called such because they are facilitated by the members themselves. They are a noncontractual form of social initiative that tap the resources of people for the common good. Members are generally motivated to secure health information and to improve well-being. Self-help groups are usually focused on particular clinical state such as chronic mental illness, a particular social state such as divorce, or on special psy-

chosocial issues such as chemical dependency. Examples include Alcoholics Anonymous (AA), Narcotics Anonymous (NA), and Overeaters Anonymous (OA). Support groups may replace or augment the family or formal health care system and generally aim to link health behaviors with everyday existence. Self-help groups foster self-reliance and are a form of healing for many.

Gender-Specific Groups

Homogeneous groups of men and women may be formed to share issues related to the members' respective gender roles. The goal of gender-specific support groups is to provide clients with peer models of connectedness, uniqueness, and power, which promote improvement of members' self-esteem and enhance relationships. Much research is currently under way to develop models for gender-specific groups, particularly those comprised of men (Hetzel et al., 1994).

Psychoeducation Groups

Education may take place within the group and may be referred to as psychoeducation (PE). Psychoeducation means combining formal educational teaching techniques with various techniques of psychotherapy. The goal of PE groups is to help both clients and families to better manage clients' symptoms through early recognition of relapse symptoms of illness and to develop better ADL and psychosocial skills (Holmes et al., 1994). Chapter 16 contains a complete discussion of the nurse's role in psychoeducation. Guidelines for developing, implementing, and evaluating client-oriented teaching in a group setting are found in Box 11-1.

Multicultural Groups

Nurses are increasingly finding themselves providing care to people from different cultures. It is a basic assumption that groups represent a social microcosm. Nurses lead groups for clients whose beliefs about health and illness differ from their own. This could create a situation that may be uncomfortable for *both* the provider and receiver of care since there is a tendency to question practices that are unfamiliar (Johnson et al., 1995). The challenge is to view differences as opportunities for learning rather than as excuses for separation. A starting point for change is openness to learning about differences. In group settings, if asked, culturally diverse clients usually enjoy sharing knowledge related to what they believe about health and illness. However, it is important to keep in mind that what is true for one client is not necessarily true for other members of that ethnic group (Campinha-Bacote, 1994).

Multicultural groups demand that their leaders prepare members for participation. Screening, selecting, and

Box 11-1

Teaching: Group

DEFINITION

Development, implementation, and evaluation of a patient teaching program for a group of individuals experiencing the same health condition

ACTIVITIES

Provide an environment conducive to learning

Include the family/significant others, as appropriate

Establish the need for a program

Determine administrative support

Determine budget

Coordinate resources within the facility to form a planning/advisory committee that can contribute to positive outcomes for the program, and provide a forum for ensuring commitment to the program

Use community resources, as appropriate

Define potential target population(s)

Write program goals

Outline major content area(s)

Write learning objectives

Write a job description for a coordinator responsible for patient education

Select a coordinator

Preview available educational materials

Develop new educational materials, as appropriate

List possible teaching strategies, educational materials, and learning activities

Train the teaching personnel, as appropriate

Educate the staff about the patient teaching program, as appropriate

Provide a written schedule—including dates, times, and places of the teaching sessions/classes—to the staff and/or patient(s), as appropriate

Determine appropriate days/times to reach maximal number of patients

Prepare announcements/memos to publicize outcomes, as appropriate

Control the size and competencies of the group, as appropriate

Orient patient(s)/significant others to educational program and the objectives it is designed to accomplish

Provide for special needs of learners (e.g., handicap access and portable oxygen), as appropriate

Adapt the educational methods/materials to the group's learning needs/characteristics, as appropriate

Provide group instruction

Evaluate the patient's progress in the program and mastery of content

Document the patient's progress on the permanent medical record

Revise teaching strategies/learning activities, if necessary, to increase learning

Provide forms for the patient to evaluate the program

Provide for further individual instruction, as appropriate

Evaluate the extent to which program goals were attained

Communicate the program's goal attainment evaluation to the planning/advisory committee

Reprinted with permission from McCloskey, J.C., & Bulechek, G.M. (Eds.). (1996). Nursing interventions classification (NIC) *(2nd ed.). St. Louis: Mosby.*

orienting clients to group behavior is particularly important. Taking time to bridge the gap between dominant group behaviors and group behavior of members of different cultures requires special skill (see Chapter 6).

Depending on the cultural background of particular clients, some traditional group behaviors may be perceived as excessively demanding or may go "against the grain" of one's cultural traditions. For example, confrontation, which is an integral part of group process, can be particularly troublesome for some clients. They may perceive the directness associated with confrontation as a personal attack, as a significant "loss of face", or as an insult. Such perceptions by clients may result in feelings of anger, resistance to becoming involved in the group, or premature termination from it.

GROUP THERAPY

Group therapy is a treatment modality in which selected clients are provided therapeutic group opportunities by a qualified group therapist in a group setting. The goals of group therapy include alleviating intrapsychic stress, reducing anxiety, and providing clients with opportunities to modify and test new behaviors in a controlled setting.

Therapy groups in inpatient settings generally use a short-term model and have open membership. Clients generally attend group daily while they are hospitalized. Outpatient therapy groups, on the other hand, are generally of longer duration, meet weekly, and have closed membership. Clients in therapy groups must be cognitively, behaviorally, and affectively capable of participation in the group and of striving for the group goals. Therefore it would be inappropriate to include clients who are acutely psychotic, manic, or profoundly depressed in intensive group therapy.

Nurses with advanced preparation are qualified to act as therapists for group psychotherapy. All nurses, however, need to understand the basic principles of group therapy to understand the impact that group therapy and group dynamics have on clients and staff in their specific work setting.

GROUP DYNAMICS

The dynamics that occur in groups contribute to the healing of participants. The goals of group therapy are curative. Curative outcomes offered to clients who participate in group therapy have been delineated by Yalom (1995) and are presented in Box 11-2. Regardless of the group type or the setting in which it occurs, some common process dynamics typically occur in therapeutic groups. These include resistance, transference, and countertransference.

Resistance

Resistance refers to the strong, usually unconscious forces that prevent group members from moving toward their goals. Individuals may not be able to understand what other group members are saying about them and may feel angry or confused. Signs of resistance include acting out, absenteeism, subgrouping, fight-flight, and dependency. Table 11-2 defines and gives an example of each.

Transference

Transference in groups occurs when clients attribute to the group leader or other group members the feelings, desires, and conflicts that were initially felt towards parents or significant others. At first this is an unconscious process. A group member will have feelings about the leader or other group members that are independent of reality. Others in the group will notice this and begin to talk about it. The member acting on the transference will be defensive at first, but when confronted repeatedly by the others, will begin to question the distortion of reality. It is at this point, that the member may remember an earlier experience with a parent or significant other that is similar to what is now being experienced. At times, other members of the group may be able to remember something about the client that is helpful in uncovering the transference. It is through this process that the client is able to perceive reality more accurately, as with the following example:

Box 11-2

Yalom's Goals of Group Therapy

INSTILLATION OF HOPE

Progress of others in the group is observed by a group member who then feels hopeful about receiving similar help.

UNIVERSALITY

A group member observes that others in the world share similar feelings or have similar problems; therefore anxiety is decreased.

IMPARTING OF INFORMATION

Interpersonal relating, developmental tasks and stages, medications and other somatic treatments, and the structure of the setting are only a few areas in which information may be shared.

ALTRUISM

The opportunity to support and to help increase self-awareness in another group member gives the helping individual increased self-esteem. It also encourages a preoccupied individual to become less self-focused.

IMITATIVE BEHAVIOR

The group leader, or a group member who has already mastered a particular psychosocial skill, can be a valuable role model.

INTERPERSONAL LEARNING

The group offers varied opportunities for relating to other people. Members test new ways of relating in a safe environment.

CATHARSIS

An outpouring of emotional tension through verbalization or display of feelings may occur in a group session. This may be a tension-reducing and growth-enhancing phenomenon.

Based on data from Yalom, I. (1995). The theory and practice of group psychotherapy (4th ed.). New York: Basic Books.

Jan, a young female client, tells Martin, the group leader, "You don't like me as much as the others in the group." This is not true and it has never occurred to Martin to think this way. Another group member, Bob, remembers and relates a previous session when Jan described her role as "scholar" in her family. She had related that she was only praised by her parents for excellent or perfect achievements in her school subjects. Margo, a friend of Jan's, gently asks, "Don't you think your reaction to Martin is a bit much? Maybe who you are really reacting to is your father?" Jan is able to explore

TABLE 11-2

Signs of resistance

DEFINITION AND FEATURES	EXAMPLE
ACTING OUT	
Acting out occurs when through actions, rather than words, an individual group member expresses unconscious feelings, desires, and conflicts. Clients do not talk directly about unconscious forces but rather dramatize them or "act out." The group leader needs to understand the symbolic meaning of the client's behavior in the acting out.	A client loudly complained of a pain in the neck because of cold air from the air conditioner in the group meeting room. The group leader asked "Who is annoying you here (or being a pain in the neck)"
ABSENTEEISM	
Absenteeism is a form of resistance exemplified by members coming late to group meetings or missing them entirely. Increases as the pressure to deal with the reality of one's behavior increases. If a member is late or absent in therapy groups, the person's vacant chair remains in place. The reason for absence or tardiness is generally explored when the member attends again.	Rita attended an outpatient therapy group. She was confronted by group members about her loud and boisterous behavior in group. She came late to the next session and quietly took her seat. The leader asked her if she saw a connection between having been confronted by the group the previous week and her lateness this week.
SUBGROUPING	
Subgrouping is the formation of smaller groups of two members (pairing) or more within a larger group. Subgroups interact among themselves rather than with the whole group. Subgroup members tend to think they are superior to the other members and frequently compete with the others or with the leader.	Vivian and Alex met in the group. They have begun a dating relationship despite a group rule that discourages interaction between members outside of group. During the next two group sessions they are quiet and interact only with each other. Frequent looks pass between them whenever other group members attempt to explore their issues. The group leader, Carol, challenges Vivian and Alex to look at their behavior and what they are avoiding by their (pairing) behavior. Carol points out that Vivian has previously related that she does not *choose* her dates but rather gets involved in relationships to avoid her loneliness. Alex is married and has told the group that he likes the variety of "affairs" but loves his wife and will not leave her.
FIGHT-OR-FLIGHT	
Fight-or-flight enables the member to avoid the anxiety of change by fighting or running away from someone or something. Action is essential in this phenomenon.	David actively engages in argument with another member of the group. He leaves the group abruptly and is absent from the next session.
DEPENDENCY	
Dependency involves obtaining security, support, and direction exclusively from the leader rather than from group members.	Group members may assume that their nurse leader is wise and strong and that they are helpless, inadequate, and dependent. They look to the nurse to "take care" of them and relieve their insecurity. When the nurse does not meet their expectations, group members become disillusioned or angry, feel betrayed, and look for a different leader, another member of the group, who will meet their dependency needs.

her tendency to distort any mild inattention as a reenactment of earlier disappointments. Jan had "transferred" her feelings of past rejection onto Martin, the parental figure in the group. "Working through" the transference enables Jan to perceive the present reality more accurately and promotes her self-growth.

Countertransference

Countertransference in groups occurs when the leader transfers onto a group member the feelings, desires, and conflicts that were originally experienced with the leader's own parents or significant others, as with the following example:

During group sessions Wilma, the group leader, consistently ignores Jeanne. Whenever Jeanne contributes her ideas or asks questions, Wilma appears angry, changes the subject, and is generally rude to her. After the fifth meeting, Jeanne asks to speak with Wilma privately about what has been happening. Wilma relates to Jeanne that she is not angry or consciously avoiding her. After a process of thoughtful self-awareness, Wilma realizes that Jeanne looks like her sister, Marilyn, from whom Wilma has been estranged since Marilyn married Wilma's former fiancé several years ago. Wilma, the leader in this case, felt about Jeanne as she did about her sister. Surfacing the countertransference enabled Wilma to deal with herself and behave objectively with Jeanne during future group sessions.

GROUP GOALS AND OUTCOMES

Formulation of specific and achievable client goals has evolved as an essential component of today's health care delivery climate. In addition to the expected individual client outcomes, the group itself needs to establish goals and achieve outcomes.

Group goals are the desired outcomes negotiated by group members and the group leader. Goals may be *formal* (explicitly stated) or *informal* (implicit to the outcome of the group), as in the following example:

Nurses on the oncology unit form and lead a group for widowed spouses. The formal goal of the group, shared with group members, is to facilitate the grieving process. The informal goal is to create a supportive environment and encourage development of a personal support system.

Group goals may be expressed in the form of a contract. This approach is especially helpful in time-limited support groups. The contract is written and signed by the leader and by each member of the group. It specifies the day, time, and location of the group meeting and the starting and ending dates. Specific rules about acceptable and unacceptable behavior are listed, and expectations of members and the leader are outlined. Each group member signs a copy of the contract, as in the following example:

Kathryn wished to join a group for women who are overweight. She met with a nurse at the health clinic. During the initial meeting the nurse explained that a group was forming the next week and would continue for 10 weeks. She asked Kathryn to sign a contract that specified (1) the day, time, and place of group meetings, as well as the fee; (2) a statement that Kathryn would need to undergo a physical examination before she began the group sessions; (3) that confidentiality was expected; (4) that Kathryn would be expected to notify the group leader if she would be unable to attend a group meeting; (5) that there would be seven other group members; and (6) that the goal of the group was to promote health.

Movement toward goals is generally on two levels. The surface level or "agenda" is the aspect that is overt, or clear, to the leader and the group membership. Other movement may be hidden below the surface and less obvious. When hidden agendas are present a sense of frustration and powerlessness is felt by group members. Hidden agendas need to be cleared before the work of the group can proceed. Hidden, or covert, agendas are dealt with in the following ways:

- Recognize the "hidden" movement
- Ask each group member to express personal feelings about the expressed goal
- Point out discrepancies between the expressed goals and those that are hidden
- Determine which hidden agendas can be changed and use problem-solving skills to plan appropriate action
- Avoid scolding the group because of the hidden agendas
- Help the group evaluate progress in handling the hidden agendas

GROUP ROLES

Roles are the "parts" individuals assume as members of a group. Roles have been termed the dynamic aspect of status, the place members hold in the eyes of others. Roles have a set of responsibilities and expected behaviors. Within the group, individuals take on roles that serve different functions. Some roles facilitate, vitalize, and produce growth in groups, whereas others inhibit the group's work. Other troublesome roles emerge in groups. A group *monopolizer* may discourage other group members from participation. The monopolizer serves other group members by allowing them to become passive and not deal with or work on the real issues. (Kottler, 1994), as in the following example:

The date and time of group meetings have been changed by the leader. Members are angry at her for the change but have not directly expressed their feelings. At the first meeting fol-

TABLE 11-3

Group roles

ROLE	BEHAVIOR
GROWTH-PRODUCING ROLES	
Initiator	Offers new ideas and suggests solutions
Information seeker	Seeks clarification of suggestions
Opinion seeker	Seeks clarification of values about an issue
Information giver	Offers facts or generalizations that are authoritative
Opinion giver	States beliefs or opinions relevant to the issues
Elaborator	Gives examples, develops meanings and explanations
Coordinator	Clarifies relationships among ideas, suggestions, and activities of individuals
Orienter	Defines the goals of a setting and orients others to them
Evaluator	Relates the standards of the milieu to a problem
Energizer	Motivates others to action and decision making
Procedural technician	Performs routine tasks
Recorder	Writes down topics, decisions, and actions resulting from discussion
VITALIZING ROLES	
Encourager	Praises, agrees with, and accepts others' ideas
Harmonizer	Mediates quarrels and relieves tension
Compromiser	Operates from within to resolve conflicts
Gatekeeper	Encourages and facilitates participation of others
Standard setter	Expresses standards for the group
Follower	Goes along passively as a friendly audience
GROWTH-INHIBITING ROLES	
Aggressor	Deflates status of others; may express disapproval of values, acts, or feelings of others; jokes aggressively
Blocker	Is negativistic and resistive in an unreasonable and stubborn manner
Recognition seeker	Tries to call attention to self, boasts about personal achievements
Self-confessor	Uses the milieu to express personal feelings and insights
"Playboy"	Displays lack of involvement and cynical nonchalance
Dominator	Asserts authority, manipulates the group of individuals
Help-seeker	Tries to get sympathy from others; expresses insecurity, confusion, or depreciation of self beyond reason
Special-interest pleader	Speaks for the underdog while masking feelings of bias and prejudice; actions are contrary to verbalizations

lowing the change, Ernest begins the group with complaints about his job. He continues talking despite efforts by other members to change the subject. In reviewing the process the leader recognizes that the group members are allowing Ernest (the monopolizer) to dominate the discussion rather than deal with their anger at her.

Scapegoating assumes that one member becomes the victimized object of conflict within the group and one or more members are persecutors. Both parties play roles in the group conflict. The scapegoat and persecutor roles are usually assumed by the members who most need the roles at the time and often reflect interpersonal conflict and avoidance of intimacy. Resolving the conflict requires the leader to remain neutral and empathetic to both sides. The leader facilitates open exchange of hostile feelings; fears about intimacy, and potential solutions to the conflict. Each person probably enacts more than one role as the life of the group evolves. Table 11-3 identifies several group roles and characteristic behaviors of each. The following is an example of how roles are enacted in a group:

An open group of older depressed women meets twice a week. During one session, members talked about losses they had experienced in their lives. Joan talked about how wonderful her family and friends had been when her husband died. Karen interrupted and began to relate in great detail how distressed she is since her husband died but how well she deals with it. Jackie responded, "I think if what you say is true, you would not be depressed like the rest of us." While the others were talking, Laurie was making jokes and displayed a lack of involvement.

Joan assumes the role of *humanizer;* Karen is the *recognition seeker;* Jackie is the *opinion giver;* and Laurie acts the *"playboy."*

GROUP LEADERSHIP

A significant role in all groups is that of the formal leader. *The* **group leader** *is the person around whom the group forms, and the person who initiates the group, provides continuity, and facilitates development of its cohesiveness. There are three kinds of formal leadership in groups: autocratic, democratic, and laissez-faire.* Each involves a leadership style and influences client outcomes and productivity. Table 11-4 lists the three common leadership styles with consequent group behaviors.

The group leader performs several tasks that facilitate group progress:

- Provides feedback and suggestions
- Elicits responses from silent members
- Clarifies feelings, thoughts, and ideas as well as non-verbal communication

- Facilitates expression of feelings and concerns
- Reflects feelings of the group
- Observes group behavior
- Summarizes progress and accomplishments
- Prepares the groups for feelings associated with ending membership in the group
- Facilitates planning of future goals

Sometimes a group has more than one leader. *Co-leadership* is shared responsibility by two leaders. Co-leaders lessen the feeling of power, even omnipotence, that group members often have about one leader. The co-leaders should have a mutual agreement about overall style and leadership, although they need not be in agreement about all issues. In fact the dynamics of co-leadership allow for the co-leaders to role model for the group how to disagree in a positive manner. A practical aspect of co-leadership is that it allows for more observation of nonverbal behavior than a single leader could achieve. In inpatient settings co-leadership provides for continuation of group meetings or activities in the event of an absence of one of the leaders. Co-leaders assist each other to maintain objectivity. They provide support and serve as a sounding board for each other.

Informal leaders are members who share the leadership tasks. An informal or *emergent leader* is generally the person who embodies group norms, who observes group needs and the wishes of the membership, and moves them in the direction of need fulfillment. There are two types of emergent or informal leaders. The first is a *task-oriented leader,* one who assumes the leadership role of assistant therapist and who is often helpful to the group leader. The *insight-oriented leader* is one who offers constructive suggestions and feedback to other group members. In both cases these individuals may be assuming the leader role as a means to avoid scrutiny of their own problems.

Nurse group leaders generally use client-centered theory as a framework for facilitating group process. A client-centered focus facilitates an increased understanding of the self by clients. The group leader is nondirective, reflecting clients' feelings. The leader facilitates member's growth and self-discovery. Characteristics of an effective client-centered group leader follow:

- The leader is a facilitator of the therapeutic process. He or she works toward becoming a participant in the group and moves back and forth between the roles of leader and participant.
- The leader is more responsive to feelings and meanings than to the details of what is being discussed in the group.
- An effective group leader accepts the group where it is *now.* This means acceptance of the individual member's degree of participation. Silence may be

TABLE 11-4

Leadership styles and client outcomes

TYPE OF LEADER	LEADERSHIP STYLE	CLIENT OUTCOMES
Autocratic	In-charge person Leader-centered Provides rigid ground rules States goals	Dependency on leader Inhibited flow of interaction Hostility, aggression, competitive, and scapegoating among members
Democratic	Shares leadership with members Uses resources of group members in the formation of goals Member-centered Facilitator of group goals, decisions	Openness to new ideas Freedom to initiate independent action Open communication problem solving and productivity among members
Laissez-faire	Nondirective Leaves group members to their own resources Indecisive about group goals	Unclear about direction of their lives Ambivalence and low morale Decreased interaction and low productivity

acceptable as long as it is not destructive to the life of the group.

- The leader provides constructive feedback without attacking a group member's defenses. The leader's own feelings are used to responsibly and therapeutically provide feedback.
- The leader uses self-disclosure in a therapeutic manner and avoids excessive use of interpretations.

STAGES OF GROUP DEVELOPMENT

The stages of development of a group are its life cycle. Following the formative pre-stage period, groups take on a life of their own. The groups are formed, express emotion and conflict, establish cohesion, accomplish tasks, and develop relatedness among members.

Pre-Group Stage

The formation or pregroup phase of a group occurs before group meetings begin and is the time when members get to know one another. In inpatient settings, potential members may have met because they live on the same unit but have not known each other in the context of a group. The formation or pre-group phase involves selection of group members and making such administrative arrangements as establishing space and time for holding meetings and deciding the length and frequency of group meetings. It is a time for goal setting by the leader, although in therapeutic groups, goals may be

renegotiated with group members during the first few sessions.

Many factors are considered in *selecting members for a group*. Deciding the number of members for the group generally depends on the group goal. The ideal group size is between seven and ten members and generally no fewer than five for task or therapeutic groups.

The *setting* for groups is arranged before the first meeting. The room in which a group meets should be large enough to accommodate the participants comfortably. In selecting the setting, consider safety, adequate ventilation, comfortable temperature, and accessibility to bathroom facilities. Adequate chairs for the leader and members are needed and are generally arranged around a table or in a circle.

In therapy groups, physical barriers such as a table are generally avoided. Arranging seats in a circle and eliminating barriers facilitates nonverbal communication and permits full observation of members by the leader. Members of task groups, however, may need to be seated around a table to accomplish their goals. Seating arrangements affect the interactions among group members. For example, those seated to the leader's right often communicate more with the leader during a meeting than those seated on the left, whereas those directly opposite the leader are most likely to challenge leadership.

Group meetings are scheduled on a regular basis. Meetings begin on time, even if some members are not present, and end as scheduled. Time boundaries are generally rigid, although some group meetings may extend beyond the allotted time if interaction is flowing or dis-

Box 11-3

Group Rules

- Attendance is expected at all group meetings.
- Prompt arrival at each group meeting is expected.
- Participation and/or attention to the group interaction is expected.
- All feelings are valid and are not to be criticized.
- Only one person speaks at a time.
- No smoking or eating during group meeting.
- Physically aggressive behavior is not allowed; no hitting or throwing of objects is permitted.
- Leaving during a group meeting will mean not being able to return during that session.
- What is discussed in group meetings remains in the group.
- Group members are expected to work together to achieve group goals.

cussion has not reached closure. Outpatient group therapy sessions occur weekly and generally last 1½ hours, whereas groups that meet every day usually last from 45 minutes to 1 hour.

Rules are guidelines for group conduct. They are the boundaries and expectations of the group. Rules are generally established before the first meeting of the group and may be spelled out in contract or protocol format. Commonly accepted rules that establish expectations of the group members are listed in Box 11-3. During the formation stage of a group, the rules for confidentiality are stated.

Confidentiality refers to the process of maintaining privacy about what goes on in a group. In task-oriented groups, members generally maintain group confidentiality until the goal of a group is accomplished, and they may pledge never to reveal the process used to accomplish the goal.

In therapeutic groups, confidentiality is the pledge of privacy that members make to each other and is a condition for inclusion of members in a group. The content revealed by members is often intimate, painful, and sometimes personal and could be used to hurt a member. Group members need to believe that they are safe and protected from reprisals by others. Group members agree to respect and protect confidentiality and pledge to "bring back" to group meetings any interaction that occurs outside the group.

Group leaders need to be clear with clients about which issues are shared with other treatment team members. Members need to be clear about what is appropriate to share with significant others who are not in the group. Suicidal and homicidal thoughts or plans are ex-

amples of issues that would have to be shared with others. Staff who participate in therapeutic and task groups usually meet to share and discuss their observations about group process and individual client progress. The purpose of meeting is to is to solve problems and plan future intervention strategies.

Initial Stage

The beginning stage of group development is characterized by testing and dependency behaviors on the part of clients. Group members hope to establish safety and security, have a need to be accepted, and sometimes strive to be "favorites" of the leader, as in the following example:

> A nurse at the local senior center forms a reminiscing group for eight elderly men who live alone. During the first meeting, Jake asked Bill, "Where did you come from?" Bill replied "New York." Tim and Peter both responded, "I'm from New York too." As the first meeting progressed, several other commonalities were sought by the members.

The initial stage of a group is the time when norms are established and rank and status emerge. *Norms are the procedures or rules accepted by the group as a whole and by each individual member of the group. Unlike prescribed rules, group norms evolve in the process of group members' interactions with one another and specify what members are expected to do in certain circumstances.* Norms describe expectations of what is appropriate or inappropriate behavior in a group and may change as the group develops and works toward its goals. Uncovering the norms of a group provides the observer with important information about group process.

Norms determine the affective relationships among group members. For example, the norm of a group might be, "Feelings are not expressed here," or "Genuine expressions of feeling for one another are permissible." Norms also determine who has control, who makes decisions, and the restrictedness or openness of relationships members have with the leader. "Group members must always defer to the group leader for a decision," "Group members do not surpass the skill of the leader," or, "It's okay to be chummy with the leader," are examples of these norms.

Norms also promote conformity. An implicit assumption is that similar behavior elicits approval. Conformity may affect who is accepted or rejected as a member. For example, the person who dresses in jeans when formal dress is the norm may not be accepted by others in the group.

In some groups, only those who are perceived as "important" are accepted, whereas in others, the underdog may be the acceptable member. Norms also dictate the boundaries in a group. In some groups the norm is to leave the minute the group meeting is over and avoid further contact with group members, whereas in others, the norm is to remain and socialize. A member who deviates from the norm risks not being accepted by the group.

Norms may be explicit or implicit. Bylaws or rules formally set forth in a contract are explicit. Informal or verbal norms are less explicit. A head nurse may not explicitly say that punctuality is the norm for team meetings, but punctuality is implicit, because all members arrive for meetings promptly. Sometimes implicit norms become overt when they are violated. For example, a new client on the unit took the chair at the group meeting usually reserved for the physician. Other members of the group say, after the violation, that the chair is reserved for the doctor.

Rank and status are concepts that describe members' positions within the group and are generally evident early in the life of the group. *Rank is the position a member holds in relation to other members of the group.* The rank of a group member determines the influence that members have on others in the group. Members who participate frequently and actively usually rank high in the group and thus have a greater influence on group behavior, as in the following example:

> Mark is a 19-year old member of a group of drug abusers. He is friendly, talkative, and creative during group sessions. The other members of his group were asked whom they "liked best" in the group. Mark was chosen.

Status is the prestige given to certain positions or individuals in a group; it is an implicit collection of rights and duties. Group members may have status from outside the group, because of their behavior within it, or because they are assigned status by the members. Status from outside the group is what the member brings with them to it. In the early stages of a group, members may overtly compete for status within the group:

> Joe, a new nurse, is on the Quality Assurance Committee. He brought with him a quality assurance project he had participated in previously. He created a high status for himself in the committee group because of expertise and status he had outside of it.

Status may also be achieved because of a member's behavior within the group:

> Mary and Elizabeth, at the first session of a newly formed group, begin to talk about having been in a group previously. They are given status by other members of the group because of their discussion of this previous experience and because other group members are impressed by it.

Individuals who have the ability to clarify issues are given the right and expectation to do so and may receive leadership status. Status may also be assigned to a member by the group. For example, the nurse has status because of the assigned leadership role.

Working Stage

The working or middle stage of group development is the time when members focus their efforts on accomplishing the group's goals. It is the time of group readiness to undertake productive work.

As the group moves into the working phase, greater concern for others' personal involvement and a sense of trust and commitment exists among the members. Members begin to confront one another, and competition among members is observed. In therapy groups, it is the phase during which individuals examine the relationship between their feelings and behavior. Therapy group members initiate behavior changes and support and encourage one another as new behaviors are tested.

During the working phase of task groups, there is a more equal sharing of power. The leader is less of a leader and more of a resource person. Empathy and cooperation are present as the group's energy is directed toward accomplishing the therapeutic goals of the group. The working or middle phase of group life is characterized by cohesiveness and competition.

Cohesiveness

Group *cohesiveness refers to the degree of ability that group members have to work together.* It may be thought of as the "togetherness" or the force acting on members to remain in the group. As a group evolves, a sense of "we-ness," or belonging, occurs. Satisfaction of the need to belong encourages members to want to stay together and to be productive.

When one member is absent from a support group meeting, another member contacts the absent member and encourages return to the group. During a group meeting, if one member verbalizes a desire to leave the group, the other members will usually encourage the individual to remain.

Group members' relationships with the leader are a factor in the development of cohesiveness. The relationship a member has with the leader encourages the members to remain in the group, to be open and comfortable during group meetings, and to work productively toward the goal of the group, as in the following:

> Mimi has been attending an insight-oriented group in the eating disorders unit. Her nurse therapist is one of the co-leaders. Whenever Mimi is confronted or experiences pain, she threatens to leave the group. At these times it helps her to recall that her nurse has told her, "No pain, no gain." Her relationship with the group's co-leader is one reason she remains in the group.

Cohesiveness may also be promoted from outside the group. Group members may join together to "defend against a foe" or because significant others are exerting pressure on them to continue in the group:

Gloria attends Alcoholics Anonymous meetings because her family has made it a condition of her living in the same household with them.

Groups "grow into" cohesiveness—it does not simply "happen." Cohesiveness is generally evident with the freedom of members to express negative or positive feelings toward one another and to express love and hate for one other and toward the group leader. Other signs of group cohesiveness include meetings outside the group "looking down" on nongroup members, and resentment of new members. The group leader promotes the development of group cohesiveness in the following ways:

- Promoting feelings of safety and a sense of support
- Permitting expression of anger and hostility toward self and others
- Clarifying observations about group or individual behaviors
- Promoting self-understanding among group members
- Teaching that all interactions can be the source of personal insight
- Pointing out how group behavior may resemble that of significant others
- Pointing out the positive qualities of unpopular group members

- Making group activities attractive
- Identifying hidden agendas that inhibit group productivity
- Supporting members who recognize issues and distortions in others
- Promoting interaction among members rather than solely with the leader
- Soliciting group members' responses to the issues
- Focusing on issues and accomplishment of group goals

Groupthink or *overcohesiveness describes a way of thinking by members of a highly cohesive group in which uniformity and agreement are important and critical thinking is impossible or unacceptable.* When groupthink exists, norms of unity and loyalty to the group as a whole must be maintained regardless of the consequences to individual members. Groupthink usually leads to ineffective group functioning because the group members never seriously consider alternative decisions or actions. Some characteristic symptoms and behaviors of overly cohesive groups are found in Table 11-5.

Self-Disclosure

Self-disclosure is a mark of a group that is working. It occurs when one person voluntarily tells things about self that another person is unlikely to know or discover. Nurses promote self-disclosure by instilling trust. They facilitate trust by clarifying group goals, tolerating the idiosyncratic behaviors of group members, acknowledg-

TABLE 11-5

Signs of overcohesiveness (groupthink)

SYMPTOM	BEHAVIOR
Invulnerability	Group members believe there are no dangers. They are overly optimistic and take extraordinary risks to accomplish goals.
Rationalization	Members collectively devise rationalizations to discount warnings and negative feedback from outsiders.
Immorality	Ethical and moral consequences of decision making are ignored by group members.
Stereotyping	Members believe that negotiation is impossible because those outside the group are weak or ineffective.
Pressure	There is pressure on individuals to conform and remain in the group.
Self-censorship	There is no deviation from what is perceived as a group consensus. Doubt and misgivings are minimized or remain unexpressed.
Unanimity	Members of the group speak in favor of the majority position, creating an illusion of unanimity. The minority position on an issue may be voiced but is never heard.
Mind guarding	Individual members of the group appoint themselves to protect the group from adverse information that may undermine the confidence the group shares about its effectiveness and morality.

ing members' needs, serving as a gatekeeper, protecting group confidentiality, and accepting members as they are.

Clients may experience conflict between genuinely "getting close" and fears of expressing their true self. Giving feedback in a respectful way facilitates trust. When nurse leaders are perceived as capable of managing behavior and assisting in goal achievement, self-disclosure is possible.

Competition

Competition occurs when there is rivalry among individuals in a group. Competition can be positive or destructive for a group. Competition can have beneficial results when it improves morale and performance of the members. It is positive when it encourages compromise, cooperation, and growth-promoting attitudes. Competition is destructive when conflict is not resolved and energy is diverted from the accomplishment of group goals or if there are angry, hostile attitudes, use of coercion or force, or intimidating communication, as in the following:

> Ann and Jim are residents at a halfway house. They are constantly competing for the housemother's attention. The interaction between them has at times been angry and intimidating to the other residents. Several have requested privately that Ann and Jim be asked to leave the house. The housemother encourages members during the weekly community meeting to discuss the competition between Ann and Jim and its destructive potential for the group.

Final Stage

The final stage, or termination phase, is the time immediately before disbanding of the group. It is the time for dissolution and disengagement. As the time of the last group meeting draws near, members begin to focus on relationships and tasks that will occur "when the group is over," as in the following example:

> A man who participated in a group for widows and widowers states, "I'm planning to ask my neighbor to dinner. She's a widow lady. We've always liked each other."

Some members may display anger rather than express the grief that is expected. Problems with dependency and competition may recur, or members may not talk about termination at all. Group leaders must take the initiative in the final stage and use reminiscing tactics to stimulate a review of group themes and facilitate discussion of group accomplishments. Ideally, at the termination of a group, therapeutic goals have been reached and tasks accomplished.

GROUP ASSESSMENT

Assessment of a group is an ongoing process that facilitates effective use of the group by its members. Evalua-

tion and retrospective assessment of the group are essential tasks of the termination phase.

The group leader is responsible for assessment of the group and ascertains whether there has been movement toward the accomplishment of group goals. The leader also evaluates group atmosphere, roles, cohesion, communication, conflict, and problem solving. Self-evaluation by the leader is essential to the process. Table 11-6 lists factors to be evaluated, assessment questions, and the expected outcomes that are present in effectively functioning groups. These evaluation factors may be used for each group meeting, periodically, or after termination of the group.

Recording Group Interaction

Assessment of a group involves some method of recording group participation. *Audiotapes* provide an accurate assessment of group participation, word emphasis, speed of speech, and hesitations. Audiotapes however, do not allow for recording of nonverbal communication. *Videotapes* give the added dimension of direct observation and viewing of the group session. Audio- and videotapes may also be used as an integral part of a group session; tapes are replayed so that the clients can become aware of their involvement in the group. Tapes are also helpful for the group when members wish to review or clarify important incidents that have happened during a group session. When either type of taping is to be used, the group members sign written permission. They are provided with a complete explanation of the reasons for taping and how the tape will be used during or outside of the group session. Members are assured that confidentiality will be maintained.

Written notes are kept by the leader. These notes contain a description of the group, its purpose, attendance, goals, and composition. Patterns of group interactions, including communication and behavior patterns, are recorded, sometimes with the use of a sociogram. Leadership patterns and techniques and progress toward goals are also noted. Issues that need follow-up in subsequent sessions may be included. In addition to the written notes, group leaders verbally communicate any issues that may influence a client's safety or the safety of others. When records are kept for third-party payers, group leaders are required to record notes about each individual member's participation.

GROUP INTERVENTION

Nurses serve as group leaders and are responsible for interventions during the life of a group. Some common interventions of a nurse leader include the following:

- Forming the group
- Stating and interpreting group objectives

TABLE 11-6

Evaluation of group

FACTOR TO BE EVALUATED	QUESTIONS	OUTCOME IN AN EFFECTIVE GROUP
Atmosphere	What is the atmosphere? Are there signs of boredom or tension?	Clients are comfortable and relaxed. Members are interested and involved. The atmosphere is conducive to productivity. Space and lighting are adequate. There is privacy, and noise is minimal.
Setting goals	Do the clients understand the purpose of the group? What are the group's stated goals? Are the goals acceptable to the members?	Group goals are clearly understood. Modification of goals occurs with participation by members.
Leadership	Who are the appointed leaders? Who are informal group leaders? In what way does the formal leader facilitate or inhibit group growth?	Leadership is assumed by different members at different times. The appointed leader is aware of group happenings and group process. The appointed leader uses a democratic style. The group's informal leaders facilitate the work of the group.
Membership	What is the level of participation of each member?	Clients participate in a manner appropriate to the circumstances.
Roles	What kinds of roles are assumed by group members? Do roles inhibit or produce group growth?	Each member has several group roles that are also shared with others. Growth-producing and group vitalizing roles predominate.
Communication	How does communication take place? Who are the listeners? Is the verbal communication compatible with nonverbal expression?	Communication is open and two-way. Ideas and feelings are expressed freely. There is congruence between verbal and nonverbal communication. There is direct communication among members and with the leader.
Conflict	What issues cause conflict in the group? Is conflict avoided, denied, or suppressed?	There is evidence that disagreement and controversy are viewed positively. Basic unresolved disagreements are accepted and tolerated. Conflict is used as an opportunity for personal and group growth.
Problem solving	What kinds of problems occur? Who solves the problems? Is there constructive criticism? Are genuine efforts made to solve problems?	Group members engage in problem solving. Constructive criticism is frank, relatively comfortable, and oriented toward goals.
Cohesion	What positive elements of cohesion are present? What evidence of trust, liking, and support among the members exists? Are there any signs of excessive cohesion?	There are high levels of trust and liking. There is mutual support for all members and conflicts are expressed and resolved. Creativity and a wide range of thinking styles are supported. Signs of groupthink are not evident.
Self-evaluation	How does each client contribute to the group goal? Are clients "growing" as a result of group participation?	Members openly examine their behavior in the group. All members participate in realistically evaluating growth toward goals.

TABLE 11-7

Communication skills in groups

TECHNIQUES OF THE LEADER(S)	GROUP MEMBER RESPONSE	OUTCOME
Giving information: "My purpose in offering this group experience is . . ."	**Further validates assumptions:** "How is this going to happen?"	Leader(s) and member(s) enter into a dialogue in which member(s) get more information to make decisions and build trust in group experience.
Seeking clarification: "Did you say you were upset with John because he said that?"	**May try to restate his thoughts or feelings:** "Yes, I guess I was upset."	Member becomes aware that he was not clear and learns to identify thoughts and feelings more precisely, at the same time taking responsibility for them.
Encouraging descriptions and exploration (delving further into communication or experiences): "How did you feel when Joann said that to you?"	**Elaborates on his message:** "I was angry."	Member deals in greater depth with an experience in the group and again takes responsibility for his reactions. (This example also places events in time or sequence, lending further perspective to group events.)
Presenting reality: "Would other members think Joann was unstable if they interviewed her for a job? You don't appear shaky to me."	**Listens and considers other possibilities.**	Member compares perception of self with others' perceptions of him.
Seeking consensual validation (seeking mutual understanding of what is being communicated): "Did I understand you to say that you feel better now than you did last week?"	**Further clarification:** "Well, yes, I'm better than last week but not as good as I'd like to be."	Group and leader(s) learn how members view progress and in which way they should receive evaluation of themselves.
Focusing (identifying a single topic to concentrate on): "Maybe we could identify one problem you have and talk more about that."	**Channels thinking:** Members may think of the most puzzling problem they have.	Group and leader(s) identify specific topics they can resolve before the meeting ends. They increase their understanding of one problem before jumping to others.
Encouraging comparison (asking members to compare and contrast their experiences with others in the group): "How did the rest of the group handle this problem?"	**Group members share their experiences** as they relate to the topic.	Group members and leader(s) place attention on significant events and can elaborate on their meanings.
Making observations: "You look more comfortable now, John, than you did at the beginning of the meeting," or, "The group has been silent for the last 5 minutes."	**Group members have something to respond to:** "I feel more at ease now," or, "I think we are quiet because we are bored."	Group members and leader(s) place attention on significant events and can elaborate on their meanings.
Giving recognition or acknowledging: "John, you are new to the group. Perhaps we can introduce ourselves."	**Feels acknowledged and included:** "Yes, I'm John, and I came here because . . ."	Members view specific instances as important, and the leaders reinforce the behavior or event they choose to notice, in this case, the desire to come to group.

TABLE 11-7—cont'd

Communication skills in groups

TECHNIQUES OF THE LEADER(S)	GROUP MEMBER RESPONSE	OUTCOME
Accepting (not necessarily agreeing with but receiving communication with openness): "Yes, I hear you say that you don't know if you want to be in the group or not."	**Feels heard and understood** without fear or attack.	Members learn that even "nonacceptable" attitudes can be talked about, and perhaps any thought is not so horrible that they cannot share it."
Encouraging evaluation (asking the group as a whole or individual members to judge their experiences): "When Marilyn gives you support do you feel better?" or, "How did we do in helping Joann with her problem?"	**Members reflect on progress made:** "Not exactly, because I don't know if I can trust her to be honest," or, "It was hard, I'd like to know from her."	The criteria for success becomes clearer to members, and new directions may be formulated as a result of the discussion.
Summarizing (encapsulating in a few sentences what has occurred): "The group discussed several issues and problems today—they were . . ."	**Members recall significant points** and close off consideration of new or extraneous topics.	Members and leader(s) place events in perspective, identifying salient points of a group session. Such a summary can lead to a better understanding of group process.

From Van Servellan, G.M. (1984). Group and family therapy. *St. Louis: Mosby.*

- Facilitating movement toward group goals
- Encouraging sharing and promoting self-expression of members
- Summarizing group progress toward goals
- Managing problematic behaviors of individual group members
- Facilitating communication among members

Nurses as group leaders carry out the principles of therapeutic communication. Communication techniques and skills, examples of client responses, and examples of outcomes in insight-oriented groups are found in Table 11-7.

Self-Intervention

Objectivity about involvement in a group is an important component of group leadership. For some nurses, managing a group can be an intimidating experience. Together with self-assessment, supervision of the process facilitates comfort. Some questions that promote self-intervention involve the following:

- What is my comfort level with this group?
- Am I meeting my personal needs or the goals of the group?
- Which group members do I like?
- Which group members do I dislike?
- How do I respond to group members who do not follow group norms?

- Is the pace of the group too fast? Too slow?
- What has been accomplished in the group?
- In what way does my leadership impede/promote accomplishment of group goals?
- Am I fulfilling the terms of the group contract? Am I failing to fulfill the terms of the group contract?

KEY POINTS

- Nurses participate in and lead many kinds of groups. Task groups are designed to achieve clearly defined goals. Support groups provide support and problem-solving opportunities for clients. Group therapy is a means of alleviating stress, reducing anxiety, and providing clients with opportunities to modify and test new behaviors in a controlled setting.
- Leadership styles influence the outcome of groups. All groups have a formal leader who has either a democratic, an autocratic, or a laissez-faire style of leadership. Informal leaders emerge from among the group membership.
- Cohesiveness in a group refers to the degree to which group members are able to work together to accomplish goals. Cohesiveness enables group members to trust and take risks as they develop and grow. Overcohesiveness, or groupthink, inhibits individual growth in groups.

- Resistance among group members may take the form of acting out, absenteeism, subgrouping, dependency, and fight-or-flight dynamics.
- The use of audio- or videotapes, process recordings, and postgroup debriefing are effective methods for assessing the therapeutic value of groups.
- Formation of a group requires the nurse to arrange the time, frequency, and place for group meetings, select the membership, establish rules, negotiate contracts, and provide for confidentiality among the membership.
- Multiple member roles emerge during the life of a group. Roles may facilitate or inhibit growth or energize the group to accomplish its goals.

REFERENCES

Campinha-Bacote, J. (1994). Transcultural psychiatric nursing: Diagnostic and treatment issues. *Journal of Psychosocial Nursing, 32*(8), 41-46.

Copp, L. & Copp, J. (1993). Illness and the human spirit. *Quality of Life: Nursing Challenge, 2*(3), 50-55.

Corey, G. (1995). *Theory and Practice of Group Counseling* (4th ed.). Pacific Grove, CA: Brooks Cole.

Crosby, G., & Sabin, J.E. (1996). A planning checklist for established time-limited psychotherapy groups. *Psychiatric Services, 47*(1), 25-26.

Hetzel, R.D., Barton, D., & Davenport, D.S. (1994). Helping men change: A group counseling model for male clients. *Journal for Specialists in Group Work, 19*(2), 52-64.

Holmes, H., Ziemba, J., Evens, T., & Williams, C. (1994). Nursing model of psychoeducation for the seriously mentally ill patient. *Archives of Psychiatric Nursing, 4*(6), 343-353.

McCloskey, J.C., & Bulechek, G.M. (Eds.). (1996). *Nursing interventions classifications* (2nd ed.). St. Louis: Mosby.

Smith, M., Hardy, K., & Riggins, O. (1996). Working with the patient with a chronic mental impairment: An activity group approach. *Journal of Psychosocial Nursing, 34*(2), 27-30.

Van Servellan, G. (1984). *Group and family therapy.* St. Louis: Mosby.

Yalom, I. D. (1995). *The theory and practice of group psychotherapy* (4th ed.). New York: Basic Books.

 CRITICAL THINKING QUESTIONS

Mrs. Phillips is a 37-year old, recently divorced registered nurse with three young children. She was admitted to the unit because of a suicidal gesture. Her supervisor at work insisted she seek treatment. The client is in debt because her ex-husband is behind in child support payments. Mrs. Phillips often finds herself working overtime because of staffing problems. During group therapy, Mrs. Phillips focuses on the problems of other clients. When asked questions about herself, she minimizes her problems and redirects the conversation. You are the group leader.

1. What is Mrs. Phillips problem?
2. What is your appraisal of Mrs. Phillips situation? Have you considered the situation from several perspectives?
3. What strategies can you use to enhance her awareness of herself in the group?
4. What roles must you assume to facilitate her participation in the group?
5. How do you choose the best option?
6. What criteria will you use to evaluate the effectiveness of your intervention?
7. Are there different ways of thinking or interacting for you to integrate into your approach as a result of this decision-making process?
8. What insights did you gain by examining this example of your critical thinking process?

Chapter 12

Working With Families

Anita Leach McMahon

LEARNING OUTCOMES

After studying and applying the concepts of this chapter, the learner will be able to:

- Analyze family systems concepts as they relate to families in the mental health care system.
- List developmental tasks and significant transitions in the life of a family.
- Examine possible coping responses of families who are faced with crisis situations.
- Explain the significance of family structure, function, and development.
- Use a genogram and ecomap to assess families.
- Interpret medical and nursing family diagnoses.
- Implement therapeutic interventions for families in the mental health care system.
- Discuss various family therapy techniques.

KEY TERMS

Blended family
Boundary
Coherence
Conflict avoidance
Differentiation of self
Disconfirmation
Disengagement
Disqualification
Double bind
Dyad
Ecomap
Emotional cutoff
Enmeshment

Extended family
Family
Family development
Family function
Family projection process
Family set
Family structure
Fusion
Genogram
Hierarchy
Multigenerational transmission
   process
Nuclear family emotional system

Overprotectiveness
Rank order
Reconstituted family
Rigidity
Scapegoat
Sibling position
Skip-generation parents
Societal regression
Stepfamily
Subsystem
System
Triangle
Triggers

As the twenty-first century approaches, drastic change is taking place in the family. The structure of the family is far from traditional and has shifted dramatically. Couples who marry are doing so at a later age. The number of children living in step-, blended, or reconstituted families is increasing by 3% annually, and it is estimated that by the year 2000, one third of all children will live with a step-parent by age 18. Of the children born in the 1990s, 22% will be born to single mothers. Two thirds of all mothers are in the work force (U.S. Bureau of the Census, 1990).

The family structure of clients in the mental health system is also being transformed. The deinstitutionalization of the last decades has shifted the primary care of clients with serious mental illness from hospital-based professionals to family members and significant others. Today's managed care climate and the health care reform movements require nurses to become creative and innovative in their approaches to the care of clients and their families (Rose, 1996). Alternative settings for care require unique mergers and alliances to maximize client stability and prevent relapse. Some families give direct care to the person with a mental illness in the home, whereas others oversee care from a distance, serving as advocates for their ill family member who must negotiate complex systems of care. Others fill the gaps that inevitably emerge in the process of a family member's recovery. Still others abandon and reject the family member with a mental disorder.

The purpose of this chapter is to describe the structures, functions, and developmental tasks of families. Theories that explain emotional processes and the development of stress in families are discussed. The chapter highlights the nursing role in family assessment and therapeutic interventions with families.

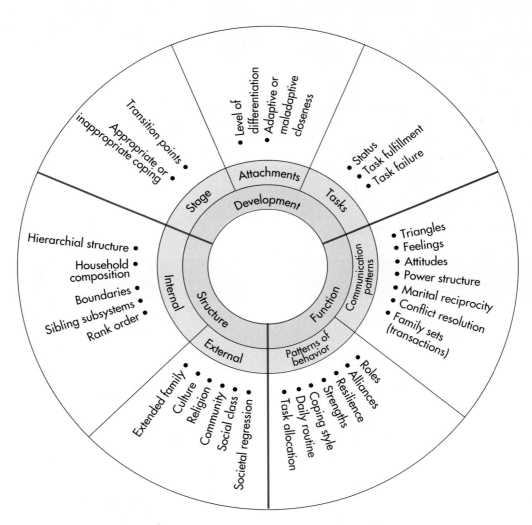

Fig. 12-1 Components of a family system.

DEFINITION OF FAMILY

A *family is a small social system made up of people held together by strong reciprocal affections and loyalties.* The traditional family begins with marriage or cohabitation; members enter the family through birth, adoption, or marriage, and leave through death, divorce, or establishment of new homes. Families are dynamic. They are systems through which and by which family heritage, as well as social, cultural, and ethnic values and beliefs are perpetuated. It is probably more accurate to describe rather then define family. Families have been labeled by their structure, level of function, and stage of development. Fig. 12-1 graphically depicts the components of family that are discussed in this chapter. The diagram illustrates the complexity of the components that make up the families and supports the idea of family as a *system, a group of people greater than the sum of its individuals but, in a unique way, constituting a whole.*

Family Systems Dynamics

Family systems theory was developed in the early 1950s by Bowen (1978) and employs a biological evolutionary perspective to describe the dynamics of a family. Two fundamental premises underlie the theory:

1. A system is a fluid, ever-changing system, and
2. A change in one part of the system is followed by a corresponding change in other parts of the system. The family is seen as a web of parts, or subsystems, that can be understood only as whole; that is, as more than and different from the sum of its parts.

Family systems theorists believe that acute and chronic stress give rise to emotional dysfunction in a family. Stress manifests itself when symptoms of mental illness appear in an individual member. Symptoms in any family member, whether physical, emotional, or social, are viewed as manifestations of dysfunction in the family relationship process.

Bowen views the family as a multigenerational system characterized by patterns of emotional interaction. Eight interlocking concepts describe the emotional patterns and interactions of the family systems approach: differentiation of self, triangles, the "nuclear family" emotional system, the multigenerational transmission process, the family projection process, sibling position, emotional cutoff, and societal regression. Table 12-1, pp. 202-204 defines each of these concepts and explains how they are used to explain dynamics in families with members who have mental disorders.

Family Structure

Families may be defined by their structure. Structure may be internal or external. *Internal structure consists of* family composition, rank order, subsystems, and boundaries. Traditional family composition, known as the *nuclear family, consists of parents and children living in the same household.*

"Skip-generation" parents, grandparents who are taking care of grandchildren, are a growing family group. More and more families are homeless and poor. As the baby boomers reach retirement age, an increase of *multigenerational or extended family* households is expected. Another emerging group is the single person choosing to remain alone or who is a young adult in transition between his or her family of origin and the formation of a new familial unit.

Another internal family's structure is rank order. *Rank order is the position of a child in a family with respect to age.* Internal structure is also defined by subsystems, or the subgroups within a family, and boundaries, the rules that define who participates and how.

The external structure of a family is its context and includes culture, religion, social class, status, mobility, environment, and extended family. Much sociological research has focused on the external structure and environmental context of families.

Structural dynamics

Salvatore Minuchin (1980) has characterized family dynamics as emerging from the internal structure of families. The theoretical foundation of a structural approach to families is the premise that a family is the social context within which individuals act and react. *Family structure, viewed from a dynamic standpoint, is an invisible set of functional demands that organize the way in which family members relate to one another.* A basic assumption is that behavior is a consequence of the organization and structure of the family and of patterns of interaction between and among family members.

According to this model, the family does not totally determine an individual's inner processes. Rather, the individual influences his or her environment, and the environment influences the individual in recurring sequences of interaction, or family sets. A person's social context, or ecosystem, includes workplace, school, neighborhood, extended family, and nuclear family. This idea is similar to the concept of societal regression. The structural model used the concepts of hierarchy, subsystems, boundaries, and family sets or transactional patterns.

Hierarchy *Hierarchy is the amount of power and status in each generational level.* In functional families the hierarchical arrangement is clear, so each family member knows who has the power. Unity and consistency exist within each generational level. On the other hand, the power in a dysfunctional system may be diluted or unclear.

TABLE 12-1

Bowen's family systems concepts

CONCEPT	DEFINITION/EXPLANATION	APPLICATION
Differentiation of Self	• *Differentiation of self is the degree to which a person defines the self as separate from others. It is described on a continuum that ranges from low levels of differentiation ("fusion") to high levels ("clearly defined sense of self").* • *It is the degree of separation or fusion between the intellectual and emotional systems of the self.* • A person's level of differentiation evolves out of the family relationship system. The level of differentiation is the background against which a family and its members live. It is quite stable and varies only slightly as it is passed from generation to generation.	• The degree to which family members differentiate from their family of origin is the degree to which they will be able to manage the stress involved in caring for a relative with mental illness. • The ability to define personal boundaries is positively related to the level of differentiation. • Family members are encouraged to develop and clarify their own values, beliefs, and goals, as well as the ability to articulate them to other family members. • Varying levels of differentiation of members within a family system explain the unique responsiveness of family members to the crisis of mental illness.
Triangle	• *Triangles are emotional configurations consisting of three members, objects, or issues. They are a way of describing relational patterns among persons, and objects or issues.* • Triangles are formed throughout the life of a family. • The major parental triangle (mother-father-child) is realigned as families expand or contract. • Triangles involve "movement." Movement in a family is related to level of differentiation and level of anxiety in the family. • Movement or rigidity reflect the closeness or distance of each of the three points on a triangle. • Individuals are at any given point in time a member of multiple triangles.	• A triangle may include a collective group such as the mental health care system. • The mental health care system becomes a point on the family triangle that also includes the identified client and the client's spouse. • The closer or more fused two points of a triangle are, the more distant the third point. If one parent is close to a child, the other parent is in a distant position. • Nurses use triangles to help families minimize triangular relationships by encouraging one-on-one relationships among family members. • If the points on a triangle are fixed and rigid, there is greater risk that when crisis occurs dysfunction will develop.
Nuclear Family Emotional System	• *A family is an emotional system in which what happens to one member influences other members of the system.* • *The nuclear family emotional system involves the patterns of emotional functioning in a nuclear family.* • The formation of the family's emotional system begins with a marriage or permanent union. • *Fusion, the emotional merging of two people into a common self,* and differentiation, the maintenance of intact boundaries around the self, are the two emotional extremes of the system.	• The stability of the marital dyad in a family with a mentally ill member can influence the degree to which the marriage is able to sustain the stress imposed on the family system by the symptoms of the client. • The emotional climate of a family determines to some extent the outcome of a family crisis. • The member of the family with mental illness may be its **scapegoat,** that is, *the person around whom family anxiety is focused.* When the family member with symptoms is removed or removes himself or herself from the system, symptoms may develop in another member of the system.

TABLE 12-1—cont'd

Bowen's family systems concepts

CONCEPT	DEFINITION/EXPLANATION	APPLICATION
	• The symptoms of fusion in the nuclear family emotional system include marital conflict, dysfunction of a spouse, and projection of anxiety onto children.	
Multigenerational Transmission Process	• *The multigenerational transmission process is the process by which patterns of interaction are passed from generation to generation.* It might be called the "apple does not fall far from the tree" phenomenon. • Each generation is linked to past and future generations through family relationships. • Family characteristics such as norms, culture, values, behaviors, problems, issues, and patterns of relationships are transmitted from one generation to another.	• A three-generation genogram (family map) is used to present information about patterns of interaction among multigenerational family members. • The genetic predisposition to mental illness within families is an example of the cross-generational transmission process. • Emotional reactivity to crisis is similar across generations of extended families. • Multigenerational family caregiving in an increasing phenomena among clients in the mental health care system. Grandparents often assume responsibility for adolescent grandchildren who have psychiatric symptoms.
Family Projection Process	• *The family projection process is a process through which parental undifferentiation impairs one or more children. It operates within the father-mother-child triangle.* • It exists in all grades of intensity and is present to some degree in all families.	• Adults who have not resolved their role in the projection process of their families of origin, tend to experience increased anxiety when coping with relatives who have symptoms of a mental disorder. • Families in which a parent is the symptom bearer have children at risk for increased levels of anxiety and lower levels of differentiation.
Sibling Position	• *Sibling position refers to the place or role one assumes or learns in a family.* • Sibling position is established by birth order and gender. • Personality profiles exist for each sibling position and are incorporated into family systems theory.	• When it is necessary for a client with a mental disorder to be cared for by a sibling, ideally the responsibility for the care should be shared by all members of the sibling subsystem. • Generally, when one sibling, to the exclusion of others in the subsystem, assumes total responsibility for the care of a relative, that sibling may be overfunctioning for other siblings in the family.
Emotional Cutoff	• *Emotional cutoff is the process of becoming physically or emotionally separated or isolated from one's family of origin, or denying its importance.* It is a dysfunctional response to fusional forces within the family. • All people have some unresolved emotional attachment to their parents.	• Adult children who have been cut off in dysfunctional ways from their family of origin may be unable to cope with parents or relatives, despite their desire or need to do so. • Individuals who are cut off from their family of origin remain emotionally connected and must confront the anxiety created by the cutoff.

Continued.

TABLE 12-1—cont'd

Bowen's family systems concepts

CONCEPT	DEFINITION/EXPLANATION	APPLICATION
	• Physical distance is not always an accurate reflection of differentiation. • There are degrees or gradation of emotional cutoff.	• Family members may cut off a mentally ill individual to preserve their own mental health or to facilitate independence by the individual who has symptoms.
Societal Regression	• *The idea that the emotional problems of families are similar to the emotional problems of society.* • Family regression and societal regression are similar and may influence each other.	• A family's health is a function of the degree to which the family system and family members are differentiated from societal and generational problems and tensions. • All families will at some time need to cope with the problems and concerns created by the growing number of people in society who develop symptoms that involve emotional responses to the environment.

From Bowen, M. (1978). Family therapy in clinical practice. *New York: Aronson.*

Subsystems *Subsystems consist of persons in reciprocal role relationships. They are the subgroups within the larger family system. Subsystems may be delineated by gender, generation, interest, or function.* Family members belong to multiple subsystems in which they hold different roles and levels of power. Generally three subsystems exist within families: the spousal subsystem (or marital dyad), the parental subsystem, and the sibling subsystem.

The spousal subsystem or *dyad involves husband and wife but may be thought of as any two individuals in the same household whose relationship is sexual.* The parental subsystem accommodates the addition of children to the family.

Boundaries *Boundaries define the separateness of a family system, subsystem, or individual from the surrounding environment.* Boundaries may be tangible, such as the family dwelling, or less tangible, as in the case of taboos that prohibit incest. Various boundaries exist around family systems and subsystems.

Clear boundaries are those that are firmly established. *Diffuse boundaries* are permeable and able to be penetrated. *Overclose boundaries* are marked by intense *enmeshment, which is an extreme form of proximity. Rigid boundaries* are inflexible and unyielding. *Disengaged boundaries* are overly rigid and prohibit interaction. *Disengagement defines extreme separateness and inappropriately rigid boundaries.* In families with a dysfunctional member, family interactions are intense and characterized by go-between communication patterns, reverberations, emotional overinvolvement, and fixed alliances.

Family sets (transactional patterns) *Repetitive sequences of behavior in families are called transactional patterns, or family sets.* Functional family sets are flexible and enable family subsystems to carry out their functions and resolve or diminish stress by accommodating to a need for change. The structure of a family (subsystems, boundaries, and hierarchical levels) unfolds in the process of these repetitive interactions.

Dysfunctional family sets include rigidity, overprotectiveness, and conflict avoidance. These maintain stress and block change in a family. *Rigidity is a conscious or unconscious attempt by family members to maintain the status quo or a public image of normality.* Issues requiring change are not allowed to surface, and the appearance of the "normal family" exists. The family describes itself as untroubled, except for the symptoms of its mentally ill member. Resistance to change prevails. *Overprotectiveness involves a high degree of mutual concern for family members and the family's welfare.* Members are hypersensitive to signs of emotional and physical distress, tension, or conflict. A lack of activity or interests outside the family exists. *Conflict avoidance is a family set aimed at maintaining family peace at any cost.* Conflictual issues remain unresolved, contributing to recycling of old problems.

Family Development

All families move through stages when they expand and grow or when they lose membership and contact. *Family development is defined as the process of progressive structural differentiation and transformation over a family's history. Family development can be thought of as family transitions that involve active acquisition and selective discarding of roles, as family members seek to fulfill the changing functional requisites for survival, and as the family adapts as a holistic system to recurring life stresses.*

Although a developmental framework is helpful for conceptualizing family processes, applicability is limited because the nuclear family structure is by no means universal, and cultural differences do exist among families. On the other hand a developmental framework can serve the nurse and families in the following ways:

- A guide for assessing family history
- A guide for setting family goals
- A means of identifying critical periods of family growth and development
- A means of predicting what a family may experience at any period in its life span
- A means of highlighting universal characteristics in families
- A means of assessing differences among families

Duvall (1977) published a family development schema that was later incorporated into the work of Carter and McGoldrick (1988). Table 12-2 identifies family developmental stages and lists the major task and emotional processes common to each stage.

A family developmental task is a responsibility, connected with emotional growth, that arises at a specific stage in the life of a family. Successful accomplishment of tasks at one stage theoretically leads to satisfaction and success with tasks that arise at later stages; failure to negotiate tasks at any point in the life of a family may leave family members vulnerable to future dysfunction.

Stages of development are sometimes determined by the age of the eldest child in a family. Stages and transition points may overlap or be repeated as successive children are integrated into the family system, and at any point a family may be considered a "multistage family." An example of a multistage family would be one with an adolescent eldest child, siblings in elementary school and parents expecting another child. All transitions are stressful, but sudden transitions between stages can be traumatic. For instance, if all the children in a family are "launched" in a short period, and simultaneously an elderly parent comes to live with his or her adult child, excessive stress would be likely.

Transition to divorce

Separation, divorce, single parenting, shifting partners, or remarriage by widowed and divorced persons affect family development and may influence the progression or transition of a family through normative developmental stages. These stages include the decision to divorce, planning the breakup, the separation, and finally the divorce (Carter and McGoldrick, 1988).

Transition points occur not only during the separation and divorce but also continue over time. The transitional process may be reactivated by graduations, marriages, or illnesses of children or by the remarriage, relocation, illness, or death of either spouse. Successful negotiation of the postdivorce stage of development involves a willingness by both parents to share financial responsibility and to maintain a parenting partnership in relation to the children.

Stepfamily transition

Another key developmental phase occurs when a **stepfamily**, or **blended** or **reconstituted family** is established. *These families may be formed because of the death of a partner or spouse, divorce of biological or adoptive parents, or abandonment by biological parents.* Stepfamilies are not static and may have children who are "his, hers, and ours." Stepfamilies are founded on loss. Their structure is formed by the emotional ties of members rather than by who lives in the reconstituted unit (Bray, 1994). The transitional tasks that need to be negotiated so that reconstituted families can be successful units include the following:

- Recovery from the loss of the first partnership and resolution of attachment
- Acceptance of all family members fears
- Acceptance of the complexity of the system
- Negotiation of acceptable, flexible boundaries.

Although divorce and step-parenting are not, in and of themselves, the cause of family dysfunction, these transitions do create stress within the family system. If a family is genetically predisposed to development of mental illness, the stress of any developmental transition may act as a catalyst for the onset of symptoms, or at the very least, worsen them.

Family Function

Family function describes how individual members behave in relation to one another. Instrumental functioning in a family refers to the mutuality needed to carry out the activities of daily living (ADLs). *Expressive functioning* refers to a family's communication patterns, problem-solving ability, family roles, power or control over one another's behavior, family beliefs, and the directionality, balance, and intensity of relationships among family members.

No family is totally functional or dysfunctional. The difference between dysfunction and function is quantitative rather than qualitative, and the degree of functioning is what counts.

The functional family is one capable of receiving, translating, and passing on historical responsibilities, fulfilling current responsibilities, and planning for an emotionally secure future for its members. It is a family that is internally selective about using information, making

TABLE 12-2

Family developmental stages

STAGE	MAJOR TASK	EMOTIONAL PROCESSES
Unattached young adult who is between families (single person)	Parent-child separation	Recognition and acceptance of self as separate from one's family of origin Achievement of emotional, social, and economic independence
New marriage/cohabitation	Commitment of two extended family systems to the newly formed system	Commitment to a new identifiable system Establishment of a workable philosophy of life as a couple Realignment of relationships with extended families to include partner Realignment of relationships with friends, associates, and community agencies Negotiation of issues such as eating and sleeping patterns, living space, finances, sexual contact, and use of time Decision making about parenthood
Postestablishment/expectant couple	Preparation for and acceptance of entrance of new members into family	Acknowledging that a child is expected. Adjusting sexual relationships to the patterns of pregnancy Acquiring knowledge about, and planning for, pregnancy, childbirth, and parenthood
Childbearing family: family with young children	Emotional integration of child into family and community	Adjustment to the stresses and responsibilities of parenthood Emotional integration of the child into the family unit Adjustment of parents and grandparents to new roles Establishment of a workable couple partnership that incorporates the new child/children into the family Planning for and incorporation of additional children into family Socialization of children Adjustment to parent-child separations Acceptance of outside influences on family Development of peer relationships by children
Family with adolescents	Fostering independence of adolescent children and support of their differentiation efforts	Maintaining flexible family boundaries. Adaptation to rapid physical, emotional, spiritual, and sociocultural changes occurring during adolescence. Recognition and acceptance of the conflict between physical dependence of adolescent children and their increasing emotional independence Reallocation of household responsibilities among older children Increasing responsibility of parents for elderly family members (grandparents)

TABLE 12-2—cont'd

Family developmental stages

STAGE	MAJOR TASK	EMOTIONAL PROCESSES
Launching and mid-life	Negotiation of multiple entrances and exits into family unit	Negotiation of shift from "parent-child" to "parent-separated adult" roles Renegotiation of couple relationship or single lifestyle Preparation of parent and adult children for the "empty nest" Negotiation of concrete plans for retirement Realignment of communication patterns with children to include their inlaws Adjustment to grandparenting role Adjustment to increased leisure time and renegotiation of roles Beginning adjustment to decreased physical energy
Later life	Acceptance of shifting societal roles and death	Adjustment to retirement Maintaining relationships with adult children, grandchildren, and great-grandchildren Realignment of physical and mental resources and energies Preparation for the death of oneself and one's partner

decisions, setting priorities, and coping with change. A mentally healthy family is capable of interacting with a larger sociocultural environmental system.

Dysfunctional families are characterized by fusion and isolation, rigid boundaries with unclear and distorted perceptions of individual members, high levels of both overtly expressed and suppressed conflict, inconsistent messages and contradictory communication patterns, unclear or rigidly held goals, an unclear power structure, fused role enactment, inadequate or dysfunctional affectional ties, enmeshment with diffuse or nonexistent generational boundaries, and isolation from the larger society.

Functional communication in families is characterized by clear, direct messages and by the requesting and receiving of feedback. Dysfunctional communication, on the other hand, is characterized by disqualification, disconformation, double binding, and pseudomutuality. Box 12-1 describes pathological communication patterns found in families and gives an example of each.

FAMILY CRISIS

The onset of psychiatric symptoms in a client can be a traumatic experience for family members. What has happened to their family member has happened to them. Many families report not knowing how to deal effec-

tively or cope with the crisis of a family member entering psychiatric treatment. Families must struggle to cope with changes and the often difficult behavior of the troubled family member. Feelings of guilt and a search for past behaviors that may have contributed to the client's condition are common responses of family members to the diagnosis of a mental disorder.

Family crisis may increase responsibilities of healthy family members and precipitate changes in routines. Feelings and attitudes about the family member with symptoms may shift from positive to negative or from negative to positive. Sympathy and understanding, confusion about the relative's behavior, helplessness, anxiety, guilt, and shame are common. Shifts in alliances may result in fragmentation or in pulling together of family members.

Family beliefs about mental illness and its cause and cure will influence reactions. Initially families express hope that the client will return to "normal." Fear of stigma and caution about the future are behaviors that evolve as the chronic nature of symptoms becomes a reality. For some, fear centers on the possibility that other family members may develop symptoms of a mental disorder.

The process of resolving a family crisis is not unlike the process of an individual crisis resolution (see Chapter 10). Families may cope well and grow with the experience or they may exhibit dysfunctional behavior patterns.

Box 12-1

Pathological Communication Patterns

DISQUALIFICATION

Characterized by contradictions, inconsistencies, changes of subject, misunderstandings, "tangentializations," incomplete sentences, obscure speech mannerisms, and literal interpretation of metaphors among family members, particularly between parents and children.

DISCONFIRMATION

Ignoring or invalidating the essential elements of another's perception of himself or herself, or of a situation that the person has experienced, by saying "You don't really feel the way you say you feel, or need what you say you need, or experience what you say you experience."

DOUBLE BIND (INCONGRUENT MESSAGES)

Two conflicting messages are delivered simultaneously. The primary injunction is negative, and punishment is alluded to. The second injunction, usually nonverbal, conflicts with the primary injunction. The receiver is in a "double bind," not knowing to which message to respond. Generally there is a third message that prohibits escape. The receiver usually is in a no-win situation. Response to either message means the receiver is either "mad" or "bad." Consistent double bind messages between parents and children result in dysfunction.

PSEUDOMUTUALITY AND PSEUDOHOSTILITY

A fixed, rigid style of relating, characterized by erratic and inappropriate distance or closeness that effects identity and which cannot be maintained. Confused expectations result, but a facade of complementarity is maintained. Energy is directed toward maintaining the false mutuality. Pseudohostility differs from pseudomutuality only in that the facade is usually a state of chronic conflict and alienation among family members.

FAMILY COPING

For clients and families, coping is a process of readjusting attitudes, feelings, perceptions, and beliefs about self and others. For some, the coping process may be painful and difficult, but healthy outcomes give rise to a greater sense of meaning and purpose in life. It can be a time of self-discovery, self-renewal, and transformation.

Coping sometimes implies struggling with issues without adequate knowledge, skills, or support. Families of clients with mental disorders must cope with disruption of family life, recurrent crises, persistence of symptoms, and sometimes loss of faith in professionals and the mental health care system. Family coping modes in times of crisis reflect family patterns of functioning. Family coping modes that have been identified include information seeking, problem solving, help seeking, reliance on religion, optimism, denial, and acceptance of crises as a way of life. Families may become angry and assertive, or take out frustrations and feelings of hopelessness on staff. Sometimes families become despairing and pessimistic and "abandon" the family member by distancing from them (Solomon, 1995).

The outcome of the coping process depends on the health of the family structure, the amount of accumulated stress among family members, the perception of and severity of the crisis event, family strengths, and the coping process itself.

NURSING MANAGEMENT OF FAMILIES

The family of a client with a psychiatric disorder is often his or her most reliable support system. For some, however, family resources and relationships may be impoverished because of the care and treatment of its member, or the family may be part of the client's problem. Nurses in psychiatric treatment settings are often the initial contact the family of a client with mental illness has with the health care system. They are in a position to assess the family and provide the interdisciplinary team with information that will be used for planning. Nurses at the basic level of education carry out therapeutic interventions with clients and those with advanced education may function as family therapists.

Family Assessment

Assessment of a family is a holistic, comprehensive process that involves evaluation of the crisis event that initiated the contact. It includes evaluation of the family coping style and the structure, functional, and developmental aspects of the family. Generally in treatment settings the goals of family assessment are as follows:

- To obtain an accurate history of the client's family
- To clarify the development of symptoms
- To determine the degree of family burden and assess family attitudes
- To assess the family's reaction to the client's symptoms

Genogram

Assessment of a family involves the use of a genogram. A *genogram is a diagrammatic historical "map" of a family over three generations that illustrates family structure, family function, and family developmental events.* Preparing a genogram begins during the initial interview with a client. Universally recognized symbols (Fig. 12-2) are used to note facts about a family. Fig. 12-3

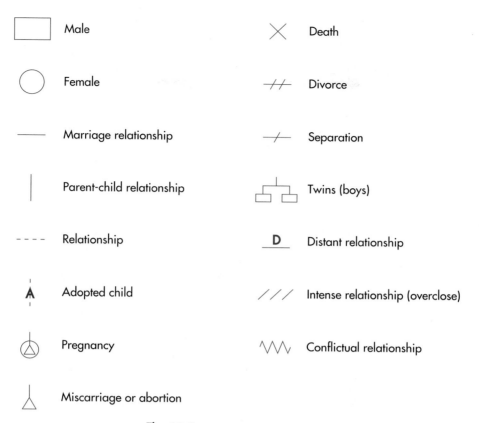

Fig. 12-2   Genogram symbols.

illustrates a three generational genogram of a family needing intervention because one of the members is a recovering alcoholic.

A genogram is generally constructed with all family members present, but nurses may also obtain the information from the clients themselves. At the beginning of an interview, the first task of the nurse is to focus on the presenting problem of the client. The detailed history needs to be connected in some way to the reason the client is seeking treatment. For instance, "The information I am asking for will help me understand how your problem developed," and "My experience has taught me that many factors contribute to the problem." Statements like these begin the process of creating a "system attitude" toward the problem. The focus of attention is shifted from the client to the family system as a whole. The information needed to prepare a genogram is outlined in Table 12-3.

The initial process of data collection generally takes two or three meetings—more if a family has been experiencing symptoms over a long period. The genogram, however, is like a "living" map that is never complete. New information is added as data collection continues and the family evolves, expands, or contracts. A useful way to include new information is to add it with the date, in a contrasting color. In a brief contact with a family not all of the genogram will be completed. Rather, the focus is placed on the structure and function that relates to the immediate crisis or symptoms.

Ecomap

An *ecomap is an overview of a nuclear family system within the context of the larger world, neighborhood, and community. It is a way of organizing the external structure of a family. It shows the relationship of family members to society and systems outside the nuclear household.*

The large circle at the center represents the nuclear family. The smaller outer circles represent significant people, agencies, or institutions that make up the family's larger environment, or context. Lines are drawn between the circle at the center and the outer circles to indicate both the strength and the direction of connections.

Ecomaps are particularly helpful for nurse case managers working with families that have multiple problems. They may also serve as a guide to networking and consolidating services for families who need and use multiple

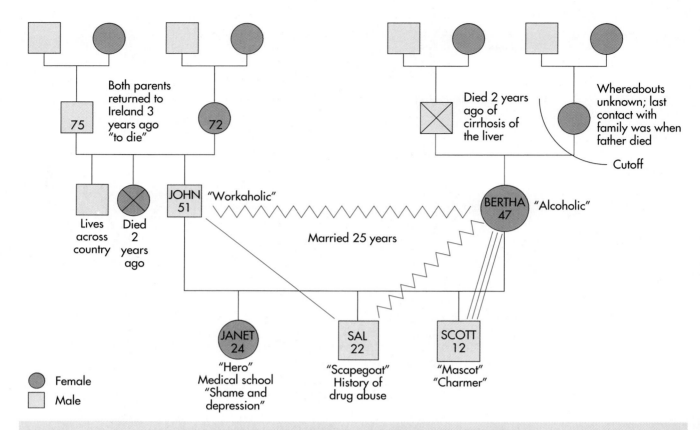

GENOGRAM CASE STUDY: FAMILY WITH AN ALCOHOLIC MEMBER

Bertha is a 47-year-old woman who has been diagnosed with alcoholism. She has been a client on the substance abuse detox unit for the past 5 days. During her hospital stay, she has received visits from John, her husband of 25 years, and one of her adult children. She complains of being unwanted and unloved by her family.

Her oldest daughter, Janet, age 24, is the family hero, an overachiever who is putting herself through medical school. Janet admits to having pulled strings to get her mother admitted but has not come to visit. As a rule, she rarely sees the family except when they need her to resolve a family crisis.

Sal, age 22, is the family scapegoat who has a history of drug abuse. Sal has refused to visit, stating that he has always been blamed for what was wrong with the family. According to Sal the real problem was his mother: "She's the drunk!"

Scott is 12 years old. The nurses on the unit refer to him as a "charmer." He states that he was unaware that his mother had a problem with alcohol until she was hospitalized. He is the family "mascot" and continues as a happy-go-lucky person, apparently unperturbed by the stress of his mother's illness.

During a recent family meeting, Bertha's husband stated that the family will be all right if Bertha stops drinking. John is the youngest of three siblings. His older sister died 2 years ago and an older brother lives across country. His parents moved back to Ireland 3 years ago "to die there." They wanted to spend their last years in their homeland.

John is described by Bertha as a workaholic who makes no money. They rarely have an argument or shout at each other, but they also never discuss important issues. John blames Bertha for Sal's problem stating that it's "all in her family. Her parents are drunks too." Little is known about other family members. Janet admits to feelings of shame and depression around her mother's illness. There is no emotional expression of feelings among family members other than a focus on Bertha's drinking, and Sal's drug abuse.

Fig. 12-3   A genogram of the family of Bertha and John, discussed in the accompanying narrative. This genogram shows the beginning assessment data.

TABLE 12-3

Genogram information

INFORMATION	MEANING OF INFORMATION
Names, nicknames, family titles	Resemblance to a family member in name and personality sets an individual up as the object of the projection process.
Ages	Coincidence of dates may render a child vulnerable to dysfunction. Oldest children are more vulnerable to stressors in the family system.
Dates of nodal events (death, births, marriages, separations, divorces, moves, promotions, jobs)	Children born after the death of a significant other are vulnerable and may become objects of the projection process. Marriages that occur after major losses in families are also known to be more vulnerable to dysfunction.
Physical location of family members	Location of family members may determine who is distant and cut off from the family or who is overly close. Family cutoffs and major losses are known to be fusional forces in families. Overcloseness or fusion may engender dysfunction when family balance is upset by crisis.
Frequency of contact between members of the extended family and the quality of emotional contact	The quality of communication among family members influences levels of function and dysfunction in families. A family strength is open communication with one another. Enmeshment or overcloseness indicates patterns of dysfunction.
Sibling position (the eldest is placed on the left in a genogram)	Sibling, spousal, and parental subsystems are identified. Position in the sibling subsystem determines vulnerability. Boundaries around each of the subsystems help determine function or dysfunction in the family.
Closeness and distance on each generational level	Family members belong to many triangles. Cross-generational triangles exist. Intense relationships move other individuals into the distant position. The degree of closeness and distance in each generation of the family system indicates the degree of fusion or differentiation that exists for each member. Boundaries that are diffuse, such as those that exist in incestual relationships, indicate dysfunctional closeness. Dysfunctional patterns of communication are passed from one generation to the next when intervention has not occurred.
Emotional cutoffs	The greater and more significant the cutoffs are in a family, the greater are the degrees of fusion and differentiation that exist. Cutoffs are more prevalant in families that are dysfunctional.
Characteristics of relationships	In functional families, degrees of closeness and distance are flexible. Dysfunctional families have extremes of closeness (enmeshment) and distance (cutoffs). In marriage, one partner is generally more of an emotional pursuer, whereas the other is an emotional distancer. Men are more often distancers, whereas women more frequently pursue their spouses. Family roles are scripts that are expected of family members. If roles and pursuit-and-distance patterns are rigid, dysfunction is likely when a family crisis occurs. Some family members remain uninvolved in family emotional issues.

service agencies. Potential networks can be sketched in one color and changed to another when actual referrals to community resources are made. Fig. 12-4 illustrates some of the actual networks of the Grass family and shows some of the potential goals planned by their nurse case manager.

Focused assessment

Although the genogram and the ecomap are useful for gathering and consolidating facts about the internal and external structures of families, it is also important to assess family function, level of family development, coping styles, and family strengths. The information-gathering process helps treatment team members gain adequate information to care for clients and their families and provides a forum for family teaching about the clients symptoms. As in any relationship, therapeutic rapport must be established before asking clients and their families questions that are potentially intrusive. Box 12-2 suggests questions that are asked to solicit the family's perception

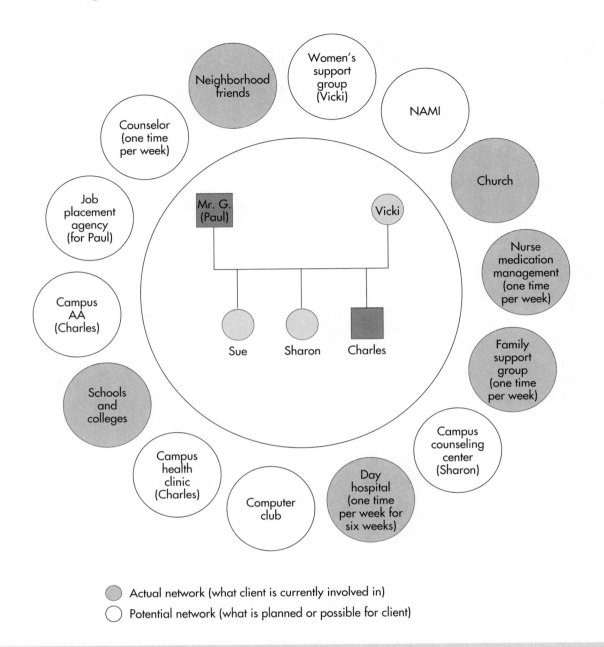

Actual network (what client is currently involved in)

Potential network (what is planned or possible for client)

ECOMAP: NETWORKING OF A FAMILY

The Grass family have been asked to have a family meeting with the nurse at the day hospital where Mr. Grass is the identified client. He attempted suicide 3 weeks ago after he lost a job he had held for 23 years. He was hospitalized briefly and has been coming to the day hospital three times a week. He is married to Vickie, and they have three college-age children, Sue, Sharon, and Charles. The purpose of the meeting is to formalize the nurse case manager's plan for his home care.

When asked about what goals the family wished to accomplish, Mr. Grass (Paul) said he needed a job. Mrs. Grass states she needs her own life back. She works full-time and is the sole provider for activities of daily living at home. The girls expressed their concern about their father's suicide attempt and fears about "catching" the illness. Charles states he is uninvolved but has sought help for himself at the campus health clinic because he began drinking too much after his father's suicide attempt.

Fig. 12-4 An ecomap of the Grass family shows the tentative plans made for the family by the nurse case manager.

Box 12-2

Focused Assessment Questions

FAMILY PERCEPTION OF CLIENT'S SYMPTOMS

- How does the family's perception of the problem differ from the client's?
- What feelings do family members have about the care of the client? How long has the family cared for the client?
- What burden has the family experienced? Emotional? Financial? How do members manage the burden?
- Do family members perceive themselves as part of the client's problem, or do they blame the client for his or her troubles?
- What future involvement with the client is expected from family members?
- To what extent are family members willing to support the client emotionally? Financially? To provide a home after discharge?

FAMILY DEVELOPMENT

- What is the expected stage of family development?
- How does the client and his or her family differ from this expected stage of development?
- Has the family completed the tasks of previous stages of development?
- What is the relationship between fulfilling, or failing to fulfill, family tasks and the client's symptoms?
- Do family members remain excessively attached to one another?
- What/who restricts freedom of development within the family system? Client? Parents? Spouse? Child? Others?

FAMILY FUNCTIONING

- How clear are family boundaries?
- What impact does the client's symptoms have on the family?
- What influence does past mental illness in the family have on the function or dysfunction of the family?
- What is the level of conflict in the family?
- What issues keep the family united/divided?
- What influence do intellectual ability and educational levels of family members have on family function?
- Are the family rules clearly defined?
- Are triangles rigid or fluid?
- What indications of fusion exist?
- Which family members are close/distant?
- What behaviors do family members describe?
- What subsystems exist within the family?
- Describe the communication patterns of family members.
- What is the predominant mood of the family?

of symptoms, stages of family development, and degree of family function.

Family Diagnosis

The issue of making a *family* diagnosis is controversial. Some third party payers only reimburse for a *Diagnostic and Statistical Manual of Mental Disorders, Fourth Edition* (DSM-IV) diagnosis that necessitates labeling the "identified client" rather than the family system. As care shifts from formal long-term family therapy to short-term therapeutic work with clients, solutions to reimbursement issues will need to be found.

DSM-IV medical diagnoses

Currently, the Axis IV psychosocial and environmental factors of the DSM-IV are usually used to determine treatment and prognosis when families of clients with psychiatric symptoms are involved. Relational problems that are the primary focus of intervention may be coded on Axis I of the DSM-IV when patterns of interaction in the family complicate or exacerbate symptoms and impair function of individual family members or the family unit itself (DSM-IV, 1994). Problems of families that have Axis IV diagnosis are found in Box 12-3.

NANDA nursing diagnoses

The formulation of a family nursing diagnosis may be approached in several ways. Many North American Nursing Diagnosis Association (NANDA) diagnoses relate to family issues, role relationships, and coping ability of families (NANDA, 1994). They include the following:

- Parental role conflict
- Parenting, altered
- Coping, ineffective family: compromised

Box 12-3

Examples of Family Problems Coded on DSM-IV Axis IV, Psychosocial and Environmental Problems

- Death of a family member
- Family health problems (spousal dysfunction)
- Separation, divorce, or estrangement of client
- Client's removal from home (cutoff)
- Remarriage of a parent (triangling)
- Sexual or physical abuse of client
- Parental overprotection (enmeshment)
- Child or elder neglect
- Sibling discord
- Death or birth of sibling

- Coping, ineffective family: disabling
- Coping, family: potential for growth
- Role performance, altered
- Family processes, altered
- Caregiver role strain
- Caregiver role strain, risk for

Typology

Another way to diagnose family function or dysfunction is to consider typology (classification by type). The Olson Model (1983) uses a continuum ranging from rigid and structural to flexible and chaotic on one axis, and disengaged and separated to connected and enmeshed on the other.

McCubbin and McCubbin (1989) developed another model based on coping styles of families. Family *resiliency* is defined by positive family flexibility and levels of bonding. *Rhythmic* family coping describes the family that values time and routines. *Regenerative* family typology describes family hardiness and coherence. **Coherence is the degree to which families value loyalty, trust, caring, and shared values in managing stressors.** Whatever system is used, determining a family's strengths and ability to cope is fundamental to planning of goals and interventions.

Family Outcomes and Goals

Nurses working with families use short-term, intermediate, and long-term outcomes when planning interventions. Usually the nurse's initial encounter with a family occurs when there is a crisis. This is particularly evident when a family member is hospitalized because of onset of symptoms. The anxiety level of family members is high, forces of undifferentiation exist, and dysfunctional thoughts, feelings, or behaviors are likely to be present in one or more family members. Family functioning may be disrupted or disorganized. In many cases the family has tried using coping mechanisms but without success. Consequently the overall initial short-term outcome for such families would include evidence of ability to function effectively on a daily basis.

Short-term outcomes reflect the immediate needs of the family to resolve the current crisis. *Intermediate outcomes* are directed toward behaviors associated with initiation of a change process. Goals would include dealing with issues of burden and family attitude toward mental illness. *Long-term outcomes* are directed toward change in dysfunctional patterns of family interaction. Such patterns, created over time, may involve multiple physical, emotional, social, and behavioral factors and therefore will take longer to resolve. These are most often the focus of family therapy.

Families themselves have identified several goals they expect to accomplish as a result of participation in treatment. Goals identified by family members of clients include the following:

- Reduction of anxiety about the client
- Learning to motivate the client to do more
- Understanding appropriate expectations
- Finding help to accept the illness of a family member
- Locating community resources
- Understanding medications and their use
- Learning appropriate responses to symptoms such as hallucinations, talking to self, paranoia
- Receiving help to gain order and control over household
- Getting client to practice better hygiene
- Finding time for personal life

Therapeutic Interventions

Nurses are often the first individuals to interact with families during home visits, at clinic appointments, at day treatment programs, during hospitalization, or in primary care settings. Interventions provided by nurses depend on their educational level and expertise. For example, nurses at the advanced practice level in child or adult psychiatric nursing may work with families on an ongoing basis doing family therapy. Nurses at the basic level of practice assess clients and identify actual or potential problems and make referrals to family therapy.

Other therapeutic interventions with families include coordination of family information with the rest of the treatment team, serving as an advocate for a client's family in legal matters, facilitating referrals and the discharge process, educating the family about the client's medications and their symptoms, and facilitating involvement of family members in a network of community support services. In addition, nurses may participate as co-therapists in direct family interventions such as multifamily groups, support groups, self-help groups for families of the mentally ill, information groups for families, and family education groups. Ability to cope is fundamental to the planning of goals and interventions.

Therapeutic use of self

Perhaps the most important factor when working with families is the nurse's ability to maintain a differentiated self, that is, to remain objective in relationships with families. Nurses, like other persons, are members of a family, and are therefore vulnerable to the way a family's characteristics, issues, and patterns of interaction can trigger their own anxieties. Failure to identify **triggers (emotional responses to a family)** may stall or interfere with building rapport with families. Engaging in self-assessment enables nurses to understand how their own family history interacts with the client's family to create triggers, raise anxiety, blur boundaries, and bring about a potential or actual impasse. The goal of self-assessment is for nurses to identify problematic issues in the management of families and to differentiate between those that belong to themselves and those that belong to the clients.

Crisis management

Crisis management for family members of an individual with a mental illness evolves around managing the crisis presented by the onset or exacerbation of the client's symptoms or the crisis created for other members of the family system. Crisis intervention with families uses the principles discussed in Chapter 10. The nurses role in crisis management is a directive one, that is, the nurse "takes charge" until the family regains its equilibrium. Strategies used by the nurse to help manage a family crisis include the following:

- Commending the strengths of the family system and its individual members
- Offering information and options
- Reframing the problem, that is, offering alternate viewpoints or facts about it
- Offering education
- Separating the symptoms from the personal identity of the family member who is the client (externalize the problems)
- Validating emotional responses
- Encouraging family members' participation in treatment and prevention of relapse
- Encouraging family caregivers to allow themselves adequate respite

Therapeutic partnerships

Therapeutic partnerships with families are the mainstay of therapeutic work with families. Before any therapeutic intervention can occur with families, rapport is established. Establishing rapport involves creating partnerships with family members aimed at supporting the recovery of clients and empowering them to thrive in their natural social environment. Therapeutic partnerships aim to reduce fear, anxiety, and guilt created by the clients symptoms. Partnerships involve agreeing on mutually acceptable goals and taking actions to achieve.

In the partnership model, mutual accessibility is expected. Clients, family members, and health team members remain mutually accessible to each other. In the initial phases of intervention, frequent contact occurs and clients and families return for reassessment or "tune-up" periodically and as the need arises.

Multifamily support groups

Several types of groups for families have been successfully used to provide social support, promote wellness, and prevent relapse of clients. Multifamily psychoeducation groups, relapse prevention groups, and national organizations are used to maintain and promote mental health (Moller and Murphy, 1996). Chapter 11 discusses some of these groups.

A unique aspect of multifamily groups is that clients, family members, and health care providers participate on an equal basis. Environmental factors for families and clients such as housing, transportation, and access to community resources are discussed. Healthly nutrition and medication compliance is stressed and case management activities are initiated (see Chapters 17, 18, 20, and 21). Among the educational needs requested by families are the following:

- Factual, honest information about the family member's diagnosis, medications, treatment plan, and prognosis.

TEACHING POINTS

Coping Strategies for a Family With a Member With a Mental Disorder

Teach the family members to:
- Believe in their own expertise.
- Value the support of other families.
- Accept limits of what can be done about symptoms.
- Learn to focus on and manage symptoms.
- Learn about medications and their side effects.
- Accept the need the symptom bearer has for quiet and alone time.
- Observe for self-destructive or suicidal behavior in the client.
- Remain calm in the face of aggression and access help immediately

- Challenge bizarre behavior and hygiene issues with firmness and gentleness.
- Know when to access the health care system for help.
- Collaborate actively with health team members.
- Take time for self and other family members.
- Learn to set limits on disruptive behavior of ill family members.
- Advocate for improved inpatient care, community services, housing, and rehabilitation.
- Identify reliable professionals in the community.
- Employ political advocacy on behalf of all people with mental illness.

- Skill training to help manage behaviors, monitor medications, and handle emergencies.
- Supportive help with the stigma, blame, and frustration of having a family member with symptoms of mental illness.

Coping strategies that may be taught to families with a member with mental illness are found in the Teaching Points box on p. 215.

National Alliance for the Mentally Ill   The National Alliance for the Mentally Ill (NAMI) is a family-centered group dedicated to advocacy for people with mental illness. The organization is made up of clients (consumers), their families, and interested health care providers, and has a network of support groups at the local, state, and national levels.

NAMI groups provide state-of-the-art information to health care professionals who treat clients and their families as well as to the consumers themselves. It provides emotional support, friendship, and treatment management tips to its members, and sponsors national and state training programs in its efforts to disseminate the latest information about symptoms and biological treatments of the symptoms of brain disease. The address of NAMI is found in the Consumer Resources box below along with those of other consumer groups that support families whose members have psychiatric symptoms. Throughout the clinical chapters of this book (Part Five),

in a feature called The Consumer's Voice, readers will find actual accounts of clients and families who are members of NAMI and who cope effectively with the symptoms of their illnesses with the support of the group.

Family therapy

Family therapy is a psychotherapeutic intervention with a family system by an individual skilled in facilitating change in the system. It implies that all members of the family participate in treatment. Family therapy explores the gestalt, or context, in which a particular emotional problem occurs and is played out among family members. It is a way of assisting family members to move their families toward a more productive way of being (Smoyak, 1995). Nurses at the basic level of practice make referrals to family therapy, whereas advanced practice nurses with special preparation in family therapy serve as family therapists or co-therapists.

Although therapeutic intervention is necessary to support all families who have members with mental illness, family therapy is not for everyone. The following sit-

CONSUMER RESOURCES

The Stepfamily Association of America
602 East Joppa Road
Baltimore, MD 21204
(301) 823-7520

National Alliance for Mentally Ill (NAMI)
200 North Glebe Road, Suite 1015
Arlington, VA 22203-3754
(703) 524-7600
Help line: (800) 950-6264

National Mental Health Consumers' Self Help Clearinghouse
c/o Community Support Programs of the Center for Mental Health Services, Substance Abuse and Mental Health Services Administration
211 Chestnut Street, Suite 1000
Philadelphia, PA 19107
(800) 553-4539

Box 12-4

Techniques Used in Family Therapy

TECHNIQUES/DEFINITION

Cotherapy: More than one therapist leads a session. Two therapists can more easily accumulate data, make observations, and keep track of interactions. Male and female, co-therapists are role models for clients.

Multiple family therapy: More than one family is seen simultaneously by one or more therapists.

Network therapy: The extended family and all social systems that interact with the family are seen together.

Operational mourning: Loss of significant members and how insufficient mourning for them has caused current problems in the family is highlighted. Mourning is reinitiated to complete the process.

Sculpting: A form of role play in which family members are arranged by others. Therapists direct family scenarios to highlight dynamics as they perceive them.

Paradoxical/Injunction: The symptom or its reversal is prescribed. The therapist instructs family members to do consciously what they are doing unconsciously. Should be used only by skilled therapists who are sure of the forces acting within the family; otherwise the family will perceive it as sarcasm, or act on the paradox.

Making assignments: Therapist assigns family members a task.

Supporting family subsystems: Subsystems within the family are overtly recognized by the therapist.

Mirroring or mimicking: The family's mood, pace, or communication patterns are matched. Allows family members insight into their behavior when with therapist.

uations suggest that family therapy would be an appropriate treatment strategy:

- Conflict occurs on the unit between the identified client and the family.
- The precipitating factor in the client's illness is embedded in the family (e.g., marital conflict, cross-generational conflicts, or extreme enmeshment).
- The client is hospitalized during a crucial developmental or transitional stage in the life of the family (e.g., during a divorce or after the death of a family member).
- Origins of the particular dysfunction cannot be separated from family interaction (e.g., clients with anorexia nervosa, alcoholism, or incest behaviors).
- Symptoms occur in another family member as the client begins to recover.
- Individual and group modalities have been nonproductive, and improved therapeutic progress is needed.

Some family therapists work exclusively using either systems, structural, or strategic models, but most take an eclectic approach. Box 12-4 lists several techniques used by family therapists and details an explanation of each.

 ## CRITICAL THINKING QUESTIONS

Mrs. Gerard, a 57-year-old Christian Scientist, was brought to the emergency room by Roy, her husband of 35 years. She had been diagnosed with breast cancer 7 years earlier but refused radiation, chemotherapy, and surgery, deciding instead to rely on her belief in God's healing power. Mr. Gerard states he can no longer comply with her wish not to seek "healing" in a hospital. As he was speaking to the nurse he began to cry and stated, "I can't take care of Prudence any longer. I can't take care of her by myself. I can't continue to watch her suffer. I'm so confused. I know this is against my faith and her wishes."

Mrs. Gerard is admitted to the oncology unit with a gaping wound of her breast. She has been incontinent of urine and stool and has had a continuous discharge of blood from her vagina for the last 4 weeks. She has been seeing the "healer" from her church for the past 7 years and continues to believe that with prayer and the help of God, she will be healed. She is passive and compliant with her husband and tells the nurse that it is time to honor his wishes and not her parents'. She is relatively pain free and makes use of meditation and imagery to manage it.

The Gerards have two grown children—a son, Daniel, and a daughter, Tara. Both are married and live nearby, but do not communicate directly with their mother. They became estranged from her several months earlier when they had an argument with her about seeking traditional medical help for her cancer. She remained persistent in her belief that God would heal her and adamantly refused to seek help from "outsiders." Her children were equally insistent that she see a doctor. Both her children had previously discontinued their membership as Christian Scientists when they married. Mr. Gerard requests that the children be called to visit.

Mrs. Gerard allows selected tests for cancer to be done but refuses any medication or treatment. After consultation with several specialists, her husband, and the healer from their church, Mrs. Gerard requests that the team just make her comfortable "Make it so my husband can take care of me," she says, "I want to go home to die." It is decided that a colostomy and indwelling catheter would effectively relieve the problems associated with Mrs. Gerard's constant incontinence. At her request the team will not do surgery on her breast.

Mrs. Gerard also agrees to a family therapy session with her children and husband, provided her healer is present and that the therapist does not try to make her change her mind about anything. Her stated goal is "to make peace in my family."

1. What reactions are you having to Mrs. Gerard's decisions about the treatment of her cancer? How will you manage your reactivity?
2. What legal and ethical issues should the nurse consider when caring for Mrs. Gerard?
3. What is your understanding of Christian Science?
4. What family diagnoses would you formulate for Mrs. Gerard and her family?
5. What family systems concepts are demonstrated in this scenario? Give examples to support your answers.
6. Should you call Mrs. Gerard's children? Why? Why not?
7. How would you integrate holistic nursing care with Mrs. Gerard's beliefs about healing?
8. What support services would you plan for Mrs. Gerard after her discharge?
9. What interventions would you implement with Mr. Gerard, Daniel, and Tara?
10. How would you form a therapeutic partnership with Mrs. Gerard and the members of her family?

KEY POINTS

- Everyone is or has been a member of a family.
- The level of function in families is related to the level of differentiation of its members, the permeability of family boundaries, and the quality of communication among members.
- The structure of a family is both internal and external and can be illustrated by means of a genogram.
- Dysfunctional families are characterized by fusion, isolation, rigid boundaries, high levels of overt and covert conflict, contradictory communication patterns, an unclear power structure, fused role enactment, and enmeshment or diffuse generational boundaries.
- Disparity between expected developmental milestones and actual task accomplishment creates vulnerability in family members.
- Therapeutic interventions with families include crisis management, forming therapeutic partnerships, referring to multifamily support groups, and referring family therapy.
- Multifamily support groups are used to promote social support, promote wellness, and prevent relapse of clients.
- The National Alliance for the Mentally Ill (NAMI) is a family-centered consumer group dedicated to advocacy for people with mental illness.

REFERENCES

American Psychiatric Association (1994). *Diagnostic and statistical manual of mental disorders, fourth edition.* Washington, DC: Author.

Bowen, M. (1978). *Family therapy in clinical practice.* New York: Aronson.

Bray, J.H. (1994). What does a typical stepfamily look like? *The family journal: Counseling and therapy for couples and families, 2*(1), 66-69.

Carter, B., & McGoldrick, M. (1988). *The changing family life cycle: A framework for family therapy* (2nd ed.). New York, NY: Gardner Press.

Duvall, E. (1977). *Marriage and family development* (5th ed.). Philadelphia, PA: Lippincott.

Hamilton-Wilson, J., & Hobbs, H. (1995). Therapeutic partnership: A model for clinical practice *Journal of Psychosocial Nursing, 33*(2), 27-30.

McCloskey, J.C., & Bulechek, G.M. (1996). *Nursing interventions classification (NIC)* (2nd ed.). St. Louis: Mosby.

McCubbin, M.A., & McCubbin, H.I. (1989). Theoretical orientation to family stress and coping. In Figley, C.P. (Ed.), *Treating stress in families.* New York: Brunner Mazel.

Minuchin, S. (1980). *Families of the slums.* New York: Jason Aronson.

Moller, M., & Murphy, M.F. (1996). Innovative treatment programs: Relapse prevention to reduce hospitalization. *Current Approaches to Psychosis: Janssen, 5*(1), 14-16.

North American Nursing Diagnosis Association (1994). *NANDA nursing diagnoses: Definition and classification 1995-1996.* Philadelphia, PA: NANDA.

Olson, D.H., Russell, C.S., & Sprenkle, D.H. (1983). Circumflex model V: Theoretical update. *Family Process, 22*(12), 69-83.

Rose, L. (1996). Families of psychiatric patients: A critical review and future research directions. *Archives of Psychiatric Nursing, 10*(2), 67-76.

Smoyak, S. (1995). Family therapy. In Anderson, C. (Ed.), *Psychiatric nursing 1974-1994: A report on the state of the art.* St. Louis: Mosby.

Solomon, P., & Draine, J. (1995). Adoptive coping among family members with serious mental illness. *Psychiatric Services, 46*(11), 1156-1160.

Toman, A. (1976). *Family constellation* (3rd ed.). New York: Springer.

U.S. Bureau of the Census (1990). Washington, DC: National Center for Health Statistics

Chapter 13

Psychobiology

Beth Harris
Anita Leach McMahon

LEARNING OUTCOMES

After studying and applying the concepts of this chapter, the learner will be able to:

- Define basic neuroanatomical and neurophysiological terminology.
- Identify the function of the blood-brain barrier.
- Explain neuroregulation.
- Discuss brain endocrine functioning.
- Explain the interrelationship between the immune and nervous systems.
- Discuss the genetic transmission of mental disorders.
- Describe the physiological effects of stress.
- Discuss rhythms and kindling as they relate to mental disorders.
- Implement a physical assessment for clients with symptoms of mental illness.
- Identify current methods of brain imaging.

KEY TERMS

Alarm response
Axon
Basal ganglia
Blood-brain barrier
Brain imaging
Brain stem
Central nervous system (CNS)
Cerebellum
Cerebrospinal fluid (CSF)
Cerebrum
Circadian rhythms
Cortex
Dendrite

Diencephalon
Enzymatic degradation
Exhaustion
Family aggregation study
Hypothalamus
Kindling
Limbic system
Medulla oblongata
Midbrain
Neuroendocrinology
Neuron
Neurotransmission

Neurotransmitter
Nuclei (nucleus)
Peripheral nervous system (PNS)
Pons
Reticular activating system
Resistance
Reuptake
Sleep architecture
Stress
Synapse
Ultradian rhythms
Ventricles

Psychiatry has changed rapidly during the last several decades and will no doubt continue to change at a rapid pace well into the next century. The increased knowledge about the psychobiology of psychiatric health and illness stems from revolutionary advances in all areas of the neurosciences. Current thinking is that psychiatric illnesses are caused by an extremely complex interplay of biological, environmental, and psychological factors.

It has been known since ancient times that mental illness stems at least in part from biological roots. The ancient Greeks believed that a person's personality and state of emotional health were derived from a balance of the basic humors (fluids) in the body. This ancient notion is remarkably similar to current beliefs that most of the major psychiatric illnesses are caused by chemical imbalances in the brain.

Somatic (i.e., biological, physical, or bodily) therapies have been one of the mainstays of treatment for psychiatric illness throughout history. Although a physical cause for psychiatric illness could not be found, physical treatment was used extensively. Persons with mental illness have been bathed, hosed, cooled, bound, chained, sedated, rendered comatose, shocked, and massaged, all in an effort to rid them of symptoms (Table 13-1). Unfortunately, it took until almost the middle of the twentieth century for electroconvulsive therapy, the first truly effective somatic treatment, to be used therapeutically. Not until the 1980s would psychobiological theories begin to approach the degree of sophistication known today.

This chapter will familiarize the learner with concepts basic to a psychobiological approach to psychiatric nursing. It includes basic knowledge about brain structure and function, neuroanatomy, and neurophysiology. Tests and neuroimaging techniques used in the diagnosis of mental illness are also included.

THE NERVOUS SYSTEM

The brain, together with the spinal cord and millions of neurons, makes up the central nervous system. Like all systems, a change in one part of the system affects the whole and becomes evident in another part of the system. Although the discussion that follows separates parts of the central nervous system, the learner needs to remember the interrelatedness of its parts.

Increasing evidence exists to support the premise that much of the behavior observed in clients with mental illness can be explained by the interplay of structural deviations and biochemical imbalances in the brain. Anatomically, the nervous system consists of two interrelated parts: the ***central nervous system (CNS),*** *comprised of the brain and spinal cord*, and *the motor and sensory nerves that are projections of the CNS, which*
are called the ***peripheral nervous system*** (PNS). The CNS, and more specifically the brain, is the part of the nervous system that is of greatest interest in psychiatry and mental illness (Color Plate 1 details the major parts of the CNS).

Neuroanatomy

The brain is comprised of eight major anatomical parts: the cerebrum, the diencephalon, the cerebellum, the brainstem, basal ganglia, the limbic system, ventricles, and neurons. Box 13-1 details the various sections of these parts. Each part of the brain has unique functions, as well as functions shared with other structures.

The ***cerebrum,*** *also called the forebrain, is the largest and uppermost section of the brain. It is divided into left and right cerebral hemispheres. Each cerebral hemisphere is composed of the outer cerebral cortex* (also known as the neocortex). *Each hemisphere is further subdivided into four lobes: frontal, parietal, temporal, and occipital,* as depicted in Color Plate 2. The cerebral ***cortex*** *is connected to various structures of the brain and is associated with uniquely human functions. Use of language, abstract thinking, perception, movement, and the ability to adapt to one's environment are all functions that derive from the cerebral cortex.* Table 13-2 lists each of the lobes found in the cerebral cortex, the functions of each, and their relation to symptoms associated with psychiatric illness.

The ***diencephalon*** *consists structurally of only 2% of the central nervous system but has major involvement in sensory and motor function and limbic pathways. It is comprised structurally of the hypothalamus, thalamus, and pineal body. The* ***hypothalamus*** *houses the pituitary gland and serves as a major control center for maintaining physiological homeostasis and regulating autonomic, endocrine, emotional, and somatic functions.* Table 13-3 lists structural components of the diencephalon, the functions of each, and some examples of their relatedness to symptoms of mental illness.

The ***cerebellum*** *is located in the posterior part of the brain behind the brain stem. It consists of two lobes and a middle section called the vermis and is linked to the brain stem. It is sometimes called the "little brain." It operates below the conscious level and coordinates voluntary muscle activity.*

The ***brain stem*** *connects the spinal cord to the brain and contains the control center for vital cardiac and respiratory functions. The brain stem houses the cranial nerve nuclei and is the "switchboard" through which all motor sensory stimuli must pass. The brain stem includes the midbrain, pons, medulla oblongata, and reticular activating system. The* ***midbrain*** *is the seat of unconscious regulation of motor activity, con-*

TABLE 13-1

Somatic therapies used in psychiatric treatment

THERAPY	WHEN USED	DESCRIPTION
Physical restraints	1700s	Clients were physically restrained and beaten when out of control.
Bloodletting	Early 1800s	Client's arm was cut and allowed to bleed freely.
The revolving chair	Early 1800s	Client was blindfolded and placed on a rapidly spinning chair.
Administration of purgatives and emetics	Early 1800s	Client was given purgatives and emetics to induce vomiting and diarrhea.
Administration of narcotics	Mid-1800s	Morphine and opium were administered.
Continuous sleep therapy	1920s to 1970s	Administration of barbiturates and other hypnotics were used to induce continuous sleep for periods of 10 days, interrupted for eating and elimination.
Surgical removal of tonsils, teeth, sections of the colon	Early 1900s	Surgery was conducted to remove "sources of mental illness caused by hidden infection."
Fever	Late 1920s, 1930s	Fever was induced by infecting the client with malaria to treat general paresis.
Narcotherapy	1930s, 1940s	Sodium amytal was administered.
Carbon dioxide inhalation	1930s	Administration of 30% carbon dioxide and 70% oxygen was given.
Hydrotherapy	Early to mid-1800s	Client was restrained in a tub of cold water with only the head above water.
Insulin coma therapy	Late 1930s to 1950s	Coma was induced by the administration of insulin.
Lobotomy	1940s, early 1950s	White matter of the frontal lobes of the brain is surgically destroyed.
Metrazol treatment	Late 1930s, 1940s	Seizures were induced by administration of pentylenetetrazol (Metrazol).
Megavitamin therapy	Late 1960s to present	Large doses of ascorbic acid, niacin, pyridoxine (B_6), folic acid (B_{12}), as well as various minerals, hormones, and dietary regimens were administered.
Electroconvulsive therapy (ECT)	Late 1930s to present	Grand mal seizures are induced by applying electrical stimulation to the brain.

Box 13-1

The Major Parts of the Brain

I. Cerebrum (forebrain)
   A. Cortex (neocortex)
      1. Frontal lobe
      2. Parietal lobe
      3. Occipital lobe
      4. Temporal lobe
II. Diencephalon
    A. Hypothalamus
    B. Thalamus
    C. Pineal body
III. Cerebellum
IV. Brainstem
    A. Pons
    B. Medulla oblongata
    C. Reticular activating system
    D. Midbrain
V. Basal ganglia
VI. Limbic system
    A. Hippocampus
VII. Ventricles
VIII. Neurons

tains the substantia nigra, which manufactures the neurotransmitter dopamine, and regulates reflexive movement of eyes and the head. The extrapyramidal side effects of medications and stereotypical movements of clients, such as those experienced by clients with tic disorders, originate at the level of the midbrain.

The **pons** contains ascending and descending nerve tracks, and is the site of production of most of the brain's epinephrine. The **medulla oblongata** is responsible for conscious control of skeletal muscle and is involved with balance and coordination. Reflex regulation of respiratory function, the cardiac system, swallowing, coughing, and sneezing are contained in the medulla.

The **reticular activating system** is a loosely organized network of neurons that receive input from other areas of the brain. Stimulation of this area activates the cortex into a state of alert wakefulness and is implicated in causing symptoms related to motivation and level of arousal (Kaplan and Sadock, 1995). The **basal ganglia** are islands of gray matter within each hemisphere of the brain. They are surrounded by the rings of the limbic system and lie between the thalamus of the diencephalon and the white matter of each hemisphere.

TABLE 13-2

Lobes of the cerebral cortex

LOBE	FUNCTION	DYSFUNCTIONAL SYMPTOMS RELATED TO MENTAL ILLNESS
Frontal lobe	• Higher order thinking • Abstract reasoning • Memory planning • Motivation • Concentration • Decision making • Speech production • Purposeful behavior	Abnormalities lead to inappropriate uninhibited behavior, labile affect, diminished motivation, and dementia
Parietal lobe	• Sensory function, including information about body position, muscles, touch and pressure, smell, hearing, vision	Abnormalities result in impaired spatial ability, denial, body image disturbance, self-care deficits (ability to dress), and left-right disorientation
Occipital lobe	• Visual function	Abnormalities cause visual illusions, hallucinations, and hysterical blindness
Temporal lobe	• Interpretation of smell • Abstract thought • Judgment • Memory • Major component of limbic system • Comprehension of sound	Implicated in aggressive and violent reactions of some clients and plays a role in olfactory and auditory hallucinations, as well as language abnormalities

TABLE 13-3

Structures of the diencephalon

STRUCTURE	FUNCTION	RELATIONSHIP TO MENTAL ILLNESS
Hypothalamus	• Regulation of hormones, eating, drinking, sleeping, waking, body temperature, chemical balances, heart rate, sex, emotions, and sexual behavior • Controls the pituitary gland • Major role in control of body rhythms and immune system regulation	• Directly involved in the stress response, psychosomatic illness, and glandular activity • Abnormalities include sleep/wake cycle disturbance, excessive eating and drinking behavior, sexual dysfunction, and mood disturbances
Thalamus	• Initiates consciousness, makes preliminary classification of external information • Influences affect, foresight, and body movement associated with fear and anger	• Implicated in lack of motivation of some clients • May be implicated in impulse control
Pineal body (gland)	• Secretes antigonadotropic hormone (melatonin), which decreases during light with subsequent increase in gonadal function. • Tumors affect sexual development • Possible regulation of biological rhythms	• Thought to be related to seasonal affective disorder, sleep architecture disturbances, and bipolar disease

Limbic System

As early as 1939, it was theorized that a reverberating CNS circuit existed that formed the pathway for emotions. Originally called the Papey circuit, it has come to be known as the limbic system. *The **limbic system** forms the limbus, or border, of the temporal lobes and is interconnected in complex and intricate ways with other brain structures. The major structures include the hippocampus, the amygdala, and a bridgelike structure called the fornix, which houses bundles of nerve fibers that connect the hippocampus to the hypothalamus.*

The limbic system is associated with subjective emotional experiences, as well as with physiological responses to emotional states. It is implicated in the moods, motivations, and sensations that accompany an individual's self-preservation response. The limbic system is involved in sexual behavior; with pleasure, memory, and learning; and with the dichotomous aggressive-submissive response.

Among the clinical symptoms that indicate dysfunction in the limbic system are absence of emotional reaction (flat affect), apathy, bulimia, hypersexuality, and visual and auditory agnosia (failure to recognize what one is seeing or hearing). This cluster of symptoms is labeled *Klüver-Bucy syndrome* and is seen in clients with dementia, brain tumors, and those who have experienced brain trauma.

The hippocampus is that part of the limbic system that consolidates information into memory. It contains numerous neurotransmitters and is the subject of ongoing neuropsychiatric research. *Korsakoff's syndrome,* associated with chronic alcoholism, represents an example of damage to the hippocampus. Clients with the syndrome have difficulty learning new information (anterograde amnesia) and often have difficulty recalling past memories *(retrograde amnesia)* even when intelligence is intact. The amygdala complex is the dorsomedial portion of the temporal lobe. It contains multiple opiate receptors and is implicated when stimulated as part of the *fear response* (dilated pupils, increased heart rate, and increased release of adrenalin).

Ventricles

Within the brain are four ***ventricles,*** *or cavities, which are filled with a cushioning fluid called **cerebrospinal fluid (CSF).*** The two lateral ventricles are located inside the cerebral hemispheres. The third lies at the midline between the two halves of the thalamus, and the fourth is in the area of the pons and medulla oblongata. The ventricles are connected both with one another and with the spinal column so that CSF circulates through the entire nervous system. The chemical contents of CSF can be examined when fluid is taken by spinal tap. Neurotransmitters and their metabolites (waste products) have been measured in cerebrospinal fluid, as well as in plasma and urine. Measurement at this time is not common practice but is conducted to advance knowledge about neurotransmitters and their relationship to mental illness (Oldham and Riba, 1994).

Blood-Brain Barrier

*The blood supply to the brain and the blood circulation of the rest of the body are kept separate by a filtering mechanism called the **blood-brain barrier**. The blood-brain barrier is an anatomic-physiologic feature of the brain consisting of "walls" of capillaries and surrounding glia-cell membranes. It protects the brain from adverse events elsewhere in the body.* The blood-brain barrier also affects the ability of compounds produced in the CNS to leave the system. The ability of a chemical to pass into the brain is based on molecular size, electrical charge, solubility, and on the presence or absence of specific transport systems and the glia cells themselves.

The blood-brain barrier plays a major role in the development of pharmacological agents used to treat symptoms of mental illness. Its protective role also prevents neurotransmitters such as epinephrine (produced in the adrenal glands) from inadvertently affecting the brain neurotransmission system.

NEUROREGULATION

On the microanatomical level, the brain is composed of several hundred billion individual *nerve cells called **neurons**.* Color Plate 3 illustrates the structure of a typical nerve cell. Each neuron has a central cell body with numerous projections that interlace extensively with projections from surrounding neurons. *The many projections that carry information into the cell body are called **dendrites**. The single projection that carries information out of the cell and onto neighboring cells or end organs is called an **axon**.* The axon can be very short or extremely long, and it may or may not have branches. A neuron's shape and its number of connections to other cells varies dramatically, depending on the location and function of the neuron. Color Plate 3 illustrates two neurons with their many dendrites in synaptic contact. *Neurons in the CNS are often grouped by function into communities called **nuclei**. More specifically, a nucleus consists of similarly functioning neuronal cell bodies.* The axons of those cell bodies reach out like vast webs into all areas of the brain and exert their influence widely.

Neurotransmission

*Sending messages to and from the multiple components of the central nervous system takes place through a complex network of neurons in a process known as **neurotransmission**. It is how the multitude of neurons communicate with each other.* Uncovering the wonder of the process has been made possible with the development of microimaging techniques. Neurotransmission regulates such human activities as consciousness, creativity, memory, and emotion.

*The process of neurotransmission takes place using chemical messengers known as **neurotransmitters**. Neurotransmitters are chemicals that affect or modify the transmission of nerve impulses between neurons. The microscopic space between neurons is called a **synapse**.* Simply stated, neurotransmitters move from the neuron by way of the axon (presynaptic cleft) into the synapse or space and is received by the dendrite (postsynaptic membrane).

It is at the synapse, the tiny space between the axon of one cell and the dendrite or cell body of another cell, that the chemical aspect of neurotransmission occurs (Zalcman, Scheller, and Tsein, 1994). Color Plate 3 illustrates this synaptic transmission.

It was once thought that neurotransmitters worked in a "lock-and-key" type of fit with specific neuroreceptors. Receptors are in fact neurochemicals on the surface of cells and may be pre- or postsynaptic. They facilitate recognition of neurotransmitters in the synaptic space. Each neurotransmitter may interact with one or more specific neuroreceptors.

The brain carries out its many diverse functions by relaying messages from cell to cell with an interplay of electrical and chemical means. Messages are carried electrically from the dendrites, along the surface of the cell body and down the axon by an all-or-nothing change in electrical or action potential at the cell membrane that, once initiated, sweeps to the end of the axon where the electrical message is converted to chemical transmission. The change in electrical potential along the axon causes storage vesicles located at the end of the axon to merge with the neuronal membrane, thereby releasing neurotransmitters into the synapse.

Neurotransmitters, once released into the synapse, bind with their specific neurotransmitter receptors on a nearby neuronal membrane. This membrane on the dendrite or cell body of the receiving neuron is called the postsynaptic receptor. By binding with the postsynaptic receptors, the neurotransmitters either increase (excite) or decrease (inhibit) its potential for electrical transmission. There are thought to be more than 100 different neurotransmitters, some primarily excitatory and some primarily inhibitory. Neurotransmitters may be biogenic amines, amino acids, or peptides. Box 13-2 lists the classical CNS neurotransmitters by chemical composition. It is at the level of neurotransmission that the various pharmacological agents used to treat clients with mental illness exert their chemical influence.

After neurotransmitter molecules act on the postsynaptic membrane receptors, they are *released back into the synapse, where they are either inactivated by enzymes in a process known as **enzymatic degradation**, or taken back up into storage vesicles in the presynaptic membrane for future use in a process referred to as **reuptake**.* One example of this process

Box 13-2

Classical Neurotransmitters Organized by Chemical Composition

Biogenic amines (monoamines)
    Catecholamines
        Dopamine
        Epinephrine
        Norepinephrine
    Indoleamines
        Serotonin
Acetylcholine
Amino acids
    Gamma amino-butyric acid (GABA)
    Glutamate
    Glycine
    Aspartate
Peptides
    Substance P
    Endorphins and enkephalins

is the enzymatic degradation of norepinephrine and serotonin by monamine oxidase (MAO). The end result of blocking both degradation and reuptake is that the neurotransmitters serotonin and norepinephrine cannot be removed as effectively from the synapse and must therefore remain and continue to act on the postsynaptic membrane receptors repeatedly. This is the way in which the MAO inhibitors (MAOIs) antidepressants work to relieve the symptoms of depression (see Chapter 15).

To make the process of neurotransmission even more complex, many neurons release more than one neurotransmitter. Furthermore, a given neurotransmitter may have a different effect on brain function depending on the location of the synapse and the condition of the postsynaptic membrane before a given neurotransmission. Some specific neurotransmitters are implicated in specific mental disorders. Table 13-4 lists selected neurotransmitters, their source (if known) in the CNS, their function, and their implication in the causation of the symptoms of mental illness.

Neuromodulation

Peptides are the newest classification of neurotransmitters. Their action is not clearly understood but it is believed that they modify or regulate the other neurotransmitters in some way. Among the peptides currently being studied by researchers are endogenous opioids, which coexist with serotonin and norepinephrine and are thought to be involved with pain sensation, stress reaction, and mood. Substance P is primarily found with

sensory neurons and is thought to coexist with acetylcholine and norepinephrine. Of current interest is the peptide, cholecystokinin, which coexists with dopamine and GABA and may be associated with the onset of eating disorders. Somatostatin, another peptide, is found with GABA and norepinephrine and has been implicated in Alzheimer's disease. As researchers uncover new neuromodulators and neurotransmitters, the complexity of the neurotransmission process becomes evident (Hyman and Coyle, 1994).

Neuroendocrinology

*The study of interactions between the nervous system and the endocrine system is known as **neuroendocrinology.*** When there is an alteration in the functioning of the brain, the pituitary gland, known as the master gland because of its role in directing the functioning of all the other endocrine glands, is directly affected by way of the hypothalamus. The pituitary, after all, is surrounded by brain tissue and responds directly to the brain's chemical influence. As can be seen in Color Plate 1, the pituitary gland is in close proximity to the hypothalamus. When the pituitary is affected by a change in the chemistry of the brain, it in turn alters the functioning of the endocrine glands, including the thyroid gland, the adrenal glands, and the gonads. Fig. 13-1 shows in schematic form the neurochemical-hypothalamus-pituitary-glandular cascade. This cascade or pathway begins with neurotransmission and ends in activating or inhibiting tissues and end organs affected by hormones.

Three brain-endocrine axes (cascades) have been identified as the following:

- Hypothalamic-pituitary-thyroid axis (HPTA)
- Hypothalamic-pituitary-adrenal axis (HPAA)
- Hypothalamic-pituitary-gonadal axis (HPGA)

Table 13-5 notes each of the brain-endocrine axes, the functions of each, and the role each plays in symptoms of mental illness.

When chemical imbalance is recognized in the brain, negative feedback loops are activated. The thyroid gland, through the hypothalamus and pituitary gland, is affected, altering the thyroid's usual response to thyroid-stimulating hormone (TSH). In similar ways, the adrenal gland, through the HPAA, can change the normal daily rhythm of cortisol production from the adrenal cortex and create a persistent overproduction of cortisol. The gonads (testes and ovaries) are affected through the hypothalamus and pituitary.

Laboratory tests measure the effects of the brain abnormalities on the three neuroendocrine axes mentioned above. The measurements of the hormones produced by the end-organs (thyroid, adrenal glands, and gonads) reflect the biochemical balance in the brain.

TABLE 13-4

Selected neurotransmitters and associated psychiatric symptoms

NEUROTRANSMITTER	MAJOR SOURCE/ LOCATION	EFFECT	IMPLICATION
Acetylcholine (Ach)	• No single major source • Synthesized from choline	• Different effects in different brain areas • Can be excitatory or inhibitory • Widespread in PNS	• Antagonism causes anticholinergic side effects of dry mouth, blurred vision, constipation, urinary hesitancy, atropine psychosis. • Underactivity implicated in Alzheimer's disease
Dopamine (DA) (Catecholamine)	• Substantia nigra and ventral tegmental area in the midbrain • Derived from tyrosine, a dietary amino acid	• Generally excitatory • Involved in motor coordination and movement, motivation, thought, emotional regulation	• Implicated in schizophrenia and other psychotic disorders • Antipsychotic medications provide dopamine postsynaptic receptor blockade and cause extrapyramidal side effects
Norepinephrine (NE) and Epinephrine (Catecholamines)	• Locus ceruleus in the brain stem • Synthesized from dopamine • Secreted by adrenal medulla	• Can be inhibitory or excitatory; different brain areas • NE supplies the noradrenergic pathways to cerebral cortex, limbic system, brain stem, and spinal cord	• Underactivity is implicated in depression • Antidepressants increase functional activity • Depleted in dementia of the Alzheimer's type (DAT) and Korsakoff's syndrome
Serotonin (5-HT)	• Raphe nucleus in the brain stem • Synthesized from amino acid • L-tryptophan metabolized as MAO; can be assayed in 24-hour urine	• Upper and caudal raphe nuclei located in pons secretes serotonin to the target areas in brain stem, limbic system, and hypothalmic-pituitary axi	• Underactivity is implicated in depression and obsessive-compulsive disorder (OCD) • Antidepressants (SSRI's) increase functional activity by blocking reuptake
Gamma-aminobutyric acid (GABA), Glutamate, Aspartate, and Glycine (amino acids)	• No single major source • Intermediate that regulates ionic conditions along axon before release at the synaptic cleft of spinal cord and PNS	• GABA and glycine are major inhibitory neurotransmitters; decreases overall excitability of the brain • Requires receptor N-Methyl D Aspartate for action. • Glutamate is excitatory and is found in all cells	• Implicated in anxiety disorders • Activity is increased by the antianxiety medications such as benzodiazepines, sedatives, and hypnotics • Transmitter-receptor action destroyed by chronic use of alcohol
Substance P Endorphins and Enkephalins (Peptides)	* Endorphins and enkephalins are widely distributed in CNS * Substance P found mainly in spinal cord and sensory neurons associated with pain	* Substance P is excitatory, and endorphins and enkephalins are generally inhibitory	* Activation and regulation of response to stress and injury * Involved in pain perceptions and reflex actions * Morphine and heroin are opioid endorphins

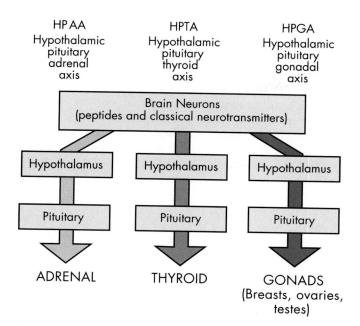

HPAA
Hypothalamic
pituitary
adrenal
axis

HPTA
Hypothalamic
pituitary
thyroid
axis

HPGA
Hypothalamic
pituitary
gonadal
axis

Brain Neurons
(peptides and classical neurotransmitters)

Hypothalamus | Hypothalamus | Hypothalamus

Pituitary | Pituitary | Pituitary

ADRENAL | THYROID | GONADS
(Breasts, ovaries, testes)

Fig. 13-1 Schematic representation of the three brain-endocrine axes (cascades).

When psychiatric symptoms occur, the biochemical alterations in the brain initiate a cascade of effects through the endocrine systems that can be measured peripherally. These laboratory tests, along with other anatomical and physiological findings, are often referred to as biological markers for psychiatric illness. Use in routine clinical practice is sometimes limited because of the expense, time, and discomfort involved, and because few of the biological markers are specific to one illness or consistently present in a given disorder. Nonetheless, the ongoing research on biological markers is uncovering new knowledge daily about psychiatric symptoms (Kaplan and Sadock, 1995). General sources of information about psychobiology of the symptoms of mental illness are listed in the Community Resources box on p. 236.

NEUROIMMUNOLOGY

Healthy functioning of the immune system is essential to well-being, since it is the immune system that protects the body from invasion by pathogens. When the immune system is sluggish or suppressed, the body becomes vulnerable to infection by viruses, bacteria, fungi, parasites, and possibly to proliferation of cancerous cells (Kaplan and Sadock, 1995). Conversely, when the immune system becomes overly responsive to pathogens or misidentifies the body's own tissues as foreign, it either fatigues the body with its overzealousness or launches an autoimmune attack against specific organs.

The CNS and the immune system have some similar characteristics. Both systems have the capacity for memory and react with greater specificity to repeated encounters with the same stimuli (Hayes, 1995). Each system is affected by the activity of the other and both are bidirectional in nature (Hayes, 1995).

TABLE 13-5

Brain-endocrine system axes

NEUROENDOCRINE AXIS	FUNCTION	RELEVANCE TO PSYCHIATRIC SYMPTOMS
Hypothalamic-pituitary thyroid axis (HPTA)	Regulation of the thyroid gland's hormone production	• Blunted TSH response to thyrotropin-releasing hormone (TRH) in depressed clients
Hypothalamic-pituitary adrenal axis (HPAA)	Regulation of the hormones of the adrenal cortex	• Entire axis hyperactive in depressed clients and in some anxious clients • Nonsuppression of cortisol by dexamethasone suppression test (DST) in depressed clients • Elevated cortisol levels in depression • Elevated corticotropin-releasing hormone (CRH) levels in depressed clients
Hypothalamic-pituitary gonadal axis (HPGA)	Regulation of the hormone production of the ovaries and testicles	• Blunted prolactin response in clients with exogenous obesity • Reduced testosterone levels in depressed clients

The immune system may also respond to the nervous system in more direct ways than were even dreamed of until recently. One of the most exciting advances in neuroimmunology was the recent discovery that white blood cells are directly affected by the nervous system. Receptors have been identified on white blood cell membranes for the neurotransmitters dopamine, serotonin, and acetylcholine, as well as for a number of hormones (Kaplan and Sadock, 1995). It has been shown that low levels of norepinephrine stimulate proliferation of a specific type of white blood cell (called a T cell) and that high concentrations inhibit T-cell proliferation.

It has also been shown that an increase in serotonin suppresses immune response, whereas a decrease in serotonin availability enhances immune activity (Kaplan and Sadock, 1995). It is logical to assume, therefore, that the immune system can respond directly to the abnormalities of the neurotransmitters systems in the brain related to mental illness. Furthermore, the tissues that create white blood cells—the thymus, bone marrow, lymph nodes, and spleen—are innervated by the sympathetic nervous system, thus rendering them responsive to the body's state of arousal.

Autoimmune diseases, in which the body misidentifies its own tissues as foreign and creates antibodies that attack them, are often triggered by viral infection. One of the theories about schizophrenia is that it may be caused in some people by an autoimmune response that focuses on the brain (Robin et al., 1989). Other studies link depression to alterations in the immune system (Herbert and Cohen, 1993). In still other studies, psychological stress has been shown to adversely affect immune function (Lutgendorf et al., 1994).

Although a great deal more research is necessary before the exact mechanisms of the immune system-CNS connection are validated, it is clear that diseases of the brain can directly affect the body's immune system and therefore the body's ability to shield itself from pathogens. Conversely, the immune system may play a role in the causation of psychiatric symptoms.

Stress Response

The autonomic nervous system (see Color Plate 4) consists of sympathetic and parasympathetic nervous systems. It prepares individuals to cope with environmental threats (stress) through either a fight (aggression) or flight (withdrawal) response. The following represents responses set up by the autonomic nervous system when fight-or-flight situations are encountered:

- Epinephrine, norepinephrine, and cortisol are released into the blood.
- The liver releases stored sugar into the blood to meet the energy needs for survival.
- Digestion slows so that blood flow may be redirected from the digestive system to the muscles and brain.
- Breathing becomes rapid and shallow to supply more oxygen to the muscles that need it.
- The heart rate increases and blood pressure rises.
- Perspiration increases to cool the body, because increased metabolism generates more heat.
- Muscles tense in preparation for fight-or-flight action, particularly the skeletal muscles of the thighs, hips, back, shoulders, arms, jaw, and face.
- Pupils dilate to let in more light. All of the senses increase their acuity.
- Blood flow to the extremities is constricted as evidenced by cold hands and feet. Blood flow is diverted to more important areas of the body.

Episodes of psychiatric illness are almost always precipitated by specific environmental triggers or by an accumulation of a number of minor stressors. Many clients can unequivocally point to the environmental "cause" of their episode of illness, known as the precipitating event.

Selye (1991) proposed that although stress itself cannot be perceived, it can be objectively measured by the structural and chemical changes that stress produces in the body. He called these changes *general adaptation syndrome (GAS)* because when stress affects the whole person, the whole person must adjust to the changes. GAS has three stages: (1) alarm reaction, (2) resistance, and (3) exhaustion.

The immediate or **alarm response** to stressful events, depicted in Fig. 13-2, *is characterized by an outpouring of hormones from the adrenal gland in response to stimulation of the central nervous system via the autonomic nervous system and the pituitary gland. The adrenal medulla, in response to direct autonomic nervous system stimulation, initially releases norepinephrine and epinephrine. As a result of norepinephrine and epinephrine release, the heart rate, breathing rate, and blood pressure rise, and glucose is released into the bloodstream for a burst of energy.*

When stress is prolonged, the adrenal cortex is stimulated by adrenocorticotropin hormone (ACTH) to release cortisol, "the stress hormone." These hormones produce bodily changes that prepare individuals to deal with the sources of stress quickly and effectively, with physical strength and mental focus. As part of the effort to rally these resources, cortisol impacts the immune system to slow it down and free the energy usually dedicated for immune functions into "fight-or-flight" reactions. Cortisol also initiates breakdown of proteins (gluconeogenesis) to supply more fuel for the body. The byproducts of this process cause a slight acidic shift in the bloodstream.

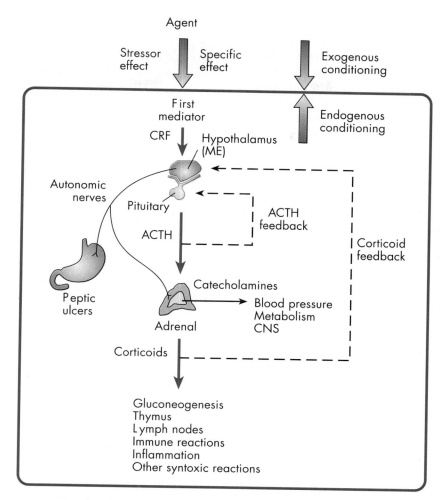

Fig. 13-2   Major pathways of the stress response.

The subjective results of this hormonal outpouring from the adrenal glands are the characteristic symptoms experienced by a person in the alarm phase: anxiety, palpitations, rapid or difficult breathing, nausea, sweating, and muscle tension. If the demands and challenges that triggered the alarm phase of the stress response cease, the body quickly returns to its normal, resting, unalarmed state. No damage has been done and hormone levels return to normal.

The stage of *resistance* represents the opposite of the alarm reaction. *Immune function returns to near normal and the characteristic symptoms of the alarm phase diminish.* The person stops feeling constantly tense and anxious. Palpitations cease, breathing returns to normal, and sweating stops. If asked, the client will guess he or she is getting used to the difficult situation. The third stage of GAS, *exhaustion, occurs when stress continues over a prolonged period of time. It also occurs when multiple stressors occur simultaneously or*

when a person undergoes repeated or overwhelming stress. In this phase, the body becomes depleted; it has exhausted its ability to maintain healthy functioning. Immune functioning is compromised and the client has a diminished capacity to fight infection. Whatever illness the client is predisposed to will either develop for the first time or will recur or worsen (Herbert and Cohen, 1993). For example, in a family with high rates of panic disorders, an individual member may develop panic attacks for the first time when exposed to stress for prolonged periods of time.

A theoretical understanding of stress can be used as a basis to plan nursing interventions (see Chapter 14). It can be used to help clients understand some of the forces that both prevent and lead to relapse. Obviously if the stress response increases the risk of relapse, prevention of the stress response or use of methods that reduce the stress response—the outpouring of adrenal hormones—will prevent or moderate relapse. This intellectual understanding of the relationship between stress and relapse can empower a client to strongly influence the cause of illness for the better by using stress management skills.

Exhaustion may be reversible if the total body is not affected and if the person is able to eliminate the source of stress. However, if stress is unrelieved, or if the body's defenses are totally compromised, the person may not have the resources to regain physiological integrity and may become physically ill or die (see Chapter 32).

Stress management skills are essential for clients recovering from an episode of mental illness. If clients are to have a strong recovery and minimal interference from symptoms, they must have a clear grasp of which stresses are most difficult and dangerous for them personally, as well as a strong repertory of stress management techniques at their fingertips. Both the most dangerous stressors and the most helpful coping techniques will vary considerably from individual to individual, so it is wise to spend time helping the client identify and deal with his or her major stressors. When stress levels are low and/or coping skills are strong, symptoms are held to a minimum and the client functions optimally. When the level of stress increases and/or there is a limited repertoire of stress management and coping skills, symptoms increase and a full-blown relapse becomes more likely. Chapter 14 presents an in-depth discussion of stress management.

GENETIC AND FAMILY CORRELATES OF MENTAL ILLNESS

It has become increasingly clear over the past several decades that specific mental illnesses run in families for both environmental and genetic reasons. Table 13-6 shows combined results from a number of twin adoption and family history studies indicating that close relatives have much higher rates of mental illness than the general population. Although the exact mechanism of genetic transmission remains unknown at present, research supports the theory that the most common mental disorders are to a greater or lesser degree genetically determined.

Genetics

Human genetic instructions are encoded on structures called chromosomes, located in the nuclei of each cell in the body. Each cell (except for sperm and the ova) contains 23 pairs of chromosomes, including a pair of sex chromosomes. The sperm and ova each contain only half a set of chromosomes. When an ova is fertilized, the half set of chromosomes from the ova and the half set from sperm unite to create a complete set of 23 pairs. Each chromosome consists of smaller units called genes, which are composed of long, helix-shaped double strands of deoxyribonucleic acid (DNA), the molecules

TABLE 13-6

First-degree relative risk for mental disorders

DISORDER	RELATIVE RISK (%)
Bipolar disorder	24.5
Schizophrenia	18.5
Bulimia nervosa	9.6
Panic disorder	9.6
Alcoholism	7.4
Generalized anxiety disorder	5.6
Anorexia nervosa	4.6
Simple phobia	3.3
Social phobia	3.2
Somatization disorder	3.1
Major depression	3.0
Agoraphobia	2.8

NOTE: *Other studies may have relative risk ratios that differ considerably from those in these studies, especially if different diagnostic criteria were used. However, the methodological soundness of studies referenced here prompted selection of them for discussion in the text and in this comparison.*

From Rieder, R.O., Kaufmann, C.A., & Knowles, J.A. (1994). Genetics. In R.E. Hales, S.C. Yudofsky, & J.A. Talbott (Eds.) The American Psychiatric Press textbook of psychiatry (2nd ed.). Washington, DC, American Psychiatric Press.

of which are arranged in precise ways to encode genetic information about every aspect of the person. Fig. 13-3 schematically depicts the structure of genes.

For some illnesses, the precise location on a specific chromosome where the genetic defect occurs is known. For example, the precise locations of the genetic defects that create Huntington's Chorea and Down syndrome have been determined. There are several possibilities why this is difficult to uncover for clients with mental disorders. Several genes or chromosomes may be involved in creating a predisposition to each specific mental illness. Some or all of the major disorders may actually be groups of disorders with similar symptoms but different causes (Rieder et al., 1994).

Research is under way to learn about the precise modes of the genetic transmission of mental disorders. The hope is that knowledge about the genetic basis of specific mental illnesses will lead to a better understanding of the nature of these disorders and to improved

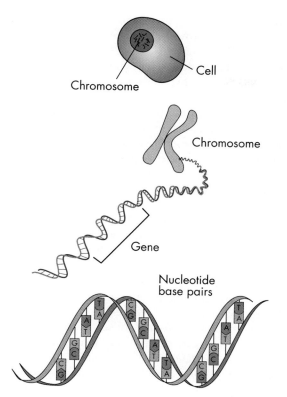

Fig. 13-3 Series of thousands to millions of base pairs form genes, the substrates—or underlying foundation—of inheritance. Genes, which are strewn along chromosomes in the cell nucleus, code for specific proteins. (From Office of Technology Assessment, Washington, D.C., 1992.)

treatments, and possibly to prevention of the disorders themselves. In the meantime, if researchers can discover prenatally or early in life whether a person is predisposed to a major mental illness, they may be able to learn what measures can prevent the genetic inheritance from expressing itself as illness.

Twin Studies

If scientists do not know *how* psychiatric illnesses are inherited, how do they know they *are* inherited? Some studies look at rates of illness in sets of identical and fraternal twins. If an illness is to any degree genetically determined, there would be higher rates of concordance (coexistence of the disorder) in identical twins than in fraternal twins. In other words, if one twin has an illness, it is expected that an identical twin would have the same illness more often than a fraternal twin if the illness is genetically determined and environmental variables remain constant.

Using twin studies methodology, anxiety disorders, substance abuse disorders, eating disorders, bipolar dis-

orders and schizophrenia have also been shown to be to some degree genetically determined. It is interesting to note that even with identical twins, the rate of concordance does not reach 100% for any of the mental illnesses. If it did, researchers would know conclusively that inheritance is the sole cause. A person would either inherit the illness and get it, or would not inherit it and would not get it. Because the concordance rate for identical twins is considerably lower than 100% for all the mental illnesses, researchers can conclude that genetics alone does not determine whether someone will develop these disorders.

Adoption Studies

Another way to discover whether illnesses are genetically determined is through studies of adopted children. The questions asked are: If a child of a parent or parents with symptoms of illness is adopted by parents with no family history of the illness, will the child continue to be at risk for the illness? If a child with no genetic history of mental illness is adopted by a family with a major mental disorder, will that child be at risk? These adoption studies have found that the influence of inheritance is stronger than the influence of the environment in which a person is raised. In other words, if a person inherits a predisposition to a psychiatric illness, he or she is likely to develop the illness even if adopted and raised by a family whose members are without symptoms. Similarly, if individuals have no family history of mental illness, they are unlikely to become ill even if raised by adoptive parents who exhibit symptoms of a major mental illness.

Family Studies

A third genetic research methodology *uses the charting of family history or pedigree. This kind of study is called a family aggregation study.* In charting the histories of families both with and without mental illness, it was found that specific illnesses are found in specific families. For example, depression expresses itself in some families and schizophrenia in others. Bipolar disorders are found in some families and eating disorders in others. Although there is some overlapping between families, the overall trend is for specific illnesses to cluster, or aggregate, in given families.

Most likely the major mental illnesses are caused by some combination of genetic predisposition and environmental stress. Not all people who are genetically predisposed will develop the illness and some who are not genetically predisposed may.

The overall conclusion of twin, adoption, and family aggregation studies is that the environment in which an individual is raised is unlikely to precipitate symptoms unless there is a genetic predisposition. Furthermore, being raised in a symptom-free environment will not necessarily prevent mental illness in a person who is genetically predisposed. Genetic inheritance in large part determines the risk for mental illness, but whether a genetically predisposed person develops a mental disorder is heavily influenced by his or her degree of environmental stress.

BIOLOGICAL RHYTHMS

The biological rhythm system can be thought of as central controlling processes by which psychological and biological changes occur in response to internal and external environmental stimuli. Rhythms, or repetitive patterns, last anywhere from seconds to years. *Daily body rhythms are referred to as* **circadian rhythms** from the Latin words, circa (about) and diem (day). Sleep and wakefulness, temperature, and neurohormonal function are examples of circadian rhythms. *Rhythms of less than 24 hours are* **ultradian rhythms.** The 90-minute sleep, dream cycle, a basic rest-activity cycle (BRAC) is an example of an ultradian rhythm.

Current theory holds that circadian rhythms are controlled by a pacemaker or internal clock. One such pacemaker is the retinohypothalamic projection in the suprachiasmatic nuclei of the hypothalamus (McEnany, 1990). Its close proximity to the eye lends credence to the idea that endogenous biological clocks are influenced by light and darkness. Although not clearly understood, it is speculated that the neurotransmitter melatonin is secreted with darkness and suppressed with light. Melatonin is a byproduct of serotonin synthesis and is excreted by the pineal body (McEnany, 1996a).

Exposure to light keeps a person's biological rhythms synchronized with the external environment. Daily exposure to natural light stimulates the brain to begin a new 24-hour cycle, thus "resetting" the biological clock and ensuring the efficient organization of various rhythms (McEnany, 1996a).

Sleep is part of a larger rhythm of rest and activity. The process of sleeping and remaining awake is expressed in a circadian pattern that varies from individual to individual but generally reflects the person's adaptation to a specific environment. *Two types of sleep alternate throughout the sleep-wake cycle, REM (rapid eye movement) and NREM (nonrapid eye movement). This is referred to as typical* **sleep architecture** (McEnany, 1996a).

REM sleep is considered active sleep and involves the CNS. Large muscles become immobile, but minute twitches of the face, fingers, or body are common. A person's eyes dart about back and forth (hence the name REM), and cerebral blood flow increases with concurrent increase in brain metabolism and temperature. During REM sleep, dreaming occurs.

NREM sleep, on the other hand, has been described as idle brain sleep. The body remains active, but the brain rests. NREM sleep consists of four stages. Stages 1 and 2 are lighter and include a "drifting off" phase. Stages 3 and 4 are deeper, occurring during early night sleep. Typically REM and NREM cycles, that is, sleep architecture, vary from 70 to 110 minutes in duration. The length of REM periods increases to as much as 60 minutes or longer as the night progresses. Sleep architecture can be identified with electroencephalography (EEG).

Sleep architecture and wakefulness are neurochemically driven. Wakefulness is influenced by norepinephrine and dopamine, as well as acetylcholine. These neurochemicals can be pharmacologically manipulated to stimulate wakefulness. For example, cocaine or amphetamines precipitate a presynaptic release of norepinephrine and dopamine and acetylcholine-altering drugs such as nicotine create hyperactive states of alertness. Histamine, aspartate, glutamate, and peptides also contribute to the experience of wakefulness. On the other hand serotonin contributes to the onset of sleep. Likewise adenosine, a neuromodulator has been implicated in both sleep and fatigue. It is also believed that there is cholinergic mediation of REM sleep and that the aminergic neurons of specific parts of the brain shut down during REM sleep (McEnany, 1996a). Chronobiology, or the study of rhythms, has been applied to clinical science.

Rhythmic pattern disturbances are well-documented in bipolar disorder and depression. Clients usually report that one of the first signs they experience when symptoms are reoccurring is disturbance in sleep-wake cycles (McEnany, 1996b).

Other internal rhythms of the body have a longer cycle. The menstrual cycle in women is approximately 28 days in length. A still longer cycle is the approximately annual cycle of mood that most people experience very subtly, becoming less energetic during winter months and more energetic during the summer. This annual pattern is greatly exaggerated in persons with bipolar disorder and seasonal affective disorder (SAD).

KINDLING

Kindling is a psychobiological process, similar to the seizure phenomenon, in which the limbic system is the recipient of repeated, daily subthreshold electrical stimulation, leading to an increased responsiveness to stable low doses of the stimulations over time. This ultimately results in covert seizurelike activity and a lower seizure threshold. Eventually the person becomes so sensitive that seizures occur from a milder stimulus or in the absence of any stimulus. Kindling is proposed to explain the recurrent nature of several neurobiological disorders including depression, bipolar disorder, chemical dependency, schizophrenia, and other disorders.

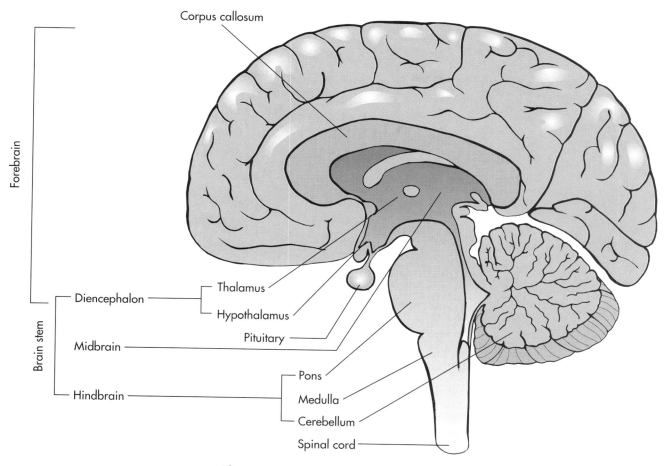

Plate 1 The major parts of the brain.

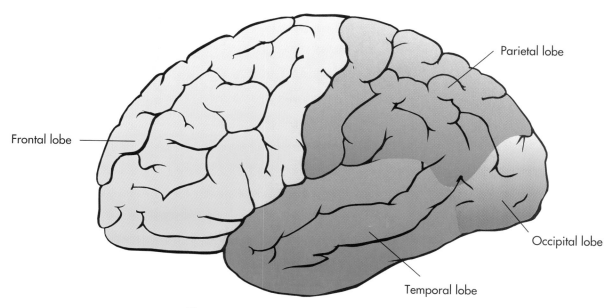

Plate 2 The lobes of the cerebral cortex.

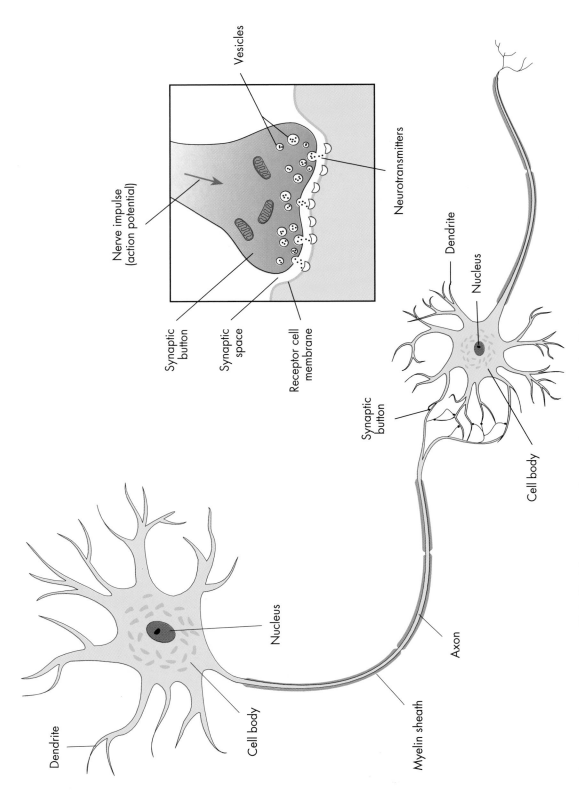

Plate 3 The structure of a typical neuron and detail of synaptic transmission.

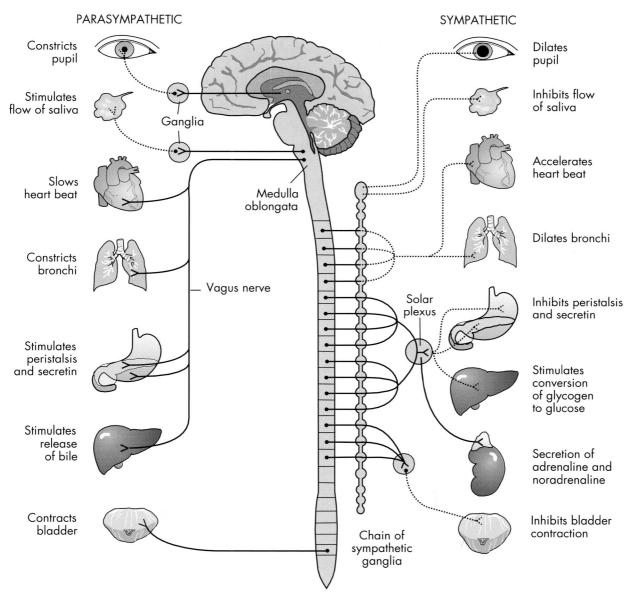

Plate 4 The autonomic nervous system and some of the organs it innervates (supplies with nerves).

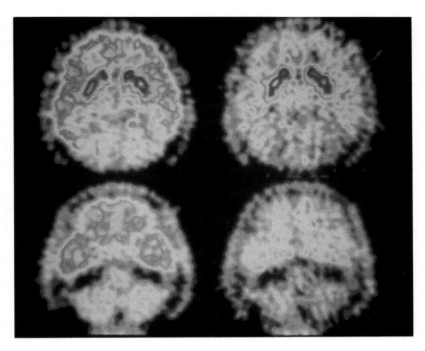

Plate 5 Positron emission tomography (PET) scan images of dopamine receptors in the human brain. Images on left show dopamine D_1 receptors, images on right show dopamine D_2 receptors. (From Farde, L., Halldin, C., Stone-elander, S., & Sedvall, G. Original investigations: PET analysis of human dopamine receptor sub-types using 11C-SCH 23390 and 11C-raclopride. *Psychopharmacology, 92,* 278-284. Springer-Verlag, New York.)

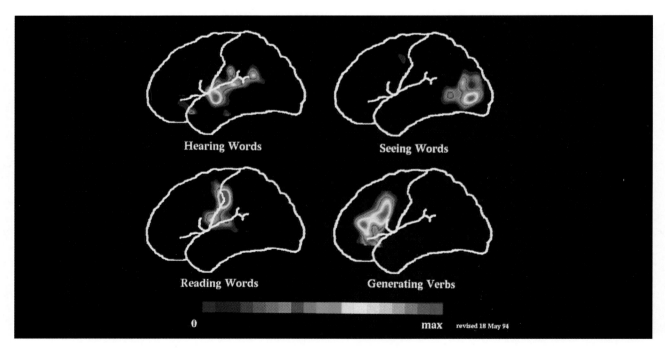

Plate 6 A positron emission tomography (PET) scan showing glucose metabolism during tasks of increasing cognitive or motor complexity. (Courtesy Marcus Raichle, M.D., Mallinckrodt Institute of Radiology, Washington University, St. Louis.)

The practical implications related to kindling are vitally important and bear repetition: clients with mood disorders do best when given effective and aggressive treatment early. It seems that a critical episode of mania or major depression establishes a pathway in the brain that allows other episodes to develop with greater ease. For example, allowing mood disorders to slip out of control because of medication noncompliance increases the risk of a poor course of illness and may subsequently render useless the medication and other interventions that controlled the symptoms initially. Kindling is thought to be responsible for the craving response described by clients addicted to cocaine (Kaplan and Sadock, 1995).

PHYSICAL ASSESSMENT OF THE CLIENT WITH SYMPTOMS OF MENTAL ILLNESS

Assessment of the client includes several basic areas: a complete physical examination and medical history; psychiatric examination, including personal and family history; and laboratory tests.

Physical Examination and Medical History

The physical examination and medical history are essential before treatment begins to rule out any non-psychiatric cause for the presenting symptoms. There are many endocrine abnormalities, neurological conditions, cancers, metabolic derangements, drug use or abuse problems, and infections that can masquerade as mental disorders because they have many symptoms in common. The physical examination, combined with laboratory testing and the client's medical and psychiatric history is used to rule out any causes for the presenting symptoms. If the assessment uncovers a potential source of the symptoms other than a neurobiological one, it should be investigated and, if necessary, treated before considering a psychiatric diagnosis. For example, if a thyroid enlargement is found in a client seeking consultation for depression, it would need full investigation and treatment since hypothyroidism can masquerade as depression.

Box 13-3

Screening Laboratory Tests Included in a Psychiatric Assessment

BLOOD

- Complete blood count (CBC)
- Electrolytes
- Venereal disease experimental laboratory (VDRL)
- Liver function tests
  - Serum glutamic-oxaloacetic transaminase (SGOT)
  - Serum glutamate-pyruvate transaminase (SGPT)
  - Lactate dehydrogenase (LDH)
  - May also include total protein (TP), albumen, globulin, alkaline phosphatase, bilirubin
- Creatinine phosphokinase (CPK)
- Thyroid function tests
  - T3
  - T4
  - TSH

URINE

- Urinalysis
- Urine for pregnancy in women of childbearing age

OTHER

- Purified protein derivative (PPD)
- ECG in adults over age 40
- Drug screening tests

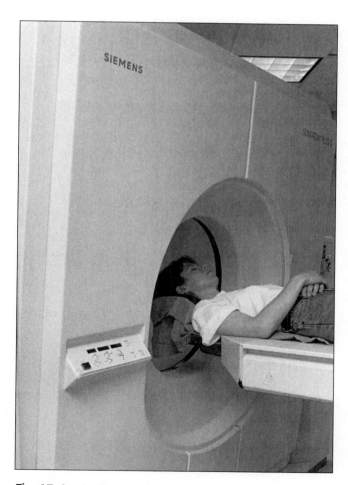

Fig. 13-4   A client undergoing a CAT scan procedure.
© CLG Photographics.

Another important reason for a thorough history and physical examination is to uncover severe stressors such as an automobile accident, rape, recent surgery, substance abuse, or domestic abuse that may be extremely important to understanding the client's current state of mental health.

A complete physical examination and medical history is also essential *before* any somatic treatment is initiated. In an emergency situation in which a client is harmful to self or others, this may be carried out in abbreviated form, but the essentials—blood pressure, temperature, pulse, respirations, baseline laboratory results, general appearance/behavior, heart/lung auscultation, and questions about recent medications/drugs taken—must *always* occur before somatic treatment begins.

In an inpatient hospital setting the history and physical are carried out either before or shortly after admission. In outpatient programs—day hospitals, partial hospitals, clinics, home care—a system for obtaining medical history and physical examination is established so that all new clients are certain to have both.

The physical examination is often embarrassing for clients. Being undressed in the presence of a person who is essentially a stranger, creates a variety of reactions in clients. Some clients may be greatly relieved to be in a place where help is available. For others cultural

TABLE 13-7

Blood and urine studies

TEST AND DESCRIPTION	PROCEDURE	FINDINGS
Dexamethasone Suppression Test (DST); used to diagnose adrenal function	Client is given 1 mg Dexamethasone PO. Blood levels are drawn at different intervals	• In the normal person: Hypothalamus reads plasma cortisol as high. The pituitary stops sending out adrenocorticotropic hormone (ACTH) to adrenal glands. Normal suppression occurs. • Dexamethasone nonsuppression in 50% of clients with depression (these are the people most likely to respond to antidepressants or ECT) DST returns to normal when recovered from depression; therefore useful in monitoring response to treatment
Urinary MHPG levels; measures a metabolite of norepinephrine in the urine	24-hour urine specimen. Dietary restrictions begin the day before: not more than 3 cups of coffee, tea, or cola; no alcoholic beverages, no psychiatric medications for 1 week (especially tricyclic antidepressants)	• Low MHPG tends to respond best to antidepressant drugs that stimulate the norepinephrine system (i.e., Imipramine [Tofranil]) • High MHPG tends to respond better to drugs that affect the serotonin system (i.e., Elavil [amitriptyline HCl] [more difficult to treat]) • Elevated in clients with affective symptoms of schizophrenia
Thyrotropin-releasing hormone (TRH) stimulation test; used to measure thyroid function	Hypothalamus produces TRH. In response, the pituitary secretes TSH. If hypothalamus fails to secrete TRH the result is reduced thyroid function. Procedure: a bolus of TRH-IV is given Blood samples measure TSH at specific intervals	• Normal response: TSH increases two times the baseline in 30 minutes Primary depression: blunted TSH response in majority of clients

TABLE 13-8

Brain imaging procedures

PROCEDURE	DESCRIPTION	USE OF FINDINGS
Electroencephalogram (EEG)	Measures and records on a graph electrical impulses or activity from the cortex of the brain. Computers may be used to enhance images.	Useful in locating tumor sites. Visualizes electrical brain activity. Normal person has short periods of REM sleep throughout night
Rapid eye movement (REM) latency measures	A biological marker for depression	Persons with depression have longer periods of REM sleep and commonly complain of insomnia.
Computerized axial tomography (CAT) Computerized tomography (CT)	Done to obtain computerized x-ray images of intracranial soft tissues and ventricles	Useful in locating brain tumor sites. Ventricular enlargement and cortical atrophy is found in clients with symptoms of schizophrenia. These clients are less responsive to treatment with drugs.
Positron emission tomography (PET)	Involves the use of radioactive substances that emit positive electrons (positrons) while CT scanning is done Provides a metabolic profile (reveals the rate at which tissue consumes biochemicals) (see Color Plate 8)	Shows biochemical abnormalities associated with mental illnesses such as schizophrenia, bipolar disorder, senile dementia, childhood autism, and ADHD (see Color Plate 7) Normal person has hyperfrontal activity. Hypofrontal activity is seen in clients with schizophrenia and autism
Single photon emission computed tomography (SPECT) Regional cerebral blood floor mapping (RCBF) Magnetic resonance imaging (MRI)	A three-dimensional imaging technique involving the detection of gamma photons emitted directly from nuclides Produces images of neurotransmitter activity and deep brain blood flow	Used to identify muscarinic acetylcholine receptors (important in diagnosis of Alzheimer's disease). In the future, it may be used to identify clients who can benefit from antidepressant medications
Regional cerebral blood floor mapping (RCBF)	A specialized scan that involves use of radioactive tracers and shows superficial blood flow regions where blood flow is high, that reflect high level of brain activity and that emit more photons (assigned brighter colors such as shades of red). "Cold" areas have less activity occurring (assigned blues and greens) (see Color Plate 11).	Research with depression has shown a patchy "moth-eaten" appearance with blue-green areas of blood flow; as treatment progresses and metabolic rate improves, perfusion clearly increases.
MRI	Uses an immense electromagnet to detect radio frequencies from the alignment of hydrogen protons in the magnetic field. A computer produces tomographic images of soft tissue and provides a three-dimensional view of the brain structure.	Useful in the early detection of cerebral pathology

influences may be at play or the stress of seeking psychiatric help may cause confusion. The presence of symptoms of mental illness may make the physical examination burdensome. Including the examination as a routine part of assessment and carrying it out as matter-of-factly and as soon as possible after the initiation of assessment is reassuring to clients. The examination is sometimes carried out by the person who will coordinate the client's treatment or sometimes by someone not otherwise involved with the client's care. If it appears that being touched or seen undressed by one's primary caretaker is a major issue for the client, bringing out strong sexual or dependency needs, it may be best to have the physical examination done by a different team member. If that is not possible, carrying out the examination matter-of-factly will be reassuring. Students are referred to a physical assessment text for the format of the physical examination.

Laboratory Tests

Laboratory tests that are routinely carried out in the assessment phase of treatment for mental illness are used to evaluate overall physical health and to rule out a nonpsychiatric cause for the client's presenting symptoms. Although presently, there are no laboratory tests used to specifically diagnose a psychiatric illness, many neurological and endocrine tests are used to make differential diagnoses.

Routine laboratory screening batteries differ from one health care agency to another, but they are likely to include the blood and urine tests listed in Box 13-3. In some settings, urine or blood is analyzed for substances of abuse. Other laboratory tests, electrocardiogram (ECG), x-rays, or pen and pencil assessment tools are used when the medical history or physical examination raise specific questions about the client's health status. Other blood and urine studies commonly used for purposes of differential diagnosis and for determining drug treatment responsiveness are found in Table 13-7 (Pagana and Pagana, 1995).

Brain Imaging

***Brain imaging** uses radiographic and electroencephalogram (EEG) techniques to identify brain structure and function.* Brain imaging techniques used in psychiatry are listed and described in Table 13-8. Much of what has been described about neuroanatomy, neuroregulation, endocrinology, and psychoimmunology earlier in this chapter was discovered through the use of these imaging techniques. Brain imaging is becoming

COMMUNITY RESOURCES

American Psychiatric Association
Division of Public Affairs
1400 K. Street, NW
Washington, DC 20005
1-202-682-6220
The Association publishes a list of brief pamphlets summarizing what is known about specific psychiatric disorders and treatments.

National Alliance for the Mentally Ill (NAMI)
200 North Glebe Road
Suite 1015
Arlington, VA 22203-3754
1-800-950-NAMI or 1-703-524-7600
Members receive quarterly newsletters that summarize recent research in psychiatry. Also has an extensive library of pamphlets, books, posters, videotapes, and audiotapes available to members at low cost on a wide variety of subjects in psychiatry.

Members receive quarterly publications that summarize recent research into the mood disorders. Numerous publications available at low cost to members.

National Institute of Mental Health (NIMH)
Room 7C-02
5600 Fishers Lane
Rockville, MD 20857
1-301-443-4513
NIMH publishes a wide variety of up-to-date summaries of research in psychiatry in the form of pamphlets on specific disorders and treatments.

Pharmaceutical Manufacturers
Many drug companies supply educational materials to practitioners for use in teaching clients about their products. The materials are generally distributed through mental health practitioners and are available on request.

increasingly common despite some risks and discomforts. However, as more emphasis is placed on containment of costs in health care, these tests are likely to be limited to use in clients for whom there is a clear indication. A good example of appropriate use would be the use of a magnetic resonance imaging (MRI) scan or computed tomography (CT) scan for a client whose physical examination shows clear indications of a space occupying lesion in the brain. Fig. 13-4 shows a client having a CAT scan. Color Plate 12 is an MRI of a client with Alzheimer's disease.

The development of positron emission tomography (PET), single photon emission computed tomography (SPECT), and other scanning technology have contributed to the current knowledge explosion about the brain and its functioning in mental illness. In many neuropsychiatric and research settings, scanners are used clinically to aid in differential diagnosis as well as treatment selection (see Color Plates 7, 9, 11, and 13).

Cost-effective ways are being explored to more widely use the technology to predict vulnerability to mental illness, to diagnose specific illnesses when symptoms have already developed, and to evaluate whether recovery has occurred in someone undergoing treatment.

KEY POINTS

- The major parts of the brain are the cerebrum, the diencephalon, the cerebellum, the brain stem, basal ganglia, the limbic system, ventricles, and neurons.
- The CNS, consisting of the brain, spinal cord, and millions of neurons is of greatest interest to mental health care providers and researchers.
- The nervous system interacts with the endocrine and immune systems in numerous ways to maintain behavioral integrity of individuals.
- Many of the major mental illnesses may be caused by a combination of genetic predisposition and environmental stress.
- Stress is a neurobiological response to external and internal threats to equilibrium. A general alarm adaptation (GAS) occurs and consists of alarm, resistance, and exhaustion.
- Research findings indicate basic neurotransmitter dysregulation and structural defects are related to causation of symptoms of schizophrenia, bipolar disorder, depression, and anxiety.
- The mood disorders are characterized by many changes in the rhythmic functions of the body but rhythm disturbances are also evident in almost all psychobiological conditions.
- Brain imaging techniques are used in psychiatric research to confirm and refine psychiatric diagnoses and to measure responses to drug treatments.

 CRITICAL THINKING QUESTIONS

Alex B. grew up in a family with numerous anxiety disorders. His mother had panic attacks and his father took antianxiety agents many times over the years because his cardiologist felt his constant high level of anxiety put him at risk for stroke from his already dangerously high blood pressure. Alex also had aunts, uncles, and cousins who had severe problems with anxiety symptoms. Alex had his first panic attack at the age of 17 while he was watching a high school football game. He had chest pain, dizziness, and difficulty breathing. He thought he was dying and had to be taken to the emergency room (ER) of a nearby hospital. His workup was normal and he was referred to the mental health clinic for an appointment the following week where he too was diagnosed with panic disorder.

1. If the nurse in the ER knows the family history of anxiety disorders, could she safely dispense with the physical examination, knowing that the symptoms are probably anxiety-related? Why or why not?
2. Would it be fair to say that Alex's anxiety disorder is his parents' fault? Does inheriting an illness from a parent or parents mean that the parent(s) are to blame? Explain your answer.
3. Some of Alex's friends think his problem is "in his head." What does that mean? If Alex were your client, how could you help him respond to that comment from his friends?
4. Mr. B's cardiologist felt his high anxiety level put Mr. B at risk for stroke because his blood pressure was already dangerously high. Discuss what the relationship might be between anxiety and blood pressure.
5. If Alex was your client in the mental health clinic, what lifestyle issues might you discuss with him as part of his treatment?
6. Having a mental or psychiatric illness is difficult to accept. Many people mistakenly view a mental illness as a sign of weakness or a moral failure. Do you think knowing there is an inherited, biological basis for panic disorder will help Alex accept having a psychiatric illness more easily? Or do you think it will make him feel even more stigmatized to have a "brain problem?" Explain your answer.
7. Are neurotransmitters or holistic approaches best for the treatment of panic disorders? Explain your answer.

REFERENCES

Goldberger, L., & Breznitz, S. (Eds.). (1993). *The handbook of stress: Theoretical and clinical aspects* (2nd ed.). New York: Macmillan.

Hayes, A. (1995). Psychiatric nursing: What does biology have to do with it? *Archives of Psychiatric Nursing, 9*(4): 216-224.

Herbert, T.B., & Cohen, S. (1993). Stress and immunity in humans: A meta-analytic review, *Psychosomatic Medicine, 55,* 364-379.

Hyman, S.E., & Coyle, J.T. (1994). The Neuroscientific Foundations of Psychiatry. In R.E. Hales, S.C. Yudofsky, & J.A. Talbott (Eds.), *The American psychiatric press textbook of psychiatry* (2nd ed.). Washington, DC: American Psychiatric Press.

Kaplan, H.I., & Sadock, B.J. (Eds.). (1995). *Comprehensive textbook of psychiatry/VI* (6th ed.). Philadelphia: Williams & Wilkins.

Lutgendorf, S.K., Antoni, M.H., Kumar, M., & Schneiderman, N. (1994). Changes in cognitive coping strategies predict EBV-antibody titre change following a stressor disclosure induction. *Journal of Psychosomatic Research, 38*(1):63-78.

McEnany, G. (1996a). Biological perspectives. Part I: Rhythm and blues revisited: Biological rhythm disturbances in depression. *Journal of the American Psychiatric Nurses Association, 2*(1), 15-22.

McEnany, G. (1996b). Psychotherapy and sleep manipulations: An examination of two nondrug biologic interventions for depression. *Journal of the American Psychiatric Nurses Association, 2*(3), 86-93.

McEnany, G. (1990). Psychobiological indices of bipolar mood disorder: Future trends in nursing care. *Archives of Psychiatric Nursing, 6*(1):29-38.

Oldham, J.M., Riba, M.B., & Tasman, A. (Eds.). 1993: *Review of Psychiatry (Vol. 12)*. Washington, DC: American Psychiatric Press.

Pagana, K.D., & Pagana, T.J. (1995): *Diagnostic and laboratory test reference* (2nd ed.). St. Louis: Mosby.

Rabin, B.S., Cohen, S., Ganguli, R., Lyble, D., & Cunnick, J. (1989): Bidirectional interaction between central nervous system and the immune system. *Critical Review in Immunology, 9*(4):279-312.

Rieder, R.O., Kaufmann, C.A., & Knowles, J.A. (1994). Genetics. In R.E. Hales, S.C. Yudofsky, & J.A. Talbott (Eds.), *The American psychiatric press textbook of psychiatry* (2nd ed.). Washington, DC: American Psychiatric Press.

Selye, H. (1991). History and present status of the stress concept. In A. Monat & R.S. Lazarus (Eds.). *Stress and coping* (3rd ed.). New York: Columbia University Press.

Selye, H. (1956). *The Stress of Life.* New York: McGraw-Hill.

U.S. Congress, Office of Technology Assessment. (1992). *The biology of mental disorders.* (Publication No. OTA-BA-538). Washington, DC; U.S. Government Printing Office.

Zalcman, S., Scheller, R. & Tsien, R. (Eds.). (1994). *Molecular neurobiology: proceedings of the second National Institute of Mental Health conference.* Rockville, MD: The Institute.

Chapter 14

Stress Theory and Interventions

Judith Haber

LEARNING OUTCOMES

After studying and applying the concepts of this chapter, the learner will be able to:
- Discuss the impact of stress and stress-related disorders on people's lives.
- Differentiate between the major concepts of the stress theories presented in this chapter.
- Discuss the role of the nurse in managing stress.
- Describe the stress management strategies presented in this chapter.
- Discuss the application of stress management strategies in psychiatric clinical settings.
- Discuss the application of stress management in non-psychiatric clinical settings.
- Analyze the significance of stress management to professional self-care.

KEY TERMS

Assertiveness training	Fight-or-flight response	Progressive relaxation
Autogenic	Hardiness	Self-hypnosis
Bioenergetics	Hassles	Stress
Biofeedback	Hope	Stress management
Cognitive appraisal	Hypnosis	Stressor
Commitments	Mantra	Therapeutic touch
Coping	Meditation	Thought stopping

tress, a buzzword of the 90s, is an everyday fact of life. It is part of being alive; people cannot avoid it! In fact a certain amount of stress is necessary for survival. *Stress refers to a broad group of experiences in which external or internal demands, or both, tax or exceed a person's resources or coping capabilities. The source of the stress, the external or internal demand, is called a **stressor***.

People usually think of stressful events such as illness, injury, or death of a loved one as negative. However, stress can also be positive, challenging us to grow in new ways. For example, buying a new home, graduating from school, or getting a promotion brings with it the stress of change of status and new responsibilities. Falling in love can be just as stressful as falling out of love; yet, too much stress, either acute or chronic, can place excessive demands on a person and interfere with their integrated functioning.

Stress is not located within a person or a particular event, rather it is a person-environment interaction. Therefore questions such as, "What is a stressful life event?" or "How much stress is too much?" are not easily answered. The most appropriate answer is based on each person's definition of the significance of an experience or life event to him or her. Whether a person's stress experience is a result of change related to major life events or the cumulative effects of minor everyday hassles, it is how he or she reacts to stressful experiences that can create a stress response.

More and more twentieth century health problems have been linked with the effects of stress. It is estimated that as many as 75% of all health complaints are stress-related. The list of these disorders is long and growing: ulcers and stomach disorders, migraine and tension headaches, high blood pressure, insomnia, back pain, muscle aches, fatigue, lethargy, and skin disorders to name a few. Research suggests that a significant proportion of stress-related health problems could be prevented by changes in lifestyle. Think about the potential savings in health care costs if stress-related health problems could be reduced. In fact, reduction of stress-related disorders is an objective identified in *Healthy People 2000* (U.S. Department of Health and Human Services [DHHS], 1995) (see Chapters 1 and 18). Industry has also become aware of the costs of stress and the potential savings when employees learn stress management skills. These savings include reduced personnel turnover, alcoholism, absenteeism, lateness, premature employee death or disability, and other symptoms of burnout.

Psychiatric nurses, as well as other health professionals, have a long history of interest in stress and the ways that people functionally or dysfunctionally cope with and manage stress. In particular, the nursing profession has a longstanding commitment to health promotion and preventive intervention. Developing a knowledge base

about stress and the behavioral, cognitive, and holistic mind-body theories that underlie stress management strategies provides a vehicle for working collaboratively with clients to help them achieve their goals to prevent and reduce stress and to achieve maximum well-being and a more rewarding lifestyle.

The purpose of this chapter is to provide a theory base about stress and present an array of stress management strategies that psychiatric nurses can use when working with clients who have a wide variety of biopsychosocial health problems. Since professional self-awareness is a central concept in this textbook, the content presented in this chapter is also appropriate for all readers to consider in understanding, assessing, and effectively managing their own stress responses.

STRESS THEORIES
The Fight-or-Flight Response to Stress

Walter B. Cannon (1963) laid the groundwork for the modern meaning of stress as a psychological problem. A psychologist at Harvard in the early part of the twentieth century, he was the first to describe the ***fight-or-flight response*** as *a series of biochemical changes that prepare people to deal with threats.* Primitive man needed quick bursts of energy to fight or flee such predators as the saber-toothed tiger. A complex part of our brains and bodies called the autonomic nervous system (see Color Plate 4 in Chapter 13), which consists of the sympathetic and parasympathetic nervous systems, prepared prehistoric humans to cope with such threats through either a fight (aggression) or a flight (withdrawal) response. Modern people have the same automatic stress responses that prehistoric humans used for dangerous jungle situations. Consider a more contemporary scenario in which a college student is leaving the library one night at 10 PM and walks down a dark deserted street. A man emerges from the shadow of a building, brandishes a knife and shouts, "Stop, or I'll get you!" Does the student try to defend himself or herself? Does the student run away? There is no right answer. Which action is taken is the result of a variety of physiological responses to extreme danger. The following represents the responses set up by the autonomic nervous system that the learner may recognize from fight-or-flight situations encountered by themselves:

1. Epinephrine, norepinephrine, and cortisol are released into the blood.
2. The liver releases stored sugar into the blood to meet the energy needs for survival.
3. Digestion slows so that blood flow may be redirected from the digestive system to the muscles and brain.

4. Breathing becomes rapid and shallow to supply more oxygen to the needed muscles.
5. The heart rate increases and blood pressure rises.
6. Perspiration increases to cool the body, because increased metabolism generates more heat.
7. Muscles tense in preparation for fight or flight action, particularly the skeletal muscles of the thighs, hips, back, shoulders, arms, jaw, and face.
8. The pupils dilate to let in more light. All of the senses increase their acuity.
9. Blood flow to the extremities is constricted as evident with cold hands and feet. This provides protection from bleeding to death quickly if hands or feet are injured and allows blood flow to be diverted to more important areas of the body.

These physiological responses are appropriate for situations of extreme danger such as those described above. However, imagine the wear and tear on the body if people responded to all stress in these ways.

Psychoneuroimmunology

The knowledge explosion in psychoneuroimmunology has contributed an expanded perspective on Cannon's (1963) theory. The neuroendocrine-immune system's interaction and its response to stress is the body's attempt to cope with its environment (McCain and Smith, 1994). As Cannon suggested, negative emotions such as anxiety and depression, which often accompany stress, may be a primary factor in influencing the immune system (Kiecolt-Glaser and Glaser, 1992). The stress response simultaneously activates the sympathetic-adrenomedullary system, resulting in the release of norepinephrine and epinephrine, and the hypothalamic-pituitary-adrenocortical system, leading to increased release of endogenous opioid peptides (e.g., endorphins), corticotropin, and cortisol (O'Leary, 1990) (see Chapters 10 and 13).

Perhaps the most important link between stress and health problems involves the effects of increased cortisol production on the immune system. Cortisol is primarily an immunosuppressive, resulting in reduction of lymphocyte numbers and function (Bennett, 1996). It is theorized that in the fight-or-flight response to stress, the body shuts down systems that are not immediately necessary to activate this response. Therefore the mechanism designed to suppress immune functioning is a survival mechanism.

However, when stress is persistent, as from the stress of unemployment or poverty, suppression of the immune system is a threat instead. The production of, and subsequent rise in, cortisol inhibits production of cytokines, which normally activate and regulate the production and functioning of lymphocytes. Therefore the rise in cortisol interferes with virtually all components of the immune system (Hayes, 1995). The relationship between stress, altered immune functioning, and the emergence of health problems leads to the belief that preventive intervention, such as stress management, contributes to self-regulation, modulation, control of stress, and reduction in stress-related health problems.

Selye's Stress-Adaptation Theory

Hans Selye, a Canadian endocrinologist, is often referred to as the "father of stress research." His pioneering work provides another framework for understanding how people respond to stress. Selye (1980, 1991) proposes that each person has a limited amount of energy to use in dealing with stress. Factors such as heredity, mental attitude, and lifestyle are among the factors that determine how quickly that energy is used and how quickly one adapts to stress.

Within Selye's (1980) framework, stress is defined as the rate of wear and tear on the body. Selye proposes that it is not just serious illness or injury that causes stress, rather any emotion or activity requires a response or change and, as such, can cause stress. Stressors can be physical, chemical, developmental, or emotional. Playing a game of basketball, walking in a snowstorm without a hat or boots, having an argument, or graduating from school are all examples of stressful events. Basically the demands and challenges of life are stressful, since they involve a process of adaptation to continuous change.

Although the experience of adaptation is stressful, it is not necessarily harmful. Think about exciting, yet stressful life events such as a job promotion or getting married. Indeed these are examples of stressful experiences to which people must adapt that can be exciting and rewarding. Since people cannot avoid the stress associated with living, they must learn to minimize its damaging effects.

Selye (1980, 1991) proposed that although stress itself cannot be perceived, it can be objectively measured by the structural and chemical changes that stress produces in the body. He called these changes *general adaptation syndrome* (*GAS*) because when stress affects the whole person, the whole person must adjust to the changes. GAS has three stages: (1) alarm reaction, (2) resistance, and (3) exhaustion (see Chapter 13).

Stress, Appraisal, and Coping

The cognitive theory of stress proposed by Lazarus and Folkman (1984) provides an interactional approach to understanding stress. Stress is a manifestation of the relationship between the person and the environment, which takes into account characteristics of the person, as well as the nature of the environmental event (Lazarus, 1966, 1976; Lazarus and Folkman, 1984). In this context, stress is defined as a relationship between the person and the environment that is appraised by the person as taxing his or her resources and endangering his or her well-being. Through a process of **cognitive appraisal,** *which refers to evaluative cognitive processes that occur between an event and the reaction to the event,* a person evaluates the significance of an event in relation to his or her well-being. The meaning, intensity, and importance of a stressful event is generated by how the event is perceived, interpreted, and the significance assigned to it by a particular person.

Cognitive appraisal

Cognitive appraisal is a central component of this stress theory. Lazarus and Folkman (1984) believe that cognitive factors play an essential role in adaptation. They affect the impact of stressful events, the choice of coping responses, and the resulting affective, physiological, and behavioral responses to stress exhibited by an individual. Cognitive appraisal mediates between the person and the environment in any stressful encounter to produce a unique interpretation of the event. This means that although certain environmental demands and pressures produce stress in substantial numbers of people, individual and group differences in the degree and type of reaction are always evident.

For example, whereas one person handles an insult by ignoring it, another feels put down, grows angry, and plans revenge. Persons and groups differ based on their sensitivity and vulnerability to certain types of events, as well as in their interpretations and reactions. Damage or potential damage is evaluated according to a person's appraisal of the situation's power to produce benefit or harm, and the coping resources the person has available to neutralize or tolerate the harm. Three types of appraisal used to evaluate stressful events are primary appraisal, secondary appraisal, and reappraisal, all of which are summarized in Table 14-1. Although the three components of primary appraisal, harm/loss, threat, and challenge are summarized separately, they are not necessarily mutually exclusive.

Secondary appraisals of coping options and primary appraisals of "what is at stake" interact with each other in shaping the degree of stress experienced by a person. Even when the stakes are high, the situation is more likely to be appraised as a challenge when a person has a sense of control over the threatening or harm/loss situation. This is because coping options are believed to be available that enable him or her to effectively face or overcome adversity.

When stressful situations are perceived as challenges, the psychological concept of hardiness may be playing a role. **Hardiness** *has been identified as a personality resource that buffers the negative effects of stress.* Persons who demonstrate hardiness are less likely to become ill under stressful situations and are more likely to perceive stressful events, like illness, as opportunities for mastery and growth (Kobasa, 1991; Pollock, 1990; Narsavage and Weaver, 1994). Hardiness appears to be consistent with resistance to stress. Research findings indicate that people high in hardiness exhibit commitment, challenge, and control.

People who are stress-resistant appear to have a specific set of attitudes toward life that includes feeling challenged by a sense of commitment to and involvement in whatever they are doing, and a sense of control over events that are happening to them (Friedman and Vanden Bos, 1992; Jennings and Staggers, 1994). Consider how such differences in cognitive appraisal affect a person's response to stressful events. People who regard stress as a challenge are more likely to perceive events in a positive light and transform them in an advantageous way thereby reducing potential stress.

Commitments and beliefs are among the most important ingredients affecting cognitive appraisal (Lazarus and Folkman, 1984). **Commitments** *express what is important to people and provide the foundation for choices people make. They guide people toward or away from situations that challenge, threaten, harm, or potentially benefit them.* Lazarus and Folkman (1984) propose that commitment is a double-edged sword. On one hand, the greater the strength of a commitment, the more vulnerable the person is to psychological stress in the area of that commitment. On the other hand, the very strength of the commitment that creates vulnerability can also propel a person toward a course of action that can reduce the threat and help sustain coping efforts in the face of obstacles.

Beliefs, such as faith in God, fate, or some natural order in the universe are general beliefs that enable people to create meaning out of life, even out of stressful, damaging experiences, and to maintain **hope** *(a response to a threat that results in the setting of a desired goal)* (Cousins, 1990; Morse and Doberneck, 1995). They determine how people evaluate events that are happening or about to happen. Beliefs about personal control are especially relevant to stress reduction, since they are positively correlated with emotions such as hope, the ability to affect the outcome of a situation, and potential coping ability.

Coping

Perhaps because of its common usage, the term *coping* has varied meaning to different people. **Coping,** as defined by Monat and Lazarus (1991), *refers to a person's efforts to master demands (conditions of harm, threat, or challenge) that are appraised (or perceived) as exceeding or taxing a person's resources.* The purpose of coping is to manage or alter the problem causing distress (problem-focused coping) and regulate emotional responses to the problem (emotional-focused coping).

TABLE 14-1

Types of stress appraisal

TYPE OF APPRAISAL	DEFINITION	EXAMPLE
Primary appraisal	Cognitive appraisal of the extent to which a stressful event is appraised as irrelevant, positive, or stressful. Stress appraisals take three forms:	A person asks, "Am I in trouble or being benefitted, now or in the future, and in what way?"
	1. Harm/loss—damage that has already occurred	A catastrophic illness or injury; loss of a loved or valued person; recognition of damage to self or social esteem (e.g., job loss)
	2. Threat—anticipation of harm or loss that has not yet occurred	After a 5-year cancer remission, a person learns that he has lung lesions and anticipates that his long-term prognosis will be poor; a 24-year-old woman recovering from her first episode of bipolar disorder worries about when the next episode will occur.
	3. Challenge—positively focuses on the potential for gain, growth, or mastery, rather than on possible risks, threats, or losses	Although a person's new job promotion carries risk of being swamped with new demands, the person focuses on the potential for gains in knowledge and skills, responsibility, recognition, and financial reward.
Secondary appraisal	Evaluation of what might and can be done to achieve an effective outcome:	
	1. What coping options are available?	A person is scheduled for a competitive job interview. This person has been out of work for 10 months and has just exhausted his severance and unemployment benefits. Although the threat of rejection is high, the person has the following internal dialogue, "As things stand now, I will probably be rejected. This would be a very damaging outcome because I have no other job prospects. If I handle the job interview effectively, I could be hired. I believe I do have the ability to handle the job effectively. I must think about what would make me an attractive candidate, rehearse, and do imagery and relaxation exercises before the interview to control my nervousness."
	2. What is the likelihood that a particular coping option will accomplish the intended outcome?	
	3. What are the consequences of using a particular coping strategy or set of strategies?	
Reappraisal	A changed appraisal made on the basis of new information from the environment or from the person's own reactions	A woman who was raped 1 month ago was feeling worthless, guilty, and isolated until she decided to attend a rape crisis support group. There she met other women who validated the seriousness of the trauma she had experienced, as well as the legitimacy of her feelings. As she listened to how they learned to cope effectively with this trauma, she began to think that, "Perhaps there was hope after all."

Problem-focused coping strategies include:

1. Defining the problem
2. Generating alternative solutions
3. Weighing the alternatives in terms of their costs and benefits
4. Choosing among the alternatives
5. Acting

Emotion-focused coping strategies are associated with altering the meaning of a situation without changing the objective facts associated with it. These strategies are equivalent to cognitive reappraisal. For example, a person might conclude that, "I have more important things to worry about," or "I don't need him (or her) as much as I thought I did." In each case the threat is decreased by changing the meaning of the situation. Other emotion-focused coping strategies do not change the meaning of an event directly, as do cognitive reappraisals. Rather, the meaning of an event remains the same even though some aspects of it are screened out or put aside temporarily. For example, behavioral strategies such as physical exercise to get one's mind off a problem, listening to music, meditating, or talking to friends can alter a person's emotional response to stress and lead to reappraisal of the situation. Expressing emotions by crying, yelling, or cursing are also examples of emotion-focused coping strategies that some refer to as "venting" or "letting off steam."

Problem-solving and emotion-focused coping are interrelated and can either facilitate or inhibit coping efforts.

EXAMPLE 1: FACILITATION OF COPING EFFORTS

A man who has been unemployed for 1 year is attending a job interview. He is very anxious as he enters the building where the interview will take place. He does some deep breathing and gives himself comforting messages to regulate the anxiety. These strategies allow him to engage in problem-focused forms of coping such as glancing over his resume and rehearsing an opening line or questions that he wants to ask his prospective employer.

EXAMPLE 2: INHIBITION OF COPING EFFORTS

A woman with a recent diagnosis of multiple sclerosis perseveres in acquiring information about her illness. The more information she gathers, the more confused and anxious she feels. She gets trapped in a cycle of problem-focused coping (information gathering and evaluation), which increases her emotional distress and interferes with the "time-out" coping strategies that she might use to reduce her emotional distress, such as physical exercise, talking to a member of the clergy, going to a movie, or going shopping.

Psychiatric nurses need to remember that influences on stress appraisal may vary from culture to culture as may coping resources.

Stressful Life Events

Stressful life events are a group of change stressors that occur in peoples' daily lives. They include catastrophes such as life-threatening health problems or death, but also include a wide array of other events that require a significant change in the ongoing life pattern of a person. Such events occur in school, work, love, marriage, childrearing, employment, finances, social activities, friendships, and health. Some life events can create anxiety, stress, and tension sufficient to affect a person's psychological and physical well-being. The experience of life events arises from an interaction between the person and the situation. The essence of the interaction is reflected in a lack of synchrony between change within the person and change within the environment.

A key assessment question related to evaluating the nature of stressful life events is, "Tell me what has been happening in your life in the past 6 months." The relationship of stressful life events to the cause, onset, course, and outcomes of psychiatric disorders such as schizophrenia, mood disorders, and anxiety disorders has been a focus of considerable research in this area (Miller, 1988, 1989).

Holmes and Rahe (1967) developed the Social Readjustment Rating Scale, which, assigns a value to each of 43 life events on the basis of the adjustment the event requires of the person. Scientists began using this scale to understand and predict susceptibility to illness. Holmes and Rahe (1967), and others multiplied the number of times an event was experienced by the readjustment value given to an event and totaled these products to find a life-change score for each person. Those who had a high life-change score were much more likely to contract an illness after the events. This suggests the importance of both the number and intensity of the events experienced by the person. The illnesses ranged widely from accidents to alcoholism, from cancer to psychiatric disorders, and from influenza to the common cold.

Current trends related to life events as stressors focus on the nature of the event and the magnitude of change it represents. Three approaches to categorizing life events are according to:

1. Social activity involving work; education; family; and educational, interpersonal, financial, health, legal, or community stressors
2. The person's social field, which includes events known as entries and exits. An entrance is the introduction of a new person into the individual's

social field; an exit is the departure of a significant other from an individual's social field

3. Social desirability as defined by the currently shared values of American society. One group of events can be considered socially desirable such as marriage, graduation, and job promotions. Another group can be considered socially undesirable such as death, mental illness, divorce, unemployment, and financial problems

Although life events theory is built on the concepts of change and magnitude of change required to adapt, research indicates that small daily **hassles** *(frustrating or irritating incidents that occur in everyday life)* or minor stresses may be more closely associated with and have a greater effect on a person's mood and health than major life events (Monat and Lazarus, 1991). Getting stuck in a traffic jam, losing a wallet or credit card, arguing with a colleague, and boredom are examples of minor hassles that represent stressful disagreements, disappointments, or unpleasant surprises. Psychiatric clients with severe and persistent mental disorders, reported rising prices of common goods, loneliness, troubling thoughts about the future, and too much time on their hands as the top four hassles that they had to confront (Segal and Vander Voort, 1993).

At this time, it is most appropriate to regard stressful life events on a continuum. At one end of the continuum are stressful life events that represent "triggers," which precipitate physical or mental disorders in predisposed people who would have developed the disorder eventually for one reason or another. At the other end of the continuum, stressful life events contribute a vulnerability factor that reduces or depletes a person's resistance and coping resources, thereby increasing their vulnerability to developing a psychiatric disorder.

THE ROLE OF THE NURSE IN MANAGING STRESS

The promotion of health through the management of symptoms has been suggested as the unique domain of nursing. Preventing and managing the symptoms of stress thereby becomes a central focus of concern for the nursing profession. **Stress management** *is a process of learning how to live with the inevitable life stressors people encounter by learning how to counteract or cope effectively with counterproductive responses to stress through enhanced self-regulation.*

Assessment

Stress assessments can be conducted in primary care settings, such as worksites, schools, primary care, pediatric, and women's health centers. Office visits and annual physicals are prime times for stress risk factor appraisals to be completed during the psychosocial assessment. Health promotion and stress-related illness prevention opportunities present themselves in broad community settings such as health fairs, screenings, home visits, and support and self-help groups. Management of stress begins with assessment of stress and stress risk factors as one component of the comprehensive psychosocial assessment. Examples of self-report instruments (paper and pencil tests) that enable health professionals to assess client stress risk factors and dimensions of stress and related variables are presented in Table 14-2. One specific example of a risk appraisal tool is the Social Readjustment Rating Scale (Holmes and Rahe, 1967).

Physiological assessment of the response to stress is accomplished by measuring the respiratory and heart rate, blood pressure, muscle activity, and skin conductance. The equipment involved may be specialized biofeedback equipment, a multichannel polygraph, or computer-assisted recording equipment. Laboratory tests may be used to test for stress-related physiological parameters such as neurotransmitter functioning and immune system functioning through use of liquid chromatography, or radioimmunoassay to measure indicators such as cortisol, and urine and plasma catecholamines or immune cell activity (Bennett, 1996). Physiological symptoms may also be assessed through direct observation, self-monitoring, and recording of symptoms using tools such as a Stress Awareness Log.

The decision to monitor physiological responses is indicated in situations where the client has identified physiological symptoms as a primary or significant aspect of the presenting problem. Primary care settings are especially appropriate clinical sites for physical assessment of stress. Physiological monitoring of symptoms is useful:

1. To determine whether a specific physiological response does occur in times of stress
2. To create a baseline against which to measure change
3. To make a differential diagnosis
4. To help select appropriate treatment techniques

Clients with physical health problems should receive health clearance before beginning a stress management program. Moreover, clients taking psychotropic medications that cause hypotension should be closely monitored physiologically when doing stress-reduction exercises.

Interventions

Stress-reduction strategies are used to help people gain control of their lives and decrease tension before it becomes unmanageable. As a result, the quality of their

TABLE 14-2

Selected stress assessment tools

ASSESSMENT TOOL	FOCUS	COMPLETED BY
Social Readjustment Rating Scale (Holmes & Rahe, 1967)	A life events scale listing more than 40 major life events, each of which is assigned a value between 11 and 100 life change units. The score has some predictive value in terms of anticipating disease or illness.	Client
Life Events Questionnaire (Pilkonis, Imber, & Rubinsky, 1985)	A 62-event scale assessing a person's appraisal of recently occurring stressful life events. The client is then asked a series of probing questions about his or her subjective response to the identified stressor.	Client and therapist
The Hassles Scale (Kanner et al., 1981)	Consists of a list of 117 irritants ranging from minor annoyances to fairly major stressors. Clients are asked to identify the hassles that have occurred in the last month and rate each one as being somewhat, moderately, or extremely severe. This scale provides an excellent complement to the major life event approach.	Client
Dysfunctional Attitude Scale (Weissman, 1980)	A 40-item scale designed to identify cognitive distortions that may be related to depression. Each item is rated on a seven-point scale, according to the extent to which the client agrees with items measuring seven value systems (love, approval, achievement, perfectionism, entitlement, omnipotence, and autonomy).	Client
Mastery of Stress Instrument (MSI) (Younger, 1993)	An 89-item Likert-type scale that contains a stress scale and four scales reflecting the concepts of mastery: certainty, change, acceptance, and growth.	Client
The Rathus Assertiveness Schedule (Rathus, 1973)	A 30-item scale consisting of statements about assertive behavior. The client is asked to rate each item on a scale from +3 (very characteristic of me) to −3 (very uncharacteristic of me). There is also a simplified version for people with low reading ability.	Client
The Symptom Checklist-90 (Derogatis & Cleary, 1977a, 1977b)	A 90-item list of symptoms that can be subdivided into five dimensions (somatization, obsessive-compulsive, interpersonal sensitivity, depression, anxiety) and rated by the client on a four-point scale. This scale is useful as a general indicator of problem areas, and as measures across time.	Client

lives is improved. As experts in health promotion, illness prevention, and health teaching, psychiatric nurses, as well as nurses in any setting, are perfectly positioned to use stress-reduction strategies to manage their own stress more effectively and collaborate with clients to teach them how to facilitate their own effective use of these techniques. From a physical and mental illness prevention perspective, stress management is recognized as a preventive intervention that potentially benefits every-body in the population (universal preventive intervention) through stress reduction. Stress management programs are also appropriate interventions for people who are above-average (selective preventive interventions) or at high (indicated preventive interventions) risk for the development of particular physical or mental disorders (Mrazek and Haggerty, 1994). For example, people who are known members of defined populations at high risk for hypertension, such as African Americans, would be appropriate candidates for a stress management program designed to increase self-regulation of blood pressure (see Chapter 18).

Stress management strategies are also used by psychiatric nurses who work in acute and rehabilitative treatment settings. In these settings, stress management strategies can be incorporated into nursing care plans or interdisciplinary treatment plans to promote effective symptom management, more effective individual and family coping, increased self-regulation, and/or relapse prevention. For example, stress management strategies such as assertiveness training, progressive relaxation, and refuting irrational beliefs and ideas may be appropriate stress management strategies to incorporate into inpatient or outpatient nursing care plans for a depressed client.

Stress management is not a magical process. The nursing interventions identified in Box 14-1 highlight nursing actions that help clients make a commitment to and follow through with using stress management activities.

STRESS MANAGEMENT STRATEGIES

The use of stress management strategies is based on the belief that mind and body are interrelated. The condition of one will necessarily affect the other. If the body is relaxed, the mind will feel relaxed as well. Many ancient Eastern philosophies provide the basis for the integrality of mind-body-spirit that is central to many contemporary stress management strategies (Chopra, 1987). Once regarded as unorthodox, therapies such as meditation, yoga, visualization, and many other approaches to self-regulation of stress, are increasingly validated as effective healing strategies. Evidence of the growing acceptance of forms of "alternative" health care approaches is the re-

cent establishment of the National Institutes of Health's Office of Alternative Medicine (Carton, 1995). Moreover, many insurance and managed care companies are beginning to reimburse health care providers for alternative health care services.

Behavioral and cognitive theories also provide a foundation for many stress management strategies. This reflects the belief of behavioral theorists in the ability of people to unlearn dysfunctional coping behaviors and learn new, more effective strategies and behaviors that reduce stress. It also reflects the perspective of cognitive theorists, which proposes that people's values, beliefs, and assumptions can be changed through cognitive restructuring, leading to reappraisal of stressful situations. Many stress management strategies are based on cognitive restructuring principles the outcome of which is a more realistic appraisal of thoughts, feelings, behaviors, and events. This increases effective coping and reduces stress. These perspectives combine to empower people, whether clients or professionals, to regulate and effectively manage the inevitable stress that accompanies modern life.

The stress management strategies presented below provide a variety of holistic, behavioral, and cognitive approaches that teach people how to reduce stress and thereby feel less tense, anxious, and more relaxed and effective. These strategies will enhance the personal and professional lives of nurses and can be taught to clients and their families in any health care setting.

Stress Awareness Log

Most people are more aware of the weather, what is playing in the movies, or their checkbook balance than they are of stress or tension in their own body. Recognizing stress through body awareness that locates where and

Box 14-1

Nursing Interventions That Promote Commitment to Stress Management Activities

- Incorporate stress management activities as a component of therapeutic staff and client programming
- Recommend stress-reduction activities to clients and their families
- Provide information about stress-reduction strategies that are consistent with a client's specific needs
- Teach stress reduction techniques to clients and/or their families. Explain the physiological rationale for these techniques
- Refer clients to community resources designed to promote effective management of stress (eg., self-help groups, health clubs, leisure organizations, book stores, libraries) and as listed in the Community Resources box on p. 250.

- Encourage clients to practice stress reduction strategies
- Reinforce the importance of self-care and devoting this time to themselves alone
- Enlist the support of family members, colleagues, and friends in meeting the client's need for uninterrupted time in a quiet setting
- Remind family members and colleagues to positively reinforce the client's stress-reduction efforts
- Schedule stress-reduction self-care activities for staff on a periodic basis

how your body stores tension is the first step in reducing stress (Cotton, 1990). Documenting stress awareness can be done effectively by keeping a Stress Awareness Log.

Some parts of the day are more stressful than others, and some stressful events are more likely to produce emotional or physical symptoms than others. It is useful for people to become aware of and identify those symptoms that are characteristic of their response to stress. For example, when stressed, Joan H. would experience painful muscle tension in her neck and left shoulder. In contrast, her sister, Diane K. got tension headaches, and another sister Bonnie P. had stomach tension associated with bouts of diarrhea. Certain types of events often produce characteristic symptoms.

A Stress Awareness Log helps people identify how particular stressful events result in particular physical and emotional symptoms by listing the particular stressful event, when it occurred, and the symptoms associated with the event. Clients should be encouraged to keep a Stress Awareness Log for 2 weeks, tracking the data daily to discover patterns that characterize their unique stress responses. They should note the time of day a stressful event occurred, document the type of stressful event and the time and description of the physical and/or emotional symptom that could be related to the stressful event. Once characteristic stress response patterns are identified in the Stress Awareness Log, appropriate stress reduction strategies are systematically applied.

Deep Breathing Exercises

Breathing is a body function that most people take for granted. It is only in recent years that people in Western cultures have become aware of the importance of correct breathing habits. For centuries, breathing exercises have been an integral part of mental, physical, and spiritual development in Asia and India. Breathing properly can reduce stress and pain. Maternity nurses, for example, who prepare women for childbirth in Lamaze classes have long recognized the importance of breathing exercises in reducing tension and discomfort associated with labor. Nurses who are pain management specialists also recognize the importance of breathing exercises in reducing pain. Many psychiatric nurses are beginning to incorporate breathing exercises in their practice as one of many available stress-reduction strategies.

The physiological benefit of deep breathing is derived from the fact that breathing calmly and deeply keeps the blood well-oxygenated and purified. Poorly oxygenated blood contributes to fatigue, lethargy, anxiety, muscular tension, mental confusion, and feelings of depression. Deep breathing is a valuable tool in preventing or alleviating these symptoms.

Although deep breathing exercises can be learned in a few minutes, and some immediate benefits are experienced, the true impact of this exercise may not be experienced until after several weeks or months of persistent practice. In fact deep breathing becomes easier with practice. Over time it may become automatic. It can be done any place, it is inconspicuous, and it gives fast results. For example, John M. had a project deadline that was rapidly approaching. Each time he looked at the clock, he noticed his tension level rising and his breathing was shallower and faster. He decided he needed a quick self-intervention to reduce his stress level. He closed the door to his office, sat back in his chair, closed his eyes, and did ten minutes of deep breathing. After 10 minutes, his breathing had slowed, he felt calmer, refreshed, and ready to get back to work with renewed energy. Psychiatric nurses can use the following guidelines to teach deep breathing to themselves or clients:

1. Stand, sit, or lie down. Lying down on the floor on a rug, mat, or blanket is the best position for performing deep breathing exercises. Make sure your spine is straight. Bend your knees and move your feet about 8 inches apart, with your toes turned outward slightly.
2. Scan your body for tension.
3. Place one hand on your abdomen and the other on your chest.
4. Inhale slowly and deeply through your nose into your abdomen to push up your hand as much as feels comfortable. Your chest should move only a little and only with your abdomen.
5. Exhale through your mouth, making a soft whooshing sound, like the wind, by blowing out gently. Keep your face, mouth, and jaw relaxed.
6. Take long, slow deep breaths that raise and lower your abdomen. Focus on the sound and feeling of breathing as you become more and more relaxed.
7. Continue deep breathing for 10 minutes at a time, once or twice a day. Once you have mastered the technique, you may want to extend this exercise to 20 minutes each time.
8. At the end of each deep breathing session, take a few minutes to scan your body for tension. Compare the tension you feel at the end of the exercise with that which you experienced when you began.
9. When you have learned to relax yourself using deep breathing, practice it whenever you feel yourself getting tense.

Visualization

People's imagination can be a powerful tool for reducing stress. Use of the imagination through visualization and imagery are not new therapeutic tools. Around the turn of the century, Emil Coué, a French pharmacist, popular-

Box 14-2

Guidelines for Effective Visualization

1. Loosen your clothing and make sure your breathing is not restricted. Lie down or sit in a comfortable, quiet place. Make sure your back is supported.

2. Close your eyes and take a full, deep breath. Exhale slowly and easily. Take a second deep breath and, again, exhale slowly. As you do, feel yourself floating down. Concentrate on your breathing . . . allow your breathing to become slow and rhythmic. Notice your heart beating strongly, but slowly.

3. Imagine that with each and every breath, you can breathe away tension and anxiety, as you allow yourself to relax more and more.

4. Let your thoughts drift through your consciousness, as you allow them to leave, floating on a white puffy cloud.

5. Form mental sense impressions that involve all of your senses and create a special place that you will be making a retreat for relaxation and guidance. The following cloud imagery provides an example:

   The sky is completely clear, except for one small, fluffy cloud that drifts alone in the gentle breeze until it is directly over you. Slowly this little cloud sinks down on you . . . it is a pleasant, delightful feeling. As the small, fluffy cloud moves across your face, you feel the cool, moist touch of it on your forehead and your cheeks. As it moves down your body, all tension slowly slips away and you find yourself letting go completely.

   The soft cloud moves across your shoulders, chest, and upper back, then across your arms as it gently brings with it a feeling of complete relaxation. It sinks down around your hips and legs, and it moves around you, surrounding you in a deep feeling of relaxation. The little cloud then sinks underneath you and you are now floating on it. The cloud gently cradles you in the sun's golden rays.

   Your body feels weightless as it drifts above the treetops. The tension has drained out of your body, arms, legs, shoulders, and neck. You no longer feel the weight of your head on your shoulders and gravity no longer ties you to the earth. The fluffy cloud supports you and the sun's gentle heat penetrates through any remaining tension.

   The little cloud begins to drift downwind, and from your safe position on the cloud, you can see the world going by below you. There is a gentle, pleasant rocking motion as you drift along. All of your cares and concerns are left behind. Whenever you are ready you may return to earth. Take a few deep breaths, becoming more aware of your surroundings as you float toward earth on your fluffy cloud. When you are ready to become fully alert, take a full deep breath and gently open your eyes as you exhale, gently resting as you feel the relaxation floating through your body.

6. Visualize one to three times a day. Visualization practice is easiest in the morning and night when lying in bed. After practice and becoming proficient, you will be able to visualize while waiting for a job interview, at the gas station, or waiting for an examination. Visualization can be combined with relaxing background music and relaxation exercises as well.

---

ized the power of positive thinking in the treatment of physical symptoms. He believed that people's thoughts become reality. If people think anxious thoughts, they become tense. Coué (1922) proposed that people can overcome anxious feelings and related tension by refocusing the mind on positive healing images. Today, Simonton and Mathews (1980) and Siegal (1986) have pioneered the use of visualization with cancer patients.

All persons engage in visualization. Daydreams, memories, and inner talk are all types of visualization. People have the ability to systematically use their visualizations and consciously apply them to train their bodies to control upsetting thoughts, achieve deep physical relaxation, and ignore stress. Positive visualizations take advantage of a person's own imagination and positive thinking to reduce stress and promote healing. Positive visualizations, which anticipate success, reduce stress. Visualization can be used in combination with deep breathing and relaxation exercises. Developing your own or working with a mental health professional to construct an effective visualization often takes time, patience, and persistence. Think about how many client populations, other than psychiatric clients, would benefit from positive visualization.

Guided visualization (imagery)

Achieving relaxation through visualization is facilitated by creating a relaxing environment in one's mind through the use of imagery. People create images complete with sights, sounds, smells, tastes, and feelings. Others visualize special scenes in detail, but omit crucial elements, waiting for their subconscious or inner guide to supply the missing pieces of their puzzle. Some people find the sounds of the seashore soothing and create a visualization about the rocky Pacific coast or a tropical island. Others imagine themselves floating above the world on a soft, white cloud or racing down a ski slope. Still others picture themselves emerging from a cool forest into a meadow of wildflowers located beside a babbling brook with a blue cloudless sky overhead. Guidelines for effective visualization appear in Box 14-2.

Progressive Relaxation

First described in 1929 by a Chicago physician, Edmund Jacobson, in his book *Progressive Relaxation*, ***progressive relaxation*** *is a deep muscle relaxation technique based on the premise that the body reponds to stressful, anxiety-provoking thoughts and events with muscle*

 COMMUNITY RESOURCES

SELF-HELP GROUPS

Alcoholics Anonymous
468 Park Avenue
New York, NY 10016

Association for Applied Psychophysiology and Biofeedback
10200 West 44th Avenue, Suite 304
Wheat Ridge, CO 80033

Divorce Anonymous
P.O. Box 5313
Chicago, IL 60680

Golden Ring Council of Senior Citizen Clubs
c/o ILGWU
1710 Broadway
New York, NY 10019

Make Today Count
514 Tama Building
Box 303
Burlington, IA 52601

Mended Hearts
721 Huntington Avenue
Boston, MA 02115

Recovery, Inc.
The Association of Nervous and Former Mental Patients
116 South Michigan Avenue
Chicago, IL 60603

Volunteers of America
340 West 85th Street
New York, NY 10024

RELAXATION TAPES

Stress Management Research Associates, Inc.
Family Relaxation and Self-Control Program
Relaxation and Stress Management Program
P.O. Box 2232-B
Houston, TX 77251

Progressive Relaxation and Breathing
New Harbinger Publications
Oakland, CA

Ten Minutes to Relax
Vital Body Marketing Company
Manhasset, NY

MUSIC

Environmental Sounds
Environments, *The Psychologically Ultimate Seashore*, Atlantic
Environments 2, *Dawn at New Hope, Pennsylvania*, Atlantic
Environments 8, *A Country Stream*, Atlantic

Meditative Listening Experiences
Paul Horn, *Inside (The Taj Mahal)*, Epic Records
Paul Horn, *Inside 2*, Epic Records
Tony Scott, *Music for Zen Meditation*, Verve Records
Tony Scott, *Tibetan Bells*, Verve Records
Walter Carlos, *The Four Seasons*, Verve Records

BOOKS

Cotton, D.H.G. (1990). *Stress management: An integrated approach to therapy.* New York: Brunner/Mazel.

Cousins, N. (1981). *Anatomy of an illness.* New York: Bantam Books.

Davis, M., Eshelman, M., & McKay, M. (1995). *The relaxation and stress reduction workbook* (4th ed.). Oakland, CA: New Harbinger.

Metcalf, C.W., & Felible, R. (1992). *Lighten up: Survival skills for people under pressure.* New York: Addison-Wesley.

tension. The physical tension, in turn, increases the subjective experience of anxiety. Deep muscle relaxation reduces physiological tension and is incompatible with anxiety. Progressive relaxation shifts people from a state of sympathetic nervous system arousal to a state of parasympathetic recuperation. Thus it decreases pulse, respiration, blood pressure, perspiration, and other physiological and psychosocial manifestations of stress. Clients with tension headaches, insomnia, lower back pain, muscle spasms, fatigue, irritable bowel syndrome, anxiety, depression, or mild phobias, are among those who can benefit from using this technique. Relaxation tapes that lead people through progressive relaxation exercises are available as listed in the Community Resources box on p. 250. Sometimes clinicians who specialize in stress management make individualized relaxation and imagery tapes for clients.

Most people do not realize which of their muscles are chronically tense. Progressive relaxation provides a way of identifying particular muscles or muscle groups and distinguishing between sensations of tension (purposeful muscle tensing) and deep relaxation (conscious relaxation of the muscles). Each muscle or muscle grouping is tensed for 5 to 7 seconds and then relaxed for 20 to 30 seconds. The cycle is then repeated until all muscle groups have gone through the relaxation process. The four major muscle groups included in the process are:

1. Hands, forearms, and biceps
2. Head, face, throat, and shoulders
3. Chest, stomach, and lower back
4. Thighs, buttocks, calves, and feet

Clients should be taught to practice progressive relaxation lying down or when seated in a chair, with all body parts comfortably supported. Calming background music such as the suggestions provided in the Community Resources box on p. 250 often enhances the relaxing experience of performing these exercises. An example of a psychiatric nurse teaching a client progressive relaxation is illustrated in the Teaching Points box on p. 252.

Meditation

Meditation has been associated with many Eastern religions for thousands of years. People who have practiced meditation believe that it provides a way of becoming one with God or the universe and finding inner peace, enlightenment, and social consciousness (Chopra, 1987; LeShan, 1974). Since *meditation is a way of uncritically focusing attention on one thing at a time,* it does not have to be associated with a religion or philosophy for people to practice this tradition. Today, it is as common for meditation to be practiced as a means of reducing stress and inner discord and increasing inner harmony and self-knowledge by suspending external vigilance and attending to sensations occurring in the moment.

A meditative state is equivalent to a state of deep rest. Electroencephalogram (EEG) tracings reveal alpha waves that characterize brain activity during relaxation. The heart and breathing rates slow down, oxygen consumption falls by 20%, and blood lactate levels, which rise with stress and fatigue, drop. It is not surprising that meditation has been effective in the treatment and prevention of insomnia, high blood pressure, strokes, migraine headaches, and autoimmune diseases such as diabetes and arthritis. It has also helped people decrease their use of drugs, alcohol, and nicotine and cope more effectively with their obsessive thinking, depression, anxiety, and hostility.

Meditation exercises are relatively easy to learn. Sometimes people experience the effect of meditation after several sessions. They feel relief from whatever emotional pain they have been experiencing. This makes sense because meditation involves attempting to focus on one object to the exclusion of others, rather than the constant ability to focus on a single thought. When meditators realize that their mind has drifted to other thoughts, they choose instead to dwell on the original object of their attention. In so doing, they realize that it is impossible to worry, fear, or hate when one's mind is thinking about something other than the object of these emotions.

Four ingredients necessary for meditation are (1) a relatively quiet environment, (2) a comfortable position, (3) a passive attitude, and (4) an object or thought on which to dwell.

- The environment should be peaceful and set aside from the hustle and bustle of everyday life.
- When choosing a comfortable position for meditating, it should be one that can be maintained for 20 minutes or longer. The traditional yoga lotus position or sitting back Japanese-fashion on one's heels are common meditation positions.
- People need to develop a passive attitude, which requires understanding that thoughts and distractions will occur and can be cleared from the mind. Thoughts and emotions are not permanent. They pass into and out of peoples' bodies and minds. They need not leave a trace.
- Most people who meditate choose an object or thought to dwell on that is called a *mantra. This is an object, a syllable, word, or name that is thought about and repeatedly chanted aloud, but not too loudly.* In fact, after about 5 minutes people shift to whispering the mantra or chanting silently as they relax more deeply. Some meditation teachers believe that the mantra chosen by a person

Progressive Relaxation Exercise

- Sit or lie down in a comfortable position, close your eyes, and take five deep breaths.
- Focus your attention on your right hand and make a fist.
- Study the tension in your fist, hand, and forearm as you clench it tighter and tighter.
- Now let go and feel the difference.
- Bend your elbow and tense your biceps, observe the feeling of tautness.
- Now let go and feel the difference.
- Repeat this procedure with your left hand and arm.
- Now focus your attention on your head; pay attention to the muscles of your forehead.
- Frown and study the tension as you frown as the strain spreads across your forehead.
- Let go of the tension and allow your forehead to become smooth again; notice the difference.
- Raise your eyebrows and hold them for a few seconds.
- Now let go.
- Tense and tighten the muscles around your eyes and cheeks.
- Now let go.
- Now clench your jaw and bite hard; notice the tension throughout your jaw.
- Relax your jaw. When your jaw is relaxed, your lips will be slightly parted.
- Let yourself appreciate the contrast between tension and relaxation.
- Now tighten the muscles in the back of your neck, feel the tension.
- Now let it go.
- Pull your shoulders back and up and tighten the muscles between your shoulders.
- Tighten and notice the tension.
- Drop your shoulders and feel relaxation spreading through your neck, throat, and shoulders—pure relaxation, deeper and deeper.

- Now tighten the muscles of your upper back.
- Tighten and let go.
- Focus your attention on tightening the muscles of your lower back. Arch your back as you tighten your muscles.
- Notice the tension and let go. Press your back into the bed, floor, or chair.
- Now tighten the muscles of your stomach and hold.
- Place your hand on your stomach. Breathe deeply into your stomach, pushing your hand up.
- Hold and then let go. Feel the contrast of relaxation as the air rushes out.
- Tighten the muscles of your buttocks. Tighten and feel the tension.
- Now let go.
- Tighten your thighs.
- Let go, noticing the difference.
- Now tense the muscles of your calves and lower legs.
- Tense them tighter and notice the difference, now let go.
- Pay attention to tensing the muscles of your feet including your toes. Point your ankle toward your knee and crunch your toes.
- Let your feet and toes relax and notice the difference.
- Lie still with your eyes closed for a few minutes. Your body should feel relaxed and loose, yet heavy.
- Now take a few moments to scan your body to notice any part of your body that feels tense and needs relaxation.
- Tense that muscle and let it go.
- Allow yourself to feel the pleasure of this relaxed feeling for a few minutes. When you are ready to bring your attention back to the present, filled with renewed energy and peace, open your eyes, stretch, and get up.

should have a special meaning, vibration, or sound to create an individual effect.

In most cases, people can learn to meditate within a few minutes. However, the best results are achieved by people who meditate 15 to 20 minutes each day for 2 to 3 weeks. As with other stress management strategies, the benefits of meditation increase with practice. People often lengthen their meditation sessions to 30 minutes. Levels of relaxation deepen; attention becomes more

steady. People become more skillful at living in the present moment and they feel more tranquil.

Yoga

Yoga, which includes meditative components, appears to have been practiced as early as 3000 BC. The practice of yoga meditation allows people to strive for the achievement of their full potential. Similar to other meditative practices, the focus of yoga is preventive rather than curative. In the most general sense, yoga is not a set of exercises, but a way of life. Eastern philosophers describe yoga as "a science by which the individual approaches truth . . . and transcends problems and suffering" (Vishnudevananda, 1960).

There are various forms of yoga practice. Hatha yoga, most familiar to people in western cultures, focuses on the physical body and progresses in stages. First is the training of the physical body itself through purification and postures that are, in effect, physical exercises that emphasize slow continual stretching movements. The difference between yogic exercises and regular physical exercise is that the latter emphasizes strenuous movements of the muscles, whereas yogic exercises focus on gradual development of elasticity, improved circulation, and mobilization of joints. The exercises are isotonic, so that contraction of one group of muscles is accompanied by relaxation or stretching of opposite muscle groups. A typical yoga exercise session involves a series of well-defined postures that focus on different parts of the body in sequence so that a balanced and comprehensive state of fitness is achieved. A session would end with a period of directed physical relaxation.

The second stage focuses on the spirit and involves controlled breathing, stilling the mind, and mental control. The third step involves meditation. Once the muscles are relaxed, the second and third stages are initiated. Breathing becomes the target of self-regulation. The person then begins a stage of sensory withdrawal and meditatively begins to narrow the focus of attention. The eventual object of focus or contemplation is a matter of personal choice, a sound or word (mantra), a flower, a candle flame, or a cloud may be selected. The final stage of yogic meditation emanates from this narrowing of awareness. The mind is said to transcend an ordinary plane of awareness. Beginners will not attain this final meditative state, this takes commitment, time, and practice. However, the earlier state of contemplation is proposed to be sufficient to restore energy and health in most people (Cotton, 1990). Unless a clinician is a yoga practitioner of the yoga philosophy in his or her own life, a referral to a yoga practitioner or program is appropriate.

Therapeutic Touch

Therapeutic touch or "laying on of hands" is an ancient tradition. Religious writings, mythology, and oral traditions of primitive tribes provide many descriptions. *Therapeutic touch is a conscious and deliberate act of voluntary, therapeutic transfer of energy from the healer to the client. Excess energy from the healer is directed to the client or energy is transferred from one place to another within the client's body.* Therapeutic touch is based on the idea that illness is a manifestation

of an imbalance of energies in the body. Krieger (1979) and MacRae (1992) propose that *prana* is the subsystem of energy that is the basis of the energy transfer in therapeutic touch. Healthy people are thought to have an excess of prana, which as a manifestation of open systems energy, can be transferred to another person. The transfer of energy is not a cure for illness. However, it provides an infusion of energy for people whose energy has been depleted by illness and helps them until their own healing powers take over. Therapeutic touch appears to be a manifestation of patterning in mutual process. Clients report feeling more relaxed and experience relief from pain following therapeutic touch. Krieger (1979) has demonstrated a significant change in the hemoglobin component of blood following therapeutic touch. However, empirical support for the efficacy of therapeutic touch is tentative at this time.

Exercise

Regular exercise has both physiological and psychological benefits. Advantages that have been associated with exercise include improved concentration, more energy, lowered risk for heart attacks, firmer appearance, reduced anxiety and hostility, elevated mood, improved immune response, and restful sleep. Exercise releases muscle tension and general physical arousal generated by the stress response. Rather than fighting or fleeing, a person can hit a punching bag, jog around the track, lift weights, use exercise machines such as a treadmill, Nordic Track or stairmaster, or attend an aerobics class. Instead of getting angry and shouting or depressed and pouting, exercise has both a tranquilizing and mood elevating effect. The release of tranquilizing endorphins and mood elevating serotonin and norepinephrine neurotransmitters during exercise results in more relaxed and optimistic persons. Exercise also clears the mind. For example, at the end of a work day it is not uncommon for people to feel that their mind is so cluttered by the events of the day that they cannot concentrate. Problems may seem impossible to solve. This is an excellent time to go for a walk, a swim, or work out. People who exercise report that time away from working diligently on a problem gives them a chance to work through everything in a more relaxed way.

When people are in good physical condition their self-image improves. They also have a greater capacity to resist stress. Physiologists have shown that regular exercise will improve endurance, reduce total peripheral resistance in blood circulation, lower blood pressure, lower cholesterol, raise the high-density lipids, and improve lung capacity, immune system functioning and muscular strength. The recommended frequency of exercise is three times per week for 35 minutes each time. For people who have not been exercising regularly, health clearance should be obtained by having a complete physical.

An exercise specialist should be consulted for an exercise prescription that systematically increases the person's exercise endurance. Clients taking psychotropic medications that cause hypotension should be closely monitored when they do stress-reduction exercise.

Self-Hypnosis

Hypnosis involves a process of achieving relaxation through narrowing of consciousness, suggestion, and attainment of a trance state. A clinician skilled in hypnosis guides a person in attaining the hypnotic trance. *Self-hypnosis, as the term suggests, is a process by which a person learns to hypnotize him or herself.* People practice self-hypnosis to achieve relaxation, to make positive suggestions for change, and to uncover forgotten events that continue to influence people's lives (Fisher, 1991). For example, self-hypnosis can be used to accomplish goals such as weight loss, smoking cessation, pain relief, and overcoming insomnia or irrational fears. Every hypnotic trance includes the following elements:

1. A reduction of muscular activity and energy output and accompanying relaxation
2. Limb catalepsy that manifests itself as muscular limb rigidity with a tendency for them to remain in any position in which they are placed; it is sometimes referred to as the "lead pipe" effect.
3. Narrowing of attention
4. Increased suggestibility

Examples of problems people experience and hypnotic suggestions that can be used to overcome them are presented in Table 14-3.

Self-hypnosis is effective in alleviating chronic fatigue, insomnia, chronic muscle tension, headaches, mild-to-moderate pain, tics and tremors, and low-to-moderate anxiety. It is a stress management strategy that can be learned quickly; most people can achieve significant relaxation in 2 days. Self-hypnosis can be self-taught through books on the subject (see the Community Resources box on p. 250). Adult education programs, wellness or holistic health centers, or hypnosis practitioners often offer courses on self-hypnosis. Self-hypnosis is a safe stress management strategy. There are no reported cases of harm resulting from self-hypnosis, even for the most inexperienced practitioners (Davis, Eshelman, and McKay, 1995).

Autogenic Training

Autogenic training (AT) is a systematic program that has its roots in hypnosis and yoga. This stress-reduction program will teach the mind and body to respond quickly and effectively to a person's verbal commands to relax and return to a balanced, normal state. The term *autogenic means self-regulation.* The principle of AT is that stress upsets the normal homeostatic balance in the body and that relaxation achieved through autogenic methods allows the body to regain the disrupted balance. In essence, AT teaches people self-regulation of the autonomic nervous system (Cotton, 1990).

Autogenic training focuses on reversing the fight-or-flight response described earlier in this chapter through achievement of six physiological outcomes:

1. Heaviness in the extremities to reduce muscular tension
2. Warmth in the extremities to induce vasodilation
3. Normalizing cardiac activity through regulation of heartbeat

TABLE 14-3

Self-hypnosis: physical and psychosocial problems and associated hypnotic suggestions

PROBLEM	HYPNOTIC SUGGESTION
Insomnia	I will gradually feel more and more drowsy. My limbs and body will feel heavy. In a few minutes, I will be able to fall asleep and sleep peacefully all night.
Chronic back pain	As I become more and more relaxed, my backache decreases. In just a few minutes, the muscles in my back will start to loosen. In an hour, they will be completely relaxed. I will feel calm and peaceful. Whenever the pain comes back, I will twist my watch a half turn to the left and my back pain will relax away again.
Low self-esteem	When I see (NAME OF PERSON) the next time, I will feel secure about myself. I can feel relaxed and at ease because I am a competent person.
Test anxiety	Whenever I feel nervous before taking a test, I can say to myself (INSERT OWN SPECIAL WORD OR PHRASE) and relax.

4. Normalizing respiratory function through regulation of breathing
5. Relaxing and warming the abdominal region
6. Cooling the forehead by reducing blood flow to the head

Autogenic exercises facilitate achievement of these outcomes. For example, to bring about warmth in the extremities through peripheral vasodilation, a person would be instructed to say, "My right hand is warm." The smooth muscles that control the diameter of the blood vessels in the right hand relax so that more warming blood flows into that hand. This helps reverse the pooling of blood in the trunk and head that is characteristic of the fight-or-flight response to stress. The person then goes on to say, "My left arm is heavy; both of my arms are heavy." several times a day. Gradually, the legs are also included, until feelings of heaviness can be induced at will. The person sequentially proceeds through the remaining six AT exercises.

Autogenic exercises are initiated by assuming a comfortable position and repeating the appropriate autogenic phrase to himself or herself, initially for 2 or 3 minutes, several times a day. These periods of practice gradually evolve into two periods of 30 minutes twice daily. In each of the six exercises the content of previous sessions is included and built on. Thus the person who has reached Exercise 4 will quickly induce heaviness and warmth in the extremities and will regulate his or her heartbeat before working on the regulation of the respiratory system (Cotton, 1990).

Autogenic training has been found to be effective in treatment of respiratory disorders (hyperventilation, bronchial asthma), gastrointestinal disorders (constipation, diarrhea, gastritis, ulcers), circulatory disorders (high blood pressure, irregular heart beat, palpitations, cold extremities, headache), and disorders of the endocrine system (some thyroid problems). It has also been demonstrated to be effective in modifying a person's response to pain and reducing anxiety, irritability, insomnia, and fatigue. Autogenic training is not recommended for children under 5 years of age or people with psychotic disorders. People who have chronic physical health problems such as diabetes or heart conditions should be under the care of an appropriate health care provider while in AT.

Thought Stopping

Thought stopping is a behavioral therapy strategy that is particularly effective in helping people who have obsessive thoughts or phobic avoidance of objects or situations. Since it is commonly accepted that negative and frightening thoughts usually precede negative and frightening emotions, if the thoughts can be controlled, over-

all stress levels can be significantly reduced (Davis, Eshelman, and McKay, 1995). *Thought stopping involves concentrating on unwanted thoughts and, after a short time, suddenly stopping and emptying one's mind.* Commands such as "STOP," a loud noise, or a distractor such as snapping a rubber band worn on the wrist or pinching oneself are used to interrupt repetitive or unpleasant thoughts. This approach is based on behavioral principles that explain the effectiveness of thought stopping:

1. The command "STOP" serves as a negative reinforcement. Behavior that is consistently punished through negative reinforcement is likely to decrease.
2. The command "STOP" serves as a distractor.
3. Thought stopping is an assertive response to an intrusive thought or feeling and followed by thought substitution of reassuring or self-accepting statements.

To illustrate thought stopping, consider a man whose wife initiated divorce proceedings. Her major complaint was that he was domineering, controlling, and smothered her with numerous phone calls each day to determine her whereabouts and make sure she had finished the list of chores he asked her to complete. During their separation, he obsessively worried about her and the children, becoming tense each time this thought crossed his mind and called his wife at least 20 times per day to alleviate his worry. Using thought-stopping techniques, he snapped a rubber band worn on his wrist to distract him from focusing on his repetitive thought each time it occurred. Snapping the rubber band also interrupted his obsessive thought about calling his wife and could be followed by a positive thought substitution such as "I'm lucky to have a competent wife and kids."

Thought-stopping techniques are most effective when they are practiced conscientiously throughout the day for 3 days to 1 week. At first the thought may return, but with practice it returns less often and in many cases, disappears completely.

Assertiveness

Assertiveness training is a behavioral strategy for reducing stress by teaching people to express personal rights and feelings. It is usually offered as a brief therapy or educational program in a community setting. Lazarus (1966) and Wolpe (1958) found that nearly all people could be assertive in some situations and yet be totally ineffective in others. The goal of assertiveness training is to increase the number and variety of situations in which assertive, rather than passive or aggressive, behavior is exhibited.

People who display relatively passive behavior do not

TABLE 14-4

Mistaken assumptions and legitimate rights

MISTAKEN ASSUMPTIONS	LEGITIMATE RIGHTS
1. It is selfish to put your needs before others' needs.	You have a right to put yourself first sometimes.
2. It is shameful to make mistakes.	You have a right to make mistakes.
3. If you can't convince others that your feelings are reasonable, then you must be wrong.	You have a right to be the final judge of your feelings and accept them as legitimate.
4. You should be flexible and adjust, it's not polite to question other people's reasons.	You have a right to protest unfair treatment or criticism.
5. Things could get even worse, don't rock the boat.	You have a right to negotiate for change.
6. You should always try to accommodate others.	You have a right to say "no."

believe that they have a right to their feelings, beliefs, and opinions. They reject the idea that people are created equal and have the right to treat each other as equals. As a result, they usually cannot find grounds for objecting to exploitation and mistreatment by others. Behavioral theorists suggest, as illustrated in Table 14-4, that such people learned as children traditional assumptions that implied that their perceptions, opinions, feelings, and wants were less important or correct than those of others. They grew up doubting themselves and looking to others for validation and guidance. Often, such people leave interactions or relationships feeling angry, resentful, ineffective, hopeless, and depressed. However, behavioral theorists believe that such learned behaviors can be unlearned and replaced by more effective satisfying assertive behavior patterns as indicated in the legitimate rights column of Table 14-4.

Assertiveness training is effective in reducing depression, anger, resentment, interpersonal anxiety, and stress. As people become more assertive, they believe in their right to their thoughts, feeling, and wants. They begin to feel entitled to relax, and spend time involved in activities important and pleasurable to them. Assertiveness training consists of eight steps that are summarized in Box 14-3. Each step is accompanied by exercises that increase the amount and effectiveness of assertive behavior. Assertiveness training groups or workshops are commonly offered in community adult education programs or at women's health, wellness, or behavioral health centers that are led by mental health professionals. Local bookstores have numerous books on assertiveness in the wellness, self-help, or psychology departments.

Refuting Irrational Beliefs

Derived from cognitive theory, the concepts of rational-emotive therapy (RET), developed by Ellis (1975), address human values and beliefs as the important compo-

nent of the personality. Rational emotive therapy is based on the assumption that a person's value system and beliefs interpret certain experiences negatively and therefore produce emotional distress. According to Ellis (1975), emotional distress is not caused by events or a person's emotional reaction to events but by his or her belief system. For example, being insulted does not cause a person to withdraw from others. Rather, it is that person's belief about being insulted that causes this particular person to withdraw.

Ellis proposes that healthy functioning is only possible when the ideas, beliefs, and values that people believe in are rational. Beliefs are defined as rational when they help people accept reality, work productively, and enjoy leisure interests. Irrationality is associated with self-destructive behavior and correlated with anxiety, anger, and depression.

According to Ellis (1975), realistic or unrealistic self-talk produces the emotions that lead people to interpret events as positive or negative. At the core of all irrational thinking are absolutist perfectionist attitudes and the assumption that others are to blame for one's problems. Two common forms of irrational self-talk are "awfulizing" and "absolutizing," which are defined and illustrated in Table 14-5.

Rational-emotive therapy helps people to dispel their irrational beliefs by educating them about this phenomenon. Reinforcement techniques are often used to help people change. People are taught to reward themselves for working to resolve self-defeating ideas and to penalize themselves if they do not. People are also taught how to speak and think more precisely and objectively, giving up the use of vague terms and overgeneralizations to define their problems in more specific terms. For example, the person is shown how the statement, "I tend to get angry easily" is more precise than, "I am an angry person." Assessment of a person's irrational beliefs, plus homework sufficient to refute one of

Box 14-3

Eight Steps of Assertiveness Training

1. Identify the three basic styles of interpersonal behavior
2. Identify those situations in which the person wants to be more effective:
   - *When* do you want to be more assertive?
   - *Who* are the people with whom you are nonassertive?
   - *What* do you want that you have been unable to achieve with nonassertive styles?
3. Describe problem scenes, those situations in which a person feels interpersonally ineffective:
   - Who is the person involved?
   - Where does the situation take place?
   - What bothers you?
   - How do you deal with it?
   - Your fear of what will take place if you are assertive
   - Your goal
4. Write your script for change. A script is a working plan for dealing with a problem assertively:
   - Look at your rights, what you want, what you need
   - Arrange a time and place to discuss the situation
   - Define the problem specifically
   - Describe your feelings using "I" messages
   - Express your request or position simply and firmly
   - Reinforce the possibility of getting what you want
5. Develop assertive body language and practice it:
   - Maintain direct eye contact
   - Maintain an erect body posture

- Speak clearly, audibly, and firmly
- Do not whine or use an apologetic tone of voice
- Make use of gestures and facial expression for emphasis
6. Learn to listen
   - Listen
   - Clarify
   - Acknowledge
7. Learn to arrive at a workable compromise that results in a win-win situation
   - My way this time, your way next time
   - Part of what I want, part of what you want
   - My way when I'm doing it, your way when you're doing it
8. Learn how to avoid manipulation
   - Broken-record technique—briefly acknowledge that you have heard the other person's point and calmly repeat your message without getting sidetracked
   - Defusing—I can see that you are angry right now, so let's discuss this later
   - Assertive delay—I hear your point, but I'll have to reserve judgement and get back to you after I've thought about it
   - Yes, but—I can understand how you think that is the solution, but I have another solution in mind

TABLE 14-5

Refuting irrational ideas

IRRATIONAL IDEA	DESCRIPTION	EXAMPLE
Awfulizing	People awfulize by making catastrophic, nightmarish interpretations of their experience. People's emotions that follow awfulizing self-talk tend to be awful because they correspond to the person's description of the world	A momentary chest pain is a heart attack A significant other being late for a date is defined as abandonment I know that if I delegate this work, the job will never get done
Absolutizing	People absolutize by expecting that things have to be a certain way and that the person also has to be a certain way. Words like "should," "ought," "must," "always," and "never" are often contained in irrational idea statements. Any deviation from that particular value or standard is bad. The person who fails to live up to the standard is bad. From a more rational perspective, it is the standard that is bad, because it is irrational	It is an absolute necessity for an adult to have love and approval from family, friends, and peers I must be unfailingly competent and almost perfect in all that I undertake Anger is automatically bad and destructive

these beliefs can take approximately 20 minutes per day for 2 weeks.

Time Management

Time management is a behavioral strategy that increases coping effectiveness and reduces stress by helping people to:

1. Establish priorities that highlight their most important goals
2. Realistically schedule time by breaking priorities into manageable steps
3. Eliminate low-priority tasks
4. Make effective decisions

Productivity increases as people spend more time and energy but only up to a certain point. Past this point, additional time and energy become counterproductive. This is the point of diminishing returns. Inappropriate use of time and ineffective decisions produce frustration, lowered self-esteem, anxiety, and stress. This results in six symptoms of ineffective time management including:

1. Rushing
2. Chronic vacillation between unpleasant alternatives
3. Fatigue or listlessness with many unfilled hours of nonproductive activity
4. Constantly missed deadlines
5. Insufficient time for rest or personal relationships
6. The sense of being overwhelmed by demands and details, and having to do what you do not want to do most of the time

Effective time management can be used to minimize deadline anxiety, avoidance anxiety, job fatigue, and burnout.

Biofeedback

Biofeedback is the use of instrumentation to become aware of normally unnoticed autonomic (involuntary) processes in the body, such as blood pressure and heart rate, to help bring them under voluntary control to increase self-regulation and thereby decrease stress (Davis, Eshelman, and McKay, 1995). Biofeedback machines give people immediate feedback about their own biological functions mediated by the autonomic nervous system including muscle tension, skin surface temperature, brain wave activity, blood pressure, heart rate, and skin conductivity (sweating). Each of these body systems influences how people experience relaxation. If a person's muscles are relaxed (electromyogram [EMG]), the person is not perspiring (galvanic skin response [GSR]), and their skin temperature is warm (thermograph), that does not mean that he or she is completely stress-free. The heart rate may still be high; an electroencephalogram (EEG) may show high brain wave activity. Biofeed-back helps people find out which components of their nervous system are and are not relaxed.

Biofeedback is based on giving continuous feedback about the results of each consecutive attempt to control an involuntary physiological function. For example, the goal of a particular biofeedback session is to decrease a person's heartrate. The person might be given feedback by biofeedback equipment that amplifies body changes and translates them into external signals such as flashing lights or bleeping sounds. A person can "see" or "hear" his or her heartbeat as it slows down or speeds up. This information gives the person the data needed to control heart rate. The person is instructed to change the external signal as it is observed. However, the person is not instructed to change the heartrate. Rather, he or she is told to change the external signal, like the bleeping sound. If the person can do this, the heart rate will be modified.

There is evidence that biofeedback is effective in treating tension headaches, migraines, hypertension, insomnia, pain and muscle spasm, asthma, stuttering, teeth grinding, anxiety, and phobic reactions.

Bioenergetics

Bioenergetics provides techniques for reducing muscular tension through the release of feelings. Bioenergetics was developed by the American psychiatrist Lowen (1967, 1976), who holds that "bioenergy," the basic life force, manifests itself on both the emotional and muscular planes. Therefore distress in one plane will manifest itself in the other. Although well-functioning people are emotionally responsive and fully alive, allowing their bioenergy to flow freely, others block expression of feelings, which then get trapped and transformed into rigid musculature. When the body is relatively unalive, perceptions and responses are diminished. People in this situation are often depressed. Making deep contact with blocked feelings and releasing tension is the key to unlocking blocked or repressed feelings and allowing resolution to occur.

Bioenergetic techniques include stressor and releaser exercises that are used to increase people's awareness of body defenses. The exercises begin with deep breathing and progress to stretching and kicking the limbs. This enables people to break through muscular rigidity and express feelings previously trapped in habitual postural modes. These modes, which are called muscular armoring, prevent the free flow of energy. The goal is to move the person to open expression of feelings, which will restore the free flow of bioenergy and enhance a sense of autonomy and aliveness.

Lowen also proposed that the study of auras, or energy fields around the body, can be used to diagnose disturbances in body functioning. For example, in the energy field of a person with schizophrenia, a bioenergetics therapist can observe characteristic alterations such as interruptions of energy flow or color changes. Different parts of each person's body radiates different kinds of feelings. For example, chronic muscle tension blocks energy, resulting in negative feelings. The head, neck, and shoulders can radiate openness and affirmation or express hostility and holding back. The legs can radiate security and balance or instability. When there are no constrictions that disturb energy flow, the feeling is positive, the personality is integrated, and the aura is bright and intense.

Psychiatric nurses have a vast array of available stress management strategies to incorporate when planning client care. Other stress management approaches such as humor (see Chapter 8), pain management (see Chapter 32), support and self-help groups (see chapters 11 and 18), and other brief treatment (see Chapter 10) and rehabilitative (see Chapters 18 and 38) approaches are presented in other chapters throughout this book.

Stress management techniques can be learned in courses that nurses take in their undergraduate or graduate education. These techniques can also be learned by attending continuing education programs or programs offered by educational institutes that specialize in behavioral health care, treatment of anxiety disorders, or holistic health. Stress management can also be learned through reading books, journals, watching psycoeducational videotapes, or through computer-assisted learning programs. Psychiatric and other nurses who wish to incorporate stress management into their clinical practice need to make sure that they have a thorough knowledge base and have had supervised practice about whichever stress management strategies they use in the delivery of safe and effective client care.

KEY POINTS

- Stress is a broad group of experiences in which internal or external demands, or both, tax or exceed a person's resources or coping capabilities. The source of the stress is a stressor.
- Important stress theories include: Cannon's fight response to stress; Selye's stress-adaptation theory; Lazarus and Folkman's stress, appraisal, and coping theory; and stressful life events theory.
- Stress assessment precedes development of a stress management program that meets the unique needs of an individual or a defined client population.
- Stress management is a process of learning how to live with the inevitable life stressors people encounter by learning how to counteract or cope effectively with counterproductive responses to stress through enhanced self-regulation.
- Stress management strategies are used by nurses working in psychiatric, primary care, and other health-related specialty settings. Nurses use stress management strategies to promote health, prevent

 CRITICAL THINKING QUESTIONS

During his annual physical, Ralph J., age 34, complained of fatigue, headaches, and a "pinching" feeling in his chest. Examination by the primary care provider (PCP) revealed elevated blood pressure, but no physical reason for the "pinching" in his chest or the headaches. In further assessment, Ralph described himself as a "workaholic" who regularly worked 12-hour days, did not exercise, was 15 lbs. overweight, and had no leisure interests. The PCP referred Ralph to the psychiatric nurse who worked at the health maintenance organization (HMO) for a stress assessment and potential involvement in the HMO's stress management program run by the psychiatric nurse.

1. Which theoretical concepts about stress are most important for the nurse to consider when assessing Ralph's symptoms?
2. What kinds of assessment questions or assessment tools would be most effective in identifying the source(s) of Ralph's stress?
3. Which stress management strategies would be most appropriate for the nurse to select to assist Ralph in modifying his stress response. What is the rationale for choosing each strategy?
4. How could the nurse most effectively explain (sell) how and why stress management is effective?
5. How would the nurse evaluate the effectiveness of the stress management interventions?

physical and mental health problems, and in the treatment and rehabilitation of physical and mental health disorders.

- Stress management strategies include Stress Awareness Logs, deep breathing exercises, visualization, progressive relaxation, meditation, yoga, therapeutic touch, exercise, self-hypnosis, autogenic training, thought stopping, assertiveness training, refuting irrational beliefs, time management, biofeedback, and bioenergetics.

REFERENCES

Bennett, C. (1996). Expanding the mind-body connection: Working women and stress. *Capsules Comments, 2:*4, 249-254.

Cannon, W.B. (1963). *Wisdom of the body.* New York: Norton.

Carter, B., McGoldrick, M. (1989). The changing family life cycle: A framework for family therapy. In B. Carter and M. McGoldrick (Eds.). *The changing family life cycle (2nd ed.).* Boston: Allyn and Bacon.

Carton, B. (1995, January 30). Health insurers embrace eye-of-newt therapy. *The Wall Street Journal.*

Charlesworth, E.A., & Nathan, R.G. (1985). *Stress management: A comprehensive guide to wellness.* New York: Ballantine Books.

Chopra, D. (1987). *Creating health: Beyond perfection, toward perfection.* Boston: Houghton-Mifflin.

Cotton, D.H.G. (1990). *Stress management: An integrated approach to therapy.* New York: Brunner/Mazel, Publishers.

Coué, E. (1922). *Self-mastery through conscious autosuggestion.* London, England: Allen and Unwin.

Cousins, N. (1990). *Head first: The biology of hope.* New York: Dutton.

Davis, M., Eshelman, E. R., & McKay, M. (1995). *The relaxation and stress reduction workbook.* Oakland, CA: New Harbinger.

Derogatis, L.R., & Cleary, P.A. (1977a). Confirmation of the dimensional structure of the SCL-90: a study in construct validation. *J Clin Psychol, 33:* 4, 981-989.

Derogatis, L.R., & Cleary, P.A. (1977b). Factorial invariance across gender for the primary symptom dimensions of the SCL-90. *Br J Social Clin Psychol, 16:* 2, 347-356.

Ellis, A. (1975). *A new guide to rational living.* Englewood Cliffs, NJ: Prentice-Hall.

Fisher, S. (1991). *Discovering the power of self-hypnosis: A new approach for enabling change and promoting health.* New York: Harper Collins.

Friedman, H.S., & VandenBos, G.R. (1992). Disease-prone and self-healing personalities. *Hosp Commun Psychiatry, 43:* 12, 1177-1179.

Hayes, A. (1995). Psychiatric nursing: What does biology have to do with it? *Arch Psychiatr Nurs, 9:* 4, 216-224.

Holmes, T.H., & Rahe, R.H. (1967). The social readjustment rating scale. *Journal of Psychsom Res, 11,* 213-218.

Jacobson, E. (1974). *Progressive relaxation.* Chicago: The University of Chicago Press.

Kanner, A.D., et al. (1981). Comparison of two modes of stress measurement: Daily hassles and uplifts versus major life events. *J Behav Med, 4:* 1-39.

Keicolt-Glaser, J., & Glaser, R. (1992). Psychoneuroimmunology: Can psychological interventions modulate immunity? *J Consult Clin Psychol, 60:* 2, 569-575.

Kobasa, M.S. (1991). *Stress and coping: An anthology.* New York: Columbia University Press.

Krieger, D. (1979). *The therapeutic touch.* Englewood Cliffs, NJ: Prentice-Hall.

Jennings, B.M., & Staggers, N. (1994). A critical analysis of hardiness. *Nurs Res, 43:* 5, 274-281.

Lazarus, R.S. (1966). *Psychological stress and the coping process.* New York: McGraw-Hill.

Lazarus, R.S. (1976). *Patterns of adjustment.* New York: McGraw-Hill.

Lazarus, R.S., & Folkman, S. (1984). *Stress, appraisal, and coping.* New York: Springer.

LeShan, L. (1974). *How to meditate.* New York: Bantam Books.

Lowen, A. (1967). *The betrayal of the body.* New York: Macmillan.

Lowen, A. (1976). *Bioenergetics.* New York: Penguin Books.

MacRae, J. (1991). *Therapeutic touch.* New York: Alfred A. Knopf.

McCain, N.L., & Smith, J.C. (1994). Stress and coping in the context of psychoneuroimmunology: A holistic framework for nursing practice and research. *Arch Psychiatr Nurs, 8:* 4, 221-227.

Miller, T.W. (1988). Advances in understanding the impact of stressful life events on health. *Hosp Commun Psychiatry, 39:* 6, 615-621.

Miller, T.W. (1989). *Stressful life events.* Madison, CT: International Universities Press, Inc.

Monat, A., & Lazarus, R.S. (1991). *Stress and coping.* (3rd. ed) New York: Columbia University Press.

Morse, J.M., & Doberneck, B. (1995). Delineating the concept of hope. *Image J Nurs Scholar, 27:* 4, 277-286.

Mrazek, P.J., & Haggerty, R.J. (1994). *Reducing risks for mental disorders.* Washington, DC: National Academy Press.

Narsavage, G.L., & Weaver, T.E. (1994). Physiologic status, coping, and hardiness as predictors of outcomes in chronic obstructive pulmonary disease. *Nur Res, 43:* 2, 90-94.

O'Leary, A. (1990). Stress, emotion, and human immune function. *American Psychologist, 108:* 2, 363-382.

Outlaw, F.H. (1993). Stress and coping: The influence of racism on the cognitive appraisal processing of African-Americans. *Issues Mental Health Nurs, 14:* 4, 399-409.

Pilkonis, P.A., Imber, S.D., & Rubinsky, P. (1985). Dimensions of life stress in psychiatric patients. *J Human Stress, Spring:* 5-11.

Pollock, S.E., & Duffy, M.E. (1990). The health-related hardiness scale: Development and psychometric analysis. *Nursing Research, 39:* 4, 218-222.

Rathus, S.A. (1973). A 30-term schedule for assessing assertive behavior. *Behavior Therapy, 4:*, 398-406.

Segal, S.P., & VanderVoort, D.J. (1993). Daily hassles of persons with severe mental illness. *Hospital and Community Psychiatry, 44:* 3, 276-278.

Selye, H. (1980). The stress concept today. In I.L. Kutash, et al. (Eds.). *Handbook on stress and anxiety.* Washington, DC: Jossey-Bass.

Selye, H. (1991). History and present status of the stress concept. In A. Monat & R.S. Lazarus (Eds.). *Stress and coping.* (3rd ed.). New York: Columbia University Press

Siegal, B.S. (1988). *Love, medicine, and miracles.* New York: Harper and Row.

Simonton, O.C., Mathews, S., & Creighton, J.L., (1980). *Getting well again.* New York: Bantam Books.

U. S. Department of Health and Human Services. (1995). *Healthy people 2000: National health promotion and disease prevention objectives.* Washington, DC: U.S. Government Printing Office.

Vishnudenanda, S. (1960). *The complete illustrated book of yoga.* New York: Julian Press.

Weissman, A.N. (1980). Assessing depressogenic attitudes: A validation study. Paper presented at the 51st Annual Meeting of the Eastern Psychological Association. Hartford, CT.

Wolpe, J. (1958). Psychotherapy by reciprocal inhibition. Stanford, CA: Stanford University Press.

Younger, J.B. (1993). Development and testing of the mastery of stress instrument. *Nursing Research, 42:* 2, 68-7-3.

Chapter 15

Psychopharmacology

Beth Harris

LEARNING OUTCOMES

After studying and applying the concepts of this chapter, the learner will be able to:
- Assess the client's medication history and current health status.
- Administer psychotropic medication safely.
- Monitor clients for therapeutic effects of pharmacological agents.
- Describe expected side effects of pharmacological agents used to treat psychiatric symptoms.
- Educate clients and their families about medications that are prescribed.
- Collaborate with the prescriber in managing side effects.
- Manage issues related to client compliance with medication regimens.

KEY TERMS

Adrenergic	Extrapyramidal side effects (EPS)	Polypharmacy
Akathisia	Hypertensive crisis	Potency
Antidyskinetics	Lag period	Psychotropic
Anticholinergic side effects	Lithium toxicity	Serotonergic
Antipsychotics	Maintenance	Tardive dyskinesia (TD)
Atropine psychosis	Mood stabilizer	Target symptoms
Compliance	Neuroleptic malignant syndrome	Toxicity
Dependence	(NMS)	Tyramine
Depot injections	Nonselective	
Dystonia	Noradrenergic	

A revolution in psychiatry began in the 1950s with the development of the major classes of *psychotropic* medications, *which exert an effect on mind and mood or modify mental activity and are used to treat symptoms of psychiatric disorders.* Knowledge about the biochemical basis of mental illnesses and their biological treatment has mushroomed. The "Decade of the Brain," a designation given to the 1990s by the National Institutes of Mental Health (NIMH), has accelerated the already rapid increase in the number and variety of drugs available to treat psychiatric symptoms.

The recent publication of the American Nurses' Association (ANA) psychopharmacological guidelines for psychiatric-mental health nursing (1994) highlights the need for all nurses to have a psychopharmacological knowledge base. As inpatient hospital stays become shorter and health care increasingly shifts its locus into the community, the responsibility of day-to-day care falls more heavily on the client and family. Therefore the need to teach clients and their family members about the knowledge and skills necessary to manage both mental illness and its treatment with medication, an ever more important role of nurses.

The brain is composed of hundreds of billions of brain cells called *neurons.* Each neuron is intimately connected to all its neighboring neurons by a vast, intertwining system of appendages called *axons* (the outgoing appendages) and *dendrites* (the incoming appendages). At each point where the nerve cells make contact (tiny spaces between the cells called *synapses*), they send communications by means of chemical messengers called *neurotransmitters.* The neurotransmitters are released by the membrane of the sending cell (presynaptic membrane) and act on receptors in the membrane of the receiving cell (postsynaptic membrane) (see Color Plate 3). There are probably at least 100 neurotransmitters, many of which have some balancing effect on others. As a result, when one or more of these neurotransmitters are either underactive or overactive, they alter the entire chemical balance of the brain (see Chapter 13).

Most psychotropic medications directly address biochemical imbalances in the brain, bringing the areas of the brain responsible for thought and emotion back into a normal, functional state. The trend with the new medications is toward greater or more rapid efficacy and fewer or milder side effects. This is possible because many of the newer medications target more specifically the brain regions or neurotransmitter receptors responsible for symptoms of mental disorders without affecting nearby or related receptors and regions that cause adverse effects. As psychotropic medications become more effective and more comfortable, the reluctance to take psychotropic medications will hopefully diminish;

clients will reap their benefits while suffering less from their side effects.

This chapter describes psychotropic medications: the antipsychotics, antidepressants, mood stabilizers, and antianxiety/sedative-hypnotics. Each class is discussed in terms of their mechanisms of action, the target symptoms for which they are prescribed, guidelines for use, side effects, contraindications, drug interactions, and nursing care.

THE ANTIPSYCHOTICS

The *antipsychotics, also called* neuroleptics *or* major tranquilizers, *are a group of medications used to treat psychotic symptoms, that is, symptoms of being out of touch with reality.* There are two major groups of antipsychotics: the classic antipsychotics and a newer group referred to as the "novel" antipsychotics. Table 15-1 lists the antipsychotics in common use along with their doses and relative side effect profiles.

Mechanism of Action

Mechanism of action of the classical antipsychotics

The classical antipsychotics block a subgroup of postsynaptic dopamine receptors, the D_2 receptors. Their blockage of the D_2 receptors in the mesolimbic pathways of the dopamine system is thought to be the mechanism of action for the treatment of positive psychotic symptoms of psychosis such as delusions, hallucinations, and paranoia. The classic antipsychotics, however, also block the D_2 receptors in the nigrostriatal pathways of the dopamine system, creating extrapyramidal or muscular side effects including muscle spasms, stiffness, restlessness, and tardive dyskinesia (TD). They also affect other neurotransmitter systems, which in turn create side effects without adding to their antipsychotic action. These actions include the following:

- Partial histamine antagonism, which causes sleepiness and weight gain
- Partial acetylcholine blockage, which causes dry mouth, blurred vision, tachycardia, constipation, nasal congestion, and a potential for atropine psychosis
- Antagonism of the alpha-adrenergic system, which causes orthostatic hypotension (Meltzer, 1992)

Mechanism of action of the novel antipsychotics

In 1989 new classes of antipsychotic medications, dibenzoxazepines and dibenzodiazepines, were introduced when the Food and Drug Administration (FDA) approved general use of clozapine (Clozaril) and loxapine (Loxitane). Another class, benzisoxazoles, was intro-

TABLE 15-1

The antipsychotics

GENERIC NAME	COMMON BRAND NAME	STANDARD DAILY DOSE (MG)	IM FORM	SIDE EFFECTS			
				SEDATIVE	EXTRA PYRAMIDAL	HYPOTENSIVE	ANTICHOLINERGIC
Phenothiazines							
Aliphatics							
Chlorpromazine HCl	Thorazine	50-400	yes	+++	+	+++	++
Trifluopromazine	Vesprin	100-150	yes	++	+++	++	++
Piperidines							
Thioridazine	Mellaril	200-600	no	+++	+	++	+++
Mesoridazine	Serentil	75-300	yes	+++	+	++	+++
Piperacetazine	Quide	20-160	no	++	++	+	
Piperazines							
Trifluoperazine	Stelazine	6-20	yes	+	+++	+	+
Acetophenazine	Tindal	60-120	no	++	++	+	++
Fluphenazine HCl	Prolixin	5-20	yes	+	+++	+	++
Fluphenazine enanthate	Prolixin enanthate	12.5-50 each 1-3 weeks	yes	+	+++	+	++
Fluphenazine decanoate	Prolixin decanoate	12.5-50 each 1-3 weeks	yes	+	+++	+	+
Perphenazine	Trilafon	8-32	yes	++	++	+	+
Thioxanthenes							
Chlorprothixene	Taractan	50-400	yes	+++	+	++	+++
Thiothixene	Navane	6-30	yes	+	+++	++	+
Butyrophenones							
Haloperidol	Haldol	6-20	yes	+	+++	+	+
Haloperidol decanoate	Haldol decanoate	50-200 each 1-3 weeks	yes	+	+++	+	++
Dihydroindolones							
Molindone	Moban	50-225	no	++	+	+	++
Dibenzodiazepine							
Clozapine	Clozaril	100-900	no	+	+	+	+
Dibenzoxazepines							
Loxapine	Loxitane	60-100	yes	++	++	+	++
Diphenylbutylpiperidines							
Pimozide	Orap	2-10	no	+	+++	+	+
Benzisoxazoles							
Risperidone	Risperdal	4-8	no	+	+	+	+
Thienobenzodiazepine							
Olanzapine	Zyprex	2.5-20	no	+	+	+	+

+ *mild*   + + *moderate*   + + + *severe*

duced when risperidone (Risperdal) came on the market. Several other atypical antipsychotics are expected to receive FDA approval. The following drugs are phase II and phase III clinical trials: quetiapine (Seroquel), sertindole (Serlect), and zinziprasidone (at present no trade name has been assigned). These new medications differ from the classic antipsychotics in several important ways that have led to their wide usage in the short time they have been available.

The novel antipsychotics, although they differ from one another to some extent, have several characteristics in common, including the following:

- They act selectively on the postsynaptic D_2 receptors
- They treat both positive and negative symptoms
- They are unlikely to cause TD
- In general, they cause fewer side effects

Clozapine, an atypical drug, interferes with dopamine receptor binding. It antagonizes or blocks not only postsynaptic dopamine D_1 receptors but also the serotonin ($5\text{-}HT_2$) alpha-1 and butamine (H_1) postsynaptic receptors, making it more active throughout the limbic system. Because of its high potential to cause agranulocytosis, its use requires careful monitoring of clients, but because of the increased costs of monitoring, its use in some settings is limited to clients who have had failed trials on other antipsychotic agents.

Risperidone (Risperdal) is the first of a new class of drugs—benzisoxazole agents. They block both dopamine (D_2) and serotonin receptors. They are absorbed well orally, metabolized in the liver, and excreted through the kidneys. Because of these drugs' strong antagonist effects on serotonin, clients who use risperidone are less likely to develop side effects caused by excessive serotonin.

Target Symptoms

Target symptoms of classical antipsychotics
Target symptoms are symptoms that the client experiences and that the drug is intended to treat. The antipsychotics are given to relieve both positive and negative symptoms of psychosis and should not be used for sedation, even though sedation is a side effect. It should be noted that the antipsychotics treat psychotic symptoms in a wide variety of disorders. They are not used to treat schizophrenia exclusively. Box 15-1 lists the psychotic symptoms best treated by antipsychotic medications.

Target symptoms of novel antipsychotics
Both risperidone (Risperdal) and clozapine (Clozaril) are effective in treating the positive and negative symptoms of schizophrenia (see Box 15-1). It is estimated that clozapine is effective in between 30% and 50% of clients with schizophrenia who do not respond to the classical antipsychotics. Consequently, many clients who continue

---

BOX 15-1

Target Symptoms for the Antipsychotics

POSITIVE SYMPTOMS

- Combativeness
- Verbal threats and aggressiveness
- Hyperactivity
- Uncontrollable hostility
- Uncontrollable negativism
- Hallucinations
- Delusions
- Insomnia related to psychosis
- Anorexia related to psychosis
- Severe agitation
- Uncontrollable rage
- Extreme sensitivity to environmental stimuli
- Paranoia/suspiciousness
- Terror
- Unclear or racing thoughts
- Ideas of reference
- Feelings of unreality

NEGATIVE SYMPTOMS

- Apathy or lack of motivation
- Social discomfort
- Lack of spontaneity
- Lack of pleasure
- Emotional withdrawal
- Poor hygiene and grooming
- Lack of insight
- Poor judgment

---

to have symptoms and were not helped before clozapine's availability are now able to manage symptoms effectively. With risperidone, the advantage is not that previously resistant clients respond but rather that clients get help with both positive *and* negative symptoms and that they experience a minimum of muscular side effects.

Because side effects are so mild with risperidone, it may well be a good choice as a first-line drug for clients experiencing their first psychotic symptoms. It is more easily and comfortably tolerated than the classical D_2 blockers (and therefore more likely to be taken), and studies show it to be at least as effective as the classic antipsychotics.

This ability of clozapine and risperidone to treat negative symptoms is one of their greatest advantages. Clients who take them find that they begin to feel well again in a way that they had not with the classical antipsychotics. Not only are clients' positive symptoms (hallucinations, delusions, paranoia, and others) softened or alleviated,

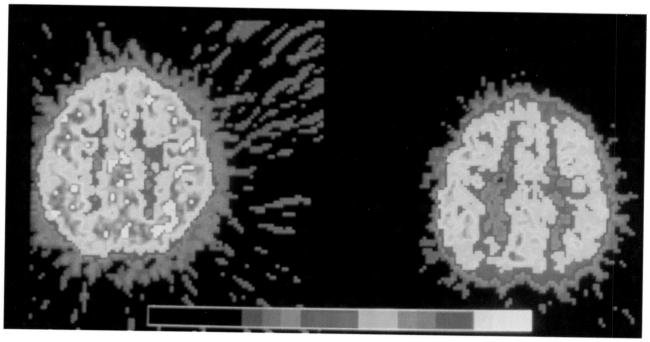

Plate 7   Brain scan images produced by positron emission tomography (PET) compare the difference in the metabolism rate in the brain of an adult with attention deficit hyperactivity disorder (ADHD) (*right*) and an adult free of the disorder (*left*). The areas of orange and white in the scan on the left demonstrate a higher rate of metabolism, while the areas of blue and green in the scan at right represent an abnormally low metabolic rate in the adult with ADHD. (From National Institute of Mental Health, Section on Clinical Brain Imaging. [1990]. Zametkin et al., Washington, DC.)

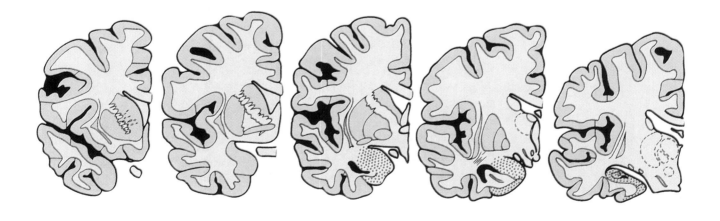

▢ reduced area/volume   ▦ disturbed brain tissure

Plate 8   Structural abnormalities in the brain involved in schizophrenia. This diagram shows regions of reduced volume and disturbed brain tissue in the brain of a person with schizophrenia. (From Roberts, G.W., Leigh, P.N., & Weinberger, D.R. (1993). *Neuropsychiatric disorders*. London: Wolfe.)

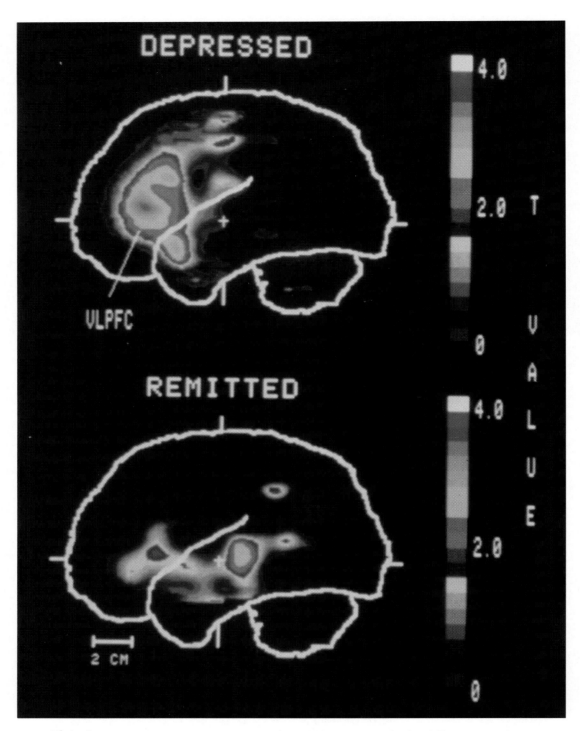

Plate 9   A positron emission tomography (PET) scan reveals the difference in the brain activity of a person while experiencing depression and when in a remitted state. The images show an entire anatomical circuit that appears to function abnormally during depression. The notation "VLPFC" refers to the ventrolateral prefrontal cortex. (Courtesy Wayne C. Drevets, M.D., Department of Psychiatry, Washington University School of Medicine, St. Louis.)

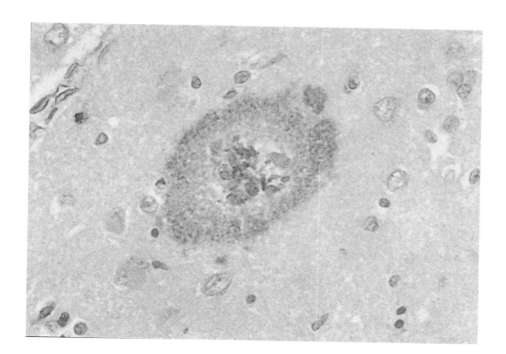

Plate 10 Amyloid plaques associated with Alzheimer's disease stained and magnified 400 times. (From Mann D.M.A., Neary, D., & Humberto, T. (1994). *Color atlas and text of adult dementias.* London: Wolfe.)

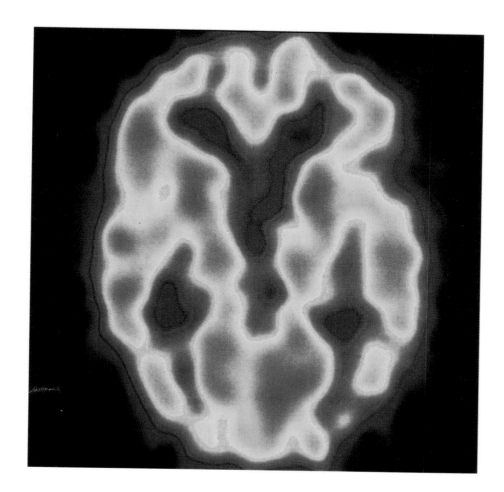

Plate 11 A positron emission tomography (PET) scan of a 67-year-old man with vascular dementia showing images of cerebral blood flow and glucose metabolism. (Courtesy of Alzheimer's Disease Diagnostic Treatment Centers, University of Southern California, Rancho Los Amigos Medical Center, Los Angeles.)

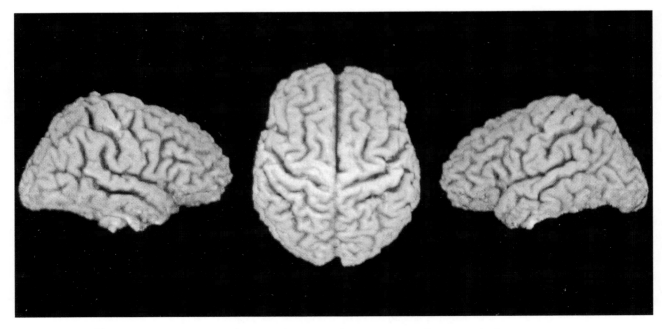

Plate 12 Cortical atrophy in Alzheimer's disease, as seen by a magnetic resonance imaging (MRI) scan. (From Roberts, G.W., Leigh, P.N., & Weinberger, D.R. (1993). *Neuropsychiatric disorders.* London: Wolfe.)

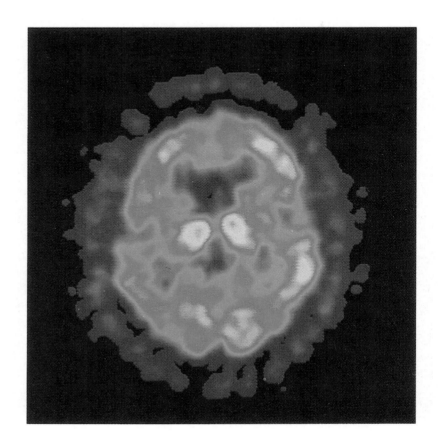

Plate 13 Hypometabolism in the frontal, parietal, and temporal regions in Alzheimer's Disease, as seen by a positron emission tomography (PET) scan. (From Roberts, G.W., Leigh, P.N., & Weinberger, D.R. (1993). *Neuropsychiatric disorders.* London: Wolfe.)

but they also begin to enjoy the company of other people and begin to develop or redevelop interests.

Guidelines for Use

The art of prescribing medications for specific clients depends on several factors. A client's age, overall health, previous response, successful use of a particular drug by a family member, and target symptoms determine the choice of drug. If a client had a favorable reaction in the past to a specific antipsychotic, that person should immediately be started on the same one if symptoms return. Antipsychotics either remove psychotic symptoms entirely, or they make them considerably less intense in about 80% of clients.

Antipsychotic effects usually begin after the first few doses of medication; but the maximum symptom relief may take several weeks or months. Treatment may begin with the liquid form to ensure compliance and progress to tablets or capsules when symptoms are under control. The short-acting IM forms are used in psychiatric emergencies when clients are dangerous to themselves or others or sometimes as alternatives to oral doses, when there is a question of adequate absorption from the gastrointestinal tract.

Depot injections, *or long-acting injections,* of haloperidol (Haldol) or fluphenazine (Prolixin) are necessary only every few weeks depending on a client's response. They are preferred by clients who would rather not deal with medications on a daily basis. They are also helpful for clients who are ambivalent about compliance because they require a decision about medication only every 2 to 4 weeks instead of every day.

Clients with psychotic symptoms continue to take maintenance antipsychotics for a minimum of 6 to 12 months after symptoms are first controlled. The medication can then be slowly and gradually tapered over a period of months to the lowest level at which symptoms remain in control. A collaborative relationship must continue between the client and the prescriber to monitor for warning signs of relapse because early identification of relapse and immediate aggressive intervention (increased dosage) can prevent a full-blown psychotic episode. Clients who have schizophrenia or persistent psychotic symptoms often take these medications continuously for many years because each attempt at reducing the dose brings a resurgence of symptoms.

Side Effects

Side effects of classical antipsychotics

Side effects are a major problem for clients who take antipsychotics. Most clients who take antipsychotics continue taking them for at least 6 months to 1 year and usually for much longer when attempts to stop them are met with symptom exacerbation. Hence, side effects must be tolerated for long periods of time. Nurses must recognize antipsychotic side effects and make every possible intervention to reduce them so clients are comfortable.

Nurses collaborate with prescribers by administering medications and carefully assessing for and monitoring both the therapeutic and side effects of each medication. When potentially dangerous side effects appear, the nurse has the responsibility to withhold the medication until the prescriber has been informed. The nurse is also responsible to teach the client about the drug and all aspects of the medication regimen. The nurse works with the prescriber to find the drug that has the greatest effect on client symptoms while simultaneously having the fewest side effects.

The individual antipsychotic agents differ from one another both in ***potency*** *(strength per milligram)* and in their side effect profiles. See Table 15-1 for the relative frequency of occurrence of sedative, ***extrapyramidal*** *(neuromuscular),* hypotensive, and ***anticholinergic*** *(parasympatholytic)* ***side effects.*** Table 15-2 lists these side effects and nursing management for each.

Three of the side effects listed in Table 15-2 require emergency intervention: neuroleptic malignant syndrome (NMS), atropine psychosis, and severe dystonia involving the inner structures of the throat. NMS and atropine psychosis can be fatal, particularly when they go unnoticed in their early stages or when mistaken for a worsening of symptoms and treated with an increased dose of an antipsychotic. It becomes essential to inform clients and their families about these dangerous side effects so that their occurrence can be prevented. Teaching Points for NMS and atropine psychoses are found in the boxes on p. 270.

In general, high-potency antipsychotics, namely chlorpromazine (Thorazine) and thioridazine (Mellaril), have more anticholinergic effects, are more sedating, and are more likely to cause hypotension, whereas the low-potency antipsychotics (all the others except novel antipsychotics) are more likely to cause neuromuscular (extrapyramidal) side effects. The neuromuscular (extrapyramidal) side effects are prevalent when clients take specific medications. The neuromuscular, or extrapyramidal side effects, are often treated by adding one of the antidyskinetic agents listed in Table 15-3. ***Antidyskinetics*** *are medications that relieve the neuromuscular (extrapyramidal) side effects of the antipsychotics,* such as dystonia, akathisia, stiffness, and tremor. They are sometimes used for preventive purposes, especially in young men who are most likely to suffer from muscular side effects. Antidyskinetics are used as needed to treat acute extrapyramidal side effects rather than as standing daily doses. When extrapyramidal side effects are severe, clients may take antidyskinetics for

Text continued on p. 271.

TABLE 15-2

Side effects of the antipsychotics and nursing management

SIDE EFFECT AND DESCRIPTION	NURSING MANAGEMENT
EXTRAPYRAMIDAL (NEUROMUSCULAR) SIDE EFFECTS	

Parkinsonism

Parkinsonism is a syndrome consisting of *akinesia* (slowness or lack of movements), muscular rigidity, alterations of posture, tremor, masklike facies, shuffling gait, loss of associated movements, hypersalivation, and drooling; can be mistaken for worsening of the underlying disorder or for depression; extremely unpleasant for the client, who may experience the akinesia and rigidity as a lack of spontaneity, lack of energy, or a zombie-like feeling

Notify the prescriber, who usually orders an antidyskinetic medication such as trihexyphenidyl (Artane) or benztropine (Cogentin) and/or reduces the antipsychotic dose.

Dystonia

Dystonia is a *muscle spasm in any muscle of the body;* may include torticollis (stiffness of the neck, which draws the head to one side and the chin to the opposite side), oculogyric crisis (an involuntary dorsal arching of the neck and/or back), protrusion of the tongue, dysphagia (trouble swallowing), and laryngeal or pharyngeal spasm with airway compromise; usually frightening and painful

Employ immediate use of an as-needed dose of an antidyskinetic, usually diphenhydramine (Benadryl) or benztropine (Cogentin), orally, IM, or IV. Provide a quiet, nonstimulating environment until the dystonia resolves. Reassure client that symptoms are benign and will resolve quickly. A standing oral dose of an antidyskinetic is usually ordered for several weeks or months, or longer after an episode of an acute dystonia to prevent a recurrence.

Tardive Dyskinesia (TD)

Tardive dyskinesia (TD) is a late-occurring, sometimes irreversible neurological side effect consisting of abnormal, involuntary movements that usually begin in the face, neck, and jaw (tongue thrusting, writhing or twisting; lip pursing; lip smacking; facial grimacing; grunting; or chewing) but can progress to or begin in any other part of the body; not to be confused with withdrawal dyskinesias, which are identical in appearance but occur only temporarily (for a few weeks or months) after antipsychotics are reduced in dose or discontinued

There is no certain cure for TD. Prevention consists of maintaining clients on the lowest possible antipsychotic dose for the briefest possible interval. Administer the Abnormal Involuntary Movement Scale (AIMS) at least every 6 months to any client taking antipsychotics to monitor for the occurrence of TD. If the AIMS score increases, the client must be informed and the dose reduced as much as possible or discontinued entirely. Clients should be taught early warning signs to help monitor for early symptoms. Clozapine (Clozaril) and risperidone (Risperdal) are extremely unlikely to cause TD. The symptoms of TD either diminish or resolve when clients are switched to novel antipsychotics.

Akathisia

Akathisia is *motor restlessness,* usually extremely unpleasant, if not intolerable, for the client, who may experience this side effect as unbearable or relentless anxiety or agitation; the inability to sit or stand still

Notify prescriber, who will usually reduce the antipsychotic dose or add an antidyskinetic such as benztropine (Cogentin) or trihexyphenidyl (Artane). If both fail, other medications have been found useful, including propranolol (Inderal), nadolol (Corgard), clonidine (Catapres), and several of the benzodiazepines, including diazepam (Valium) and lorazepam (Ativan).

TABLE 15-2—cont'd

Side effects of the antipsychotics and nursing management

SIDE EFFECT AND DESCRIPTION	NURSING MANAGEMENT
ANTICHOLINERGIC SIDE EFFECTS	
Blurred vision	Reassure client that this usually resolves untreated 1 or 2 weeks after the final dose adjustments. Provide large-print books or magazines in the interim.
Dry mouth	Reassure client that this usually resolves untreated 1 or 2 weeks into treatment. In the meantime, teach the client to carry a cup of water and take occasional sips; or moisten the mouth with mouthwash, sugarless gum, or hard candies. When severe or prolonged, it can cause an increase in dental caries or gum disease. The client may respond to use of a saliva substitute. A cholinergic agent such as bethanechol (Urecholine) may be prescribed.
Nasal congestion	Reassure client that this usually resolves untreated 1 or 2 weeks into treatment. In the meantime, increasing fluid intake may help. The prescriber may order a nasal decongestant spray.
Constipation	The client should increase dietary intake of fiber and fluid intake. Recommend an increase in exercise, if possible. The prescriber may order a bulking agent such as psillium (Metamucil or others), a stool softener (Colace or others), or a mild laxative. Infrequently, a paralytic ileus will develop and require emergency surgical intervention.
Urinary hesitancy or retention	Palpate or percuss the bladder for fullness. Use methods of inducing voiding. If unsuccessful, catheterization may become necessary. The dose may be reduced, changed to a less anticholinergic agent, or a cholinergic agent such as bethanechol (Urecholine) may be added.
Atropine Psychosis *Atropine psychosis (also called anticholinergic delirium) is an emergency situation in which a psychosis caused by the anticholinergic properties of the antipsychotics develops, especially when the antipsychotic drugs are used in combination with other anticholinergic medications such as antidepressants. Symptoms include purposeless overactivity, agitation, confusion, disorientation, dry, flushed skin, tachycardia, sluggish and dilated pupils, bowel hypomotility, difficulty speaking, and memory impairment.*	Withhold the antipsychotic and other anticholinergic medications. Inform the prescriber, who usually discontinues the medications and may order a cholinergic agent such as physostigmine (Antilirium) if symptoms are severe. Reorient and reassure the client. Reduce the amount of stimulation in the environment.

Continued.

TABLE 15-2—cont'd

Side effects of the antipsychotics and nursing management

SIDE EFFECT AND DESCRIPTION	NURSING MANAGEMENT
OTHER SIDE EFFECTS	

Sedation

Sedation is an induced state of quiet, calmness, or sleep

Usually resolves untreated in a week or two. Reassure the client and encourage getting up and moving in the morning. Keep the client involved in activities to prevent sleep during the day. The prescriber may reduce the dose or change to a less-sedating antipsychotic.

Orthostatic Hypotension

This side effect is characterized by a fall in blood pressure upon arising from a lying down or sitting position; often accompanied by nausea, light-headedness, palpitations, and, in the elderly, by falling

Teach the client to get out of bed and up from chairs slowly, adjusting position gradually and holding on to a stable object until symptoms pass. Dehydration accentuates symptom, so increase client's fluid intake. Monitor blood pressure when dose is increased or when symptoms occur.

Alterations of Sexual Functioning

May include reduction in sex drive, inability to achieve orgasm, inability to achieve an erection or retrograde ejaculation, breast enlargement (in men or women), production of milk from the breast, or amenorrhea

Teach the client that sexual problems are common during periods of intense stress including psychiatric hospitalization. Changing the medication may be helpful. Reassure the client that these side effects are reversible and benign. Menses will usually return in several months with or without a change in antipsychotic. Remind the client that contraception is necessary even if the period has temporarily stopped.

Increased Appetite

Increased desire to eat with consequent weight gain

The client responds best to a moderately calorie-restricted diet. Suggest basic methods of weight management, including exercise. Provide low-calorie snacks.

Decreased Tolerance to Alcohol and Other Sedative Drugs

Clients become quickly and easily sedated by alcohol or other sedatives while taking antipsychotics

Inform clients of this effect. Teach them to limit alcohol intake to no more than one or two drinks per day or to abstain.

Allergy

Pruritic maculopapular rash, usually on the face, neck, and chest

Usually benign and does not require treatment; teach clients to consult prescriber if symptoms persist.

Cholestatic Jaundice

An allergic response; early symptoms are malaise, fever, nausea, and abdominal pain followed in a week or so with itching and jaundice; usually benign and self-limiting

Withold medication. Notify the prescriber. Initiate bed rest, increase fluids, and apply topical preparations for itch.

Phototoxicity

Extreme sensitivity of the skin to sunburn

Recommend that the client use strong sunscreen and wear clothes and/or hats that cover most of the skin.

TABLE 15-2—cont'd

Side effects of the antipsychotics and nursing management

SIDE EFFECT AND DESCRIPTION	NURSING MANAGEMENT
OTHER SIDE EFFECTS	

Agranulocytosis

Severe reduction in the number of granulocytes (basophils, eosinophils, and neutrophils); clients have abnormally low white blood counts

This is a potentially lethal side effect. It is suspect if severe sore throat, fever, malaise, and/or sores in the mouth develop in the first 2 months of treatment. Initiate reverse isolation if agranulocytosis is confirmed.

Pigmentation of the Skin or Eyes

The skin takes on a golden brown coloration, changing to gray, blue, or purple with long-term antipsychotic use

Inform client that this is caused by the antipsychotic and is not permanent.

Pigmentary Retinopathy

A rare, irreversible, degenerative retinopathy that may cause blindness

Because this is usually caused by using thioridazine (Mellaril) in doses higher than 800 mg per day, it can be prevented by avoiding doses above that limit.

Hyperglycemia

A greater than normal amount of glucose in the blood

Known diabetics who were previously stabilized may begin to show higher levels of glucose in the blood and urine. Carefully check glucose levels and monitor for symptoms of hyperglycemia.

Cardiac Changes

There are usually mild electrocardiogram (ECG) changes that result from the anticholinergic properties of the antipsychotics. Chlorpromazine (Thorazine) can have a direct depressant action on the heart and a vasodilating action and may increase coronary blood flow. It may also have an antiarrhythmic effect. Thioridazine (Mellaril) causes a high incidence of T wave changes.

Clients with preexisting cardiovascular disease need periodic monitoring of ECG and vital signs throughout dosage adjustment and course of treatment. Clients with preexisting cardiovascular disease usually do better on low-potency antipsychotics.

Neuroleptic Malignant Syndrome

Neuroleptic malignant syndrome (NMS) is an emergency state consisting of altered consciousness, unstable blood pressure and pulse, fever, severe muscular rigidity, severe diaphoresis, severe tremors, and drooling. It is fatal in an estimated 15% to 20% of cases.

Withhold and notify the prescriber immediately. Treatment usually consists of supportive measures, including cooling blankets for fever, IV fluids for hydration, an airway if necessary, range-of-motion exercises or frequent changes in position for severe muscular rigidity, and frequent monitoring of blood pressure, pulse, temperature and respirations. Somatic interventions include administration of bromocriptine (Parlodel) or dantrolene (Dantrium).

Seizures

There may be an increased incidence of seizures in clients with seizure disorders

Increase dosage of anticonvulsant and initiate seizure precautions in clients with preexisting seizure disorders. If seizures develop in a client with no prior history of seizures, an antiseizure medication is usually given for 6 to 8 weeks, and the dose of the antipsychotic is reduced.

Gastrointestinal Distress

Heartburn or nausea

Give medication during mealtimes or with food.

TEACHING POINTS

Client Experiencing Neuroleptic Malignant Syndrome (NMS)

Teach the client, family, and/or significant others the following:

1. NMS can happen to anyone taking antipsychotic medications at any time during the course of treatment.

2. Early symptoms of NMS are stiffness, fever, sweating, and tremors.

3. Stop taking the antipsychotic medication immediately if NMS is suspected, and contact the prescriber or emergency health care provider immediately.

4. NMS is rapidly progressive and can be fatal if undetected. If untreated, the following symptoms quickly develop: severe stiffness, difficulty moving, difficulty swallowing, profuse sweating, strong tremors, and high fever.

5. NMS, when detected early and treated aggressively, resolves within several days and causes no permanent harm.

TEACHING POINTS

Client Experiencing Atropine Psychosis

Teach the client, family, and/or significant others the following:

1. Atropine psychosis can happen to anyone taking antipsychotic or antidepressant medications at any time during the course of treatment. It is most likely to occur when more than one medication is being taken.

2. Signs and symptoms of atropine psychosis include agitation; sudden disorientation to person, place, and/or time; tachycardia; dilated pupils; drug skin; and flushed skin.

3. Stop taking all medications immediately, and contact prescriber or emergency health care provider immediately if atropine psychosis is suspected.

4. Atropine psychosis, when detected early and treated aggressively, usually resolves within several hours or days and causes no permanent harm.

TABLE 15-3

Antidyskinetics

GENERIC NAME	MOST COMMON TRADE NAME	USUAL DAILY DOSE (MG)	PARENTERAL FORM AVAILABLE?
Anticholinergics			
Benztropine	Cogentin	1-6	Yes
Trihexyphenidyl	Artane	2-15	No
Procyclidine	Kemadrin	5-30	No
Biperiden	Akineton	2-10	Yes
Antihistamines			
Diphenhydramine	Benadryl	25-100	Yes
Others			
Amantadine	Symmetrel	100-300	No

several weeks or even months.

The most serious long-term risk of taking the classic antipsychotics is the development of TD, a late-developing side effect consisting of faulty, involuntary movements (see Table 15-2). The most widely accepted examination to test for the presence of TD is the Abnormal Involuntary Movement Scale (AIMS). Although it is believed that TD will not result from long-term use of novel antipsychotics, currently, there is little research about the development of neuromuscular side effects after long-term use.

Side effects of novel antipsychotics

Minimization of extrapyramidal or neuromuscular side effects is a major advantage of the novel antipsychotics. Clients who take these antipsychotics rarely experience stiffness, dystonias, akathisia, tremors, or tardive dyskinesia. Clozapine (Clozaril) has an important drawback—a risk of causing agranulocytosis in slightly less than 1% of those who take it. Because of the life-threatening nature of this side effect and the deaths it has caused in both Europe and the United States, clients who take clozapine must have a weekly white blood count (WBC) that is within normal limits before the next week's prescription is filled.

The amount of time, effort, and money involved in this monitoring makes clozapine one of the most costly and labor-intensive of the psychotropics—both for the client and for the staff who prescribe and monitor it. In 1995 dollars an average dose of clozapine costs the client or insurer about $11,000 per year, excluding the cost of physician visits, laboratory testing, or the time required for the necessary paperwork and office, laboratory, and pharmacy visits. Risperidone (Risperdal) costs one half to one third this amount.

Clozapine cannot be given concomitantly with any other medications that cause bone marrow suppression, because the combination of two medications that suppress bone marrow would greatly increase the risk of agranulocytosis. Because of potential liability, an informed consent must be obtained by clients who receive clozapine. Clients and their families need to be carefully educated about potential agranulocytosis. The Teaching Points below outlines information for clients who take clozapine. In addition to constipation, drowsiness, hypotension, nausea, seizures, anticholinergic side effects, and weight gain, clozapine has some unique side effects, which are presented in Table 15-4, along with the nursing management for each.

The side effect profile of risperidone (Risperdal) is the same as that for the classic dopamine blockers, except that the severity of side effects is considerably less. TD is theoretically possible, because risperidone creates a D_2 postsynaptic receptor blockade, but it is not as common. When doses are kept below 8 mg per day, efficacy is comparable to all the other antipsychotics, and side effects are minimal by comparison.

Contraindications

The only absolute contraindications for the antipsychotics are a history of severe blood dyscrasia or severe central nervous system (CNS) depression. The antipsychotics should also be avoided during pregnancy and lactation, whenever possible. If a client has a history of NMS, an alternate drug should be used.

TEACHING POINTS

Agranulocytosis for Client Taking Clozapine (Clozaril)

Teach the client, family, and/or significant others the following:

1. There is a 1% risk of developing agranulocytosis for clients taking clozapine (Clozaril).

2. The risk of agranulocytosis is greatest from week 4 to week 18; the risk is almost nonexistent before week 4 and after week 18.

3. To minimize the risk of agranulocytosis, a weekly blood test will be taken to measure the WBC.

4. Each week a new prescription will be written, only if the WBC is normal; if the WBC is low or falling too rapidly, the clozapine (Clozaril) may be stopped or more frequent blood tests may be ordered.

5. Agranulocytosis can be fatal.

6. Signs of a falling WBC include sore throat, sudden high fever, malaise, or infection in any part of the body. If these signs appear, the prescriber must be contacted immediately, and no more clozapine (Clozaril) should be taken.

7. When agranulocytosis occurs, it is a medical emergency and requires immediate hospitalization to protect against infection.

8. If agranulocytosis develops, the client will not be able to take clozapine (Clozaril) safely again at any time.

TABLE 15-4

Side effects of clozapine (Clozaril) and nursing management

SIDE EFFECT AND DESCRIPTION	NURSING MANAGEMENT
Fever Chronic low-grade temperature	This is most common in the first few weeks. If fever remains below 100.5°F, it is considered benign. If it rises to 100.5°F (38°C) or above, it should be worked up like any other fever. Because a high, spiking fever can be a symptom of agranulocytosis, an emergency WBC should be drawn for fever accompanied by sore throat.
Hypersalivation Excess salivation with drooling is most pronounced at night during sleep	Cover pillow with a towel at night. If severe or embarrassing, it can be treated with benztropine (Cogentin).
Tachycardia Pulse rate over 120; may be asymptomatic or may be experienced as palpitations	If client is asymptomatic and has no coronary risk factors, wait to see if heart rate returns to normal. If symptomatic or coronary risk factors are present, client may be treated with a beta-blocker.
Agranulocytosis Reduction in granulocyte count below 500 per mm³. Leukopenia is a WBC below 3,500, and neutropenia is a neutrophil count below 1,000 per mm³.	Prevention includes a weekly WBC for the duration of clozapine therapy. Teach clients to observe for signs of high, spiking fever, sores in the throat or mouth, or other signs of infection. For a WBC below 3,500, get complete blood count (CBC), two times per week and continue clozapine. For WBC below 3,000 or granulocyte count below 1,500, stop clozapine and get CBC every other day. When WBC returns to 3,500, restart clozapine. For WBC below 2,000 or granulocyte count below 1,000, discontinue clozapine immediately and do not restart at anytime.

Interactions

Important drug interactions occur with the antipsychotics. Some of the most common interaction effects include the following:

• When antipsychotics are given with another sedating medication, including alcohol, depression of the CNS is compounded.
• Antacids impede the absorption of the antipsychotics.
• Concentrated liquid antipsychotics should never be combined with liquid lithium preparations (lithium citrate) because an insoluble precipitate forms, rendering both medications unabsorbable.
• Concentrated elixir forms of perphenazine (Trilafon) and fluphenazine (Prolixin) should never be mixed with apple juice, coffee, tea, or other caffeinated beverages because a precipitate forms, making absorption of the medication erratic at best.

• Combining an antipsychotic with other anticholinergic medications increases the risk of atropine psychosis.
• Cigarette smoking or heavy consumption of alcohol or barbiturates increases hepatic metabolism, requiring larger doses of the antipsychotics.
• When added to a stable regimen of antidepressants, an antipsychotic can raise the plasma level of the antidepressant.
• When combined with an antihypertensive, an antipsychotic can cause profound hypotension.
• The antihypertensive effect of guanethidine monosulfate (Ismelin) is blocked by chlorpromazine HCl (Thorazine), haloperidol (Haldol), and thiothixenes (Navane).
• Antipsychotics lower the seizure threshold and may necessitate an increase of anticonvulsant medication for clients with seizure disorders.
• Antipsychotics may potentiate the effects of anesthetics.

THE ANTIDEPRESSANTS
Mechanism of Action

Antidepressants, as their name suggests, are most commonly used to treat major depression. They are extremely effective in alleviating the symptoms of depression for about 70% of those who take them. The antidepressants alleviate depression by increasing the activity of norepinephrine and/or serotonin in the synapses (or more specifically at the postsynaptic membrane receptors) in the part of the brain that controls mood. The non-monoamine oxidase inhibitor (MAOI) antidepressants (trycyclics and selective serotonin reuptake inhibitors [SSRIs]) accomplish this by blocking the reuptake (i.e., the removal) of norepinephrine and/or serotonin from the synapse. The MAOI antidepressants increase both norepinephrine and serotonin activity by inhibiting the enzyme (monoamine oxidase) that normally breaks down these two neurotransmitters chemically in the synapse itself.

TABLE 15-5

The antidepressants

GENERIC NAME	MOST COMMON TRADE NAME	USUAL DAILY DOSE (MG)	NEUROTRANSMITTER ACTIVITY*
Tricyclic Antidepressants			
Amitriptyline	Elavil	100-300	N,S
Amoxapine	Asendin	150-450	N,S
Desipramine	Norpramin	100-300	N
Doxepin	Sinequan	100-300	N,S
Imipramine	Tofranil	100-300	N,S
Maprotiline	Ludiomil	100-200	N
Nortriptyline	Pamelor	50-150	N,S
Protriptyline	Vivactil	15-60	N,S
Trimipramine	Surmontil	100-300	N,S
SSRI† Antidepressants			
Clomipramine	Anafranil	100-250	S
Fluoxetine	Prozac	40-80	S
Sertraline	Zoloft	50-200	S
Paroxetine	Paxil	20-50	S
Nefazodone	Serzone	200-400	S
Fluvoxamine	Luvox	100-300	S
Other Non-MAOI Antidepressants			
Trazodone	Desyrel	150-300	S
Bupropion	Wellbutrin	200-450	N,S
Venlafaxine	Effexor	75-300	N,S
Mirtazapine	Remeron	15-45	N,S
MAOI‡ Antidepressants			
Phenelzine	Nardil	15-90	N,S
Tranylcypromine	Parnate	10-30	N,S
Isocarboxazid	Marplan	10-30	N,S

*N-norepinephrine; S-serotonin   †Selective serotonin reuptake inhibitor   ‡Monoamine oxidase inhibitor

The majority of antidepressants increase both serotonin and norepinephrine activity, but many work on just one neurotransmitter. Antidepressants that activate only serotonin are called **serotonergic**. *Antidepressants that activate only noradrenalin (norepinephrine) are called* **noradrenergic** *or* **adrenergic**. *Antidepressants that activate both of these neurotransmitters are called* **nonselective**. Table 15-5 lists the subclasses of the antidepressants, and their dosages and neurotransmitter action.

Blood levels

Therapeutic blood levels of many of the tricyclic antidepressants can be measured with blood level assay. When an antidepressant is effective, there is little need to measure blood levels. However, when there is a lack of response, blood levels help guide the best intervention. The following are selected therapeutic blood levels:

- Nortriptyline (Pamelor): 50-150 ng/mL
- Desipramine (Norpramin): > 125 ng/mL
- Imipramine (Tofranil): < 180 ng/mL (combined imipramine and desipramine level)

Except for nortriptyline, blood levels of the tricyclics should be at least 100 ng/mL to be effective. Upper limits are 250–300 ng/mL, at which point side effects usually become intolerable. Blood levels are drawn in the morning before the first dose of antidepressant.

Target Symptoms

There are several subgroups of antidepressants: tricyclic antidepressants, SSRIs or serotonergics (serotonin enhancing), MAOIs, and others that do not fit into any of these categories. Regardless of class, antidepressants are used to treat symptoms of mood alteration.

Symptoms that are targeted for treatment by antidepressants are discussed in detail in Chapter 30 and include sleep and appetite disturbances, sad or anxious mood, hopelessness, helplessness, guilt, persisting loss of energy and sex drive, anhedonia, psychomotor agitation and/or retardation, trouble concentrating, and preoccupation with death or suicide. It should be noted that symptoms of disorders other than mood disorders are effectively treated with these pharmacological agents. For example, symptoms of obsessive-compulsive disorder (OCD) respond well to serotonin-enhancing drugs such as paroxetine (Paxil) and nefazodone (Serzone). Imipramine (Tofranil) is used in the management of severe pain.

Guidelines for Use

The choice of a particular drug for treatment of depression is determined by a client's target symptoms, differences in side effects of the drugs, and whether a close relative has had a positive response to a particular drug. Clinically, antidepressants are generally used in oral forms, although injectable forms are available for several.

As a general rule, antidepressant dosing begins low and builds to therapeutic levels. The initial dose is usually the smallest available oral tablet or capsule. The dose is raised slowly, usually twice a week, until it is within the therapeutic dosage range. Once a therapeutic range is reached and if there is minimal discomfort from side effects, the dose should remain stable for 6 to 8 weeks. If symptoms diminish, clients usually remain on the drug for longer periods.

In clients with a positive history of heart disease or in elderly clients at risk for stroke or myocardial infarction (MI), antidepressants must be used in smaller, divided doses, with cautious increases monitored by serial ECGs. These clients also need to be monitored continuously by a cardiologist or internist and are usually hospitalized to initiate and stabilize antidepressant treatment. Antidepressants should be avoided in clients with known cardiac conduction defects or histories of recent MIs. The best alternative for clients with cardiac disease may be electroconvulsive therapy (ECT) (see Chapter 30).

When clients have a good response to antidepressants, their depressive symptoms sometimes disappear abruptly. Clients with this kind of response will one morning report their amazement that overnight they have returned to their normal, nondepressed state. More commonly, the antidepressant response is gradual. Clients first begin to appear better to others as their grooming and affect improve. Others compliment them on their improvement, and they protest that they do not feel better. Gradually, as time passes, they regain the ability to sleep and eat normally, and eventually, they experience a subjective feeling of improvement in mood. Full recovery for some severely depressed clients may take 6 months to 1 year or more, and many clients remain on medication for life.

One of the hardest features of the antidepressants for clients to tolerate is the **lag period** *of 1 to 6 weeks (sometimes even longer in the geriatric population) between starting the medication and feeling symptom relief.* Because clients usually try all other means of obtaining relief before entering the health care system and accepting antidepressants, they are usually extremely depressed and desperate at the time they begin the medication. When they learn that they will only feel side effects for the first few weeks without any lifting of the depression, they often feel overwhelming despair and hopelessness and should be monitored carefully. The suicide risk for clients on antidepressant therapy is greatest when therapeutic effects increase energy levels.

Side Effects

Side effects of non-MAOIs

Side effects of antidepressants can be troubling for clients. Some of the side effects of the non-MAOI antidepressants are caused by the medications' effects on the same neurotransmitter systems that cause relief from depression. For example, serotonergic antidepressants cause nausea specifically because of the postsynaptic serotonin blockage. On the other hand, most of the antidepressants also affect neurotransmitter systems that cause side effects without adding to their antidepressant effects. A good example is the anticholinergic side effect cluster that includes dry mouth, nasal congestion, blurred vision, constipation, and urinary hesitancy. The highest incidence of anticholinergic effects occurs in clients who take amitriptyline (Elavil), protriptyline (Vivactil), trimipramine (Surmontil), and doxepin (Sinequan).

Like the antipsychotic agents, the non-MAOI antidepressants can cause atropine psychosis. Use of tricyclic antidepressants may also exacerbate chronic (wide angle) glaucoma or precipitate acute (narrow angle) glaucoma. The latter requires emergency and ongoing treatment with cholinergic eye drops or other miotic agents.

Several other side effects of non-MAOI antidepressants are similar to those of the antipsychotics. Table 15-6 lists these side effects and the drugs that most often cause them. Nursing management is found in Table 15-2.

The side effects of the non-MAOI antidepressants appear in the first 1 to 2 weeks of treatment and/or after a dose increase. They are tolerable to most clients and diminish over a period of a few weeks or months until the client barely notices them.

The development and use of the SSRIs have a higher incidence of compliance, in part because of their low side effect profiles. They may cause agitation or anxiety, headache, nausea, vomiting, and insomnia. Of note is serotonin syndrome, a potentially life-threatening condition that occurs when there is inadequate washout between trials of MAOIs and SSRIs or when a client is extremely sensitive to the increased serotonin activity from SSRIs. Symptoms include restlessness, agitation, diaphoresis, hyperreflexia, myoclonus, tremor, rigidity, nausea, diarrhea, abdominal cramping, insomnia, fever, and autonomic instability. When severe, it can progress to delirium and coma. Cyproheptadine (Periactin), a serotonin antagonist, is used to counteract these side effects when they occur.

Side effects of MAOIs

The most common side effects of the MAOI antidepressants are weight gain, orthostatic hypotension, sedation, anticholinergic side effects, and insomnia. However the most severe side effect is *hypertensive crisis, a sudden, severe increase in blood pressure caused by high*

TABLE 15-6

Side effects of antidepressants and the drugs that cause them

SIDE EFFECT	DRUGS
Sweating	Imipramine (Tofranil)
	Buproprion (Wellbutrin)
Alterations in sexual functioning	All SSRIs, all MAOIs
Cardiac effects (palpitations, dysrhythmias, heart blockage, and congestive heart failure)	Amitriptyline (Elavil)
	Trimipramine (Surmontil)
	Imipramine
	Other tricyclics that have quinidine-like effects
Orthostatic hypotension	Imipramine
Sedation	Amitriptyline
	Trazodone (Desyrel)
	Amoxapine (Asendin)
	Doxepin (Sinequan)
Seizures	Maprotiline (Ludiomil)
	Buproprion
	Clomipramine (Anafranil)
Weight gain	Amitriptyline
	Doxepin

tyramine levels, which occurs when prohibited foods or medications are ingested. Without immediate measures to control blood pressure, intracranial hemorrhage and death may result. Warning signs of hypertensive crisis include throbbing occipital headache, stiff neck, chills, nausea, flushing of skin, fever, apprehension, retroorbital pain, pallor, sweating, chest pain, and palpitations. Emergency treatment for hypertensive crisis usually consists of IV administration of phentolamine (Regitine) repeated as necessary to control blood pressure. Alternatives include beta-blockers and one of the calcium channel blockers, nifedipine (Procardia), both of which have shown promise in the treatment of hypertensive crisis. Any client having this reaction should rest in a quiet, darkened room, disturbed only for frequent vital signs. Fever is managed with external cooling techniques.

Occasionally, outpatient clients are given a small oral dose of chlorpromazine (Thorazine) to carry at all times in case they accidentally ingest a forbidden food and experience the symptoms of hypertensive crisis. The chlorpromazine will temporarily reduce the blood pressure until the client can reach professional help. The danger with this particular approach is that the client may have rebound hypotension that makes it dangerous to travel for help.

Contraindications and Interactions

Absolute contraindications to antidepressant use are severe CNS depression, including coma or near-comatose states; unstable cardiac dysrhythmias; and severe cardiac conduction defects. With the MAOI antidepressants, rarely the antidepressant of first choice because of interaction of MAOIs and tyramine, the client must faithfully adhere both to a restrictive low-tyramine diet and to some important medication restrictions. Because of these requirements, MAOI antidepressants are usually used only when trials of other antidepressants fail.

BOX 15-2

Tyramine-Restricted Diet for MAOI Antidepressants

The following foods must be avoided:

DAIRY FOODS

Cheese pizza, sour cream, yogurt, and all cheeses except cream and cottage cheese

MEATS AND PROTEIN-RICH FOODS

Beef and chicken livers, unrefrigerated fermented sausage, summer sausage, bologna, salami, pepperoni, tofu, pickled fish, pickled herring, lox, caviar, dried salted herring, and other smoked fish

VEGETABLES AND FRUITS

Broad bean pods, fava beans, Italian green beans, snow pea pods, sauerkraut, avocados

DESSERTS, SWEETS

Chocolate cake, cookies, ice cream, pudding, or chocolate candy

ALCOHOLIC BEVERAGES

Chianti wine, sherry, red wine, burgundy, ale, beer, vermouth, sauterne, Reisling, liqueurs

FATS

Avocados, salad dressings with cheese or monosodium glutamate (MSG)

OTHERS

Food containing brewer's yeast or yeast extract (i.e., some soups, sauces, relishes, gravies); monosodium glutamate; meat tenderizers; yeast vitamin supplements; hydrolyzed protein extracts used as a base for soup, gravy or sauce; soy sauce

---

BOX 15-3

Medications To Be Avoided When Taking an MAOI Antidepressant

- Sympathomimetics including amphetamines, ephedrine, pseudoephedrine, norephedrine, phenylephrine, all catecholamines, L-dopa, and methylphenidate
- General anesthetics
- Local or spinal anesthetics that contain epinephrine or levonordefrin (e.g., Novocaine, Xylocaine)
- Over-the-counter cough, cold, and sinus medications (tablets, capsules, or sprays) that contain sympathomimetics (e.g., Actifed, Sudafed, Contact, Dristan, Neosynephrine spray, Afrin, NyQuil, Dimetapp, Coricidin, Triaminic, and so on)
- Meperidine (Demerol) and narcotic pain killers that contain codeine, morphine, or hydrocodone (e.g., Percocet, Percodan)
- Cocaine
- Reserpine (Serpasil), alpha-methyl-dopa, and guanethidine monosulfate (Ismelin)
- Other antidepressants and MAOIs including pargyline (Eutonyl), nitrofurantoin (Macrolantin) antibiotics, and procarbazine (Matulane)
- Serotonergic antidepressants (e.g., clomipramine [Anafranil], fluoxetine [Prozac], sertraline [Zoloft], paroxetine [Paxil], fluvoxamine [Luvox], nefazodone [Serzone], and venlafaxine [Effexor])

Tyramine is a substance that occurs naturally in a variety of foods. It is a pressor substance, which is a chemical that elevates blood pressure to a normal level. In most persons, it is degraded by the enzyme monoamine oxidase so that it does not cause hypertension. However, when monoamine oxidase is inhibited by an MAOI, an increased amount of tyramine is available and raises blood pressure inexorably, causing a potentially fatal hypertensive crisis. Box 15-2 lists the foods that must be eliminated for clients taking MAOIs. In addition to avoiding the specific foods listed, it is important for clients to restrict aged, pickled, smoked, or overripe foods of any kind. All foods must be refrigerated and eaten when they are fresh, because poor refrigeration and aging increase the tyramine content of foods that already contain it. Box 15-3 lists the medications that must be avoided to prevent similar life-threatening interactions. These food and medication restrictions can be very inconvenient for clients and usually require extensive teaching.

MOOD STABILIZERS

Two types of drugs are currently used as mood stabilizers: lithium, one of the oldest drugs used in psychiatry, and the anticonvulsants, drugs used to treat seizure disorders. Each is discussed separately.

All mood stabilizers perform what seems to be a dual function: they elevate mood when a client is experiencing depression and they dampen mood when a client is in a manic episode. In other words, mood stabilizers target the symptoms of a major depressive episode when a client is in that state, and they target the symptoms of a manic or hypomanic episode when a client is experiencing that mood state. When the client is in a normal mood state, the mood stabilizer prevents instability in the direction of either mania or depression.

For any one medication to perform these seemingly opposite functions is counterintuitive. Yet mood stabilizers become more understandable if normal mood is seen as the stable condition and both mania and depression are seen as the result of a dysregulation or instability caused by a failure of the mood to automatically revert to normal when temporarily altered by life events. *Mood stabilizers keep the mood regulated. By chemically stabilizing the membranes in the brain, they allow the mood to regulate itself properly; that is, they allow the mood to automatically revert to normal when temporarily too high or low.* Some clients who fail on all mood stabilizing agents have benefited from the calcium channel blocker verapamil (Calan).

Lithium

Lithium is a medication that is like no other in psychiatry. It is a natural salt found in the form of lithium carbonate and used in that same form medicinally. It exists in most lakes, rivers, and streams and can be found in heavy concentration in rock formations around the world. Because it is so widespread, most persons have at least trace amounts of lithium in the bloodstream.

Mechanism of action

When persons take lithium as a medication, it has many different effects on their bodies. It alters or stabilizes neurotransmitter activity in their brains. More specifically, it normalizes or stabilizes synaptic transmission of norepinephrine, serotonin, and dopamine. Lithium also inhibits the release of thyroid hormone and testosterone and rebalances disturbed circadian rhythms. Its effectiveness as a mood stabilizer is likely to be the result of several of these factors.

When any lithium preparation is absorbed by the body, the lithium ion splits off, distributes evenly throughout the body via the bloodstream, and is excreted by the kidneys. The serum half-life under ordinary conditions is about 24 hours.

Target symptoms

What is known about lithium is that it is a powerful mood stabilizer. Lithium is used primarily in the treatment of bipolar I and II disorders, both in the acute manic and depressive episodes, and as prophylaxis against further episodes. In bipolar disorder, it either stops manic and depressive episodes altogether, or makes them milder, shorter, and less frequent. Chapter 30 lists target symptoms and discusses nursing management of them.

Lithium is also used to treat major depression, either by itself or in small doses combined with one of the antidepressants. In addition to its use in treating bipolar disorder, lithium is known to reduce the severity and frequency of rage outbursts in intermittent explosive disorder and to reduce impulsivity and mood lability in personality disorders. It is used to stabilize mood in schizoaffective disorder and occasionally to treat schizophrenia in combination with an antipsychotic.

Guidelines for use

Lithium is available in several forms: tablets and capsules that are regular or slow-release, and in liquid form. Lithium is not available in injectable forms. The solid form is lithium carbonate, and the liquid form is lithium citrate. The liquid form is used for persons who are unable to swallow solid forms and occasionally in the beginning of treatment to ensure compliance in clients who "cheek" or "tongue" their medications, that is, they hide the tablets or capsules under their tongues or in their cheeks to avoid swallowing them. Lithium citrate, the liquid form, should not be mixed with any other antipsychotic liquid medication because a precipitate forms that renders both drugs ineffective.

The solid form is the most commonly used. When

BOX 15-4

Baseline Workup for the Client Beginning Lithium Therapy

Medical and psychiatric history
Physical examination
Thyroid function tests: T3, T4, and/or thyroid-stimulating
  hormone (TSH)
• Kidney function tests: serum creatinine in the elderly
• Fasting blood sugar (FBS)
• Electrocardiogram (ECG)
• Chest X ray
• Serum electrolytes
• Complete blood count (CBC)
• Blood urea nitrogen (BUN)

standard lithium carbonate causes severe side effects within 1 to 3 hours after the dose is taken (the time when the blood level peaks), it sometimes helps to change to a slow-release form. Slow-release forms cause a more gradual increase in blood level without the intense peaks that cause discomfort for some persons.

Before lithium therapy is begun, a baseline workup is completed (Box 15-4). These tests are usually repeated every 6 months to 1 year throughout the course of lithium treatment to detect any changes resulting from prolonged lithium administration. If the client has a history of heart disease or any other condition that affects electrolyte balance, further pretesting is required. Lithium is started at a low dose. Young and middle-age adults begin with between 600 mg and 1,200 mg per day and the elderly with 150 to 300 mg per day. The dose is gradually increased by 300 mg every few days until a therapeutic blood level is reached. For most persons, lithium becomes effective at a blood level somewhere between 0.5 and 1.5 mEq/L.

Lithium is usually given in divided doses throughout the day, although some persons can take it in a single dose, usually at bedtime. For clients who can tolerate the peak in blood level after a large single dose, it is thought that the lithium may be less likely to impair the kidney's ability to concentrate urine. Many clients find the side effects of a single daily dose uncomfortable or even intolerable and prefer divided doses.

Lithium takes at least 1 week to begin working, but may take 4 weeks or more before a stable therapeutic level is achieved and a symptom-free state occurs. Because many clients are in severely abnormal mood states when lithium is begun, they may need to receive adjunctive medications until the lithium begins to work. It is common to treat clients in a manic state either with a sedative-hypnotic such as lorazepam (Ativan) or with an antipsychotic such as haloperidol (Haldol) until such

time as the lithium stabilizes the mood. Once the mood is stabilized, the adjunctive medication(s) can be discontinued.

When clients have a favorable response to lithium, they continue to take it indefinitely. The disorders treated by lithium are lifelong illnesses and require lifelong treatment. Because most of lithium's side effects are either reversible or treatable, a long course of treatment is almost always safe, if carefully monitored.

Compliance may be especially difficult when lithium is used to treat bipolar disorder. Clients describe missing the excitement, the inflated sense of self-esteem and well-being, the creativity, and the extraordinary energy of the hypomanic state. Many clients either discontinue their lithium or reduce the dose hoping to achieve a hypomanic state without sliding into true mania. During full-fledged mania, most clients agree, there is far too much turmoil and chaos to be creative or productive or even to feel good. The problem with trying to lower the lithium dose to achieve hypomania is that very few persons can manage to remain in the hypomanic state. Persons who attempt it either become depressed or fully manic in a short time.

Lithium serum levels In an acute manic or depressive state the lithium serum level should range from 1.0 to 1.5 mEq/L for symptoms to abate. Once symptoms are under control, the dosage and blood level can be lowered for stabilization and prevention of future episodes. Higher dosages are needed by young clients and clients with high body weight. However, elderly clients whose renal functions have slowed with age, clients with low body weight, and clients with renal impairments need a far smaller dose to maintain therapeutic blood levels.

Initially, the lithium level is measured once or twice per week. Later, when the lithium dose and serum level are stabilized, lithium levels only need to be drawn every few months. Blood levels are always drawn about 12 hours after the last dose of lithium. If they are drawn at a time any closer or farther away from the last dose, the level will be erroneously high or low and will not be a helpful guide for adjusting the dose.

Side effects

Lithium is considered a safe and effective drug for the treatment of bipolar disorders. Like all drugs, it has troublesome side effects. The most common side effects of lithium and the nursing management for them are listed in Table 15-7. Many involve kidney function, because the drug is excreted through the kidney. Bipolar disorders are chronic illnesses, and mood stabilizers are used by clients for a lifetime. Long-term use of the drug has an impact on body systems other than the brain. The most common risks of long-term lithium use are hypothyroidism and inability of the kidney to concentrate urine.

TABLE 15-7

Side effects of lithium and nursing management

SIDE EFFECT AND DESCRIPTION	NURSING MANAGEMENT
Polyuria, with possible progression to nephrogenic diabetes insipidus—urine output is large in volume and so dilute that it may be colorless; client may complain of urinating so often that it interferes with activities of daily living (ADLs), including sleep	Inform client that increased urination is common and benign. Urine volume may diminish if the prescriber reduces the lithium dose or changes to a slow-release form, or a single daily dose. When severe, polyuria is often treated with a thiazide or potassium-sparing diuretic, and the lithium dose is reduced.
Increased thirst (polydipsia)	Recommend that clients quench their thirst and maintain a fairly stable intake of 8 cups or glasses of liquids per day. The best thirst quencher is water or a low-calorie beverage that will not cause weight gain. Gum or hard candies may help moisten the mouth.
Fine hand tremor: Worsens with intentional movements; it can make writing, drinking hot beverages, and many other motor tasks difficult	Tremors are persistent in some clients. When tremors are severe or incapacitating, the prescriber may treat them with a beta-blocker. Recommend to reduction or elimination caffeine-containing beverages.
Nausea, abdominal discomfort, diarrhea, or soft stools	Recommend that client take lithium with meals, a glass of milk, or a snack.
Muscle weakness or fatigue	Because this is not a common side effect of lithium, ascertain if it is being caused by another medication. Encourage client to remain active and get regular physical exercise.
Edema of the feet, hands, face, or other body parts	A moderate salt restriction may reduce the edema. If moderate salt restriction is undertaken, the serum lithium level usually rises somewhat, and toxicity may occur
Hypothyroidism	Inform client that this is reversible and treatable. The prescriber usually orders thyroid hormone replacement, such as levothyroxine (Synthroid) or dessicated thyroid.
Weight gain	Moderate calorie restriction and increased exercise usually help. Advise against fluid restriction or sodium restriction, unless undertaken with knowledge of prescriber.
Hair thinning or loss	Because hair loss can be a symptom of hypothyroidism, inform prescriber so thyroid functioning can be checked. If hair does not return, lithium is usually stopped so hair can regrow.
Benign, reversible granulocytosis	This side effect is the basis for use of lithium treatment in some granulocytopenic conditions.
Mild hypoglycemia	This may mask mild diabetes mellitus and is usually treated with diet and exercise. Lithium is usually continued.

Lithium toxicity One of the risks of lithium administration is *lithium toxicity, which refers to the toxic effects that occur when the serum lithium level becomes too high.* The level that is therapeutic differs from person to person, but for all clients, the difference between the therapeutic and toxic levels is small. During the acute manic phase, the serum level often has to be as high as 1.0 to 1.5 mEq/L to terminate the manic episode. Once a person is stabilized and being maintained, the level can often be as low as 0.6 to 0.8 mEq/L or lower and still provide excellent mood stabilization. When the serum level goes higher than what is normal for an individual client, signs of toxicity begin to appear. The signs of lithium toxicity are listed in Box 15-5 and range from milder symptoms at slight levels of elevation to grand mal seizures, collapse, and death at higher serum levels (2.5 to 5.0 mEq/L and higher). Fortunately, severe lithium toxicity is rare and can be prevented with careful education of the client.

The serum half-life of lithium is approximately 24 hours, so the level comes down rapidly when no more lithium is taken. Therefore clients taking lithium need to be taught that missed doses should be skipped altogether and never made up. Hemodialysis is an effective method of removing lithium from the bloodstream. When toxicity becomes that severe, it is important to monitor vital signs, intake and output, and fluid and electrolyte balance. Bed rest is essential at higher levels because of clouded consciousness, and it is helpful even with mild toxicity.

One of the most common causes of toxicity is an abrupt change in serum sodium. Lithium competes with sodium for reabsorption in the proximal tubules of the kidney, so when sodium is scarce, the kidneys reabsorb lithium in its place. It is important to keep the intake of liquids and salty foods at a consistent level to maintain a stable lithium level. Lithium toxicity can also result from anything that causes hemoconcentration, such as prolonged vomiting, diarrhea, and dehydration, by some drug interactions or by intentional or accidental overdose. Clients and families require careful teaching about lithium toxicity and its symptoms and management. Teaching Points for educating clients and their families are presented on p. 281.

Contraindications

Lithium is contraindicated in acute renal failure. It is used cautiously in chronic renal failure, cardiovascular disease, cerebellar disorders, diabetes mellitus, electrolyte imbalance, and hypertension. It may aggravate the course of myasthenia gravis, Parkinsons disease, ulcerative colitis, psoriasis, acne, goiter, and osteoporosis. As a general rule, it should be avoided during pregnancy and lactation. When it is taken by a woman during the first trimester of pregnancy, a slight increase in cardiac abnormalities in the fetus has been reported.

Interactions

When a client takes an antipsychotic and lithium concomitantly, a neurotoxic picture of either lithium toxicity (from the lithium) or NMS (from the antipsychotic) may be diagnosed. It was once thought that this neurotoxic syndrome was an interaction between the two medications. Current thinking is that antipsychotics and lithium combine well and have no significant interaction. Clients should be examined for both NMS and lithium toxicity, diagnosed with one or the other, and treated accordingly.

Lithium does, however, interact in potentially dangerous ways with several other medications. The most important interactions seen clinically are the following:

- When liquid antipsychotics and liquid lithium citrate are combined, they form an insoluble precipitate from which neither medication can be absorbed.
- Ibuprofen (Advil, Motrin) raises the lithium level to the point of toxicity in some persons.
- The lithium level can rise as high as twice its level if a diuretic is added. The result is lithium toxicity. Exceptions to this rule are osmotic diuretics and aminophylline, both of which reduce the lithium level.

BOX 15-5

Signs of Lithium Toxicity

Diarrhea
Nausea and vomiting
Difficulty walking or inability to walk
Poor motor coordination
Sluggishness, lethargy, drowsiness
Slurred speech
Ringing in ears
Blurred vision
Marked tremor
Muscle weakness
Frank muscle twitching
Involuntary cyclical movements of eyeballs
Difficulty speaking
Muscle twitching
Increased deep tendon reflexes
Visual or tactile hallucinations
Oliguria, anuria
Confusion or seriously impaired consciousness
Jerking or snakelike movements of the extremities
Grand mal seizures
Coma or death

Signs and Symptoms That May Indicate Lithium Toxicity

Teach the client, family, and/or significant others the following:

1. Lithium toxicity is an uncommon but potential side effect of lithium.

2. Early signs and symptoms of lithium toxicity include diarrhea, nausea, vomiting, poor coordination, drowsiness, slurred speech, tremor, weakness, muscle twitching, and confusion.

3. Lithium toxicity can be fatal when it is severe.

4. If there is suspicion of lithium toxicity, no doses of lithium should be taken until prescriber is reached for advice. If toxicity is suspected, prescriber should be called immediately.

5. Lithium toxicity is best prevented by maintaining a stable amount of sodium in the diet and by drinking at least 8 cups or glasses of liquids every day—more if thirst persists. Liquid intake should be fairly stable from day to day.

6. A client should tell all health care providers that he or she takes lithium so that no other medications are prescribed that interact with lithium in such a way as to cause toxicity.

7. Avoid ibuprofen (Advil, Motrin) because it raises lithium levels in some persons.

• When alcohol intake is limited to two drinks, it has minimal effect on lithium level. Drinking alcohol in excess reduces lithium levels because of alcohol's diuretic action. This is a considerable risk for persons who ordinarily drink in excess of one or two drinks, because lithium masks the signs of alcohol intoxication.

• Tetracycline, methyldopa (Aldomet), phenylbutazone, indomethacin (Indocin), or piroxicam (Feldene) can raise lithium levels.

• Lithium can prolong the neuromuscular blockage of succinylcholine and pancuronium and should therefore be discontinued before any surgical procedure involving muscular relaxation by these agents.

• Neurotoxicity can result from combining calcium channel blockers with lithium, so the combination should be prescribed cautiously.

• When combined with carbamazepine (Tegretol), lithium clearance is decreased, and lithium toxicity may result.

• When combined with verapamil (Calan), neurotoxicity may occur.

Anticonvulsants

There is a large group of clients who cannot, for one reason or another, benefit from lithium. For these clients, who either are not helped by or cannot tolerate lithium, the most common alternatives to lithium are the anticonvulsant medications listed in Table 15-8.

Carbamazepine (Tegretol) is the most commonly used alternative to lithium, although sodium valproate (Depakote) is more comfortable in terms of side effects for many people, and it too is widely used. Valproic acid (De-

pakene) is rarely used, not because it is less effective than the others, but because it is more likely than sodium valproate to upset the stomach. Valproic acid and sodium valproate are often spoken of collectively as valproate.

Clonazepam (Klonopin) is an anticonvulsant member of the benzodiazepine family (see the antianxiety agents section that follows). It may have mood stabilizing properties, and it certainly is an effective sedative-hypnotic for clients either in a manic state or an agitated depressed state. Clonazepam is rarely used alone as a mood stabilizer. It is almost always combined with either lithium, carbamazepine, or valproate. It is often necessary for sedation in the treatment of acute episodes of mania or depression because the other mood stabilizers do not begin to work for at least 1 week. Because it is a benzodiazepine, there is the risk of **dependence (physiological addiction)** and the danger of abrupt withdrawal symptoms. Nonetheless, some clients with bipolar disorder continue to take it as a part of their long-term regimen of prophylaxis because their mood is most stable when clonazepam is included as part of the regimen.

Mechanism of Action

It is not clear what the exact mechanism of action is for the anticonvulsant mood stabilizers, but there is an interesting theory. These medications may work to stabilize mood using the same mechanism they use to prevent seizures but in a different part of the brain.

A seizure is a rapid and uncontrolled spread of an electrochemical message or impulse in the brain. It can be compared with a huge lightning bolt that originates from a small electrical event but spreads rapidly and forcefully into the surrounding area. Essentially, anticonvulsant medications prevent seizures by preventing the

TABLE 15-8

Anticonvulsants

GENERIC NAME	MOST COMMON TRADE NAME	USUAL DAILY DOSE (MG)	SERUM LEVEL (μ/ML)
Carbamazepine	Tegretol	800-1,200	4-12
Valproic acid	Depakene	750-5,000	50-100
Sodium valproate	Depakote	750-5,000	50-100
Clonazepam	Klonopin	1.5-20	—

lightninglike spread of small impulses in the motor areas of the brain. They do this by stabilizing the membranes in the brain, that is by changing the electrochemical balance in the cell membranes of the brain so that electrical impulses cannot spread easily. If electrochemical impulses cannot spread, then there can be no seizure.

When a client is switched from lithium to another mood stabilizer, the lithium must be discontinued slowly and gradually over a period of several weeks. At the same time the lithium is reduced, either carbamazepine or valproate is started and the dose is slowly and gradually raised. Starting doses are generally 200 to 400 mg per day for carbamazepine and 500 to 1,500 mg per day for valproate. If these doses are tolerated well, the dose is raised once or twice a week as tolerated until blood levels are within therapeutic range. Doses are divided at the beginning of treatment and usually remain divided into at least two doses per day to minimize discomfort from side effects. The bulk of the dose can be given at bedtime to prevent daytime sleepiness and to enhance nighttime sleep.

Target symptoms

Target symptoms for the anticonvulsant mood stabilizers are identical to those for lithium. Like lithium, they treat the symptoms of acute episodes of depression or mania and also provide prophylaxis against future manic episodes. In addition to treating bipolar disorders, mood stabilizers are used extensively to treat aggression and control seizures.

Guidelines for use

The use of anticonvulsant drugs presents a contemporary option for the treatment of mood disorders. Lithium is effective in about 70% of persons who take it. There is evidence that in clients with rapid cycles, that is, clients who have four or more cycles of abnormal mood per year, lithium is less effective. Lithium is less effective for

persons with pronounced mixed states—states with features of severe depression and mania either coexisting or rapidly alternating with one another. Finally, some clients with bipolar disorders find that lithium is effective in the early stages of illness, but that as the years progress, lithium by itself no longer provides the stability it did earlier in life.

There are also a number of clients who cannot take lithium because they cannot tolerate one or more of the side effects, for example, a severe exacerbation of psoriasis or nephrogenic diabetes insipidus that does not respond to the usual treatments.

Side effects and interactions

Side effects of carbamazepine includes nausea, vomiting, sedation, dizziness, light-headedness, clumsiness, ataxia, rash, blurred vision, dry mouth, urinary retention or hesitency, and bone marrow suppression. The nursing management of most of these side effects can be found in Table 15-2. The most serious side effect is bone marrow suppression, which, because it can be life-threatening, must be the subject of careful teaching (see Teaching Points on p. 283). With carbamazepine, platelet and white and/or red cell counts can be suppressed.

The side effects of valproate include nausea, vomiting, sedation, weight gain, tremor, temporary hair thinning or loss, diarrhea, and reduced platelet count (thrombocytopenia). With valproate, the platelet count is the most likely element to be suppressed. Symptoms of decreased platelet count include easy bleeding, bruising, and petechiae.

Nurses need to be aware of the drug interactions that occur with the anticonvulsants. Interactions with carbamazepine and valproate include the following:

- They cannot be combined with another bone marrow-suppressing medication (e.g., clozapine) because the risk of agranulocytosis and other syn-

Signs and Symptoms of Bone Marrow Suppression with Carbamazepine (Tegretol) and Valproate (Depakote)

Teach the client, family, and/or significant others the following:

1. Bone marrow suppression can occur at any time during treatment.

2. Bone marrow supression can be life-threatening.

3. If bone marrow suppression is suspected, avoid taking another dose until prescriber is contacted for advice.

4. Three kinds of blood cells that can be suppressed are produced by the bone marrow: red blood cells, white blood cells, and platelets.

5. If too few red blood cells are being produced by bone marrow, anemia results with symptoms of pallor, weakness, tiredness, and fatigue.

6. If the white blood cell production is suppressed, it is difficult to fight infection. Symptoms usually include sudden onset of a high fever (over 100.4°F [38°C]), sore throat, and malaise.

7. If platelet production is affected, blood clotting is slowed. Symptoms include easy bruising or bleeding, usually most noticeable as bleeding gums after tooth brushing, or bruises or petechiae on the arms and legs.

dromes of profound bone marrow suppression increase dramatically.

- When they are combined with erythromycin, cimetidine (Tagamet), isoniazid, or propoxyphene (Darvon), plasma carbamazepine levels may rise.
- When they are combined with verapamil (Calan), plasma carbamazepine levels rise.
- When they are combined with lithium, the lithium level may increase. Phenobarb, phenytoin, or primidone may decrease carbamazepine effects.

ANTIANXIETY AGENTS

There are many classes of drugs used to treat anxiety. These include benzodiazepines, barbiturates, and oth-

ers. Historically, these classes of drugs were referred to as minor tranquilizers because of their sedative-hypnotic effects. Although the use of benzodiazepines has declined in the last decade, they are still among the most widely used of all drugs. They are prescribed most often in primary care settings (85% of their use) rather than in psychiatric settings. Some of these drugs are marketed specifically for their antianxiety, sedative, or hypnotic effects, but in practice, any of these drugs can be used interchangeably for anxiety, sedation, or sleep simply by increasing or decreasing the dose. The drugs are classified by their chemical structures. Table 15-9 lists each of the commonly used classes, the medications, and their hypnotic and sedating doses.

Mechanism of Action

Antianxiety agents are CNS depressants. The most commonly used members of this class of medications are the benzodiazepines. They work by potentiating a major inhibitory neurotransmitter called gamma-aminobutyric acid (GABA). As a result, the overall excitability of the CNS is reduced in a safe and effective way.

Benzodiazepines

Although benzodiazepines are all equally effective in their sedative-hypnotic actions, they differ from one another in their metabolism, speed of onset, and half-life. The onset of action seems to depend on their rapidity of absorption, which can vary from less than 1 hour for diazepam (Valium) to 6 hours or more for prazepam (Centrax). Once they are absorbed, most undergo transformation in the liver to one or more active metabolites with a range of half-lives. Exceptions are lorazepam (Ativan), oxazepam (Serax), and possibly alprazolam (Xanax), which have no active metabolites and are, therefore, more easily metabolized and excreted. It is this property that makes these three agents safer for clients who have difficulty with the metabolism and excretion of drugs, such as the elderly, and those with severe liver disease.

Barbiturates

The barbiturates are a large, fairly old and well-known group of drugs that are derived from barbituric acid. Phenobarbital is the barbiturate most often prescribed because of its common use as an anticonvulsant. Barbiturates have been used far longer than other psychotropic medications in current use; consequently, for many years they were used as general sedatives for anyone in need of behavioral control.

Like the other members of this drug class, the barbiturates are CNS depressants. They have a number of disadvantages in comparison to the benzodiazepines and

TABLE 15-9

Antianxiety agents

GENERIC NAME	MOST COMMON BRAND NAME	HYPNOTIC DOSAGE (MG)	SEDATIVE DOSE (TOTAL DAILY DOSAGE IN MG)	ORAL ABSORPTION	HALF-LIFE (HRS)
Benzodiazepines					
Alprazolam	Xanax	—	0.75-4	Intermediate	12
Chlordiazepoxide	Librium	25	15-60	Intermediate	18
Clonazepam	Klonopin	1.5-10	1.5-10	Slow to intermediate	34
Clorazepate	Tranxene	—	15-60	Rapid	100
Diazepam	Valium	10	5-40	Rapid	60
Flurazepam	Dalmane	15-30		Intermediate	75
Halazepam	Paxipam	—	20-120	Slow	
Lorazepam	Ativan	2-4	1-6	Intermediate	15
Oxazepam	Serax	10-30	45-120	Slow to intermediate	8
Prazepam	Centrax	10-20	20-60	Slow	100
Quazepam	Doral	—	7.5-15		
Temazepam	Restoril	15-30	15-30	Slow to intermediate	10
Triazolam	Halcion	0.125-0.5	0.125-0.5	Intermediate	3
Barbiturates					
Amobarbital	Amytal	100-200	60-150	Slow	8-42
Butabarbital	Butisol	50-100	45-120	Slow	34-42
Pentobarbital	Nembutal	100-200	90-120	Intermediate	15-48
Phenobarbital	Luminal	100-200	30-90	Rapid	24
Secobarbital	Seconal	100-200	90-200	Intermediate	19-34
Nonbenzodiazepine, Nonbarbiturate Propanediols					
Meprobamate	Equanil	800	400-1,600		10
Tybamate	Solacen	—	500-1,500		
Quinazolines					
Methaqualone	Quaalude	150-300	250-300		10-42
Acetylinic Alcohols					
Ethchlorvynol	Placidyl	500-1,000	200-600		10-25
Piperidinedione Derivatives					
Glutethimide	Doriden	250-500	125-750		5-22
Methyprylon	Noludar	200-400	150-400		
Chloral Derivatives					
Chloral hydrate	Noctec	500-2,000	500-1,000		4-10
Chloral betaine	Beta-Chlor	870-1,000			
Triclofos	Triclos	750-1,500			
Monoureides					
Paraldehyde	Paral	3,000-8,000	1,200-6,000		
New compounds					
Buspirone	BuSpar		15-25		2-11
Zolpidem	Ambien	5-10			2.5

are, therefore, less commonly used. Their disadvantages include the following:

- *More rapid development of tolerance and physical dependence (phenobarbital is an exception to this rule)*—When used as hypnotics, there is conclusive evidence that the barbiturates are effective for a maximum of 7–14 consecutive nights.
- *Narrow margin of safety*—The hypnotic dose is only three to four times the sedative dose. As tolerance develops, the effective dose approaches the lethal dose. This does not occur with the benzodiazepines. Barbiturates are also far more likely than benzodiazepines to be fatal in overdose.
- *Greater degree of sedation and hangover*
- *Induction of hepatic enzymes, causing marked interference with the metabolism of many other drugs including but not limited to anticoagulants and other psychotropic drugs*—This occurs to a much lesser degree with the benzodiazepines.
- *Suppression of REM sleep with rebound after discontinuation, characterized by intense dreaming or nightmares*—This is far less pronounced with the benzodiazepines.

Nonbenzodiazepines, nonbarbiturates

There is another large group of fairly old drugs that is being prescribed less since the advent of the benzodiazepines. The National Institute of Drug Abuse (NIDA) takes the position that although these drugs are as effective as other antianxiety agents, they offer no advantage over barbiturates or benzodiazepines and may lead to serious ***toxicity*** *(a condition resulting from ingesting a substance that results in poisoning)*. The disadvantages of this group include the following:

- They present a high risk of abuse and physical dependence.
- They have a narrow margin of safety.
- They suppress REM sleep.
- With the exception of chloral hydrate (Noctec), they activate the hepatic microsomal enzymes and, therefore, interfere markedly with the effectiveness of many other drugs.
- Chloral hydrate (Noctec) causes distressing gastrointestinal side effects and can displace and, therefore, potentiate other protein-bound drugs.
- Methaqualone (Quaalude) was widely abused for years and can no longer be prescribed. It can still be obtained illegally.

Zolpidem (Ambien), which was released for use in 1994 is one relatively new member of this group. It is neither a barbiturate nor a benzodiazepine, thus its inclusion in this group. In doses of 5 to 10 mg, it is recommended as a hypnotic. However, as with all the medications in this class, it could also be used as a sedative or to reduce anxiety. Addiction potential is equivalent to other drugs in this class, and side effects are similar.

Buspirone (BuSpar)

Buspirone (BuSpar) is an antianxiety agent that differs from all the others in several significant ways. It is not a CNS depressant and does not produce sedation or euphoria. It seems to have no potential for causing tolerance or physical dependence, and there is no withdrawal syndrome. It has little or no muscle relaxant property. It is not cross-tolerant with the other antianxiety agents and does not interact in any appreciable way with alcohol. Yet it does seem to be an effective antianxiety agent. Its mechanism of action is unclear, but it is known to have some dopamine-blocking and serotonin-blocking activity. Unlike other antianxiety agents, there is a lag period of 1 week or more before the antianxiety effects begin. This effectively eliminates its usefulness as an as-needed drug for anxiety. The usual daily dose is 15 to 30 mg. Side effects are usually mild and may include hypotension, tolerance to the antianxiety effects, nausea, vomiting, dry mouth, constipation, fatigue, headache, decreased libido, or impotence.

Target Symptoms

Clients with anxiety have a variety of symptoms. Some of the target symptoms that are successfully treated with antianxiety agents are discussed in Chapter 22. Although the treatment of anxiety is the major reason to prescribe these drugs for clients, there are multiple indications for their use. Box 15-6 lists symptoms and disorders for which antianxiety agents may be indicated.

Prescriber or client preference and duration of action/half-life determine the choice of drug. Unless the need for sedation is overwhelming, it is wise to try such conservative measures as listening to the client's problem, providing reassurance where appropriate, and/or teaching relaxation techniques, yoga, or meditation. Clients who suffer from sleep disturbance can be helped to decrease caffeine and alcohol intake during the afternoon and evening and to create a relaxing routine before bedtime. Increasing exercise during the morning or afternoon can be helpful. These measures alone may be successful, but a drug may also treat insomnia.

Anxiety or insomnia may be symptoms of other conditions. For example, both sleep disturbance and anxiety can be results of depression. When anxiety and sleep dis-

BOX 15-6

Indications for Use of Antianxiety Agents

Generalized anxiety disorder
Situational or anticipatory anxiety
Panic disorder; alprazolam (Xanax) may be especially useful
Agoraphobia and other phobias; alprazolam (Xanax) may be especially useful
Sleep disorders
Detoxification from alcohol or other sedative-hypnotics
Anxiety associated with physical illness or with depression
Clonazepam (Klonopin) for bipolar disorder and possibly panic disorder
Seizure disorders (especially clonazepam, diazepam, and phenobarbital)
Muscle relaxation (benzodiazepines)
Acute toxic psychoses from lysergic acid diethylamide (LSD) and phencyclidine (PCP) (benzodiazepines)
Akathisia, a side effect of the antipsychotic medications (benzodiazepines)
Preoperative or operative medication
Diazepam or lorazepam can be used intravenously to control laryngeal dystonia unresponsive to anticholinergics
Short-term sedation in mania or psychosis
Stress-related conditions
Anxiety secondary to dementia

turbance are caused by treatable primary conditions, they often dissipate when the primary condition is treated. It is precisely because anxiety and sleeplessness are so often secondary to a treatable condition that all clients who have these symptoms should undergo a thorough history and physical examination, as well as a careful psychiatric evaluation. When a primary disorder cannot be found or quickly treated, particularly if the anxiety and sleeplessness are severe or intolerable, the use of a drug may be indicated. It may be that drugs are needed temporarily until the primary condition responds to its more specific treatment.

Sometimes, when an anxiety disorder such as generalized anxiety disorder or panic disorder is the primary condition, medications may be needed for an extended period of time. In these cases, it is preferable to avoid the risk of addiction by treating the client with antidepressants.

Guidelines for Use

There is overwhelming agreement among psychopharmacologists that when any of these agents are used to treat anxiety or sleep disturbance, the course of treatment should be brief and/or intermittent whenever possible. It is generally recommended that when used as hypnotics, the dosing pattern should be every other or every third night, or for a maximum of 3 to 7 straight days followed by an equally long drug-free period. None of these agents has been shown to be helpful as a hypnotic for any longer than 28 consecutive nights, and many are helpful only for less.

On the other hand, when a client has a disabling, chronic anxiety disorder such as severe generalized anxiety disorder, panic disorder, or agoraphobia, benzodiazepines have been successfully used continuously over a long period of time (for longer than 6 months) with little decrease in effectiveness and little or no need for dose increase. Such client needs should be considered on an individual basis.

Benzodiazepines with long half-lives have the disadvantage of possible toxic buildup with chronic administration. When used as hypnotics, they are more likely to cause hangover sedation the following day. They have the advantage of a milder but sometimes more delayed withdrawal syndrome on discontinuation.

Shorter-acting agents, when used as hypnotics, have the advantage of a diminished risk of hangover sedation and the disadvantage of a more abrupt withdrawal picture on discontinuation. When ultra–short-acting benzodiazepines are used to induce sleep, they may cause early morning awakening when their effect wanes at the end of the night.

Chlordiazepoxide (Librium), diazepam (Valium), and lorazepam (Ativan) are available in parenteral forms. Only lorazepam is recommended for IM use because no other benzodiazepine is evenly and predictably absorbed by that route. Lorazepam is also rapid-acting when given sublingually.

The benzodiazepines are often used in detoxification regimens to safely withdraw clients from any of the antianxiety, sedative, and hypnotic agents to which they have become addicted. Commonly, a test dose of chlordiazepoxide (Librium) 25 mg or an equivalent dose of any other member of this drug class is given to a client who shows withdrawal signs or who is known to be addicted. An hour later, if the client is sound asleep, the addiction is judged to be mild or absent. On the other extreme, if 1 hour later the client still shows signs of withdrawal, the addiction is judged to be severe and a detoxification regimen is established based on how many more doses are required at 1-hour intervals to stop the withdrawal syndrome. Whatever total amount is required to stop withdrawal is then administered every 4 hours for one 24-hour period. Each subsequent 24-hour period, the dose is reduced by 20% of the original dose. In 5 days the detoxification is complete.

This 5-day withdrawal is effective in most cases with a few notable exceptions. Clients who are addicted to alprazolam (Xanax) and triazolam (Halcion) often find it difficult to detoxify this quickly, so when they must be withdrawn from their medication, they usually require a much slower, much more gradual withdrawal over a period of several months or more. Because nonbarbiturate, nonbenzodiazepine antianxiety agents have multiple toxicities and effects on other organ systems, detoxification is usually most comfortable when carried out with the same drug to which the person is addicted.

Side Effects

In small doses, antianxiety agents create a calming, relaxing, antianxiety effect and a decrease in activity and excitement—the sedative effect. In larger doses the CNS depression is greater, and the client shows signs of intoxication, similar to alcohol intoxication, including slurred speech, ataxia, dizziness, diplopia, and blurred vision. At this point, if clients are in a quiet, comfortable environment, they will fall asleep—the hynoptic effect. These therapeutic effects should be differentiated from side effects and effects of tolerance and withdrawal. Table 15-10 lists the side effects of the antianxiety agents and suggests nursing management strategies for each.

Tolerance to the sedative and hypnotic effects eventually develop with all of these drugs except buspirone (BuSpar), which does not appear to be addictive. As tolerance develops, the client finds that the dose of the drug that provided relief a few days earlier no longer works. The client may resort to increasing doses of the drug to produce the desired effect. Tolerance to the antianxiety effect, particularly with the benzodiazepines, develops more slowly and in many cases, may not develop to any clinically significant degree.

All of these drugs (except buspirone), if taken in large enough doses or long enough, can lead to physical and emotional addiction or dependence. Once physical dependence has developed, there are characteristic signs of

TABLE 15-10

Side effects of antianxiety agents and nursing management

SIDE EFFECT	NURSING MANAGEMENT
Daytime sedation and drowsiness with a decrease in mental and physical responsiveness and efficiency; can be accompanied by dizziness, light-headedness, uncoordination or impaired performance, judgment, and attention	The most important intervention is to inform the client that this will occur and will be most pronounced during the first month of treatment. Advise client to avoid driving or operating dangerous machinery while feeling sedated. Encourage client to arrange for brief rest periods during the day for the first 2 to 4 weeks of treatment.
Paradoxical excitement with symptoms of excitement, hostility, rage, confusion, depersonalization, and/or hyperactivity	Teach client that this is a possibility, particularly among the elderly. If this occurs, the medication is stopped.
Anterograde amnesia	Advise client that he or she may have difficulty learning new information.
Headache	Teach client to use relaxation techniques, warm or cold compresses, or to take a mild analgesic such as acetaminophen (Tylenol) for the first few weeks of treatment, after which this problem usually abates.
Nausea, vomiting, epigastric discomfort, or diarrhea	Encourage client to avoid taking this medication on an empty stomach. These problems often abate after the first few weeks of treatment.
Weight gain	Advise client to moderately increase physical activity and moderately reduce caloric intake.
Temporary rebound of symptoms when these medications are stopped, including symptoms of insomnia, anxiety, nightmares, or bizarre dreams	Inform client that these problems are likely to occur during and after withdrawal. Encourage client to tolerate these symptoms as a necessary part of withdrawal.

withdrawal if the drug is abruptly discontinued. Shortly after the last dose (24 hours to 10 days, depending on the half-life of the drug), the client will exhibit any or all of the following:

- Insomnia
- Weakness
- Muscle tremors
- Anxiety
- Irritability
- Sweating
- Anorexia
- Fever
- Nausea and vomiting
- Headache
- Uncoordination
- Restlessness

After a few days of these milder symptoms, more severe signs and symptoms of withdrawal may develop, including the following:

- Postural hypotension
- Tinnitus
- Incoherence
- Delirium
- Psychosis
- Convulsions
- Status epilepticus
- Cardiovascular collapse
- Loss of temperature-regulating mechanism
- Death

Contraindications

Absolute contraindications to the use of antianxiety agents include severe respiratory compromise, known hypersensitivity to individual compounds, and acute intermittent porphyria (a rare metabolic disorder characterized by excessive excretion of porphyrins).

These drugs should be avoided whenever possible in clients with a history of drug or alcohol abuse or suicide attempts by overdose because of the increased risk of abuse. Clients with a history of peptic ulcers should avoid chloral hydrate (Noctec) because of its irritation of the gastrointestinal tract. In clients with uremia or hepatic insufficiency, hypnotics can precipitate coma as a result of inadequate metabolism and excretion of the drugs. These clients can often be treated with smaller doses of short-acting compounds.

The safe use of these compounds in pregnancy and breastfeeding has not been established. There is inconclusive evidence of an increased incidence of cleft lip and palate after diazepam (Valium) use in the first trimester. In the last trimester, antianxiety agents can produce physical dependence in the fetus and/or neonatal depression, evidenced by poor sucking, hypotonia, and hypothermia. Barbiturates and benzodiazepines are excreted in small amounts in human breast milk and can cause lethargy and weight loss in the breastfed infant. Most authorities agree that antianxiety agents should be avoided when possible during pregnancy and breastfeeding.

Interactions

There are many potential drug interactions with antianxiety agents. Clinically significant ones are as follows:

- Antianxiety agents combined with each other or any other CNS depressant, including alcohol, can cause profound sedation.
- The nonbarbiturate, nonbenzodiazepine antianxiety agents activate the hepatic enzymes and therefore reduce blood levels of many other medications.
- Benzodiazepines taken concomitantly with oral contraceptives can cause contraceptive failure by reducing blood levels of the contraceptives and may increase the effects of the benzodiazepine.
- Cimetidine (Tagamet) and disulfiram (Antabuse) inhibit benzodiazepine metabolism, causing increased and prolonged effects.
- Diazepam (Valium) prolongs the neuromuscular blockage with gallamine or succinylcholine.
- When benzodiazepines are given with digoxin, the half-life of digoxin is lengthened.

OTHER CLASSES OF PSYCHOTROPIC MEDICATIONS

Clients who have psychiatric symptoms may be taking other classes of drugs for unrelated illnesses. Others may have some "nonpsychiatric" classes of drugs prescribed to treat target behaviors of their psychiatric illnesses. Beta-blockers are one such group of drugs.

Propranolol (Inderal) and other beta-blockers such as atenolol (Tenormin) and pindolol (Visken) have a number of uses in the treatment of mental disorders. These include the following:

- Tremor secondary to lithium or antidepressants
- Akathisia
- Tachycardia secondary to clozapine or antidepressants
- Treat situational anxiety or performance anxiety (stage fright)

The usual daily dose of propranolol is 80 to 120 mg in divided doses or a single dose of 20 to 40 mg taken for situational anxiety, or performance anxiety (stage fright) 30 to 60 minutes before performing. Propranolol side effects are usually mild but may include bradycardia, hypotension, light-headedness, giddiness, ataxia, or dizziness.

THE NURSE'S ROLE IN PSYCHOTROPIC MEDICATION ADMINISTRATION

Psychiatric-mental health nursing's *Standards* (1994) carefully describe the nurse's role in psychopharmacology, both for the psychiatric nurse with basic preparation and for those in advanced practice. What the profession's standards make clear is the need for a high degree of skill and knowledge about pharmacological agents. With the rapidly increasing numbers of new medications and the constant evolution of knowledge in psychiatry and related fields, nurses need to be current in their knowledge of psychotropic medications. In basic practice the nurse's role centers on working with the prescriber to make the medication regimen as safe, effective, comfortable, and understandable as possible for the client. The advance practice nurse assumes the role of prescriber.

Assessment

The role of the nurse in psychopharmacology begins with assessment of the client's physical state, medical and psychiatric history, history of medication use, and knowledge of medications. The physical examination and medical and psychiatric history are essential in making or validating the diagnosis of the illness for which the client seeks treatment. Only by ruling out a nonpsychiatric basis for the client's symptoms can health care professionals be certain that symptoms are not secondary to a nonpsychiatric problem.

Working with the client and family, as well as with the other professional disciplines, and drawing from whatever written records exist, the nurse collects information about the following:

- *Current drug use.* Medications the client currently takes (psychotropic and nonpsychotropic, prescription, and over-the-counter medications, as well as illicit drugs), including name, dose, schedule, experienced side effects, effectiveness, and length of time prescribed. When working in an inpatient setting, the nurse should search the client's belongings and confiscate all medications at the time of admission to prevent self-administration during hospitalization
- *History of effectiveness/response to prior medication.* All the psychotropics the client has ever taken regularly, including the name, indication, dose, schedule, experienced side effects, effectiveness, length of time prescribed, reason for discontinuation, and the effect of discontinuation on the client's symptoms
- *Patterns of use.* Whether the client took each medication regularly and as prescribed; if not, the reason(s); if the client stopped a medication without consulting the prescriber, the reason for discontinuing the medication
- *Therapeutic response of first- and second-degree (biological) family members.* Any close family member's response to psychotropic medications; both good and bad responses to these medications tend to run in families
- *Client preferences.* The client and client's family's perceptions about what the medications are supposed to do; any preferences for a route of medica-

tion, frequency of taking medication, schedule of administration, or any other aspect of the medication or medication regimen
- *Medication allergies.*
- *Pattern of alcohol use (if any).* Whether the person uses alcohol to relieve anxiety or other symptoms; whether alcohol induces extreme or uncontrollable behavior; whether the person is alcoholic
- *Caffeine and nicotine use.* Include all forms of nicotine use, including chewing tobacco
- *Social variables.* Age, physical condition, socioeconomic status, job, and financial considerations

After collecting this information, the nurse ascertains clients' attitudes toward medications and their level of knowledge about them. The nurse also assesses the client's knowledge about the psychotropic medication(s) currently being taken. The information gathered in the nurse's assessment is synthesized and shared with colleagues for use in formulating nursing diagnoses and planning future pharmacological interventions.

Intervention: Treatment Phases

Initiation

The initiation or beginning stage of drug therapy uses the information gathered by the treatment team during the assessment process. In settings where a professional team is involved in treatment such as in inpatient, partial hospital, day hospital, or outpatient settings, team members collaborate on the diagnosis and choice of treatment. In home care settings, private practice, group practice, and some HMOs and clinics, the individual practitioner makes these decisions, sometimes in consultation or with supervision by other professionals.

The choice of a specific medication is based on the client's symptoms and diagnosis, the side-effect profile of each medication, the client's overall state of health, other medications the client is taking, family history of medication response, and personal history of past response.

When there is difficulty determining the diagnosis or exact nature of a client's problem, the multidisciplinary team or colleagues of the prescriber who are consulted sometimes recommend avoiding medicating the client until a more complete assessment can be made. If that option is taken, the client is usually hospitalized so that nurses' observations of behaviors and symptoms can occur firsthand. Hospitalization may provide the basis for clarification of the client's diagnosis.

In most instances, only one medication from each class of the psychotropic drugs is chosen, but it may be necessary to combine medications from several different groups to bring symptom relief.

Once a medication is chosen, it is started at a low dose, usually lower than the lowest dose in the standard range of therapeutic doses. The dose is gradually increased every few days until the dose is in the standard range or therapeutic blood levels are achieved. If the target symptoms are improving, dose increases stop. If at any point side effects, which should be monitored continuously by the nurse, become intolerable or dangerous, the medication dose is reduced to the point where the side effects are tolerable. The basic principle, therefore, is expressed as *start low—go slow.*

Any time side effects are a problem, the first option for altering the medication regimen is for the prescriber to reduce the dose of the offending agent. Unfortunately, this may result in an exacerbation of symptoms. If so, the dose can then sometimes be more gradually raised back to the previous level. Sometimes the side effect diminishes when the prescriber either combines or divides the doses in a different way.

For some side effects, adding another medication that treats the side effect will help. For example, clients with severe lithium tremor can be helped by adding propranolol (Inderal) to their regimens. The final alternative is to change to another agent within the same family that causes less of the specific side effect that troubles the client. When this is done, the ineffective medication is usually tapered slowly, while at the same time, the new medication is started and gradually increased. Some medications such as MAOIs and tricyclic antidepressants may require complete withdrawal before beginning a different group of drugs.

Simultaneously prescribing more than one medication within the same class of drug to the same client is referred to as **polypharmacy.** This is discouraged by most psychopharmacologists. The only exception to this general rule applies to mood stabilizers, which are sometimes combined to achieve a satisfactory effect.

For many of the psychotropic medications, it is necessary for the client to have baseline and periodic blood levels drawn. The nurse should clearly and simply state the reason for the blood test and, when possible, have a trusted staff member present during the venipuncture.

Stabilization

Stabilization of the medication regimen may take place in inpatient settings, but as psychiatric care moves out of hospitals and into communities, more clients are being started and stabilized on psychotropic medications in less restrictive settings.

For most psychotropic medications there is a lag period between the onset of treatment and symptom remission. During this difficult time the client may have some side effects but virtually no relief from the psychiatric symptoms. It is the nurse's role to support clients and assure them that a delay in response is normal and has a time limit.

Use of as-needed medications

The nurse is sometimes given the option of using as-needed medications. It is best to agree with the client's family and other team members about the precise indications for such doses. Many studies completed in the last decade have shown that with antipsychotics, it is as fast and as effective to give standing divided doses as it is to raise the dose precipitously by using multiple, as-needed medications. Certainly, once the client is stabilized on a medication, the continuing use of antipsychotic as-needed medications is rarely helpful. Using as-needed dosages of lithium, other mood stabilizers, or antidepressants is never helpful and, in fact, only increases the client's risk of intolerable or dangerous side effects such as lithium toxicity, anticholinergic delirium, or extreme sedation.

Use of as-needed antianxiety agents is at times helpful, particularly during the beginning of treatment for psychotic, bipolar, or depressive symptoms. Because of the tendency to develop tolerance for the antianxiety agents, some clients want higher doses than those prescribed and learn behaviors to manipulate the nurse into providing as-needed medications. Under these circumstances, it is especially important to have agreed upon, measurable, objective indications for the as-needed drug.

Joan was being treated in the psychiatric day hospital with alprazolam (Xanax) for severe anxiety associated with an exacerbation of obsessive-compulsive disorder (OCD). The OCD was being treated with nefazodone (Serzone), but until it brought the disorder's symptoms of OCD under control, it was agreed that Joan should have as-needed alprazolam available for a maximum of 3 times per day for 3 months. During the first week at the day hospital, she came to the nurse at least once each hour complaining of feeling anxious and asking for one of the as-needed alprazolam ordered by her prescriber. In collaboration, the nurse, the client, and the physician specified concrete parameters for administering alprazolam: a pulse rate higher than 100, absence of relief from 5 minutes of deep breathing exercises with a partner, and absence of relief from 10 minutes of listening with headphones to a tape of relaxing classical music that had been produced for purposes of relaxation by the staff of the day hospital. All three criteria have to be met before the as-needed alprazolam is dispensed.

Maintenance

After the client has been stabilized, the target symptoms controlled, and the medication causes only mild or no side effects, the client continues the regimen in what is called the **maintenance** phase. *During this phase the dose is stable and is usually smaller than what was needed for symptom control during the acute phase of illness.* Clients are not hospitalized during this phase of treatment and ideally are functional, both socially and vocationally.

The major issue for the nurse and client during this phase is usually **compliance,** *or taking medications as prescribed.* To prevent relapse, clients continue to take psychotropic medications for a long time, sometimes for a lifetime. The major exception to this rule is the antianxiety agents, which are usually stopped as soon as is clinically possible. The rate of noncompliance with psychotropics is the same as for all other medications; about half of clients fail to take the medication as prescribed. For psychotropic medications, stopping the medication prematurely doubles the risk of relapse. What can be done to improve the client's ability to take the medication accurately and successfully? See Box 15-7 for the factors that increase or decrease medication compliance.

One of the first considerations when a drug does not seem to be working is the possibility of noncompliance. Sometimes when clients are unwilling or unable to voice their complaints about their medication, or when they have been ordered by a court to take medications, they find ways to discard them, even when each dose is administered in the hospital. Clients taking tablets or capsules can hide them under their tongues ("tonguing") or in their cheeks ("cheeking") until the staff member is out of sight, and they can safely discard the dose. Others may spit the tablets or capsules into the cup of water used to wash down the medication, then discard the medication with the used cup. Clients taking liquid medications sometimes spit the liquid medication into the water cup and discard it with the cup.

Nurses should be suspicious that noncompliance might occur if clients have a history of noncompliance, complain about their medications but continue to accept them at medication time, have very low blood serums levels despite an adequate dosing schedule, or experience no discernible therapeutic or side effects despite a standard dose. When clients are suspect, they should be informed about staff observations. The client may be started on liquid form of the medication, or the medication can be crushed and mixed with a palatable food or liquid. Medication is administered in front of the nurse, with care being taken to see that both containers are empty before they are discarded. If solid forms are used, both the client's mouth and the water cup should be checked immediately after the medication is taken. When checking

---

BOX 15-7

Factors Related to Medication Compliance

FACTORS THAT INCREASE COMPLIANCE

Client's perception that the illness is severe and medication is needed

Client's feeling of being personally susceptible to the illness or personally at risk for relapse

Client's knowledge of the illness and treatment

Client's perception of the importance of the regimen

Moderate level of anxiety (useful worrying)

Family stability and support for compliance

Well-established relationship between client and caregiver

Continuity and length of relationship with caregiver

Structured, professional relationship between client and caregiver

Optimism on the part of the caregiver about a medication's efficacy

Medication's importance stressed by caregiver

Provision of explicit, consistent, written information

Access to help when questions about medication or its side effects arise

Return of unpleasant symptoms immediately on stopping a medication or other treatment

FACTORS THAT DECREASE COMPLIANCE

Need for too many changes in lifestyle or habits

Increasing number or complexity of recommendations (e.g., too many doses per day, doses arranged in specific ways around meals, different medication schedules on different days of the week, directions to hold doses for a variety of reasons, and others)

Medication side effects that cause discomfort or distress

Fear of drug dependence

Lack of support from family or friends for compliance

Long course of treatment in which symptoms are controlled (reduces perceived need for medication)

Client who is hostile, aggressive, or pathologically stubborn (reduces ability to collaborate in treatment)

Lack of immediate return of symptoms if medication or other treatment is stopped

Client who enjoys a return of symptoms (e.g., grandiosity or elation)

Fear of independence and responsibility that comes with recovery

Equating taking medications with being ill

Persistent delusion that medications are harmful or poisonous

the client's mouth, the nurse uses a tongue blade to look under the tongue and in both cheeks.

If a client is taking medication, and target symptoms of an antidepressant, a mood stabilizer, or an antipsychotic have not responded within 4 to 6 weeks, the medication is considered a failure. A decision is then made about an alternative treatment, either another medication or a nondrug alternative. Again at this point, it is the nurse's role to support clients and educate them about the next alternative. Clients are often discharged before the full therapeutic effects of drugs are evident. In these circumstances the need is greater than ever to monitor clients carefully by following them in a day program or with home or outpatient visits. The nurse must ensure that problems with medications are uncovered and addressed quickly and effectively, before the client despairs of finding a drug regimen that relieves symptoms without undue discomfort.

At some point during the transition between inpatient treatment, partial hospitalization, halfway house, day program, home care, or outpatient treatment, clients begin assuming the responsibility for self-administration of medication. The sooner this process can begin, the better. Even while medications are being dispensed, clients can be asked to identify the tablets and capsules they are receiving and describe their target symptoms and potential side effects. Many clients can self-administer medications safely even when they are quite symptomatic, and they should be encouraged to do so whenever possible to maintain or develop their skills at managing their own medications.

Before clients begin administering their own medications, it is important to teach that many medications are manufactured by several different pharmaceutical companies. The same medication will often be given a different brand or trade name by each company that makes it and will be a different size, shape, and color. Clients need to know that when they use a different pharmacy, medication may have a different appearance and name. They should be told to ask about the change and make sure they receive the same generic name medication in the same dose despite the change in appearance.

Client Education

Once a medication has been chosen, it becomes the nurse's responsibility to provide the client with information about the medication(s). In many settings, this process of informed consent is formalized, and both the nurse and client sign a formal statement that indicates that the client understands basic, specific information about medication alternatives, indications, target symptoms, side effects, long-term risks, and self-management. See Chapter 16 for suggested methods on educating clients about medications. Because most clients take their medications independently for at least part, if not all, of their course of treatment, they need to know how to manage them effectively. When there are misunderstandings or fears about the medication(s), it is the nurse's responsibility to correct misinformation and help the client deal with the fears. In fact, the first step in teaching clients about medications is to explore the client's perceptions and feelings about them.

Teaching changes the client's behavior in ways that are measurable. Box 15-8 lists the expected outcomes (measurable behavior changes) for clients who have been taught about their psychotropic medications. Often it is advisable to teach the client's family using the same outcome measures.

The teaching methods for reaching outcomes can be varied. Nurses can teach clients informally while they dispense medications or in small informal groups that occur spontaneously. Nurses in outpatient settings often run medication management groups, family groups, and groups for clients with similar disorders (e.g., a group of clients with mood disorders). Some settings offer formal nurse-led medication teaching groups and classes. In other settings, more of the teaching is done on a one-to-one basis. In all settings, verbal teaching can be supple-

---

BOX 15-8

Expected Outcomes of Medication Teaching

At the conclusion of a teaching session about medication, the client will be able to do the following:

- State the name of the medication.
- Identify the dosage and schedule.
- State why the medication is needed.
- List the target symptoms that the medication will treat.
- Choose a method to remember to take the medication as scheduled.
- Describe activity, food, or medication restrictions, if they apply.
- Describe the procedure for blood monitoring, when necessary.
- List the side effects that must and need not be reported immediately to the prescriber.
- Describe side effects and how to manage them if they occur.
- Describe the course of treatment.
- Indicate what to do if a dose is missed.
- Select a form of identification to wear or carry that lists the medication(s) prescribed.
- State that the prescriber should be informed before increasing or decreasing the dose.
- Discuss the social use of alcohol.
- Recognize exacerbation of symptoms, even when medications are being taken; know what action to take.

mented by written material. The NIMH and other public and private agencies concerned with health issues publish written material for clients (see the Consumer Resources box on at right).

Legal and Ethical Issues in Psychopharmacology

Prescribing, administering, and monitoring psychotropic medications are extremely powerful interventions. Nursing efforts are directed toward making the medications work for the client's good. Sometimes, however, they can make the client uncomfortable or even ill. Sometimes they create life-threatening problems for the client. Informed consent is the client's right (see Chapter 3). The following guidelines list client rights and nursing responsibilities regarding psychopharmacological treatment:

- A client has the right to a thorough physical and psychiatric assessment before pharmocological treatment begins.
- At a minimum, the client has the right to be informed of the name of the medication, the target symptom(s), and potentially dangerous side effects before a medication is given.
- The issue of medicating clients against their will in an emergency situation is governed by state law. Nurses should be aware of the state law as it applies to their practice.
- The client, together with the nurse and the prescriber, has the right to collaborate on all issues related to medication: the decision to take medication and the choice of agent(s), dose, schedule, treatment of side effects, and length of treatment.
- If clients self-administer medications, they have the right to be informed about over-the-counter drug interactions, including alcohol, potential side effects, food or medication restrictions, danger signs that would warrant an immediate call to the prescriber, and long-term risks.
- Nurses have a legal responsibility to systematically update themselves about new drugs and new research findings about existing drugs.

KEY POINTS

- The prevailing belief is that the major mental disorders are caused by a combination of genetically determined brain abnormalities (chemical imbalances in the neurotransmitter systems, structural abnormalities, or both) and the influence of stress in the environment. Psychotropic medications provide symptom relief by acting directly on the neurotransmitter systems of the brain.

CONSUMER RESOURCES

National Institute of Mental Health (NIMH)
Room 7C-02
5600 Fishers Lane
Rockville, MD 20857
(301)443-4513
NIMH publishes a wide variety of up-to-date summaries of research in psychiatry in the form of pamphlets on specific disorders and treatments. Ask for a form to apply for the mailing list to receive copies of all their new publications as they are produced.

Lithium Information Center
OCD Information Center
The Dean Foundation for Health, Research, and Education
8000 Excelsior Drive, Suite 302
Madison, WI 53717-1914
(608)836-8070
Publishes pamphlets and books about lithium, the other mood stabilizers, and a variety of other medication and nonmedication topics in psychiatry.

National Alliance for the Mentally Ill (NAMI)
200 North Glebe Road
Suite 1015
Arlington, VA 22203-3754
(800)950-NAMI or (703)524-7600
Members receive quarterly newsletters that summarize recent research in psychiatry. NAMI also has an extensive library of pamphlets, books, posters, videotapes, and audiotapes available to members at low cost on a wide variety of subjects in psychiatry.

American Psychiatric Association (APA)
Division of Public Affairs
1400 K Street, NW
Washington, DC 20005
(202)682-6220
Publishes a list of brief pamphlets summarizing what is known about specific psychiatric disorders and treatments.

Pharmaceutical companies
All drug companies that manufacture psychotropic medications make information available to professionals. Many also have information specifically written for lay persons. The phone number for each drug company is listed in the front of the PDR. By calling the consumer information number listed, clients can inquire about written materials for consumers.

CRITICAL THINKING QUESTIONS

Ellen, age 22, is a brilliant woman and has always done well at most everything she attempts. Her mother, her grandmother, and two of her uncles have been diagnosed with bipolar I disorder and are functioning well with ongoing treatment with lithium and carbamazepine (Tegretol). Now she, too, is beginning to show signs of the disorder. After finishing college last year, she took a job at an advertising firm. Ellen's work has been good, brilliant at times, but this month when working especially long hours to sign a large, important account, she began feeling elated. Her speech was pressured, and she began to feel she knew more than anyone else in her firm. She discovered she needed only 1 or 2 hours of sleep at night—much less than usual—and she was becoming more irritable at work, and less tolerant of her coworkers' ideas and opinions. One day in an important meeting, she screamed at her boss, calling his ideas "stupid" and left the meeting abruptly. This was uncharacteristic of her past work behavior and caused a great deal of concern and surprise among her peers, and consternation on the part of her boss. He suspended her for 2 days and asked her to report to his office on her return.

Later that day, she spoke to her mother on the telephone. Her mother had been concerned that Ellen had seemed so restless and short-tempered lately. She worried that Ellen may be developing the same illness she and her mother had. On hearing about the day's events and Ellen's sleeplessness, she became even more concerned. When she shared this worry with Ellen, Ellen became enraged. She denied being ill and defended her position that her boss's ideas were the real problem. Only after several calls and visits both from her mother and grandmother did Ellen agree to see a counselor at her firm's Employee Assistance Program. The counselor called in a psychiatrist for consul-

tation who issued the diagnosis of bipolar disorder. The recommended treatment was lithium.

1. In a family such as this, where there is a pattern of inheritance of bipolar disorder, what do you think would be the best way to deal with the issue of vulnerability to the illness? Should the matter be discussed? Would it be better to ignore the issue unless it surfaces?
2. Is it helpful or harmful for persons to know they have increased risks of developing such a disorder?
3. Could there be any relationship between Ellen's successes and her illness? If so, what?
4. If Ellen does have bipolar disorder and is treated with lithium, she may fear what many successful persons who take mood stabilizers for bipolar disorder fear—that their creativity and energy will be adversely affected by the medication. How could a nurse help a client deal with such a fear?
5. Ellen has always wanted to have children. She knows that lithium is best avoided during pregnancy and wonders how she is ever going to have children if she, like her mother and grandmother, will need to continue to take lithium throughout her lifetime. Furthermore, she wonders if she, too, would pass this illness to future generations. How would you deal with these concerns?
6. If lithium stabilizes Ellen's illness, allowing her to return to her normal mood state without the irritability, sleeplessness, and grandiosity she experienced when she was ill, is there a need for her to seek psychotherapy? If mental illness is chemical or anatomical in nature and well-treated with a medication, why might there be a need for psychotherapy? Would the need be any greater than for a major nonpsychiatric illness? Why or why not?

- Psychotropic medications effectively treat specific psychiatric symptoms and disorders. They do not cure; they control symptoms, much as antihypertensives control hypertension and insulin controls diabetes.
- Antipsychotic medications treat psychotic symptoms by reducing the activity level of dopamine (and in some cases, serotonin) in the brain. They are symptom-specific rather than illness-specific.
- Antidepressant medications control depression, OCD, and panic disorder by increasing the activity level of norepinephrine and serotonin in the brain.

- Mood stabilizing medications include lithium and two anticonvulsants: carbamazepine and valproate. These medications create greater stability in the membranes of the brain so that mood can be more effectively regulated, that is, returned to baseline normal mood more easily and automatically after a temporary derangement of mood.
- Antianxiety agents work by increasing the activity of GABA, one of the major inhibiting neurotransmitters in the brain.
- The nurse's role in psychopharmacology includes assessing clients, administering medication, monitor-

ing for therapeutic and side effects, educating clients, managing side effects, and managing compliance issues. In some states, advance practice nurses prescribe medication.

REFERENCES

American Nurses' Association. (1994). *Psychiatric mental health nursing psychopharmacology project.* Washington, DC: Author.

American Nurses' Association. (1995). *A statement on psychiatric-mental health clinical nursing practice and standards of psychiatric-mental health clinical nursing practice.* Washington, DC: Author.

American Psychiatric Association. (1994). *Diagnostic and statistical manual of mental disorders* (4th ed.). Washington, DC: Author.

Gilman A.G., Goodman L.S., Rall T.W., & Murad F. (Eds). (1993). *Goodman and Gilman's the pharmacological basis of therapeutics* (9th ed.). New York: Macmillan.

Meltzer H. (Ed) (1992). *Novel antipsychotic drugs.* New York: Raven Press.

McCloskey J.C., & Bulechek E.M. (1996) *Nursing interventions classification (NIC)* (2nd ed.). St. Louis: Mosby.

Skidmore-Roth, L. (1996). *Mosby's drug guide for nurses.* St. Louis: Mosby.

Sprague R.L., & Kalachnik J.E. (1991). Reliability, validity, and a total score cutoff for the dyskinesia identification system: Condensed user scale (DISCUS) with mentally ill and mentally retarded population. *Psychopharmacology Bulletin, 27:*51-58.

Wilson H.W., & Classen A.M. (1995). 18-month outcome of clozapine treatment for 100 patients in a state psychiatric hospital. *Psychiatric Services, 46(4):*386-389.

Chapter 16

Health Teaching

Barbara Krainovich-Miller

LEARNING OUTCOMES

After studying and applying the concepts of this chapter, the learner will be able to:

- Discuss the relationship between health teaching as an American Nurses Association (ANA) (1994) standard of care and as a role of the basic level psychiatric-mental health nurse.
- Discuss the role of the basic level psychiatric-mental health nurse in relation to health teaching and psychoeducation programs for clients, families and significant others, client groups, and communities.
- Discuss the relationship between health teaching as an implementation standard and the implementation standards of the following: counseling, milieu therapy, self-care activities, psychobiological interventions, case management, and health promotion and health maintenance.
- Determine the use of teaching strategies of the following learning theories: cognitive, behavioral, social cognitive, and adult.
- Determine outcomes related to the cognitive, affective, and psychomotor domains.
- Discuss assessment of the learner who has a psychiatric-mental health disorder.
- Develop realistic outcomes and a plan for health teaching a client with a major psychiatric-mental health disorder.
- Determine the similarities and differences between health teaching and psychoeducation programs.
- Discuss the major goals of current psychoeducation programs.
- Discuss the use of health teaching and psychoeducation programs of the basic level psychiatric-mental health nurse in relation to the following client therapies: individual, group, family, community/milieu, crisis intervention, and biological or psychopharmacology therapies.

KEY TERMS

Behavioral theory
Cognitive theory
Health teaching
Learning
Learning outcomes

Locus of control
Mnemonics
Motivation for learning
Need to learn
Psychoeducation programs

Readiness to learn
Reinforcement
Teaching strategies

Since the time of Florence Nightingale, health teaching has been one of nursing's most important roles. It differentiates nurses from physicians and other health care professionals such as social workers and psychologists. Many nurse theorists include health teaching as an essential concept in their theories/models (e.g., Henderson, Orem, Peplau, Watson). There is widespread agreement that health teaching is an important psychiatric-mental health nursing role, yet it is often neglected in undergraduate and graduate curricula (Ferguson, 1991; Redman, 1991, 1993). Given this perspective, this text devotes a chapter to health teaching to emphasize its importance for psychiatric-mental health nursing's future.

The purpose of this chapter is to discuss the relationships among the teaching/learning process, the nursing process, and health teaching as one of psychiatric-mental health nursing's *Standards* (ANA, 1994) and as one of its roles. The necessary knowledge, skills, and teaching strategies for providing quality health teaching to clients with mental disorders and their families, significant others, and communities will be discussed. In addition, psychoeducation programs are presented from interdisciplinary and nursing frameworks.

Although nurses value health teaching, few research studies describe how nurses carry out their teaching activities with clients (Kuipers et al., 1994). A major treatment for psychiatric client's symptoms is medication, yet client adherence to medication regimens continues to be a tremendous problem (Kuipers et al., 1994). Noncompliance is often viewed as a lack of teaching effectiveness, and nurses tend to blame themselves (Antai-Otong, 1989). There is a relatively small body of nursing literature on patient education for clients with mental disorders compared with other clients. The majority of theoretical and research nursing literature related to clients with mental disorders focuses on medication compliance, yet few discuss specific strategies for implementing medication education (Antai-Otong, 1989; Batey and Ledbetter, 1982; Cohen and Amdur, 1981; Coudreaut-Quinn, Emmons, and McMorrow, 1992; Davidhizar and Powell, 1987; Harmon and Tratnack, 1992; Hart, Craig-Williams, and Gladwell, 1985; Heyduk, 1991; Kucera-Bozarth, Beck, and Lyss, 1982). This literature represents various client groups in the United States, Ireland, and the United Kingdom.

LEARNING PRINCIPLES AND THE TEACHING PROCESS

Thus far in your education, you most likely have been exposed to the following teaching/learning theories in psychology, sociology, education, and nursing courses: classical conditioning, operant conditioning, Gestalt-field social/cognitive, adult learning, and critical thinking. Some of these theories are discussed in various clinical chapters throughout this text. However, in relation to teaching/learning, these theories fit into two major categories: behavioral and cognitive (Knowles, 1990). Central to *behavioral theories is the premise that all behavior is learned and the focus is on conditioning or reinforcing behaviors, with motivation coming from people and environmental conditions. Cognitive theory focuses on reframing beliefs, values, assumptions, and ideas so that individuals think differently, thereby setting the stage for the development of insights or understandings to change behavior.* Linking these theories to principles of learning and teaching is important to health teaching. "*Learning is any change in cognitive, psychomotor, or affective behavior [learning domains] that is a result of*" exposure to health teaching (Van Hoozer et al., 1987).

THE RELATIONSHIP BETWEEN HEALTH TEACHING AND THE NURSING PROCESS
Health Teaching: The Psychiatric-Mental Health Nursing Role

You might be thinking at this point, "Why is health teaching being explained here? Isn't it the same regardless of the type of client or setting?" The answer is yes and no. Yes, teaching clients with mental disorders requires the basic principles of teaching, so in that respect it is the same. However, teaching clients with mental disorders is not the same because the application of the teaching/learning theory, or the teaching strategies used with this population, is different. If nurses are to succeed in teaching clients with mental disorders, they must develop and use specific teaching strategies. According to the ANA, health teaching is a role function of the psychiatric-mental health nurse. *Health teaching may be referred to as client education or client teaching. Health teaching is used as a formal or informal intervention by all nurses in their everyday clinical practice.* Now more than ever before, health teaching is an essential power tool of the psychiatric-mental health nurse working with clients in a variety of settings.

Health teaching is most effectively implemented in relation to a North American Nursing Diagnosis Association (NANDA) nursing diagnosis rather than as a separate teaching plan or teaching intervention protocol for an isolated clinical problem, such as the need for medication teaching. Box 16-1 illustrates an example of one type of teaching plan or intervention protocol for a specific clinical problem. This particular example is also referred to as a Nursing Interventions Classification (NIC) teaching intervention protocol for medications, which is a research-based practice protocol (McCloskey and Bulechek, 1996). As explained in Chapter 5, NIC inter-

BOX 16-1

Teaching: Prescribed Medication

DEFINITION

Preparing a patient to safely take prescribed medications and monitor their effects

ACTIVITIES

Instruct the patient to recognize distinct characteristics of the medication(s) as appropriate

Inform the patient of both the generic and brand names of each medication

Instruct the patient on the purpose and action of each medication

Instruct the patient on the dosage, route, and duration of each medication

Instruct the patient on the proper administration/application of each medication

Evaluate the patient's ability to self-administer medications

Instruct the patient to perform needed procedures before taking a medication (e.g., check pulse, glucose) as appropriate

Inform the patient what to do if a dose of medication is missed

Instruct the patient on which criteria to use when deciding to alter medication dosage/schedule as appropriate

Inform the patient of consequences of not taking or abruptly discontinuing medication(s) as appropriate

Instruct the patient on specific precautions to observe when taking medication(s) (e.g., no power tools) as appropriate

Instruct the patient on possible adverse side effects of each medication

Instruct the patient how to relieve and/or prevent certain side effects as appropriate

Instruct the patient on appropriate actions to take if side effects occur

Instruct the patient on the signs and symptoms of over- and under-dosage

Inform the patient of possible drug/food interactions as appropriate

Instruct the patient how to properly store medication(s)

Instruct the patient on proper care of devices used for administration

Provide the patient with written information about the action, purpose, side effects, etc., of medications

Assist the patient to develop a written medication schedule

Instruct the patient to carry documentation of his/her prescribed medication regimen

Instruct the patient on how to fill his/her prescription(s) as appropriate

Inform the patient of possible changes in appearance and/or dosage when filling generic medication prescription(s)

Warn the patient of the risks associated with taking expired medication

Caution the patient against giving prescribed medication to others

Determine the patient's ability to obtain required medications

Provide information on medication reimbursement as appropriate

Provide information on cost saving programs/organizations to obtain medications and devices as appropriate

Provide information on medication alert devices and how to obtain them

Reinforce information provided by other health care team members as appropriate

Include the family/significant other as appropriate

Reprinted with permission from McCloskey J.C., & Bulechek G.M. (Eds.). (1996). Nursing interventions classification (NIC) *(2nd ed.). St. Louis: Mosby.*

ventions can be used to augment nursing care plans or for individual clinical problems. The illustrated NIC intervention for teaching medications is a generic practice protocol that can be used with an individual client or groups of clients. For example, using the nursing process as the framework for health teaching, the most common nursing diagnosis, based on the assessed data of the client not taking his or her new medication risperidone, (Risperdol) would be the NANDA nursing diagnosis of knowledge deficit of medication related to change in medication from haloperidol (Haldol) to Risperdol. In this case, the NIC could be used by the nurse as a practice guideline to make sure that the appropriate content was covered when teaching about Risperdol. Yet what is missing is the "how to teach" or the specific teaching strategies needed to teach this client about his or her medications. ***Teaching strategies*** *refer to the specific techniques, methods, or activities used in applying teaching/learning theories to bring about planned learning outcomes.* Teaching strategies turn giving information or covering the content into teaching. Examples of teaching strategies are discussed on p. 303 and pp. 305-310 of this chapter.

Health teaching is often an implied aspect of any nursing care plan for clients with psychiatric-mental health disorders. The nursing care plan in Chapter 5 presented the nursing diagnosis of moderate anxiety related to fear of presentations. Almost all interventions listed required the nurse to teach the client.

For example, a nurse needs to teach the client about anxiety-reducing methods, such as recognizing beginning signs of anxiety and when to use the prescribed medication. Almost every nursing or interdisciplinary therapy prescribed for clients with mental disorders requires health teaching. Health teaching is an integral part of the health care needs of individuals, families, and community populations at risk. Although specific goals of health teaching depend on the client's individualized learning outcomes, overall *learning outcomes include changing clients' health-related behaviors and empowering clients to take as much control of their own health as possible.*

Health Teaching as an Implementation Standard of Care

In psychiatric-mental health nursing's *Standards,* health teaching is viewed as "implementation." Measurement criteria is used to determine if this standard is met. To implement health teaching, the nurse needs to use principles of teaching/learning, as well as relevant theories related to the diagnosis and treatment of mental disorders. The complex assessment process is emphasized, as well as the need for teaching strategies (methods). A number of teaching strategies that are essential to teaching this population are derived from principles of learning. All the areas of client assessment, are used to provide ap-

propriate health teaching for clients and their families or significant others.

For example, a client with a history of a severe and persistent mental disorder may be admitted for an acute schizophrenic episode (see Chapter 29). A comprehensive psychiatric-mental health nursing assessment results in the client's NANDA nursing diagnosis of ineffective management of health regimen related to lack of understanding regarding the need for daily medication even when symptom-free. In this situation the nurse would include specific, planned health-teaching nursing interventions related to the effect of medications on symptoms and the need to continue medication even when feeling well, along with other appropriate interventions. In addition, the nurse would include methods or specific teaching strategies to be used.

Health Teaching and the Other Implementation Standards of Care

Health teaching is one of seven implementation *Standards of Care* (ANA, 1994) (see Appendix A). The other six are as follows:

- Counseling
- Milieu therapy
- Self-care activities
- Psychobiological interventions
- Case management
- Health promotion and health maintenance

Table 16-1 illustrates that although health teaching is a separate standard, it is also embedded in each of the other implementation standards. Health teaching is

TABLE 16-1

Psychiatric-mental health nursing's implementation standard and required health teaching	
STANDARD OF CARE	**REQUIRED HEALTH TEACHING**
Counseling	Problem solving, stress management, relaxation techniques, assertiveness training, conflict resolution, and behavior modification
Milieu therapy	Norms and rules that govern behavior and ADLs
Self-care activities	Assuming personal responsibility for ADLs
Psychobiological interventions	Opportunities are provided for the client and significant others to question, discuss, and explore his or her feelings about past, current, and projected use of therapies
Case management	Services are based on a comprehensive approach to client's physical, mental, emotional, and social health problems
Health promotion and health maintenance	Interventions are designed for clients identified as at-risk for mental health problems

required for the selected measurement criteria to be met. For example, for nurses to meet the measurement criterion for counseling, they will have to perform health teaching. The psychiatric-mental health nurse might use teaching strategies such as role modeling, positive feedback, active listening, homework, and rehearsal to effectively teach the client activities of daily living (ADL) survival skills of problem solving, stress management, and/or behavior modification.

Perhaps in your clinical learning experience you have performed health teaching such as teaching a middle-age male client about his blood pressure medication and a teen-age female client how to use a nasal inhaler. Which principles of teaching/learning theory did you use? Did you use different strategies for each client? Did they work? Now imagine the challenge of an adult client with mental illness whose reality testing is impaired. What strategies would you use and when? How much information should you give? Do you teach this client as you would a groggy, fresh postoperative client who was recently medicated for pain? As you study this chapter you will gain the necessary knowledge and skills to teach such clients. The complexity of this type of health teaching is tremendous. The task of developing and using appropriate teaching strategies requires critical thinking (Krainovich-Miller, 1995).

Fig. 16-1 illustrates the relationship between health teaching as an essential role and as an essential measurement criterion for psychiatric-mental health nursing's *Standards.* The very nature of these standards assumes that clients need health teaching. Clients seek nursing care to bring about a change in health status; for psychi-

atric-mental health clients, this usually means a change in behavior. Health teaching, delivered by the basic level psychiatric-mental health nurse, is aimed at bringing about cognitive and behavioral changes in the client or learner. *The client or learner may be an individual client and/or family member or significant other, or a group of clients and/or family members or significant others.* Effective client education requires that the nurse use the power tools listed in Box 16-2.

THE RELATIONSHIP BETWEEN THE NURSING PROCESS AND THE TEACHING PROCESS
Assessment

Table 16-2 presents the similarities and differences between health teaching as a teaching process model of client education and the nursing process. The psychiatric-mental health nurse must identify the client or learner needs by assessing (1) the need to learn and (2) the cognitive and noncognitive "readiness to learn."

The teaching process parallels the use of diagnostic reasoning in the nursing process in terms of a comprehensive client assessment. For client health teaching, the **need to learn** *refers to a client's request for information or interest in learning how to perform a task related to his or her health condition.* This is not the typical situation with clients with mental disorders.

Assessment variables

In nonpsychiatric settings, the client is usually better able to describe to the nurse his or her need to learn. However, variables such as the acuteness of the illness, pain, mental and physical handicaps, language spoken, and age all affect the nurse's ability to assess the client's learning needs and ability to learn (Craft, 1987). The challenge in the psychiatric setting is that a client may have many of the previously described variables, plus variables that reflect significant difficulties in mental or cognitive functioning and related behaviors that may mask evidence or prevent the client from expressing the need to learn.

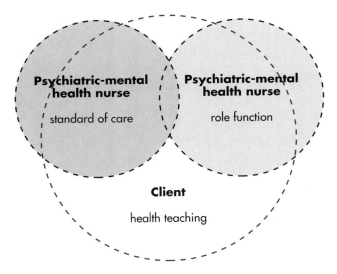

Fig. 16-1   The relationship of psychiatric-mental health nursing's *Standards* and the role of health teaching.

BOX 16-2

Power Tools of Teaching

Psychiatric-mental health nursing standards of care (nursing process)
The nurse-client relationship (establishing trust)
Therapeutic communication techniques
Teaching/learning strategies

TABLE 16-2

Relationship of assessment aspects of the teaching process to the nursing process

ASSESSMENT	DIAGNOSIS	OUTCOME IDENTIFI-CATION	PLANNING	IMPLEMEN-TATION	EVALUATION
Nursing Process					
Comprehensive nursing assessment	NANDA nursing diagnosis related to learning needs (e.g., ineffective management of health regimen related to lack of understanding regarding the need for daily medication)	Short-term outcomes reflect learning goals, are measurable, and are on a time line	Individualized plan prescribes specific health teaching interventions to attain expected outcomes	Specific health teaching interventions are carried out with other interventions and are documented	Outcomes met, partially met, or not met
Teaching Process					
Specific assessment of learner in relation to learning needs and readiness	Learning diagnosis (e.g., lack of understanding of prescribed medication)	Development of specific learning goals	Develop a specific plan to teach medication	Use multiple teaching strategies	Learning outcomes achieved or not achieved

Adapted from Redman, B.K. (1993). The process of patient education *(7th ed.). St. Louis: Mosby.*

Readiness to learn

Because clients are hospitalized for shorter and shorter periods of time, the nurse must assume that they need to learn and move on to developing their **readiness to learn.** *Readiness to learn refers to an individual's mental age/maturity, emotional development, and motivation for learning* (Tyler, 1964). **Motivation for learning** *refers to individuals' inner drives that causes them to learn new behaviors* (Redman, 1993; Knowles, 1990).

Motivation for learning

Cultural and related socioeconomic factors (see Chapter 6), as well as the emotional responses of the individual in general and in relation to their psychiatric disorder, influence a client's motivation for learning. A number of theories offer explanations of the role of motivation in learning (Redman, 1993). For example, behavioral theory connects motivation to **reinforcement,** that is, a *behavior that was learned through positive reinforcement will be repeated*; or, using Maslow's theory, basic needs for food, shelter, and even self-esteem can be great motivators. **Locus of control,** a concept derived from social learning theory, *considers a person's motivation closely linked with his or her attributions or beliefs.* Individuals with an *internal locus of control* are more likely to seek out the needed information in a usual life situation,

yet are less likely to adapt in a health crisis (i.e., take on new behaviors in a situation beyond their control) because they need and are used to controlling the situation. Individuals with an *external locus of control* do not perceive control over their environment and yet are more adaptive when presented with "control" in a health crisis situation, especially by someone in authority (Craft, 1987). Here, control refers to what needs to be learned to restore health. There are standardized internal-external locus of control scales for assessing this variable. When possible, this variable should be assessed in determining the best way to enhance clients' motivations to learn.

The motivation to learn includes an individual's psychological, emotional, and physiological readiness to learn (Craft, 1987). For example, the emotional threat that a person perceives as a result of a psychiatric disorder results in an increased anxiety level and subsequently begins a chain of physiological reactions that then decrease his or her readiness to learn. Overall the general practice of developing a collaborative teaching/learning environment helps to enhance readiness to learn.

Benefit to the client versus benefit to the learner

Helping to motivate the learner is often discussed in terms of the benefits the learner derives. Presenting these benefits is a teaching strategy used to motivate the learner to do well. For example, in the academic setting the benefit to the learner is the reward, such as a grade of "A" or a diploma. Nurses do not have these typical benefits to offer their clients. The challenge for nurses is to motivate their clients, through the use of teaching strategies, so that they see, feel, and know that the "feeling better" outcome is a worthwhile reward.

Competency and incompetency

Both the need to learn and readiness to learn are affected by a client's competence (see Chapter 3). Competency is not easily determined. It is easier to describe mental incompetence in terms of the client's behavior that reflects his or her difficulty in intellectual reasoning secondary to psychoneurobiological stresses. In clinical practice, determining mental incompetence is often based on objective criteria and subjective judgment (Fulbrook, 1994). The nurse must consider the following:

- The client's right to know
- The client's psychiatric diagnosis and treatment
- The client's right to refuse treatment

In addition, in terms of teaching/learning, is the right of the client to refuse health teaching.

Comprehensive nursing health assessment

A comprehensive nursing assessment usually provides all the information a nurse needs to determine the client's need and readiness to learn. Box 16-3 lists crucial assessment areas or variables that the nurse must consider and evaluate; most are usually included in a standard nursing assessment tool (see Chapter 5). During the assessment, cognitive impairment and inappropriate behavior may leave gaps in data that are important to an accurate assessment of the learner's needs. As with implementing the nursing process, the nurse often uses other resources to complete the assessment. For example, the nurse may need to question the client's family or significant others, or other health care professionals, as well as review previous medical records to determine the following:

- What was taught before?
- How successful was it?
- What was the client's learning style?
- Which strategies worked best?
- If placed on similar medication, how long did it take before symptoms decreased and readiness to learn increased?

The nurse's level of experience and intuition influences the amount and accuracy of the data (Benner, 1984) and the way the data will be used in the development of appropriate teaching strategies for the best learning outcomes (Krainovich-Miller, 1995).

A low level of anxiety can be a motivator for learning, but anxiety can be a deterrent at a moderate level and can make learning nearly impossible at high and panic levels (Brenners, Harris, and Weston, 1987). The section on crisis intervention in Chapter 10 reiterates this point. Consider the single factor of anxiety level along with the other areas listed in Box 16-3, and the complexity of

---

BOX 16-3

Assessment Model: Need to Learn and Readiness to Learn

MENTAL STATUS INCLUDING THE DEGREE OR LEVEL OF THE FOLLOWING:

Mental competence (judgment and insight)
Mental age
Emotional maturity or response
Degree of appropriate behavior
Speech or communication pattern
Perceptual disturbance
Thought process
Sensorium and cognition
Impulse control
Reliability
Risk to self and others
Anxiety level
Coping ability or problem-solving ability
Coping resources

Understanding of psychiatric diagnosis and perceived threat
Physical abilities, including reading and hearing abilities
DSM-IV diagnosis; acute or chronic
Chronologic versus mental age
Occupation
Educational background, including reading level
Usual learning style or preference

MOTIVATION TO LEARN INCLUDING THE FOLLOWING:

Gender, race, cultural, and ethnic background preferences
Emotional responses
Locus of control assessment
Needs
Prior positive reinforcement behavior
Prior knowledge and skills related to what is to be learned

From Krainovich-Miller, B. (1995). Teaching/learning strategies used with the psychiatric-mental health client (unpublished manuscript).

BOX 16-4

General Strategies to Enhance Teaching the Anxious Client

- Self-evaluation criteria of the nurse: How anxious am I?
- Evaluation of nurse-client relationship: At what stage are we? Is there any trust?
- Evaluation of experience as a nurse: Do I have any past client examples on which to draw?
- Evaluation of the environment: Is the environment adding to the client's anxiety? How can I decrease it?
- Evaluation of the client: Is medication needed for the anxiety or agitation? How long since medications were initiated?
- Evaluation of client's support system: Is a family member or significant other available for the teaching session?

BOX 16-5

Variables that Negatively Impact the Teaching Process

Lack of teaching tools
Lack of space
Lack of privacy
Lack of time
Lack of client readiness to learn (motivation)

teaching this type of client becomes self-evident. Box 16-4 lists questions the nurse might ask when assessing the learning needs of an anxious client. The answers may help the nurse develop the appropriate climate to teach the client.

Other nonclient assessment variables that negatively affect learning

Box 16-5 lists other variables that negatively affect a client's readiness to learn. Some of these are out of the nurse's control; some are simply viewed as part of the clinical environment in which nurses teach rather than an ideal academic setting. For example, it may be determined that a particular client with a severe and persistent mental disorder is a visual learner (i.e., learns best through symbols, drawings, or viewing a film) rather than a "reading" learner (learns best by reading the printed word). Therefore it makes sense to use a videotape on the side effects of the client's medications rather than to provide literature. Psychiatric-mental health nurses rarely find themselves in such a simple situation. More typically, this type of client lives in a shelter without access to a videocassette recorder, and funds are usually not available for purchasing videotapes or VCRs or for making a client-oriented teaching videotape. Ongoing challenges for nurse and client include: lack of space, privacy, and time.

Teaching time is becoming an even more scarce commodity because clients may be discharged before teaching is completed or before they are capable of comprehending and retaining the information (e.g., medication effectiveness reached). One of the most important assessment factors is the answer to the last question of Box 16-4. A nurse may have only one or two formal opportunities to teach clients and their support systems during

an episode of care. Add to this the fact that clients' cognitive abilities are not at an optimal level for teaching. Including the clients' support systems becomes essential; they are a natural reinforcement resource for the nurse.

Other teaching strategies include simple things the nurse does, such as showing respect and courtesy by calling the client by name, using touch when appropriate, or including a family member or significant other during a teaching session. Such strategies help develop trust, decrease anxiety levels, or may even serve to make clients "feel good or cared about" so that learning can take place.

From a critical thinking framework, the nurse uses the teaching and nursing processes simultaneously when assessing clients. The importance of linking the teaching process with the nursing process will become evident as you read the clinical chapters and become familiar with commonly occurring behaviors of clients with severe and persistent mental disorders. Because nursing diagnoses are derived from comprehensive assessments, the need to learn may first be determined by the nurse rather than verbally identified by the client. The psychiatric-mental health nurse may often assess that a client's need to learn and readiness to learn are not at the best level for teaching but that teaching must be initiated because of previously mentioned ethical and legal guidelines. Proceeding with teaching without the criterion of "readiness to learn" is very similar to elementary school learning, which cannot always wait for childrens' readiness to learn (Tyler, 1964). For example, the nurse may determine the diagnosis of medication knowledge deficit related to cognitive impairment. Although the client is unable to identify a learning need and readiness to learn is not at the most opportune level, the psychiatric-mental health nurse begins to teach the client about the medications. Through the nurse-client relationship and implementation of the plan of care, the client will hopefully realize the need to learn about neuroleptic medication(s) and expected side effects, once the desired or therapeutic effect is reached.

The teaching process with clients with mental disorders does not proceed in a linear fashion and is similar to

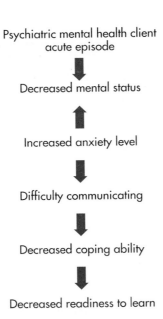

Psychiatric mental health client
acute episode

↓

Decreased mental status

↑

Increased anxiety level

↓

Difficulty communicating

↓

Decreased coping ability

↓

Decreased readiness to learn

Fig. 16-2   Readiness-to-learn challenge.

the nursing process described in Chapter 5. For example, the psychiatric-mental health nurse rarely conducts a complete physical health assessment. It is important that all necessary data are collected to formulate an accurate nursing diagnosis. In terms of the teaching process, it is important to understand that teaching principles, such as the client identifying the need to learn and having a sufficient degree of readiness to learn, may not always be present to the desired degree, yet the nurse cannot wait for "readiness" to happen. Fig. 16-2 illustrates the challenge of teaching clients with mental disorders of developing teaching strategies that provide, support, or build both readiness and the need to learn so that the client's learning outcomes are achieved.

Critical Thinking and Documenting Health Teaching

The nursing process and the teaching/learning process require critical thinking. As illustrated in Table 16-2, although the terminology differs slightly, understanding the similarities and differences between the two processes is important. A major difference from a nursing perspective is the manner in which the processes are documented. Documenting health teaching within the nursing process, in the form of a written nursing diagnosis and a related nursing care plan that includes outcomes related to health teaching, is extremely important. This type of nursing care plan supports a comprehensive nursing assessment to derive a nursing diagnosis that requires the use of health teaching for outcomes to be met. It labels what psychiatric-mental health nurses do in re-

lation to health teaching and supports that standards of care are met. In light of restructuring and downsizing in most mental health care settings and from a clinical and perhaps more practical perspective, it is unrealistic to conceive that a nurse will develop a separate teaching or learning plan each time he or she teaches a client. The nursing care plan in Chapter 5 illustrates this point. An overall teaching plan or protocol may be developed for a specific teaching situation such as when teaching groups of clients about their medications, an NIC intervention protocol for teaching medication would be an appropriate guideline. Chapter 11 discusses this type of health education group.

Learning Outcomes

How much can persons with mental disorders learn, especially those who are not in touch with reality or able to control their behavior? The answer is more than you might think but not as much as desired. As expected, the major outcomes of learning for clients with mental disorders focus on clients' adherence to treatment, especially with medications, and/or the development of necessary support and survival skills. The fact that nonadherence is still high remains a substantial problem to psychiatric-mental health nurses, other health care professionals and clients' families and significant others (Harmon and Tratnack, 1992; Heyduk, 1991; Kuipers et al., 1994). *Learning outcomes should reflect exactly what a client will learn and should be documented in measurable behaviors.*

The assessment model in Box 16-3 reflects the multifaceted considerations used to determine a nursing diagnosis related to the learning needs of the client, which in turn determine realistic learning outcomes. Similar to nurses in other settings, psychiatric-mental health nurses strongly encourage their clients, within ethical/moral guidelines, to learn the new behaviors needed to comply with treatment. For example, a psychiatric-mental health nurse may spend much teaching time stressing the need to take neuroleptic medication even though the client is experiencing unpleasant side effects. In other situations, the nurse may determine that other behaviors also need to be taught as the client's symptoms continue to interfere with his or her ability to comprehend the importance of the teaching goal. For example, the nurse may teach a family member or significant other, and the learning outcome is for that person to acquire the knowledge and/or behavior in place of the client until the client is able to acquire it.

Box 16-6 lists the essential teaching strategies or tools of the psychiatric-mental health nurse. When used within the context of the previous discussion, these strategies help bring about the following learning outcomes for teaching adherence to medication compliance:

BOX 16-6

Essential Teaching Strategies

Conduct a comprehensive assessment:
Know clients' learning styles.
Find out what client already knows about the topic to be taught.
Decrease anxiety.
Show respect and caring.
Develop trust through the nurse-client relationship.
Use therapeutic communication techniques.
Keep noise and distracting stimuli, when possible, to a minimum.
Provide a stimulating, positive environment.
Use a one-on-one and/or group format.
Make the learning process fun and interesting.
Be an active listener.
Be creative: use color, drawings, symbols.
Be flexible.

Provide outcomes that client can meet.
Conduct frequent, short sessions, no longer than 15 minutes.
Keep content simple; use short sound bytes.
Provide activities that develop self-esteem.
Repeat information, using multiple media: verbal, printed word, pictures, mnemonics.
Actively involve the learner.
Give homework.
Provide consistent feedback, first positive then constructive.
Rehearse with clients on how to use the information and in what context.
Seek ideas from clients, family members, or significant others on what works and does not work.
Use family members or significant others or even other clients during teaching sessions.

• Client takes medication as scheduled, as measured by the following:
  -Client reports taking medication even though he or she "feels better"
• Client "feels better" when taking the medication, as measured by the following:
  -Client reports a decrease in the disturbing symptom of hearing voices.
  -Client is able to shop at local supermarket.
• Client does not experience relapse symptoms, as measured by the following:
  -Client reports no relapse of symptoms of hallucinations or delusions.
  -Client attends and participates in day treatment program activities.
  -Significant others agree that client meets outcomes.

The extremely important role that family or significant others play in the health education of the client is further discussed in this chapter's section on psychoeducation programs. *Psychoeducation programs are structured, focused, and prescribed sessions that combine formal educational teaching techniques with various techniques of psychotherapy, which are primarily for assisting families prevent relapse in the care of clients with severe and persistent mental disorders* (Anderson, Reiss, and Hogarty, 1986; Watkins, 1985). Using the framework of the psychiatric-mental health nursing's *Standards* (ANA, 1994), *health teaching is education of the client with a mental disorder based on assessment of learning needs, which occurs mainly outside the psychotherapeutic modalities (i.e., psychotherapy); family or significant others may or may*

not be included. It is usually initiated on a one-on-one basis, but may be done in a group format.

Teaching Strategies and Processing Information

Box 16-2 presents teaching strategies as one power tool of teaching. Table 16-3 offers examples of learning domains and an example of a client learning outcome. Table 16-4 presents the principles derived from behavioral and cognitive theories and an example of a related teaching strategy to be used with a client with a mental disorder. From a nursing process framework, these strategies are helpful whether they are used one-on-one or in a group teaching session. The goal for the nurse in the teacher role is to strive for a supportive, conversational, though professional, attitude—one that conveys to the client that the information to be learned is important and instructional (i.e., the nurse strives to develop client's need and readiness to learn).

Applying teaching strategies

While reading the clinical chapters on the nursing management of mental disorders, it will become clear that clients with major disorders such as schizophrenia, mood disorder, and/or delirium and dementia experience great difficulty in processing information and verbally communicating information, especially during an acute episode. For example, they experience decreased concentration and are easily distracted. In turn, this limits their abilities to attend to tasks. Box 16-6 summarizes a number of essential teaching strategies for use with clients with mental disorders. Table 16-5 lists some com-

TABLE 16-3

Domains of learning		
DOMAIN	**TYPE OF LEARNING**	**EXAMPLE OF CLIENT OUTCOME**
Cognitive	Knowledge and intellectual abilities	Describes at least three side effects of prescribed neuroleptic medication
Psychomotor	Physical skills	Measures intake and output to monitor for complication of water intoxication
Affective	Attitudes and values	Cooperates during drawing of blood for blood lithium level

mon problems and general strategies that may assist the nurse in initiating a teaching session.

Strategy: sound bytes An essential strategy to use with a client with a mental disorder is to *teach in small or brief sound bytes and repeat information often over time*, especially until a client's medication reaches a therapeutic level and symptoms that disrupt his or her cognitive abilities subside. A costrategy with sound bytes is the use of **mnemonics**, or *methods of presenting material that assist in retaining and retrieving the material.* For example, Box 16-7 represents teaching tips in the form of important sound bytes of "teaching don'ts" that may be used with clients with mental disorders in regard to medications. In Box 16-8 the sound bytes are presented as the "4 Ss" of health teaching tips. In the in-

BOX 16-7

Strategy: Client Medication Don'ts

Don't mix your medication with any other over-the-counter medication.
Don't mix your medication with alcohol.
Don't stop taking your medication when you experience unpleasant side effects.
Don't stop taking your medication once you start feeling better.

BOX 16-8

Health Teaching: "4 Ss" Sound Bytes

Summer: Think ticks in the countryside.
Sun: Think sunscreen and hat.
Smoking: Think "No, I'll try gum."
Side effects of medication: Think "I'll discuss them with my nurse before I stop taking the medications."

patient setting, these teaching tips can easily be incorporated in all medication teaching. A related strategy is to use them on index cards and post them on bulletin boards, at the medication station, and at various locations on the unit. This strategy is enhanced by using colorful index cards and catchy drawings or symbols or neon markers. This is further enhanced by the creativity of the nurse and input from clients. Clients and families or significant others can be taught to do the same at home (e.g., place cards on the refrigerator, in the medicine chest, or in their wallets, pocketbooks, or pockets).

Strategy: short, frequent sessions Breaking up content into a tolerable and easily retrievable format enables the basic level psychiatric-mental health nurse to implement multiple teaching interventions listed in Box 16-1, as well as implement any other nursing care plan that addresses the need for medication teaching or the need to learn overall health teaching survival skills. For example, most clients with mental disorders could not tolerate being taught the NIC in one or even two sessions. It would take much more than 1 hour for each session. It would be much better for clients if the nurse planned four to six 15-minute sessions thus employing the strategies of keeping sessions short and interesting and planning frequent sessions over time.

Strategy: involving all possible resources Nurses have a number of teaching resources they can use, such as clients, family, significant others, and pharmaceutical and health product companies. As discussed, clients are important resources for finding out what they already know and to determine their learning styles. Families and significant others are also extremely important not only for helping to determine clients' learning styles when clients are unable to provide this information but also as reinforcers of content. Box 16-9 illustrates another aspect of this strategy, which is to "actively" involve client and family or significant others in teaching sessions. Some of the resources listed need to be adapted to the situation. For example, there are a number of videos on

TABLE 16-4

Application of learning principles and related teaching or learning strategies

PRINCIPLE	TEACHING/LEARNING STRATEGY AND EXAMPLE
It is best to provide partial positive, satisfying, and beneficial reinforcement/feedback as soon as possible after clients perform desired behavior.	Know what is satisfying to the client and how he or she will react to reinforcement such as praise (e.g., "You knew all the side effects, great job," or "I am really proud of your progress, your blood levels show that you are taking your medication as scheduled."); or make a point of smiling when a desired behavior is shown.
Positive actions should remove an undesired behavior, feeling, or stimulus.	Teaching the client to relieve dry mouth by rinsing mouth, drinking small amounts of water often; chewing on ice chips, etc.
Immediate negative reinforcement will help to decrease or extinguish nonpositive behavior.	If client displays unacceptable behavior, point out the behavior immediately (e.g., if a client goes to throw a cup of water at another client, take the cup from the client and state immediately that such behavior is not allowed and why).
In selected situations, withdrawing positive reinforcement for negative behaviors by ignoring the situation may extinguish the behaviors.	Do not focus attention on client's negative behaviors as long as others are not harmed or disturbed by client. In young children, do not call attention to a tantrum. After unacceptable display of behavior, decrease the amount of time spent with client.
New learning can interfere with prior learning.	If a client is new to your agency but has been on medication a long time and is now having a problem related to the medication, explore what the client knows before trying to teach new information that may be contradictory to what was previously taught.
Ideas are remembered for a long time, facts are not. It is important to help clients find meaning in what is being learned. Offer information, but always relate it to client's ADLs.	Nurse: "Jane, I know you enjoy going to the park and watching the birds. Taking your lithium on a daily basis even when you are feeling OK will keep your symptoms under control so that you can go to the park."
Rehearse with client.	Nurse: "Peter, it sounds like you get very scared when you go into the supermarket, and you think everyone is making terrible faces at you. Tell me out loud what you are going to say to yourself silently next time you go to the supermarket and you hear the same voices."
Visual imagery is viewed as a relaxation technique as well as a learning technique. Visual imagery can help clients retain information.	Nurse: "Ann, let me tell you about a technique that will help you to remember some of the things about your medication that you are concerned about not remembering. First close your eyes; I want you to visualize. . . ."
Suggest learning for shorter periods over a long period of time.	Nurse: "James, there is a lot to learn about your medication. I would suggest that you spend 5 to 10 minutes each day reviewing this information rather than spending 1 hour once or twice a week."

Continued.

TABLE 16-4—cont'd

Application of learning principles and related teaching or learning strategies

PRINCIPLE	TEACHING/LEARNING STRATEGY AND EXAMPLE
The ability to recall information is helped by using shorter words and shorter sentences.	Nurse: "Sandy, your new antidepressant drug is called Paxil." *rather than* "Sandy, your psychiatrist put you on a very good new selective serotonin reuptake inhibitor, referred to as an SSRI, antidepressant drug called Paroxetine or Paxil."
Use discrete categories.	Nurse: "Sandy, take one Paxil pill every morning."
Repetition of selected information increases retention.	Each time the nurse sees a client, she or he determines what information the client recalls and then repeats the most essential aspects of the medication. (e.g., "Jim, name me your medications," or, "Tell me how you will know if you are experiencing a side effect from your medication.")
Concrete, specific examples are remembered better than general, abstract examples.	Nurse (after assessing that client drinks 3 to 4 cups of coffee per day but has no tea, soda, or chocolate): "Ralph, while you are taking Ativan, drink only 1 cup of caffeinated coffee per day; caffeine decreases the effect of your medicine." *rather than* "Ralph, while you are taking your intermediate-acting benzodiazepine, Ativan, avoid caffeine of any sort."
Proceed from simple content or activities to the more complex.	Nurse (after client receives medication for the first time): "Jane, the medication I am giving you is the same medication you took the last time you became sick. It is called Haldol. It will help you think more clearly and help stop the voices." *rather than* "Jane, this medication is a neuroleptic called Haldol. It will decrease your hallucinations. You will need a blood level drawn."
Learning is context-dependent.	Nurse (same Jane as above, a few days later): "Jane, when you were home, what time did you take your medication?"
Use client contracting.	Develop realistic, measurable short-term goals in collaboration with client and write a contract.
Problem solving is a principle, a strategy, and an outcome; it is essential for ADL personal/social skill outcomes (i.e., the nontalking head teacher allows creativity and participation).	Help the client describe problem and resources or solutions for changing the situation.
Give client homework in relation to what is being worked on. It can be reviewed collaboratively at the next meeting. Client takes responsibility for own problem solving.	Nurse: "John, I want you to write down each day any side effects you experience."
A progressive relaxation technique (cognitive/biological theory) is viewed as a principle/strategy used to produce an outcome in self or may be used to help client decrease pain, anxiety, and stress to increase readiness to learn. The nurse can use aspects of the processes.	Use with a client who is capable of learning the steps of the process, is able to keep notes, and will perform the exercise. Use many of the previously listed strategies: discussion, role modeling, rehearsal, homework, tape recordings, quiet environment, mind clear of stressful thoughts; relaxed muscles; and response to a sound, word, or phrase that is repeated silently or aloud that allows for mental relaxation to occur.

TABLE 16-4—cont'd

Application of learning principles and related teaching/learning strategies

PRINCIPLE	TEACHING/LEARNING STRATEGY AND EXAMPLE
Visualization/guided imagery (cognitive/biological theory) is viewed as a principle and a strategy and is used to produce an outcome in self, or may be used to help client decrease pain, anxiety, and stress to increase readiness to learn. The nurse can use aspects of the process.	Requires a client who is able to tolerate the process and able to communicate clearly. Also, as noted previously, client must be able to indicate what is relaxing and what type of image is relaxing for them.
Schema-focused cognitive therapy techniques (combine cognitive, behavioral, interpersonal, and experiential techniques) help the client reframe the past and obtain a healthful self.	Requires client who is able to tolerate the processes and able to communicate clearly. Also as noted previously, client must be able to indicate what is relaxing and what type of image is relaxing for him or her.

TABLE 16-5

Expected behaviors that negatively impact teaching/learning process and strategies

CLIENT PROBLEM	TEACHING SESSION STRATEGY
Difficulty processing information, poor concentration, easily distracted, limited attention span for task	Use short, focused sessions.
	Give directions in small, simple steps. For example, if the goal is "Comb your hair," break it down into steps such as, "Go to your room, get the comb from the top drawer, go to the mirror, and start combing your hair."
Memory deficits and difficulty retrieving information previously learned (e.g., forgets what it was like when not taking medications, so when feeling better stops taking medications).	Have client make cards to keep in wallet or pockets or on refrigerator and medication cabinet that describe in own words the feelings and symptoms experienced when not taking medication. Use mnemonics.
Thought content impaired (e.g., delusions)	Use short, focused sessions; determine best time based on when medication initiated.
Language impaired	Use short, focused sessions; use written and other visual materials such as videos.
Impaired decision-making ability as seen in lack of insight, problem-solving skills, and ability to initiate tasks	Use above strategies, and determine time and effect of medication.
Moderate to panic-level anxiety	Decrease anxiety level through presence and use of the following, as appropriate: touch; silence; walking with client; supportive, short, informative statements; and/or medication.
Psychomotor retardation	Use short sessions and stimulating teaching tools.
Does not perceive reality in normal way, from simplest example of not hearing a doorbell as a doorbell but instead as a phone ringing.	Decrease stimuli. Use short, focused sessions. Use simple material.

symptoms and medications that nurses can use for self-education, but the nurse, with some modification, can also use them for client and family or significant others. Many of the videos are 45 to 60 minutes long, too long for a client teaching session. However, if they are carefully reviewed by the nurse, certain segments may be found to be useful for a short session.

Strategy: videotaped teaching sessions Videotaping a client during a survival skills session can be a rapid and powerful way to offer feedback to the client. For example, the nurse could videotape a social skills session consisting of clients who pair up to learn how to appropriately introduce themselves and shake hands. Replaying the videotape and discussing it can give clients immediate feedback. This type of session would have a number of outcomes for the clients, including the following:

- Clients will evaluate their own performances, as well as each others.
- Clients will devise alternative "introduction" approaches that fit their own styles.
- Clients will learn social skills through active participation.
- Clients will learn problem solving through active participation.

Each institution and situation may require a different approval process for videotaping. This should be explored before implementing this strategy.

BOX 16-9

Involvement Strategies for Client, Family and Significant Others

- Use teaching modules, such as print and computer-assisted instruction (CAI) with feedback.
- Distribute print (size, language, and level appropriate) information and discuss it.
- Show transparencies, slides, or videotape; stop and discuss at intervals.
- Videotape and view with feedback during session.
- Role model using clients.
- Rehearse using the context with nurse or other clients.
- Have clients repeat major points of previous session.
- Assign homework with discussion at next session.
- Have clients make their own teaching cards during the session or as homework.
- Initiate client discussion after short viewing of educational videotape.
- Form client groups to discuss experiences of symptoms.

HEALTH TEACHING VERSUS PSYCHOEDUCATION
Differences Between Health Teaching and Psychoeducation Programs

The previous discussion focused on the use of teaching/learning principles in teaching the client with a mental disorder in one-on-one or in a group health teaching sessions. The overriding framework was the nursing process; health teaching was embedded in the nursing care plan related to a nursing diagnosis. Teaching in a group format is the norm in many psychiatric and nonpsychiatric settings. Psychoeducation was defined at the beginning of this chapter as structured, focused, prescribed teaching sessions that combine formal educational teaching techniques with various techniques of psychotherapy primarily for assisting families who care for clients with severe and persistent mental disorders to prevent relapse. Table 16-6 illustrates the similarities and differences between health teaching sessions and psychoeducation programs. There is little strict agreement on the term *psychoeducation* in psychiatry (Goldman, 1988). However, there is agreement that psychoeducation programs should do the following:

- Use a variety of cognitive, behavioral, and psychosocial approaches.
- Involve a group of families or significant others in caregiver roles for individuals with major mental disorders to develop problem-solving and survival skills.
- Be part of a therapy process (traditional or purist view) and/or an orientation program.
- Provide research-based information about the mental disorder, with a particular emphasis on neurobiological etiological factors and treatments, as well as the various ways the family or significant others can adapt to the client's experience of them.
- Provide symptom management strategies for clients and families or significant others.
- Have relapse prevention as the ultimate goal.

The trend over the last three decades has been to decrease the length of hospital stay and increase the community treatment of clients with mental disorders, especially those with severe and persistent disorders (Bernheim and Lehman, 1985; Mannion, Mueser, and Solomon, 1994). The goal of psychoeducation programs is to help both clients and families to do the following:

- Manage clients' symptoms at home better
- Recognize early "relapse" symptoms
- Develop better ADLs and psychosocial skills (Holmes et al., 1994)

The original focus of psychoeducation programs was on family members, mainly because they were being asked

TABLE 16-6

Similarities and differences between health teaching sessions and psychoeducation programs

HEALTH TEACHING SESSIONS	TRADITIONAL PSYCHOEDUCATION PROGRAMS
Based on learning theory; individual assessment of client learning needs; need to learn and readiness to learn determined to develop teaching plan	Based on learning theory and theories related to psychotherapy; assume that need to learn and readiness to learn are affected; proceed with family or significant others
Uses educational (teaching/learning) strategies	Uses educational strategies and techniques of psychotherapy
Usually includes informal sessions conducted on a one-on-one basis (nurse and client, may include family/significant others); may also take place in a client group setting	Psychoeducation sessions are always part of a formal program that has a structured number of sessions and specific goals; usually group format, there are some exceptions of one-on-one with clients with severe impairments
May use formal teaching protocols in conjunction with above, or some group sessions may be structured using protocols	Originally sessions were with families, now may be groups of clients, as well as families and significant others
Takes place in a variety of settings	Takes place in a variety of settings
Goal is related to the individual assessment of the learning needs of the client, family, and significant other's learning needs related to promotion and prevention, care, maintenance, and prevention of relapse	Goals are to assist in client's posthospital or episode of care readjustment and long-term management of illness and relapse prevention
Depending on the particular need, may not focus on biologic/biochemical etiology	Focus is always on biological or biochemical explanation of the etiological factors of mental disorders and includes the latest research and stress management; some programs also include psychodynamic
In structured hospital or community program, length of session is usually short, 10 to 15 minutes; 50 to 60 minutes with a group session	Sessions in structured hospital settings are shorter than in other settings; length of time varies from 1 hour to four 1-hour sessions, to six 3-hour sessions, to 25 hours a week for 3 weeks to 1 year
May use didactic or process format, or a combination	Uses a didactic format rather than process-oriented format
Choice of content is determined by nurse's philosophy and assessment of the readiness of learners. Clients' degrees of affective and cognitive functioning are always major considerations	Choice of content is determined by the health professional's (i.e., group leader) orientation, as well as degree of patient affective and cognitive functioning
Used with any client with a mental disorder	Usually used with a client with a severe and persistent mental disorder who is prone to relapse
Outcomes depend on the specific learning need assessed (e.g., knowledgeable about specific medications and side effects, able to dress self, and so on).	Outcomes include that the family or significant others and client are knowledgeable about diagnosis, and client experiences less stigma and reduced isolation; they develop ways to cope with chronic illness and increase hope and self-esteem

to accept the role of long-term primary caregivers. In these beginning programs the client was only indirectly included (Hayes and Gantt, 1992). When the focus was family members, psychoeducation programs helped prepare them for discharge of the client.

Today, the psychoeducational movement embraces both a biological and psychodynamic explanation of mental disorders and related treatments (Gingerich et al., 1992), and the focus is not only on the family but also on the client and significant others (Hayes and Gantt, 1992). The newer models that have this extended philosophy use psychoeducational programs for clients on admission and throughout their episode of care, regardless of the setting (Maynard, 1993; Siegmann and Long, 1995; Sorensen et al., 1994).

Psychiatric-Mental Health Nurses and Psychoeducation

There are a number of psychoeducational models. Providing psychoeducation means that client "illness," survival information, and supports are provided to client, family, or significant others in a nonjudgmental manner through a formal educational and psychotherapy framework (Anderson, Reiss, and Hogarty, 1986; Gingerich et al., 1992; Keefler and Koritar, 1994. Therefore from the above perspective, psychoeducation programs are health teaching sessions that occur in groups, but not all group health teaching sessions are psychoeducation programs.

According to Williams (1989), most psychiatric nursing texts do not usually emphasize client and family education concerning clients' mental disorders, nor is it stressed in basic undergraduate curricula. Traditionally, basic-level psychiatric-mental health nurses did not formally teach client and family or significant others about the latest research related to the etiological factors, epidemiology, prognosis, and treatment of the particular DSM-IV mental disorder. They also did not focus on developing the caregiving skills of the family. This type of education usually occurred in a more informal manner (Daley, Bowler, and Cahalane, 1992) or in a formal manner by the advanced practice nurse. However, as clients continue to have shorter hospital stays, psychiatric-mental health nurses will play an increasingly significant role in formal psychoeducation programs.

Psychiatric-mental health nurse psychoeducation models

A number of nurses have adapted the major concepts of psychoeducation and developed structured programs, as well as informal sessions, that can be used with clients and families or significant others. However, they do not always adhere to the purest view of psychoeducation (Basolo-Kunzer, 1994; Collins, Given, and Given, 1994; Daley, Bowler, and Cahalane, 1992; Holmes, Ziemba,

Evans, and Williams, 1994; Huddleston, 1992; Kane, DiMartino, and Jimenez, 1990; Mohr, 1993; Moller and Wer, 1989; Williams, 1989). The overall goals of these programs remain in concert with traditional nonnursing psychoeducation programs in that they assist in the client's posthospital/episode of care readjustment and long-term management of the illness and relapse prevention, but they are not conceived within the framework of the family psychotherapy process. The principles and related strategies illustrated in Table 16-4 are certainly applicable to nursing and nonnursing psychoeducation groups, whether the group consists of clients who are experiencing acute phases of severe and persistent mental disorders and/or their families or significant others.

An essential goal of nurse-adapted psychoeducation programs is the development of survival or coping skills. Box 16-10 lists an example of the basic psychoeducation content for families or significant others of clients experiencing schizophrenia. The strategies listed in Box 16-6 can be used to implement this type of curriculum. The same program could be adapted for clients with this or any major disorder.

The important role nurses play in psychoeducation programs is obvious. It is an extremely important treatment modality for bringing about the desired outcomes of decrease in relapse and rehospitalization. Psychoeducation has been recommended by both mental health practitioners and consumers, including the National Alliance for the Mentally Ill (NAMI), as an essential way to assist those with severe and persistent mental disorders to manage their illnesses (Hayes and Gantt, 1992).

BOX 16-10

Basic Psychoeducation Content

Latest research on the disorder, emphasizing the following neurobiological issues:
- Etiological factors, epidemiology, prognosis
- Symptoms
- Treatment alternatives
- Medications and side effects
- Relationship of illness and stress and relapse
  Home-management coping strategies including the following:
- Communication techniques
- Monitoring stress
- Stress-management techniques
- Problem-solving techniques
- Early warning signs of relapse and how to cope with symptoms
- Developing ADL survival skills including social/leisure
- Living with the stigma

Health Teaching and Psychoeducation for the Community

As clients with mental disorders are moved more quickly into the community, there will be an even greater need for health teaching for community groups. The nurse-adapted psychoeducation framework will be an appropriate group format. The goals of psychoeducation could be refined for community groups to teach them about the neurobiological and psychodynamics of major mental disorders and their prevention, promotion, treatment, and relapse prevention. The more educated the consumers, the more empowered they are to assist each other in accepting clients with mental disorders in their communities. This in turn can make it less stressful for the client returning to the community. Psychiatric-mental health nurses have a prime opportunity to continue their leadership in this arena.

KEY POINTS

- Health teaching is a standard of care and an essential role of the psychiatric-mental health nurse and is performed with individuals, families, and community groups.
- Health teaching requires that the nurse integrate knowledge of the principles of teaching and learning with knowledge of health and illness. It is carried out in formal and informal sessions with individuals and groups. The nurse uses multiple teaching strategies depending on the learning needs and readiness of the learners.
- Health teaching is embedded in the interventions related to a nursing diagnosis and is documented within the nursing care plan.
- NIC teaching interventions supplement the nursing care plan or are used as individual research-based practice protocols.
- The "need to learn" refers to a client's request for information on how to perform some task related to his or her health condition.
- "Readiness to learn" refers to an individual's mental age or maturity and emotional and motivational level for learning.
- A comprehensive nursing assessment is critical in determining a client's learning needs and readiness to learn.
- Learning outcomes reflect measurable behaviors.
- Learning needs can be embedded in a nursing diagnosis and documented by a nursing care plan.
- Nurses need to evaluate their reactions to client behavior, the stage of the nurse-client relationship, and clients, families, and significant others to teach successfully.
- A number of factors that may negatively affect client learning needs may be out of the control of the nurse.

CRITICAL THINKING QUESTIONS

Walter, a 50-year-old male bus driver is admitted to your floor. He speaks English and has a 20-year history of chronic schizophrenia. His wife states that he stopped taking his medication. Walter is mildly agitated and states he is hearing voices. You do not hear these voices and notice that he has a decreased attention span.

Answer the following questions from the framework of meeting the goal of health teaching for this client.
1. What information do you need to assess Walter?
2. What areas of assessment are still needed?
3. What is one possible nursing diagnosis?
4. Who would you teach?
5. Discuss short- and long-term goals based on your nursing diagnosis that relate to health teaching.
6. What type of content would you teach?
7. Discuss the essential teaching strategies you would use.

- Specific goals of health teaching depend on individualized learning outcomes, as well as overall learning outcomes including changing clients' health-related behaviors and empowering clients to take as much control of their health as possible.
- Medication noncompliance is a major teaching need of clients with mental disorders.
- Psychoeducation programs are structured, focused, prescribed sessions that combine formal educational teaching techniques with various techniques of psychotherapy. They are used primarily for assisting families in the care of clients with severe and persistent mental disorders as a way of preventing relapse.
- Psychoeducation programs include health teaching; however, not all health teaching sessions include the primary goals of psychoeducation.

REFERENCES

American Nurses Association. (1994). *A statement on psychiatric-mental health clinical nursing practice and standards of psychiatric-mental health clinical nursing practice.* Washington, DC: Author.

Anderson, C.M., Reiss, D.J., & Hogarty, G.E. (1986). *Schizophrenia and the family: A practitioner's guide to psychoeducation and management.* New York: Guilford.

Antai-Otong, D. (1989). Concerns of the hospitalized and community psychiatric client. *Nursing Clinics of North America, 24*(3), 665-673.

Basolo-Kunzer, M. (1994). Caring for families of psychiatric patients. *Nursing Clinics of North America*(1), 73-9.

Batey, S., & Ledbetter, J. (1982). Medication education for patients in a partial hospitalization program. *Journal of Psychosocial Nursing and Mental Health Service, 20*(7), 7-10.

Benner, P. (1984). *From novice to expert: Excellence and power in clinical nursing practice.* Menlo Park, CA: Addison-Wesley.

Bernheim, K.F., & Lehman, A.F. (1985). *Working with families of the mentally ill.* Norton: NY Guilford Press.

Brenners, D. K., Harris, B., & Weston, P. S. (1987). Managing manic behavior. *American Journal of Nursing, 5,* 620-623.

Cohen, M., & Amdur, M.A. (1981). Medication group for psychiatric patients. *American Journal of Nursing, 2,* 343-345.

Collins, C.E., Given, B.A., & Given, C.W. (1994). Interventions with family caregivers of persons with Alzheimer's disease. *Nursing Clinics of North America, 29*(1), 195-207.

Coudreaut-Quinn, E., Emmons, M.A., & McMorrow, M. (1992). Self-medication during inpatient psychiatric treatment. *Journal of Psychosocial Nursing and Mental Health Services, 30*(12), 32-36.

Craft, M. J. (1987). Selecting and using teaching strategies, resources, and materials for client education. In Van Hoozer, H. L., Bratton, B. D., Ostmoe, P. M., Weinholtz, D., Craft, M. J., Gjerde, C. L., & Albanese, M.A. (Eds.), *The teaching process: Theory and practice in nursing.* Norwalk, CT: Appleton-Century-Crofts.

Daley, D. C., Bowler, K., & Cahalane, H. (1992). Approaches to patient and family education with affective disorders. *Patient Education and Counseling, 19,* 163-174.

Davidhizar, R., & Powell, M. J. (1987). Patient medication education groups. *Hospital Topics, 65*(1), 21-24.

Dinkmeyer, D. (1991). Mental health counseling: A psychoeducational approach. *Journal of Mental Health Counseling, 13*(1), 37-42.

Falloon, I. R. H., et al. (1982). Family management in the prevention of exacerbations of schizophrenia. *New England Journal of Medicine, 306,* 1437-1449.

Fulbrook, P. (1994). Assessing mental competence of patients and relatives. *Journal of Advanced Nursing, 20,* 457-461.

Gingerich, E., Golden, S., Holley, D., Nemser, J., Nuzzola, P., & Pollen, L. (1992). The therapist as psychoeducator. *Hospital and Community Psychiatry, 43*(9), 928-930.

Goldman, C. R. (1988). Toward a definition of psychoeducation. *Hospital Community Psychiatry, 39,* 666-668.

Harmon, R. B., & Tratnack, S.A. (1992). Teaching hospitalized patients with serious, persistent mental illness. *Journal of Psychosocial Nursing and Mental Health Services, 30*(7), 33-38.

Hart, C.A., Craig-Williams, G., & Gladwell, C. L. (1985). A deliberative and group approach to inpatient consumer medication education. *JOURNAL, NYSNA, 16*(1), 33-42.

Hayes, R., & Gantt, A. (1992). Patient psychoeducation: The therapeutic use of knowledge for the mentally ill. *Social Work in Health Care, 17*(1), 53-67.

Heyduk, L. (1991). Medication education: Increasing patient compliance. *Journal of Psychosocial Nursing, 30*(3), 27-32.

Holmes, H., Ziemba, J., Evens, T., & Williams, C. (1994). Nursing model of psychoeducation for the seriously mentally ill patient. *Issues in Mental Health Nursing, 15,* 85-104.

Huddleston, J. (1992). Family and group psychoeducational approaches in the management of schizophrenia. *Clinical Nurse Specialist, 6,* 118-121,

Kane, C., DiMartino, E., & Jimenez, M. (1990). A comparison of short-term psychoeducational and support groups for relatives coping with chronic schizophrenia. *Archives of Psychiatric Nursing, 4*(6), 343-353.

Keefler, J., & Koritar, E. (1994). Essential elements of a family psychoeducation program in the aftercare of schizophrenia. *Journal of Marital and Family Therapy, 20*(4), 369-380.

Knowles, M. (1990). *The adult learner: A neglected species* (3rd ed.). Houston, TX: Gulf.

Krainovich-Miller, B. (1995). Teaching strategies for positive learning outcomes for the psychiatric client. Submitted for publication.

Kucera-Bozarth, K., Beck, N. C., & Lyss, L. (1982). Compliance with lithium regimes. *Journal of Psychosocial Nursing and Mental Health Services, 20*(7), 11-15.

Kuipers, J., Bell, C., Davidhizar, R., Cosgray, R., & Fawley, R. (1994). Knowledge and attitudes of chronic mentally ill patients before and after medication education. *Journal of Advanced Nursing, 20*(3), 450-456.

Malow, R. M., West, J. A., Corrigan, S. A., Pena, J. M., & Cunningham, S. C. (1994). Outcome of psychoeducation for HIV risk reduction. *AIDS Education and Prevention, 6*(2), 113-125.

Mannion, E., Mueser, K., & Solomon, P. (1994). Designing psychoeducational services for spouses of persons with serious mental illness. *Community Mental Health Journal, 30*(2), 177-190.

Maynard, C. (1993). Psychoeducational approach to depression in women. *Journal of Psychosocial Nursing, 31*(12), 9-35.

McCloskey, J. C., & Bulechek, G. M. (Eds.). (1996). *Nursing interventions classification (NIC): Iowa intervention project* (2nd ed.), St. Louis: Mosby.

McFarlane, W. R. (1991). Family psychoeducational approach: New applications of treatment. In A. S. Gurman & D. P. Kniskern (Eds.). *Handbook of Family Therapy Vol. II* (pp. 363-395) New York: Brunner/Mazel.

Mohr, W. K. (1993). Nurse-led psychoeducational programs in psychiatric settings: Developing a curriculum. *Journal of Psychosocial Nursing, 31*(3), 34-46.

Moller, M., & Wer, J. E. (1989). Simultaneous patient/family education regarding schizophrenia: The Nebraska Model. *Archives of Psychiatric Nursing, 3,* 332-337.

Redman, B. K. (1991). Courses in patient education in masters programs in nursing. *Journal of Nursing Education, 30*(1), 42-43.

Redman, B. K. (1993). *The process of patient education* (7th ed), St. Louis: Mosby.

Siegmann, R. M., & Long, G. M. (1995). Psychoeducational group therapy changes the face of managed care. *Journal of Practical Psychiatry and Behavioral Health 1*,(1), 29-36.

Sorensen, J. L., London, J., Heitzmann, C., Gibson, D. R., Morales, E. S., Dumontet, R., & Acree, M. (1994). Psychoeducational group approach: HIV risk reduction in drug users. *AIDS Education and Prevention, 6*(2), 95-112.

Tyler, F. T. (1964). Issues related to readiness to learn. In E. R. Hilgard (Ed.). *Theories of learning and instruction.* Chicago: The National Society for the Study of Education.

Van Hoozer, H. L., Bratton, B. D., Ostmoe, P. M., Weinholtz, D., Craft, M. J., Gjerde, C. L., & Albanese, M. A. (1987). *The teaching process: Theory and practice in nursing.* Norwalk, CT: Appleton-Century-Crofts.

Watkins, C. (1985). Psychoeducational training in counseling psychology programs: Some thoughts on a training curriculum. *The Counseling Psychologist, 13*(2), 295-303.

Williams, C. (1989). Patient education for people with schizophrenia. *Perspectives in Psychiatric Care, 25*(2), 14-21.

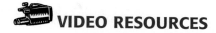 **VIDEO RESOURCES**

Mosby's Community Health Nursing Video Series: *Patient Teaching in the Community*

Part Four

Continuity of Care

Chapter 17

Psychiatric Case Management

Beverly J. Farnsworth
Anicia S. Biglow

LEARNING OUTCOMES

After studying and applying the concepts of this chapter, the learner will be able to:

- Discuss the historical perspectives of case management in relation to health care restructuring.
- Discuss the use of the term *case management* in a variety of settings and contexts.
- Differentiate between case management and managed care.
- Discuss the major requirements for cost-effective quality case management care.
- Discuss the major goal of the case manager of clients with mental disorders.
- Describe the four generic models of case management: full support, personal strengths, rehabilitation, and expanded broker.
- Discuss three major case management approaches.
- Analyze the differences among the following tools of case management: interdisciplinary treatment plan (ITP)/ critical paths, nursing care plans, research-based practice guidelines, and assessment measures.
- Describe similarities and differences in the goals of the psychiatric-mental health nurse case manager who functions in agencies that use the generic models and approaches of case management.

KEY TERMS

Assessment tools	Critical path	Nurse case manager
Brokers	Interdisciplinary treatment plan (ITP)	Variance
Case management		

Case management, although not a new concept in the field of mental health nursing (Baier, 1987), is viewed as a positive strategy for the delivery of health care to all, especially to high-cost, high-volume, and high-risk populations. In a climate of fragmentation, limited access, and underfinancing of mental and physical health care services for clients with mental disorders, case management is an essential strategy for delivering cost-effective, quality mental health nursing care. *Case management is a method of providing cost-effective quality care (cost, process, outcomes) by managing the holistic health concerns of clients (individuals, families, and groups) who are in need of extensive services (Girard, 1994). It requires integrating, coordinating, and advocating for complex mental and physical health care services from a variety of health care providers and settings, within the framework of planned health care outcomes (Bower, 1992).*

The purpose of this chapter is to explore the important issues surrounding case management and its application to the mental health care field. The basic principles, models and approaches, goals and outcomes, and tools of case management, as well as the role of the case manager, is presented. The role of the psychiatric-mental health nurse as a case manager is discussed here in relation to generic models and approaches of case management.

Understanding and applying case management principles during your educational clinical experiences will help prepare you for the tremendous changes occurring today and in the next millennium in the field of mental health nursing.

HISTORICAL PERSPECTIVE IN THE CLIMATE OF HEALTH CARE RESTRUCTURING

In the 1980s the public became increasingly aware of health care costs and the difficulties in obtaining health care for persons with and without health care insurance. Many clients had unmet physical health care needs, especially those with severe and persistent mental illnesses. Multiple factors contributed to this ineffective and costly health care delivery system, including the following:

- Advances in medical and communication technologies
- An increasing chronically ill aging population
- Disregard for the cost of resources
- Misuse of resources
- Undetermined and undefined outcomes
- Undetermined and long lengths of stay for treatment

- Similar services provided by multiple agencies

Restructuring payment systems for health care and decreasing lengths of stay, regardless of type of illness or setting, were initial attempts to rectify the ills of costly care. However, most people agreed that services remained fragmented, and most were dissatisfied with the care, including—most importantly—the consumer. Employers, insurers, and the health care industry began to explore methods to help health care become more cost- and value-effective.

The 1990s brought direct focus on health care through heated debates about various health care restructuring proposals discussed on the national, state, and local levels. The nursing profession participated in these debates by offering public testimony and publishing *Nursing's Agenda for Health Care Reform* (American Nurses Association [ANA], 1991). This landmark document clearly indicated that case management is one of the basic components of nursing's "core of care."

CASE MANAGEMENT AND NURSING

Although case management has a long tradition in social work (Stanhope and Lancaster, 1996), it also has its roots in public health nursing. At the turn of the century, public health nurses "coordinated community services" as part of the delivery of nursing care through a primary nursing approach (Bower, 1992; Cohen and Cesta, 1993; Girard, 1994). The need for a more sophisticated method of coordinating services, or "case management" evolved as a way for communities to handle the influx of clients with mental disorders during the period of deinstitutionalization in the 1960s. In today's highly technological world, case management has a much broader and more sophisticated approach than public health nursing's earlier coordination of community services. However, community health nurses who work in this arena continue to evolve; today they are considered natural case managers (Worley, 1991a).

PRINCIPLES OF CASE MANAGEMENT
Basic Principles

As a cost-saving, process- and outcome-oriented system, the basic principles of case management include the following:

- Continuity of care, reflecting appreciation of clients' needs for support and treatment over an extended period

- Use of the case management relationship to develop collaborative relationships with the client, family, or significant others, and other caretakers

- Determining needed mental and medical support and services that facilitate personal development and prevention of mental illness
- Flexibility in the frequency, duration, and location of interventions, reflecting an appreciation of a client's individual needs
- Facilitating client's resourcefulness with a focus on personal strengths and assets rather than needs and deficits (Kanter, 1989)

Although case management, as defined, seems simple and straightforward, it is actually a quite complex concept that is sometimes confusing to a newcomer to the field of nursing. From a nursing perspective, case management can be used directly and indirectly in the practices of all health care professionals and paraprofessionals and the clergy, as well as in almost any type of health care-related setting (Bower, 1992; Stanhope and Lancaster, 1996). In fact, it is the most often used "nursing care delivery system" in these settings (American Hospital Association Survey, 1990). Case management is also implemented from different perspectives. It is often described in the literature or used in communications among and between nurses, other health care professionals, and the consumer as a system, role, and/or service.

The promotion and maintenance of mental health, as well as the prevention and treatment of mental disorders, is a complex process that requires multiple providers and services (see Chapter 18). The delivery of mental health care requires that programs of care be implemented through a case management framework that addresses the characteristics listed in Box 17-1.

Case Management and Managed Care

In addition to case management being viewed from a number of perspectives by a variety of professional and paraprofessional health care providers in multiple settings, it is sometimes used synonymously and incorrectly with the term *managed care*. Managed care refers primarily to strategies employed by purchasers of health care services to influence aggregate utilization levels of various types of services to maintain quality and control costs. Managed care arrangements such as health maintenance organizations (HMOs) and preferred provider organizations (PPOs) do not emphasize the individual, client-level care coordination, as does case management (Bower, 1992), although the ultimate goal of quality, cost-effective care may be the same. In general, consumers are familiar with managed care. Many talk about it as a "place" where they must go for their health care, such as an HMO, because their insurance company holds a contract with the HMO. In this context the client receives "managed" health care through a negotiated, prepaid, discounted arrangement (Hicks, Stallmeyer,

> **BOX 17-1**
>
> ## Characteristics of Case Management
>
> Care is episode-based
> - Does not focus exclusively on the care provided within one area/specialty
> - Promotes continuity of the plan and provider across the continuum of care
>
> Care is longitudinally based
> - Client followed along the trajectory of illness
> - Client referred to the most appropriate provider
> - Provides most cost-effective complement of treatment services for desired outcomes
> - Promotes effective utilization of health care resources and provides for an optimum level of rehabilitation/restoration
>
> Care is provided to targeted or selected client populations
> - Clients are from high-cost, high-volume, or high-risk categories
>
> Care focuses on coordinating services and transitions
>
> Care is outcome driven
>
> Providers are fiscally aware and responsive
> - There is a cost-quality link for clients and organizations
> - Management of the costs of care is an important function of case managers
>
> Central focus of care is on clients and their families
>
> Nurse case managers:
> - Assess the full range of needs and issues
> - Advocate for clients and their families
> - Foster decision making, independence, and growth
> - Establish an effective relationship with client/family nucleus
> - Educate client/family and support them in moving toward self-care
> - Collaborate to tap expertise of all providers/disciplines; secure input and active involvement
>
> Care is benchmarked by the ability to procure and enhance the accessibility of services
>
> Care is proactive
> - Providers try to prevent problems and issues
> - One goal of care is to interrupt cyclic patterns
>
> *From Bower A.K. (1992).* Case management by nurses. *Washington, DC: American Nurses Association.*

and Coleman, 1993). Some of the newer managed care programs may use the previously described case management philosophy, but these concepts are not interchangeable (Bower, 1992; Hicks, Stallmeyer, and Coleman, 1993). See Chapters 1 and 2 for further discussion of managed care.

Case Management and the Role of the Case Manager

Case management is implemented through the role of the case manager. From this perspective, *case management is a method of assigning responsibility for systems coordination to one person (case manager) who works with a client in accessing and coordinating the necessary multidisciplinary services; it provides a mechanism to help the client navigate through the health care system* (Merrill, 1990). Therefore the principle function of a case manager is the coordination of care and services. Who makes the best case manager—the clinician, the professional, or the paraprofessional—is continually debated in the literature (Bower, 1992). However, it is the perspective of this book that nurses are best suited for this role by their broad-based education and skills, their professional licenses, *Standards of Care* (ANA, 1991), biopsychosocial clinical expertise and experience, as well as the profession's rich history of coordinating services (Bower, 1992).

MODELS AND PHILOSOPHICAL APPROACHES OF CASE MANAGEMENT

The implementation of case management services varies within program designs. Most programs use components of four generic case management models: full support, personal strengths, rehabilitation, and/or expanded broker. Table 17-1 describes these models in terms of the role of the case manager. The team specialty functions of nursing, medicine, psychiatry, social work, and vocational rehabilitation and the generic functions of advocacy, collaboration, and monitoring are parts of the full support model. However, all models implicitly address these functions by the very definition of case management. Later in the chapter, case studies are presented that reflect some of these generic models and the role of the psychiatric-mental health nurse.

TABLE 17-1

Generic case management models: role of case manager

FULL SUPPORT	PERSONAL STRENGTHS	REHABILITATION	EXPANDED BROKER
Active clinical case management that utilizes team support in providing specialty and generic functions	Focuses on developing individual strengths of clients rather than pathology to obtain basic necessities; actively creates personal and environmental situations where success can be attained	Focuses on the client and family in identifying and enhancing strengths of clients to become successful and satisfied in the social environment of their choice with the least amount of professional help	Focuses on linking the client with community resources
Teaching of coping skills such as symptom self-management and symptom education, and implementing clinical services such as supportive psychotherapy, symptom management, crisis intervention with client/case management	Has two underlying assumptions: • Individuals with severe and persistent mental illness have difficulty organizing and interacting with their environment in obtaining basic necessities • These deficits are directly related to their difficulty to secure resources essential for human growth and development, such as employment, housing, social support, and medical services	Services are determined by individual client goals and needs rather than pre-established system goals	Major functions include assessment, planning, linking, and advocating on behalf of client

Data from Modroin, M., Rapp, C., & Chamberlain, R. (1985, June). Case management with psychiatrically disabled individuals: Curriculum and training program. *Lawrence, KS: University of Kansas School of Social Welfare; Robinson, G. (1990). Choices in case management.* In-site, 3, 1, 4-6, 11; *and Solomon, P. (1992). The efficacy of case management services for severely mentally disabled clients.* Community Mental Health Journal, 28, *163-180.*

OUTCOMES OF CASE MANAGEMENT

Outcomes of case management are directly related to the goal of providing cost-effective, quality health care. Important to the process of documenting outcomes is the identification of factors that have demonstrated effectiveness in lowering costs and improving client outcomes and satisfaction. These include the following:

- Enhanced communication with and education of clients and their families, which enables them to better plan for and make more fully informed decisions about care
- Early identification of discharge needs, resulting in the development of plans to address potential or real barriers
- Identification of client problems and barriers to care within a time frame that allows them to be addressed proactively or concurrently, rather than retrospectively
- More effective and efficient communication among the disciplines involved in client care, as well as with clients and their families
- Reduction or elimination of duplicate or overlapping care, tests, and treatments through improved sequencing and coordination of care activities
- Minimized or eliminated delays in required tests, treatments, or care
- Enhanced knowledge among providers regarding the financial aspects of care
- Attention to the needs of clients and the issues and problems encountered in providing efficient, effective care at both the individual and aggregate client levels (Bower, 1992)

As discussed in Chapter 4, ongoing quality improvement outcomes evaluation audits and outcomes research are identifying variables that affect length of stay, appropriate timing of interventions such as client education, the influence of individual practice patterns on outcomes, the impact of management decisions, the effects of other department's policies and procedures on nursing, and client and family perception of quality (Zander, 1988). An often-cited study conducted at the New England Medical Center used the system-administrative, or primary nurse case management model (Cohen and Cesta, 1993). Its case management system decreased length of stay by 1 day for most clients and reduced costs by 40% in major clinical departments (Bower, 1992; Zander, 1988).

The Case Manager's Role and Outcomes

Cost effectiveness and success of case management systems are enhanced when the case manager has the following:

- A financial interest in the solution

- A role in designing service options
- Multiple service options
- Authority to choose services most appropriate for a client
- Access to financial resources to link the client to needed services
- Regularly scheduled clinical supervision
- Automated data and tracking systems for clients and outcomes
- Available outside consultants who can look objectively at issues such as system barriers and resources
- Available continuing education and training programs (Alloy, 1990; Merrill, 1990)

GENERAL TOOLS OF CASE MANAGEMENT WITHIN THE CONTEXT OF MENTAL HEALTH

Case management tools include interdisciplinary treatment plans (ITPs), nursing care plans, research-based practice protocols, and assessment tools. The case management documentation systems originated in the acute care hospital setting. However, the system is being adapted or developed in community and home care settings. Regardless of setting or discipline orientation, these tools provide guidelines for assessing, documenting, and providing intervention guidelines, as well as for bringing about planned outcomes in a timely, cost-effective manner.

Interdisciplinary Treatment Plans

Interdisciplinary Treatment Plans (ITPs) *are essential documentation systems. They are also referred to as the master interdisciplinary care plan, managed care plans, case management plans, multidisciplinary action plan (MAP), Care Maps, critical paths, or clinical pathways.* The generic term *ITP* will be used for this discussion. ITP simply refers to the documentation system that reflects the case management model of the institution. The name for the tool is often institution-specific. A typical ITP *is used to manage the comprehensive care of the client. The framework of the plan integrates the dimensions of care of all members of the health care team. It is directed by the case manager, who uses the tool to facilitate and minimize interruptions to the set timing and sequencing within the care system* (Bower, 1992). In most hospital settings, regardless of whether a formal case management system is in place, the nurse is usually in the role of managing the ITP.

The development of the ITP revolves around the primary medical/psychiatric diagnosis and is linked to the prospective payment system through the diagnosis-related group (DRG) code. For example, most ITPs use

BOX 17-2

Home Care Nurse-Adapted ITP With Nursing Diagnosis for Bipolar Disorder

ASSOCIATED NURSING DIAGNOSES

Noncompliance, ineffective family and individual coping skills, knowledge deficit, and sleep pattern disturbance; service skills identified

Skilled assessment of the client with psychiatric registered nurse two times per week for the following:
- Teach antidepressive medication and side effects
- Monitor medication regimen and compliance with lithium therapy
- Obtain venipuncture for lithium level per physician order
- Teach client and family about disease and management
- Provide individual and family psychotherapy related to overwhelming anger and fragmentation in family support
- Monitor client's mental status for signs and symptoms of depression or mania
- Evaluate home safety and teach precautions to ensure safety
- Assess sleep patterns, factors contributing to sleep disturbance, and effectiveness of sleep medication regimen, and teach behavior modification plan to stabilize sleep patterns
- Explore support groups in the community that are available to the client and family
- Observe and assess all systems

Skilled assessment of the client with occupational therapist (OT) for evaluation of diversional deficit
- Assess activities of daily living
- Assess safety in home
- Plan, implement, and supervise therapeutic activity program

REASON FOR HOMEBOUND STATUS

Unsafe for client to be out of hospital without supervision

Nurse short-term goals
- Client adheres to prescribed medications and other regimens
- Family taught to effectively care for client
- Client maintained safely in home
- Lithium level within normal limits

OCCUPATIONAL THERAPIST SHORT-TERM GOAL

Initiate therapeutic activity program

Nurse long-term goals
- Client cared for safely with home as the therapeutic environment
- Decrease in identified problem behaviors or behaviors are controlled
- Sleep patterns stabilized
- Symptoms stabilized; increased or enhanced coping skills

Occupational therapist long-term goal
Home therapeutic activity program adhered to by client and family

Discharge plans
Discharge client when client-centered goals that were agreed upon by the client with the psychiatric home care team are achieved.

Courtesy Anicia S. Biglow, HUG, 1995, Atlanta.

the DRG/ICD9 code number (Cohen and Cesta, 1993). The use of an ITP in the psychiatric setting, especially in the community home care setting, is relatively new. Most ITPs do not include the use of nursing diagnoses but do indicate the various nursing interventions and teaching activities implemented by the nurse. However, like the medical/psychiatric diagnosis, the use of a specific nursing diagnosis on the ITP can be an effective way of addressing teaching and therapy needs and developing interventions and strategies to meet client goals, which are supported by members of the interdisciplinary team. Box 17-2 provides a nurse-adapted ITP used with a client with an affective mental disorder that includes the nursing diagnosis, outcomes, and interventions. The code number 296.2X.3X refers to both the ICD9 and DSM-IV code number for bipolar I disorder, most recent episode depressed. This type of ITP assists in the documentation process and is an important aid in reimbursement from third-party payers (Marrelli, 1994).

The essential design features of most shortened one- to two-page or longer version ITPs include the following:

- Specific ICD9 code diagnosis linked to prospective payment system by DRG
- Critical events (multidisciplinary treatment interventions) for each day of an episode of care
- Specified timeline of outcomes
- Variance tracking

Critical path refers to the idea that for the particular client problem, the plan includes the essential treatment interventions that must be performed each day to meet the expected time-specific client outcomes. The client problem usually reflects a specific DRG. The critical path traces the client from first treatment encounter to final exit from the system. Critical paths were first used by the New England Medical Center in Boston (Zander, 1988, 1991) who adapted the term *Care Maps*. Usually ITPs are several pages long, but in many areas of the country, there is a movement toward the following changes:

- Shortening the case management ITP to a one-sided, single-page or two-sided, single-page tool
- Creating ITPs that cover the client for the entire episode of care in the hospital and community/homes

Another essential aspect of the critical path is ***variance,*** which refers to "anything that does not happen when it is supposed to happen" (Cohen and Cesta, 1993). Examples of variances that might occur include the following:

- *Operational* (e.g., broken equipment, such as a magnetic resonance image unit not working)

- *Health care provider* (e.g., a physician that does not order an MRI)
- *Client* (e.g., a client refusing to have an MRI)
- *Clinical indicator* (e.g., a client does not meet the expected stated/documented outcome in the specified timeline)

A one-page version of a critical path that charts the nursing and physician processes that are identified in the case management plan is presented on p. 325. It shows the exact mapping of all significant incidents that must happen for the client to achieve the standard outcome in accordance to the maps (Zander, 1988). The use of critical paths in acute care settings decreases fragmentation of care by anticipating care activities; lowering unforeseen omission of needed care; increasing quality care, because client outcomes are addressed; and increasing the client's satisfaction because they know when and where events will happen (Girard, 1994). It is projected that the same will hold true for community-based or home care settings.

Nursing Care Plans

Nursing care plans are another effective case management tool (Townsend, 1994). As discussed in Chapter 5, nursing care plans are based on an individual assessment of the client with a derived North American Nursing Diagnosis Association (NANDA) nursing diagnoses. They include specific client outcomes with timelines. Because of the brevity of ITPs, case management plans, and critical paths, and/or their nonnursing diagnosis focus, the need for individualized nursing care plans becomes imperative. An interdisciplinary documentation format guideline cannot replace the nursing care plan and vice versa. A nursing care plan is an adjunct; it allows for further specific guidelines and documents evidence for tracking client outcomes. Although, as indicated in the characteristics of case management in Box 17-1, the focus of episode-based care does not exclusively focus on the care provided by one area/speciality. The fact is that the medical diagnosis, in the form of an ICD9 code/DRG/DSM-IV, and the related treatment predominate on most tools. Therefore it is extremely important for nurses to document their care for particular client problems and their contributions to case management outcomes. As the one-page critical path is linked to the ITP, the nursing care plan can be linked to the critical path through the use of the nursing diagnosis. This is important in carrying out the nurse case manager role of coordinator of care and services on an interdisciplinary team. Standardized nursing care plans can decrease duplication of services. See Chapter 5 for examples of nursing care plans that are standardized, computerized, and can easily be individualized.

INTERDISCIPLINARY TREATMENT PLAN

Critical Pathway: Major Depression   296.2X.3X; 300.40; 311.00

Patient Name: _____   Case Manager: _____   Physician: _____   Medical Record # _____

Admit date: _____   Expected LOS: _____   UR days certified: _____   Discharge Date: _____   Actual LOS: _____

Day/Date:	0–8 Hours	8–24 Hours	Day 2	Day 3	Day 4	Day 5
ASSESSMENTS & EVALUATIONS	Nursing Nutritional screen Admit note Precautions	H & P, Social HX, RT/TA; Dr: Initial TX Plan/Admit Note Prec. Eval.; AIMS Scale	Precaution Evaluation	Psych Eval done Social Hx on chart Precaution Evaluation Assess for level of care	Assess for readiness for discharge	Assess for goals achieved Assess client support network
PROCEDURES	Lab ordered-Admit profile UA, UDS, UCG, EKG, Other:	Lab done: UA, UDS, UCG, EKG Other:	Lab results checked Abnormals called to Dr.	Follow-up for abnormal lab results		
CONSULTS	IT ordered Y/N FT ordered Y/N GT ordered Y/N Psych Testing Order Y/N	GT started Psych Testing done	Schedule MTP meeting	IT started FT started Psych Testing Results Home Contract		
TREATMENT PLANNING	N1: _____ Axis III: _____		RT/TA started School started (youth)	Master TX Plan Updated RT/TA entry		
INTERVENTIONS	Assess Suicidal potential	Monitor sleep pattern	Encourage identification of causative factors	Identify strengths and accomplishments	Help develop and rehearse problem solving skills	Encourage pt. participation in D/C plan
MEDICATIONS	Meds ordered, Informed Consent		Drug interaction checked by Pharmacist/Dr. signs informed consent	Meds evaluated/ readjusted		Discharge instructions for medication self-admin
LEVEL TEACHING	Level ordered Patient Rights Orient to Unit	Orient to Program	Re-evaluate Medication Teaching Stress Reduction; Goals	Re-evaluate for PHP Meds reinforced; Positive coping mechanism	Re-evaluate for D/C Decision making; Assertiveness training	Re-evaluate Promote self-reliance & diversional activities
NUTRITION/DIET CARE CONTINUUM	Diet Ordered: _____ Initial D/C Plans	Chart daily intake Outcome survey	Chart daily intake Evaluate support system	Weight, chart intake D/C Plan update/ revise	Chart daily intake After Care Plan written	Diet D/C instruction Outcome survey
PATIENT OUTCOMES	Controls self-harm	Attentive in group therapy	Expresses feelings	Makes + self statements	Uses problem solving skill	Verbalizes hope for future

Strategic Clinical Systems, PsychPaths™ © 1994. All Rights Reserved. Darla Belt, RN & Vickie Pflueger, RNC: Authors

Research-Based Practice Protocols

Research-based practice protocols, such as the Agency for Health Care Policy and Research (AHCPR) guidelines for depression or nursing intervention classification (NIC) (McCloskey and Bulechek, 1996) for multiple commonly occurring client problems, are examples of case management tools that provide valuable and reliable intervention information that can be used in the development of ITPs, case management critical paths, and nursing care plans. Chapter 5 and each of the clinical chapters provide examples of how to use a NIC with a standardized nursing care plan.

Assessment Tools

Although not usually referred to as a case management tool, from a multidisciplinary perspective the assessment process is critical to properly diagnosing the client, monitoring a response to interventions, and addressing the client's on-going needs, all of which are essential to case management. *Assessment tools perform two purposes: (1) they give credibility and make evasive concepts such as anger and agitation more concrete and (2) they serve as a baseline for establishing outcomes* (Carson, 1994). Examples of standard assessment tools used by psychiatric home care nurse case managers are the mini-mental examination for cognitive abilities; the Sheehan Anxiety Scale for anxiety; and the Visual Analogue Scale, Zung Depression Self-Rating Inventory Scale, or the Global Assessment of Functioning Scale for depression. See Chapter 5 and clinical and population at-risk chapters for additional assessment tools.

Resource and Services Tools

Examples of community resources from a case management framework are the Department of Health, the Department of Mental Health social service agencies, insurance agencies, educational systems, religious institutions, public health programs, rehabilitation centers, community mental health centers, and volunteer organizations. Nurse case managers use agencies from the federal, state, and local levels to provide case management. The case manager needs to be knowledgeable of these resources and access them directly and/or make them available for clients with mental disorders and their families or significant others. The use of such tools by the nurse case manager is vital to the process of effectively and efficiently linking the client to appropriate services, especially those who have severe and persistent mental disorders. Examples of additional resources can be found in the clinical and population at-risk chapters. Case studies provided at the end of this chapter demonstrate the use of such community resources.

The nurse case manager uses case management tools to coordinate the assessment, diagnosis, outcomes, planning, and related interventions, as well as the documentation of clinical and social environmental mental health needs of clients. These tools guide clinical approaches, define staff accountability, link resources, and establish and monitor outcomes. The effectiveness and utilization of these tools are influenced by the knowledge, skill, and educational preparation of the nurse case manager. In many settings, these tools are computerized for ease of use and accuracy of documentation.

CASE MANAGEMENT AND THE NURSE CASE MANAGER WITHIN THE MENTAL HEALTH FIELD

Case management, organized through the nurse case manager role, extends nurses an opportunity to demonstrate their leadership and clinical roles on multidisciplinary health care teams by providing coordinated health care. The *nurse case manager combines the principles of case management with the nursing process in monitoring and managing the care of clients with mental disorders who have complex acute health care needs and those with severe and persistent mental health disorders to bring about planned health care outcomes* (Box 17-3).

BOX 17-3

Knowledge and Skills of a Nurse Case Manager

- Updated knowledge of the health care system and parameters for reimbursement
- Solid clinical knowledge of psychiatric disorders and clinical skills in physical and psychosocial assessment, medications, and interventions
- Knowledge of community, home care, and institution resources
- Effective discharge planning skills and timeliness in linking resources
- Management skills, especially in areas of communication, facilitation, collaboration, negotiation, problem solving, consultation, and organization
- Skills in family and community assessments
- Skills in collaboration and facilitation of team-building strategies
- Skill in quality improvement strategies, program evaluation, outcome development/monitoring, and research
- Skills in teaching, counseling, education, and goal setting

Based on data from Bower, K.A. (1992). Case management by nurses. *Washington, DC: American Nurses Association; Zander, K. (1988). Managed care with acute care settings: Design and implementation via nursing case management.* Health Care Supervisor, *6:27-43.*

Psychiatric-Mental Health Nursing's *Standards*

As discussed in Chapter 5, psychiatric-mental health nursing's *Standards* (ANA, 1994) mandates the use of its standards of care, which are the components of the nursing process, for the delivery of quality nursing care. Connolly (1992) demonstrated the importance of psychiatric nursing standards in identifying the components and functions of the case manager. Table 17-2 further illustrates this point. The ANA's implementation standard of case management is as follows: *the psychiatric-mental health nurse provides case management to coordinate comprehensive health services and ensure continuity of care* (1994). This correlates to the basic characteristics of the case manager as indicated in Box 17-1. All of the standards of care guide nurse case managers in carrying out the goals of case management in relation to their client populations.

Educational Preparation of the Nurse Case Manager

Psychiatric-mental health nursing's Standards (ANA, 1994) recommend that a baccalaureate in nursing be the minimum preparation for nurse case managers and that a master's in science degree is desired. However, in the midst of health care restructuring, the reality is that a case management model/approach is becoming the norm in almost all mental health care settings across the United States. Nurses, regardless of their educational preparation or speciality, are finding themselves in the case manager role. All nurses, regardless of their educational preparation, can use the ANA standard of case management as a guide for carrying out the nurse case manager role. Many settings offer in-service education programs on the role of the nurse case manager when implementing a case management model, as well as the "how to" of developing critical paths (Cohen and Cesta, 1993).

Goals of the Nurse Case Manager

The goals of the nurse case manager include the following (ANA, 1991):

- Reduce the fragmentation of the present mental health care system
- Promote the mental health consumer's active participation in decisions about their health care
- Provide an advocate on the behalf of clients with mental disorders and their family or significant others
- Bring about planned mental and physical health care client outcomes

Coordinator of Care and Services

The principle role of the nurse case manager is that of coordinator of care and services; it is this core function that brings about the goal of case management. Essential coordination of care is the development of relationships among the client, family members, and other health care providers. Through effective communication techniques and collaborative skills, the nurse case manager builds trust and support that fosters these relationships. The nurse case manager is the bridge that links community services with clients' needs. To be successful, nurse case managers must secure the input, cooperation, and active involvement of all providers essential to clients' care (Bower, 1992; Pittman, 1989). Nurse case managers act as brokers. *Brokers obtain the necessary services needed for their clients.* Fig. 17-1 illustrates the coordination process of the nurse case manager broker.

Collaboration and Empowerment of Clients

The nurse case manager develops a collaborative system in which clients and their families/significant others play active roles in decisions that affect them, such as changes in medication or living arrangements. From this type of collaboration emerges clients and families/significant others who are empowered to continue as active participants in their health care. The full support model case

TABLE 17-2

Collaborative principles

PRINCIPLE	GOAL
Family consultation	To educate and support families to successfully cope with their caregiving responsibilities
Family education programs	To emphasize family coping rather than family pathology
Advanced practice nurse consultation	To assist staff within a case management system in planning a comprehensive treatment plan that includes attention to the physical health care needs, nutrition, self-care deficits, and medication compliance of clients with mental disorders

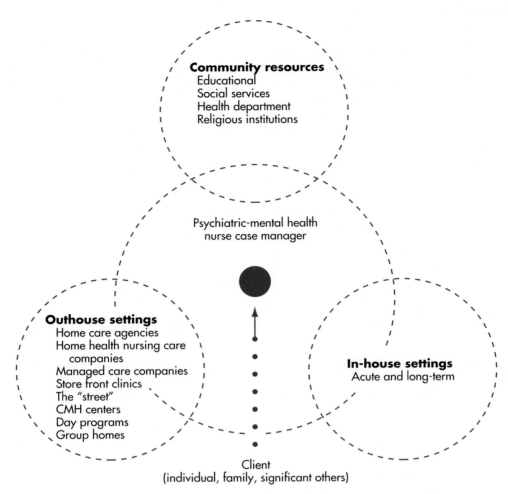

Fig. 17-1 The coordination process of a nurse case manager broker.

study that follows illustrates this important aspect of the nurse case manager role.

Table 17-2 illustrates collaborative principles and related goals that the nurse case manager uses in daily formal and informal communications with clients and caregivers. In turn, all contribute their expertise and resources to support clients with mental disorders (Reinhard, 1994). The collaborative role of the nurse case manager allows for the redistribution of control from the professional caregiver system to the client, family, and informal care systems.

A psychiatric-mental health nurse may work in a health care agency that implements case management from the perspective of a system, role, process, technology, service, or a combination of some or all of these perspectives. Box 17-4 lists a number of positive outcomes nurses experience in this role.

APPLICATION OF THE NURSE CASE MANAGER ROLE
Full Support Model Case Study

History and assessment
John is 35 years old and has a diagnosis of schizophrenia, paranoid type. He has had a long history of hospitalizations since the age of 24. After his last hospitalization, John was referred by the discharge planning nurse to the Dedicated Case Management Program (DCMP) at the local mental health center. During the initial meeting at the DCMP, the nurse case manager observed some tongue wiggling, restlessness, and pacing. The nurse case manager referred John to the psychiatrist for medication evaluation because of extrapyramidal side effects from his present neuroleptic medications. The psychiatrist changed his medication from haloperidol (Haldol) to

risperadone (Risperdal). After the change in medication, the nurse case manager made a home visit assessment and observed that his apartment was dark and cluttered with dirty dishes, cans, and clothes. John acknowledged that he had difficulty keeping things organized but felt overwhelmed with where to begin. He spent most of his time in his room, only leaving his apartment for cigarettes and food. The nurse case manager reviewed his records further and uncovered that for the past 2 years, since his mother died, John had been noncompliant with his treatment regimen.

Nursing diagnoses

Impaired home maintenance management and ineffective management of therapeutic regimen were derived, and outcomes and a plan were developed.

Nurse case manager interventions

Part of the plan was to make referrals to the social worker, residential staff, and day treatment program staff for evaluation of services. A team meeting was then scheduled to develop an ITP and implement strategies to address medication teaching and management, symptom identification and management, ADLs, safety of environment, diversional and social needs, and crisis management. During the past year, since the nurse case manager implemented the full support model of case management, John has not needed rehospitalization.

BOX 17-4

Positive Outcomes of the Nurse Case Manager Role

Nurse case managers have multiple opportunities to experience the following:
• Challenged
• Empowered
• Independent

Nurse case managers have opportunities to do the following:
• Use and demonstrate depth and breadth of skills and knowledge in leadership and clinical abilities
• Develop new experiences and knowledge in other areas
• Take risks in managing the quality and cost of health care in meeting the needs of clients
• Develop collegial and collaborative relationships with other disciplines, as well as professional relationships with clients/families/significant others

KEY POINTS

• Modern-day case management has its roots in social work and public health nursing.
• Cost-effective quality care requires not only cost savings but positive processes and outcomes for the client.
• The four generic case management models are full support, personal strength, rehabilitation, and expanded broker.
• Models of case management tend to have three areas of approach: the system-administrative approach, the administrative approach and the professional case management approach.
• Tools used by case managers include ITPs, case management plans with critical paths, nursing care plans, clinical guidelines (Agency for Health Care Policy and Research and NIC), assessment measures, and resource agencies.
• The case manager's principle function is coordination of care and services, which is brought about through collaboration and advocacy.

 CRITICAL THINKING QUESTIONS

Referral to psychiatric home health care nurse case management was made by the social worker for discharge services for a 76-year-old depressed woman. As an inpatient the client received electroconvulsive therapy (ECT) and was started on paroxetine (Paxil). The client also has uncontrolled hypertension. The staff and physician recommended posthospital transition to a retirement or assisted living environment as a result of confusion and some delusional thinking. However, the client and her 52-year-old son refused the recommendation for alternative living but agreed to the home health care services and day treatment program. According to the social worker, the client has a long history of depression. She has been independent most of her life and is a retired nutritionist. A major concern expressed by the social worker relates to a long history of an abusive relationship with her son. Her son moved in with her about 15 months ago during his divorce and also has chronic depression.
1. How would you begin assessing the abusive relationship?
2. If you find that the son is once again abusing his mother, what actions should you, as the case manager, take?
3. What are the client education priorities?
4. Who do you need most to maintain a degree of care coordination?

- Experienced psychiatric-mental health advanced practice registered nurses are the most qualified to perform case management functions; however, all nurses, regardless of educational preparation, with in-service education are able to carry out the activities of case management.
- Case management is shown to be useful for clients with mental disorders.
- Nurse case managers and clients experience positive outcomes as a result of case management.

REFERENCES

Alloy, V. (1990). Case management: A design for the '90s. *Insites, 3,* 10.

American Hospital Association Survey. (1990). *Report of the hospital nursing personnel survey—1990.* Chicago, IL: Author.

American Nurses Association. (1991). *Nursing's agenda for health care reform.* Kansas City, MO: Author.

American Nurses Association. (1994). A *statement on psychiatric-mental health clinical nursing practice and standards of psychiatric-mental health clinical nursing practice.* Washington, DC: Author.

American Psychiatric Association. (1994). *Diagnostic and statistical manual of mental disorders, fourth edition,* Washington, DC: Author.

Baier, M. (1987). Case management with the chronically mentally ill. *Journal of Psychosocial Nursing and Mental Health Services, 25,* 17-20, 33, 35.

Borland, A,. McRae, J., & Lycan, C. (1989). Outcomes of five years of continuous intensive case management. *Hospital and Community Psychiatry, 40,* 369-376.

Bower, K. A. (1992). *Case management by nurses.* Washington, DC: American Nurses Association.

Carson, V. B. (1994, June). Psychiatric home care documentation: Doing psych but talking med-surg language. *Caring Magazine,* 32-41.

Cohen, E. L. (1991). Nursing case management: Does it pay? *Journal of Nursing Administration, 21,* 20-25.

Cohen, E. L., & Cesta, T. G. (1993). *Nursing case management: From concept to evaluation.* St. Louis: Mosby.

Connolly, P.M. (1992). What does a nurse need to know and do to maintain an effective level of case management. *Journal of Psychosocial Nursing and Mental Health Services, 30,* 35-9.

Dittbrenner, H. (1994, June). Psychiatric home care: An overview. *Caring, 13,* 6, 26-29.

Ethridge, P. (1991). A nursing HMO: Carondelet St. Mary's experience. *Nursing Management, 22,* 22-27.

Ethridge, P., & Lamb, G. (1989). Professional nursing case management improves quality, access, and cost. *Nursing Management, 20,* 30-35.

Girard, N. (1994). The case management model of patient care delivery. *AORN Journal, 60,* 403-405, 408-412, 415.

Hicks, L. L., Stallmeyer, J. M., & Coleman, J. R. (1993). *Role of the nurse in managed care.* Washington, DC: American Nurses Publishing.

Kanter, J. (1989). Clinical case management: Definition, principles, components. *Hospital and Community Psychiatry, 40,* 361-367.

Kozlak, J., & Thobaben, M. (1992). Treating the elderly mentally ill at home, *Perspectives in Psychiatric Care, 28,* 31-35.

Marrelli, P. N. (1994). *Handbook of home health standards and documentation and guidelines for reimbursement.* (2nd ed.). St. Louis, MO: Mosby.

Mechanic, D., & Aiken, L. H. (1987). Improving the care of patients with chronic mental illness. *The New England Journal of Medicine, 317,* 1634-1638.

Mellon, S.K. (1994). Mental health clinical nurse specialists in home care of the '90s. *Issues in Mental Health Nursing, 15,* 229-37.

Merrill, J. (1990). Jeffrey Merrill on case management. *Insites, 3,* 2.

Modroin, M., Rapp, C., & Chamberlain, R. (1985, June). *Case management with psychiatrically disabled individuals: Curriculum and training program.* University of Kansas School of Social Welfare, Lawrence.

Mound, B., Gyulay, R., Khan, P., & Goering, P. (1991). The expanded role of nurse care managers. *Journal of Psychosocial Nursing and Mental Health Services, 29,* 18-22.

O'Connor, F., & Eggert, L. (1994). Psychosocial assessment for treatment planning and evaluation. *Journal of Psychosocial Nursing, 32,* 31-42.

O'Connor, F. W., Sprunger, J. E., & Petry, S.D. (1992). A clozapine treatment program for patients living in the community. *Hospital and Community Psychiatry, 43,* 909-11.

Pittman, D.C. (1989). Nursing case management: Holistic care for the deinstitiutionalized chronically mentally ill. *Journal of Psychosocial Nursing and Mental Health Services, 27,* 23-7, 33-4.

Reinhard, S.C. (1994). Perspectives on the family's caregiving experience in mental illness. *Image: Journal of Nursing Scholarship, 26,* 70-4.

Robinson, G. (1990). Choices in case management. *Insites, 3,* 1, 4-6, 11.

Smith, G.B. (1994). Hospital case management for psychiatric diagnoses: Focusing on quality and cost outcomes. *Journal of Psychosocial Nursing and Mental Health Services, 32,* 3-4.

Solomon, P. (1992). The efficacy of case management services for severely mentally disabled clients. *Community Mental Health Journal, 28,* 163-180.

Stanhope, M., & Lancaster, J. (1996). *Community health nursing: Process and practice for promoting health* (4th ed.). St. Louis: Mosby.

Taylor, G.L. (1988). Public health nursing documentation and case management. *Journal of Community Health Nursing* 5(1):11-18.

Townsend, M. (1994). *Nursing diagnoses in psychiatric nursing: A pocket guide for care plan construction.* Philadelphia, PA: F. A. Davis.

Van-Dongen, C.J., & Jambunathan, J. (1992). Pilot study results: The psychiatric RN case manager. *Journal of Psychosocial Nursing and Mental Health Services, 30,* 11-4, 35-6.

U.S. Department of Health and Human Services. (1993). *Depression in Primary Care: Vols. 1 and 2.* (AHCPR Publication No. 93-0550). Rockville, MD: U.S. Government Printing Office.

Worley, N. (1991a). Born in the USA . . . case management of people with long-term mental illness part 1. *Nursing Times, 87,* 32-4.

Worley, N. (1991b). Adviser to the team . . . role of the nurse in the case management for people with mental illness part 2. *Nursing Times, 87,* 38-40.

Worley, N.K., Drago, L., & Hadley, T. (1990). Improving the physical health-mental interface for the chronically mentally ill: Could nurse case managers make a difference? *Archives of Psychiatric Nursing, 4,* 108-113.

Zander, K. (1988). Managed care within acute care settings: Design and implementation via nursing case management. *Health Care Supervisor, 6,* 27-43.

Zander, K. (1992). Physicians, Care Maps, and collaboration. *The New Definition, 7*(1), 1-4.

Chapter 18

Health Promotion and Maintenance and Preventive Interventions

Claire Griffin-Francell

LEARNING OUTCOMES

After studying and applying the concepts of this chapter, the learner will be able to:

- Discuss the significance of a wellness approach to the delivery of mental health care.
- Discuss the *Healthy People 2000* objectives that pertain to mental health and mental disorders.
- Evaluate similarities and differences among the three prevention models for mental disorders presented in this chapter.
- Discuss the components of the Mental Health Intervention Spectrum Model.
- Identify examples of preventive, treatment, and maintenance intervention programs.
- Describe the role of psychiatric nurses in preventive, treatment, and maintenance intervention programs.
- Discuss the significance of the mental health consumer movement.
- Discuss community action as a vehicle for creating change.
- Identify linkages between community action and preventive intervention.
- Describe the role of psychiatric nurses as participants in community action.

KEY TERMS

Community action	Primary prevention	Tertiary prevention
Indicated preventive interventions	Secondary prevention	Treatment interventions
Maintenance interventions	Selective preventive interventions	Universal preventive interventions

n the 1990s, more Americans are concerned about their health than ever before. An emphasis on healthy life choices has intensified as environmental disease factors make headlines more frequently. Motivation to stay well has also become a concern as health care costs remain an issue. The general public—the consumers of health care—has become much more aware that maintaining health applies not only to physical health, but mental health as well. Providers of physical and mental health care are shifting from an illness-cure to a wellness-prevention approach to health care services. Consumer-provider coalitions are catalysts for promoting community action that facilitates change in the nature and location of health care services available to individuals, families, and communities.

It is estimated that 50% of health problems seen in primary care practices are mental health in nature. This is consistent with the fact that the National Institute of Mental Health has estimated that 20% of adults suffer from a mental disorder each year, and 32% will have a mental disorder in their lifetime (Robins and Regier, 1991). It is increasingly clear that prevention of mental disorders is a necessity rather than a luxury.

Promotion of mental health focuses on enhancement of well-being and strengthens life-enhancing and life-sustaining activities such as school achievement, employment, and effective parenting. Preventive interventions are designed to reduce the risk for mental disorders, thereby increasing the cost-effectiveness of mental health treatment resources. Maintenance interventions for persons with severe and persistent mental disorders are integral with psychiatric rehabilitation and focus on reducing relapse and recurrence of mental disorders, which create an immense financial and emotional cost to American society (Rice, Kelman, and Miller, 1990).

The purpose of this chapter is to discuss how key concepts such as risk reduction, consumerism, community action, and preventive and maintenance interventions can be used to promote mental health and decrease disability from mental disorders.

PREVENTION OF MENTAL DISORDERS

A national trend that highlights the value of illness prevention is captured by the slogan "an ounce of prevention is worth a pound of cure." Integral with health care restructuring and the movement toward capitated health care financing within a managed care system is a greater economic incentive to prevent illness rather than treat it. However, a report issued by the Institute of Medicine (1994) concludes that while the prevention of mental disorders can play an important role in alleviating the incalculable financial and social burden imposed by these disorders, little evidence exists that any specific mental disorder can be prevented. Nevertheless, research aimed

---

BOX 18-1

Healthy People 2000 Objectives Related to Mental Health and Mental Disorders

To reduce mental disorders by the year 2000, objectives target the following:
- Reducing mental disorders among adults
- Reducing adverse health effects from stress
- Reducing uncontrolled stress
- Reducing suicide
- Reducing suicide attempts among children and adolescents
- Increasing use of treatment by people with major depressive disorders
- Increasing the proportion of people who seek help for personal and emotional problems
- Increasing the use of community support programs by people with mental disorders
- Increasing workplace stress management programs
- Increasing appropriate suicide prevention strategies in jails
- Increasing the number of states with established mutual help clearinghouses
- Increasing routine review of mental functioning by primary care providers for both children and adults

From U.S. Department of Health and Human Services, (1995). Healthy People 2000, Review 1994. (DHHS Publication No. (PHS) 91-50212). Washington, DC. U.S. Government Printing Office.

---

at reducing risk factors associated with specific disorders should be conducted and rigorously evaluated (IOM, 1994).

Consistent with this trend, the U.S. Public Health Service has sponsored a national incentive, *Healthy People 2000,* to promote health and prevent disease in this country (USDHHS, 1995). The *Healthy People 2000 Review 1994* objectives that pertain to mental health and mental disorders are listed in Box 18-1. The objectives provide direction for nursing as well as multidisciplinary services that aim to reduce the incidence of mental disorders by increasing available preventive and maintenance interventions.

It is important to keep in mind that although the idea of promoting mental health and preventing mental illness is sensible and proactive, the vastness and vagueness of this goal can be overwhelming. Conceptually, everything has implications for reducing emotional disorders and promoting mental health. Defining measures that accurately evaluate the short- and long-term benefits of preventive intervention programs is difficult. For example, successful teaching of parenting skills to parents of children with conduct disorders may fulfill short-term goals, but the long-term effectiveness of this intervention in relation to the children's mental health as adults may be unclear and unsupported by empirical evidence.

Another problem relates to the concepts and definitions associated with prevention. For example, what is the difference between health promotion and disease prevention? According to the IOM (1994), health promotion is not driven by an emphasis on illness, but rather by a focus on the enhancement of well-being. It is provided to individuals, groups, or large populations to enhance competence, self-esteem, and a sense of well-being rather than to try to prevent psychological or social problems or mental disorders, which is the distinguishing characteristic of prevention. An agreement on what is being promoted or prevented is of paramount importance to best determine what action should be taken and to whom the action should be directed, an entire population or only people believed to be at risk for developing a disorder.

MODELS FOR PREVENTION OF MENTAL DISORDERS

The prevention models used for many years were originally based on an approach to controlling infectious disease. Historically, most nurses and physicians accepted the Public Health Model of Prevention as useful and relevant for conceptualizing mental health intervention programs. Caplan (1964) discussed basic concepts underlying preventive mental health in his classic book *Principles of Preventive Psychiatry.* Since that time, research has advanced the understanding of the complexity of the association between risk factors and health outcomes, which led to the development of the Mental Health Intervention Spectrum Model (IOM, 1994). This model has created a paradigm shift in conceptualizing a spectrum of preventive intervention for mental disorders.

The Public Health Model of Prevention

In 1957 the Commission on Chronic Illness distributed a classification system of disease prevention (Commission on Chronic Illness, 1957). The Public Health Model, originally based on a communicable disease approach, was adapted for a broad range of prevention efforts in chronic physical disease and noninfectious diseases. It consisted of the following three types of prevention:

- ***Primary prevention** seeks to decrease the number of new cases of a disorder or illness (incidence).*
- ***Secondary prevention** seeks to lower the rate of established cases (prevalence).*

- ***Tertiary prevention** seeks to decrease the amount of disability associated with an existing disorder or illness.*

This model views mental illnesses as diseases in the medical-model tradition and thereby uses the epidemiological approach associated with the public health model to develop preventive intervention, treatment, and rehabilitation programs. In relation to primary prevention intervention, the model consists of the following steps:

1. Identify a disease (e.g., schizophrenia) of sufficient importance to substantiate the need for a preventive intervention program.
2. Develop reliable diagnostic methods so that persons can be divided into groups according to whether they have the disease.
3. Conduct a series of epidemiological and laboratory studies to identify the most likely cause of the disease.
4. Initiate and evaluate an experimental preventive intervention program based on the results of those studies.

This model has been effective for a wide range of causative agent communicable diseases such as chicken pox, measles, tuberculosis, and polio, as well as nutritional diseases such as scurvy, rickets, and pellagra. It has also been effective for mental disorders caused by single agents such as poisons, toxins, electrolyte imbalances, nutritional deficiencies, or licit or illicit drugs. However, most mental disorders are multicausal in nature. It is therefore difficult to target the removal of one causative agent through a mental health preventive intervention program, thereby reducing the risk for development of a specific mental disorder.

The Caplan Mental Health Prevention Model

Based on the public health model of prevention, Caplan (1964) described three levels of preventive intervention in relation to mental illness and emotional disturbance.

- *Primary prevention* consists of decreasing the incidence of mental disorders or reducing the rate at which new cases of a disorder (e.g., depression) develop.
- *Secondary prevention* consists of reducing the prevalence of a disorder by reducing the number of existing cases. Early case finding, screening, and immediate treatment are secondary prevention activities.
- *Tertiary prevention* consists of activities that attempt to reduce the severity of a disorder (e.g., schizophrenia) and related disabilities through rehabilitation programs (e.g., social skills training and intensive case management programs).

Mental health prevention activities obviously address an array of services that range from the prevention of mental illness to minimizing the negative sequelae of existing mental disorders. In the United States the thrust of funding and the allocation of economic resources for mental health services has been in secondary prevention activities.

The Mental Health Intervention Spectrum Model

The Mental Health Intervention Spectrum Model for Mental Disorders (IOM, 1994) is based on the work of Gordon (1987), who proposed an alternative classification system to the public health model. In Gordon's risk reduction model, the risk of getting a physical disease was weighed against the cost, risk, and discomfort of the preventive intervention.

The Committee on Prevention of Mental Disorders of the IOM (1994) presents an alternative system, based on much of Gordon's (1987) work, which emphasizes prevention but recognizes the importance of a whole spectrum of interventions for mental disorders, from prevention through treatment to maintenance, as illustrated in Fig. 18-1. This chapter focuses on the prevention and maintenance components of this model, which are described in the following sections.

Universal preventive interactions

Universal preventive interventions are targeted to the general public or a whole population group that has not been identified as being at risk for a particular mental disorder. A public health promotion program that advocates early, regular, and comprehensive prenatal care is an example of a universal preventive intervention program that may be effective in promoting healthy brain development. This universal preventive intervention may be linked to an important mental health outcome: reduction in the incidence of schizophrenia (McEvoy, 1995). Safe-sex education programs represent another universal preventive intervention program. This one is aimed at reducing the risk for human immunodeficiency virus (HIV), acquired immunodeficiency syndrome (AIDS), and other sexually transmitted diseases.

Community agencies offer other types of universal preventive intervention programs that enhance well-being and quality of life, including assertiveness training, parenting effectiveness, couple-relationship enhancement programs, mastery learning, and other competency building programs.

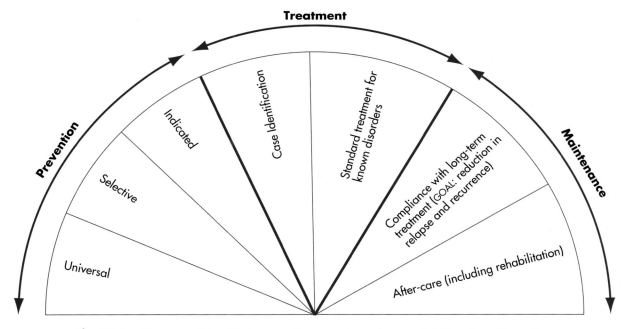

Fig. 18-1   The mental health intervention spectrum for mental disorders. From *Reducing Risks for Mental Disorders.* National Academy of Sciences, 1994.

Selective preventive interventions

Selective preventive interventions are targeted to individuals or subgroups of the population whose risks of developing mental disorders are significantly higher than average. Risk groups may be identified on the basis of biological, psychological, or social risk factors that are known to be associated with the onset of a mental disorder (IOM, 1994).

Many selective preventive interventions target children because of their increased vulnerability. For example, the Women, Infants, and Children (WIC) program, administered by the Department of Agriculture and community health nurses, provides supplemental food to low-income mothers with infants and toddlers. Normal brain development requires good nutrition. Classroom teachers know that hungry children are often sleepy, restless, or inattentive to learning. They may also be at risk for conduct disorders and depression.

Other selective preventive intervention programs include family bereavement programs, children-of-divorce intervention programs, caregiver support groups, and academic skills and social skills training programs. Examples of support groups include Alzheimer's disease support groups, local National Alliance for the Mentally Ill (NAMI) groups for caregivers of people with schizophrenia and affective disorders, Parents without Partners, and bereavement groups such as Compassionate Friends (for parents who have lost a child through death), widow-to-widow, and suicide survivor support groups.

These programs help people master developmental and situational crises. During major life changes, some individuals have difficulty navigating life's transitions and responding effectively to unexpected events. A phone directory contains numerous listings for mental health providers who work with persons of all ages who have problems with sexual dysfunction, marital conflict, divorce, bereavement, infertility, unplanned pregnancies, child abuse, and learning problems. The risk for dysfunction can be reduced through selective preventive intervention programs.

Indicated preventive intervention

Indicated preventive interventions are targeted at high-risk individuals who are identified as having minimal but detectable signs or symptoms that foreshadow mental disorders or who have biological markers that indicate a predisposition for a mental disorder. Sometimes referred to as early intervention programs, indicated preventive interventions include parent-child interaction training programs, which provide interventions for children whose parents have identified them as having behavior problems. Another indicated program could be aimed at a child who has a parent with a neurobiological disorder such as schizophrenia. Indicated interventions can also be designed to reduce violent behavior in young adults. Community leaders can mobilize neighborhood residents, the criminal justice system, community health nurses, and school staff to reduce the risk of violent and criminal behavior. An example of this is a "Stop the Violence" initiative begun in 1994 in Atlanta. Table 18-1 provides other examples of preventive intervention programs, the associated risk factors, and program outcomes.

Psychiatric nurses, like all nurses, have always been committed to a wellness health care delivery model that is integral with health promotion and illness prevention. Psychiatric nurses may design, secure funding for, and/or implement universal, selective, or indicated preventive intervention programs. They often may delegate to and/or supervise mental health personnel who participate in the implementation of such programs. They also may function as a member of an interdisciplinary mental health team within a variety of community-based health settings.

TREATMENT INTERVENTIONS

Treatment interventions focus on case identification and treatment protocols for known mental disorders, which include interventions that:

- Identify the mental health problem as early as possible
- Reduce the time the mental health problem exists
- Halt the progression of severity or co-occurance of other mental health problems
- Decrease the likelihood of relapse

Much of the psychiatric nurse's work has been focused in this category. Psychiatric nurses who work in hospitals, community mental health centers, home care, work sites, schools, and group homes participate in case-finding activities. Those who work in mobile outreach teams visit shelters, the streets, and store-front facilities to identify cases. Nurses who work in primary care settings are in a prime position to identify mental health problems in clients who initially have physical health problems.

The chapters in this textbook present treatment guidelines for persons with different types of mental disorders. Whenever possible, there are preferred practice guidelines for each disorder or treatment modality that are derived from research findings. For example, *Nursing Intervention Classification* (NIC) by McCloskey and Bulechek (1996) contains research-based practice protocols used in many of the chapters that provide standardized approaches to dealing with specific clinical problems such as hallucinations (see Chapter 29), crisis intervention (see Chapter 10), pain management, and grieving (see Chapter 32). The guidelines developed by the Agency for Health Care Policy Research (AHCPR) are another example of research-based practice protocols that are used to develop practice guidelines for mental

TABLE 18-1

Preventive intervention programs, associated risk factors, and program outcomes

STUDY/PROGRAM	RISK FACTORS	OUTCOMES
Infants and Toddlers Selective Infant health and development program	Low birth weight, poor family management practices, early behavioral problems	↑Cognitive competence ↓Behavioral problems
Young Children Indicated Parent-child interaction training	Economic deprivation, early behavior problems, ineffective parenting skills, maternal depression	↓Rates of attention deficit disorder (ADD) ↓Rates of conduct problems
Elementary School Age Selective Family bereavement program	Child bereavement, poor family management practices, early behavior problems	↓Symptoms and levels of depression ↓Conduct disorder
Adolescent Universal Adolescent alcohol prevention trial	Social influences to use drugs, early onset of drug use, attitudes favorable to drug use	↓Rates of alcohol, tobacco, and cannabis use ↓Prevalence of problem alcohol use and drunkenness
Adult Selective Peer and professionally led groups to support family caregivers	Caregiver burden, anxiety, depression	↓Levels of psychiatric symptoms ↓Anxiety, depression ↑Coping skills
Elderly Selective Widow-to-Widow, a mutual help program for the widowed	Widowhood, bereavement, depression, anxiety, social isolation	↓Depressive symptoms ↑Social involvement

disorders such as depression (USDHHS, 1993) (see Chapter 30).

The era of distinct treatment choices based on personal experience, tradition and authority, and trial and error is ending rapidly. Treatment effectiveness is now determined through outcome evaluation, including cost-benefit analysis and consumer satisfaction indicators (see Chapter 4). The psychiatric nurse's role in providing competent, skilled care to clients, their families, and communities is integral with achieving effective treatment outcomes. This role will be discussed in succeeding chapters of this book.

MAINTENANCE INTERVENTIONS

Maintenance interventions target populations who need continuing and coordinated treatment manage- *ment, such as those individuals with severe and persistent mental disorders such as schizophrenia, major depression, bipolar disorder, panic disorders, and the pervasive developmental disorders of childhood.* The goal of maintenance interventions is to decrease disability, prevent relapse, and promote optimal functional status and quality of life (IOM, 1994; Moller and Murphy, 1996). Psychiatric rehabilitation provides the umbrella concept for the spectrum of psychoeducation, support, and psychobiological interventions appropriate for these individuals, their families, and their communities (Keefler and Koritar, 1994; Sharfstein, Stoline, and Koran, 1995).

Psychiatric Rehabilitation

The aim of psychiatric rehabilitation is to increase the functioning of persons with mental disorders through

BOX 18-2

Psychiatric Rehabilitation Interventions

- Increased coping skills
- Focus on strengths
- Skill coaching in new settings
- Development of supports
- Self-determination
- Skills teaching
- Focus on the present
- Promotion of choices
- Humanistic-focused approach

BOX 18-3

Principles of Community Support

- Self-determination
- Personal dignity
- Individualization
- Normalization
- Comprehensive
- Available and accessible
- Flexible
- Consumer and family involvement
- Least restrictive setting
- Indefinite duration
- Coordination
- Natural support systems
- Mutual self-help

symptom control. This allows them to be more successful and satisfied in their environments of choice, thereby reducing the likelihood of relapse (Anthony, 1993; Francell, 1994; Meltzer, 1992). The two branches of psychiatric rehabilitation are development of social skills and development of environmental supports (Palmer-Erbs and Anthony, 1995). Recovering a satisfactory quality of life accompanied by reduced relapse rates is possible when appropriate community supports exist.

Successful maintenance interventions require an accurate needs assessment for survival in the community. This must be followed by the development and implementation of a comprehensive plan of services appropriate for each individual that includes interventions such as those listed in Box 18-2. When consumers are asked what they need to survive, they often reply, "I need a job, an apartment, and a friend." Services to support these needs include day treatment sites, which are now becoming vocational rehabilitation sites; psychoeducation centers; and locations for case management programs that provide community psychiatric rehabilitation support services.

Vocational Rehabilitation and Psychoeducation

Vocational rehabilitation programs promote vocational choice, supported employment, community job development, and job coaching. Education of clients and their families or significant others is an essential component of symptom control. Maintenance medication regimens play an important role in ongoing psychiatric treatment. Nurses are challenged to develop and use teaching/learning strategies that help clients understand the need to continue to take medications that have unpleasant side effects. Equally important are educational programs for clients and their significant others about the mental disorders that affect them, symptom management strategies, relapse prevention, and intervention strategies. Many families who struggle to care compe-

tently for family members with mental disorders benefit from coaching about how to become more competent in this role. Nurses can use educational materials published by organizations such as NAMI and other specialty organizations listed in the Consumer Resources box on p. 339 and the Community Resources boxes in Parts Five and Six of this text. Pharmaceutical companies and libraries are another valuable source of educational materials about mental disorders (see Chapter 16).

Community Support

In 1977 the U.S. Congress established the Community Support Program (CSP) that initially provided $3.5 million for community rehabilitation services. Some advocates saw this as a long overdue acknowledgment that persons with severe mental disorders needed social supports in the community to prevent further disability (Parrish, 1991). In 1986, Public Law 99-660, the State Planning Grant for Comprehensive Services for Persons with Severe Mental Illness, was signed into law. This law mandated that state mental health divisions develop a range of needed support services. It tied future federal block grant funding to this plan. The staff at NIMH designed and disseminated the Model Plan that gave direction to state planning agencies. A system of care, using the principles of community support listed in Box 18-3, that included comprehensive support services delivered through case managers was to be established in local communities close to the client's residence (NIMH, 1987). Coordinating agencies were to make available all components of the model plan; case managers were to help clients access these resources. Public Law 99-660 also mandated that case managers develop educational outreach programs to educate and support families, so they could

CONSUMER RESOURCES

The National Alliance for the Mentally Ill (NAMI)
200 North Glebe Road, Suite 1015
Arlington, VA 22203-3754
Also publishes *The Advocate Newsletter*

National Depressive and Manic Depressive Association
North Franklin Street, Suite 501
Chicago, IL 60610

National Mental Health Consumer Self-Help Clearinghouse
South Juniper Street, Suite 502
Philadelphia, PA 19107

Recommended Videotapes
"Hospital Without Walls" (PACT Model)
Box 3173
Duke University Medical Center
Durham, NC 27710

Understanding Relapse: Managing the Symptoms of Schizophrenia
NurSeminars, Inc.
Sunridge Drive
Nine Mile Falls, WA 99026

Suggested Readings
Gorman, J.M. (1991). *The essential guide to psychiatric drugs.* New York: St. Martin.

Papolpos, D., & Papolos, J. (1992). *Overcoming depression.* New York: Harper Perennial.

Torrey, E.F. (1995). *Surviving schizophrenia,* (3rd ed.). New York: HarperCollins.

Woolis, R. (1992). *When someone you love has a mental illness.* New York: Jeremy P. Tarcher/Perigee Books.

function as primary caregivers. They also helped clients obtain federal and state entitlements, if needed.

Considering that in 1986 the majority of mental health providers engaged in either office-based psychotherapy or inpatient treatment, a massive retraining effort had to be undertaken to achieve this goal. New service roles such as case manager and job coach have been developed to facilitate the provision of community support services. Intensive community case management programs such as the Program in Assertive Community Treatment (PACT) have provided community support services such as those listed in Box 18-4. Psychiatric nurses are excellent intensive case managers and supervisors of case management services (Pittman, 1989; Van Dongan and Jambunathan, 1992).

THE MENTAL HEALTH CONSUMER MOVEMENT

In the past, public and private sector hospitals and community mental health centers failed to meet the ongoing, comprehensive needs of persons with mental health problems, particularly those with severe and persistent mental disorders. Societal stigma about having "mental health" problems has existed since the beginning of time. Differential insurance benefits for mental health care has also been a reality for those who sought reimbursement for mental health services such as psy-

chotherapy or hospitalization. For those with severe and persistent mental disorders, stabilization and discharge from a psychiatric hospital was followed only by a community mental health center (CMHC) appointment and a prescription for medication. Goldfinger (1994), a community psychiatrist, described this disaster succinctly: "We designed an appointment-driven system for people who don't wear wristwatches."

Recipients of mental health services have participated in creating the shift from a provider-driven to a consumer-driven mental health delivery system, one that could no longer ignore, mistreat, or neglect them. Collective anger fueled some militant attitudes as clients asserted their consumer rights in mental health treatment decisions (Deegan, 1993; Freese, 1992). The consumer movement has had a long struggle, beginning with the formation of the National Mental Health Association in 1909, to get where it is today. The highlights of this movement are presented in Box 18-5.

The concept of empowerment has unified consumers who once felt that their opinions, feelings, and strength were discounted by mental health providers and policymakers. Consumer representatives now meet with mental health decision makers at every level. They have helped develop provider sensitivity to client and family needs and have educated legislators and policymakers about mental health needs (Hatfield and Lefley, 1993). Consumer organizations such as NAMI, the National

BOX 18-4

Intensive Community Case Management Support Services

MEDICATION SUPPORT

- Deliver medications
- Educate about medications
- Monitor medication compliance and side effects

FAMILY INVOLVEMENT

- Intervene with crisis management
- Provide counseling and psychoeducation
- Coordinate with family services agencies

PROMOTION OF SELF-CARE SKILLS

- Demonstrate grocery shopping and cooking strategies
- Educate on use of transportation
- Encourage purchase and care of clothing
- Reinforce personal hygiene

ENTITLEMENTS

- Assist with documentation
- Accompany to entitlement offices
- Manage food stamps
- Assist with determination of benefits

HEALTH PROMOTION

- Provide preventive health education
- Perform health screenings
- Schedule health maintenance visits
- Serve as liaison for acute medical care
- Provide reproductive counseling and sex education

FINANCIAL MANAGEMENT

- Plan budget
- Troubleshoot financial problems
- Assist with bills
- Increase independence in money management

COUNSELING

- Use problem-oriented approach
- Integrate into continuous work
- Develop goals with client and team
- Assist with development of communication skills
- Educate about legal rights

HOUSING ASSISTANCE

- Find suitable shelter
- Secure leases and pay rent
- Purchase and repair household items
- Develop relationship with landlord
- Improve housekeeping skills

VOCATIONAL REHABILITATIVE APPROACH

- Secure vocational rehabilitation opportunities as appropriate
- Offer support in finding volunteer and vocational opportunities
- Serve as liaison with and educate employers
- Serve as job coach

Mental Health Consumers Organization, the Manic-Depressive Organization, the National Mental Health Clearinghouse, the Ex-Patient/Survivors Association, and others mentioned throughout this text affect mental health service delivery in most states.

Many psychiatric nursing leaders collaborate on a regular basis with mental health consumer groups and have developed partnerships with NAMI leaders to reform mental health care.

Psychiatric nurses who have contributed to the development of the psychoeducation field now function as family and consumer advocates. For example, an advanced practice psychiatric nurse served on the board of directors of NAMI. During her 6-year term, she traveled to 45 states, using her psychiatric nursing and political skills to organize families of the mentally ill into a powerful consumer advocacy force. Another psychiatric nurse coordinates the NAMI Curriculum and Training Network, which influences the training of mental health professionals at many universities.

COMMUNITY ACTION

Communities have a variety of political structures; socioeconomic levels; cultural and ethnic groups; and natural, human, and financial resources. *Community action involves taking action to create change in a particular community.* Creative use of available resources increases the likelihood of achieving change. Community action is a form of population-focused preventive intervention. An example of community action might be the formation of a coalition consisting of school, health care, political, and corporate representatives whose goal is to secure state grant funding for the development and implementation of a community-wide adolescent alcohol and drug prevention program, sponsorship of which would be located in a center for teens funded by local corporations. The membership of the coalition would be typical of a community action team, that is, composed of both consumer and provider representatives.

Many psychiatric nurses function in the role of change agent, playing leadership roles in community ac-

BOX 18-5

Consumer Movement Highlights

EVENT

The National Mental Health Association (NMHA) was founded in 1909 by a group that included Clifford Beers, a former client who achieved noteriety as the author of the autobiography, *A Mind That Found Itself* (1908). Originally known as the National Committee for Mental Hygiene, this organization was involved in advocating mental hospital reform after World War I.

Purpose

The NMHA has a broad agenda of advocacy activities related to promoting mental health, preventing mental disorders, and reducing severe forms of mental illness. It provides public education materials and programs and recently conducted a wide-scale education campaign on depression. The NMHA is collaborating with organizations such as NAMI to improve mental health services for those with severe and persistent mental disorders.

EVENT

The National Alliance for the Mentally Ill (NAMI) was founded in 1979 by parents, siblings, primary consumers of mental health care, and interested professionals who were committed to addressing the inadequacies of the mental health delivery system. Their mission was to "eradicate mental illnesses and to improve the quality of life of all affected by these illnesses" (NAMI, 1992). However, the NAMI target population included those with severe and persistent mental disorders such as schizophrenia, major depression, bipolar disorder, post-traumatic stress disorder (PTSD), and anxiety disorders.

Purpose

An action-oriented group, NAMI established offices in Washington, D.C., so it could vigorously pursue advocacy activities with policymakers and legislators. Major NAMI con-

cerns included: (1) parity in insurance coverage for neurobiological disorders in relation to physical disorders (Coates, 1990); (2) assistance to caregivers that would enable them to be integral members of the decision-making process that affects their lives (Griffin-Francell, 1994; Griffen-Francell, Conn, and Gray,1988), including practical help that would make the 24-hour-a-day caregiving responsibility for disabled adult children more tolerable; (3) elimination of societal stigma and blame for families, particularly in terms of having "caused" their family member's "mental illness"; (4) increased NIMH funding for research dollars targeting severe and persistent neurobiological disorders; and (5) legislative action that focused on federal and state protection and advocacy laws for persons with mental illness, revisions in vocational rehabilitation acts, and community support programs. Examples of NAMI-supported legislation are the Americans with Disabilities Act, the State Plan for Comprehensive Services for Mentally Ill Persons Act, the Children's and Mental Health Improvement Act, and the Projects for Assistance in Transition from Homelessness (PATH) bill in the McKinney Homeless Assistance Act.

EVENT

The First Annual Mental Health Consumers Conference took place in Atlanta, in 1984. With financial and technical assistance from NIMH, consumer organization membership grew at a rapid rate.

Purpose

Consumerism in mental health organizations resulted in a change in terminology for former clients. Most decided to be called "consumers," whereas others decided to be called "survivors." The new terminology signified a new assertive position taken by the consumers of mental health care and their families.

---

tion. Many nurses serve on interdisciplinary planning and advisory boards, which develop health policy, allocate resources, or design implementation plans. Those nurses bring knowledge and expertise to interactions with community leaders who exercise considerable political power (Fox, 1993).

As change agents responsible for initiating community action programs, psychiatric nurses influence the physical and mental health of the communities in which they live and work (Dunn, 1993; Connolly, 1991). For example, school nurses collaborated with parents of children who were refused admission to public schools because of

physical and emotional disabilities. They formed a powerful consumer-provider coalition, which became a national force that successfully advocated for enactment of the 1975 Public Law 94:142, The Special Education Act for All Disabled Children (Norris, 1989). This law changed discriminatory practices toward disabled children, including those with severe emotional disorders (SED). Although the movement began at the local, grassroots level in different communities throughout the country, the scope of influence was national. University schools of education changed curricula to meet the needs of this target population.

Community action programs provide a powerful vehicle for creating community population-based change. Linkages between community action and consumer participation and the establishment of preventive and maintenance intervention programs are essential. Psychiatric nurses, as change agents and program implementers, can indeed play a pivotal role in enhancing the mental and physical health of the United States citizens.

KEY POINTS

- Models for prevention of mental disorders include the Public Health Model of Prevention, the Caplan Mental Health Prevention Model, and the Mental Health Intervention Spectrum Model.
- The Mental Health Intervention Spectrum Model focuses on universal, selective, and indicated preventive interventions; treatment interventions, including case finding and treatment protocols for known disorders; and maintenance interventions, the umbrella concept of which is psychiatric rehabilitation.
- Three components of psychiatric rehabilitation are vocational rehabilitation, psychoeducation, and community support services.
- Psychiatric nurses are defining significant roles as providers of preventive intervention services in a variety of health care settings.
- The mental health consumer movement represented the shift from a provider-driven to a consumer-driven mental health delivery system in which the recipients of mental health care, and their families, formed consumer organizations; asserted their consumer rights in mental health treatment decisions; advocated for parity in mental health insurance benefits, increased mental health research dollars, and legislative change; and crusaded for destigmatization.
- Community action involves taking action to create change in a particular community and is a form of population-focused preventive intervention.
- Psychiatric nurses function in the role of change agent, playing leadership roles in community action.

 ## CRITICAL THINKING QUESTIONS

John C., a 34-year-old man diagnosed with schizophrenia, paranoid type, is about to be discharged from a public mental hospital after his fifth hospitalization in 2 years. He has a history of not adhering to his medication regimen. He has had a variety of side effects to the 11 different medications he has taken in the past. His only family is a 73-year-old mother who lives in a small apartment and is in poor physical health. In the past, John has lived on the streets, where he has been arrested and jailed three separate times for stealing food and disturbing the peace. Shelters refuse to allow him in because of his noisy response to his hallucinations. In preparation for a city wide event, city councilmen, the mayor, and small business owners want to "sweep" panhandlers from the downtown park where John spends his days.

A nearby community mental health center offers psychotherapy at scheduled times. Most of these office-based therapists have caseloads of more than 100 clients. Several case managers are at the center, and only a few of them are nurses, but their caseloads are about 40 clients each. A state-funded intensive community case management program does exist. An outpatient commitment statute is approved by the legislature, but it is rarely used. Three universities near the downtown area prepare mental health clinicians.

The office of NAMI's state affiliate has a membership of 1,000 families.

1. What conclusions can you draw about the effectiveness of John's previous treatment intervention? Discuss your rationale.
2. How would you develop a community action plan to change the social and health care environment for John and his peers?
3. Explain whether this person is a candidate for preventive intervention. If not, then what would be the appropriate intervention focus within the Mental Health Spectrum Intervention Model?
4. Within a maintenance intervention framework, how would you handle John's refusal to adhere to his medication regimen if he is discharged to the streets?
5. What is the significance of the university's presence in relation to persons like John? Do university preprofessional schools have any obligation to homeless mentally ill persons like him?
6. What role would the local NAMI chapter play?
7. Does the city have the right to want to "clear the streets of panhandlers" in preparation for the city event? What is the most constructive approach to dealing with this client population?

REFERENCES

Anthony, W.A. (1993). Recovery from mental illness. *Psychosocial Rehabilitation Journal, 16*(4), 11-23.

Caplan. (1964). *Principles of preventive psychiatry.* New York: Basic Books.

Coates, R.C. (1990). *A street is not a home.* Buffalo, N.Y.: Prometheus Books.

Connolly, P.M. (1991). Services for the underserved: A nurse managed center for the chronically mentally ill. *Journal of Psychosocial Nursing and Mental Health Services, 29*(1), 15-20.

Deegan, P.E. (1993). Recovering our sense of value after being labeled mentally ill. *Journal of Psychosocial Nursing and Mental Health Services, 31*(4), 7-11.

Dunn, J.K. (1993). Medical skills and knowledge, how necessary are they for psychiatric nurses? *Journal of Psychosocial Nursing and Mental Health Services, 31*(12), 25-28.

Fox, J. (1993). The role of nursing in public policy reform. *Journal of Psychosocial Nursing and Mental Health Services, 31*(8), 9-12.

Francell, E.G. (1994). Medication: The foundation of recovery. *Innovations & Research, 3*(4), 32-40.

Freese, F.J. (1992). The movies and the mentally ill. *The Journal.* California Alliance for the Mentally Ill, *4*(1).

Goldfinger, S. (1994). Quote from a presentation at NAMI convention in Miami.

Gordon, R. (1987). An operational classification of disease prevention. In J.A. Steinberg & M.M. Silverman (Eds.), *Preventing mental disorders.* Rockville, MD: Department of Health and Human Services.

Griffin-Francell, C. (1994). A message from NAMI: Thirteen things families want professionals to do. *Community Psychiatrist, 8*(1), 7.

Griffin-Francell, C., Conn, V. & Gray, P. (1988). Families' perception of burden of care for chronic mentally ill relatives. *Hospital and Community Psychiatry, Vol.* 39(12). 1296-1300.

Hatfield, A., & Lefley, H. (1993). *Surviving Mental Illness.* New York: The Guilford Press.

Institute of Medicine. (1989). *Research on children and adolescents with mental, behavioral, and developmental disorders.* Washington, DC: National Academy Press.

Institute of Medicine. (1994). *Reducing risks for mental disorders.* Washington, DC: National Academy Press.

Keefler, J., & Koritar, E. (1994). Essentials of a family psychoeducation program in the aftercare of schizophrenia. *Journal of Marriage and Family Therapy, 20*(4), 369-380.

McCloskey, J., & Bulechek, G. (1995). *Nursing Intervention classification (NIC)* (2nd ed.). St. Louis: Mosby.

McEvoy, J. (1995, February). An update on the neurobiology of psychosis. Lecture delivered at *Progress in psychoses: Seratonin-dopamine antagonists* symposium. Atlanta.

Meltzer, H. (1992). Dimensions of outcome with clozapine. *British Journal of Psychiatry, 160* (Suppl. 17), 46-53.

Moller, M.D., & Murphy, M. (1996). Symptom management and relapse prevention: A wellness approach. *Directions in Psychiatric Nursing, 3.*

National Alliance for the Mentally Ill (NAMI), Board of Directors (1992). *Public policy platform of NAMI.* Arlington, VA: Author.

National Institute for Mental Health. (1987). *Toward a model plan for a comprehensive, community-based mental health system.* Rockville, MD: Alcohol, Drug Abuse, and Mental Health Administration.

Norris, R.F. (1989). Fighting back from tragedy. In R.E. Friedman, A.J. Duchnowski, & E.L. Henderson (Eds.), *Advocacy on behalf of children with serious emotional problems.* Springfield, IL: Charles C. Thomas.

Palmer-Erbs, V.K., & Anthony, W.A. (1995). Incorporating psychiatric rehabilitation principles into psychiatric-mental health nursing practice: An opportunity to develop a partnership among nurses, consumers, and families. *The Journal of Psychosocial Nursing and Mental Health Services, 33*(3).

Parrish, J. (1991). CSP: Program of firsts. *Innovations & Research, 1*(1), 8-9.

Pittman, D.C. (1989). Nursing case management: Holistic care for the deinstitutionalized chronic mentally ill. *Journal of Psychosocial Nursing and Mental Health Services, 27* (11), 23-27.

Rice, D.P., Kelman, S., & Miller, L.S. (1990). *The economic costs of alcohol and drug abuse and mental illness.* San Francisco: Institute for Health and Aging, University of California DHHS.

Robins, L.N., & Regier, D.A. (1991). *Psychiatric disorders in America: The Epidemologic Catchment Area Study.* New York: The Free Press.

Sharfstein, S.S., Stoline, A.M., & Koran, L. (1995). Mental Health Services. In A.R., Kovner (Ed.). *Jonas's Health Care Delivery in the United States.* New York: Springer.

U.S. Department of Health and Human Services. (1991). *Healthy People 2000.* (DHHS Publication No. (PHS) 91-50212). Washington, DC: U.S. Government Printing Office.

U.S. Department of Health and Human Services. (1993). *Depression in primary care: Detection and diagnosis. Vol 1. Clinical Practice Guideline no. 5.* (DHHS Publication No. 93-0550). Rockville, Md.: Public Health Service, Agency for Health Care Policy and Research.

Van Dongan, C.J., & Jambunathan, J. (1992). Pilot study results: The psychiatric RN case manager. *Journal of Psychosocial Nursing and Mental Health Services, 30*(11), 11-14.

Chapter 19

Psychiatric Nursing in Inpatient Settings

Mary Walker

LEARNING OUTCOMES

After studying and applying the concepts of this chapter, the learner will be able to:

- Define milieu therapy.
- Explain both content and process levels of communication.
- Identify examples of transference and countertransference in therapeutic relationships.
- Describe selected unconscious primitive dynamics that are acted out in the psychiatric inpatient unit.
- Relate five milieu functions.
- Verbalize nursing standards of milieu management.
- Describe nursing process roles in inpatient settings.
- Explain the collaborative role in the team approach to treatment.

KEY TERMS

Containment	Milieu therapy	Therapeutic community
Content	Process	Transference
Countertransference	Structure	Validation
Involvement	Support	

There is a relationship between the environment and a person's health. Florence Nightingale was the first nurse to emphasize environmental modifications such as fresh air and light as important components of treatment.

In the 1950s, Jones developed the concept of a ***therapeutic community,*** *a setting based on the premise that the interaction between persons and their environments positively or adversely affects their behaviors* (Jones, 1953). Although few acute inpatient units today incorporate all of the components of the therapeutic community, using the environment as a treatment in and of itself is still a strong therapeutic modality.

Milieu *(or environment)* ***therapy*** *is the systematic management of the socioenvironment as a treatment modality for the benefit of clients.* The socioenvironment includes physical, interpersonal, and treatment dimensions of the treatment setting. Milieu therapy is a complex, challenging nursing responsibility that is a nursing standard of care, as well as a collaborative function with other team members. Every interaction that the nurse has with a client is seen as a potentially healing opportunity. The physical environment encompasses such elements as the use of rooms, furniture, and sound to be calming and esthetically pleasing and therefore therapeutic. The treatment dimension of the socioenvironment implies that scheduled activities occur on time and meet their objectives. Nurses, by virtue of their close contact with clients, are the persons responsible for milieu management. No other health care providers are present as consistently as nurses, especially in the inpatient setting. Even in outpatient settings, nurses are responsible for much of the continuity of a client's care.

The three major goals in milieu therapy include the following:

- Resocialization, where a client is able to learn or relearn more functional ways of relating to others
- Ego development, in which therapeutic milieu strengthens a person's ability to cope when problems can be handled with the support of staff and other clients
- Prevention of regression, in which clients who are placed in the dependent position of client can actually begin to rely on the hospital too much. Thoughtful milieu interventions can help foster or maintain independence

With increasingly shorter inpatient stays, it is more challenging to use the milieu to meet these original goals. However, milieu therapy can still be used to promote elements of these goals, as well as crisis intervention, symptom stabilization, and some restoration toward a person's previous functioning (LeCuyer, 1992).

The purpose of this chapter is to define the responsibility of the nurse as an active agent in managing the inpatient milieu. Dynamics and functions of a healthy milieu are explored. Issues affecting a milieu are also addressed. Finally, nursing standards and roles in milieu therapy are reviewed.

MILIEU PROCESSES

Several important processes occur in an inpatient setting, and they must be recognized and acted on if the milieu is to be therapeutic. The milieu processes to be explored are content and process, transference-countertransference, and primitive dynamics.

Content and Process

To understand the challenge of analyzing the milieu, the nurse should first know that there are two levels occurring in any communication (see Chapter 8). These two levels occur simultaneously and are equally important in analyzing the milieu. The two levels are referred to as content and process.

Content *refers to what is actually being said or done with the client,* such as the topic of conversation or an activity. ***Process*** *refers to the underlying dynamics of the communication, a series of behaviors for which the goal is communication of a message.* The process may be congruent or incongruent with the content level of the message. For example, when the nurse conducts an assessment of the client, a standard series of questions is asked. The questions comprise the content level of the communication. The nurse's posture, tone of voice, eye contact, sequencing of questions, attitude, and other nonverbal behaviors convey an even more powerful communication to the client. This represents the process component of the communication.

Content and process are evident in the communication patterns between individuals, as well as among group members and among all persons interacting with each other in the milieu. The nurse must not only be "tuned in" to individual interaction patterns but also to group and milieu patterns. In fact, patterns that appear at individual or group levels will often appear in the larger environment in what is called a "parallel" process (Kahn, Sturke and Schaffer, 1992). For example, staff anger about hospital reorganization and aggressive behavior among clients in a therapy group may be related. The client group could be acting out the staff's anger.

The nurse needs to be aware of the process issues being played out in the inpatient unit and understand that group dynamics are always operating either therapeutically or antitherapeutically (Kahn and White, 1989). One of the first questions a nurse needs to ask if there is negative behavior among clients is, "What might be happening among the staff that could be contributing to these negative behaviors?"

Transference-Countertransference

Another process related to the milieu is the psychodynamic principle of transference (see Chapters 8 and 9). *Transference refers to an unconscious process whereby a client perceives the nurse as someone from the client's past.* Transference can be positive or negative. For example, if a client has an antagonistic relationship with his or her spouse, the client may communicate aggressively with the nurse because of the similarity. The nurse may have no idea why the client is communicating aggressively. If the client's reaction to the nurse seems to be without foundation, it is likely that transference is present. An example of a positive transference occurred with Jan and her nurse. The nurse reminded Jan of her Aunt Millie, a kindly woman who treated Jan with love and respect, quite often pointing out her positive qualities. Jan responded warmly to the nurse, and rapport was easily established between Jan and the nurse. Again, the nurse may have no idea why a client is communicating warmly.

Countertransference is the unconscious process whereby the nurse perceives and relates to the client as someone from the nurse's past. Negative transference and countertransference need to be assessed in the inpatient milieu, because these issues can hinder the goal of symptom stabilization. Although they are both clues to understanding a client's past relationships and how his or her current interaction in the milieu contributes to present problems (Bonnivier, 1992), delving into these issues may worsen symptoms. Therefore the nurse needs to understand these issues, to reduce additional relationship difficulties, and to focus on stabilization of symptoms.

Primitive Dynamics

In addition to transference reactions, clients may also act out dynamics from childhood. The milieu provides a microcosm of the outside world, and clients may recreate past conflictual relationships with other clients or staff (Bonnivier, 1992). Issues such as power, response to authority, dependency, self-worth, identity, and acceptance are some areas that might be problematic for clients. If these issues developed in childhood and were never resolved, they may be reenacted in the client's home and work environment, as well as the treatment milieu. The nurse's assessment should include the client's usual interactions in the environment, because these can provide clues to problems the client may be experiencing in the outside world (Tuck and Keels, 1992). For example, the nurse might observe a client vying for staff attention when another client is interacting with the nurse. This may represent a primitive dynamic of sibling rivalry and provide insight into how the client may seek attention and interact with other authority figures at work.

Because a typical inpatient stay is short, the nurse does not use knowledge of the client's primitive dynamics with the goal of providing client insight into their behavior. However, each interaction the nurse has with the client helps the nurse keep abreast of the changing dynamics of individuals and groups in the milieu.

MENTAL HEALTH CARE DELIVERY

Deilvery of mental health services in the inpatient setting is undergoing revolutionary change. Presently, the average length of stay in general hospital psychiatric units is less than a week, and it is growing shorter. In 1994, statistics for private psychiatric hospitals indicated an average length of stay for adults of 12.4 days and an overall length of stay, including children and elders, of 15.2 days (National Association of Psychiatric Health Systems [NAPHS], 1995). Thus there is limited time to use the milieu as a therapeutic agent.

In addition, clients are admitted and discharged daily, so the atmosphere of the unit is constantly changing. What may have been a tranquil, therapeutic unit milieu at 3 PM, may be tense and disorganized at 10 PM. Newly admitted clients with their psychiatric crises are quite challenging for the nurse to assess, develop an initial care plan, and assimilate into the ongoing milieu with other clients. Scrutiny of the milieu processes enables the nurse to keep abreast of the changing dynamics of individuals and groups in the milieu.

Functions of the Milieu

Because the environment influences thinking, feelings, and behavior, the nurse may exert a powerful therapeutic effect through everyday interactions with clients and through thoughtfully changing aspects of the milieu to meet therapeutic goals. A milieu is successful to the degree to which clients and staff have goal-directed interactions and are involved in decisions (Gunderson, 1980), and the staff holds expectations for normal functioning of the client (Ellsworth, 1983).

There are five functions of a therapeutic milieu; each one parallels client needs at a particular point in treatment. These five functions include containment, support, structure, involvement, and validation (Gunderson, 1978).

Containment
Containment refers to sustaining the physical well-being of clients and those around them. Containment encompasses the control of clients' behavior when destructive impulses are overwhelming (Gunderson, 1978). Containment activities include providing food, shelter, seclusion, locked areas, and legal commitment to a hospital. Containment is the primary function of treatment

on an acute inpatient unit, since most clients are hospitalized because they pose a danger to themselves or others. The nursing objective is to prevent assaults, self-harm, accidents, or physical deterioration in those clients who lack impulse control or good judgment. The milieu temporarily bolsters internal controls until clients regain their own internal controls. The containment function also acts to diminish environmental stimuli, so clients are not overwhelmed with processing information (Walker, 1994).

Safety is a critical nursing consideration for clients who need containment aspects of the milieu. For example, frequent monitoring of clients who are in restraints or seclusion is a common method of providing safe containment. Elopement or suicide precautions, equipment checks, and unit policies restricting a client's freedom are other examples of how the nurse provides containment measures.

The nurse also works toward helping clients to assist in providing containment for the group. Peer pressure to conform to healthy milieu norms is encouraged by regular unit meetings where clients discuss problems and resolve group issues nonaggressively.

When the nurse does not provide appropriate containment, there may be negative consequences for clients. For example, Mark, who was diagnosed as psychotic, was receiving command hallucinations to injure another client. Mark needed to be secluded to protect the other clients and to provide external control until he was able to control himself. The nurse needed to make a timely decision about whether to seclude Mark. If the decision was not appropriately made, the unit would not be contained, and the environment would be unsafe.

Containment can, however, be overused. If clients do not need external controls, containment becomes punitive or coercive. It may suppress initiative by giving clients the message that they are unable, or not expected, to control their behavior.

Support

A second function of the therapeutic milieu is to provide *support, the promotion of a sense of well-being and self-esteem in clients* (LeCuyer, 1992). In a supportive milieu, clients feel comfortable and secure and have lowered anxiety (Gunderson, 1978). Clients receive support through respectful interventions, which may include encouragement, advice, reality testing, praise, positive reinforcement, and a communicated belief that there is hope for them. More formally, the nurse can build support into the milieu by providing opportunities for success and by structuring interactions with other clients. For example, the nurse may organize a group outing or a card game among clients to facilitate less threatening verbal exchange. Scheduling time to sit with clients and listen to their concerns is another supportive intervention. A

postdischarge telephone call by the nurse also demonstrates support.

Support should be high for those clients who are anxious, depressed, or in crisis. An overemphasis on support, to the exclusion of structure or validation, may not be helpful to clients with borderline or paranoid personality features. Clients with these diagnoses have problems with self-boundaries and may feel confused or disorganized without external structural boundaries. For these clients, highly supportive interactions may be misconstrued or mistrusted (Gunderson, 1978).

Structure

Structure pertains to all aspects of a milieu that provide an organized, predictable environment. Examples of structure include scheduling client's time; maintaining a pleasing, uncluttered physical environment; providing unit programs and policies, classes, groups; and client contracts. Structure is important for those clients whose lives are "disordered" and is an important precondition to other therapeutic work (Kahn, Sturke, and Schaffer, 1992).

Formal mechanisms of providing order may involve highly structured token economies, hierarchical staff organization, mandatory expected behaviors, and regulation of aspects of daily living such as eating and sleeping. Nurses working in prison systems or with clients who have antisocial personality disorder provide a highly structured milieu to effect therapeutic change. Other formal structures are an adequate client-staff ratio and staff stability.

When unit order in the inpatient setting is too low, there is an increased likelihood of social conflict. Clients who have difficulty with loss of control may perceive a low-structure setting as disorganized and threatening; they may become defensive and decrease their engagement in the milieu (Kahn, Sturke, and Schaffer, 1992). A poorly structured milieu may be too few activities for clients, inconsistent implementation of a schedule, or inconsistently applied consequences for functional or dysfunctional behavior (Walker, 1994).

In acute inpatient units, highly structured milieus with low environmental stimulation have been found to produce more rapid improvement in psychotic symptoms than open, unstructured units (Cohen and Kahn, 1990). However, for clients who are not psychotic, milieus with a more moderate emphasis on structure and a moderate level of environmental stimulation tend to be correlated with more positive client outcomes (Emrich, 1989).

Informally, nurses increase structure by emphasizing unit policies and expectations of appropriate behavior. These may be posted on the unit or written down and given to clients. The nurse may often reorient clients with psychoses as part of a plan of care or engage others in the milieu to assist new clients in learning positive norms and rules. Reviewing daily schedules with a client group is another example of providing boundaries and organization so the clients can focus on internal reorganization. Daily activities then can be reviewed in the evening to determine how well the clients participated in the scheduled activities and their views of any therapeutic benefits.

Highly structured environments can also be problematic. Too much structure can mask client symptoms, because assessing how the client manages discretionary time can reveal dysfunctional behavior. If free time is not managed well, transition to a less-structured world may be more difficult (Gunderson, 1978).

Involvement

Passivity or disengagement is often a problem among persons with mental illness. An important function of a healthy milieu is to encourage clients to be active partners in their treatments and social environments. *Involvement refers to mobilizing clients with activities that encourage attendance to and interaction with others* (Gunderson, 1980).

Highly involved clients give input into their treatment, but they also are open to feedback from the staff about symptoms and issues. Examples of how involvement may be used are found in Table 19-1. Problem solving is achieved through discussion, negotiation, and consensus (Jack, 1989). The nurse actively seeks client participation by being open to a client's expression of feelings. The client, in turn, is responsible for behaviors on the unit. Staff assist clients by helping them achieve an awareness of how they interact on the inpatient unit and how their behaviors may affect others (Tuck and Keels, 1992). The goal is to help clients realize the effect their behaviors have on persons outside the hospital.

Staff also role model aspects of effective involvement by demonstrating the same behaviors that staff expect of clients (Puskar et al., 1990). This could consist of assertively denying inappropriate requests or discussing irritations instead of behaving aggressively.

High levels of involvement are particularly helpful for withdrawn or nonparanoid clients with schizophrenia. Too much involvement, however, may make some clients feel intruded on (Gunderson, 1978). For example, a client with severe paranoia might suspect ulterior motives in the staff if extensive involvement is encouraged. When the levels of involvement are too low, there may be few opportunities in the milieu for clients to make decisions or interact with others.

Validation

The fifth function of a milieu, *validation, refers to interventions that affirm a person's uniqueness* (Gunderson, 1980). This is done primarily through individualizing treatment plans, but it can also be brought out in one-on-one interventions by staff. Validation is an essential ingredient for healing when it is done with open acceptance and confirmation from the client (Emrich, 1989). When validation is high in the milieu, clients feel affirmed, even if their behaviors are not acceptable (Walker, 1994).

Clients who may benefit especially from high unit validation are those with paranoid or borderline traits. If validation is high, but structure and involvement are low, very passive clients may feel neglected or confused about treatment (Gunderson, 1978). When client validation on a unit is low overall, clients may become defensive and controlling if their personal decisions are not taken into account. This affects a client's sense of worth.

A therapeutic milieu would ideally incorporate all five functions into its operation. However, a milieu is usually

TABLE 19-1

Nursing strategies related to involvement

CLIENT BEHAVIOR	NURSING STRATEGY
Nonassertive communication	Encourage client to state preference to the client group about the movies the clients will watch on Saturday night.
Domineering toward others	Include client in a group activity, such as volleyball, where success depends on collaboration with others.
Psychotic	Initially, have client avoid unit meetings. When able to sit quietly for about 20 minutes, have client attend a unit meeting when no participation is expected. Increased participation as tolerated.
Depressed	Initially, pair client with one other stable client for activities. Then move client into triads and groups as energy increases. Insist that client attend all activities.

not able to provide strength in all functions simultaneously. The challenge for the nurse is to show flexibility in bolstering those functions that are needed most by the group. Examples of common milieu interventions can be found in Table 19-2.

Role of the Nurse

Although all the roles defined in psychiatric-mental health nursing's *Standards* (American Nurses' Association [ANA], 1994) are enacted in the inpatient setting, three roles are specifically delineated in this chapter. Standards of milieu management, as well as process roles and collaboration with other disciplines are discussed.

Standards of milieu management

Specific standards have been developed related to environmental management (ANA, 1994). Overall, the nurse is expected to provide, structure, and maintain a therapeutic environment in collaboration with clients and other health care providers (ANA, 1994).

Length of stay in inpatient psychiatric care has become dramatically shorter as emphasis has shifted from increasing a client's ability to function to stabilization through pharmacological therapy (Cohen and Kahn, 1990). This shift to shorter inpatient stays creates some pressure on the nurse to refer clients to community services that continue therapies initiated in the hospital. Good discharge planning requires that the psychiatric-mental health nurse conduct the following:

- Build rapport quickly with clients
- Engage clients in therapy in a way that encourages a commitment to continue treatment on an outpatient basis
- Demonstrate a comprehensive knowledge of appropriate community resources for a variety of client needs
- Work with the client, family, and significant others to formulate a discharge plan tailored to the client's unique situation
- Coordinate services to be communicated to all key interdisciplinary team members

Box 19-1 provides a list of community resources that may be helpful to discharged clients.

TABLE 19-2

Examples of common milieu interventions

INTERVENTION	EXAMPLE
Role modeling	The nurse keeps commitments made to a client. The nurse comes to work neatly groomed with professional attire.
Confrontation	A staff nurse explains to a client that his off-unit privileges are revoked because he had a positive drug screen.
Seclusion	A client shouting threats to others is escorted to a locked room until her behavior is under control.
Suicide precautions	The charge nurse assigns a psychiatric technician to stay within arm's reach of an actively suicidal client.
Peer pressure	During a unit meeting, the nurse encourages other clients to sensitively share how a client's refusal to take a shower and wash his clothes affects other members of the community.
Positive reinforcement	The nurse praises efforts toward a goal, even if it was not achieved.
Structured interactions among clients	A nurse introduces and seats a withdrawn client next to a more verbal client during lunch.
Therapeutic schedule of activities	The nurse develops and coordinates a monthly schedule of client education topics.
Consistent expectations	The nurse follows through on limits set with clients.
Unit meeting	There is an attempted suicide on the unit, so the nurse calls clients and staff together for a meeting to process feelings related to the event.

Box 19-1

Examples of Community Resources

SERVING INDIVIDUALS
Rape crisis centers
Churches and synagogues
Job-training agencies
Art shows
Recreation clubs
Adult education programs
Literacy programs
Employment agencies
Mediation groups
Meals on Wheels
Colleges and universities
Mental health agencies
Day-treatment centers
Partial hospitalization programs

SERVING FAMILIES
Women, Infants, and Children (WIC)
Nutritional services
Community "Welcome Wagon"
Sex-counseling agencies
Family planning agencies

Recreation centers
Children's groups (such as Girl Scouts)
Church groups
Day care centers for children, the disabled, and the elderly
Family recreation centers and groups
Shelters for victims of domestic violence

SERVING THE COMMUNITY
Environmental groups
Education groups (such as American Lung Association)
Supportive housing
Self-help groups
Community emergency shelters
Government agencies
Police departments
Fire departments
Fair-housing bureaus or agencies
Mental health home care agencies
Prisons
Performing arts centers
Public forests and parks

Process roles

In addition to milieu management, nurses enact specific roles that have a powerful impact on clients within the treatment environment. These roles are performed to a greater or lesser extent by the nurse, depending on current milieu dynamics. A list of these roles and examples of each can be found in Table 19-3.

Collaboration with other disciplines

Nursing practice can be thought of as occurring in two contexts: within particular settings and within a multidisciplinary team. The four mental health disciplines that have traditionally provided services to clients with mental illness are nursing, medicine, social work, and psychology. Disciplines to whom referrals for clients with mental illness are made include dietary, physical therapy, biofeedback, chaplaincy, pharmacy, activities therapies, and others. Definitions for each discipline differ slightly from state to state. General definitions and functions of the health care team members are found in Chapter 5.

Working together is a challenge for any two individuals, no matter what the task. Increasing the number of persons with different educational backgrounds, vocabulary, priorities, methods of problem solving, goals, and communication styles adds to the challenge of working together. The multidisciplinary team comes together for a common purpose—to plan, implement, and evaluate the treatment of individual clients. The client is considered a member of the team. Each person on the team is treated with mutual respect because each has a vital contribution to make. Though team members may overlap in some areas of knowledge and responsibility, each one has a unique contribution to make that must be communicated for effective treatment planning to occur. Decision making usually occurs by consensus, and all members specify the activities they will pursue. Any team member can coordinate client care, but the nurse usually provides this service, because nurses are always present in the inpatient environment. Though working in a team context is often difficult and energy-consuming, the outcome for the client is great, with more focused interventions, which are implemented consistently across activities, shifts, and disciplines. This kind of teamwork is very powerful on behalf of the client.

KEY POINTS

- Milieu therapy is the systematic management of the socioenvironment as a treatment modality for the benefit of clients.

TABLE 19-3

Nursing process roles in the milieu

PROCESS ROLES	DEFINING CHARACTERISTICS AND EXAMPLES
Nurturer	• Caregiver • Source of unconditional acceptance • Promoter of growth EXAMPLE: A nurse listens attentively to a client with depression and then gently but firmly encourages the client to join other clients in the dining room for lunch
Coordinator	• Organizes client-care activities • Oversees implementation of the care plan EXAMPLE: A client may need assistance in adjusting daily schedule to participate in a special recreational outing.
Socializing agent	• Helps clients establish norms for behavior. • Teaches clients how to relate to others • Suggests uses for unstructured time EXAMPLE: Using behavior modification and modeling techniques, the nurse teaches the client how to initiate and sustain a conversation.
Counselor	• Evaluates client and family processes of problem solving • Helps clients develop more functional coping skills EXAMPLE: A nurse assists a client who mutilates herself when she is anxious to develop alternative tension-reducing methods.
Educator	• Teaches behavior that promotes health EXAMPLE: A nurse holds a daily medication-education class for clients.
Technician	• Provides specialized skills EXAMPLE: A nurse obtains blood pressure readings in standing and supine positions.
Advocate	• Intercedes for, acts on behalf of, or speaks for clients when they are unable to provide these services for themselves or are unaware of other options EXAMPLE: The nurse explores with the client financial options of obtaining a new, more costly medication.
Collaborator	• Functions as a member of the interdisciplinary team to plan and implement care • Communicates client progress with team members EXAMPLE: The nurse, as a case manager, shares assessment data about the client with other team members.

• The nurse must be attuned to the content (what is actually being said), as well as the process (the meaning) levels of communication.

• Transference occurs when the client unconsciously perceives and reacts to the nurse as someone from the client's past. Countertransference occurs when the nurse perceives the client as similar to someone in the nurse's past.

• Clients tend to act out early problematic developmental issues in the milieu.

• Five important functions needed in a healthy inpatient milieu are containment, support, structure, involvement, and validation. The nurse must modify each of the five functions to meet individual and group needs.

• The ANA standard related to milieu states that the psychiatric-mental health nurse provides, structures, and maintains a therapeutic environment in collaboration with the client and other health care providers.

• The process roles of the psychiatric-mental health nurse are nurturer, coordinator, socializing agent, counselor, educator, technician, advocate, and collaborator.

CRITICAL THINKING QUESTIONS

You are just beginning your 3 PM-to-midnight shift on an acute inpatient psychiatric unit. The offgoing shift nurse explains that there has been one incident of client self-mutilation during the day and an adolescent attempted to run away. The unit atmosphere feels tense.

1. In light of the day's incidents, what milieu functions might you increase to promote safety on the unit? Give your rationale.
2. What are some ways to assess the unit's atmosphere?
3. Another client comes to you and tells you that you are a terrible nurse because of the two earlier incidents. What are two processes that might be present in this interaction? How might you respond to this client?
4. Discuss three factors that you would evaluate to determine if a parallel process was operating at the staff as well as of the client level?
5. How could you mobilize the client group to decrease tension in the milieu?
6. Discuss the possible effects of the admission of several new clients with varying diagnoses on the unit during your shift.

• Collaboration, or working closely with other mental health care team members for the purpose of increasing quality of care, increases the likelihood of meeting client outcomes.

REFERENCES

American Nurses Association. (1994). *A statement on psychiatric-mental health clinical nursing practice and standards of psychiatric-mental health clinical nursing practice.* Washington, DC: American Nurses Publishing.

Bonnivier, J. (1992). A peer supervision group: Put countertransference to work. *Journal of Psychosocial Nursing, 30*(5), 5-8.

Carveth, J. (1995). Perceived patient deviance and avoidance by nurses. *Nursing Research, 44,* 173-178.

Cohen, S., & Kahn, A. (1990). Antipsychotic effect of milieu in the acute treatment of schizophrenia. *General Hospital Psychiatry, 12,* 248-251.

Ellsworth, R. (1983). Characteristics of effective treatment milieus. In J. Gunderson (Ed.), *Principles and practice of milieu therapy.* Northvale, NJ: Jason Aronson.

Emrich, K. (1989). Helping or hurting? Interacting in the psychiatric milieu. *Journal of Psychosocial Nursing, 27*(12), 26-29.

Gunderson, J. (1978). Defining the therapeutic processes in psychiatric milieus. *Psychiatry, 41,* 327-335.

Gunderson, J. (1980). A reevaluation of milieu therapy for nonchronic schizophrenic patients. *Schizophrenia Bulletin, 6*(1), 64-69.

Gutheil, T. (1985). The therapeutic milieu: Changing themes and theories. *Hospital and Community Psychiatry, 36*(12), 1279-1285.

Jack, L. (1989). Use of milieu as a problem-solving strategy in addiction treatment. *Nursing Clinics of North America, 24*(1), 69-80.

Johnson, J., & Parker, K. (1983). Some antitherapeutic effects of a therapeutic community. *Hospital and Community Psychiatry, 34*(2), 170-171.

Jones, M. (1953). *The therapeutic community.* New Haven, CT: Yale University Press.

Kahn, E., Sturke, I., & Schaffer, J. (1992). Inpatient group processes parallel unit dynamics. *Journal of Group Psychotherapy, 42*(3), 407-418.

Kahn, E., & White, E. (1989). Adapting milieu approaches to acute inpatient care for schizophrenic patients. *Hospital and Community Psychiatry, 40*(6), 609-614.

LeCuyer, E. (1992). Milieu therapy for short-stay units: A transformed practice theory. *Archives of Psychiatric Nursing, 6*(2), 108-116.

National Association of Psychiatric Health Systems (NAPHS) (1995). *Trends in psychiatric health systems: 1995 annual survey.* Washington, DC: Author.

Ng, M. (1992). The community meeting: A review. *The International Journal of Social Psychiatry, 38*(3), 179-188.

Puskar, K., McAdam, D., Burkhart-Morgan, C., Isadore, R., Grimenstein, J., Wilson, S., & Jarrett, P. (1990). Psychiatric nursing management of medication-free psychotic patients. *Archives of Psychiatric Nursing, 4*(2), 78-86.

Rosenbaum, M. (1991). Violence in the psychiatric wards: Role of the lax milieu. *General Hospital Psychiatry, 13,* 115-121.

Tuck, I., & Keels, M. (1992). Milieu therapy: A review of development of this concept and its implications for psychiatric nursing. *Issues in Mental Health Nursing, 13,* 51-58.

Walker, M. (1994). Creating a therapeutic inpatient milieu. *Perspectives in Psychiatric Care, 30*(3), 5-8.

Yurkovich, E. (1989). Patient and nurse roles in the therapeutic community. *Perspectives in Psychiatric Care, 25,* 18-22.

Chapter 20

Psychiatric Nursing in Community Settings

Pam Price-Hoskins

LEARNING OUTCOMES

After studying and applying the concepts of this chapter, the learner will be able to:
- List the characteristics of a healthy community.
- Analyze health resources needed in a community.
- Identify resources supportive of persons with mental disorders in a community.
- Recommend referrals that are appropriate for a client's needs in the community.

KEY TERMS

Advocacy	Community mental health resources	Least restrictive environment
Case management	Community resource	Primary care provider
Community	Deinstitutionalization	Single room occupancy hotels
Community health resources	Foster care	Supported housing

community has many characteristics, one of which is health status. A community's health status influences the health status of the individuals living in that community. The values held by the community members also influence the health status of the community. For example, the citizens of Lonecliff, a very small town, value individuals' right to choose. In Lonecliff, there are several churches, a brothel, two bingo parlors, and a liquor-free dance hall. The community has several factions of citizens, among whom there is little communication. It is difficult to pass community bond issues to improve schools or health facilities, because "people make choices and must live with them." The health status of Lonecliff citizens is affected by the value system, the variety of choices, the isolation among different groups, and the difficulty in improving community services through taxes.

The community value of most concern in this chapter is the value of freedom. The corporate and community values in the United States uphold, defend, and legitimize freedom: freedom of speech, freedom of movement, freedom to own property, freedom to choose what happens to one's body, and freedom from confinement. Freedom from confinement and freedom of movement are especially important for persons with severe and persistent mental disorders, who, in the past, were confined to hospitals for decades at a time. Today, however, it is accepted that all persons who live without harming themselves or others have a right to freedom from confinement and freedom of movement. Many communities still struggle with where persons with severe and persistent mental disorders may live. The attitude often is: "They can live anywhere but in my community or in my neighborhood."

Even if these individuals have difficulty with judgment or impulse control, for example, they still have a right to live in the least restrictive environment possible. A *least restrictive environment provides a place to live with just enough structure and supervision to provide the assistance needed,* no more and no less. A healthy community creates an atmosphere within which a continuum of least restrictive environments can be provided for persons in the community. These least restrictive environments include places for all citizens: infants and young children, the elderly, persons with disabilities, persons with severe and persistent mental disorders, and even those who are violent or have committed crimes. Infants and young children live in the highly supervised and nurturing environment of the family and quite often in day (or night) care centers. Elderly persons may live with spouses, independently, with relatives, with friends, or in community living settings. Persons with disabilities may live independently, independently with part-time or full-time assistance, in group homes, in foster care, and in institutions designed to meet their health and supervision needs. Persons with mental disorders may live indepen-

dently, with their families, in group homes, with friends, in halfway houses, or in the highly structured, supervised environment of a subacute care center or a hospital. Persons who are violent may live in highly supervised 24-hour treatment environments, in highly structured living centers, or at home with highly structured supervision. Persons who have committed crimes may live in private or state-run prisons, in prerelease centers, or in their own homes with 24-hour monitoring devices.

To provide both for the safety of all community citizens and for the least restrictive environment for the needs of various populations within the community, a continuum of care must be available. The continuum is organized along the lines of restriction of personal freedom (from most restrictive to no restrictions) and along the lines of health support (from maximum to minimum support). Therefore the purpose of this chapter is to explore the parameters of healthy communities, to examine the continuum of restrictive environments, and to outline the resources healthy communities may provide to prevent mental illness, promote mental health, and to provide treatment for persons with mental disorders in the community. Although inpatient treatment is an important part of the continuum of treatment and restriction, it is explored thoroughly in Chapter 19 and is only mentioned briefly here.

EPIDEMIOLOGY

An American family untouched by mental illness is rare. One in three American adults will be diagnosed with a mental disorder sometime in life, and 20% have a mental disorder at any given time (Institute of Medicine [IOM], 1994). Higher prevalence rates were found in communities with social disintegration (Leighton et al., 1963) than in healthy communities. Chaotic, or unhealthy, communities have high rates of homocide, suicide, teen pregnancy, gangs, rapes, and rampant fear. Therefore the health of the community in preventing mental illness and in adequately treating and supporting persons with mental illnesses cannot be overemphasized.

Before the discovery of chlorpromazine HCl (Thorazine), virtually every person with a mental illness was institutionalized, except those who were cared for at home by family members. Few were ever discharged, and length of stay often lasted for decades. Thousands of persons per year were admitted only to die in the institution years later. On the brink of the twenty-first century, only hundreds of people are hospitalized for more than 1 year, and long-term inpatient treatment is considered to be approximately 30 days. Brief hospitalization may be 12 hours.

The psychiatric treatment of persons with mental illnesses occurs in the community. As community mental health and illness resources continue to be developed, preliminary studies indicate that, with intensive community case management and adequate community resources, clients can be maintained in the community with a higher quality of life than that available in a hospital. However, the cost is nearly two times the cost of maintaining the same person in a hospital (Okin, 1995; Rapp and Moore, 1995). The cost is greater because, for a person with a mental illness to live in the community, many health resources are needed to maintain the person in that unstructured environment. Intensive case management, payment for housing, and supervision of medication, group therapy, job skills training, and so forth are examples of resources one individual might need to live in the community. The values of freedom of movement, freedom from confinement, and the least restrictive environment are costly. In addition, about the same number of persons are institutionalized today as in 1955, about 1% of the population (Shore, 1989). Those institutions are not restricted to mental hospitals and include supported housing, nursing homes, long-term residential treatment centers, prisons, and others. However, even the institutions that treat mental illness are less restrictive than in the past.

HISTORY OF COMMUNITY MENTAL HEALTH

Until the time of the American Revolution, when the era of moral treatment began, persons with mental illness were kept at home, lived on the streets, or were incarcerated. Philippe Pinel in France and William Tuke in Great Britain are credited with developing the asylum, a rural haven for those afflicted with mental illness. Moral treatment was brought to the United States in 1783 by Benjamin Rush, who is considered to be the father of American psychiatry. In the 1850s, when the states started taking responsibility for the asylum care of persons with mental illnesses in the United States, the era of custodial care began. The first community-based service, a boarding house for persons with mental illnesses, was begun in Massachusetts in 1885. Few community services were established until a change in societal values together with the discovery of chlorpromazine HCl (Thorazine) in the 1950s made the deinstitutionalization movement possible. This change first began in 1908 with the publication of *A Mind That Found Itself* (Beers, 1981). A concern for children with mental illness first sparked the change, and the movement developed momentum through funding provided in the 1963 Community Mental Health Centers Act. President John F. Kennedy articulated the vision of community mental health in 1963, which led to the establishment of community mental health centers in the late 1960s and early 1970s.

There is controversy about the success of the community mental health movement thus far. However, the length of treatment in institutions is much shorter, fewer persons are ever admitted (there is even a population of young persons with chronic mental illnesses who have never been hospitalized), and many more persons are receiving services in the community. However, some believe that all the changes have not sufficiently improved the care provided to persons with mental illnesses (Shore, 1989). This belief has some validity because of the number of persons with severe and persistent mental disorders in insitutions other than hospitals and the number of homeless persons with mental illnesses. Others believe that, although the vision of John F. Kennedy has not been fully realized, the redirection of resources from institutions to community services has improved the quality of life for those served, and thus positive change has occurred.

The movement to the community has placed persons with severe and persistent mental disorders intimately among us and has fueled a prejudice that has always existed against persons with mental illnesses. This prejudice has been addressed by a variety of community groups. However, there is little evidence that it has been replaced with a more enlightened understanding of mental illness and the realities of living with a mental illness. Nurses have the opportunity to learn about mental illness and to work with persons with mental illnesses, and may help change community values concerning persons with severe and persistent mental disorders living in their communities and neighborhoods.

HEALTHY COMMUNITIES

Community *is defined as an identifiable group of people living in the same locality under similar conditions and having common interests.* Healthy communities are identifiable groups of individuals living in healthy conditions, which include:

- Operative democratic processes for all members of the community, not equally but equitably
- Protection of human rights
- Orientation of members to significant aspects of the life of the community
- Consistent, fair rules
- Opportunities for persons to participate in government
- Clean environment that is free of emotional, social, and physical toxins

Communities exist on a continuum of most healthy to least healthy; in addition, the health status is dynamic, as is the health status of individuals and families living in communities. Individuals and families must be networked and supported by adequate resources to be considered a community.

In healthy communities, a respect for individuals and families within the community is reflected in the following:

- A tolerance of a wide range of behaviors, as long as the behaviors do not hurt self or others
- Concern for one another while respecting boundaries such as personal property, privacy, and cultural expression
- Community members striving to optimize the community's physical, emotional, spiritual, and environmental attributes
- Working together to achieve a higher standard of living and health status
- Citizen empowerment to identify the health needs of the community
- The citizens' valuing of diversity and appreciation of cultural differences
- Community leaders who foster individual and collective responsibility for the community's well-being

Community Resources

A *community resource is an available supply of a necessary commodity that can be used by members of a particular group or location when needed.* Community resources are supportive services that promote, maintain, and restore individual, family, and community well-being and thereby make a contribution to health and mental health. Community resources must be available, accessible, affordable, and provided in a culturally sensitive manner. Examples of community resources are education, clean air and water, safe streets and roads, police protection, mail service, and waste disposal.

Community Health Resources

Although community resources support community health, only some resources directly influence community health. *Community health resources are needed commodities that directly affect the health of the community.* Examples of community resources that are also community health resources are clean air, clean water, and waste disposal.

A *primary care provider (PCP),* is also a community health resource. PCPs are *persons specially educated to provide health promotion, disease prevention, and early disease intervention services and to assist persons in maintaining their health as they manage chronic diseases.* These professionals may be physicians, clinical nurse specialists (CNSs), nurse practitioners (NPs), or physician's assistants (PAs). Many are vying for the insurance dollar and the federal and state dollars for reimbursement for health care services. Thus there may be many other providers who will offer primary care in the future.

At least 50% of the problems that clients bring to a PCP are mental health in nature, and about 75% of these are misdiagnosed as physical issues. Because primary care providers are the "front door" to the health care system in a great majority of cases, current knowledge about mental health and mental illness is critical in treating clients. One of the contributions psychiatric-mental health nurses make to primary care is to function as educators and consultants to PCPs to ensure that they maintain a current knowledge base about mental illness and mental health (Krauss, 1993). For example, much of the education of clients treated with psychotropic medications prescribed by PCPs is carried out by nurses working with these providers.

Emergency services are another health resource for the community. Emergency services are designed for true emergencies, in which clients have no time to see their PCPs, or the resources needed for treatment are not available in an office or clinic. However, emergency services have been deluged for the past 20 years with clients who have no PCP and/or no resources to pay for the services received. Therefore emergency services have a second thrust, that of a primary care clinic. Some emergency services have established a clinic, open 24 hours a day, as part of their services to meet the needs of the indigent community. The clinic concept has dramatically reduced the cost of the service provided while maintaining an accessible service for emergencies.

Another community health resource is support groups and self-help groups. There are community groups concerned with community problems such as preservation of the environment; advocacy groups are an example. There are also groups with the goal of changing the community. One example is a group of professionals and people with physical disabilites, whose goal is to create a barrier-free society. Mothers Against Drunk Drivers (MADD) and the National Association for the Advancement of Colored People (NAACP) are other community groups that promote community health. Some groups such as Children of Aging Parents (COAP) and groups for relatives of people with Alzheimer's disease are concerned with the health of individuals in the community, thereby promoting the health of the entire community. The majority of funding for these groups is community fundraising for charitable organizations. Community charities such as United Way or Community Chest may also provide some operating funds for organizations that influence the health of individuals, families, and the whole community.

Community Mental Health Resources

Community mental health resources are services specifically designed to prevent mental illness and to promote, maintain, and restore mental health of indi-

viduals, families, and the community. Community mental health centers, community support programs, and independent mental health services are described here.

Community mental health centers

The most comprehensive community mental health resource is the community mental health center (CMHC). CMHCs are required to offer the 10 services listed in Box 20-1. A community mental health center may, for example, have 10 beds for inpatient treatment and a partial night program. The staff that works with the clients who occupy the 10 beds also provides emergency services during the night and on weekends, offering crisis stabilization, and evaluation services. During the day, a multidisciplinary team may offer a course on parenting, run a day-treatment program, continue the emergency services as clients present themselves, and conduct consultations for providers in the community. The CMHC may own a small apartment building that houses clients who need the supervised care of a halfway house and who are able to maintain themselves in this environment. The clients may come to the center for weekly therapy, medication evaluation, and support group meetings, while holding part-time jobs.

Local communities were expected to take over funding of CMHCs from the federal government once the importance of the centers to the communities was established. Funding has now shifted to states and local communities, and every state has maintained the commitment to funding CMHCs. A few areas in the United States are still not covered by the CMHC system.

Community support programs

Another community mental health resource, established by the U.S. government in 1980, is the Community Support Program. The program's goal is to promote physical and mental health, emotional and financial independence, and personal and societal status for persons with severe and persistent mental disorders. The services provided by community support programs are found in Box 20-2 (see Chapter 18).

A community support program, housed within a local CMHC, may hire a group of case managers who work closely with and under the supervision of a psychiatric-mental health clinical nurse specialist. Clients are assigned to case managers, depending on their needs and the case managers' skills. The case manager is responsible for accessing and coordinating services (see Chapter 17). If the client needs financial assistance, the case manager goes with the client to complete forms, complete interviews, and follow up with the agencies. The client may go to a neighborhood church to attend a lithium support group and pick up food stamps. The case manager ensures that the service providers are expecting the client and addresses as much paperwork as possible.

The services of community support programs are congruent with the mission of CMHCs, and the programs are often housed together. However, just as funding for CMHCs moved from the federal level to the state and community levels, the same is true of community support programs. In many communities the spectrum of community support services has not yet been developed, and funding is a primary reason.

Independent mental health services

A generic name, independent mental health services is used to encompass the myriad of treatment options developed outside the federal, state, and local governments.

Box 20-1

Services Provided by Community Mental Health Centers

- Inpatient care
- Outpatient care
- Partial hospitalization
- Emergency care
- Consultation and education services
- Services for children and the elderly
- Alcoholism and drug abuse services
- Screening before admission to state hospitals
- Follow-up care for discharged clients
- Transitional housing

Box 20-2

Services Provided by Community Support Programs

- Identification of target populations in both the hospital and the community
- Assistance in applying for social services
- Crisis intervention in the least restrictive environment, with inpatient hospitalization available
- Psychosocial rehabilitation services, with major components being social skills training (see Chapter 38) and psychoeducation (see Chapter 16)
- Long-term support services in living and work settings
- Integrated mental health treatment and medical care
- Support services for family, friends, and significant others
- Efforts to encourage concerned individuals to develop and provide opportunities for employment and housing
- Protection of clients' rights
- Case management (see Chapter 17)

These services are developed within the private enterprise system and remain unintegrated or loosely networked into a web of other services available for clients needing mental health services. Examples of psychiatric-mental health service providers are psychiatric-mental health clinical nurse specialists, advanced nurse practitioners, psychiatrists, psychiatric social workers, clinical psychologists, and licensed professional counselors. Examples of psychiatric-mental health services are day care centers and support groups for clients and their families, such as Alcoholics Anonymous (AA) and lithium support groups. Examples of services provided are individual, group, and family therapy; skills training; and psychoeducation. Fees for independent mental health services may be paid by clients themselves, insurance, or community funding sources. Many support groups have little organizational structure and are supported by member donations.

INTERVENTION AND REHABILITATION (HOSPITAL WITHOUT WALLS)

One of the most exciting events in mental health has been *deinstitutionalization, the movement of clients from the hospital to the community.* The factors influencing this move were outlined above. Persons with mental illnesses need a broad spectrum of treatment settings, work and leisure opportunities, as well as living situations to individualize treatment for their current mental health needs. A "hospital without walls" is one name that captures the flexibility and fluidity of the community movement today. This concept includes treatment, living, and work and leisure.

Treatment

The hospital used to be the central component of a poorly developed mental health care system. The hospital was the best developed and best funded, and was thought to provide the best outcomes. The thrust of community mental health care is to have the hospital as one essential component, used as little as possible, for the shortest duration possible, with stabilization, not treatment, as its primary purpose. (See Chapter 19 for more information about the hospital setting and the nursing role.) In addition to hospitals, treatment may occur in partial programs, in outpatient treatment, in psychiatric home care, and through case management.

Treatment in partial programs
Treatment in partial programs is intense therapy offered for part of a day and/or part of a week. Treatment in partial programs may follow inpatient care; clients may also be admitted directly to partial treatment. Often, clients will start treatment in a partial program to evaluate

whether they can manage in a program less structured than the 24-hour hospital environment.

Clients in partial programs need considerable support and opportunity to work through daily issues and to learn to manage their psychiatric and medical conditions. Clients in partial treatment are either able to manage part of their day independently (e.g., they are able to work, or they have family support systems available when they are not in treatment). Length of treatment in partial programs may vary from a few days to several months. Partial treatment options include the following:

- *Day treatment,* in which clients spend daytime hours engaged in therapeutic treatment programs and spend evenings, nights, and weekends at home, halfway houses, room-and-board homes, or other shelters
- *Night treatment,* in which clients spend the day, usually weekdays, at work or school and spend evenings, nights, and weekends in the treatment facility
- *Structured outpatient treatment,* in which particular services and hours are chosen to meet a client's particular clinical and daily living needs; structured outpatient treatment is usually less than 8 hours per week
- *Respite care,* in which clients are cared for 24 hours or more so that full-time caregiving family members may have time away from a loved one who has a mental illness

The role of the nurse in partial treatment programs is similar to that of inpatient care. Nursing and other treatments are provided, evaluated, and documented in relation to stated client goals. Nurses monitor physical needs of clients because of the close connection between emotional and physical problems. The focus of nursing care is geared toward promotion of healthy behaviors and is supportive of stabilization of illness. The nurse should teach clients new patterns of interaction, which clients need to nurture and expand. There is a collaborative relationship between nurses and the client because the client has increased freedom to make decisions in the nurse-client relationship (see Chapter 9). This freedom gives the client the responsibility to choose which goals are most important and to pursue those with the assistance of the nurse and other health care team members. The nurse is less directive in the partial treatment setting and uses a problem-solving approach. Clients are thus assisted to discover ways of managing their lives successfully.

A vital nursing role in partial programs is medication monitoring and teaching. Compliance with a medication regimen is one of the greatest problems clients face. This problem is related to the uncomfortable side effects of some medications, as well as clients' feelings that they do not need medication. The nurse in this setting has the challenge of working with clients to diminish side effects as much as possible and to help the clients make a commitment to taking prescribed medication.

The nurse's role in working with individuals and groups in a socializing, normative fashion is important to the outcome of partial treatment programs. In addition, fostering healthful roles and relationships in groups and between individuals is usually performed by the nurse.

Outpatient treatment

Clients need services or are referred for psychiatric treatment to agencies and clinics for outpatient treatment. Outpatient treatment usually consists of one or two services for 1 to a few hours per week. Criteria for outpatient treatment include the following:

- Diagnosis of mental illness
- Psychiatric stability
- Ability to function at home and at work or school

Outpatient agencies provide various services, such as individual psychotherapy, group psychotherapy, marital and family therapy, socialization and occupational groups, and medication clinics. Clients may attend only one session, may engage in brief therapy of two to six visits, or may engage in long-term insight therapy, group therapy, or support therapy. Services are rendered by a variety of mental health care providers, including psychiatrists, psychiatric nurses (basic and advanced), psychiatric social workers, and mental health care workers or psychiatric technicians.

Typically, clients with certain acute mental illnesses (such as acute anxiety, some forms of depression, post-traumatic syndromes, multiple personality, and adjustment disorders such as marital conflict and conduct disorder) are treated in outpatient settings or by a provider connected with the agency or clinic. Clients with chronic uncomplicated illnesses are also treated in outpatient settings, in groups, and in medication clinics. Clients are referred to inpatient treatment if relapse occurs and the client is considered dangerous to self or others (see Chapter 19).

A psychiatric nurse providing services in an outpatient setting is able to do crisis intervention and engage in problem solving that would help maintain clients in the community and out of the hospital.

Mary J., RN, received a phone call from a client with schizophrenia who demanded admission to the hospital. He was complaining of shortness of breath, the walls closing in, and a concern that the neighbors were watching him. He had been receiving injections of antipsychotic medication in the mental health clinic. This client had maintained a functional lifestyle with structured activities for the past 4 months. A large snowfall had kept the client from his usual routine. The nurse discussed the situation with the client and planned activities with him to structure his day until he could resume his regular schedule. The structure included morning and afternoon telephone appointments to maintain contact. The client was able to implement the structure as planned, and hospitalization was avoided.

Psychiatric home care

A recent trend in community services is the provision of psychiatric-mental health services in the client's home. Psychiatric home care was developed to fill a gap in services between hospitalization and outpatient treatment. Visiting nurse associations and home health care agencies are two resources available for home-based psychosocial interventions (see Chapter 21). These services may be reimbursed by Medicare, Medicaid, private insurance companies, and prepaid health plans. Medicare and third-party payers require a bachelor's or master's degree in nursing for reimbursement for these services. Because clients almost always have medical, as well as psychiatric, problems, home care nurses may be expected to provide medical care in addition to psychiatric-mental health care. However, social workers, bachelor's-level counselors, and others may also provide services in the client's residence.

Case management

Case management is the coordination of services for clients whose medical and psychiatric needs are complex and for clients who do not have the resources, personally or within their support networks, to coordinate the needs and services. For clients with mental illness, the need for coordination includes environmental as well as medical and psychiatric issues (see Chapter 17).

Living

Living arrangements are independent of but intimately related to the treatment the client receives. For clients with severe and persistent mental disorders who need structured community residential settings, about half return to the hospital within the year for further treatment; 16% return to live in an institution for longer term. However, 28% move on to more independent living, and 57% are able to maintain themselves in the structured community residential setting. There are 94% who prefer to live in the community rather than in a hospital. Research has indicated that during clients' tenure in a structured community setting, their cognitive and social functioning significantly improved. Areas unaffected by community residential living were activities of daily living (ADLs), vocational and educational functioning, and positive psychiatric symptoms (Okin et al., 1995). (See Chapter 38 for a further exploration of treatment options for persons with severe and persistent mental disorders.)

The opinions of clients differ markedly from those of their treatment teams in regard to housing preferences. Ordinarily, clients assess themselves as needing less-structured environments and wanting to live more independently than treatment team assessments. The success of a placement in work, play, and living depends on a client's willingness to make a placement work. Therefore the views of treatment teams and clients need to be reconciled (Minsky, Riesser, and Duffy, 1995).

Supported housing is becoming acceptable among consumers, and is being viewed as effective among providers. *Supported housing is the provision of housing of the client's choice, in community housing rather than mental health programs, and the provision of services and supports required to maximize the client's opportunities for success over time* (Carling, 1993). Supported housing is based on the belief that people, regardless of their disability, know what is best for them (Howie the Harp, 1993).

As stated earlier, living arrangements and treatment settings are independent but intimately related. For example, a client may participate in a partial program 5 days per week, 6 hours per day, and live at home with family, in a halfway house, in an apartment, or in a shelter. The various living options available to persons with mental illnesses and persons with severe and persistent mental disorders are explored in this section. They include independent living, living with family, transitional living, and permanent housing arrangements.

Independent living

When clients are able to function effectively in caring for themselves and their living quarters, can pay their bills and fulfill the role of a good neighbor, and are single, the usual choice of living is independent living. Many clients, both with acute and severe and persistent mental disorders, are able to live independently.

Living with family

Often families of origin become a refuge for clients with mental illnesses who are not able to maintain adequate adult-role functioning or may not be able to maintain full-time employment. Clients most often live with parents but also live with siblings, aunts, uncles, and others.

Clients who are married most often stay in their marital home. Spouses and children often need support, encouragement, and coaching to deal with the changing roles and relationships that mental illness, acute or persistent, may precipitate. There may be a need for a temporary placement in another living arrangement while family dynamics, roles, and relationships are sorted out after the advent of a mental illness or a relapse.

Transitional living

Clients with mental disorders may not be able to live independently or with their families for various reasons. Therefore either transitional or permanent living arrangements must be available. Transitional living arrangements include quarterway, halfway, three-quarterway housing, foster care, and shelters.

Quarterway housing refers to the extent to which the dwelling is supervised and the therapeutic milieu maintained by trained staff. A quarterway house is staffed 24 hours a day with persons licensed to give medications and provide crisis intervention, social skills training, and ADL coaching. This is considered residential treatment when certain governmental housing standards and therapy requirements are met.

A halfway house is supervised 24 hours per day by support personnel, but medications are maintained by the clients, and therapeutic activities are limited to support and development of living skills. Three-quarterway housing has intermittent visiting supervision to check the status of the household and its residents. Members of the household provide their own planning and entertainment and negotiate roles and relationships.

Foster care, or *placement with a selected family,* is another supportive living arrangement designed to enhance skills of cooperative living. Persons who provide foster care are paid for each client for whom they care. In most states, foster caretakers are expected to attend specialized training classes and to meet certain minimum requirements (e.g., a high school diploma and no police record). A foster home may become a permanent living arrangement.

Shelters are considered temporary housing arrangements. Shelters are provided by voluntary and government agencies for persons who have no place to live. The qualifications the applicant must meet vary from shelter to shelter, as do the stipulations for remaining in the shelter. For example, Shelter Sanctuary requires that the person be homeless and have no employment. The Shelter Sanctuary provides a bed in a dormitory setting, with communal bathrooms and showers. To remain a maximum of 21 days, the resident must be in the building by 7:30 PM showing no signs of alcohol or drug use, must attend a chapel service, and must participate in the employment coaching services provided.

Permanent housing arrangements

Permanent housing arrangements include group homes, nursing homes, room-and-board facilities, and single-room-occupancy dwellings (SROs). These are used when clients recognize that independent living is unavailable and unrealistic for them or unacceptable to them.

Group homes or apartments provide permanent living arrangements in which residents share responsibilities associated with home life, such as cooking, cleaning, maintenance, and yard work. A group home may be supervised full-time or part-time, depending on the residents' needs and availability of funding for supervision.

Nursing homes provide permanent living arrangements in which residents have no responsibility for tasks associated with home life; residents, however, may have an opportunity to participate in some work as part of their treatment program. Nursing homes may be locked skilled nursing facilities or may allow more freedom for clients. In nursing homes, paraprofessional staff members are supervised by registered nurses, and physicians make visits to the home when needed by the residents. A nursing home may be the first step out of a hospital on the way to a permanent living experience; in such a situation, a nursing home is considered a temporary placement.

Room-and-board facilities (as the term implies) provide room and board. Some states require supervision of the managers of room-and-board facilities; no responsibilities are expected of residents beyond courteous behavior.

Single-room occupancy hotels provide a room and bathroom but no meals and usually require residents to vacate the premises by a certain time in the morning and to return after a certain time at night. Persons may keep their belongings in their rooms but may not have access to them during the day.

Work and Leisure

All adults, regardless of health status, need meaningful work. The challenge for all persons is to find work that matches their personal skills, gifts, energy levels, patterns of concentration, and other characteristics. For persons with mental illnesses, finding the match may be more challenging than it is for others.

Vocational rehabilitation is a generic term for programs for or approaches to clients who need assistance in identifying, training for, and maintaining employment congruent with their skills, education, limitations, and opportunities. Vocational rehabilitation is often appropriate for clients whose lives have been significantly altered by mental illness. Clients can be referred for assessment and evaluation by health care professionals who have assessed a need for significant change in employment for a client.

Work hardening may be needed by clients as part of their continuing care for mental illness. The purpose of work hardening is to assist clients in developing skills to maintain employment, taking into consideration the work environment and issues created by their illnesses.

Leisure is a critical part of the equation for healthful living: a balance between work and leisure. For clients with mental illness, leisure activities may be difficult to plan or afford. Developing and maintaining friends with whom to relax may also be challenging. Nevertheless, leisure is necessary. In the community, leisure activities that are free or low-cost and require little interaction with others are helpful. Libraries and other community resources often have free lectures where people who have common interests can gather.

ROLES OF THE NURSE IN THE COMMUNITY

Although all of the roles outlined in the psychiatric-mental health nursing's *Standards* are applicable in the community, treatment roles, case finding and referral, and advocacy are explored here.

Treatment Roles

The clinical roles for an RN in the community are many and varied. The nurse in the community may work in a clinic, a halfway house, an apartment complex, or under a bridge. The nurse in any of these settings is responsible for thorough assessment, diagnosis, treatment planning, implementation, and evaluation of the effectiveness of the nursing treatment. The nurse's clients may be individuals, families, the community as a whole, or a segment of the community with a specialized need. Role opportunities for nurses may depend on educational preparation, as shown in Table 20-1. Nursing roles often encompass multiple settings and several clients, as in the following example:

Kelly T. works for the Cherokee Nation and spends 2 days per week in the health department giving human immunodeficiency virus (HIV) pretesting counseling, testing, and post-testing counseling. He screens and conducts case finding for other sexually transmitted diseases as well. Two half-days per week, Kelly goes to the two tribe schools and teaches mental health classes, stress management, and social skills. He also administers vision and hearing screenings and immunizations, and facilitates a peer support group for children with learning disabilities. Kelly spends 1½ days at the Salvation Army and the Day Center for the Homeless working with Native American homeless persons with mental illnesses conducting assessment and referral. He also gives influenza injections and hepatitis vaccines, provides teaching for high-risk persons, and helps solve the everyday problems of caring for mental health and medical conditions of the homeless. Much of his time in all of these settings is spent making phone calls to other health care providers, giving rides, and contacting teachers, employers, and families. He also coordinates resources needed by clients (e.g., homeless persons), groups (e.g., school children and their teachers), families (e.g., a family with a member with HIV), communities (e.g., attending a tribal council meeting where mental health issues are being discussed), or community segments (e.g., teenagers with alcoholism).

Other roles that are important in the community are medication evaluation, documentation, and administration. Relapse is a common problem with all chronic illnesses, including severe and persistent mental illness. Conducting classes through a community education program, working with individual families, and teaching

classes through a client or family support group are examples of ways to meet this role in the community.

Case Finding and Referral

Case finding and referral roles dovetail with the prevention and promotion aspects of the nursing role. Whatever the setting, whether at work or during leisure time, a nurse is asked many interesting, often unusual questions: "Oh, you're a nurse. Maybe you can help me figure out

TABLE 20-1

Examples of mental health nursing roles by educational preparation

NURSING ROLE	ASSOCIATE DEGREE	BACHELOR'S DEGREE	MASTER'S DEGREE
Counseling	Therapeutic communication	Problem solving	Psychotherapy
Milieu management	Implements interventions for improving the milieu	Assesses milieu and implements interventions for improving the milieu	Designs milieu; alters systems based on systems assessment
Self-care activities	Assesses self-care needs; assists clients in meeting self-care needs; supervises nursing assistants in carrying out self-care needs	Develops intervention strategies for clients with complex self-care needs; teaches clients and works in a problem-solving framework to address barriers clients experience in relation to self-care	Develops programs for the development of self-care skills for specific populations; tests the programs in an evaluation framework to generate baseline and quality improvement data
Psychobiological interventions	Administers medications, evaluates side effects, and teaches clients and their families about medications	Develops nursing protocols related to medication side effects and issues of noncompliance	Teaches clients who refuse to take medications about other ways to respond to relapse symptoms and illness management; in some states, prescribes medications
Health teaching	Teaches individuals and groups about antidepressants from a standardized protocol	Develops a treatment regimen for clients with personality disorders concerning boundary maintenance	Develops teaching protocol for social skills for clients with severe and persistent mental disorders
Case management	Participates in the decision making and implements decisions of the treatment team; represents the client's viewpoint when the client is unable to do so	Acts as primary case manager, communicating with other team members, accessing resources needed for client	Serves as consultant for primary case managers, working on complex issues, including the professional relationship between client and case manager
Health promotion/health maintenance	Includes healthy lifestyle principles in nursing care plan and teaching plan	Considers long-term view of client's illness, strengths, and resources available in working toward the client's commitment to a healthy lifestyle	Works with community groups to include principles of stress management and early signs of mental illness and relapse in planning a family health fair

what to do about my. . . ." The issues and problems of life that are queried so casually must be responded to with sensitivity; the nurse does not give advice but instead provides useful direction for actions. Providing information and education is within the scope of nursing practice and must be handled with care. For example, a person discusses at a party her concern for her grandmother, who is becoming more forgetful and is not managing her money well. Listening, empathizing, and reflecting the concerns of the person is appropriate. If asked questions that have factual answers, giving the information is appropriate. Telling her she ought to tell her

grandmother's physician that the medication is not working or telling her to file for an incompetency hearing and become the grandmother's guardian is not appropriate. Referring the person to the Elder Protection Agency in her city for further information and options is appropriate. The guidelines for making referrals are found in Box 20-3.

The purpose of the case finding and referral role is to assist in decreasing the level of illness by early identification and referral of persons in need of treatment. Each professional, regardless of discipline, has a knowledge base that sensitizes that person to information a lay per-

---

Box 20-3

Guidelines for Making a Referral

STEP 1

The referral process begins with the identification of a specific need that the nurse is unable to address adequately.

STEP 2

The nurse validates the existence of the need with the client and asks the client to determine a priority for meeting that need. For example:

A nurse, Ms. N., who has a BSN degree, identifies a need for sex counseling for a client, Ms. O., but recognizes that sex counseling is beyond the scope of her role as nurse. Ms. N. shares her recognition of this need with Ms. O., who agrees that she is sexually dysfunctional and that the problem is creating a severe strain in her marriage. Ms. O. asks Ms. N. to identify some services available to address the problem.

STEP 3

Match the client's need with the appropriate community service. If need and service are ill-matched, the client will not be helped and will feel frustrated and hopeless, and the community service will be wasted. (For the O. family, for example, sex education will not meet the need; agencies that provide sex counseling are therefore the only agencies considered by Ms. N.)

STEP 4

Determine whether a client is eligible for the community service that seems most appropriate. Every agency has some criteria, and it is useless for a nurse to refer clients to services for which they are ineligible.

STEP 5

The nurse makes contact with the agency to be sure that it provides the needed service and to confirm that the client is eligible. This step is particularly important if the nurse is unfamiliar with the agency. While discussing the possibility of making a referral, the nurse also ascertains whether there are other resources available to deal with the problem and

obtains specific information about fees, hours, kinds of therapy offered, and protocols or forms for referrals. At this point, the client's identity is not revealed to the agency.

STEP 6

The nurse shares the information gathered with the client and identifies up to three resources that will effectively meet the client's need. The nurse encourages the client to consider the information and make an informed decision. (In the case of Ms. O., her husband may need to be involved in the decision.)

STEP 7

Once the client has made a decision, the nurse and the client decide which of them will approach the agency. If the agency requires paperwork or disclosure of information by the nurse, the nurse asks the client's permission to comply with this requirement and then gives the client a copy of the information provided. When possible, however, the client should be the one who discloses information, although the nurse may accompany the client to the agency or be available for moral support.

STEP 8

If the client is able to contact the agency independently, the nurse should stay out of the situation entirely, ascertaining only that the client's problem is being addressed.

STEP 9

Follow up with the client to find out how the referral is working. If the client is dissatisfied, the nurse asks the client's permission to contact the agency or to arrange a three-way meeting to address the problem and achieve a more workable solution. (Agencies are usually willing and sometimes eager to receive feedback about their services.) It may turn out, however, that a referral to some other service is needed; if so, assessment, contact, and follow-up should ensure a better outcome. The more nurses learn about community resources, the more effective their referrals will be.

son may miss. This professional can help a person get needed assistance as quickly as possible. There is some evidence that early intevention may actually prevent the development of illness. In other situations such as normal developmental crises (see Chapter 7), assistance with a rough transition may promote that person's overall health. Referral to a school counselor or church youth director costs little, if anything, and may significantly impact a person's health.

Advocacy

Many problems in the community are social, political, and economic but have influence on the health status of individuals, families, and the community. Nurses deal with and help clients deal with conditions beyond the nursing profession's control. However, the lack of control does not exonerate nurses from the responsibility to influence those larger problems beyond purely health matters. *Advocacy is speaking up for persons who cannot, at the moment, speak for themselves.* Methods of advocacy include the following:

- Voting
- Becoming active in a political party
- Running for office
- Endorsing a candidate
- Offering testimony to governmental, regulatory, and voluntary agencies

Although political involvement in the community may seem a little farfetched to be considered as part of the nursing role, the contrary is true. Advocacy in any form is a central component to the effectiveness of the nursing profession's responsibility to society. The nurse's role in

CRITICAL THINKING QUESTIONS

Amy is 35 years old and has been treated sporadically by the mental health system, both publicly and privately, since she was 16 years old. Her medical diagnosis has consistently been alcohol and drug dependence. In the last 5 years, she has been treated for borderline personality disorder as well.

Amy has been assigned to your caseload. You are her sixth case manager. On assessment, she tells you the following:

- She lives in three places: jail, hospitals, and the streets.
- When she is cold and hungry, she goes "home" to her parents' house in a very nice part of the community. She is always welcome there, but she is expected to remain sober and to let them know where she is at all times. She finds the rules too restrictive, so she drops in only occasionally, usually on weekends and holidays.
- She has been to the state hospital five times for detoxification from alcohol. She uses speed and lots of downers, but mostly she buys alcohol. She gets money by begging in the street and occasionally through prostitution.
- She does not enjoy working and cannot understand why anybody would work. She receives food stamps and a small monthly stipend check from investments her parents made in her name.
  1. As Amy's case manager, you are expected to help her find permanent housing and a steady income, preferably from private enterprise. These are long-term goals that are established for all persons being served by your agency.

  a. If you could develop an idealistic plan for Amy, and she would support it, what plans would you develop?
  b. In your plan, in what ways did you account for her two illnesses?
  c. In your plan, what assumptions did you have to make about Amy?
  d. What would your timeline be for the achievement of the two goals? Provide a rationale for your decision.
  2. Amy tells you she would like to live with some of her friends from the streets. They would like to live without hassle and would be willing to provide half the cost of the housing, including bills.
  a. What are your thoughts and feelings about Amy's desires? Assume that you would not share these with Amy.
  b. Would you or would you not support Amy in trying to negotiate some aspect of her desires for housing? Why or why not? What are your values and beliefs that support this decision? What conflicts did you have to resolve to come to this decision?
  3. At the minimum, what community resources does Amy need to live in any community? List at least seven resources and label them as community resources, health resources, or mental health resources as they would serve Amy's specific needs.

community mental health care emphasizes and highlights that responsibility, but the responsibility exists, regardless of what position the nurse holds in the community.

KEY POINTS

- The community is the context within which the greatest part of health, mental health, and treatment for mental illness is carried out.
- The community is defined as an identifiable group of people living in the same locality under similar conditions and having common interests.
- In healthy communities, there is respect for individuals and families within the community, reflected in (1) a tolerance of a wide range of behaviors as long as the behaviors do not hurt self or others; and (2) a concern for one another while respecting boundaries such as personal property, privacy, and cultural expression.
- The adequacy, availability, and appropriateness of community resources directly affects the health of the community.
- Mental health resources depend on a solid network of general community resources.
- Community mental health centers, community support programs, emergency and crisis clinics, private practitioners, and partial programs all comprise the mental health resources of the community. Each community develops its own set of resources.
- The needs of clients with mental illnesses include treatment, living, work, and leisure. Treatment and living arrangements are independent, yet related issues that need to be addressed by the client in conjunction with the treatment team.
- Besides traditional nursing roles, the roles that are strongly developed in the community include the nursing process, medication evaluation and teaching, case finding and referral, health promotion and disease prevention, and advocacy.

REFERENCES

American Nurses Association (1994). *Statement on psychiatric-mental health clinical nursing practice and standards of psychiatric-mental health clinical nursing practice.* Washington, DC: American Nurses Publishing.

Beers, C. (1981). *A mind that found itself.* Pittsburgh: University of Pittsburgh Press.

Carling, P. J. (1993). Housing and supports for persons with mental illness: Emerging approaches to research and practice. *Hospital and Community Psychiatry, 44*(5), 439–449.

Howie the Harp. (1993). Taking issue: Taking a new approach to independent living. *Hospital and Community Psychiatry, 44*(5), 413.

Institute of Medicine. (1994). *Reducing risks for mental disorders: Frontiers for preventive intervention research.* Washington, DC: National Academy Press.

Krauss, J. (1993). *Healthcare reform: Essential mental health services.* Washington, DC: American Nurses Publishing.

Leighton, C.D., et al. (1963). *The character of danger.* New York: Basic Books.

McCarty, D., Argeriou, M., Huebner, R.B., & Lubran, B. (1991). Alcoholism, drug abuse, and the homeless. *American Psychologist, 46,* 1139-1148.

Minsky, S., Riesser, G.G., & Duffy, M. (1995). The eye of the beholder: Housing preferences of inpatients and their treatment teams. *Psychiatric Services, 46,* 173-176.

Okin, R.L., Borus, J.F., Baer, L., & Jones, A. L. (1995). Long-term outcome of state hospital patients discharged into structured community residential settings. *Psychiatric Services, 46,* 73-78.

Okin, R.L. (1995). Testing the limits of deinstitutionalization. *Psychiatric Services, 46,* 569-574.

President's Commission on Mental Health (1978). *Report to the President from the President's Commission on Mental Health, vol 1.* Washington, DC: U.S. Government Printing Office.

Rapp, C.A., & Moore, T. (1995). The first 18 months of mental health reform in Kansas. *Psychiatric Services, 46,* 580-585.

Shore, J.H. (1989). Community psychiatry. In H.I. Kaplan & B.J. Sadock (Eds.), *Comprehensive textbook of psychiatry.* Vol 2, (5th ed.). Baltimore: Williams and Wilkins.

Strole, L. et al. (1962). *Mental health in the Metropolis: The Midtown Manhattan Study.* New York: McGraw-Hill.

Chapter 21

Psychiatric Home Care

Judith Haber

LEARNING OUTCOMES

After studying and applying the concepts of this chapter, the learner will be able to:
- Define home care and psychiatric home care.
- Identify types of agencies that provide psychiatric home care.
- Discuss reimbursement sources for psychiatric home care.
- Identify psychiatric home care referral sources.
- Identify client populations that require psychiatric home care services.
- Describe factors contributing to the expansion of psychiatric home care.
- Compare the advantages and disadvantages of psychiatric home care models.
- Discuss assumptions about psychiatric home care.
- Discuss the role of the nurse in psychiatric home care.
- Apply theories relevant to the delivery of effective psychiatric home care services.
- Apply the nursing process to the delivery of psychiatric home care services with selected client populations.

KEY TERMS

Home care	Psychiatric home care

Skyrocketing health care costs coupled with a philosophical shift to community-based health care have increased the demand for mental health care services delivered in the home. Psychiatric nurses have become important members of the multidisciplinary home care team. As home care nurses, psychiatric nurses provide skilled nursing services to clients and their families in their homes within a community context.

The purpose of this chapter is to highlight an exciting and expanding community role for psychiatric nurses. This chapter presents theoretical and economic foundations of psychiatric home care nursing, current issues and trends, and the role of the nurse in the provision of psychiatric home care.

DEFINITION OF PSYCHIATRIC HOME CARE

Home care, including psychiatric home care, is one component of comprehensive health and mental health care delivery (Mellon, 1994). *Home care provides a spectrum of health-related services to clients and their families in the home setting.* Home settings include residential care facilities such as senior citizen residences and congregate housing, group homes, halfway houses, as well as private homes, apartments, and boardinghouses. *Psychiatric home care is the delivery of mental health and related physical health care in a home setting.* Essential to this care are social and environmental health care services.

Clients requiring psychiatric home care often have complex health care needs that are truly biopsychosocial in nature. Psychiatric nurses, as major providers of psychiatric home care, function as direct care providers and as case managers who develop, coordinate, and implement the care plan. This requires accessing a broad range of the physical, mental, and social services presented in Box 21-1.

TYPES OF AGENCIES THAT PROVIDE PSYCHIATRIC HOME CARE SERVICES

Home care services, which include psychiatric home care, are provided by multidisciplinary teams that include psychiatric nurses at the basic and advanced levels of practice, in the following types of agencies:

- *Public or official agencies operated by federal, state, or local governments.* The Veterans Administration, a federally funded health care system, includes home care services. On the state level, county health departments in rural counties often have a certified home care agency.
- *Private and voluntary nonprofit agencies.* The Visiting Nurse Service of Greater New York is an example of a private nonprofit home care agency.

Box 21-1

Physical and Mental Health Services Available to Psychiatric Home Care Clients

Counseling
Psychological testing
Medication monitoring/management
Social work services
Medical services
Skilled nursing
Occupational therapy
Physical therapy
Vocational therapy
Speech therapy
Recreational therapy
Nutritional services
Intravenous/parenteral therapy
Home health aide/homemaker services
Transportation services
Laboratory services
Medical supplies
Pharmacy services
Wound care/enterostomal services
Pain management
Entitlement services
Legal services

- *Combinations of public and private nonprofit agencies operated by both sources or a new board of directors.* The Community Nursing Service of Philadelphia is an example of a combined public-private nonprofit agency.
- *Hospital-based agencies administered by a hospital's board of directors.* The Montefiore Home Health Agency is an example of a hospital-based agency.
- *Proprietary (for-profit) agencies administered by a private owner, which can include franchised home care agencies that are part of a state, regional, or national chain.* Staffbuilders, Inc., is an example of a proprietary national home care company that franchises individual Staffbuilders home care agencies based on regionally identified needs.
- *Individual or group partnerships of nurses and/or other health care professionals who provide home care services, or a specific type of home care service, on a contractual or private basis.* HUG, Inc. (Help Us Grow) is a psychiatric home care service developed by advanced practice psychiatric nurses, which provides psychiatric home care services on a private basis or through contracts with HMOs or other health care organizations.

Typically, clients are referred for psychiatric home care during the discharge planning process, as they make the transition from inpatient settings to community-based treatment programs such as day treatment programs, halfway houses, community mental health centers, group homes, or family residences. Psychiatric home care services provided by the previously listed agencies complement the services offered by such community-based treatment programs. Box 21-2 presents a detailed list of possible referral sources for psychiatric home care.

REIMBURSEMENT SOURCES

Eligibility for psychiatric home care services, including skilled psychiatric nursing services, is based on the client having a primary psychiatric diagnosis, homebound status, and identified need for treatment that requires intermittent skilled nursing care (Health Care Financing Administration [HCFA], 1989). Primary psychiatric diagnoses include major depression, bipolar disorder, schizophrenia, anxiety disorders, borderline personality disorder, and substance abuse disorders.

Homebound status is based on the client not leaving the home except for physician visits, medical care, or attendance at therapeutic programs such as day treatment centers that are part of the care plan. Some clients may be homebound because they refuse to leave their homes. Geropsychiatric clients often have medical conditions that impair mobility and necessitate home care. Justifying homebound status for younger clients can be more difficult in clients with psychiatric disabilities. However, many of these clients have paranoia, agoraphobia, or generalized anxiety about new situations, which render them essentially homebound (Hellwig, 1993). Need for treatment is indicated through written orders by a psychiatrist working with the psychiatric nurse and

other team members to implement the care plan. Reimbursement for psychiatric home care services are obtained from the four sources identified in Table 21-1.

PSYCHIATRIC HOME CARE CLIENT POPULATIONS

Psychiatric home care is a feasible, cost-effective alternative to hospitalization for several client populations including the elderly, persons with severe and persistent mental disorders living at home, and people with medical illnesses. These people and their families are appropriate psychiatric home care clients for the following reasons:

- Of persons age 65 to 74, 95% are living in the community. As many as 25%, or more, of the 3 million elderly have significant mental health problems. It is estimated that 15% to 30% of older adults are clinically depressed; persons over age 65 account for 20% of all suicides (Harper, 1989). Approximately 20% of the elderly show mild to severe signs of cognitive impairment from irreversible dementia disorders or other organic disorders (Kozlak and Thobaben, 1992). Yet less than 6% of those seen at community mental health centers are elderly and only 2% to 7% of persons over age 65 are seen by psychiatrists, psychologists, or advanced practice psychiatric nurses (Buckwalter and Stolley, 1991).
- Home care provided by a psychiatric nurse, which includes assessment for depression, medication interactions, confusion, cognitive impairment, and dementia; counseling; implementation of home-based assistive self-care resources; and referral to appropriate community support services, may allow the person additional years of independent living in the home environment (Harper, 1989).
- Approximately 2.5 to 5 million persons in the United States have serious and persistent neurobiological disorders (Krauss, 1993). It is estimated that 70% (1.75 to 3.5 million) of these individuals live in the community, with many living at home with their families. Psychiatric nurses provide essential services to this vulnerable population. They provide direct services to clients in the home setting, including medication monitoring, counseling, relapse monitoring, and crisis intervention, and they access and coordinate rehabilitative services. Psychiatric nurses also work with family members to establish appropriate structures and provide psychoeducation and encouragement to relieve caregiver burden.
- Persons with chronic and debilitating illnesses such as multiple sclerosis, Parkinson's disease, cancer, chronic obstructive pulmonary disease (COPD), and human immunodeficiency virus/acquired immunodeficiency syndrome (HIV/AIDS) often become anx-

Box 21-2

Referral Sources for Psychiatric Home Care

Hospital discharge planners
Nurses, physicians, social workers
Insurance companies including health maintenance organizations (HMOs) and preferred provider organizations (PPOs)
Clients and former clients
Family members
Employee assistance programs
Clergy
Health departments
Landlords, neighbors
Community agencies
Long-term and intermediate care facilities

TABLE 21-1

Reimbursement sources for psychiatric home care services

REIMBURSEMENT SOURCE	EXAMPLE
1. Medicare, a federal reimbursement program, provides funds for psychiatric home care for clients who have a primary psychiatric diagnosis, are homebound, and have been evaluated by a psychiatrist and are reevaluated every 60 days. Homebound status is defined by the client's inability to leave home as a result of a physical illness or injury, or because a mental illness makes it unsafe to leave home unattended or the client refuses to leave the residence (HCFA, 1989).	John G., 87, has been hospitalized with a primary diagnosis of depression. Never married and with no relatives living near by, John lives alone in a small apartment in a two-family house. He describes himself as :". . . not very sociable; I like to be by myself. I never had any trouble passing the time until I got too depressed to read. Even though I feel better, I don't know how I will shop, cook, or do my laundry." The discharge planner on the psychiatric unit is concerned about John's ability to manage independently in his apartment. The discharge planner refers John to a proprietary home care agency for evaluation regarding skilled nursing and home health aide services.
2. Medicaid, a federal- and state-funded program, includes reimbursement for psychiatric home care. Each state has specific criteria for determining eligibility and reimbursement for psychiatric home care. Usually, establishment of financial need, based on specific criteria such as income, savings, and other sources of support are key criteria, in addition to the psychiatric diagnosis and evidence of disability.	Vannie R., 46, has a 25-year history of bipolar disorder and alcohol dependence. He has not held a job in 10 years; public assistance is his only source of support. Vannie does not take his lithium reliably. He lives in an apartment that is so filthy, it nearly was condemned. He rarely eats anything except toaster pastries and cream-filled cakes because he spends all his money on vodka and beer. Vannie intermittently attends the outpatient mental health clinic. He is referred for home care services by the social worker at the clinic.
3. Many private indemnity, PPO, and HMO insurance plans provide third-party payment for psychiatric home care services. Often company- or plan-specific rules and regulations related to home care and/or psychiatric home care benefits are established. Private payers vary on whether they cover psychiatric home care services, the types of reimbursable services, and the number of visits covered annually or per illness. Some health insurance companies pay for psychiatric home care services on a case-by-case basis. As home care services are increasingly viewed as a cost-effective alternative to hospitalization (Hellwig, 1993; Miller and Duffey, 1993), psychiatric home care will become a standard component of all health insurance plans.	Marie S., 24, has a primary psychiatric diagnosis of schizophrenia. She has a 6-year history of repeated hospitalizations and is awaiting placement in an apartment in her community. Marie has been referred to the psychiatric home care program of the Visiting Nurse Service for an evaluation of activities of daily living (ADLs), medication monitoring, and coordination of community-based services, including day treatment, vocational counseling, and occupational therapy. The psychiatric nurse will function as the case manager.
4. Self-pay, where clients pay for psychiatric home care services, occurs when individuals are not eligible for Medicare or Medicaid benefits, when their insurance plans do not cover home health care services, or if they do not have health insurance. Sometimes clients choose to pay for psychiatric home services when the limits on those benefits have been reached, and they wish to continue home care services beyond the period authorized by a private insurer or government program.	Harvey G., age 77, has degenerative disease of the spine, Parkinson's disease, and major depression. He had been receiving home care services from a psychiatric nurse who coordinated services including a home health aide, physical and occupational therapy, and a day care program. Improvement in Mr. G.'s nutrition, ambulation, exercise tolerance, dexterity, hopelessness, medication managment, and his wife's care-giver burden were the focus of services. When Mr. G. reached his maximum level of function, Medicare reimbursement terminated. However, the family wanted to continue the home care services on a self-pay basis, feeling that the services of the psychiatric nurse and home health aide were central to maintaining Mr. G's progress.

ious and/or depressed. The physical component of their illness is often so overwhelming that emotional problems such as depression and anxiety are often overlooked or too readily accepted by family and physicians as an untreatable sequelae of the medical illness. The fact that mental and physical health have a strong reciprocal relationship is easily forgotten. Medical-surgical home care nurses are often in the best position to detect and then consult with psychiatric home care nurses who are knowledgeable about physical and psychiatric disorders. Home care nurses make consultation visits to assess, treat, and/or refer to appropriate resources the secondary mental health problems of clients with primary medical diagnoses. They may also suggest psychosocial strategies for medical-surgical nurses to implement in their roles as direct care providers and case managers, thereby improving the functioning and quality of life of these clients and their families.

FORCES INFLUENCING THE EXPANSION OF PSYCHIATRIC HOME CARE

In the arena of mental health care, there is no greater question than how to address the care of individuals and families in the community. As the delivery of mental health care services increasingly shifts to community-based settings, the need and demand for psychiatric home care is projected to increase exponentially (Mellon, 1994). Some of the factors contributing to the increased demand include the following:

- Home care services are cost-effective alternatives to hospitalization or long-term institutional care.
- Shortened hospital length of stay for a client with mental illness, shifting from a treatment to a stabilization focus, has increased the need for community-based treatment programs, with initiation and maintenance of treatments at home, which were formerly performed only within the hospital.
- Many people prefer to remain in their homes, living as independently as possible.
- The deinstitutionalization of clients with mental disorders has resulted in an increasing number of clients with complex physical and psychiatric problems residing in the community.
- Approximately 50% to 80% of persons with HIV/AIDS have some degree of cognitive impairment related to AIDS Dementia Complex (ADC), and at least 80% experience anxiety and depression (Pessin et al., 1993).
- An aging American population is producing a four-generation society in which the frail elderly (86 to 100 years of age) and centenarians (100 and older) are the fastest growing cohorts (Krauss, 1993).

Ninety-five percent of the elderly, many of whom have complex physical and emotional problems, live in the community without adequate support systems.

- Fifty percent of women who have been the primary caretakers of elderly family members now must work or choose to work outside the home. They are unavailable to care for elderly family members.
- The traditional support system provided by the extended family has been almost eliminated by the increasing mobility of society and an increase in small family units and single heads of household.
- There is a greater need for respite care for family members of clients who live at home. This care can prevent hospitalization, institutionalization, caregiver overload and burnout, and client abuse.

OUTCOMES OF PSYCHIATRIC HOME CARE

Psychiatric home care, as illustrated in Fig. 21-1, is one component of the continuous circle of psychiatric care available to clients with mental disorders and their families in a community context. Psychiatric home care has the following four desired outcomes: (1) promotion, maintenance, or restoration of clients' optimal level of health, realistic functioning, and independence; (2) minimized disability and maximized physical and psychiatric rehabilitation; (3) provision of treatment in the least restrictive environment that preserves a person's func-

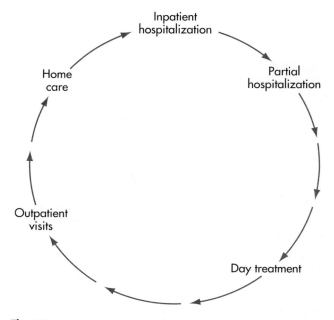

Fig. 21-1 Continuous circle of psychiatric care within the community.

tional position in the family and community; and (4) prevention of relapse and hospitalization.

To achieve the above outcomes, plans for psychiatric home care services must consider the whole individual in the context of the family and community. Services must be allocated in a cost-effective, coordinated, and integrated manner and be designed to achieve projected outcomes.

PSYCHIATRIC HOME CARE PROGRAM MODELS

Psychiatric home care programs are generally structured in one of two ways. Some agencies develop a separate psychiatric home care team staffed by specially trained psychiatric nurses, advanced practice psychiatric nurses, psychiatric social workers, rehabilitation staff, and home health aides. They do not interact with the general home care staff or clients, unless they are asked to conduct evaluations with and consult on medical-surgical clients who exhibit behavioral or psychosocial problems along with their primary medical problems. An advantage of this organizational approach is the development of a cohesive and effective psychiatric home care team. However, a disadvantage of the separate-team approach is that services may be underused as a result of built-in barriers (Miller and Duffey, 1993). For example, a separate psychiatric team may add to the perceived stigmatization of mental illness, and mental health issues may not be integrated into the care of clients with general medical diagnoses. Likewise, input from team members specializing in physical health problems would not be as readily available to the psychiatric home care team whose clients have numerous concurrent physical health problems.

Other agencies prefer a matrix system in which each home care office is staffed with psychiatric nurses who are members of the interdisciplinary home care team. The general home care multidisciplinary staff is used to provide physical therapy, occupational therapy, social services, and other supportive home care services, such as a home health aide or homemaker services, to clients with mental disorders. As members of the interdisciplinary team, psychiatric home care nurses are highly visible and participate in early case finding. Miller and Duffey (1993) propose that this approach increases the skill of all team members in delivering home care services to this complex and challenging population. It also increases the integration of mental health services for all home care clients. Consequently, there may be less room for client manipulation because of a more consistent and well-informed approach. Moreover, specially trained individuals working as a team can produce a comprehensive biopsychosocial interdisciplinary treatment plan with clear goals and expectations for psychiatric and other

home care clients. For example, the AIDS Mental Health Program, sponsored by the Visiting Nurse Service of New York (VSNY), integrates mental health and physical home care services for homebound clients with AIDS, resulting in a more comprehensive treatment regimen (Pessin et al., 1993). Through home-based psychiatric intervention and support that maximizes psychiatric functioning, this program improves the quality of life of clients with AIDS and their caregivers (see Chapter 32).

THE ROLE OF THE NURSE IN PSYCHIATRIC HOME CARE

Psychiatric-mental health nursing's *Standards, Standards of Community Health Nursing Practice,* and *Standards of Home Health Nursing Practice* (ANA 1986a; 1994) define the role of the psychiatric nurse in the delivery of home care services to clients with mental disorders and their families in community settings.

Psychiatric nurses are important members of the home care team. Psychiatric home care nurses play a pivotal role in assisting clients to more effectively adapt to the community setting (Hellwig, 1993). Unlike other nurses whose clients receive care in an "institutional" setting, the psychiatric home care nurse has the unique opportunity of working with clients and their families on their "own turf," that is, in the home setting. The home setting is part of a larger community and social system in which other health care professionals and multiple services required by home care clients are located.

The nurse is essentially a "guest" in the client's home, which is an empowering position for the client and family. In fact, the client has the right to refuse the nurse's admittance to the home. For example, persuading clients with paranoia to allow the nurse into the home requires patience, tact, and a gentle expression of concern for the client. Another difference between the role of the psychiatric nurse in a hospital-based versus a home care setting is the increased need to structure the home care environment and greater autonomy in doing so. For example, assessing clients with mental disorders and intervening in their problems require psychiatric home care nurses to demonstrate sensitivity and versatility. The nurse must be alert to the nuances of behavior and adapt the treatment plan to meet the client's multiple and often rapidly changing needs. Consider a situation in which a psychiatric home care nurse had to work by phone with the client's landlord to lock up the insulin that the client was threatening to use to commit suicide, until the nurse could drive to the client's apartment to assess the situation and take appropriate action.

The ability to collaborate is another hallmark of psychiatric home care nursing. The psychiatrist relies on the nurse's expertise in assessing and intervening with clients with mental disorders. Thus nurses must be confident about their skills and abilities to intervene. For example, Rhonda, a client diagnosed with major depression, expressed feelings of increasing hopelessness about her future to her psychiatric home care nurse. Further assessment indicated that Rhonda did have suicidal feelings that had become increasingly stronger, but which she had not revealed to her psychiatrist. After assessing her lethality, the nurse developed and coordinated a treatment plan with the psychiatrist and Rhonda that included (1) an adjustment in the dosage of her anti-depressant, (2) increased skilled nursing visits and home health aide services, (3) a no-suicide contract with Rhonda, and (4) a plan to work on structuring her future. The nurse succeeded in reducing Rhonda's depressive and suicidal symptoms by working closely with the psychiatrist to develop and implement an effective treatment plan.

Psychiatric nurses who work in home care programs operationalize a variety of roles depending on their qualifications, agency organizational structure and policies, and client needs. These roles include direct caregiving activities such as counseling (see Chapter 9), crisis intervention (see Chapter 10), psychotherapy (see Chapter 9), and health teaching including psychoeducation (see Chapter 16). It also includes referral, health promotion and preventive intervention (see Chapter 18), case management (see Chapter 17), and consultation with family members and other direct care providers who need to expand their knowledge base about the principles of psychiatric care (see Chapter 32).

Nurses who provide psychiatric home care are expected to have an in-depth knowledge base (Hellwig, 1993). Psychiatric nurses function as both generalists and specialists on multidisciplinary home care teams, depending on the complexity of clients' problems. They must have training and/or experience beyond the standard education required for initial licensure. Masters level preparation in psychiatric mental health nursing and/or experience in the specialty generally meet the minimum qualifications necessary for approval to practice in a home setting (Kozlak and Thobaben, 1992).

The Psychiatric Home Care Nurse: Basic Level of Practice

As indicated in Standards III through VII of the psychiatric-mental health nursing's *Standards* and *Standards of Home Health Nursing Practice* (ANA, 1986a; 1994), psychiatric home care nurses at the basic level of practice are qualified to provide direct clinical services to clients and their families. In this capacity, they function as case managers who conduct comprehensive assessments (Standard III), formulate nursing diagnoses (Standard IV), develop and implement plans of care (Standards V and VI), and evaluate client outcomes (Standard VIII). Essential to their role is the provision of psychoeducational services and coordination of multiple services

required by psychiatric home care clients to achieve continuity of care (see the Case Study box at right).

The psychiatric home care nurse is in an ideal position to provide the interface between clients and the many providers who manage various aspects of their care. The psychiatric home care nurse is in an ideal position to discuss overt or covert changes in behavior that signal that the client is decompensating psychiatrically and/or medically and arrange for intensification of outpatient services or earlier rehospitalization. Such foresight can help to avoid rehospitalization or result in a shorter length of stay. If rehospitalization is necessary, the home care nurse, following discharge, can then continue helping clients to readjust to community living. Psychiatric home nurses also discuss client medications, treatments, and psychiatric interventions with family members as well as other members of the interdisciplinary team. This keeps them apprised of the "big picture" as it relates to particular clients (Duffey, Miller, and Parlocha, 1993; Hellwig, 1993).

The Psychiatric Home Care Nurse: Advanced Practice Level

At the advanced practice level, clinical nurse specialists in psychiatric-mental health nursing function as expert clinicians in the provision of direct care to clients and their families in home settings. They also operationalize other important role components as teachers, consultants, and researchers.

As expert clinicians, advanced practice psychiatric home care nurses conduct comprehensive psychosocial assessments; evaluate mental status; conduct individual, group, and family psychotherapy; perform medication management and psychoeducation; and function as case managers who can access and coordinate client services and providers for vulnerable populations who are often isolated and unable to access the intervention they need (Klebanoff and Casler, 1986). The following case study illustrates how an advanced practice psychiatric home care nurse works with other mental health care professionals to provide psychiatric and physical care in the home setting (see the Case Study box on p. 374).

Advanced practice psychiatric home care nurses also function in a consultative role (Klebanoff and Casler, 1986). In that capacity, they may supervise the delivery of psychiatric home care by other nurses, and, they may consult with staff about medical-surgical or psychiatric cases in which there is a psychosocial problem that needs to be handled more effectively. These nurses engage in a variety of other consultative activities including quality improvement, research, and performance appraisals. As change agents, advanced practice psychiatric home care nurses develop and implement new home care programs. For example, outreach mental health services for targeted populations with mental health needs are a fertile area for

Case Study

Edith W., age 65, is a client with a 30-year history of bipolar disorder and rheumatoid arthritis. Psychiatric home care services were initiated after discharge for hospitalization related to a manic episode. Edith lived in a senior citizen residence where she had a reputation of being "very difficult to get along with." She often berated the nurses who administered her multiple medications, placed numerous calls to the psychiatrist about being given incorrect medications, lashed out at other residents and her daughter, and refused treatment for a chronic leg ulcer. The psychiatric home care nurse, in her role as case manager, was responsible for conducting a comprehensive assessment, formulating nursing diagnoses, determining needed services, developing a treatment plan, and implementing specific nursing interventions. The only problem was that Edith would not let the nurse into her apartment, despite repeated phone calls, planned appointments, and actual visits. Finally, Edith agreed to speak to the nurse from the doorway of her apartment; the initial assessment was conducted with Edith sitting in her doorway and the nurse sitting in the hall.

Apparently, the nurse's persistence paid off, she passed the test and was, thereafter, permitted to make home care visits to Edith. The nurse obtained Edith's consent to have home health aide services, paid for by Medicare, to assist her with meeting hygiene, exercise, and ambulation needs, as well as providing cognitive stimulation. She worked with a new psychiatrist (Edith had "fired" the previous one) to initiate an effective medication regimen that eliminated numerous medications and sought to stabilize her on lithium and carbamazepine (Tegretol). The nurse coordinated laboratory follow-up of CBC with differential for agranulocytosis and drew blood for required lithium levels. She acted as a liason with the residence nurses who administered Edith's medications, suggesting approaches to increase her cooperation in taking her medications. The nurse also educated and assessed Edith regarding her response to and side effects of lithium and Tegretol and assessed Edith as she was weaned off her previous psychotropic medications.

Once a trusting relationship was established, the psychiatric home care nurse was also able to convince Edith to allow her to examine her leg ulcer and initiate a referral to a vascular specialist. In collaboration with the physician, the nurse provided follow-up dressing changes and kept him apprised of Edith's progress between visits. Finally, the long-term goal of decreasing social isolation was met when Edith agreed to and the nurse arranged for her to access a community resource by attending a senior citizen day program three times per week. Edith's daughter, the only relative still talking to her, was given telephone counseling by the nurse to help her deal with her mother more effectively through constructive confrontation, limit setting, and brief visits. At the end of 6 months, psychiatric home care services were terminated.

---

home care program development. In urban areas where the incidence of AIDS is high, an AIDS mental health program that provides home-based mental health services for homebound clients with AIDS and their formal and informal caregivers (including nurses, home health aides, family members, and significant others) meets an important community health need. By helping clients remain at home whenever possible and maximizing their psychiatric functioning, this program improves the quality of life for clients with AIDS and their caregivers (Pessin, et al., 1993). The advanced practice psychiatric home care nurse could be the change agent who conceptualizes, designs, markets, and coordinates implementation of the program.

Advanced practice psychiatric home care nurses also enact a teaching component. Typically, they develop and teach in-service classes to the professional psychiatric home care nursing staff as well as to assistive personnel. For example, one nurse developed and taught a mini-course on the psychoeducational needs of clients and families with severe and persistent neurobiological disorders and related psychoeducational strategies for meeting these needs, including providing relevant health information, skills training, and psychosocial support (Holmes et al., 1994; Keefler and Koritar, 1994).

APPLICATION OF THE NURSING PROCESS TO PSYCHIATRIC HOME CARE

In home care, documentation is a legal necessity, as it is in all other practice settings. This supports the use of the nursing process, as guided by the ANA (1986) *Standards of Home Health Nursing Practice* listed in Box 21-3, to develop treatment plans for psychiatric home care clients.

Assessment

Psychiatric home care nurses conduct comprehensive assessments that include collection of biopsychosocial data, as outlined in Box 21-4, including cultural data as presented in the Cultural Highlights on p. 374. The psy-

Case Study

Ralph is a 68-year-old divorced man who was referred to the psychiatric home care program before discharge from an acute inpatient psychiatric unit for management of his schizophrenia, an acute depressive episode, diabetes, and hypertension. He was returning to his apartment to live alone, with his daughter checking in periodically. Ralph had been hospitalized at the state psychiatric hospital 20 times over the last 40 years. The psychiatrist was concerned about Ralph's ability to function independently at home and about his compliance with psychotropic medications in addition to his other medical problems, including self-administration of insulin. Ralph had had intermittent contact with the community mental health center after previous hospitalizations, but refused to go to day-treatment programs or senior citizen programs. He preferred to stay at home with intermittent visits to the psychiatrist and internist.

The advanced practice psychiatric home care nurse became the case manager. Direct services included close monitoring of Ralph's psychotropic medications, which included intramuscular fluphenazine decanoate (Prolixin), as well as benztropine mesylate (Cogentin) and paroxetine (Paxil). Adjustment of dosages to deal with his auditory hallucinations and education about the purposes and side effects of the medications were essential interventions. Helping Ralph to understand the disease process of schizophrenia was a major focus of intervention for both Ralph and his family, who had a poor knowledge base about his illness. Moreover, determining Ralph's competence to self-administer insulin, test his blood sugar, and plan meals within his diabetic meal plan was another major treatment focus. Increasing his functional level and developing social networks for his recovery were other components of intervention.

Collaboration with Ralph's psychiatrist and internist and other agencies for meeting his complex needs involved referrals to the regional Council on Aging and senior centers, which could accomodate clients with severe and persistent mental disorders and provide the essential social networks, day activities, and health supervision Ralph needed to prevent relapse and rehospitalization. Ralph was also referred to a diabetic self-care group that met weekly at the local hospital diabetic clinic, which provided nutritional counseling and insulin administration and skin- and foot-care classes. Before termination, linkages were established with the necessary community agencies and community mental health center to ensure that Ralph had the support he would need to maintain himself in the community. Without the establishment of such linkages, clients such as Ralph are intimidated by and have trouble navigating a complex health care system and, as a result, often do not seek appropriate health care. Home visits by the advanced practice psychiatric nurse were an essential part of the delivery of mental health services to Ralph, who might otherwise have "fallen through the cracks."

 CULTURAL HIGHLIGHTS

Essential Cultural Factors to Assess When Initiating Psychiatric Home Care Services

- Race and ethnic origin
- Country of origin and countries resided in
- Length of time residing in the United States
- Family structure
- Dietary patterns
- Religious and spiritual practices
- Communication patterns, primary language, and secondary language
- Integration of art, music, drama, and literature in the home
- Dress and clothing practices
- Health and illness beliefs and practices

- Mental health and mental illness beliefs and practices
- Native health and mental illness beliefs and practices
- Perceptions of health care providers
- Family beliefs, values, customs, and rituals about health, mental health, illness, and mental illness as well as the health care delivery system
- Use of ethnic or cultural healers
- Availability of cultural and ethnic health resources
- Risk factors, vulnerabilities, or resistances

Box 21-3

ANA Standards of Home Health Nursing Practice

STANDARD I: ORGANIZATION OF HOME HEALTH SERVICES

All home care services are planned, organized, and directed by a master's-prepared professional nurse with experience in community health and administration.

STANDARD II: THEORY

The nurse applies theoretical concepts as a basis for decisions in practice.

STANDARD III: DATA COLLECTION

The nurse continuously collects and records data that are comprehensive, accurate, and systematic.

STANDARD IV: DIAGNOSIS

The nurse uses health assessment data to determine nursing diagnoses.

STANDARD V: INTERVENTION

The nurse develops care plans that establish goals. The care plan is based on nursing diagnoses and incorporates therapeutic, preventive, and rehabiliatative nursing actions.

STANDARD VI: INTERVENTION

The nurse, guided by the care plan, intervenes to provide comfort; to restore, improve, and promote health; to prevent complications and sequelae of illness; and to effect rehabilitation.

STANDARD VII: EVALUATION

The nurse continually evaluates the client and family's responses to interventions to determine progress toward goal attainment and to revise the data base, nursing diagnoses, and plan of care.

STANDARD VIII: CONTINUITY OF CARE

The nurse is responsible for the client's appropriate and uninterrupted care along the health care continuum and therefore uses discharge planning, case management, and coordination of community resources.

STANDARD IX: INTERDISCIPLINARY COLLABORATION

The nurse initiates and maintains a liaison relationship with all appropriate health care providers to ensure that all efforts effectively complement one another.

STANDARD X: PROFESSIONAL DEVELOPMENT

The nurse assumes responsibility for professional development and contributes to the professional growth of others.

STANDARD XI: RESEARCH

The nurse participates in research activities that contribute to the profession's continuing development of knowledge of home care.

STANDARD XII: ETHICS

The nurse uses the code for nurses established by the American Nurses Association as a guide for ethical decision making in practice.

From American Nurses Association. (1986). Standard of home health nursing practice. *Kansas City, MO: Author.*

chiatric home care nurse collects data in a standardized, succinct, and systematic manner, regarding the biopsychosocial indicators for home care services and related resources needed by the client and/or family. Data are collected through history taking, interviewing, physical assessment, mental status examination, and documentation of diagnostic tests that have been performed and show relevant findings (see Chapter 5). The termination of suicidal risk is also an essential component of the psychiatric home care assessment. Home care agencies usu-

ally provide standardized assessment forms, flow sheets, checklists, progress notes, and other documentation forms for the psychiatric home care nurse's use.

Data sources for conducting the asessment include the client and family members or other significant persons (e.g., neighbors, clergy, friends, health care providers) who become the primary sources for the collection of subjective and objective data. The home environment also provides essential assessment data as presented in the checklist in Box 21-5.

Box 21-4

Psychiatric Home Care Assessment Categories

- Physical, emotional, cognitive, psychological, social, cultural, religious, spiritual, community, and environmental history
- Support systems, lifestyle factors, and stressors
- Developmental patterns of the client and family, family risk factors, dynamics, and current and past coping strategies
- Sleep, rest, and activity patterns; appetite and nutritional patterns; elimination patterns; sexuality and reproductive patterns; and other habits affecting health, knowledge, and motivation
- Self- and role-relationship patterns, socialization patterns
- Mental and emotional status including thought processes, cognitive functioning, and perceptual patterns
- Understanding and receptivity to psychiatric home care and expectations of the psychiatric home care program

Nursing Diagnosis

A nursing diagnosis identifies actual or potential health problems. With the previous example, nursing diagnoses should reflect the broad array of actual or potential psychosocial as well as physical health problems. Box 21-6 highlights common psychosocial nursing diagnoses for psychiatric home care clients.

Outcome Identification

Expected outcomes for clients receiving psychiatric home care services must consider the needs of the individual client in the context of the family and resources, as well as the community in which the person lives. Because the majority of clients eligible for psychiatric home care services have mental health and physical problems of a severe and persistent nature, goals must be realistic if clients and care providers are to achieve effective outcomes.

For example, Harvey G., who is described in Table 21-1, Example 4, is markedly incapacitated by degenerative disc disease of the spine and Parkinson's Disease. Depressed by his incapacitation, he spends most of his days lying in bed staring at the ceiling, demanding that his wife assist him in all his ADLs. Although Harvey will never run a 4-minute mile, it is realisitic to develop short- and long-term goals that would increase his activity level, exercise capacity, ADL independence, cognitive function-

Box 21-5

Home Environment Checklist

- Type of housing
- Number of rooms
- Condition of residence
  Furnishings
  Privacy
  Sleeping arrangements
  Adequacy of bathroom facilities
  Adequacy of kitchen facilities (e.g. refrigeration, cooking, cleanliness, table and chairs for eating)
  Adequacy of water supply or source
  Waste or garbage disposal
  Lighting
  Heating, cooling, ventilation
  Laundry facilities
  Telephone
- Safety features
  Smoke alarms
  Emergency telephone numbers
  Crime prevention
  Ramps and other safety devices (e.g., grab bars)
- Safety hazards
  Noise level
  Crowding
  Storage of medicines, cleaners, and poisons
  Unsafe toys
  Loose rugs
  Clutter
  Tools
  Swimming pool
  Traffic
  Air pollution
  Fire hazards
  Plants, shrubs, and flowers
  Cars
  Stairways
- Accessibility of resources (e.g. transportation, grocery, stores, pharmacy, physicians, hospital)

ing, and overall level of functioning; decrease his depression; and provide respite for his wife. The psychiatric home care nurse and Harvey, in collaboration with his home health aide and physical and occupational therapists to whom he was referred, developed weekly goals for him to achieve. At the end of 2 months the outcomes attained included the following: Harvey was able to walk 1 mile twice a day while accompanied by the home health aide, accompany his wife to the supermarket and pharmacy, spend 14 hours per day out of bed, sit at his desk doing paperwork for 2 hours a day, and be 90% self-sufficient in his ADLs. Harvey's depression improved significantly.

Box 21-6

Nursing Diagnoses: Actual and Potential Health Problems for Psychiatric Home Care Clients and Their Families

- Altered comfort/pain
- Altered elimination
- Altered environmental conditions
- Altered health maintenance
- Altered perception
- Altered sleep, rest, or activity pattern
- Anger
- Anxiety: mild, moderate, severe, panic
- Caregiver role strain
- Chemical dependency: alcohol, drugs, prescription medications
- Communication, impaired verbal
- Coping, ineffective family: compromised
- Coping, ineffective individual
- Delayed developmental level
- Denial, ineffective
- Family dysfunction; impaired dynamics, structure, or support systems
- Grieving, anticipatory, normal bereavement, dysfunctional
- Home maintenance management, impaired
- Impaired cognition
- Impaired nutrition
- Impairment in socialization
- Knowledge deficit
- Mobility, impaired physical
- Parental role conflict
- Role performance, altered
- Self-care deficit
- Self-esteem, chronic low
- Self-mutilation, high-risk for
- Sensory/perceptual alternations (visual, auditory, kinesthetic, gustatory, tactile, olfactory)
- Spiritual distress
- Values/belief conflict

- Mental health status changes
- Health status changes
- Need for ongoing health care services after discharge from an inpatient treatment program
- Changes in the home environment
- Family changes
- Changes in support systems
- Need for health or medication teaching
- Need for anticipatory guidance
- Changes in leisure or diversionary activities
- Need to access community services that provide an alternative to hospitalization
- Psychiatric crisis or emergency

Planning and developing a nursing care plan for psychiatric home care clients should encompass identification of all applicable nursing diagnoses, outcomes, and interventions. An example of a nursing care plan for a psychiatric home care client is presented on pp. 378-379).

Implementation

The goals of intervention in a psychiatric home care context are improvement, stabilization, and restoration of physical and mental health and social functioning, as well as improvement of the physical environment of the client and family. Psychiatric home care nurses strive to promote health and prevent complications and long-term illness sequelae (Harvey and Seelman, 1991; Morris, 1996). See Box 21-7 for direct interventions used in the home by psychiatric home care nurses.

Evaluation

Psychiatric home care nurses continually evaluate the client's and family members' responses to interventions by determining outcome attainment and needed revisions to the assessment data base, nursing diagnoses, and plan of care. Discharge from psychiatric home care programs occur when the nurse and the client and family determine whether the identified outcomes have been achieved. As the client is increasingly able to engage in self-care and/or the family is able to assume increased responsibility for the client's care, the psychiatric home care nurse and other home care team members decrease the intensity and frequency of their visits. Discharge from psychiatric home care includes plans for aftercare, if needed, as well as continuation of participation in community programs and use of community resources that were initiated as part of the treatment plan. Sometimes clients require other types of case management programs such as those located in social welfare agencies or community mental health centers.

Because home care services and their reimbursement are regulated by federal and state agencies, as well as cer-

Planning

The most common population groups requiring psychiatric home care services are the elderly, persons with severe and persistent mental disorders, and persons with psychosocial responses to their health conditions, particularly those with chronic health problems such as multiple sclerosis, chronic obstructive pulmonary disease (COPD), cancer, or AIDS.

Indicators of the need for psychiatric home care services include the following:

NURSING CARE PLAN

Psychiatric Home Care

NURSING ASSESSMENT DATA

Subjective: Her son states: "For the past 3 months my mother has been increasingly demanding. She has been calling us as many as 20 times a day with physical complaints. She says she feels a knot in her stomach and cannot eat and, as a result, she has lost 20 lbs." Her daughter-in-law says, "She doesn't want to leave her home and refuses to go to the senior citizen program at her church. She and her sister used to attend this program every day until her sister started to have hearing problems and memory loss severe enough to make her feel embarrassed to participate in social activities." Yolanda is worried that her sister will have to go to a nursing home because of her increasing cognitive impairment and that she, Yolanda, will be "left alone to die." She describes her chest as "feeling heavy" and her heart as "racing," and she feels so "weak" she can hardly get out of bed and has no energy to do her cooking or housecleaning. *Objective*: Yolanda F. is an 87-year-old caucasian woman who was born in Italy but was living in the United States for 60 years. She lives in and maintains her own home; her 94-year-old sister lives across the street. Widowed for the past 20 years, Yolanda has no previous psychiatric history, but was just discharged from the psychiatric unit at the local hospital for treatment of depression. She is taking fluoxetine (Prozac) 20 mg every day in the morning. Her family has "had it with her demandingness." The social worker contacted a local home care agency to initiate psychiatric home care services.

NANDA Diagnosis: Grieving, dysfunctional related to perceived loss of sister as a lifelong significant other as evidenced by depressed feelings, social withdrawal, weight loss, and other somatic symptoms.

Outcomes	Interventions	Rationale	Evaluation
Short term ***Within 1 week*** 1. Will consume 1,800 calories of food per day 2. Will discuss feelings of loss and worry about sister and self 3. Will take antidepressant daily 4. Will decrease telephone calls to son and daughter-in-law to four per day	• Develop nurse-client relationship. • Use therapeutic communication techniques to elicit grief-related thoughts and feelings. • Explore client's knowledge base about and adherence to medication regimen.	• Presence of the nurse has been shown to elevate mood, promote optimism, and develop trust. • Therapeutic communication strategies will facilitate the client's expression of grief. • A major reason for nonadherence to medication regimen is lack of adequate knowledge about the medication, its therapeutic value, its side effects, and related management strategies.	**Short term** 2, 3. Met in 1 week 1, 4. Met in 2 weeks **Long term** 1, 2, 3. Partially met. Reports less constant sadness and worry, gained 4 lbs. in 1 month, fewer somatic symptoms. 4. Not met: Has not returned to senior citizen program despite four phone calls to make pick-up appointments that were then broken before pick-up time. 5. Met. Phone calls to son have decreased to two per day.
Long term ***Within 1 month*** 1. Will report feeling less sadness and worry 2. Will gain 5 lbs 3. Will report less "heaviness in chest," "heart racing," and fatigue, and more energy 4. Will return to the senior citizen program one time per week without her sister	• Explore relationship between client's somatic symptoms and potential side effects of fluoxetine. • Teach deep breathing and muscle relaxation and encourage use at first signs of somatic symptoms. • Encourage discussion of preferred foods and accept offer of tea and homemade pastry.	• Major roles of the nurse in relation to medications are teaching medication management strategies and monitoring side effects. • Encourage use of competing stimuli as a functional coping strategy. • Consider age and culturally appropriate foods and hospitality norms.	

NURSING CARE PLAN

Psychiatric Home Care—cont'd

Outcomes	Interventions	Rationale	Evaluation
5. Will decrease telephone calls to son and daughter-in-law to two per day	• Plan weekly menus—1,800 calories per day—six small meals per day.	• Sufficient calories to initiate weight gain; small frequent meals minimize likelihood of gastric distress	
	• Initiate home health aide services—2 hrs. at lunch and at dinner—to assist with food preparation, meal intake monitoring, and meal companionship.	• ADL supervision increases likelihood of goal attainment.	
	• Confer with staff at senior citizen program about withdrawal from program and strategies for reentry.	• Collaborate with interdisciplinary team to develop and assess effectiveness of socialization strategies.	
	• Discuss client's preferred time for calling son and daughter-in-law and expanding telephone network.	• Encourage assumption of control (choice) about calling relatives within defined limits and expanding relationship options.	

Box 21-7

Psychiatric Home Care Interventions

- Comprehensive in-home assessment
- Crisis intervention
- Individual/family/group therapy
- Counseling
- Verbal and/or written contracts with clients
- Medication administration, monitoring, teaching
- Health guidance/teaching/referral
  - Diet/special diet/nutrition
  - Rest/sleep/wake activities
  - Management of illness symptoms
  - Stress management
  - Risk factor reduction
  - Safety measures
  - ADL management
  - Social skills training
  - Emergency measures
  - Functional coping strategies
  - Obtaining entitlements
- Client advocacy
- Mental, spiritual, emotional, physical observation, interpretation, and evaluation

- Correction of actual and/or potential environmental safety hazards
  - Heating, cooling, ventilation
  - Stairways, ramps, safety bars, and bannisters
  - Sanitation
  - Storage of medications
  - Mats and throw rugs
  - Gas and electrical hazards
  - Cooking and bathing facilities
  - Sleeping facilities and arrangements
  - Neighborhood
- Case management
  - Communicating with physician about client status, progress, and treatment plan
  - Accessing and coordinating team and community resources
  - Communicating with and supporting members of the interdisciplinary team
  - Supervision of professional and nonprofessional nursing personnel
- Role modeling

COMMUNITY RESOURCES

American Hospital Association
Division of Ambulatory and Home Care Services
840 North Lake Shore Drive
Chicago, IL 60611
(312)280-6000

American Association for Continuing Care
1101 Connecticut Avenue NW
Washington, DC 20036
(202)857-1194

American Federation of Home Health Agencies
1320 Fenwick Lane, Suite 500
Silver Spring, MD 20910
(301)588-1454

American Nurses Association
600 Maryland Avenue SW, Suite 100 West
Washington, DC 20024
(202)554-4444

Council of Community Health Services
National League for Nursing
350 Hudson Street
New York, NY 10014
(212)989-9393

Home Health Services and Staffing Association
2101 L Street NW
Washington, DC 20037
(202)547-7424

National Association of Home Care
205 C Street NE
Washington, DC 20002
(202)547-7424

National Homecaring Council
67 Irving Place
New York, NY 10003
(212)674-4990

Box 21-8

Examples of Home Care Agencies Providing Psychiatric Home Care Services

American Home Care, Inc.
Homestaff Health Care Services, Inc.
Interim Health Care
Olsten Kimberly Quality Care
Priority Care, Inc.
Staffbuilders Health Care Services
US Homecare
Visiting Nurse Service of America

---

tifying organizations, psychiatric home care records are evaluated regularly by external reviewers such as those listed in the Community Resources box above. Chart audits, reviews by regulatory agencies, peer reviews, and home care agency accrediting and certification organizations such as HCFA also evaluate the quality and effectiveness of psychiatric home care services. Examples of some home care agencies providing psychiatric home care services are presented in Box 21-8.

KEY POINTS

• Psychiatric home care is the delivery of mental health and related physical health care in the home setting.
• Agencies providing psychiatric home care services include public or official agencies, private and voluntary agencies, a combination of public and private nonprofit agencies operated by both sources or a board of directors, hospital-based agencies, proprietary agencies, and individual or group partnerships.
• Reimbursement sources for psychiatric home care services are Medicare, Medicaid, private insurance plans, and self-pay monies.
• Psychiatric home care populations consist of the elderly, clients with severe and persistent mental disorders living at home, and persons with catastrophic and chronic medical illnesses.
• Forces driving the expansion of psychiatric home care are changes in the structure of health care delivery including a shift to community-based care, shortened lengths of hospital stays, cost-containment, and changes in family structure and function.
• Psychiatric home care nurses provide direct care to clients and their families in a community context. They function as case managers who coordinate

CRITICAL THINKING QUESTIONS

Alexa Z., age 34, has a history of bipolar disorder, which has been treated in the past with lithium carbonate, periodic hospitalizations, and attendance at a day-treatment program. Hospitalizations have occurred approximately every 2 years since Alexa was first diagnosed as having bipolar disorder in her early twenties. Recently her husband filed for divorce, and Alexa became suicidal. They have no children and have been married for 9 years.

Alexa was hospitalized after a car accident in which she sustained a ruptured spleen and a broken shoulder. She had stopped taking lithium before the accident, because she "missed the highs and was bored with the evenness of her current mood." During the hospitalization, she was given phenothiazines. Shortly before discharge, she was again started on lithium carbonate. Her spouse moved out of their condominium while she was in the hospital, but he agreed to help with her care at home until she was more independent.

The hospital-based discharge planner made the referral to a home care agency that had a psychiatric home care program.

1. What would be priority assessment factors to consider in Alexa's case?
2. Given Alexa's physical and mental status, what kinds of home care services would the psychiatric home care nurse access and coordinate?
3. What kinds of referrals would be appropriate for Alexa's husband, given Alexa's psychiatric disorder and their recent separation?
4. What would be appropriate interventions for Alexa?

services, make referrals, advocate on their clients' behalf, and function as consultants.

- Psychiatric home care nurses conduct comprehensive assessments; formulate nursing diagnoses; develop realistic goals, outcomes, and treatment plans; and implement interventions that improve and/or restore physical and mental health and social functioning and ameliorate the physical environment of the client and family. Psychiatric home care nurses promote physical and mental health, and prevent complications and long-term illness sequelae.

- Psychiatric home care nurses continually evaluate the client and family members' responses to interventions by determining outcome attainment and needed revisions to the assessment data base, nursing diagnoses, and plan of care.

REFERENCES

American Nurses Association. (1986a). *Standards of community health nursing practice.* Kansas City, MO: Author.

American Nurses Association. (1986b). *Standards of home health nursing practice.* Kansas City, MO: Author.

American Nurses Association. (1994). *A statement on psychiatric-mental health nursing practice and standards of psychiatric-mental health nursing practice.* Washington, DC: Author.

Buckwalter, K.C., & Stolley, J. (1991). Managing mentally ill elders at home. *Geriatric Nursing,* 136-139.

Duffey, J., Miller, M.P., & Parlocha, P. (1993). Psychiatric home care. *Home Health Care Nurse, II, 2,* 22-28.

Harper, M.S. (1989). Providing mental health services in the homes of the elderly. *Caring Magazine, 8*(6), 4-53.

Harvey, S., & Seelman, M. (1991). Development of a mental health home care program. *Caring Magazine, 10*(3), 20-22.

Health Care Financing Administration (1989). *Medicare home health agency manual.* (Publication No. 11, Revision 222, Retrieval Title P11R222). Washington, DC: Author.

Hellwig, K. (1993). Managing patients in the community setting. *Journal of Psychosocial Nursing, 31*(12), 21-24.

Holmes, H., Ziemba, J., Evans, T., & Williams, C.A. (1994). Nursing model of psychoeducation for the seriously mentally ill. *Issues in Mental Health Nursing, 15*(1), 85-104.

Keefler, J., & Koritar, E. (1994). Essential elements of a family psychoeducation program in the aftercare of schizophrenia. *Journal of Marriage and Family Therapy, 20*(4), 369-380.

Klebanoff, N. & Casler, C. (1986). The psychosocial clinical nurse specialist: An untapped resource for home care. *Home Health Care Nursing, 4*(6), 36-40.

Kozlak, J., & Thobaben, M. (1992). Treating the elderly mentally ill at home. *Perspectives in Psychiatric Care, 28*(2), 31-35.

Krauss, J. B. (1993). *Health care reform: Essential mental health services.* Washington, DC: American Nurses Publishing.

Mellon, S.K. (1994). Mental health clinical nurse specialist in home care for the 90s. *Issues in Mental Health Nursing, 15*(3), 229-237.

Miller, M.P., & Duffey, J. (1993). Planning and program development for psychiatric home care. *Journal of Nursing Administration, 23*(11), 35-41.

Morris, M. (1996). Patients' perceptions of psychiatric home care. *Archives of Psychiatric Nursing, 10*:3, 176-183.

Pessin, N., et al. (1993). Integrating mental health and home care services for AIDS patients. *Caring Magazine, 12*(5), 30-34.

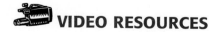

VIDEO RESOURCES

Mosby's Community Health Nuring Series:
The Home Visit

Part Five

Nursing Management of Mental Health Disorders

Chapter 22

Anxiety Disorders

Barbara Krainovich-Miller

LEARNING OUTCOMES

After studying and applying the concepts of this chapter, the learner will be able to:
- Discuss levels of anxiety and its affect on learning behavior.
- Discuss the epidemiological risk factors related to anxiety disorders.
- Discuss the biological and psychosocial relevant theories related to anxiety disorders: biological and psychosocial.
- Describe the usual signs and symptoms of anxiety for the following domains: affective, cognitive, physiological, and psychomotor.
- Describe the use of focused assessment questions in relation to a comprehensive nursing assessment for a client admitted for an anxiety disorder.
- Describe the common nursing diagnoses used for clients with anxiety disorders.
- Identify the most frequently used nursing diagnoses related to clients with anxiety disorders who are admitted to the inpatient setting.
- Discuss interventions of the implementation standard in relation to the hospitalized and nonhospitalized client with an anxiety disorder.
- Evaluate the outcomes of an established nursing care plan for the nursing diagnosis of altered role performance.

KEY TERMS

Agoraphobia	Normal anxiety	Social phobia
In vivo desensitization	Pathological anxiety	Specific phobia

Anxiety is a phenomenon that humankind has always recognized. Anxiety can be defined as a feeling, a mood, an emotional response, a syndrome, a symptom, or an illness (Krainovich-Miller, 1988). Anxiety is generally an unpleasant experience that is similar to fear. However, in this chapter it will become clear that the anxiety a student might experience in relation to an upcoming test and the anxiety experienced by a client with an anxiety disorder differs significantly in terms of its duration and intensity of the symptoms, as well as its affect on a person's activities of daily living (ADLs). You will truly understand how it must feel to "wish you could jump out of your body."

Although the last 10 years of the twentieth century have been called the "Decade of the Brain," describing them as the "Age of Anxiety" still fits (Cattell, 1963). Almost every day, at least one television talk show focuses on some aspect of anxiety and how it affects the lives of people, especially those with an anxiety disorder. For example, a popular 2-hour news program has run a week-long special spot on phobias.

Several celebrities have publicly discussed their difficulties with anxiety and anxiety disorders. Actress and comedian Roseanne Barr, diagnosed with obsessive-compulsive disorder (OCD), described standing in her shower for hours unable to break this ritual and resume her life. The popularity of this topic is understandable when anxiety disorders are viewed as a major public health concern and not as a trivial matter. The four most commonly occurring mental health disorders in the United States are (1) phobias, (2) substance-related disorders, (3) major depressive disorder, and (4) OCD (Kaplan and Sadock, 1995). Phobias and OCD are anxiety disorders. These disorders are often misdiagnosed or unrecognized in primary care settings (Liebowitz and Barlow, 1995; National Institutes of Mental Health [NIMH], 1994).

Anxiety is a universal phenomena that is discussed from several different perspectives. One type of anxiety has been labeled ***normal anxiety***. *It is defined as a normal response to an observable threat, which some call fear* (May, 1977). There is also the concept of ***pathological anxiety*** (previously termed *neurotic anxiety*), which is the type of anxiety experienced by those with anxiety disorders and is differentiated from fear. This type of "not normal" anxiety is *defined as an affective/cognitive/behavioral/physiological response to an internal or external threat, real or imagined, during which the person experiences a "felt" unpleasant emotional state* (Freud, 1936).

An in-depth understanding of anxiety is needed by nurses, especially those who work with clients with mental health disorders. First, to handle their own normal anxiety in response to a variety of situations such as a client's acting-out (physical and verbally aggressive behaviors) and second, to intervene in a client's anxiety.

Anxiety is considered one of the most important concepts in psychiatric nursing (Peplau, 1963).

The purpose of this chapter is to clarify the concept of anxiety and present the framework for nurses to implement a plan of care for those diagnosed with anxiety disorders. Box 22-1 lists the DSM-IV anxiety disorders. All of the listed disorders except acute traumatic stress disorder, post-traumatic stress disorder (PTSD), and anxiety disorders related to a medical condition are discussed in this chapter. The other disorders are discussed in Chapters 23 and 24. Table 22-1 presents the definitions of the anxiety disorders to be discussed throughout this chapter. Throughout the remainder of the chapter, except where specified, the term anxiety refers to "not normal" anxiety.

EPIDEMIOLOGY

The high rate of anxiety disorders reflect the epidemiological statistics regarding anxiety disorders found across cultures in Africa, Asia, and Europe. Phobias are considered the most common mental health disorder in the United States. A conservative estimate is from 5% to 10%; others report up to 25%. Specific phobia is more common (5% to 10%) than social phobia (2% to 3%) (Kaplan and Sadock, 1995). It is believed that the incidence of this disorder is greater than reported because many individuals with phobias do not come to the attention of the clinician or are misdiagnosed.

Women are diagnosed more often with anxiety disorders, except with OCD, where men and women are equally affected. Studies reveal that the incidence of OCD is probably much higher than reported (2% to 10%) (Kaplan and Sadock, 1995). Some estimate that about

---

Box 22-1

DSM-IV Anxiety Disorders

Panic disorder without agoraphobia
Panic disorder with agoraphobia
Agoraphobia without history of panic disorder
Specific phobia
Social phobia
Obsessive-compulsive disorder (OCD)
Posttraumatic stress disorder (PTSD)
Acute stress disorder
Generalized anxiety disorder (GAD)
Anxiety disorder due to a medical condition
Anxiety disorders NOS

Reprinted with permission from American Psychiatric Association. (1994.). Diagnostic and statistical manual of mental disorder, *Fourth edition. Washington, DC: Author.*

TABLE 22-1

Anxiety disorders

DEFINITION	CLINICAL EXAMPLE
Panic attack: Intense, discrete episode of anxiety that occurs unexpectedly and on an intermittent basis (Four attacks in 1 month, or one or more attacks followed by 1 month of persistent fear, first attack usually before age 30; lasts 5-30 minutes; demonstrates at least four of the signs and symptoms of anxiety noted for panic attack in Table 22-3; an organic factor is ruled out; person lives in constant fear of another attack; tension becomes a part of the anticipatory pattern, and when coupled with the attacks, sets up a pattern of avoidance of places, people, and situations associated with the attack, which leads to a restricted lifestyle (NIMH, 1994).	Margo I. is 25-year-old mother of four young children. Her husband John is a long-distance truck driver who is away from home for weeks at a time. While shopping with the children she experienced a sudden "dizzy spell" accompanied by shortness of breath and chest pain. The storekeeper called an ambulance and she was taken to a nearby hospital. During the admission interview Margo reported that she had experienced several similar episodes during the past 4 months. She described a sense of dread immediately before, during, and for a short time after each episode. She stated, "I thought I was going crazy, like my body could jump through my skin and out a window." During these episodes she also experienced numbness followed by tingling in her extremities, nausea, and hot and cold flashes that produced profuse sweating followed by chills. She also indicated that these episodes occurred without warning, at various times during the day, and under different circumstances.
Phobias: Irrational fears of some discrete object or situation that presents no real threat, or the magnified and distorted perception that does not fit with the actual degree of danger; exposure evokes anxiety response; person knows fear is unreasonable; avoidance or endurance with intense anxiety; interferes with ADLs (i.e., restricted lifestyle). *Specific phobia: Above characteristics in relation to a fear of something specific (e.g., animals, blood, heights, flying). Social phobia: same characteristics in relation to fear of one or more social or performance situations; fear of acting in an embarrassing way. Agoraphobia: Fear of being incapacitated by, forced into, or trapped in a situation from which there would be no easy escape, and there is a possibility of experiencing a sense of helplessness or embarrassment should a panic attack occur.* Examples of places that escalate such attacks are restaurants, theaters, and malls or crowded social gatherings; and being away from home, in a relatively confined area, or in a crowd.	**Specific phobia:** Randy T. is a 25-year-old male graduate law student who has an irrational fear of needles. He has missed two appointments, and previously fainted twice when he had his blood drawn during a routine physical. He tells his girlfriend that he is afraid of getting acquired immunodeficiency syndrome (AIDS) and is trying to protect himself. He also tells her that he knows his fear is irrational but he is unable to control it. He becomes very anxious at the sight of a needle and worries intensely at the thought of making an appointment with his physician.
Obsessive-compulsive disorder (OCD): *Individual has recurrent, intrusive, and anxiety-producing obsessions (ideas, impulses, or images) or compulsions (repetitive behaviors or mental acts) that a person must perform, are excessive and time-consuming (more than 1 hr/day), and cause distress and impairment of ADLs.*	Laura M.'s 3-year-old daughter died of an inoperable brain tumor. Two years later, Laura gave birth to Erica, a healthy baby girl. Laura sought reassurance from her pediatrician and several neurologists that this child had no increased risk of developing a brain tumor. Despite their reassurances she continued to experience thoughts about being a "bad mother" and that she would once again fail to recognize the symptoms "soon enough" and her baby would die. Shortly after Erica's second birthday, her husband noticed that before she dressed or bathed the child, she conducted the systematic neurological assessment she had observed the doctors perform on their first daughter. The process took

TABLE 22-1—cont'd

Anxiety disorders

DEFINITION	CLINICAL EXAMPLE
	more than 2 hours and she did it several times a day, leaving little time for any other household and social activities. He shared his observation with her, but she did not respond and left the room. Several months later, after waiting impatiently for her to finish dressing Erica so that they could go out, he went to the bedroom and observed Laura ritualistically conducting the neurological examination. When he interrupted her, she became very angry, told him to leave the room, and began the assessment from the beginning.
Generalized anxiety disorder (GAD): Characterized by unrealistic or excessive anxiety about two or more life experiences, lasting over days for at least 6 months; it is accompanied by sustained and pervasive feelings of distress and physiological changes that contribute to the discomfort, and the person has great difficulty controlling the worry and anxiety that are associated with three or more of the symptoms indicated for generalized anxiety disorder in Table 22-3, significant distress and impairment in ADLs.	Jane R. is enrolled in a graduate educational psychology research course designed to help her develop her dissertation proposal. She chooses the sex-education needs of elementary school children as her topic and begins the literature search. She is highly productive in conducting the search and collection of reprints and texts. Several weeks into the course she begins to read these materials and evaluate them for relevancy to her topic. Over the past 6 months she has been feeling keyed up and on edge and has had a great deal of difficulty concentrating. She is irritable and has difficulty staying asleep. She becomes concerned about these symptoms, which leads to further symptoms of palpitations and light-headedness. She perceives that these symptoms contribute to her inability to complete her dissertation work. She seeks medical help from the university health center, where a physical basis for the symptoms is ruled out and GAD is diagnosed. Further assessment interviews revealed that as a child she had been sexually abused by a teacher.

10% of outpatient psychiatric diagnoses are OCD (Fifer et al., 1995). The OCD Foundation reports that over 5 million people have OCD in the United States. It is common for clients with OCD to have another mental health disorder, the common comorbid diagnoses is depression, which is found in about 67% of the cases (Spitzer et al., 1995).

Current studies offer prevalence rates that are higher than those indicated by the reported national statistics (e.g., 3.8% for panic disorder and 5.6% for panic attacks). It is thought that GAD is less common now because the new DSM-IV criteria are more restrictive. Another reason for low frequency rate for GAD is that almost all clients with GAD have another mental health disorder (Kaplan and Sadock, 1995). However, community surveys report a prevalence of 4.1% to 6.6% for the general population; higher rates are reported in women, African Americans, and persons under the age of 30 (Andreasen and Black, 1995).

THEORETICAL FRAMEWORK

Biological and psychosocial correlates of anxiety are discussed. It is an exciting time in psychiatric-mental health nursing because of the challenging implications of the neurobiological theories in terms of psychopharmocolgical treatment. The concept of stress is closely aligned with anxiety. Some theorists see anxiety as a consequence of stress and others see it as a cause, (see Chapter 14).

Biological Correlates

Autonomic nervous system

An early theory stated that peripheral stimulation of the autonomic nervous system, or ANS (e.g., increased heart rate, pulse, respirations, perspiration), was responsible for the subjective experience of anxiety. Currently it is thought that in most cases, the peripheral nervous system manifestations follow central nervous system (CNS) anxiety. For instance, in panic disorder, it is thought that ANS's alarm system (fight-or-flight) responds excessively and unnecessarily when there is no danger (NIMH, 1993) (see Chapters 13 and 14).

Unexpected, traumatic, and intensely stressful catastrophic events may alter physiological functioning. The physiological changes that occur and persist as a result of these situations have not been clearly delineated. They are, however, reflected in the development of an exaggerated startle response, dissociative experiences, and reexperiencing (flashbacks) of the event long after it has occurred (Bremner, et al., 1990). (See Chapters 23 and 24 for more information).

Neurotransmitters

Norepinephrine, serotonin, and the GABA (gamma-aminobutyric acid) system are the major neurotransmitters being studied in relation to anxiety through pharmacological intervention (see Chapter 15). The role of norepinephrine in individuals who have anxiety disorders, specifically panic disorders, suggests that these individuals have a malfunctioning noradrenergic system that has a low threshold for arousal and unpredictable increased activity, and is responsible for the anxiety symptoms. Norepinephrine is released through increased midbrain activity as a result of increased heart rate, blood lactase levels, and oxygen use in an individual; increases in norepinephrine increase anxiety. Researchers and clinicians have found that various drugs can initiate a panic attack and others decrease the anxiety symptoms. The role of serotonin was discovered through observations of individuals with OCD who had a favorable response from selective serotonin reuptake inhibitor (SSRI) antidepressants such as clomipramine (Anafranil) (see Chapter 15). Evidence suggests that a drug that has serotonin and nonserotonin properties combined with a drug that releases serotonin can produce anxiety in those diagnosed with anxiety disorders. Selective reduction of serotonin levels appears to restore normal functioning (Bowery, 1991). The role of the GABA neurotransmitter, through its GABA receptor, is that of a major inhibitory neurotransmitter in the brain. Psychopharmacological intervention and observations support this role, however, the exact pharmacology of GABA receptors is very complex.

There is clear evidence that the benzodiazepines and barbiturates have their activity at the GABA receptors. Their action is to enhance GABA activity, that is, to have a therapeutic effect in some of the anxiety disorders by inhibiting arousal thereby decreasing anxiety. Benzodiazepines block the reuptake of the modulator neurotransmitter GABA and enhances GABA binding at the receptor sites. This drug results in a calming and sedative effect. For instance, high-potency benzodiazepines such as alprazolam (Xanax) have been found to be useful in panic disorders.

Neuroanatomical studies

Studies of neuroanotomical structures of this population have shown an increase in the cerebral ventricles, defects in the right temporal lobe, and asymmetrical right and left hemispheres. Further study is needed to determine if psychopharmacological intervention plays a role in any of these changes, if these changes are the result of the anxiety symptoms, or if the changes are what causes the anxiety syndromes. Functional studies suggest that individuals with anxiety disorders have some abnormalities in the cerebral cortex, which may contribute to the anxiety symptoms (Kaplan and Sadock, 1995). For example, among people with some forms of OCD, positron emission tomography (PET) scans have identified abnormalities in the frontal lobes and basal ganglia (Jenike, 1992). Prefrontal leukotomy and cingulotomy result in a decrease in OCD symptoms. An increase in symptoms occurs after electrical stimulation of the cingulum, head trauma, and Von Economo's encephalitis.

Genetic studies

Marks (1986) proposed the genetic theory of anxiety. This theory, includes all organisms, stating that humans are selectively bred to defend against anxiety. Susceptibility to threats of anxiety are genetically determined. The strongest biological correlate, based on study data, is the role of genetics. More than 50% of individuals with a panic disorder have a relative with the disorder. There is similar evidence for the other anxiety disorders.

Twin studies also suggest that anxiety disorders are to some degree inherited (Kaplan and Sadock, 1995). Although there is some controversy regarding early twin studies because mixed groups of patients with anxiety disorders were used; a later study does report that anxiety disorders with panic attack were five times as frequent in monozygotic twins (Andreasen and Black, 1995). There is a higher incidence of phobia among members with a history of phobia in the family (almost three times higher). In addition, there is a higher incidence of phobias in monozygotic twin studies, but the specifics of social versus specific phobias have not been studied (Andreasen and Black, 1995). A few studies have reported up to 20% of first-degree relatives of persons with OCD also have OCD.

Psychosocial Correlates

Psychodynamic theories

The psychoanalytic, or Freudian, school of thought proposes that anxiety is the response of the ego to unconscious, unacceptable thoughts, feelings, and impulses that threaten to emerge into consciousness. The ego attempts to protect the self from being overwhelmed by the anxiety through the use of defense mechanisms. Defense mechanisms maintain such thoughts and feelings, and impulses out of awareness in the unconscious. The commonly used defense mechanisms are listed in Table 22-2.

What is stored in the unconscious continues to influence the behavior of the individual and contributes to the development of the symptoms associated with anxiety disorders. For example, anxiety signals the ego that unacceptable thoughts are rising to consciousness; this is a signal to the ego to protect itself. If anxiety continues past its "alerting" or mild level, it may advance to a severe or panic level. It is proposed that the defense mechanism of repression, if successful, should preserve the ego and prevent symptom formation. If this mechanism is unsuccessful, anxiety will manifest itself as symptoms reflected by the clinical descriptions found in Table 22-1 and the symptoms listed in Table 22-3.

Text continued on p. 393.

TABLE 22-2

Defense mechanisms

DEFENSE MECHANISM/DEFINITION	IMPACT ON FUNCTIONING	CLINICAL EXAMPLE
Compensation An unconscious "making-up" for a limitation or defect through an exaggerated presentation of self or accomplishment	Protects the self from recognizing a personal limitation, results in exaggerated responses that reflect a lack of self-awareness and self-acceptance and increase the risk of dysfunctional behavior.	Joe has inadequate social skills and difficulty making friends. He compensates for this inadequacy by becoming the "class brain" through overinvolvement in the pursuit of academic accomplishment.
Denial An unconscious ignoring or insufficiently perceiving and appreciating intolerable perceptions	There is failure to recognize what is occurring in a situation or in one's life and how one's own participation in the situation interferes with effective functioning; failure to recognize what is happening generates inappropriate behavior, complicates existing problems, and escalates a simple difficulty into a major crisis.	During group meetings, Ned states he cannot eat chocolate or cheese or drink wine while on his medication. He comes back from a pass with a cheeseburger and a bag of chocolate candies.
Displacement An unconscious process of substitution; a feeling or emotion is transferred from its actual object or focus to a substitute object or focus	An uncomfortable or distressing affect such as anger that is generated in one situation/relationship is ventilated in another, unrelated situation toward an uninvolved person. The original source of the affect is never addressed or resolved, and problems are created where the inappropriate ventilation occurred.	Jack has a hatred toward his father but perceives this as unacceptable and dangerous. He manages this hatred by unconsciously displacing it onto a younger sibling and acting out aggressively and assaultively toward this sibling.
Dissociation An unconscious process by which a portion of the personality that is associated with emotional distress is cut off from conscious control and kept out of awareness	The use of this mechanism fragments the personality and interferes with the ability to function as an integrated person. The person experiences unaccounted periods during which what	Dora experiences somnambulism (sleepwalking). When this occurs, she gets up and engages in complicated activities. These activities are under the direction of a disconnected fragment

Continued.

TABLE 22-2—cont'd

Defense mechanisms

DEFENSE MECHANISM/DEFINITION	IMPACT ON FUNCTIONING	CLINICAL EXAMPLE
	is said or done occurs outside of awareness and is not recalled afterward. This mechanism is implicated in the development of dual or multiple personalities.	of her personality and outside the awareness of the major part of her personality, which remains asleep. When she is awake, this fragment also directs her automatic writing behavior.
Fixation Some aspect of the personality is halted or stuck at an incomplete stage of human development	Protects the immature self from a threat to physical or psychological survival; results in arrested development. The person's way of perceiving, thinking, feeling, and behaving continues to operate at the level of development where the traumatic event occurred and does not mature as the person becomes chronologically older. This immaturity interferes with the ability to function effectively as an adult and meet needs appropriately.	Amy has never learned how to delay gratification for any length of time. Her demanding behavior is comparable to that of a 2 year old. When she wants something, she wants it immediately, and when it is not provided on demand, she throws a tantrum and becomes assaultive and violent.
Identification An unconscious process by which one assumes the attitudes and behavior patterns of an authority or parent figure, differentiated from the conscious process of role modeling or imitation	This psychological mechanism formulates identity. It is an attempt at wish fulfillment. The person aspires to the strength and desired qualities and traits of another. The person using this mechanism exhibits the desired traits. Use may promote growth and development when the focus of identification provides a positive model, or dysfunction if the model is negative, self-destructive, or antisocial.	Betsy, an adolescent client, develops a positive identification with the student nurse. She verbalizes a desire and interest in becoming a nurse. Her school performance improves and she begins to sound like the nurse in group therapy.
Intellectualization Thinking is disconnected from feeling; interactions with others and situations are dealt with at only a cognitive level, and the emotional aspect is avoided, ignored, or significantly lessened	The holistic person experiences life, relationships, and situations from the thinking and feeling perspectives. When the emotional dimension of the person is diminished or excluded, perception is distorted, relationships with others impaired, and the imbalanced perspective contributes to the selection of inappropriate solutions to problems and an inability to give or receive social support.	During a group therapy session, Alice tearfully discloses the physical abuse she experienced as a child and having been thrown out of the home by her father to live on the streets at age 13 after her mother died. Clare, a client in the group, responds to this disclosure. She tells Alice that at least she survived and that she needs to stop crying and just forget about the past and get on with her life. Clare's response fails to acknowledge the acute emotional distress experienced by Alice and reflects a lack of empathy.

TABLE 22-2—cont'd

Defense mechanisms

DEFENSE MECHANISM/DEFINITION	IMPACT ON FUNCTIONING	CLINICAL EXAMPLE
Projection An unconscious process, a form of displacement that is closely related to denial and repression; it is the process of disowning and attributing to another person those objectionable or unacceptable traits, attitudes, motives, and desires that the person does not wish to acknowledge possessing; it is a transfer of possession of the unacceptable from self to another	The disowning and attributing process enables a person to remain blind to important aspects of his or her own personality and behavior and distort his or her perception of the other person. What is projected is an echo of his or her own unconscious. The person casts the blame and shame onto another and denies his or her ownership to protect his or her self-image. This disowning interferes with his or her self-awareness and personal growth. When parents use this mechanism, they also interfere with their offspring's development.	Nora has unacceptable feelings of rage and urges to lash out at others. She baits and provokes her adolescent daughter's anger. When the daughter responds by yelling back angrily, Nora describes the behavior as rageful and impulsive.
Rationalization An unconscious process in which the individual uses excuses based on an unfounded belief that one's behavior is the result of thoughtful deliberation, unbiased judgment, and full awareness of motives ignoring information to the contrary	When threat to the value of self is perceived, this mechanism helps the person maintain self-respect, prevent feelings of guilt, explain behavior, and provide socially acceptable motives for actions. If used pervasively and not recognized as an excuse, then it becomes a barrier to increasing self-awareness and personal development.	Hal tends to avoid taking responsibility for his offensive and inappropriate behavior by acting blasé and indifferent. When confronted about his behavior, he has given the following excuses: "I know I was restricted to the unit, but I had to leave because I had to make a phone call in private. It isn't fair to expect me to use a pay phone where everyone can hear what I say," or, "I can't control my temper because both my parents said it was okay to blow off steam," and, "I hit Bob because I found him in my room, and I have the right to protect my property."
Reaction Formation An unconscious process in which the individual exhibits behavior in a way that is directly opposite to a person's unacceptable personality trait or impulse	To maintain the repression of an unacceptable impulse, the person denies or disguises a personality trait. This process may impair functioning if the motivation is out of awareness and the person becomes internally estranged from the real self.	Elaine is a recovering alcohol abuser who controls her impulse to drink by becoming an activist in a program for preventing drunk driving and working with others to help them maintain sobriety.
Regression An unconscious process by which the personality loses developmental achievements and reverts to an earlier level of functioning	Interferes with the use of mature coping. Problems result from immature behavior, feeling, and thinking.	Carla's husband divorces her and remarries. Her emotional reaction to the divorce is characterized by bouts of tearfulness and violent rages that in-

TABLE 22-2—cont'd

Defense mechanisms

DEFENSE MECHANISM/DEFINITION	IMPACT ON FUNCTIONING	CLINICAL EXAMPLE
		volve destruction of furniture and clothing. She returns to her parent's home with the expectation that they will take care of her.
Repression An unconscious process whereby unacceptable desires, impulses, thoughts, wishes, motivations, and behaviors that are incompatible or disturbing to the person are excluded from awareness and pushed into the unconsciousness. An unconscious process of disconnecting thoughts, feelings, and behavior from one another and from awareness is used when threats and situational events generate intense anxiety.	The unconscious repressed thoughts continue to influence behavior. Repressed feelings may erupt at inappropriate times and interfere with functioning and relationships. Problems arise because of the unavailability of what is repressed for resolution through logical analysis and problem solving. The unawareness contributes to rigid and constricted perceptions, thinking, and behavior. A positive use occurs when a potentially overwhelming threat occurs and its use protects against overwhelming anxiety.	Annie is experiencing night terrors. Over the past year she has developed increasing fear of leaving her house. She has forgotten (repressed) the date and circumstances of a traumatic mugging and rape that had occurred in the past.
Restitution The "making-up-for" activities meant to relieve guilt for personal behavior that the person perceives as neglectful, reprehensible, or mean	Use may contribute to the person's choice of a career in a helping profession or through the promotion of a cause that will help others. Problems arise when the use interferes with a realistic perception of the needs and desires as required or perceived by the recipient of the care or help. The person's perception of self-worth and self-esteem become heavily or exclusively invested in "making-up," so the loss of this role becomes a loss of self-worth.	Louise is a workaholic parent who relieves her guilt associated with extensive absence from home and failure to participate in special events with her children by providing them with unlimited spending money and expensive gifts.
Splitting The tendency to categorize people and situations dichotomously into right or wrong or good or bad related to an inability to accept the coexistence of contradictory feelings and tolerate these conflicted ambivalent feelings or perceive the gray areas in a situation	The use results in perceiving and labeling people and situations as either all good or all bad and behaving accordingly. The behavior is inappropriate or an overreaction to situations. Needs are not sufficiently satisfied and relationships with others are difficult to maintain.	Pat perceives the nurse as helpful, warm, and supportive. Smoking on the unit is restricted to one area. Pat violates the smoking rule, and the nurse suspends her smoking privilege for 24 hours. Pat has no insight into her behavior and, using splitting, declares the nurse as bad and her enemy and the psychiatrist as the only one who understands her problems.

TABLE 22-2—cont'd

Defense mechanisms

DEFENSE MECHANISM/DEFINITION	IMPACT ON FUNCTIONING	CLINICAL EXAMPLE
Sublimation Transformation and channeling of unacceptable impulses, desires, and behaviors into socially acceptable behaviors	Effective in providing motivation for participation in vocational and recreational activities that enhance self and may help others by transforming the unacceptable into the socially acceptable; the use may help people find and maintain a positive place in society.	Tom experiences his angry impulses as unacceptable. These impulses and desires involve the dissection of animals. He transforms and channels this energy and desire into becoming a physician and the coroner for a large city.
Substitution An alternative or substitute gratification comparable with the one that would have been enjoyed if it were available	May help the person negotiate a difficulty for the short term, but because the material is stored in the unconscious it is out of awareness and becomes an impediment to personal growth and development.	Irene perceives her husband as cold, indifferent, and distant. She feels deprived and wants to experience the good feelings she had when they were dating and first married. She substitutes food and the feelings associated with eating for the good-relationship feelings and becomes a compulsive eater.
Symbolization The use of words, ideas, or objects to symbolically represent repressed thoughts, feelings, and impulses that are relegated to the unconsciousness	The person treats the symbol as if it were real and directing behavior; consequently there is impairment of the ability to self-responsible, and behavior tends to be inappropriate in relation to the situation. This mechanism is used by psychotic clients and by grieving people when grieving is difficult to resolve.	Zane has a panic attack when he loses a good luck charm because he believes that he is safe only if the object is in his possession.
Undoing An unconscious symbolic act directed toward reversing a previous unacceptable act	The failure to recognize the connection between current behavior and the past unacceptable action promotes unproductive and inappropriate behavior. A persistent obsessive thought pattern and compulsive ritualistic behavior result and interfere with current functioning.	Kim was an abusive parent. This behavior was experienced as unacceptable and a source of emotional pain. After surrendering her child in a divorce custody battle, she worked in a child psychiatric unit and developed overclose relationships with children who were victims of abuse and gave them special attention.

Interpersonal theorists such as Sullivan (1953), May (1972), and Peplau (1963) attribute the development and maintenance of anxiety disorders to dysfunctional relationships with family, significant others, and influential people in family, social, and work environments rather than as a response to instinctual drives. Anxiety responses in reaction to interactions with influential people result in inadequate and distorted communication with others, which then interferes with the ability to cope effectively in ADLs.

TABLE 22-3

Signs and symptoms of anxiety

AFFECTIVE	PHYSIOLOGICAL	BEHAVIORAL	COGNITIVE
Focus on self-awareness of physiological sensations	**Sympathetic**	Restlessness (pacing)*	Distortions of perceptions (time, space, people, and meaning of events)
Fear of unspecific consequences	Cardiovascular excitation: superficial vasoconstriction	Insomnia	Diminished learning ability
Expressed concerns as a result of change in life event	Heart pounding†	Glancing about, scanning and vigilance	Diminished ability to problem solve
Sleep disturbance pattern (difficulty falling or staying asleep, or restless unsatisfying sleep)*	Chest pain or discomfort†	Poor eye contact	Decreased perceptual field
	Increased blood pressure	Extraneous movements (e.g., foot shuffle, hand/arm movements, fidgeting)	Difficulty concentrating*
	Increased pulse (increased heart rate)†	Tendency to blame others	Blocking of thought
Easily fatigued	Increased respiration	Rumination (repeating things over and over)	Mind going blank*
Increased wariness	Respiratory difficulties (e.g., shortness of breath or smothering sensation)†	Extremely active or inactive	Impaired attention
Irritability*		Crying	Reduced recall (forgetfulness)
Apprehension painful and persistent	Increased perspiration (sweating)†	Running	Selective attention
Increased helplessness	Choking†	Combative	Forgetfulness
Uncertainty	Dry mouth		Difficulty relating one thing to another (i.e., make associations)
Fearful of dying†	Increased reflexes		
Fear of going crazy or of doing something uncontrolled†	Twitching		Preoccupation
	Trembling or shaking†		Confusion
Scared	Weakness		Impaired verbal communication
Regretful	Anorexia		Depersonalization or derealization†
Overexcited	Pupil dilation		
Rattled	Muscle/facial tension*		
Distressed	Voice quivering		
Jittery	Facial flushing (hot flashes) or chills†		
Feeling of inadequacy	**Parasympathetic**		
Feeling keyed up or on edge*	Decreased pulse, blood pressure		
Shakiness	Faintness or dizziness†		
Anxious	Abdominal pain/distress		
Anguish	Nausea†		
Unsteady feelings†	Diarrhea		
	Urinary urgency, frequency, and hesitancy		
	Numbness or tingling sensations (paresthesias)†		

*At least three of these symptoms are necessary for a DSM-IV designation of generalized anxiety disorders (see Table 22-1).
†At least four of these symptoms are necessary for a DSM-IV designation of panic attack (see Table 22-1).

Both the psychoanalytic and the interpersonal theorists consider the experiences and responses of anxiety in the early years of growth and development as influencing the development of mental health disorders. The theories of Sullivan and Peplau consider the experience of anxiety as an opportunity and a challenge for learning and development.

Nurses find their theories useful in the clinical setting because the concept of anxiety is a nursing diagnosis that nurses often identify and intervene in with their clients in a variety of settings (Krainovich-Miller, 1988). In particular, nurses use Peplau's interpersonal theory successfully in the clinical setting. In this theory, anxiety is viewed as a concept that is interpersonally communicated. Anxiety affects the client's ability to perceive a situation as it is and generate ways of handling the situation. Nurses have the opportunity to help clients recognize and deal with anxiety so that they can grow from the experience. The nursing care plan in Chapter 5 illustrates this point.

Behavioral theories

Traditional behavioral or learning theories hold a different view of the development of anxiety in relation to anxiety disorders. This theory starts from the basis that all behavior is learned; this would include mental disorders. Therefore this theory proposes that anxiety is a learned behavior, an internal conditioned response to a perceived threat or stimuli in the environment. The focus of this theory is on the client's actions rather than psychodynamic models that would concentrate on the client's emotional/developmental state as in the following example.

Mary Jo T. was a passenger in a car and was severely injured in an accident. Once recovered, she arranged to return to work using her usual car pool. Her colleague came to pick her up one morning. At the sight of the car (i.e., exposure to traumatic stimuli), Mary Jo became sick (i.e. an anxiety reaction began). Through the process of generalization Mary not only stopped going to work with her colleague, who was the original person driving when the accident occurred, but eventually stopped going in any cars. She would have a panic attack even at the thought of going in a car. The sight, and later the thought, of taking a car ride was the altering signal of the previous painful traumatic experience. It is also proposed that anxiety is a learned behavior from

parents (i.e., the individual imitates parental anxiety responses) (Kaplan and Sadock, 1995).

The previous example highlights that in this theory, anxiety is a learned response to an unpleasant stimuli, and avoiding the stimulus reduces the anxiety for the person; the person learns to avoid the unpleasant stimuli. Clinicians using this theory use behavior modification as the main vehicle for changing behavior.

Learning theory proposed systematic desensitization as a method for eradicating the anxiety in relation to stimuli such as those just described. This method was later refined and is referred to as ***in vivo desensitization.*** *In vivo is a systematic method for sequentially and progressively exposing the person to the anxiety-producing situation, usually with a therapist present. Over a period of time, the client becomes desensitized to the anxiety-producing situation or event.* This technique can be used for external stimuli, as well as internal sensations (e.g., increased heart rate) or even the anticipation fear of having a panic attack (Kaplan and Sadock, 1995).

Cognitive theories

Cognitive theories propose that anxiety is a result of faulty or distorted thinking patterns that occur or precede maladaptive behaviors and emotional disorders such as anxiety disorders. One model suggests that individuals diagnosed with anxiety disorders do not perceive the threat accurately (overestimate the threat and underestimate their ability to cope with the situation). This model would explain a panic disorder as a person's faulty thinking evokes physiological anxiety symptoms (e.g., increased heart rate and palpitations) followed by thoughts of loss of control and fear of dying that occur before and during the anxiety escalating to a panic level. The faulty thinking trigger may be a worry, an unpleasant mental image, exercise, or even a minor illness. For example, an individual with a panic disorder may have a typical beginning thought such as "I have that terrible feeling," then experience almost simultaneously increased heart rate, tightened chest muscles, or a queasy stomach; the person is now anxious. The person's thoughts quickly escalate to catastrophic proportions such as "This feeling is getting worse," "I am going to have a panic attack," or "I am going to die; I am having a heart attack." (See Chapters 13 and 15 for an in-depth presentation of cognitive theory.)

The *Nursing Process*

Assessment
Clinical Profile

Table 22-3 lists the usual signs and symptoms of anxiety. These are experienced by individuals in varying degrees and combinations depending on their particular DSM-IV diagnosis. It is essential for those with anxiety disorders, especially clients who experience panic attacks and general anxiety disorders (GAD) who often "feel" as though they are having a heart attack to have a comprehensive health assessment. The case study presented with the Critical Thinking Questions at the end of the chapter illustrates this point. Box 22-2 lists the numerous coexisting conditions that may accompany panic disorder; these same conditions are seen in many of the other anxiety disorders. This list of coexisting conditions emphasizes the importance of conducting the comprehensive health assessment to determine if any of these conditions exist, as well as to rule out, for example, that the person is experiencing a heart attack rather than a panic attack.

Many clients diagnosed with anxiety disorders are not admitted to the inpatient setting for treatment unless they pose a danger to themselves and/or are so severely restricted by their anxiety reaction that they are unable to meet their ADL needs. As previously discussed, many have had their condition for a long time before they seek or receive the right care from the appropriate clinician. Since about one third of clients with OCD have a comorbid diagnosis of major depression, suicide is considered a risk. It is important to review the major symptoms

Box 22-2

Coexisting Conditions with Panic Disorder

Simple phobias
Social phobias
Depression
OCD
Alcohol abuse
Drug abuse
Suicidal tendencies
Irritable bowel syndrome
Mitral valve prolapse

From National Institute of Mental Health. (1993). Understanding panic disorder. *Rockville, MD: Author.*

of depression and indicators of the risk of suicide as presented in Chapter 30.

Psychiatric nurses, regardless of the setting, are usually presented with a client who already has a DSM-IV anxiety disorder diagnosis. The nurse considers the client's DSM-IV diagnosis as part of the health assessment data. Table 22-1 presents the clinical profiles, including a clinical example, for the anxiety disorders discussed in this chapter. Some general goals the nurse might consider while conducting the nursing health assessment are as follows (Liebowitz and Barlow, 1995):

Psychoeducation such as letting the client know that he or she is not going crazy

Counteract the fear, hopelessness, and demoralization that often characterize the patient with various anxiety disorders

Present positive and hopeful attitude because prognosis is good related to the number of successful treatments (both medication and cognitive-behavioral therapy)

According to the DSM-IV, panic attack and agoraphobia are defined as separate entities but are not considered a disorder in themselves. Fear of animals, storms, heights, illness, injury, and death are the most common type of phobias to objects and situations in specific phobias (APA, 1994). Examples of compulsions, or repetitive behaviors, are hand washing, ordering, checking; examples of obsessions, repetitive mental thoughts, or mental activities are praying, counting, repeating words silently.

Focused Assessment

Table 22-4 presents a number of important questions to be used for a focused assessment of a client with an anxiety disorder. In addition, the nurse needs to determine the level of anxiety of the client. This can be done through observations of the client's verbal and nonverbal behavior, or by asking the client to rate his or her own anxiety level, when appropriate. Peplau's levels of anxiety are presented in Table 22-5. The nurse can use this guide to determine the client's anxiety level. If the client's anxiety level is above a mild level, he or she may have difficulty responding to the focused questions. Essential to completing an assessment is determining the client's degree or level of anxiety and implementing measures to decrease it.

The Nursing Process

TABLE 22-4

Focused assessment of persons with anxiety disorder

ASSESSMENT	CLIENT RESPONSE
When did you first notice the symptoms?	I got off a plane and started walking toward the baggage area, when I suddenly got this horrible attack.
What was the "attack" like?	It was dreadful. I felt like I was dying. I couldn't breath, I was hot and then cold; felt like vomiting, my heart was racing. I never felt that scared before in my life. I wanted to run, but I didn't know where I would go. It seemed to last forever. I just sat down in the nearest chair.
How long did it last?	I don't know. I lost track of time. It was a long time. I never looked at my watch. I don't even know what time I got home. I just went right to bed and told my family that I thought I had caught some virus.
What was happening in your life at that time?	I had been away on a business trip when they called and told me that the company was sold and that the new owners were going to lay off all the sales executives. My job was gone. The flight home was bad; all I did was think about what would happen to my family.
Was this the only time that the attack happened?	No way, I get them so bad that I can't even go on job interviews.
Tell me about some of the other times that you have had an attack.	At first they were only bad if I tried to get on a plane to go for an interview, but then they started happening when I was making an appointment for an interview. Now they just happen. I never know when they will strike.
Tell me about what you were thinking just before you had your last attack.	I was thinking about what I would do if I ever got an attack during a job interview. What could I do? I can't talk to people or even sit when I get one. I kept wondering if I could recognize it coming on and make an excuse to leave.
Tell me about what you were feeling just before your last attack.	Worried, of course. I need a job and I have these attacks. What's going to happen to my family?
Tell me about what you were doing just before your last attack.	My wife had gotten a newspaper and I was just sitting there quietly thumbing through it when Wham! it hit me all of a sudden.
What is it like for you when these symptoms occur?	I think I'm going crazy. I've got to be alone. I don't want my family to see me this way. I lock myself in the bathroom or bedroom. I pace or go to bed.
What do you do to prevent the symptoms?	I've tried everything. I even went on a weekend binge. I tried to stay drunk. It worked, but then on Monday I had the worst attack ever.
What else have you tried?	I don't go out of the house much anymore. I don't watch TV either because I have had some bad attacks just sitting watching a movie.
What do you think brings on the symptoms?	I have no clue.
What would happen if you had to live with these symptoms for the rest of your life?	I don't want to even think about that. This isn't living. It's like being a tortured hostage.
What do you think first caused these symptoms?	I don't know. I had the first one in an airport, but I've never been afraid of flying and even liked traveling, and now I get them everywhere.
What do you think will make them go away?	Maybe if I took tranquilizers on a regular basis it would help.

The Nursing Process

TABLE 22-4—cont'd
Focused assessment of persons with anxiety disorder

ASSESSMENT	CLIENT RESPONSE
What do the people around you say or do about the symptoms?	My wife is very sympathetic. She has gone back to work, and I am kind of a "house-husband." She's doing real well, and it's easier for her with me home to watch the kids, and they like me home. My parents were more supportive in the beginning, and they helped us financially. We don't need the help anymore. They keep telling me to stop complaining and go to work.
How do the symptoms affect your life?	I can't go on job interviews and I can't go out with friends because I might have an attack. My wife still sees our friends, but I don't. I'm even afraid to play golf because I don't know what I would do if I had an attack.
Who else in your family had or has these symptoms?	Nobody, really. My sister has always been nervous in strange places and stays home most of the time, but she has never talked about any attacks. She's just a stay-at-home person, and that's okay.

TABLE 22-5
Assessment of levels of anxiety

LEVEL/DEGREE	OBSERVATION	FOCUS ATTENTION	LEARNING AND ADAPTATION
+ Mild	Alert (sees, hears, grasps more than previously)	Aware and alert	If has well-developed skills and is able to use all steps in learning (observe, describe, analyze, formulate meanings and relations, validate with another person, test, integrate, use learning product)
+ + Moderate	Perceptual field narrowed (sees, hears, grasps less but can be directed (selective inattention)	Selective inattention, fails to notice what goes on in situations peripheral to the immediate focus but can notice if attention is pointed there by another observer	As above
+ + + Severe	Perceptual field greatly reduced, focus is on detail or on many scattered details	As above, plus dissociating tendencies operate to prevent panic, that is, the person does not notice what goes on in a situation (specifically communication with reference to self). There is inability to do so even when attention is pointed in this direction by another observer.	With or without skill the behavior of the person will be oriented toward getting immediate relief; adaptive patterns (i.e., automatic behavior that does not require thought) are used to relieve, reduce, or prevent greater anxiety

From Peplau, H. (1963). A working definition of anxiety. In S.F. Burd, & M.A. Marshall (Eds.). Some clinical approaches to psychiatric nursing (pp. 323-327). New York: Macmillan.

The Nursing Process

TABLE 22-5—cont'd

Assessment of levels of anxiety

LEVEL/DEGREE	OBSERVATION	FOCUS ATTENTION	LEARNING AND ADAPTATION
+ + + + Panic	Awe, dread, terror, uncanniness—detail previously focused upon is "blown up", i.e. exclusive focus plus elaboration; or speed of the scatter is greatly increased.	Unable to focus	As above plus, with or without skill the behavior of the person will be oriented toward getting immediate relief; adaptive patterns (i.e., automatic behavior that does not require thought) are used to relieve, reduce, or prevent greater anxiety

Assessment Tools

Whenever possible, valid and reliable tools should be used to rate and/or determine the client's anxiety level and or general symptoms of their particular anxiety disorder. Such standardized tools collect data not only for the assessment to determine a valid and reliable diagnosis but can also serve as baseline data to measure client outcomes. These data are used in determining the diagnosis and later in determining outcomes. Asking clients to rate their symptoms on a standardized tool is an essential part of data collection, but it also can be used by clients as part of their own ongoing data collection.

Another standardized assessment tool is the Hamilton Anxiety Scale. The clinician rates the presenting signs and symptoms of anxiety on a 0 to 4 scale, 4 being severe and grossly disabling. Often, when OCD is suspected, the Yale-Brown Obsessive-Compulsive Scale is used. Box 22-3 illustrates one of the 10 questions of this self rating-scale. Box 22-4 lists simple Graphic Anxiety Scales (GASs) that can be used to determine state and trait anxiety levels of an individual. The trait level of anxiety refers to a person's usual anxiety level and the state anxiety level refers to the clients transient level and intensity of anxiety related to a specific situation (Spielberger, et al., 1983). For example, in the discussion of behavioral theory of anxiety the clinical example of Mary Jo illustrates the difference between state and trait anxiety levels. On history and after her accident, Mary Jo rated her usual anxiety level as moderate or at a level 3. When she thought about going for a car ride, she self-rated her anxiety as severe to panic, or at a 5.

Often, medication is needed to decrease the client's anxiety level for the assessment to be completed. This is common when a client is brought to the emergency room experiencing a panic attack that he or she may be describing as having a heart attack. If the presence of

Box 22-3

Example of the Yale-Brown Obsessive-Compulsive Scale Rating Scale

DISTRESS ASSOCIATED WITH COMPULSIVE BEHAVIOR

How would you feel if prevented from performing your compulsions?

How anxious would you become? How anxious do you get while performing compulsions until you are satisfied they are completed?

0 = None

1 = Mild, only slightly anxious if compulsions prevented or only slightly anxious during performance of compulsions

2 = Moderate, reports that anxiety would mount but remain manageable if compulsions prevented or that anxiety increases but remains manageable during performance of compulsions

3 = Severe, prominent and very disturbing increase in anxiety if compulsions interrupted or prominent and very disturbing increases in anxiety during performance of compulsions

4 = Extreme, incapacitating anxiety from any intervention aimed at modifying activity or incapacitating anxiety develops during performance of compulsions

From Goodman, W.K., et al. (1989). The Yale-Brown obsessive-compulsive scale. Archives of General Psychiatry, 46, 1000-1011. © AMA, 1989

the nurse alone does not decrease the client's anxiety, continuing to question the client or to complete the comprehensive examination when a client is highly anxious will only increase the anxiety (Peplau, 1963). Appropriate measures must be taken so that the com-

The Nursing Process

Box 22-4

Graphic Anxiety Scales

Date _____ Patient Code # _____ MR # _____

Directions Part I: The following question relates to your current state of anxiety. Please circle the number (0-4) that best corresponds to the question: HOW DO YOU FEEL RIGHT NOW?

0	1	2	3	4
calm	slightly anxious	moderately anxious	very anxious	extremely anxious

Directions Part II: The following question relates to your usual state of anxiety. Please circle the number (0-4) that best corresponds to the question: HOW DO YOU USUALLY FEEL?

0	1	2	3	4
calm	slightly anxious	moderately anxious	very anxious	extremely anxious

Comment(s):

From Levin, R. F., & Mullooly, V. M. (1986). Anxiety assessment: The graphic rating scale. *Unpublished manuscript.*

prehensive assessment can be completed within a reasonable (i.e., according to agency protocol and sound clinical judgement) amount of time. This includes reviewing the results of routine electrocardiogram (ECG) tests and blood chemistries to rule out any medical problem. Once the nurse completes both the comprehensive and focused assessment, a nursing diagnosis(es) is formulated.

Nursing Diagnosis

Box 22-5 lists the possible nursing diagnoses that are derived with clients with anxiety disorders. The many possible diagnoses relates to the fact that many of these individuals tend to keep these disorders a secret and do not seek the appropriate help until the disorder has disrupted their ADLs and/or they pose a threat to themselves. Examples of related to factors, based on the individual assessment (see Chapter 5), are found in Box 22-6.

Outcome Identification

Outcomes must be realistic and measurable for clients with anxiety disorders. Clients with OCD are highly sensitive to treatment (Kaplan and Sadock, 1995). Up to 90% of clients can be treated for panic disorders, and early treatment can prevent the disorder from progressing to various phobias (NIMH, 1993). For example, the nursing

Box 22-5

Common Nursing Diagnoses Used With Clients With Anxiety Disorders

Moderate to severe anxiety
Fear
Powerlessness
Hopelessness
Acute confusion
Altered thought processes
Altered role performance
Altered family process
Ineffective individual coping
Impaired adjustment
Social isolation
Risk for self-directed violence
Self-esteem disturbances
Altered health maintenance
Impaired verbal communication

care plan on p. 412 and Table 22-6 indicate outcomes for the listed nursing diagnoses.

Planning

Planning related to the derived nursing diagnoses for clients with anxiety disorders is a challenging opportu-

The Nursing Process

Box 22-6

Common Nursing Diagnoses and Related Factors for Clients With Anxiety Disorders

Powerlessness related to negative self-representation of coping abilities

Ineffective individual coping related to fear of not completing doctoral program

Social isolation related to need for repetitive hygiene activies

Moderate anxiety related to fear of making professional presentation

nity for nurses both at the entry level and the advanced practice level. Most clients with anxiety disorders are not treated in the patient setting unless they pose a danger to themselves overtly and/or by a severely restricted ADL lifestyle.

A nursing care plan for the nursing diagnosis moderate level anxiety for a client with a phobia is presented in Chapter 5. A nursing care plan for the nursing diagnosis social isolation for a client with OCD is presented on p. 412.

Interdisciplinary Treatment Plan

Chapter 24 presents an example of a 5-day critical pathway used for clients with anxiety disorders in the inpatient setting on p. 447. As noted earlier the main reason for hospitalization relates to self-harm and/or toward others and restricted ADLs. Interdisciplinary treatment

plans (ITPs) for OCD and phobias for the community setting are being developed. Regardless of whether there is an actual form to reflect an ITP, the concept of an ITP is essential for treating clients with anxiety disorders regardless of setting. The nurse in the case manager role is often the one to coordinate the client's care. This is discussed further in the following section.

Implementation

The most successful treatments for clients with anxiety disorders are psychopharmacology in conjunction with behavioral/cognitive therapies (Andreasen and Black, 1994; Kaplan and Sadock, 1995).

Counseling

In the hospital setting the nurse-client relationship, from a formal and informal context, is an essential format for counseling the client with an anxiety disorder (Box 22-7). The presence of the nurse is key to decreasing the client's anxiety and establishing trust. Nurses functioning in the basic role must be knowledgeable about the basic cognitive and behavioral therapies used with these clients. As discussed previously under behavioral theories of anxiety, in vivo exposure is the primary behavior treatment for clients with panic disorder. Cognitive therapy strategies, applied relaxation, respiratory training, and other techniques to decrease anxiety and stress are explained in Chapters 8, 9, 11, and 14. All of these can be used in counseling the client with an anxiety disorder. The Research Highlight on p. 403 discusses the implications of a cognitive-behavioral approach.

TABLE 22-6

Nursing diagnoses and examples of outcomes and interventions

NURSING DIAGNOSIS	OUTCOME IDENTIFICATION	GENERAL INTERVENTIONS
Powerlessness related to negative self-representation of coping abilities	Will verbally recognize two coping skills useful during the beginning of a panic attack	Identification of strengths Cognitive reframing
Ineffective individual coping related to fear of not completing doctoral program	Will use relaxation techniques before attending classes	Review and rehearse relaxation techniques and problem-solving strategies
Social isolation related to need for repetitive hygiene activities	Will be able to leave home and go to work at least twice a week	Explain the rationale of in vivo desensitization
Moderate anxiety related to fear of making professional presentation	Will take medication a half hour before presentation	Review and rehearse relaxation techniques Discuss the purpose and use of medication

The Nursing Process

Box 22-7

Counseling

DEFINITION

Use of an interactive helping process focusing on the needs, problems, or feelings of the patient and significant others to enhance or support coping, problem-solving, and interpersonal relationships

ACTIVITIES

Establish a therapeutic relationship based on trust and respect

Demonstrate empathy, warmth, and genuineness

Establish the length of the counseling relationship

Establish goals

Provide privacy and ensure confidentiality

Provide factual information, as necessary and appropriate

Encourage expression of feelings

Assist patient to identify the problem or situation that is causing the distress

Use techniques of reflection and clarification to facilitate expression of concerns

Ask patient/significant others to identify what they can/cannot do about what is happening

Assist patient to list and prioritize all possible alternatives to a problem

Identify any differences between patient's view of the situation and the view of the health care team

Determine how family behavior affects patient

Verbalize the discrepancy between the patient's feelings and behaviors

Use assessment tools (e.g., paper and pencil measures, audiotape, videotape, or interactional exercises with other people) to help increase patient's self-awareness and counselor's knowledge of situation, as appropriate

Reveal selected aspects of one's own experiences or personality to foster genuineness and trust, as appropriate

Assist patient to identify strengths, and reinforce these

Encourage new skill development, as appropriate

Encourage substitution of undesirable habits with desirable habits

Reinforce new skills

Discourage decision making when the patient is under severe stress

Reprinted with permission from McCloskey J.C. & Bulechek G.M. (Ed.).(1996). Nursing interventions classification (NIC). *(2nd ed.). St. Louis: Mosby.*

One important strategy is to teach the client to compare his or her own trait anxiety level with their state anxiety level at the time of an anxiety attack. The Graphic Anxiety Scales (GASs) is one tool that can easily be used by clients (see Box 22-4) for this purpose (Krainovich-Miller, 1988). This is an important homework assignment for the client. For instance, the client is asked by the nurse to keep a record of how often the anxiety attack occurs, what symptoms are experienced, the events surrounding the attack, and to rate their current anxiety level or state, for the particular episode. At each counseling session the nurse and client can use this information to chart the client's progress. This also serves as outcome measurement data.

Box 22-8 lists a number of general interventions and/or goals that the nurse may implement during formal counseling sessions or general interactions with the client; these are described in Chapter 9. For example, it is essential when dealing with a client that is beginning to experience a panic attack that the nurse says to the person, "I will stay with you; you will not lose control," "I will not let you lose control; you are not losing your mind," or "I am here; you are not having a heart attack. I know it feels like you are having one." Chapter 14 includes a number of interventions for panic level anxiety. Some important examples from this list are that the nurse should offer simple clear statements using a reassuring calm and confident tone; such interventions are invaluable to this type of client (Schweitzer et al., 1995).

This same strategy is equally effective when a client with OCD begins a ritual process because many times the client knows that he or she should not be doing it, or feels it is not right, or that it is "crazy." Once the behavior is started, the nurse does not stop it. The nurse can stay with the client and give nonjudgmental recognition. Often, a nurse may be working with a client with OCD who is on medication and in therapy is being taught to use the behavioral/cognitive "thought stopping" technique. In this case the client is taught to snap an elastic band or even say out loud, *"Stop!"* when a compulsive idea, or "unwanted thought," comes to mind on which he or she feels compelled to act, as in the following example:

The Nursing Process

RESEARCH HIGHLIGHT

Schweitzer, P. B., Nesse, R. M., Fantone, R. F., & Curtis, G. C. (1995). Outcomes of group cognitive behavioral training in the treatment of panic disorder and agoraphobia. *Journal of the American Psychiatric Nurses Association, 1*(3), 83-91.

Summary

The purpose of this study was to determine the differences in the severity of symptoms of clients with panic disorder and agoraphobia before and after a 6-week group cognitive behavioral training program.

This prospective clinical study used a convenience sample of 40 subjects who received a 6 week consecutive training cognitive behavioral therapy by nurse-facilitators. Before and after completing the training program, subjects completed the Symptom Check List-90-Revised and the Weekly Ratings Scale, which measured variables such as intensity of panic symptoms, phobic avoidance, generalized anxiety, and depression.

Significant differences between baseline and endpoint means scores of the group participants were found. No significant differences in progress were noted between subjects who were taking medications and those who were not, nor did a concurrent diagnosis of depression or any other anxiety disorder contribute to different outcomes.

Implications for Nursing Practice

- Nurse-run cognitive behavioral group therapy can significantly reduce symptoms of clients with panic disorder and agoraphobia.

- Nurses have a significant role to play in using cognitive behavioral strategies with clients with anxiety disorders.

- Data from standardized assessment tools can be used as baseline data and to determine outcomes.

Sue was a market analyst for a company that required her to travel extensively. Her obsession about taking overnight business trips coincided with her upcoming divorce. Her worrying thoughts of someone coming into her hotel room in the middle of the night kept her awake most of the night and when at home, her anxiety would increase just thinking about the next trip. Her nurse therapist taught her how to use the thought stopping technique using her jogger's stop watch that had an alarm. She practiced the following at home before trips. She would set the alarm for 3 minutes, she would start to visualize the following: being in a strange hotel room in a new city, unpacking, anticipating going to bed, the room being dark, and the door opening as she is lying in bed. At that point the alarm would go off and she would shout out loud, *"Stop!"* and at the same time snap her fingers. She would continue to say *"Stop!"* and snap her fingers if the thought occurred before 30 seconds.

Gradually she taught herself to say stop in a normal voice, in a whisper until she was finally able to say it silently to herself. Over time, it required only a few stops for the phobic thought to leave completely; the phobic experience would last only a few minutes. After a time, she was able to say stop silently and use a rubber band instead of snapping her fingers. Then she made her own tape recording of saying, *"Stop!"* at intervals of 4, 6, 3, 7 minutes; she would play this in her hotel room while unpacking. She noticed over the next few months that she was having fewer obsessions about sleeping in a strange room and was more focused on the challenge of her business of the day.

It is extremely important to inform this type of client that it takes time for the medication to work and that it is important to practice the cognitive/behavioral therapies as discussed. Because a great number of clients with OCD have a comorbid diagnosis of major depressive disorder, the nurse must assess for the risk of suicide.

Useful treatments for clients with phobias include exposure therapy to desensitize the client to the phobic object; hypnosis, which enhances the therapist's suggestion that the object is not dangerous, and supportive therapy and family therapy that help to actively confront phobic objects during treatment. Behavior therapy is considered the most effective for individuals with phobias, especially in combination with psychopharmacology, insight-oriented therapy and group approaches are useful. Groups that have been found useful for clients with phobias are psychoeducation, insight-oriented, and social skills training. The nursing care plan in Chapter

The Nursing Process

Box 22-8

General Goals and Interventions for Counseling Clients With Anxiety Disorders

The nurse must do the following

1. Assess own level of anxiety before and during interactions.
2. Assess client's level of anxiety and use techniques to decrease at lowest level, including medication as ordered and needed
3. Let the client know he or she will be safe and is not "going crazy."
4. Help the client to do the following:
   • Identify current level of anxiety.
   • Identify ideas/events/persons that increase their level of anxiety
   • Identify activities that decrease their level of anxiety.
   • Work on one problem at a time
5. Teach the client a variety of relaxation techniques (see Chapter 14)
6. Set limits on environmental stimuli
7. Reinforce the goals established in group or individual therapy
8. Encourage activities that decrease the client engaging in destructive activities

5 offers one example of a client with a phobia related to performance. Thought stopping, refuting irrational ideas, and coping skills training can also be used successfully with this type of client. Various homework assignments can be used with each technique.

Coping skills training focuses on giving the client more self-control for the particular anxiety-provoking situation (Davis, Eshelman, and McKay, 1995) (Box 22-9). As discussed in Chapter 14, there are multiple steps to coping skills training. For example, once the client is taught and has mastered progressive relaxation techniques, then they can be applied to the stressful anxiety-producing event. However, they are first applied to imaginary scenes rather than the actual situation, as in the following example:

Mary lives in the city and has a specific phobia regarding heights. Yet she is a salesperson who must visit different clients at their offices. Many such clients have offices in skyscraper buildings, most have the typical office with walls of glass. So even when she got through the elevator experience, she then was confronted with the anxiety-producing

situation of looking out through a window and seeing the ground from 40 flights up. Mary has been working on her deep muscle relaxation and was at the point of being able to do it almost automatically.

When Mary first started this process she had difficulty visualizing the scene. She found it helpful to practice the technique for 15 minutes in the morning and 15 in the evening. Next she learned to achieve deep diaphragmatic or abdominal breathing. Although she knew what triggers her major anxiety (i.e., fear of heights), one of her homework assignments was to make a hierarchy of stressful events, up to or as close to 20 items as possible. After doing that, she placed them in priority order least to most stressful. Then she practiced her relaxation techniques on a lesser anxiety-producing event such as thinking about speaking up at a staff meeting. She continued to practice with each event she listed, she did the list over and over until she became more confident about confronting her height phobia. Her next assignment was to create a personal list of anxiety-coping thoughts, thoughts designed to stop the painful emotions. Mary was instructed on the following four components of an emotional response for her painful emotions:

1. The stimulus situation: You have to visit a client in an all window office which is located on the fiftieth floor.
2. Physical reactions: Your autonomic nervous system produces symptoms such as a hand tremor, sweating, dry mouth, palpitations.
3. Behavioral response: You attempt to deal with the situation by calling and asking your client to come to your office or changing the meeting to another day.
4. Thoughts: Your interpretations of the situation, predictions, and self-evaluations are what create emotions. If, at this point, you say to yourself, "I can't do this . . . I will panic, . . . " "I'm going to fall apart," then the emotional response will be anxiety. If your self statements or fear-conquering statements to yourself are, "I'm going to stay calm . . . I've done it before . . . Relax now . . . I don't have to look outside . . . I can't get hurt." You are literally telling your body it does not have to get aroused and then you can relax.

Mary practiced this until she was able to stop the physiological arousal much quicker, that is, she did not get into the fight-or-flight response mode. Mary used the following monologs:

• Preparation: "I'm going to be all right."
• Confronting the stressful situation: "I can do this, I'm doing it now"
• Coping with fear: "Just breathe deeply."
• Reinforcing success: "I am able to relax away anxiety."

The Nursing Process

BOX 22-9

Coping Enhancement

DEFINITION

Assisting a patient to adapt to perceived stressors, changes, or threats which interfere with meeting life demands and roles

ACTIVITIES

Appraise a patient's adjustment to changes in body image, as indicated

Appraise the impact of the patient's life situation on roles and relationships

Encourage patient to identify a realistic description of change in role

Appraise the patient's understanding of the disease process

Appraise and discuss alternative responses to situation

Use a calm, reassuring approach

Provide an atmosphere of acceptance

Assist the patient in developing an objective appraisal of the event

Help patient to identify the information he/she is most interested in obtaining

Provide factual information concerning diagnosis, treatment, and prognosis

Provide the patient with realistic choices about certain aspects of care

Encourage an attitude of realistic hope as a way of dealing with feelings of helplessness

Evaluate the patient's decision-making ability

Seek to understand the patient's perspective of a stressful situation

Discourage decision making when the patient is under severe stress

Encourage gradual mastery of the situation

Encourage patience in developing relationships

Encourage relationships with persons who have common interests and goals

Encourage social and community activities

Encourage the acceptance of limitations of others

Acknowledge the patient's spiritual/cultural background

Encourage the use of spiritual resources, if desired

Explore patient's previous achievements of success

Explore patient's reasons for self-criticism

Confront patient's ambivalent (angry or depressed) feelings

Foster constructive outlets for anger and hostility

Arrange situations that encourage patient's autonomy

Assist patient in identifying positive responses from others

Encourage the identification of specific life values

Explore with the patient previous methods of dealing with life problems

Introduce patient to persons (or groups) who have successfully undergone the same experience

Support the use of appropriate defense mechanisms

Encourage verbalization of feelings, perceptions, and fears

Discuss consequences of not dealing with guilt and shame

Encourage the patient to identify own strengths and abilities

Assist the patient in identifying appropriate short- and long-term goals

Assist patient in breaking down complex goals into small, manageable steps

Assist the patient in examining available resources to meet the goals

Reduce stimuli in the environment that could be misinterpreted as threatening

Appraise patient needs/desires for social support

Assist the patient to identify available support systems

Determine the risk of the patient's inflicting self-harm

Encourage family involvement, as appropriate

Encourage the family to verbalize feelings about ill family member

Provide appropriate social skills training

Assist the patient to identify positive strategies to deal with limitations and manage needed life-style or role changes

Assist the patient to solve problems in a constructive manner

Instruct the patient on the use of relaxation techniques, as needed

Assist the patient to grieve and work through the losses of chronic illness and/or disability, if appropriate

Assist the patient to clarify misconceptions

Encourage the patient to evaluate own behavior

Reprinted with permission from McCloskey J.C., & Bulechek G.M. (Ed.). (1996). Nursing interventions classification (NIC). (2nd ed.). St. Louis: Mosby.

The Nursing Process

Mary's final step in coping skills training was coping in the real life situation. Mary finally reached this point after a number of weeks, and she was able to apply what she had learned in an actual appointment with a client rather than just in the imagined scenes. During the process, Mary thought of many more positive monolog statements. She even made file cards with the phrase, "Turn off your worry and do something." She put one on the refrigerator, another in her bathroom, and one in her purse. She looked at these often, and they became reinforcement for the success she had experienced.

Chapter 14 presents an in-depth explanation of the various relaxation and cognitive strategies that are used in group and individual therapy sessions with such clients. Review this section of the text, since it is imperative that nurses familiarize themselves with these techniques. Table 22-7 summarizes a number of behavioral and cognitive techniques that are used in therapy with clients with phobias and OCD. In vivo was previously explained in the assessment section. Another useful cognitive technique in reframing would be to help the client say to himself or herself, "I can get through this attack; it will only last 5 minutes," instead of thinking or even saying out loud, "I am going to die! I have to get out of here; I can't take it." Successful outcomes depend on the client being (Kaplan and Sadock, 1995):

- Committed to the therapies including medication
- Involved in the establishment of the goals for the his or her problems, and

TABLE 22-7

Specific counseling interventions	
ANXIETY DISORDER	**COGNITIVE/ BEHAVIORAL TECHNIQUES**
Client phobias	In vivo desensitization
	Cognitive reframing
	Social-skills training
Client with OCD	Exposure and response prevention
	Desensitization
	Role model appropriate Behavior
	Thought stopping of unwanted ideas that produce the unwanted behavior

- Offered multiple strategies for dealing with uncomfortable and unwanted feelings and behaviors

Milieu Therapy

The definition and examples of milieu therapy were presented in Chapter 5. For clients with anxiety disorders who are not hospitalized, the major milieu nursing intervention would be directed toward helping clients manage their own environment. For example, cognitive reframing and relaxation techniques would be important skills for the nurse to teach an individual with an anxiety disorder so that the client can create his or her own supportive environment. The example presented in the counseling section of the woman managing her phobic obsessions would be an example of helping the client manage and create a supportive environment. In this case, teaching the client the cognitive strategy of "thought stopping" is both a counseling and a milieu management intervention.

As a major reason for in-hospital treatment is that the person is a threat to self, the major goal of milieu therapy for this type of client would be to provide a safe environment and to contract with the client for this goal. The example presented in the nursing care plan on p. 412 includes interventions and rationales reflecting the milieu goals of creating an emotionally safe and supportive environment. In such a climate the nurse would assure the client that the other clients would not ridicule her repetitive behavior of hand washing. Goal-oriented contracting is an essential part of milieu therapy. For those clients with anxiety disorders with co-morbid depression, it is important to contract for not harming self. The client must establish his or her daily schedules for all activities, especially those activities that increase self-esteem such as dressing and grooming yourself.

Homework assignments such as asking the client to keep their own daily log of their anxiety reactions (e.g. signs and symptoms, as well as the events preceding their reaction) are not only cognitive therapy techniques that can be used in counseling but also can be viewed as milieu therapy interventions. Another milieu therapy intervention is reinforcing what the client learns in individual therapy/counseling and group sessions.

Self-Care Activities

Clients with anxiety disorders, specifically phobias and OCD, often require assistance with self-care activities. The nursing care plan on p. 412 offers a typical example of an individual whose compulsive behavior of hand

The Nursing Process

washing may prevent her from meeting other self-care activities of eating, working, or even dressing. The nurse has a unique opportunity to assist the client with such activities in the in-hospital setting, as well as to guide family or significant others with this goal for clients being treated in the nonhospital setting. The goals of the nursing care plan demonstrate that desensitization is a useful strategy for helping the client decrease the lengthy hand-washing behavior to take care of necessary self-care activities.

Psychobiological Interventions

Psychopharmacology in conjunction with behavioral therapy is the recommended treatment of choice for clients with anxiety disorders (Laraia, 1991). Table 22-8 offers some examples of the common drugs used with the various anxiety disorders based on clinical trials. As emphasized in Chapters 5 and 15, any client placed on medications, especially SSRIs, requires a complete medical history and physical examination, including appropriate laboratory tests for baseline data. In this age of neurobiology, this is usually being accomplished on admission to determine the appropriate DSM-IV diagnosis. See Chapter 15 for a presentation of the antianxiety drugs and an in-depth understanding of antianxiety drugs, dosage, side effects, interactions, use with the el-

derly or during pregnancy, and vulnerable populations, as well as the nursing implications and teaching points. Medication Tips on page 408 highlight selected teaching for clients taking antianxiety medications.

Individuals with panic attacks are usually given a combination of an antidepressant and a benzodiazapine, for example, imiprimine HCl (Tofranil) and alprazolam (Xanax). The benzodiazepine relieves the person of the excruciating pain of the panic attack and/or the anticipatory anxiety and phobic avoidance, which sometimes is more restrictive for the individual and the actual attack. The client is started on low doses, which are gradually increased until the panic attacks do not occur; slow titrating is used to minimize side effects. The client may be kept on the benzodiazepines from 6 months to a year; however, some providers slowly withdraw the drug after a few months to determine the affect of the antidepressant, which may by then have reached its therapeutic effect.

Withdrawal symptoms are one drawback of the benzodiazepines, such as weakness or malaise. Clients should always be tapered off a benzodiazepine to avoid such symptoms. Some practitioners avoid using the benzodiazepines if at all possible because of the problem of dependency or abuse and cognitive impairment. This is of special concern with clients who have a dual diagnosis of alcohol or drug abuse. In other cases in which co-

TABLE 22-8

Pharmacotherapy for anxiety disorders

DISORDERS	TYPE	GENERIC AND TRADE NAMES
Panic	Tricyclics	Clomipramine (Anafranil) or imipramine (Tofranil)
	Monoamine oxidase inhibitors (MAOIs)	Phenelzine (Nardil)
		Tranylcypromine (Parnate)
	SSRIs	Fluoxetine (Prozac), sertraline (Zoloft)
		Paroxetine (Paxil)
	Benzodiazepine	Alprazolam (Xanax)
		Clonazepam (Klonopin)
		Lorazepam (Ativan)
	Beta-blockers	Propanolol (Inderal)
OCD	Tricyclic	Anafranil
	SSRIs	Prozac, Zoloft, Paxil
		Carbamazepine (Tegretol)
Social phobia	MAOIs	Nardil
	Benzodiazepine	Xanax or Klonopin
GAD	Benzodiazepine	Diazepam (Valium)
	Azapirone (anxiolytic action)	Buspirone (BuSpar)

The Nursing Process

MEDICATION TIPS

Antianxiety Drug Therapy

1. Caution client not to increase dose or frequency of ingestion without prior approval of provider.

2. Caution client that these medications reduce ability to handle mechanical equipment such as cars, saws, and machinery.

3. Caution not to drink alcoholic beverages or take other antianxiety drugs because depressant effects of both will be potentiated.

4. Caution women to avoid becoming pregnant because taking benzodiazepines and anticonvulsants increase risk of congenital anomalies.

5. Caution clients to avoid beverages containing caffeine because it decreases desired effect of drug.

6. Caution new mothers not to take benzodiazepines if breastfeeding because the drug is excreted in the milk and will have adverse effects on the infant.

7. Teach clients taking MAOIs the details of a tyramine restricted diet.

8. Teach clients taking anticonvulsants about regular blood work schedule's to monitor occurance of blood dyscrasias.

9. Teach client about physical effects of benzodiazapines and not to stop them abruptly to avoid withdrawal symptoms (which can occur with 3 to 4 months of daily use).

10. Instruct clients to take at mealtime to avoid gastrointestinal distress; avoid antacids that will delay absorption.

morbid depression accompanies the panic disorder a practitioner may choose the antidepressant treatment over a benzodiazepine as the primary treatment for both disorders (Hyman, Arana, and Rosenbaum, 1995). For those clients who are not on a benzodiazepine, and for whom depression is not a problem, it is important for the nurse to teach the client to let the practitioner know if they are experiencing the intolerable pain of the panic attack and request the appropriate medication be ordered. The neurobiological cause of anxiety disorders supports that medications can relieve these symptoms. See Chapter 15 for potential dependency or addiction problems with benzodiazepines and the need to withdraw in a detoxification manner.

As much as addiction to benzodiazepines is a potentially serious problem, so is adherence to medication, making it similar to many of the other mental health disorders. For example, the most common reason a client with a panic disorder does not take the antidepressant cyclic drug clomipramine (Anafranil) is because of overstimulation when first started on the drug; a slow dose titration schedule will usually avoid this side effect. It is also important to indicate to the client that it may require 8 to 12 weeks to have a response to the drug, which is longer than it would take if he or she were taking it for depression (Kaplan and Sadock, 1995). Providers are reporting less side effects with the SSRIs, and some are therefore using them as a first choice. How-

ever, because jitteriness and anxiety reaction are common and have similar side effects as trycyclics, low initial doses are also recommended.

Controlled studies and practitioners report that 50% of clients with OCD in the United States respond significantly to only one of the cyclic drugs, clomipramine, and SSRIs. Yet other smaller studies and case reports are positive for the trycyclic antidepressants, MAOIs, and high-potency benzodiazepines; benzodiazepines are usually reserved for those clients with OCD and panic attacks; however, benzodiazepines are generally not effective in treating clients with OCD. Further data are needed to support their wide use with clients with OCD (Hyman, Arana, and Rosenbaum, 1995). There is evidence to suggest that those individuals who mainly have obsessions respond best to psychopharmacology, whereas those who present predominantly with compulsive rituals with behavior therapy; a combination is usually prescribed (Hyman, Arana, and Rosenbaum, 1995).

Clients with OCD who are placed on an antidepressant such as Anafranil (clomipramine) should be informed that it may take from 4 to 6 weeks or as long as 16 weeks to register a response to the drug. Another important intervention is to teach the client that he or she will not be as disturbed by some of the side effects of Anafranil if it is taken before bedtime. If a tricyclic such as imipramine (Tofranil) is used, the client will be started on a small dose that is gradually increased until

The Nursing Process

the most effective dose is reached. This is done to decrease side effects such as dry mouth, constipation, and blurred vision. If a daily dose is prescribed, it should be taken at bedtime. Most clients will be on a tricyclic for several weeks, months, or even 1 year. Once the drug is no longer needed, use will be tapered off over a period of several weeks.

As illustrated in the nursing care plan in Chapter 5, a beta-blocker such as propranolol (Inderal) is often prescribed and found effective for those individuals diagnosed with a social phobia such as performance anxiety. The client is taught to take the medication at least 45 minutes before the performance so that the anxiety symptoms will be decreased.

Although many practitioners find benzodiazepines helpful for clients with GAD, because of the lack of research on treatment outcomes with these clients, psychopharmacology is usually combined with cognitive or behavioral therapy. A low-potency, long-acting benzodiazepine such as diazepam (Valium) is safer, more effective, and carries a lesser risk of dependence than a high-potency, short-acting one such as Xanax (Alprazolam). Some clients have improvement within a 2 to 6 week period, but most have recurrences if not treated long term (i.e., for 6 months or more). It is usually recommended that periodically the practitioner should taper the client's medication to determine the status of the anxiety symptoms; this also requires that the symptoms are carefully evaluated to determine if they are symptoms of the GAD versus rebound or withdrawal symptoms (see Chapter 15).

The nurse may find that other clients with alcoholism with GAD as a comorbid diagnosis are frequently placed on buspirone (BuSpar) because of its potentially nonaddictive qualities. Unlike the benzodiazepines, BuSpar has no direct effect on GABA receptors, has a slow onset, and does not cause sedation. If a client is being switched from a benzodiazepine to BuSpar, the benzodiazepine must still be tapered to prevent withdrawal symptoms (Hyman, Arana, and Rosenbaum, 1995). BuSpar has not been found effective for clients with panic disorder.

Health Teaching

Biological theories need to be considered in conjunction with the psychosocial theories in developing psychoeducation programs for clients, families, and significant others. These theories are viewed not only as etiological factors but also as risk factors. Psychoeducation programs (see Chapter 16) include teaching the client and family or significant others about the latest theories and

research related to the etiologic factors, prognosis, symptoms, treatment, and outcomes. For instance, the nurse would stress the role of psychopharmacology for anxiety symptom reduction in conjunction with various cognitive or behavioral treatments but would also counsel regarding the possible familial pattern of anxiety disorders. It is apparent that health teaching as an intervention is used by the nurse to implement all of the interventions of the implementation standard. Box 22-10 presents considerations for family members that the nurse can use with family or significant others.

B O X 2 2 - 1 0

What to Do if a Family Member Has an Anxiety Disorder

1. Do not make assumptions about what the affected person needs; ask them.
2. Be predictable; do not surprise the person.
3. Let the person with the disorder set the pace for recovery.
4. Find something positive in every experience. If the affected person is only able to go partway to a particular goal, such as a movie theater or party, consider that an achievement rather than a failure.
5. Do not enable avoidance: negotiate with the person with panic disorder to take one step forward when he or she wants to avoid something.
6. Do not sacrifice your own life and build resentments.
7. Do not panic when the person with the disorder panics.
8. Remember that it is all right to be anxious yourself; it is natural for you to be concerned and even worried about the person with panic disorder.
9. Be patient and accepting, but do not settle for the affected person being permanently disabled.
10. Say: "You can do it no matter how you feel. I am proud of you. Tell me what you need now. Breathe slow and low. Stay in the present. It is not the place that is bothering you, it is the thought. I know that what you are feeling is painful, but it is not dangerous. You are courageous."

Do not say: "Relax. Calm down. Do not be anxious. Let's see if you can do this (i.e., setting up a test for the affected person). You can fight this. What should we do next? Do not be ridiculous. You have to stay. Do not be a coward."

From National Institute of Mental Health. (1993). Understanding panic disorders. *Rockville, MD: Author.*

The Nursing Process

The Teaching Points below and Medication Tips on p. 408 can be used with family or significant others, as well as the client. The use of these "seemingly" simple techniques allows the individuals to validate their own feelings, yet at the same time, gives clients permission to tell themselves that they are not going crazy even though they are experiencing the symptoms. This type of intervention empowers the client by letting him or her know that he or she has the power to control this situation, that no harm can come to the client by the symptom experience, and that he or she will in fact survive the ordeal. The nurse can teach and encourage the client and family/significant others to make use of the Community Resources box listed on p. 411.

Case Management

The role of case manager is essential for clients with anxiety disorders. First, in the inpatient setting the nurse case manager coordinates the necessary testing so that differential diagnoses related to the physical health problems are ruled out. Second, the nurse case manager monitors the planned treatment activities to ensure that they are provided and that therapy is arranged for posthospitalization. Third, whether client's are in the in-hospital or community setting, a special effort is needed to make sure they stay in treatment because clients with anxiety disorders, especially those with panic disorder and ago-

raphobia, tend to have a high dropout rate for maintaining successful treatment.

The nurse case manager is also the best health professional to address psychopharmacology adherence. A simple intervention is to let clients know at the very beginning of treatment that adherence is a problem and that the nurse case manager needs their cooperation. For example, an intervention addressing this issue is the nurse telling the client to talk with him or her or another health care professional, regardless of the type or magnitude of the side effect of a medication or the treatment modality. It is sometimes the unpleasant yet safe side effects that prompt a client to stop medication.

Another key objective for the nurse case manager is to be knowledgeable about community resources (see Community Resources box on p. 411) available to clients with various anxiety disorders and to encourage the client, as well as family or significant others, to make use of such resources. Including psychoeducation of the client, family, and significant others is a crucial case management intervention.

Health Promotion and Health Maintenance

Health promotion and health maintenance interventions are extremely important for clients with anxiety disorders, especially because of the high incidence of nonadherence to treatment regimen, especially medication. En-

TEACHING POINTS

Clients with anxiety disorders need to be taught using a psychoeducation framework: Teach the client, family, and significant others the following:
1. Provide information regarding the latest research on their diagnosis, symptoms, treatment, prognosis.
2. Focus on the individual's strengths, in particular coping skills.
3. Adherence to medication and other treatment strategies agreed on in individual and/or group therapy/counseling (i.e., reframe her or his cognitive distortions [assumptions], use of relaxation techniques).
4. Contract for the goal of adherence to medication, treatment regime, and nonthreatening behavior toward self or others.
5. Rehearse various coping/relaxation skills with the client in regard to anxiety producing

event/situation (e.g., use a stopping thought technique when anxiety starts, focus on another simple task, count backwards from 100 by threes).
6. *Client with panic disorder:* Keep a fear/anxiety level journal; label it 0 to 10; keep telling yourself the following; "Although I feel very frightened and it seems like I am going to die, these feelings are not dangerous or harmful to me, I am not going to die, it will stop in about ten minutes, I can get through this horrible episode."
7. *To families of a client with an anxiety disorder:* Do not tell the person to be calm, relax or that he or she is being ridiculous. If dealing with a client with OCD, do not try to stop their behavior, it will only increase their anxiety.

The Nursing Process

couraging the client, as well as the family or significant others, to learn more about the anxiety disorder through formal psychoeducation programs, self-help groups, and community organizations such as those listed in the Community Resources box below. This can be an empowering nursing intervention. Health promotion and health maintenance nursing interventions emphasize informing the clients that they must take care of their general health by having yearly routine checkups by primary health care providers, as well as the need to "not ignore" symptoms that occur by assuming they are part of anxiety reactions. The nurse should encourage the client to note any anxiety symptoms and events surrounding the symptoms in a journal or log. Such information will help the client and nurse learn if what the client is experiencing is part of an anxiety disorder or is in fact reflective of another physical disorder.

May 1 is National Anxiety Screening Day. The purpose of that day emphasizes the magnitude of the problem and to help more individuals to seek appropriate treatment. The previous discussion in the sections on epidemiology and the role of genetics support that health promotion for those not diagnosed and for those at risk is paramount. Most of the discussions in all the

previous interventions of the implementation standard can be used as health promotion and health maintenance interventions. For example, the teaching points on p. 410 can be used by the nurse to help the family cope with the family member with an anxiety disorder. In this case the focus is on the health maintenance of the client; however, these teaching strategies also focus on the health promotion of the family or significant others.

Evaluation

The nurse continually evaluates the client's progress toward achieving the identified outcomes whether the client is in-hospital and or in the community setting. The length of stay for a client with an anxiety disorder is related to identified outcomes and of course, reimbursement issues. The nursing care plan on p. 412 indicates that evaluation is a continual collaborative process. Those clients who are hospitalized because of a threat to self are carefully evaluated and not discharged until it is evaluated that the threat no longer exists. An overall criterion for evaluating outcomes is the ability of the client to function in ADLs at a comfortable level of anxiety. Evaluation is also a collaborative process. The journal or

COMMUNITY RESOURCES

Anxiety Disorders Association of America (ADAA)
6000 Executive Blvd.
Rockville, MD 20852
(301) 231-9350

Association for the Advancement of Behavior Therapy
305 7th Avenue, Suite 16A
New York, NY 10001
(212) 647-1890

Freedom From Fear
308 Seaview Ave.
Staten Island, NY 10305
(718) 351-1717

National Alliance for the Mentally Ill (NAMI)
200 North Glebe Road, Suite 1015
Arlington, VA 22203-3754
(800) 950-6264

National Anxiety Foundation
3135 Custer Drive
Lexington, KY 40517
(606) 272-7166

National Institute of Mental Health (NIMH) Panic Disorder Education Program
Room 7c-02
5600 Fishers Lane
Rockville, MD 20857
(800) 64-PANIC

The Obsessive-Compulsive Foundation
P.O. Box 70
Milford, CT 06460-0070
(800) 639-7462 or (203) 878-5669

The Nursing Process

NURSING CARE PLAN

Anxiety Disorders

NURSING ASSESSMENT DATA

Subjective: states, "I know I should go to work and school and see friends and that it is silly to wash so much, but I have to or I get too anxious." *Objective:* 28 year old female, doctoral student, overly concerned about hygiene, not able to fulfill work or school commitments; *DSM-IV diagnosis:* OCD.

NANDA Diagnosis: Social isolation related to need for repetitive hygiene activities before work and socialization.

Outcomes	Interventions	Rationale	Evaluation
Short term 1. Client will attend group *within 1 day.* 2. Client will spend no longer than 2 hours/day washing hands *within 5 days*	• Initiate nurse-client relationship • Contract for attendance at group therapy, adherence to medication regimen and homework assignments • Assist with self-care as needed	• Establishes trusting, safe environment. • Contracting is a basic principle of cognitive therapy. • Ritual may prevent client from sleep and rest.	**Short term** 1. Met 2. Met **Long term** 1. Partially met. Spending more than 2 hours, will discuss medication adherence
Long term 1. Client will spend no longer than 2 hours washing hands *within 2 weeks.* 2. Client will spend no longer than 1 hour washing hands *within 3 weeks.* 3. Client will spend no longer than 5 minutes washing hands before leaving the house *within 4 weeks.*	• See Boxes 22-7 and 22-8 for nursing interventions related to coping enhancement and counseling • Initially do not interfere with rituals • Allow time for rituals • Do not interrupt ritual once it has started • Reinforce one-on-one and therapy goals • Discuss purpose and side effects of medication	• Encouraging social interacting through counseling and coping enhancement interventions decreases social isolation. • Interrupting ritual can send client into panic-level anxiety. • Presence of the nurse can decrease anxiety. • Increases client adherence with medication regimen.	2. Not met. Will reevaluate with interdisciplinary team 3. Not met because client has not yet met previous long-term outcomes; will discuss with interdisciplinary team

log technique of noting signs and symptoms, frequency, and intensity of the symptoms of anxiety and the events are important indicators or data that are used to evaluate how outcomes are met. The standardized assessment tools indicated in this chapter can also be used as baseline data and repeated after a certain length of treatment to determine if a decrease in symptoms was achieved.

KEY POINTS

- Anxiety is considered one of the most important concepts in psychiatric nursing (Peplau, 1963). To work with clients with anxiety disorders, nurses must have an in-depth understanding to handle their own normal anxiety in response to a variety of situations such as a client's acting-out (physical and

verbally aggressive behaviors) and second, to intervene in a client's anxiety.
- Phobias and OCD represent two of the four most common mental health disorders in the United States. These same statistics are found across cultures in Africa, Asia, and Europe. Women are diagnosed more often with anxiety disorders, except for OCD, where men and women are equally affected.
- The strongest biological correlate, based on study data, is the role of genetics. More than 50% of individuals with a panic disorder have a relative with the disorder. There is similar evidence for the other anxiety disorders. Twin studies also suggest that anxiety disorders are to some degree inherited.
- Psychodynamic, cognitive, and behavioral theories have contributed to an understanding of the

The Nursing Process

THE CONSUMER'S VOICE

Panic Attack

Steven Kaplan

My heart is racing; the muscles in the back of my neck tighten. A cold, clammy feeling envelops my body. No, I am not tuned into Baywatch; I am having a panic attack. A full-blown attack doesn't last too long, but its effects have led to drastic changes in my existence.

My panic attacks caused my world to contract tighter and tighter until I became agoraphobic. Agoraphobia can best be described by thinking of the radio shock collars that keep a dog from straying. As the dog experiences the jolt from the shock collar and learns where the boundaries of the "fence" lie, he learns to avoid those areas. Likewise, as I experienced panic attacks in a movie theater, restaurant, or mall, I learned to avoid these places at all costs. (Well, the mall was no loss. I never liked to shop anyway.)

How about a "three-for-the-price-of-one sale"? That's what I got. The panic attacks and the agoraphobia led to depression. When it all started in the early 1970s, I didn't know what was happening to me or where to go for help. I felt ashamed and scared. I was fortunate to have a friend with a newly acquired masters degree in social work, who listened to me and recommended that I seek professional help.

My psychiatrist, along with my own determination (and I can't forget my friendly neighborhood pharmacist), helped me understand and cope with my disorder. Understanding from employers, friends, and family, however, was mixed at best. My brother, with whom I was working at the time, was hostile and derisive. My father and mother didn't know what to think. My wife saw my condition as a weakness, not an illness. Her attitude was a factor in our divorce.

I joined a support group 15 years after I first had symptoms. That group, and the one I am now in, have been invaluable in my continuing struggle to be well and functional. For the first time ever I didn't have to explain what I felt. In the groups I found acceptance, understanding, support, and friendship.

I am now at the point of "coming out of the closet" about my disorder. I still don't fully disclose my condition, but I do tell selected parts of my story. I find this partial candor to be helpful, and I look forward to the day when mental health will be treated the same as physical health.

---

anxiety disorders. The role of the psychosocial theories are important to the care and treatment of individuals with anxiety disorders, since no single biological theory has been validated as a definitive cause of any one of the anxiety disorders.

- Traditional behavioral or learning theories propose that anxiety is a learned behavior, an internal conditioned response to a perceived threat or stimuli in the environment.
- Cognitive theorists propose that anxiety is a result of faulty or distorted thinking patterns that occur or precede maladaptive behaviors and emotional disorders such as anxiety disorders.
- Self-assessment of the nurse's own anxiety level, as well as the client's, is essential to decreasing the client's anxiety level.
- A comprehensive health assessment should be conducted on clients who experience panic attacks and general anxiety disorders, since they often "feel" as though they are having a heart attack, as

well as those diagnosed as having an anxiety disorder related to a medical condition.
- Many clients diagnosed with anxiety disorders are not admitted to the inpatient setting for treatment unless they pose a danger to themselves and inability to meet their ADLs.
- One third of the clients with OCD have a comorbid diagnosis of major depression for whom suicide is considered a risk.
- Fear of animals, storms, heights, illness, injury, and death are the most common type of phobias to objects and situations in specific phobias.
- Examples of compulsion behaviors are hand washing, ordering, and checking; examples of mental acts are praying, counting, and repeating words silently.
- Essential to completing an assessment is determining the client's degree or level of anxiety and implementing measures to decrease it.
- The most successful treatments for clients with anxiety disorders are psychopharmacology in conjunction with behavioral or cognitive therapies.

CRITICAL THINKING QUESTIONS

Mary Ann T. is a 29-year-old woman who has episodes of shortness of breath and chest discomfort. She is afraid she is having a heart attack. She is in a "holding room" in the emergency room with an initial rule out diagnosis of panic attack. Mary Ann has received no medication and was only seen briefly by the house physician. She appears frightened and confused, her eyes are wide open, and she is holding her hand over her heart and sweating profusely. As you (the nurse) enter the room, she states, "I can't stay here. Help me! Let me get up and walk. I can't stay on the stretcher. I feel like I am going to die!" Answer the questions in the role of this nurse, who is the initial emergency room nurse assessing her.

1. What data in the chart would you review?
2. What data would be essential for you to collect?
3. What criteria were used to determine the preliminary diagnosis of panic attack?
4. Are there any other rule out diagnoses the physician might consider? What laboratory tests would you expect to be ordered?
5. What initial nursing interventions would you use to collect data on this client?
6. Knowing that you will conduct a comprehensive nursing assessment, what are three expected nursing diagnoses?
7. What nursing interventions to decrease the client's anxiety would you be able to use if medication was not available and why?
8. What criteria would you use to continue or stop the assessment process?

REFERENCES

American Psychiatric Association. (1994). *Diagnostic and statistical manual of mental disorders, fourth edition.* Washington, DC: Author.

Andreasen, N.C., & Black, D.W. (1995). *Introductory textbook of psychiatry,* (2nd ed.). Washington, DC: American Psychiatric Press.

Bowery, N.G.P. (1992). GABA receptor pharmacology. *Annual Review of Pharmacology Toxicology, 33,* 109.

Bremner, et al. (1992). Dissociation and posttraumatic stress disorder in Vietnam combat veterans. *American Journal of Psychiatry, 149,* 328-332.

Cattell, R.B. (1963). The nature and measurement of anxiety. *Scientific America, 63(3),* 96-104.

Davis, M., Eshelman, E.R., & McKay, M. (1995). *The relaxation and stress reduction workbook* (4th ed.). Oakland, CA: New Harbinger.

Fifer, S.K., Mathias, S.D., Patrick, D.L., Mazonson, P.D., Lubeck, D.P., & Bueschling, D.P. (1995). Untreated anxiety among adult primary care patients in a health maintenance organization. *Archives of General Psychiatry, 51,* 740-750.

Freud, S. (1936). *The problem of anxiety.* New York: The Psychoanalytic Quarterly Press.

Hyman, S.E., Arana, G.W., & Rosenbaum, J.F. (1995). *Handbook of psychiatric drug therapy,* (3rd ed.). Boston: Little, Brown.

Jenike, M.A., (Ed.). (1992). Obsessional disorders. *Psychiatric Clinics of North America, 15,* 743.

Kaplan, H., & Sadock, B. (1995). *Comprehensive textbook of psychiatry,* (6th ed.). Baltimore: Williams and Wilkins.

Krainovich-Miller, B. (1988). *The clinical validation of the nursing diagnosis preoperative state anxiety.* Unpublished doctoral dissertation. Columbia University, Teachers College, New York.

Laraia, M.T. (1991). Biological correlates of panic disorder with agoraphobia: Practice perspectives for nurses. *Archives of Psychiatric Nursing, 5(6),* 373-381.

Liebowitz, M.R., & Barlow, D.H. (1995). Panic disorder: The latest diagnosis and treatment. *Journal of Practical Psychology and Behavior, 5,* 10-19.

May, R. (1977). *The meaning of anxiety* (rev. ed.). New York: W.W. Norton.

National Institute of Mental Health. (1993). *Understanding panic disorder.* Rockville, MD: Author.

National Institute of Mental Health. (1994). *Panic disorder in the medical setting.* Rockville, MD: Author.

Peplau, H. (1963). A working definition of anxiety. In S.F. Burd, & M.A. Marshall (Eds.), *Some clinical approaches to psychiatric nursing.* New York: Macmillan.

Schweitzer, P.B., Nesse, R.M., Fantone, R.F., & Curtis, G.C. (1995) Outcomes of group cognitive behavioral training in the treatment of panic disorder and agoraphobia. *Journal of the American Psychiatric Nurses Association, 1(3),* 83-91.

Spielberger, C.D., et al. (1983). *Manual for the state-trait anxiety inventory.* Palo Alto, CA: Consulting Psychologists Press.

Spitzer, R.L., et al. (1995). Health-related quality of life in primary care patients with mental disorders: Results from the PRIME-MD 1000 study. *Journal of the American Medical Association, 274(19),* 1511-1517.

Sullivan, H.S. (1953). Interpersonal theory of psychiatry. New York: W.W. Norton.

Chapter 23

Dissociative Disorders

Suzanne Lego
Barbara Krainovich-Miller

LEARNING OUTCOMES

After studying and applying the concepts of this chapter, the learner will be able to:
- Identify the least and most common forms of dissociative disorders.
- Describe the characteristics of dissociative identity disorder (DID).
- Discuss the epidemiological risk factors related to DID.
- Discuss the relevant biological, sociocultural, and psychodynamic theories related to DID.
- Discuss the role of trauma in the development of DID.
- Discuss the relationship among risk factors and relevant theories of the development of DID.
- Describe the use of focused assessment questions in conjunction with comprehensive health assessment of a client with DID.
- Describe the following interventions of the implementation standard in relation to hospitalized clients with DID: counseling, milieu management, self-care, psychobiological interventions, health teaching, case management, health promotion, and health prevention.

KEY TERMS

Abreaction
Alternate feeling states
Alternate identity(ies)
Alternate personality states
Alters
Amnesia

Blank spell
Cognitive restructuring
Core personality
Dissociation
Fabrication
Fugue behavior

Host personality
Hypnosis
Main personality
Personality
Switching

Before 1994 the most common dissociative disorder was known as multiple personality disorder (MPD). The learner may be familiar with MPD from television film versions of *Three Faces of Eve* and *Sybil* or various talk show interviews of individuals claiming to have from two to ten or even more personalities. However, in recent years, dissociation has come to the attention of the public in two other ways. First, MPD is now called dissociative identity disorder (DID), and it has been used as a legal defense by defendants who claim they themselves did not commit the crime, but rather the event took place when an alternate personality took charge of them (Appelbaum and Greer, 1994). Second, many persons are uncovering long-buried, repressed or dissociated memories of traumas such as child abuse.

Dissociative disorders are thought to arise from a trauma that disrupts the conscious memory and results in a psychological retreat from reality—a retreat from a person's "primary" identity or perception of self. The *Diagnostic and Statistical Manual, Fourth Edition* (DSM-IV) lists five dissociative disorders of amnesia, fugue, identity disorder, depersonalization disorder, and dissociative disorder not otherwise specified (NOS). Box 23-1 defines three of the five dissociative disorders that are rarely seen.

A majority of this chapter focuses on the most commonly seen form of dissociative disorder, DID. DID "is the fragmentation of the psyche into dissociated personality states who mistakenly believe themselves to be separate people" (Ross, 1994). The purpose of this chapter is to provide a framework for the learner to understand and plan nursing care for those clients experiencing DID and those who experience dissociation.

EPIDEMIOLOGY

There is an increase in the rate of occurrence of dissociative identity disorder. Available statistics in North America indicate that 45% of all psychiatric admissions involve some form of dissociative disorder and that 5% of these meet the diagnostic criteria for DID (Kaplan, Sadock, and Grebb, 1994; Sewter, 1995). For those reported cases of DID, from three to nine times more adult women experience DID than men. Female clients with DID have an average of 15 or more identities, compared with an average of only eight identities for male clients with DID (American Psychiatric Association [APA], 1994).

In addition, the literature reveals a debate over the importance of and reasons for the increased incidence of DID. It is suggested that it is because of an increased awareness of the diagnosis by health care professionals, resulting in increased case identification. Others argue that the high incidence is a result of overdiagnoses by health care professionals in highly suggestible clients (APA, 1994; Spiegel and McHugh, 1995), and perhaps it is even because of artificially " . . . culturally driven misdirection of psychiatry and psychotherapy" (Spiegel and McHugh, 1995). Furthermore, the literature suggests that this high incidence may be related to the overlapping symptoms between, for example, DID and some demonstrations of acute post-traumatic stress disorder, that these statistics reflect the reporting of more than one diagnosis per individual, or that the reported dissociative symptoms are in fact not that of a dissociative disorder but of a person experiencing a major psychotic disorder with comorbid dissociative symptoms (Offringa and Goff, 1995). Putnam (1991a) reported that borderline personality disorder (PD) and schizophrenia are two common misdiagnoses made in clients with DID. The links or relationships between and among symptoms of dissociative disorders, in particular DID, PTSD, and PD need to be determined. In the future the use of valid and reliable assessment tools and systematic use of the DSM-IV criteria by all health care professionals will yield more accurate statistics (Putnam, 1991a).

Epidemiology data support that dissociative disorders are common and that health care professionals must become more familiar with the trauma model, which is discussed later in this chapter, to provide appropriate treatment through early and accurate diagnosing of DID (Putnam and Lowenstein, 1993; Ross, 1994).

Box 23-1

Rarely Seen Dissociative Disorders

DISSOCIATIVE AMNESIA

A disorder characterized by "one or more episodes of inability to recall important personal information, usually of a traumatic or stressful nature, that is too extensive to be explained by ordinary forgetfulness."

DISSOCIATIVE FUGUE

A disorder characterized by "sudden, unexpected travel away from home or one's customary place of work, with inability to recall one's past."

DEPERSONALIZATION DISORDER

A disorder characterized by "persistent or recurrent experiences of feelings detached from, and as if one is an outside observer of, one's mental processes or body (e.g., feeling as though one is in a dream)."

From American Psychiatric Association. (1994). Diagnostic and Statistical Manual of Mental Disorders, *Fourth Edition. Washington, DC: Author.*

THEORETICAL FRAMEWORK

Although there is no definitive explanation of the development of DID, or any of the dissociative disorders, Kaplan, Sadock, and Grebb (1994) report that in almost 100% of cases there is a history of trauma. A number of theories account for some of the development of the symptoms experienced by these individuals. Biological, sociocultural, and psychodynamic correlates are discussed.

Biological Correlates

Heredity
Studies suggest that there is a higher incidence of DID in individuals who have a first-degree biological relative with the same disorder (APA, 1994). In general, dissociative disorders center around familial lines and develop across generations. Further clinical studies are needed to definitively support the familial transmission of these disorders.

Autonomic nervous system activity
Other studies report differences in physiological measures such as skin temperature, heart rate, and respiration in clients with DID compared with the control group (Putnam, Zahn, and Post, 1990). Changes in vision have been reported as one of the most common physiological differences noted in clients with dissociative disorders (Miller, 1989).

Abnormal electroencephalogram (EEG) activity has been reported in some clients with DID, and it is hypothesized that epilepsy is involved as a causative factor (Putnam, 1984). However, EEG research studies have not revealed evidence of epileptic activity in individuals with dissociative symptoms. A few studies have reported temporal hyperfusion in clients with DID, a hypothesis suggested early in the nineteenth century (Putnam, 1991b). Thus the temporal lobe/complex partial epilepsy/kindling model of DID needs further investigation.

Learning and memory
As noted in the definition at the start of this chapter, memory is affected in dissociation. Learning and retrieval of information are dependent on identifying in which state of consciousness the information was learned. As early as the nineteenth century, Pierre Janet and Jean-Martin Charcotte noted the phenomenon of alter personality state-dependent learning and retrieval. In fact, this hypothesis was proposed as early as 1891 and was considered "the basis for MPD, [it stressed] . . . that state-dependent physiology, bodily sensations, and other organic cues served to differentially encode memories and behaviors in dissociating patients" (Putnam, 1991b).

Another area that has not been studied well in clients with DID is the psychophysiological reactivity during **switching**, *the transition process from one identity state to another.* It has been observed that responses to stresses in the environment, as well as psychological triggers, contribute to switching. Putnam (1991b) suggests that little is known about the underlying neurobiological mechanisms that may contribute to switching, and therefore they need to be studied. The behavioral states of consciousness model has the most supportive data to date. Collectively the findings from studies past and present suggest that amnesia and other memory disturbances in DID are very complex, and further study is needed to validate this theory.

Role of trauma
In the early 1900s, Janet first identified the connection between dissociation and trauma (physical and sexual) (Putnam, 1991b). Most studies of survivors of natural disasters link dissociative symptoms as a strong indicator of later PTSD symptoms (Spiegel and McHugh, 1995). Although trauma and its effect on the neurological system have not been specifically studied in clients experiencing dissociative disorders, there is evidence that suggests that trauma can cause alterations in an individual's neurological response to stress even years after the original insult. When a person is threatened, multiple neurobiological systems are activated. The activation of various brain regions and neurotransmitter systems represents an adaptive response that is a factor in the development of anxiety and fear, as well as the subsequent behavioral fight-or-flight response that protects the person from impending danger. Alterations in other neurobiological systems may further contribute to multiple symptoms, such as the dissociation phenomena. The role of trauma in the development of DID is usually linked with the later untreated PTSD. In fact, this supporting data contributed to the development of the new DSM-IV category of acute stress disorder (Spiegel and McHugh, 1995).

Memory studies and those related to the role of trauma tentatively support that memory problems and amnesia are the major problems of most dissociative disorders (Putnam, 1991b). The relatively small number of studies that focus on the neurobiological causes of the development of DID, the learning/memory paradigm, and trauma in relation to dissociative disorders, as well as the researchers' identified limitations such as small sample sizes, single case studies, and different findings among variables, suggest that caution should be exercised when drawing any cause-and-effect conclusions. Although the role of trauma in the development of DID is controversial and difficult to study in a controlled "laboratory," studies continue to present findings that support this premise (van der Kolk and Fisler, 1995). The role of trauma is discussed later in this chapter.

Sociocultural Correlates

A history of physical and sexual abuse is reported in almost all clients experiencing DID. Dissociation from this perspective is seen as a long-term adjustment disorder in reaction to the abuser and abusive environment. Further evidence supports that dissociation occurs in those individuals who do not seek psychotherapy after experiencing this type of trauma (Chu, 1994).

Putnam (1986) studied 100 clients with DID. All reported childhood trauma including one or more of the following: sexual abuse, physical abuse, physical and sexual abuse, extreme neglect, witness to violent death, other abuses, and extreme poverty.

A number of studies report a higher correlation between individuals with DID with a history of the above abuses and high scores on the Dissociative Experiences Scale (DES), a specific dissociative screening instrument that has high discriminant validity (Putnam, 1991).

There seems to be some resistance to accepting the trauma/sociocultural theory because it requires the acknowledgment of the high incidence of childhood sexual and physical abuse in society. In addition, nurses across the country have reported caring for clients with DID who describe cult abuse experiences, yet it has been nearly impossible to trace the cults or even prove that they exist. Although there is overwhelming evidence

that serious trauma is a causative factor, a cause-and-effect connection has not been established.

Psychodynamic Correlates

The development of DID from the psychodynamic framework necessitates the understanding of dissociation. Dissociation is a process used by all human beings to protect themselves against anxiety. A common example is when people "forget" information they do not want to hear. In its most powerful use, dissociation removes the individual from the self in such a way that a new identity is adopted temporarily. In the formation of DID, dissociation begins early in childhood and continues through life as a child so that various alternate personalities come into being (see definitions below). From this psychodynamic view, Lego (1988a) described the etiological factors of dissociation disorder as follows:

- The individual has the potential to dissociate.
- The individual experiences overwhelming life experience(s) [trauma].
- The individual is not provided with soothing, restorative experiences.
- The individual dissociates the [traumatic] experience(s).
- The dissociated experiences or aspects of them (e.g., feeling states) appear later in personality formations.

The *Nursing* *Process*

Assessment
Clinical Profile

The previous chapter discussed the role of "avoidance of anxiety" in the development of anxiety disorders. The avoidance of anxiety is also a major issue for individuals diagnosed with a dissociative disorder. For these individuals, dissociation is a powerful defense mechanism used against the severe trauma and resulting anxiety they have experienced. ***Dissociation*** for these individuals is *a "psychological" separation from the body during a traumatic event accomplished by taking their inner "self" unconsciously away so that the traumatic event cannot be seen, heard, felt, or experienced in any way* (Ross, 1994). ***Personality*** *is an established, enduring*

pattern of perceiving, thinking, feeling, and relating to the environment and to others. ***Alters*** *or* ***alternate personalities*** *refer to the co-presence of two or more distinct personalities within an individual; each personality is unique. Alters are also referred to as* ***alternate identities, alternate personality states*** *or* ***alternate feeling states.***

Mental health literature supports the perspective that dissociation exists along a continuum and is present in a number of mental disorders (Putnam, 1991b). Dissociation is discussed from a similar context in subsequent chapters about post-traumatic stress disorder (see Chapter 24) and personality disorders (see Chapter 26).

The Nursing Process

One of the main reasons for changing MPD to DID was to emphasize that the problem for clients experiencing DID is one of "failure to integrate various aspects of identity, memory, and consciousness, rather than a perliferation of personalities; . . . where there is a *presence* rather than existence of more than one identity or personality states" (Spiegel and McHugh, 1995). The term *presence* is used in the definition, because it refers to the client's experience of this phenomenon rather than the "reality" or existence of the multiple identities or personality states. This is similar to the individual diagnosed with an acute schizophrenic episode who "experiences" the presence of delusions rather than the delusions actually "existing." Another important factor in the name change from MPD to DID is that amnesia was reintroduced as a criterion. *Amnesia refers to an inability to recall important personal information that is too profound and pervasive to be blamed on ordinary forgetfulness. Language, factual knowledge, and general intellectual functioning remain intact. Memory is usually lost for the period of time surrounding a significant event . . . sometimes accompanied by a sense of acting automatically rather than voluntarily* (Grinspoon, 1992).

Clients admitted to the hospital usually present in some type of crisis situation such as suicidal ideation, gestures, or attempts; severe anxiety or depression; evidence of fugue behaviors; self-inflicted injury; threats of violence; or violent behaviors of alters. (Kluft, 1991; 1993). The majority of clients who are ultimately given the diagnosis of DID seek help from a practitioner in private practice or at a community health agency for symptoms of depression and time loss. Clients may describe odd happenings in their lives, for example, awakening in a strange city with no idea how they got there. This is an example of a *blank spell,* a sign of amnesia, *which refers to a period of time that the presenting identity cannot account for; these spells may last minutes, hours, or days. The experiences during that period are held by the presenting alter* (Curtin, 1993). Blank spells are part of the syndrome referred to as fugue behaviors. *Fugue behavior is defined as the unconscious process of taking on a new identity, and amnesia replaces the old identity; the fugue states often entail traveling to a new situation or environment* (Kaplan, Sadock, and Grebb, 1994). The following example illustrates such behavior:

Marie T., age 33, was referred for a differential diagnosis to a psychiatrist by her neurologist who thought she was experiencing panic attacks rather than seizure spells. The consultanting physician gave her the diagnosis of DID and clarified that the episodes were blank spells. During the consultation, her boyfriend described the spells, as he observed them many times during the course of a week. They seemed to increase in number when Marie was under more stress. When Marie would lie down to rest, her boyfriend would hear talking coming from her room. When he went to see what was happening, he would find Marie tossing and turning in bed, seemingly talking in her sleep. After a few minutes, the spell would end. Sometimes she would wake, behave as usual, and not recall anything of the spell. Other times she would awaken frightened, speak in French, not recognize him, and later behave normally and not recall the spell. He also described other times in which he thought she blanked out, because she would come in a room where he was and would have injuries on her arm or leg and not be able to recall how they happened (Ross, 1994).

Clients describe hearing voices inside their heads. These voices are the alters talking to each other and to the main personality. The *main personality refers to the host or core personality of the client before dissociating; the main personality is the personality seeking treatment and is often unaware of the alternates* (Ross, 1994). Clients are often very upset when confronted with these lapses and voices. They may think they are going crazy. Others respond to the anxiety with *fabrication, or making up stories to fill in gaps in their memories,* or they do not let others know that they hear voices (Curtin, 1993). Still others diagnose themselves and seek help but are not believed and do not receive treatment, or they fear help because they think they will be diagnosed as "insane" (Anonymous, 1994; Anderson and Ross, 1988).

Comprehensive Nursing Assessment

Often, the assessment of a client with DID may reveal the following patterns of alternate identities or personality states (Lego, 1988):

- Healthy-appearing, cordial person with various "neurotic" problems
- Prim, proper identity
- Sexually promiscuous "id" identity
- Angry identity, prone to violence

The following clinical example illustrates the presence of several of the above identities:

Eleanor P. is a suicidal client admitted to the psychiatric hospital after treatment for self-inflicted razor slashes on her arms and legs. During the admission assessment interview, she sat quietly slumped in the chair with her head down. On several occasions she said, "Why did *she* do this" and cried softly. Otherwise, she was nonresponsive. The second morning after admission, Eleanor exited her room by shoving

The Nursing Process

aside the nurse assigned to her for close observation. She loudly and aggressively demanded breakfast. When the nurse told her that meals would be served within the next half hour, she attempted to assault the nurse and was placed in restraints. Three hours later, she appeared calm and responded to questions quietly. During the nursing assessment interview later that day, Eleanor stated that she was sorry about the attack on the nurse. Suddenly, her posture, facial expression, and tone of voice changed, and she said aggressively, "Shut up, Eleanor, you wimp! You better be quiet, or I'll cut you up again." The nurse asked, "What is your name?" Eleanor replied, "I'm Blaze—what's it to you?"

The anger and lack of impulse control observed in clients with DID is similar to the demonstration of these behaviors by clients with impulse disorders (see Chapter 25) or PD (see Chapter 26) (Grame, 1993).

During an assessment, it is important to understand the relationships among alternate personalities and the main (host or core) personality. The main personality is usually the last one to become aware of the alternates. Box 23-2 illustrates the varied relationships between the host personality and among the alternates and which relationships can be identified as barriers to a therapeutic relationship. The previous example of Eleanor P., illustrates the harmful nature of some alternates, as indicated in the last point of Box 23-2. Table 23-1 illustrates the differences between Eleanor P. and Blaze Danger, two of the developed alternates of a 25-year-old client.

During the history-taking part of a comprehensive nursing assessment it is not uncommon for clients with long histories of DID to relate that they were aware for a long time that something was not quite right, yet even when given the diagnosis they did not accept it, as in the following example:

A 39-year-old woman, after a number of years of therapy, was finally correctly diagnosed as experiencing DID. She denied the diagnosis for a long time. She related that for many years she was totally unaware of ever doing anything wrong. After completing school with great difficulty, she married a handicapped man. On their first Christmas Eve as newlyweds, she went into a sudden rage, smashing things and screaming at her husband. During the incident, she did not know why she was having a "fit" and was shocked watching her husband watch "her" in total disbelief. In therapy, she continued to deny her diagnosis, and only after a number of years of therapy did she become aware of how hostile some of her alters were toward her therapist. She had one alter who made her husband her daddy, another was married to him, one hated him, and the host personality was ashamed during sex with him (Anonymous, 1994).

Box 23-2

Relationships Among Host and Alternate Identities

- The host personality may have no knowledge of alternates (barrier)
- The host personality may know of some alternates but not others (barrier)
- The alternates may have knowledge of the host when the host knows nothing of the alternates (barrier)
- The alternates may be antagonistic toward one another and torment or injure one another (barrier)
- The alternates may know of one another and work cooperatively

It is essential that the nurse use all the theories, principles, techniques, and strategies discussed in Chapters 5, 8, and 9 during assessment. The nurse is usually the first person the client comes in contact with, and the nurse needs to see the assessment as the first opportunity to establish a trusting bond, which is crucial to the client's recovery. Box 23-3 illustrates the major clinical manifestations the nurse might assess during a comprehensive nursing assessment, which would include a focused assessment as discussed below.

Focused assessment

To derive accurate nursing diagnoses for clients with DID during assessment, the nurse must include focused questions related to time loss, depersonalization or derealization, common life experiences, flashbacks, and especially whether the client hears voices in his or her head. Answers to these questions provide validation for the diagnosis of DID. In other outpatient settings the derived data contribute to the diagnosis of DID. The Dissociation/Impulsivity Scale (DIS) (Sewter, 1995), a nurse-developed scale, can be used by the nurse to assess the degree of control the client is experiencing. The client can also use this as a self-assessment.

In some community settings, nurses, especially in advanced practice roles, may administer the Dissociative Experiences Scale (DES). The scale is usually used for an initial screening of a client where DID is suspected. The tool consists of 28 items, scored 0-100. The average time needed for the client to complete the items and for it to be scored is 15 minutes. Construct validity and reliability are at acceptable norms as compared with many other self-report tools used to screen many other disorders (Ross, 1994). In a review of a client's record, the nurse may also examine the results of more detailed instru-

The Nursing Process

TABLE 23-1

Differences among alternate personalities in a client with DID

CLIENT: A 25-year-old woman with two fully developed copresent personalities named Eleanor P. and Blaze Danger and one undeveloped personality named Babe

AREA OF DIFFERENCE	ELEANOR P.	BLAZE DANGER
Dress	Conservative navy suit, white blouse; small gold earrings and neck chain; low heeled navy shoes, no makeup; hair brushed and worn straight	Short skirt, low-cut blouse studded with faux jewels; high spiked-heel shoes; large dangling glitter earrings, several large heavy necklaces
Vocabulary	Chooses words carefully and precisely, is refined, reflects education; avid reader of nonfiction	Coarse, vulgar, uses obscenities often; misuse of words reflects lack of knowledge about meaning; reads comic books
Voice tone, affect	Soft-spoken, sad	Loud, angry
Behavior	Controlled, socially appropriate, sits with legs crossed and hands folded	Restless, sprawled in chair; dramatic and aggressive gesturing
Social relationships and perception of others	Shy; has difficulty making friends, and reaching out to others; afraid of rejection, has no boyfriends	States that "only stupid people are trusting"; has drinking buddies and guy friends
Perception of situations	"My job is challenging; I have had bonuses and they have offered to pay my tuition if I go back to school"	"I don't work; she's a slave and nobody is going to boss me around; she ain't going to no school either"
Style of relating, coping style	Nonassertive, self-blame	Aggressive, blames others; fights
Handwriting	Neat, cramped; uses script, correct spelling	Careless; uses large block letters; frequently misspells words
Somatic complaints	Migraine headaches	"Feet hurt from too much dancing"
Memories of the past	Memories begin in grade school	Memories begin with adolescence
Awareness of other personalities	Aware of Blaze; unaware of what Blaze does except when confronted with the consequences	Aware of Eleanor; aware of most of Eleanor's actions except when she is at work, when Blaze claims to be sleeping
Appearance of Babe, an undeveloped personality	Unaware of Babe, a small child with the memories of early childhood and abuse and who is chronically terrified and cries often; Babe is unaware of Eleanor and Blaze	Unaware of Babe
Management of time gaps	Aware of gaps; believes gaps occur when Blaze is in control Babe is unaware of gaps	Ascribes gaps to being asleep
Control of personalities	No control: Babe takes over both when they are anxious	Takes over from Eleanor; emerges after Babe has been out

The Nursing Process

BOX 23-3

Common Clinical Manifestations of Dissociative Identity Disorder

- History of medical and psychiatric diagnoses, misdiagnoses, treatment failures
- History of violent trauma: verbal and physical/sexual abuse
- Inconsistencies in accounts of elapsed time (i.e., evidence of amnesia or ongoing blank spells)
- Inconsistencies in physical behaviors such as switching right- or left-handedness, voice changes, or marked differences in clothing and hairstyles on different occasions (directly observed or recounted by client or significant others)
- A pattern or psychophysiological complaints (e.g., severe headaches, chest pain, or a fluctuation in pain threshold
- Experiences of voices *inside* the head talking to one another or to the client; context and content are different from a client experiencing psychotic delusions or hallucinations that come from outside, such as an auditory hallucination
- An individual referring to self as "we" rather than "I"
- Complaints of multiple symptoms associated with anxiety, eating disorders, depression, psychosomatic disorders, sexual dysfunctions, sleep disorders, substance abuse, and even symptoms that imitate a schizophrenic episode

BOX 23-4

Common Nursing Diagnoses for Clients With Dissociative Identity Disorder

Role performance, altered
Body image disturbance
Violence, risk for: self-directed
Coping, ineffective individual
Self-esteem disturbance

Assessment occurs throughout an episode of treatment. On the basis of these assessments, one or several diagnoses and related goals or outcome identification statements are formulated on first encounter with the client, and revised or new ones are developed throughout an episode of care. Box 23-4 lists other nursing diagnoses often seen in clients with the diagnosis of DID. A nursing care plan for the diagnosis of risk for violence, a common nursing diagnosis for a client with DID admitted to an inpatient unit, is presented on p. 423.

Outcome Identification

The overall outcome for clients with DID focuses on consolidation or integration of all of the alternate personalities into one person who can experience the full range of life's emotions and personal and social relationships while carrying out activities of daily living (ADLs). This usually requires long-term treatment (Lego, 1995; Ross, 1994). Outcomes for these clients often evolve over time. For example, until the main personality is aware of the alters, it is difficult for the person to agree on goals related to these alters, but all alters are included in the goal formation.

Several difficulties exist in relation to the establishment of short-term outcomes including: (1) enduring patterns of dysfunctional behavior, (2) short hospital stays for acute crisis, and (3) the need for long-term therapy. These difficulties make establishing timelines a challenge for all members of the interdisciplinary team. Box 23-5 offers a mnemonic, a memory word or phrase hint (see Chapter 16) that was developed by a nurse (Sewter, 1995) as a guide for formulating realistic goals with a client with DID. Box 23-6 offers a nurse-developed safety contract for clients with DID in the hospital setting; the parentheses show ways of adapting the contract to other settings. This type of contract is an example of a mutually agreed on, realistic, short-term outcome.

As discussed in Chapter 5, long-term goals are projections of what might occur with the client if all indicated

ments that help verify the diagnosis of DID, for example, the Dissociate Disorders Interview Schedule (DDIS) or the Dissociative Experience Scale. Regardless of whether the nurse performs this aspect of the assessment, it is important to review the results of these screening tools, as well as any other relevant indirect client data (see Chapter 5). It is important for the nurse to become familiar with test results of screening methods used for accurate diagnosing of DID.

Nursing Diagnosis

Answers to assessment questions assist the nurse in deriving accurate nursing diagnosis(es) for clients with DID. Although the nurse always considers the available indirect data such as the established DSM-IV diagnosis, the most important data are the actual direct assessment data and the comparison of this data with the established defining characteristics for the particular North American Nursing Diagnosis Association (NANDA) nursing diagnosis under consideration. Although the length of stay for clients with dissociative disorders continues to decrease, DID is the most frequently treated diagnosis in the inpatient setting (Ross, 1994).

The Nursing Process

NURSING CARE PLAN

Risk for Violence, Self-Directed

NURSING ASSESSMENT DATA

Subjective: states "I don't know how long I have been with him (boyfriend)" and "She should die." Later states, "No! Don't hurt me!" *Objective:* A 32-year-old married woman with two children is admitted to the inpatient unit after repeatedly telling her live-in boyfriend that she is going to kill herself. She was brought to the ER with a lacerated arm by her boyfriend. She does not know how she got hurt. She indicates that she is not living with her husband and that her mother is taking care of her children in another state. She has had multiple admissions for panic states, rage reactions, and other diagnoses. Treatment has been unsuccessful. There is a history of sexual abuse. She admits hearing voices inside her head. She is agitated and confused. *DSM-IV diagnosis:* dissociative identity disorder.

NANDA Diagnosis: Potential for violence (directed at self) related to history of panic states, rage reactions, and suicidal behavior

Outcomes	Interventions	Rationale	Evaluation
Short term 1. Client will talk about feelings that preceded the suicide ideation *within 3 days.* 2. Client will agree not to harm self *within 6 hours* 3. Client will demonstrate nonviolent behavior *within 1 week.*	• Establish nurse-client relationship and trust. • Determine that client understands unit policies, structure, expectations, and requirements for privileges. • Develop a contract with the client in which she agrees to nonviolence.	• Establishes boundaries so that the significance of deviations can be immediately processed. • Contracting, a basic principle of cognitive therapy, signals volitional agreement to not act destructively.	**Short term** 1. Not met *in 3 days* 2. Met in 4 hours 3. Met within 2 days
Long term Alter personality #1 will agree to "not harm" main personality *within 1 month.*	• See Box 23-7. • Pose questions that help the client to reflect on internal feelings and thoughts • If the client engages in destructive behavior and cannot respond to "talking it out," immediately interrupt the behavior by whatever appropriate means is available (e.g., quiet or seclusion rooms, physical restraints, or medication). • When using external controls, explain the rationale for doing so and continue to talk with the client. • During interaction, observe for alter behavior. • Give recognition to alters.	• Being able to put into words, rather than actions, her internal feelings will help her to think before she acts, thereby enhancing coping skills. • Assuming the ego function of impulse control for the client prevents destructive behavior and provides the possibility that the client will learn to internalize this function for herself. • Presence of the nurse can decrease anxiety. • Establishing trust helps alters to come out; nurse must convey belief that the alters exist for the person; client must feel safe.	**Long term** Partially met. Alter personality talks with primary therapist during sessions, and main personality is now aware of alter #1 will be monitored at community referral

The Nursing Process

BOX 23-5

Goal Formulation Guide

I CARE MNEMONIC

I   *Identify* the problem
C   *Confront* it
A   Bring it to the *attention* of the client
R   *Reframe* it
E   *Encourage* the client to use new coping skills

From Sewter, M.J. (1995, October). Psychological trauma and dissociation: From PTSD to DID. *Presented at the ninth annual conference of American Psychiatric Nurses Association, Philadelphia.*

BOX 23-6

Safety Contract

I/We (all alters), known or unknown, agree not to harm myself or the body in any way. I/we also agree not to exhibit any behavior considered inappropriate by this unit [insert setting]. I/We agree to use my/our dissociation/impulsivity scale to ensure my/our safety. I/We agree to come to staff [to call if not in an hospital setting] prior to acting on impulses if I/We feel unable to follow this contract.

Modified from Sewter, M.J. (1995, October). Psychological trauma and dissociation: From PTSD to DID. *Presented at the ninth annual conference of American Psychiatric Nurses Association, Philadelphia.*

resources are available and, most importantly, if the client consistently engages in the plan. As study continues on the validity of DID (Ross, 1994), it is hoped that early diagnosis and treatment will contribute to more realistic outcome identification.

Planning

Planning refers to the establishment of a standardized nursing care plan and integrating it with the interdisciplinary treatment plan (ITP). A nursing care plan related to a client with DID admitted to the hospital setting is presented on p. 423. Box 23-7 lists interventions associated with violence prevention in the environment. The majority of clients with DID are treated on an outpatient basis by a private practice health care professional or one associated with a community-based, mental health agency. Those who are treated in an inpatient hospital, partial day hospital program, or a community outpatient

program require an interdisciplinary team effort (Putnam and Lowenstein, 1993). Team members share the same goal—that of helping the client to integrate and to function at the most optimal level possible. Multiple interdisciplinary techniques are used with most clients with DID, such as psychoeducation, mapping alters, negotiating to identify alters, and multiple contracts. It is essential that discharge criteria from an inpatient setting include that the primary therapist continue treatment on discharge (Kluft, 1991). Interdisciplinary treatment for hospitalized clients with DID usually consists of contracts, psychotherapy, hypnosis, psychopharmacology, homogeneous group therapy, and various videotape techniques. Nursing staff members bring to the team the unique perspective of the psychiatric-mental health nurse (American Nurses' Association [ANA], 1994). This means that for nurses to carry out their standards of care, their own assessments and plans must be integrated with the total plan of care. ITPs specifically for dissociative disorders are in development. An ITP for an anxiety disorder is often used for a client with a dissociative disorder. See the ITP for anxiety disorders in Chapter 5 and 24.

Implementation

Hospital staff members who are not familiar or who do not have the expertise in the care of clients with DID can have difficulty dealing with this client population (Kluft, 1993). Where clients with PD (see Chapter 26) divide the staff, in many situations, it is the staff that divides itself over the controversial nature of DID. Staff members may feel inadequate or helpless in dealing with this type of client, may be angry at the person admitting the client (usually a psychiatrist), may feel frightened or overwhelmed when alters appear and switch, or may be manipulated by the client. Staff members may be uncertain about whether to believe the presence of alters or the history of abuse. They may feel uncertain about how to treat the client and address the alters. (Kluft, 1993). Although most clients with DID, unlike those with PD, do not initially accept or even "like their diagnoses," when they sense that staff members do not believe them, they actually try to convince the staff that they are genuine. In turn staff members feel manipulated, and a rejection cycle is set into motion (Kluft, 1993).

Table 23-2 summarizes a number of nursing interventions for working with clients with DID. Rationales and examples are included. These interventions are also evident in the previous discussion as well as in the nursing care plan. Each intervention of the implementation standard of care is discussed below.

The Nursing Process

BOX 23-7

Environmental Management: Violence Prevention

DEFINITION

Monitoring and manipulation of the physical environment to decrease the potential for violent behavior directed toward self, others, or environment

ACTIVITIES

Remove potential weapons from environment (e.g., sharps and ropelike objects)

Search environment routinely to maintain it as hazard free

Search patient and belongings for weapons/potential weapons during inpatient admission procedure, as appropriate

Monitor the safety of items being brought to the environment by visitors

Instruct visitors and other caregivers about relevant patient safety issues

Limit patient use of potential weapons (e.g., sharps and ropelike objects)

Monitor patient during use of potential weapons (e.g., razor)

Place patient with potential for self-harm with a roommate to decrease isolation and opportunity to act out self-harm thoughts, as appropriate

Assign single room to patient with potential for violence toward others

Place patient in bedroom located near nursing station

Limit access to windows, unless locked and shatterproof, as appropriate

Lock utility and storage rooms

Provide paper dishes and plastic-utensils at meals

Place patient in least restrictive environment that allows for necessary level of observation

Provide ongoing surveillance of all patient access areas to maintain patient safety and therapeutically intervene, as needed

Remove other individuals from the vicinity of a violent or potentially violent patient

Maintain a designated safe area (e.g., seclusion room) for patient to be placed when violent

Apply mitts, splints, helmets, or restraints to limit mobility and ability to initiate self-harm, as appropriate

Provide plastic, rather than metal, clothes hangers, as appropriate

Reprinted with permission from McCloskey, J.C., & Bulechek G.M. (Eds.) (1996). Nursing interventions classification (NIC) *(2nd ed.). St. Louis: Mosby.*

Counseling

Counseling is essential for the client with DID. Counseling is conducted by psychiatric nurses who are prepared at the basic and advanced levels. Staff nurses often provide counseling within the framework of the nurse-client relationship (see Chapter 9). Counseling in the form of individual psychotherapy or family therapy (see Chapters 11 and 12) is most often performed by the advanced practice nurse, psychiatrist, psychologist, or social worker.

For counseling to be successful, the nurse must collaborate with the primary therapist and be aware of the psychotherapy goals. A primary goal is the establishment of trust. This is accomplished by the nurse demonstrating mutual respect and creating an open and safe environment. Often these clients have had past traumatic experiences with an authority figure; these experiences have been inconsistent, unreliable, and rigid, which heightens mistrust (Stafford, 1993). Alters do not always

show themselves in dramatic ways. There can be subtle changes in gestures, voice, or dress that indicate an alter is communicating rather than the main personality. Developing a trusting nurse-client relationship enables the nurse to know the client so well as to notice such subtle changes in behavior.

Counseling in the form of long-term psychotherapy (individual sessions twice a week) combined with hypnosis is usually the treatment of choice for clients with DID. Insight-oriented psychotherapy in conjunction with hypnosis or drug-assisted interviewing techniques is considered the most effective. Medications for overt symptoms of anxiety or depression are seen as having an adjunct role by most therapists (Kaplan, Sadock, and Grebb, 1994; Putnam and Lowenstein, 1993).

There is an interrelationship between the goals of psychotherapy and hypnosis. *Abreaction refers to the release of emotion after recalling painful experiences that*

TABLE 23-2

Nursing interventions and rationales for working with the client with DID

NURSING INTERVENTION	RATIONALE AND EXAMPLES
Do not ask for other alternates, even when the client wants others to take over.	Nurse must take care not to further the dissociation. Instead, the client is told he or she (more are female than male) can speak for themselves.
Remind alters they are part of the host personality, even though this may seem confusing to the client on a conscious level.	Discourages dissociation and encourages integration. "It seems to you, you are 4 years old, but you are 34 now. The things that happened then are over and can never happen again."
Encourage clients to experience openly the feelings that have been dissociated, rather than asking for alternates.	Discourages dissociation and encourages integration. "Tell me about feeling angry" is better than "Is one of you angry?"
Emphasize the multiplicity of feelings in all of us—nurses, clients, families.	Fosters integration. For example, the client says, "I bet you never get angry." Nurse: "We all get angry sometimes."
Help alters to understand one another and the purpose of each by pointing out the host will one day be able to tolerate all feelings.	Fosters integration. For example, when one alter complains about how "good" another is, "Someday (host's name) will be able to tolerate anger." This is preferable to the more mechanistic approach: "Someday you will all merge."
Do not reassure calm alters that they will be protected from angry alters.	Tends to strengthen the angry alters. Setting alters against one another fosters and strengthens dissociation.
Keep a chart of all the personalities and what they represent in the client's record. This is not discussed with or shared with the client.	Helps nurses recognize alters when they appear. Clients are not involved in this process, since this may be seen as encouragement to produce more alters, furthering dissociation. If all nurses know about all alters, they will be able to offer quiet reassurance when angry alters appear.
Help alters to understand one another and the purpose of each by pointing out that the host will one day be able to tolerate all feelings.	The client must feel safe to abreact. It fosters integration to say "You are (the core) and (the core) is you. When you hurt (the core) you hurt yourself." This may confuse clients consciously but will be reassuring on an unconscious level.
If client is secluded or restrained, and calmer alter appears, proceed and explain that it is for protection, not punishment.	Reassures that client is in a safe environment.
When child alters appear, keep client on the unit and away from others.	Protects client from embarrassment.
Avoid situations that may be seen by the client as intrusive or assaultive.	These clients have often been abused and are sensitive to situations where they are overpowered.
Help the client combat loneliness by remaining emotionally available.	Because of their bizarre and sometimes unpredictable behavior, these clients are often avoided and shunned by others.
When clients request as-needed medications, help clients explore the feelings that may have led to the symptoms or the history that is being abreacted.	When clients remember or abreact abuse, they feel the same pain they felt earlier. The nurse might say, "It's OK to remember what happened without feeling the pain."

From Lego, S. (1995) The client with dissociative identity disorder. In S. Lego (ED.). Psychiatric nursing: A comprehensive reference. Philadelphia: J. B. Lippincott.

The Nursing Process

have been repressed because the thoughts and feelings were not tolerable (Edgerton and Campbell, 1994). It is the painful process of reexperiencing, both physically and emotionally, the memories of that experience as if it were happening again (Anderson and Ross, 1988). This process is necessary to achieve integration (Ross and Gahan, 1988). Box 23-8 outlines the therapeutic process of abreaction. Abreactions may happen spontaneously but are usually planned in stages by the primary therapist. When the nurse observes a client experiencing an abreaction, the following interventions are appropriate:

- Allow the process to continue for the client to learn and integrate information.
- Use comforting techniques to assure the client that the environment is safe.
- Let the client know that you are there and that you know he or she is experiencing what happened in the past.
- After the abreaction, help the client to cognitively process the abreaction by understanding and accepting the feelings attached to the experience.

For example, if the abreaction reveals sexual abuse, the nurse helps the client understand her or his involvement in the abuse but stresses that the total responsibility for the abuse is with the abuser. The goal is to help the client keep the memories in the context of the past but not dissociate them.

Hypnosis in this context refers to the use of various verbal and/or audio techniques to create a state of decreased general awareness similar to sleep; including heightened attention but constricted awareness, inertia, and passivity. However, unlike sleep, the person does not lose complete awareness. During the process, the person is in a highly relaxed and suggestible state and usually able to respond to repetitive suggestions to reveal thoughts and feelings from memory that are out of conscious awareness. An added benefit includes the ability to regress in age so as to relive something in the distant past (Davis, Eshelman, and McKay, 1995). Clients with DID have a high hypnotic capacity and are therefore candidates for hypnosis (Bowers, 1991).

Within the context of therapy, videotape techniques have been used to "introduce" the client to alters that may be unknown. Unknown alters are a barrier to the therapeutic process. See Box 23-2 for other barriers within the host and alter relationship. The use of this technique gives clients the opportunity to understand more about the traumas they have experienced and their reactions to them. Clients are also helped to see and accept what others have seen about them and to communicate internally across dissociate barriers, that is, alter to alter.

To accomplish the overall goals of counseling clients with DID, especially those with a history of abuse, the nurse helps the client work through varied feelings such as shame, guilt, betrayal, and anger. Working through anger is usually an essential part of therapy. The client needs to be given permission to be angry in socially acceptable ways. Punching pillows, writing letters, writing in journals, and engaging in creative movement and occupational therapy are some different techniques for releasing anger. See Chapter 30 for a further discussion of these and other techniques.

Cognitive restructuring is an important technique for the nurse to use in *helping clients reframe their beliefs about themselves (and alters) and their past experiences.* Box 23-9 lists eight assumptions made by clients with DID that the nurse can help clients reframe. A working relationship is necessary for the nurse to challenge these beliefs and help clients perceive these beliefs in nongeneralized ways and work toward unifying themselves (Anderson and Ross, 1988).

Group therapy is advocated by some but not all therapists (Ross and Gahan, 1988). Homogeneous group therapy has been found to be far more helpful than heterogenous group therapy. Homogenous groups in this context are groups that consist of only clients with DID. It has been found that in heterogenous groups (i.e., those with clients with DID, as well as other diagnoses) that the clients that do not have DID feel frightened by and hostile toward those with DID. The advantage of homogeneous groups of clients with DID is that they can provide a safe atmosphere to explore past traumas and deal with some of the upsetting or frightening behaviors of the alters.

Through the therapeutic process of psychotherapy, trust must be established for the client with DID to achieve the following (Anderson and Ross, 1988):

- Become educated
- Break through amnesic barriers
- Experience abreaction

BOX 23-8

Therapeutic Process of Abreaction

- Signals of abreaction
  - Partial memory awareness
  - Nightmare or repetitive dreams
  - Intense hallucinations (visual, auditory, or tactile)
- Recovery of information or blocked-out memories
- Education and reeducation
- Release of repressed trauma and pent-up emotions

From Anderson, G., & Ross, C. (1988). A model for psychiatric nurses who have multiple personality disorder. Canadian Journal of Psychiatric Nursing, Oct/Nov/Dec, 13-18.

The Nursing Process

BOX 23-9

Core Assumptions of Clients With Dissociative Identity Disorder

Different parts of the self are separate selves.
The victim is responsible for the abuse.
It is wrong to show anger.
The past is the present.
The main personality cannot handle the memories.
I love my parents but she (alter) hates them.
The main personality must be punished.
I can't trust myself or others.

Based on data from Ross, C., & Gahan, P. (1988). Techniques in the treatment of multiple personality disorder. American Journal of Psychotherapy, 42(1), 40-51.

BOX 23-10

Essential Aspects of a Limit-Setting Protocol

- Contract for nondisruptive behavior on admission and review of protocol.
- Set boundaries/rules of the protocol.
- Explain the rationale for the protocol.
- Offer specific information about the consequences that will occur if rules are not followed.
- List options for dealing with anger and other physically violent behaviors.
- At the beginning of each shift, designate a member of the staff to be the "communicator" during the implementation of the limit-setting protocol.

- Work through feelings
- Cognitively restructure
- Experience the safety of structure through limit setting and boundaries
- Develop new coping skills

Milieu Therapy

The aim of milieu therapy is the creation of an optimal environment for growth and change. Most experts agree that a milieu is therapeutic to the degree that clients are involved with each other. Thus the unit is structured for high client-client contact, as well as for high client-staff interaction. The nurse directs efforts at creating a milieu in which norms of honesty, openness, curiosity, respect, and self-reflection predominate. Whether the client is in the inpatient or community/private office setting, providing a safe environment is very important for the client with DID (Anderson and Ross, 1994).

The inpatient unit in particular needs to provide a caring atmosphere where clients with DID can feel safe to talk about past traumatic experiences, reveal alters, receive support and reassurance, and begin to integrate fragmented identity states into the main or host personality. Consistency in the milieu is extremely important; boundaries must be clear and predictable yet nonpunitive.

Clients with DID are not known for their manipulative behaviors, but they can be misunderstood by staff members when they are not believed. However, clients with DID may have some difficulty with staff members who are in authoritative roles. Many clients have had inconsistent, as well as traumatic, experiences with authority figures. (Stafford, 1993). Clients' reactions to the nurse carrying out the rules of the milieu may vary. For example, a nurse who wakes up a client for breakfast may be seen as too authoritarian, or if the nurse lets the client sleep, the

client may consider the nurse uncaring. It is important to expect varied reactions. A nondefensive, matter-of-fact, caring style is usually most effective (Stafford, 1993). Negotiating and contracting (see Box 23-6) are important strategies, especially for self-mutilating behaviors. There is often no warning to the outburst of some clients, yet stimuli in the environment does contribute to alters switching. Even groups of clients or staff members on the unit can trigger flashbacks of varying traumas.

The nurse, as a key member of the treatment team, is often responsible, with staff input, for establishing, implementing, and evaluating a limit-setting protocol for negative behaviors. Box 23-10 lists the essential aspects of a limit-setting protocol that can be used for a variety of behaviors. It is important that staff be consistent in setting limits on all negative behaviors. Often, when limit setting is inconsistent, negative behaviors escalate to a crisis level. Another helpful strategy is to have staff members review and rehearse the general limit-setting protocol with a focus on various clients' behaviors that disrupt the milieu setting. The mere presence of clients with DID can disrupt the unit. It can be upsetting to staff and clients when sudden switching takes place, and a "violent" alter threatens oneself or others. Rehearsing how to address the alter during such an episode can be very helpful to staff members so that they can respond in a firm, sensitive, consistent manner to the violent alter, any other alters, or the host personality from the smallest infraction of the milieu's rules to the most threatening, unsafe violent act.

Self-Care Activities

Depending on the frequency of switching and type of behaviors of the alters, some clients may need help with ADL. The nurse may assist the client with ADL skills in

The Nursing Process

terms of hygiene/grooming, nutrition, and/or rest. For example, on arising, a client's "sexual" alter may have dressed in an inappropriate and unacceptable way for the rules of the unit. The nurse notices that the client is dressed inappropriately and uses this opportunity to intervene. It is important that the nurse does not assume that the main personality did the dressing or will be present during their interaction. In fact, quite often even if the main personality is present, that personality may be unaware of their dress style. The nurse needs to assess who is present to determine how to best handle the situation. One way might be to ask the client to look at the dress style and wait for a reply. The response of the client will direct the nurse's next communication. The client may be shocked by the attire and say "I don't know how or why I dressed this way; I am going to change." Or another client might say, "She did it," or "we did it."

Nurses who are not conducting therapy with such a client or who have less experience working with alters may find it more comfortable to use the term "you" rather than figuring out whether to call the person Mrs. J. or Jane, when in fact by the response the nurse knows it was the "sexy" alter Mary who did the inappropriate dressing. Firmly stating to the client "you" (meaning one or all alters and host) will have to change before eating can be an effective way of handling this situation. Interventions related to self-care activities are often carried out through counseling related to a one-on-one or group activity.

Psychobiological Interventions

Psychobiological intervention (treatment using medication) is usually prescribed by the physician in combination with some other form of therapy. Nurses have the essential collaborative role in psychobiological intervention with clients with DID. Most often, medication is prescribed for clients with DID who demonstrate symptoms of anxiety or depression. Studies have shown that antianxiety drugs have some efficacy for symptoms of anxiety, and a variety of antidepressants have moderate efficacy for clients with symptoms of depression. Medication use with clients with DID is mainly viewed as an adjunct to psychotherapy (Putnam and Lowenstein, 1993). Neuroleptics are rarely indicated for clients with DID.

Health Teaching

Health teaching, especially using a psychoeducational framework (see Chapter 16), can be very effective in helping clients with DID achieve an integrated personality and live more satisfying, productive lives. Although clients with DID initially are in disbelief regarding their diagnoses (Ross, 1994; Ross and Gahan, 1988) and do not

embrace their diagnoses as do clients with personality disorders (see Chapter 26), the psychoeducation framework helps clients with DID become more open to learning about their own illnesses. One of the major goals of psychoeducation is teaching the clients about their diagnoses and the role of abuse. Clients with DID go through a process of accepting and rejecting their diagnoses. The process often involves experiences of increased fear/anxiety, during which various coping skills are revealed. Some of their coping skills are more effective than others. This is an excellent opportunity to teach clients new coping skills to deal with their diagnoses, alters, and stress (Anderson and Ross, 1988). Clients with DID previously handled stress by forming alters; the goal of fusion or unity requires the formation of different types of coping skills. Often this aspect of teaching is practiced and rehearsed through the safety, trust, and security of counseling sessions, either in the form of the nurse-client relationship and/or psychotherapy (see the Teaching Points on p. 430).

Case Management

There is concern that in this era of health care cost containment, clients with DID will be negatively affected through decreased hospital length of stay, inadequate funding for third-party reimbursement, and decreased community resources. Often these clients have few if any insurance benefits left by the time the correct diagnosis of DID is made (Putnam and Lowenstein, 1993; Ross, 1994). As with all clients, case management interventions are based on a comprehensive approach to the client. The role of nurse case manager is extremely important with these clients. The nurse manages the therapeutic process, which involves the client, all of the client's alters, the therapist, the multidisciplinary team, the clients' support system, and significant others (Anderson and Ross, 1993).

Health Promotion and Health Maintenance

Clients with mental health disorders are at risk for other disorders. Hence health promotion and disease prevention interventions are aimed at identifying at-risk clients before diagnosis. In addition, recent studies have indicated that there is a relatively alarming incidence of comorbidity, chemical dependence, and eating disorders among clients with DID (Kolodner and Frances, 1993; Levin and Spauster, 1994). The plan of care for clients with DID must include opportunities for health promotion and health maintenance activities. Many of these psychoeducation programs for clients and significant others, as well as education of other nurses and health

The Nursing Process

TEACHING POINTS

Clients with DID need to be taught within a psychoeducation framework. The nurse should teach the client, family, or significant others to do the following:

1. Provide information regarding the latest research on the client's diagnosis, symptoms, treatment, and prognosis
2. Focus on the strengths of the main personality, in particular coping skills

3. Help the client reframe cognitive distortions (assumptions)
4. Contract for the goal of integration and nonviolent behavior toward self or others
5. Rehearse various coping skills with the clients in regard to alter behavior

RESEARCH HIGHLIGHT

Putnam, F., & Lowenstein, R. (1993). Treatment of MPD: A survey of current practices. *American Journal of Psychiatry, 150* (7), 1048-1052.

Summary
The purpose of the study was to determine types and efficacy of treatment modalities for clients with DID among a variety of clinicians. A cross-section survey design rendered a 49% return rate. Analysis was based on a sample of 305 subjects.

Results/Discussion
The largest group of clinicians to respond were psychologists, followed by psychiatrists, social workers, and other therapists including nurses. Psychiatrists had significantly more experience treating these clients than any of the other clinicians. In keeping with epidemiologic data, clients were predominately female, caucasian, and well-educated. The majority of clients were seen in private practice, outpatient settings; psychiatrists used the inpatient setting more often. Regardless of the type of clinician, the average length of time for treatment was almost 4 years, with an average of almost 2 sessions per week. Most clients sought professional help for 6 to 7 years before an ac-

curate diagnosis of DID was made. Reimbursement sources were the same for all clinicians. The average outpatient cost of treatment was $14,400, which did not include in-hospital stays. The eight most common treatment modalities, listed in frequency order, were as follows: psychotherapy, hypnosis, medication, art therapy, family therapy, group therapy mixed diagnoses, behavioral modification, and group therapy DID only.

Implications for Nursing Practice
- DID is more common than previously thought. Nurses as well as other clinicians need to be better educated about clients with DID.
- Nurses need to understand the psychobiology of trauma in the development of DID, as well as the relevant principles of psychodynamic psychotherapy, hypnosis, and pharmacology in treating clients with DID.
- Nurses have the ability to affect the prognosis of clients with DID through early case finding of abused or neglected children and adolescents.

care professionals about the disorder. Psychoeducation programs include the development of new coping skills to handle life's stresses, past and present. Such programs are essential to health promotion and health maintenance interventions.

Evaluation

The plan of care requires the formal process of evaluation in which the identified outcomes are assessed continuously and at selected times. Theoretically, the length of stay for a client with DID is related to identified goals. For

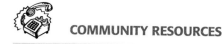

COMMUNITY RESOURCES

Incest Survivors Anonymous
P.O. Box 1745
Long Beach, CA 90807-7245
(310)428-5599
For survivors of abuse

MARS Station Computer Bulletin Board
P.O. Box 038
Rockville, MD 20848-0038
(301)649-2347

National Alliance for the Mentally Ill
200 North Glebe Road, Suite 1015
Arlington, VA 22203-3754
(800)950-6264

Sexual Assault Recovery Anonymous (SARA)
P.O. Box 16
Surrey, British Columbia
CANADA V3T4W
(604)584-2626

SUGGESTED READINGS

Blume, E.S. (1990). *Secret survivors.* New York: John Wiley & Sons.

THE CONSUMER'S VOICE

Dissociative Identity Disorder

Anonymous

Having a dissociative disorder is like living life on a roller coaster—an abundance of serious lows without too many real highs. The major symptom I experience is frequent loss of time, that is, someone will tell me something about what I've said or done, and I'll have no recollection of the transaction. When I am in a more acute state, I hear voices commenting negatively on what I say or do, or what others say or do. I experience periods of severe depression where I become obsessed with doing harm to myself or others. I become very fearful and hyper alert. I can't sleep at night, and my job performance falls. I then begin to think more harshly about myself and my thoughts become disorganized. My psychiatrist has called it "cognitive slippage," and I believe that's accurate. I know something is wrong, but I cannot control my symptoms, so then I am hospitalized.

The impact on my life has been severe. I have not been able to maintain a long-term relationship, and it is a struggle for me to work and pursue graduate studies. I have experienced stigma. It is why I feel I must remain anonymous. I am a registered nurse (RN) with a respected position in the mental health field, and I have listened to many professionals speak with ignorance and disdain of persons with dissociative disorders. If my disorder were known, I would lose all credibility. The very fact that I have been hospitalized has caused people to treat me differently.

I cope with the disorder by taking medications that help my moods, help me sleep, and keep my thoughts in order. I have also been in individual therapy for many years before and since receiving this diagnosis. In addition, I spend time with friends, have many pets, enjoy going hiking, and also keep a journal.

Psychiatric nurses have been of essential help to me during my hospitalizations. I have had the good fortune to be hospitalized on a dissociative disorders unit at a hospital in Baltimore. The nurses there are knowledgeable about dissociative disorders. They have been great reality testers, taught me excellent skills for focusing and grounding myself, but most of all, the RN most frequently assigned to me has believed in me and helped me believe in myself.

Coping with this disorder has been possible (1) because I have good therapy, (2) the hospital has been there when I needed it, and (3) I have some good, supportive friends. I've been able to keep myself from feeling disabled by holding a job, managing my affairs, and using leisure time to relax. These are elements that have helped me effectively cope.

My suggestion to future and current psychiatric nurses would be to keep learning as much as you can about the range of psychiatric disabilities but never, ever leave your heart behind.

CRITICAL THINKING QUESTIONS

Jane was a well-educated, attractive, caucasian woman. She was a freelance artist, who also ran a business as an art teacher in a nearby community. Two years ago, Jane sought psychiatric help for subtle complaints of depression and feelings of "losing her mind." Antidepressant medications did not help. Two days ago she was found wondering about in her local supermarket, saying, "Why am I here? Where am I?" After a short time, she would say, "She is going to kill me." When asked about her bleeding wrist, Jane seemed unaware that she was bleeding. She was brought by police to the local ER and later admitted to the psychiatric unit.

Answer the following questions as if you were the admitting nurse on the unit.

1. How you would conduct your comprehensive health assessment of Jane?
2. What are two possible nursing diagnoses for Jane?
3. What type of contracts would you develop with Jane?
4. A staff member asks you, "Are you going to talk to her alters?" How would you respond?
5. Today the primary therapist initiated hypnosis with intensive insight-oriented therapy with Jane. At the end of the day, Jane says to you, "Hypnosis is ridiculous. Why do they want to use it on her?" How would you respond to this question?

many clients with DID there are repeated hospitalizations over a long period. Meeting identified outcomes in the designated hospital length of stay, which is usually set by reimbursement guidelines, is difficult given the projected length of required treatment (Kluft, 1991). The nursing care plan presented on p. 423 indicates that the nurse evaluate the selected outcomes during a client's brief hospital stay and document these outcomes in the evaluation column of the care plan. The Research Highlight on p. 430 reflects the complex nature of this disorder.

KEY POINTS

- Dissociation is a "psychological" separation from the body during a traumatic event by taking the inner "self" away somewhere, where the abuse cannot be seen, heard, felt or experienced in any way (Ramsgard and Shook, 1995).
- Dissociative disorders are thought to arise from a trauma that disrupts the conscious memory and results in a psychological retreat from reality, a retreat from the "primary" identity or perception of self.
- Dissociate identity disorder (DID) is the most common reported form of dissociative disorder in the

United States. It was previously known as multiple personality disorder.

- *Personality* is an established enduring pattern of perceiving, thinking, feeling, and relating to the environment and to others. Alternate identities, or personality states, refer to the copresence of two or more distinct personalities within an individual; each personality is unique.
- DID is a failure of integration of various aspects of identity, memory, and consciousness, rather than a proliferation of personalities. There is a presence rather than existence of more than one identity or personality states.
- About 45% of all psychiatric admissions involve some form of dissociative disorder, and 5% of these meet the diagnostic criteria for DID.
- Clients admitted to the hospital setting with a diagnosis of DID usually present in some type of crisis situation.
- Blank spells are a common symptom of DID. They are a sign of amnesia and refer to a period for which the presenting identity cannot account. These spells may last minutes, hours, or days. The experiences during that period are held by the presenting alter and are part of the syndrome referred to as *fugue behaviors*.
- The *main personality* is the host or core personality of the client before dissociating. The main personality is the personality seeking treatment and is often unaware of the alternates.
- A focused assessment is part of a comprehensive nursing assessment. It often reveals the following: a healthy appearing, cordial person with various "neurotic" problems; a prim, proper identity; a sexually promiscuous "id" identity; and an angry identity prone to violence.
- A common nursing diagnosis for a client with DID admitted to an inpatient unit is high risk for violence.
- The major overall outcome for clients with DID focuses on consolidation or integration of all alternate personalities into one person who can experience the full range of life's emotions and personal and social relationships while carrying out ADLS.
- The usual and most effective treatment for DID is long-term, insight-oriented psychotherapy (individual sessions twice a week) combined with hypnosis or drug-assisted interviewing techniques. Medications for overt symptoms of anxiety or depression have an adjunctive role.

REFERENCES

American Nurses Association. (1994). *A statement on psychiatric-mental health clinical nursing practice and standards of psychiatric-mental health clinical nursing practice.* Washington, DC: Author.

American Psychiatric Association. (1994). *Diagnostic and statistical manual of mental disorders, fourth edition.* Washington, DC: Author.

Anonymous. (1994). Living and working with MPD…multiple personality disorder (MPD). *Journal of Psychosocial Nursing and Mental Health Services, 32*(8), 17-22, 48-29.

Anonymous. (1993). Coming out: My experience as a mental patient. *Journal of Psychosocial Nursing and Mental Health Services, 31*(5), 17-20, 34-35.

Anderson, G., & Ross, C. (1988, Oct/Nov/Dec). A model for psychiatric nurses working with clients who have multiple personality disorder. *Canadian Journal of Psychiatric Nursing, 4*:13-18.

Appelbaum, P.S., & Greer, A. (1994). Who's on trial? Multiple personalities and the insanity defense. *Hospital and Community Psychiatry, 45*(10), 963-966.

Bowers, K.S. (1991). Dissociation in hypnosis and multiple personality disorder. *International Journal of Clinical and Experimental Hypnosis, 39*(3), 155-176.

Chu, J. (1994). The rational treatment of multiple personality disorder. *Psychotherapy, 31*(1), 94-100.

Curtin, S. (1993). Recognizing multiple personality disorder. *Journal of Psychosocial Nursing, 31*(2), 29-33.

Davis, M., Eshelman, E.R., & McKay, M. (1995). *The relaxation & stress reduction workbook* (4th ed.). Oakland, CA: New Harbinger.

Edgerton, J.D., & Campbell, R.J. (Eds). (1994). *American psychiatric glossary,* (7th ed.). Washington, DC: American Psychiatric Press.

Grame, C. (1993). Internal containment in the treatment of patients with dissociative disorders. *Bulletin of Menninger Clinic, 57*(3), 355-361.

Grinspoon, L. (1992). Dissociation and dissociative disorder, part 1. *Harvard Mental Health Letter, 8*(9), 1-4.

Kaplan, H.I., Sadock, B.J., & Grebb, J.A. (1994). *Synopsis of psychiatry: Behavioral sciences, clinical psychiatry,* (7th ed.). Baltimore, MD: Williams & Wilkins.

Kolodner, G., & Frances, R. (1993). Recognizing dissociative disorders in patients with chemical dependency. *Hospital and Community Psychiatry, 44*(11), 1041-1043.

Kluft, R.P. (1991). Hospital treatment of multiple personality disorder: An overview. *Psychiatric Clinics of North America, 14*(3), 695-718.

Kluft, R.P., & Fine, C. (Eds.) (1993). *Clinical perspectives on multiple personality disorder.* Washington, DC: American Psychiatric Press.

Kluft, R.P. (1992). Enhancing the hospital treatment of dissociative disorder patients by developing nursing expertise in the application of hypnotic techniques without formal trance introduction. *American Journal of Clinical Hypnosis, 34*(3), 158-167.

Kluft, R.P. (1993). Multiple personality disorder: A contemporary perspective. *Harvard Mental Health Letter, 10*(4), 5-7.

Lego, S. (1988). Multiple personality disorder: An interpersonal approach to etiology, treatment, and nursing care. *Archives of Psychiatric Nursing, 2*(4), 19-24.

Lego, S. (1995). The client who has dissociative identity disorder. In S. Lego (Ed.), *Psychiatric nursing: A comprehensive reference.* Philadelphia: JB Lippincott.

Levin, A., & Spauster, E. (1994). Inpatient cognitive behavioral treatment of eating disorder patients with dissociative disorders. *Dissociation, VII*(3), 178-184.

McHugh, P.R. (1993). Multiple personality disorder. *Harvard Mental Health Letter, 10*(3), 4-6.

Miller, S. (1989). Optical differences in cases of multiple personality disorder. *Journal of Neurological and Mental Disorders, 177,* 480-486.

Offringra, G.A., & Goff, D. (1995). Dissociative disorder, psychosis, or both? *Harvard Review of Psychiatry, 3*(4), 22-226.

Putnam, F.W., & Lowenstein, R. (1993). Treatment of MPD: A survey of current practices. *American Journal of Psychiatry, 150*(7), 1048-1052.

Putnam, F.W. (1991a). Recent research on multiple personality disorder. *Psychiatric Clinics of North America, 14*(3), 489-501.

Putnam, F.W. (1991b). Dissociative phenomena. In A. Tasman (Ed.), *Annual review of psychiatry* (pp. 159-174). Washington, DC: American Psychiatric Press.

Putnam, F.W., Zahn, T., & Post, R. (1990). Differential autonomic nervous system activity in multiple personality disorder. *Psychiatry Research, 31,* 251-260.

Putnam, F.W. (1989). *Diagnosis and treatment of multiple personality disorder.* New York: Guilford Press.

Putnam, F.W. (1986). The scientific investigation of multiple personality disorder. In J.M. Quen (Ed.) *Split minds: Split brains.* New York: New York University Press.

Putnam, F.W. (1984). The psychophysiologic investigation of multiple personality disorder. *Psychiatric Clinics of North America, 7,* 31-39.

Ross, C.A., & Gahan, P. (1988). Techniques in the treatment of multiple personality disorder. *American Journal of Psychotherapy, 42*(1), 40-51.

Ross, C.A. (1989). *Multiple personality disorder. Diagnosis, clinical feature, and treatment.* New York: Wiley.

Ross, C.A. (1994). *Osiris complex: Case studies in multiple personality disorder.* Toronto: University of Toronto Press.

Sewter, M.J. (1995, October). *Psychological trauma and dissociation: From PTSD to DID.* Presented at the ninth annual conference of American Psychiatric Nurses Association, Philadelphia, PA.

Spiegel, D. & McHugh, P. (1995). The pros and cons of dissociative identity (multiple personality) disorder. *Journal of Practical Psychiatry and Behavioral Health, 9,* 158-163.

Stafford, L. (1993). Dissociation and multiple personality disorder: A challenge for psychosocial nurses. *Journal of Psychosocial Nursing, 31*(1), 15-20.

van der Kolk, B.A., & Fisler, R. (1995). Dissociation and the fragmentary nature of traumatic memories: Overview and exploratory study. *Journal of Traumatic Stress, 8,* 505-525.

Chapter 24

Post-Traumatic Stress Disorder

Carolyn Maynard
Sara Torres

LEARNING OUTCOMES

After studying and applying the concepts of this chapter, the learner will be able to:

- Identify situations, personal vulnerabilities, and cultural factors that increase the risk of traumatic stress.
- Recognize the biopsychosocial symptoms associated with the clinical profile of post-traumatic stress.
- Use epidemiological information and theories about post-traumatic stress and coping in risk identification and intervention.
- Identify some common psychotropic medications used to treat post-traumatic stress disorders (PTSD), including their side effects.
- Apply the nursing process to care of clients with PTSD.
- Use current theories about post-traumatic stress disorder in the formulation of nursing diagnoses and outcome criteria that reflect realistic progress toward resolution of distressing symptoms and in the selection of nursing interventions for clients with symptoms of post-traumatic stress.

KEY TERMS

Behavioral sensitization
Betrayal guilt
Comorbidity
Covictims
Depersonalization
Dissociation

Environment support
Fear conditioning
Flashback
Hyperarousal
Learned helplessness
Moral guilt

Psychogenic amnesia
Psychogenic fugue
Spiritual guilt
Stimulus generalization
Survivor guilt

Symptoms of post-traumatic stress disorder (PTSD) have been described since the earliest records of war. During the Civil War PTSD symptoms were labeled "soldier's heart" or "irritable heart." In World War I, these same symptoms were called "shell shock," and in World War II they were labeled "battle fatigue." The importance of post-traumatic stress was brought to the attention of the health care system and the public through the persistent symptoms, distress, and problems of Vietnam veterans. Clinical work and research with these veterans has contributed to an understanding of the situations, personal vulnerabilities, and symptoms associated with PTSD. Rarely were these symptoms related to exposure to other types of trauma, and little attention was paid to identifying and responding to such symptoms outside periods of war. Only over the past decade have trauma-related symptoms been clustered and applied to civilian trauma (Tomb, 1994).

There is an increasing understanding that PTSD occurs more often in the general population than first thought. The work of psychiatric nurse, Dr. Ann Burgess, on rape trauma victims has expanded the disorder beyond the wartime experience. As more communities experience violence, understanding the syndrome of feelings and behaviors that make up PTSD becomes increasingly important. Problems associated with PTSD extend beyond the individual client. All members of a family are affected when an individual develops post-traumatic symptoms.

The term *post-traumatic stress disorder* was created in the third edition of the *Diagnostic and Statistical Manual of Mental Disorders* (American Psychiatric Association [APA], 1980). The diagnosis was subsumed under the category of anxiety disorders (Tomb, 1994). The conceptualization of PTSD has evolved to include specific patterns of psychological responses to severe trauma of all types, including civilian catastrophes. PTSD generally refers to a syndrome of symptoms that occur in response to a perceived severe physical or emotional trauma. Anxiety is a pervasive aspect of life associated with a wide variety of human experiences and is usually manageable. Some events that involve death or threat of serious injury to the self or others may result in stress that is so intense, threatening, and severe that the individual may experience both an immediate crisis and a post-traumatic stress response. Reaction to the traumatic event includes intense fear, helplessness, or horror. Individuals experiencing PTSD report reexperiencing the event in a painful manner, with little control over the emergence of the memories. Generally there is avoidance of any reference or reminder of the trauma, and the individual attempts to numb the emotions to ward off the negative feelings associated with the situation. In an effort to identify and avoid any approaching reminders, persons with PTSD remain in a state of **hyperarousal** with persistent symptoms of increased arousal (not present before the trauma) in which there may be difficulty achieving relaxation due to increased anxiety. Although, acute anxiety is immediately associated with the traumatic event, the symptoms that lead to a diagnosis of PTSD may not develop for days, weeks, months, or even years after the event (Tomb, 1994). PTSD is typically managed on an outpatient basis. Hospitalization may be necessary if symptoms become severe or when there is a risk of severe depression with suicidal or other violent ideation or episodes. Inpatient care may also be prescribed if other problems such as substance abuse coincide with the PTSD symptoms.

The purpose of this chapter is to help nurses apply the nursing process to persons experiencing PTSD. Theories used to explain the development of the post-trauma phenomenon are discussed. Primary and co-morbid psychiatric diagnoses are presented. A clinical profile of characteristic symptoms is described with methods of assessment and interventions.

EPIDEMIOLOGY

Statistics on the extent of PTSD are not very accurate, because individuals involved in traumatic situations are not always identified and diagnosed. Some community-based studies have indicated that in the United States, there is a lifetime prevalence rate of PTSD ranging from 1% to 14% of the general population (APA, 1994). The group in which PTSD has been most widely studied and reported is combat veterans of the Vietnam War, although the disorder occurs in all age groups and follows traumatic events such as rape, physical abuse, accidents, catastrophic illnesses, major losses, community violence, and all types of natural and human origin disasters. Box 24-1 lists risk factors associated with the development of post-traumatic stress disorder (Ullman, 1994).

The incidence of chronic, persistent PTSD in Vietnam War veterans ranges from 2% to 15% (Vargas and Davidson, 1993). Findings from the congressionally mandated National Vietnam Veterans Readjustment Study estimated the lifetime prevalence of PTSD to be 30.9% among male combat veterans and 26% among female veterans. A lifetime prevalence of partial PTSD raised the percentage to 53.4% and 47.2% respectively (Weiss et al., 1992). Estimates of current prevalence are 15% for men and 8.5% for women (Friedman et al., 1994). Nearly 500,000 Vietnam veterans have been found to have PTSD 15 years after their military experiences (Schienger et al., 1992).

Prevalence rates of PTSD in Vietnam veterans differ among race/ethnic subgroups. A 13.7% current prevalence rate was found for caucasian and other men, whereas the rate rose to 20.6% among African-American men and 27.9% among Hispanic men (Schienger et al., 1992). Veterans who were more involved in combat were

Risk Factors Associated With the Development of Post-Traumatic Stress Disorder

Age—the young or old are more vulnerable
Unstable or problematic family
Domestic violence
Early separation from parents
Family history of anxiety or antisocial behavior
Physical and/or sexual abuse as a child
Problems with authorities and behaviors indicative of a
    conduct disorder
Depression
Ethnic minority status
Background of academic failure
Psychiatric treatment or hospitalization as a child
Substance abuse
Pretrauma emotional, cognitive, and behavioral problems
Blaming self for situations outside own control
Combat exposure
Prisoner of war during combat
Rape or sexual assault
Physical assault
Cultural and environmental factors
Lack of coping skills or resources

more likely to experience PTSD, regardless of race or ethnicity. Among prisoner of war (POW) veterans captured during the Korean War, nine out of ten survivors continue to experience PTSD 35 years after their release. The greater risk of PTSD among POWs is attributed to the exposure to forced marches, starvation, random killings, torture, and solitary confinement (*Emotional trauma haunts Korean POWs,* 1991).

Events that may precede traumatic stress symptoms include a wide variety of stressors. Although these stressful situations have a direct impact on the victims, there is also a traumatic effect on those who are indirectly involved. *Covictims are individuals who are more indirectly involved with catastrophic events but are also at risk for developing PTSD.* Covictims may receive exposure to traumatic situations through relationships with a victim, being an eyewitness to an occurrence, or while rescuing victims or providing care to them. Covictims include family members and friends and emergency medical, rescue, and police personnel who provide services during catastrophes. Nurses who care for traumatized clients on a regular basis may also be at risk of becoming covictims.

In general the degree of risk for covictims is determined by the intensity of their exposure to catastrophic events and their involvement with the victims. Children

often witness or experience acts of violence in their homes, streets, schools, and communities. Based on conservative estimates, more than 3 million persons are exposed to some type of traumatic event each year (Schwarz and Perry, 1994). A 6-month follow-up study found symptoms of PTSD among 33% of neighborhood women not directly involved in an incident in which 21 people were massacred and 15 were wounded (Hough et al., 1990).

THEORETICAL FRAMEWORK

There is no single theoretical explanation for the development and persistence of post-traumatic stress symptoms. There are theories that account for some but not all of the symptoms experienced by survivors. These include biological, behavioral, cognitive, and psychodynamic theories.

Biological Correlates

Long-standing alterations in the biological response to stress may contribute to a number of complaints commonly expressed by patients with PTSD. Biological theories of PTSD developed from both preclinical studies (animal models) and measures of biological variables of clinical populations with PTSD. The most common biological studies that correlate to PTSD focus on hormone and neurotransmitter deregulation in PTSD: neurobiological response to danger, norepinephrine, hypothalamic-pituitary-adrenal axis (HPA), and opiates (Kolb, 1993).

Trauma can cause alterations in an individual's neurological response to stress even years after the original insult. When a person is threatened, multiple neurobiological systems are activated. The activation of various brain regions and neurotransmitter systems represents an adaptive response that is critical for survival. Many neurotransmitters and hormones are important mediators in the development of anxiety and fear, as well as the subsequent behavioral fight-or-flight responses that protect an individual from impending danger. The neurotransmitter norepinephrine and adrenaline play a role in hyperarousal, as does endogenous opioids in reexperiencing traumatic events. Both have been implicated in the development of symptoms of PTSD. Measurements of heart rate, skin conductance, frontalis electromyogram, and urinary catecholamine, as well as studies of sleep, all suggest that PTSD has a biological basis (see Chapters 13 and 14).

For example, increased sensitivity and sensitization of the noradrenergic system may leave the individual in a hyperaroused, vigilant, sleep-deprived, and at times explosive state that worsens over time. To quiet these symptoms of hyperarousal, clients with PTSD often withdraw and use substances, particularly central nervous system depressants, that suppress peripheral and central catecholamine functions. Alterations in other neurobiological systems may further contribute to multiple symptoms such as intrusive memories, dissociation phenomena, and even numbing.

Finally, norepinephrine appears to play an important role in stimuli, selective attention, hypervigilance, autonomic arousal (i.e., increased blood pressure and pulse), and fear. The acute neurobiological response to trauma generally serves a protective role; it appears that for some individuals chronic responses may become maladaptive (Dinan et al., 1990). For example, it has been suggested that PTSD-related symptoms such as chronic hyperarousal, recurrent intrusive memories, passivity, and numbing develop in response to trauma-induced deregulation of multiple neurobiological systems.

Although it is normal for norepinephrine to increase under conditions of acute stress, there is evidence that certain types of stress, especially uncontrollable stress, can cause chronic maladaptive alterations in catecholaminergic systems. Exaggerated increases in heart rate and a rise in blood pressure, subjective distress, and plasma epinephrine during stress have been reported in combat veterans with PTSD (Blanchard et al., 1991).

Levels of endogenous opiates increase markedly during acute uncontrolled stress. This release of opiates causes a substantial degree of analgesia in both animals and humans (Pitman, 1990). Elevated levels of opioids during acute stress contribute to the observation that pain is often muted during the acute states of an injury. In fact, some combat veterans report feeling little or no pain when wounded in battle. With regard to chronic PTSD, it has been hypothesized that deregulation of endogenous opioids may contribute to avoidance and numbing symptoms.

Changes in catecholamine transmission have also been implicated in the disturbed sleep, nightmares, flashbacks, and startle reaction experienced by clients with PTSD (Kolb, 1993). Catecholamine alterations, which may have been triggered by the traumatic event, contribute to decreased dreaming (REM sleep) and deep sleep (stage four sleep), as well as increased dreaming during REM sleep (see Chapter 13). Based on this theory, flashbacks can be explained as waking nightmares caused by neurochemical derangements involving catecholamine transmission.

Characterization of the biological causes of PTSD relies on available neurobiological technology. With further advances in neurobiology technology in areas such as brain imaging, it soon will be possible to better delineate acute and long-term stress-induced changes in central and peripheral nervous system functioning.

Bioinformational processing and emotional network theories that encompass the interaction among sensory, affective, and cognitive information may, through future research, provide further insight into the relationship between the impact of a catastrophic event and development of post-traumatic symptoms. These theories currently propose that the intense bombardment of sensory stimuli, the excessive arousal of the sympathetic nervous system, the emotional response generated by the event, and the interpretation of the event are linked. The trauma forces this linkage by producing changes in cellular functioning and receptivity to information and altering neurochemical and hormonal substances and neurotransmitters. A persistent physiological learning and habituation (the pattern is engraved and consequently occurs automatically) is the result of these alterations. Hyperarousal and hyperactivity are established by these sudden and dramatic physiological changes associated with the trauma and thereafter are sustained by triggering mechanisms that arise from memories, emotions, and the environment.

The psychobiological patterns that develop predispose survivors to symptoms such as flashbacks, startle responses, persistent intrusive thoughts, sleep disturbances, and nightmares. The biologically habituated excessive arousal and neurochemical changes are reinforced by the linkage to the emotional system. Hyperarousal and hyperreactivity to emotional states interfere with the ability to discriminate among and interpret perceptual stimuli arising from the environment and those coming from memories of the traumatic event (Boudenyne and Hyer, 1990; Litz et al., 1992).

Cognitive/Behavioral Correlates

The major cognitive theories are the information processing model and the shattering of the assumptive world. Behavioral theories are based on both classical conditioning paradigms and two-factor learning theory. Learning theory has been used to explain the persistence of symptoms of anxiety, avoidance, and biological hyperarousal associated with PTSD.

Cognitive theory of stress, coping, and adaptation proposes that what one thinks and feels influences behavior. Cognitive appraisal is a powerful predictor of whether coping is focused on the regulation of emotions or on problem solving (Lazarus and Folkman, 1984). Managing emotions that severely limit or exclude cognitive problem solving predisposes survivors to dysfunctional coping. The interpretation of an event that flows from cognitive appraisals is a subjective process that may or may not reflect the objective reality. If the cognitive appraisal is distorted by prior experiences that produced psychobiological changes, the emotional and behavioral responses tend to be inappropriate (Lazarus and Folkman, 1984). A distorted appraisal of the traumatic experience may interfere with the ability to attach a meaning to the event, which allows for healing the psychological wounds of trauma, and may limit the use of personal and social resources that would facilitate resolution of the trauma.

The information processing model emphasizes the impact of trauma on cognition and control (defenses) in regulating the processing of information. This theory proposes that until the traumatic event can be integrated into existing cognitive schema, the psychological representations of the event are stored in inactive memory, which has an intrinsic property of repeated representation.

The *shattering of the assumptive world* theory postulates that individuals hold the following major assumptions disrupted by trauma:

- The belief in personal invulnerability
- The perception of the world as meaningful
- The perception of the self as positive

The disruption of these assumptions destabilizes the entire personality, producing a state of disequilibrium characterized by symptoms of PTSD. For example, to reestablish equilibrium, the individual must develop a modified set of assumptions that can assimilate the trauma. The cognitive/behavioral processes that appear to be particularly related to PTSD include the following:

- Fear conditioning
- Behavioral sensitization
- Memory
- Learned helplessness

Fear conditioning is a response that occurs when an individual experiences a life-threatening trauma in which a wide variety of stimuli present at the time of the trauma become related or conditioned to the attendant feelings of terror and extreme anxiety. As a result, previously neutral stimuli become capable of evoking these same feelings of terror (Orr, 1990). For example, the smell of burning firewood—a neutral stimulus—can become a conditioned stimulus for a survivor of a life-threatening fire. After the fire, the smell of burning wood no longer evokes feelings of comfort and peace but instead of fear and terror. Both specific (e.g., the location or time of the trauma) and nonspecific cues associated with the traumatic event are capable of becoming conditioned stimuli. It also appears that *stimuli similar to those associated with the trauma, can at times become conditioned stimuli referred to as* **stimulus generalization.** Furthermore, it is possible for a conditioned stimulus to condition other neutral stimuli that are present when the conditioned stimulus evokes a state of terror or fear (higher order conditions). The result may be an individual who becomes fearful and anxious in response to a wide variety of stimuli (Butler et al., 1990).

Behavioral sensitization refers to an enhanced response to repeated presentations of stimuli. The time interval between the initial stimuli and subsequent stimuli still appears to be an important variable. If sufficient time has passed between the initial presentation and subsequent reexposure, a single stressful stimulus can elicit behavioral sensitization (Antelman, 1988).

Exposure to a potent stressor increases the capacity of a subsequent stressor to increase dopamine formation in the forebrain. Clinically, increased arousal, hypervigilance, insomnia, poor concentration, autonomic hyperactivity, and exaggerated startle response are all seen in clients with chronic PTSD. For some clients these symptoms do not diminish over time but instead increase. It has been suggested that this increase may constitute a form of behavioral sensitization.

PTSD is in large part a disorder of memory. Intrusive recollections of trauma in the form of recurrent daytime memories, nightmares, and flashbacks are characteristic of the disorder (Squire, 1991). These intrusive recollections often remain vivid for the individual's lifetime and can be reawakened or triggered by a variety of stimuli. Most individuals who have PTSD find these intrusive recollections highly distressing and in some cases, tormenting. Traumatic events cause an overstimulation of endogenous stress-response hormones and neuromodulators, and these substances cause an overconsolidation of memory or superconditioning. This overconsolidation may account for subsequent recurrent intrusive memories.

It has been suggested that overconsolidation or indelible memories may have survival value (McGaugh, 1990). For self-preservation, it is critical to remember events that occur during an aroused state of alarm. Failure to remember such situations makes one vulnerable to similar dangers in the future. The intrusive nature of memories, nightmares, and flashbacks seen in PTSD may be an unfortunate side effect or consequence of a neurobiological mechanism that essentially serves a protective role. Dangerous situations are remembered but unfortunately, in some cases, cannot be forgotten. Although at times these traumatic memories intrude for no apparent reason, they often occur in response to particular stimuli that evoke the memory.

A learned helplessness paradigm has often been used as a way of conceptualizing post-trauma reactions that include chronic depression, passivity, and futility. **Learned helplessness** *results when persons believe or expect that their responses will not influence the future probability of environmental outcomes.* Helplessness reduces the motivation to control an outcome and leads individuals to conclude that they have no influence on outcomes. Mere exposure to an uncontrollable event is not sufficient to produce helplessness, rather the perception that future events are uncontrollable results in learned helplessness. Depression may develop as the result of feeling powerless to control events.

The *Nursing Process*

Assessment

Clinical Profile

Acute PTSD is diagnosed if symptoms occur 1 month after exposure and last less than 3 months. Symptoms lasting 3 months or longer are termed *chronic*. If onset of symptoms occurs at least 6 months following the traumatic event, the diagnosis specifies "delayed onset" (APA, 1994). The immediate post-trauma symptoms are usually classified as part of a crisis stress response and may be labeled as an acute stress disorder if symptoms occur within 4 weeks and are resolved within that period. If symptoms persist for more than 1 month and other criteria are met, the diagnosis is changed to PTSD (APA, 1994). Acute stress disorder, during the first month after a trauma, can appear identical to the PTSD that occurs after 1 month (Tomb, 1994). There is some evidence that a diagnosis of acute stress disorder carries an increased risk for a later diagnosis of PTSD (Koopman et al., 1995).

Events that precipitate PTSD are outside the range of typical human experiences. The circumstances of traumatic events are so overwhelming, unpredictable, horrifying, and sometimes life-threatening that they generate feelings of fear, confusion, powerlessness, and helplessness. The traumatic aspects of the event bombard the victim's senses, information-processing capacities, emotional system, and coping resources. The intense and excessive flood of sensory stimuli and the life-threatening aspects of the event affect the person's physical, cognitive, emotional, physiological, behavioral, and spiritual dimensions.

Symptoms of Post-Traumatic Stress Disorder

Box 24-2 highlights the symptoms that may be observed in persons with PTSD and which encompass the cognitive, affective, physiological, behavioral, and relational domains (APA, 1994; Shaley, 1990). Clients with post-traumatic stress tend to have a low level of stress tolerance. Their sense of self is impaired, their personalities are fragmented, and they have difficulties with role and social functioning (Shives, 1994). Recognizing PTSD may be complicated by the fact that symptoms of post-traumatic stress persist over time or do not develop until some time after the trauma. In some instances, symptoms may remain latent for many years. Often, the symptoms wax and wane over time when avoidance is operative (Blank, 1994). Some of the symptoms accompanying PTSD, which may be particularly problematic, include hypervigilance and physiological arousal, guilt, dissociation (depersonalization, psychogenic amnesia and fugue, and flashbacks), and avoidance of situations, sounds, and persons who might trigger PTSD symptoms.

Hypervigilance and physiological arousal

Survivors of life-threatening traumatic events are often left with a continuing sense of being in danger. Because traumatic events tend to occur without warning, these persons behave physiologically and psychologically as if another such incident might be waiting to happen. Unprepared and overwhelmed at the time of the traumatic incident, survivors attempt to prepare themselves for the next catastrophic event by being hypervigilant to signs of impending danger. Their conscious or unconscious intention is to ward off such events. The hypervigilance exhibited by survivors is accompanied by psychological and physiological arousal. Survivors are always ready to activate a fight-or-flight response. This readiness and defensive wariness are evident in their startle response to noise or any stimuli associated with the traumatic event. Fireworks elicit an exaggerated startle response in the combat veteran exposed to life-threatening gunfire on the battlefield.

The traumatic experience transforms the response to the perceived threat into a pattern of constant arousal, regardless of whether an actual threat is present (Blank, 1994). Pervasive anxiety is another consequence of this hyperalertness (see Chapter 22). The legacy of the traumatic event and of its unexpected occurrence appear to alter the physiological stress response, resulting in sleep difficulties and problems with memory and concentration. Irritability often is a presenting symptom with outbursts of temper and periods of aggressiveness. The following clinical example illustrates these symptoms:

> Adam survived a terrorist bombing of a cafe. Since that experience, he has been continuously anxious and hyperalert. When in any type of public restaurant or bar, he insists on being seated near the door. While eating, he continuously scans the room and entryway. He eats rapidly, watching the room and only occasionally glancing at his food. He leaves immediately and will not sit and socialize.

Guilt

In addition to the pervasive anxiety experienced by survivors of traumatic situations, guilt is an important and

The Nursing Process

Box 24-2

Post-Traumatic Stress Symptoms

COGNITIVE SYMPTOMS

Difficulty concentrating

Recurrent and intrusive recollections of traumatic experiences

Sudden reliving traumatic experiences: illusions, hallucinations

Dissociative experiences: psychogenic amnesia (inability to recall important aspect of trauma)

Anniversary reactions associated with traumatic event

Avoidance of thoughts associated with traumatic event

Impaired future orientation related to career, marriage, family

Recurring vivid dreams/nightmares

Perception of reality that is unconventional and often distorted

Self-blame

Lack of cognitive integration of traumatic event

Perceived vulnerability: perception of threat and danger in innocuous/neutral situations

Absolutist thinking

Problem solving overridden by anger and anxiety

AFFECTIVE SYMPTOMS

Irritability, explosive angry outbursts

Intense distress when confronted with events that symbolize or resemble some aspect of traumatic experience

Avoidance of feelings associated with traumatic event

Restricted range of affect

Unable to experience loving feelings

Diminished or constricted responsiveness: emotional anesthesia (psychic numbing)

Emotional liability

Feelings of guilt

Inability to enjoy activities

Feelings of depression

Symptoms of anxiety: nervousness, jumpiness, jitters, panic attacks

Feelings of alienation or detachment

Phobias

PHYSIOLOGICAL SYMPTOMS

Difficulty falling or staying asleep

Exaggerated startle response

Physiological reactivity in the presence of stimuli that reactivate memories, feelings, or sensations associated with trauma

Hypervigilance/hyperalertness

High resting heart rate and blood pressure, increased urinary catecholamine

BEHAVIORAL SYMPTOMS

Phobic avoidance of situations that elicit recall of traumatic event

Diminished interest and participation in significant activities

Psychogenic fugue: unexpected travel away from home, assumption of a new identity

Restlessness

Impulsiveness: sudden trips, unexplained absences, changes in lifestyle or residence

Difficulty completing tasks

Episodes of unpredictable aggressiveness

Substance abuse: alcohol, street drugs

Chemical dependency on prescribed antianxiety or pain relief medications used to treat emotional distress and/or physical pain after traumatic event

Self-mutilation: attempt to end feelings of depersonalization

Sexual dysfunction

RELATIONSHIP SYMPTOMS

Detachment, estrangement, and isolation from others

Impaired ability to experience intimacy, tenderness, and sexuality

Impaired marital relationships

Impaired parent relationships

Excessive interpersonal distance from others, related to fear of betrayal that was experienced in the past with an officer who put a patrol in unnecessary danger or a physically or sexually abusive parent, husband, mugger, or rapist

Avoidance of personal disclosure related to mistrust of others and fear of rejection

The Nursing Process

distressing aspect of the post-traumatic response. The factors that generate post-traumatic guilt may be related to real or perceived harmful actions or a failure to use actions required to survive. When guilt negatively influences thinking, feelings, behavior, and relationships with others, it impairs the survivor's ability to resolve the post-traumatic stress response. There are three types of guilt associated with post-traumatic stress: survivor, moral or spiritual, and betrayal (Opp and Samson, 1989).

Survivor guilt is characterized by self-blame and regret consequent to losing a significant person in combat, a disaster, or an accident. It is related to the life-threatening nature of the traumatic situation that may lead to a distortion of reality and regression to magical thinking. Survivors struggle with the meaning of their being alive while others died. It is sometimes difficult for individuals to recognize and accept that their escape from disaster and their survival were by chance and not necessarily something they caused or an abandonment of those who were unable to make their way to safety (Opp and Samson, 1989). A clinical example of survivor guilt is illustrated in the following case study of Lucy.

Lucy was at work when a dam broke and flooded the area around her home. Her children and husband were at home when the dam broke. Because there had been no warning of the impending catastrophe, they were swept away by the wall of water that destroyed their home. Lucy experienced acute guilt after the loss, based on her perception that had she been home she could have helped her family reach safety. She has difficulty accepting the reality that she would not have been able to make a difference and would have also perished in the flood.

Moral or spiritual guilt is characterized by self-blame and regret generated by actions that caused harm or death in a catastrophe. *Moral or spiritual guilt may occur when persons sought their own safety first and made no effort to help others, particularly family members, when such help was possible or perceived as possible during a catastrophe* (Opp and Samson, 1989). A clinical example of moral guilt follows:

Tom was on a train when it derailed. His immediate reaction after the train stopped careening down a slope into a gully was to get out. He escaped with minor bruises and lacerations caused by pushing out a window in his escape. After escaping, he discovered that the woman and child sitting opposite him were trapped, and when a fire broke out, they died in the fire. Tom, because he felt he should have rescued them, experienced moral guilt.

Betrayal guilt is characterized by self-blame and regret consequent to a deliberate harmful action toward another during a traumatic situation that involved violation of trust. For example, hostages or POWs who align with their captors and spy on other members of their group to gain special treatment or privileges experience betrayal guilt, particularly when their actions are harmful or deadly. In a rape situation, the covictim survivor may feel guilty for not being home when the rapist broke in (Opp and Samson, 1989). The following case study of Sam illustrates betrayal guilt:

Sam fell asleep while on guard duty in Vietnam. As he slept, the enemy was able to sneak up on his unit and open fire. The other personnel in his unit were killed. After his discharge from the Army, he suffered distressing guilt about exposing his friends to mortal danger.

Dissociation

Dissociation involves the disconnection or separation of one part of memory from another. In dissociation, specific memories are inaccessible because they are associated with very negative and painful feelings (Yates and Nasby, 1993). Persons who experience dissociative episodes may have feelings of unreality. Some sexual abuse and rape survivors report floating out of their bodies and looking down at the traumatic situation. Post-traumatic stress symptoms that are particularly disturbing involving dissociative experiences are depersonalization, psychogenic amnesia and fugues, and flashbacks.

Depersonalization

Depersonalization is characterized by an alteration in the perception or experience of the self in which the usual sense of one's own reality is temporarily lost or changed. The person feels detached from the self. Persons may feel as if they are outside themselves and able to observe their own actions and mental processes. Some describe the experience as feeling outside their bodies, feeling like a robot, or as if in a dream. A sense of not being in complete control of one's actions, including speech, may be experienced. Reality testing remains intact, however. During a depersonalization episode, perception of the environment may be altered in relation to the size or shape of objects. These episodes may occur spontaneously, beginning and ending abruptly. They are usually precipitated by anxiety or depression, which may be related to a person, place, or thing that triggers memories of the trauma. The following clinical example illustrates depersonalization:

Karen was a guest in a resort hotel when a fire broke out and raged rapidly through the first floor and upward through the elevator shafts and stairwells. She was able to escape through

The Nursing Process

a broken window. She received lacerations and burns that were serious but not life-threatening. While making her way toward safety and waiting for medical attention, she observed other guests screaming in pain because their clothes were ablaze, leaping to their deaths from upper-story windows and being carried out and put into body bags. Her husband, who had been attending a meeting in a room without windows, was unable to escape and died in the fire.

About 5 months after the disaster, Karen sought psychiatric help. During the admission interview she stated, "I'm losing my mind." She described being on a business trip and checking into a hotel, when suddenly she felt as if she were floating above her body and watching herself go through the motions of signing the registry and requesting a particular room. The episode ended as suddenly as it began. While getting ready for bed later that evening, she suddenly saw the room ablaze. She could smell smoke, but the flames were not consuming the furnishings. She ran into the hallway screaming and was comforted by other guests. She returned to her room. The house physician was called, who prescribed and administered an antianxiety medication.

Psychogenic amnesia
Psychogenic amnesia, which is associated with post-traumatic stress, *tends to be localized. It usually involves the loss of memories of a specified period related to a traumatic event or circumstance. The memory loss is sudden, unrelated to organic mental disorder, and too great to be explained as simple forgetfulness. The person is usually aware of the inability to recall what occurred.*

Psychogenic fugue
Psychogenic fugue is characterized by sudden unexpected travel, usually away from home to another geographical area; assumption of a new identity; and the inability to recall one's real identity and the event that precipitated the trip and relocation. In some instances the person may manifest a personality that is diametrically opposed to the previous identity. The quiet person becomes outgoing, and the gregarious person becomes withdrawn and socially isolated. The following is an example of psychogenic fugue:

John was a passenger on a plane that developed problems and was forced to land before reaching its destination. During the landing, the plane veered off the runway, causing injury and death among the passengers including John's business partner, who was seated next to him. John walked away from the plane unharmed. He rented a car, refusing to continue the trip by plane, and drove away in the opposite direction of his original destination. During the next 3 days he

traveled until nightfall and stopped at motels where he paid cash and signed the register "Albert Smith." On the morning of the third day he located a furnished room, turned in the rental car, and applied for a job as the night manager in a small seedy hotel. John worked at this job for the next 6 months. Before the accident he had been an outgoing and successful salesman. Since leaving the scene of the accident, he avoided talking with others and isolated himself. He awoke one morning, feeling confused about where he was and how he had gotten there.

Flashbacks
Flashbacks are vivid images of experiences of a traumatic event or circumstance that force their way unbidden into a person's awareness. These images may or may not be accompanied by related emotions. Affect flashbacks consist of sudden "pangs" of emotion that are related to the event (Blank, 1994). The following is a clinical example of flashbacks:

Carl was in a restaurant when a terrorist bomb exploded, killing several patrons. He received severe injuries but recovered without complications or disabilities. Three months after the incident he began to have nightmares that were violent, bloody portrayals of the bombing. Shortly thereafter, vivid memories of the explosion and its aftermath occurred while he was at work, watching television, and socializing with friends. The intrusiveness and unpredictability of the recollections became so real that on several occasions, while at work, Carl dove under his desk for protection. After these flashbacks, his work and social life became increasingly impaired.

Avoidance of triggers
Avoidance of the triggers that activate negative feelings is an important dimension of the post-traumatic stress response. Persons with PTSD have intense emotions such as horror, grief, and shame related to the traumatic situation. These feelings are often kept outside of the awareness by avoidance of places, persons, and things that trigger memories, feelings, or flashbacks about the traumatic event. Persons who develop PTSD may experience acute distress when flashbacks and intrusive memories occur. They sometimes go to any length to protect themselves from exposure to situations reminiscent of the original trauma. The avoidance behavior and numbing of emotions are demoralizing and contribute to social isolation. As individuals numb their emotions, they lose interest in current events, and their abilities to feel or experience normal emotions decrease. This response is often associated with depression (Tomb, 1994). The following clinical example illustrates how avoidance of trig-

The Nursing Process

gers manifested itself in Carl, who was discussed in the preceding clinical example:

> Carl refused to go to a restaurant. He experienced acute episodes of physiological arousal, hyperalertness, and fear if he walked by a restaurant. To prevent this from happening, he established a pattern of deliberately choosing to walk blocks out of his way, taking a route that would keep him from passing a restaurant.

Comorbidity

Comorbidity, which is the coexistence of disorders, often occurs with PTSD. The comorbid conditions found most often include substance abuse, generalized anxiety disorder, unipolar major depression, suicidal ideation, atypical psychosis, antisocial and borderline personality disorders, dissociative symptoms, obsession-compulsion, and intermittent explosive disorder (Bremner et al., 1992; Brown and Wolfe, 1994; Goodwin, Cheeves, and Connell, 1990; Keane and Wolfe, 1990; Kramer et al., 1994; Machell, 1993). Almost half of persons with PTSD also have symptoms of major depression, and 80% of combat veterans with PTSD have alcoholism (Post-traumatic Stress: Part I, 1991).

Addiction to prescribed antianxiety drugs has also been found among survivors of traumatic events. Individuals with PTSD often report having more general health problems (Litz et al., 1992). More research is needed on the prevalence and incidence of comorbid disorders among survivors of trauma.

Environmental Factors

Environmental support refers to individuals who support victim's and covictims of trauma. Such individuals can be family members, significant others, and/or professionals and nonprofessionals in the community. Ideally, survivors need to talk about traumatic experiences immediately after the event. Crisis intervention is essential (see Chapter 10). The risk of persistent or delayed onset of post-traumatic stress symptoms increases when the debriefing process is postponed or absent (Walker, 1990). Children and adults with impaired intellectual capacities may be unable to articulate what happened to them because they lack the vocabulary or understanding. Adolescents and adults may be inhibited from disclosing the incident because of shame, humiliation, or fear.

One of the most influential factors that increases the severity and persistence of the post-traumatic stress response is the victim's or co-victim's inability to talk about the event or circumstances and associated feelings. Inadequate or perceived lack of supportive family and social relationships may also impair both immediate and long-term coping (Green et al., 1990; Moss, Frank, and Anderson, 1990). Among Vietnam veterans, personal factors that predispose them to persistent and distressing post-trauma symptoms and have a negative impact on adjustment include the following: having grown up in a family that had a "hard time making ends meet," having had symptoms of drug abuse or dependence before entering the military, having had symptoms of an affective disorder before entering the service, and having had behavior problems during childhood. These factors probably also predispose nonmilitary persons who are exposed to traumatic events (Buydens-Branchey, 1990; Moss, Frank, and Anderson, 1990).

Community and societal support for survivors of traumatic events are also important in treating PTSD. Survivors who lack accessible, supportive crisis follow-up and outreach mental health care services have an increased risk of PTSD. Recovery is also hampered by unrealistic expectations that recovery time will be brief and negative societal attitudes that ignore or blame the survivors for their residual problems.

Conducting an Assessment

The nurse should begin the assessment process with statements that facilitate disclosure ("Tell me about") and questions that help clients describe their symptoms and problems. Information is collected about the following:

- The circumstances that precipitated the symptoms
- Description of the event and its impact
- The timeframe for onset of current symptoms
- Coping strategies immediately after the trauma

Specific symptoms should be identified along with subjective statements about perceptions of and feelings about their symptoms. The nurse identifies whether the symptoms have persisted since the traumatic event, have occurred periodically, or appeared at a later time. If there was a delay, the circumstances of their appearance are explored to determine if they were precipitated by an anniversary reaction and occurred shortly before or at the time of year when the traumatic event occurred. The nurse should elicit information about interpersonal relationships and feelings toward others.

Numbing may lead to emotional isolation, so it is important to identify the client's feelings of estrangement and whether there is a perceived support system. The nurse should identify whether the client has been able to discuss the event and symptoms with others and exam-

The Nursing Process

ine whether the client has experienced trauma in the past. Conducting an assessment of whether domestic abuse or any type of victimization has occurred is strongly emphasized.

Other important actions to take during the assessment process include the following:

- Assist the client to recognize that feelings about the catastrophe are normal.
- Encourage the client to share with others who have experienced similar situations.
- Identify client's perceptions of fear and feelings of powerlessness.
- Discuss problems and methods of coping the client used prior to the traumatic event.
- Assist the client to label feelings and experiences; this is the first step in acquiring control.

Cultural issues

The assessment and treatment of PTSD in different cultural groups is complicated by several factors. One is acculturation, the process of assimilating into the host culture. This may be undermined by past violence and current adverse conditions, which may lead to biopsychosocial maladjustment. Another factor is the expertise of the nurse because working with individuals from diverse groups requires special education, experience, and supervision. There are several issues to consider in assessing PTSD in diverse cultural groups, including the following:

- The basic symptom picture of PTSD across cultures is similar to that observed in American trauma victims.
- Where, when, and how to work with translators is an important first step.
- Methods for establishing rapport across cultures require special training and supervision

The Cultural Highlights box below provides important cultural assessment data to be considered in the treatment of refugees.

Screening Tools

Common screening tools used for PTSD include self-report measures, structured interviews, and objective

CULTURAL HIGHLIGHTS

Assessment of Post-Traumatic Stress Disorder Symptoms in Refugees

1. Preflight occupation, social status, coping mechanisms, psychiatric disorders

2. Reasons for initiating the flight from the mother country

3. Client's willingness to leave, along with the amount of care and deliberation given to the decision (i.e., many leave unwillingly because family members of fellow villagers are leaving; decisions may be careful and balanced after due deliberation or precipitously made in a moment of fear)

4. Nature and duration of the flight; with losses, traumatic events, injuries, and other experiences during the flight

5. Experiences (positive and negative) in countries of refuge

6. Losses as a result of the flight (e.g., relationships, social roles and status, property, vocations and avocations, and daily activities)

7. Elements of continuity from preflight to postflight life (e.g., language, household members, religion, occupation, sports, and hobbies)

8. Problems in the new country (e.g., language, finances, marital or family disruption, affiliation with expatriate community, and security from assault and theft)

9. Behaviors and affiliations in the new country (e.g., number of indigenous friends, citizenship, and use of indigenous resources and institutions such as banks or political parties)

10. Feelings about the new country, its culture and people, and prospects of living out one's life in the new country (e.g., clarification about wanting to return to country-of-origin and location and content of any dreams).

Based on data from Westmeyer, J. (1989). Journal of Traumatic Stress, 2(4), 515-547.

The Nursing Process

measures. Two of the most common tools are the Mississippi Scale Post-Traumatic Stress Disorder and the Clinician-Administered Post-Traumatic Stress Disorder. One of the most commonly used is the professionally administered Weschler Adult Intelligence Scale-Revised (WAIS-R), which is used to assess difficulties such as learning, attention, memory, and concentration. Most of these tools focus on the DSM-IV criteria for PTSD. It is important to recognize that the scores on any one instrument are not sufficient to make a diagnosis of PTSD. Assessment of PTSD needs to include evaluations of developmental, social, familial, educational, vocational, medical, cognitive, interpersonal, behavioral, and emotional functioning. An individual's pretrauma functioning, as well as assessment of the trauma experience and the subsequent symptom picture, must also be explored. Repeated assessments over a period of time are helpful because of the longitudinal fluctuations seen in the development of PTSD.

Much work remains to be done, especially in adapting the instruments well-known in a combat-related PTSD setting to civilian-related trauma. Possible gender and racial/cultural influences on the assessment of PTSD need to be explored. In addition, it is important to conduct a complete physical examination, since general medical conditions may occur as consequences of trauma (e.g., head injury or burns).

Nursing Diagnosis

Post-trauma response is the primary nursing diagnosis used with survivors of catastrophes who experience persistent symptoms or a delayed reaction. A nursing care plan for this nursing diagnosis based on specific client data is presented on p. 446. The two DSM-IV diagnoses used for these individuals are PTSD and acute stress disorder.

Outcome Identification

Although the nursing care plan lists specific outcome criteria for the client, a discussion of overall client outcome criteria is warranted. The immediate goals of nursing interventions are to help clients experience some degree of relief from their symptoms and initiate the healing process. Both long-term and short-term goals are identified. Evidence of progress toward effective coping and resolution of symptoms is reflected in the following outcome criteria:

- Makes a contract to talk with family or significant others and health professionals or staff about feelings of frustration rather than act on them

- Has increased episodes of reexperiencing event
- Verbalizes the relationship between episodes of anxiety and exposure to sounds and circumstances symbolic of the traumatic event
- Demonstrates mastery of two coping strategies
- Verbally acknowledges self-imposed social isolation
- Initiates grieving process by talking about losses incurred by the traumatic event
- Describes how logical thinking and problem solving revised perception of fear-inducing thoughts
- Uses problem-solving and decision-making skills in the assignment of meaning to the traumatic event
- Verbally acknowledges the choice of behaviors that reinforce feelings of estrangement and alienation
- Makes future plans
- Specifies aspects of past and current situations that contribute to a sense of powerlessness
- Replaces self-blame with acceptance of the unpredictability of the traumatic event
- Shares feelings with significant others
- Gets sufficient sleep and rest
- Actively participates in social groups

Each of these general outcome criteria is individualized for clients based on assessment data.

Planning

The intervention section of the nursing care plan found on p. 446 illustrates the interventions of the planning aspect of the nursing process. The interdisciplinary treatment plan presented on p. 447 details the contributions of all members of the health care team.

Implementation

Nursing care of clients who experience post-trauma response include both independent and collaborative interventions. Such interventions are implemented according to the nurses level of basic or advanced practice as discussed in Chapters 2 and 5.

Counseling

Counseling is an essential nursing intervention for clients with PTSD. Clients must feel that the nurse is accepting and nonjudgmental. Mutual respect and openness are essential. The nurse carefully monitors evolution of the relationship to ensure that development of dependence on the nurse is not fostered.

Interventions include verbal recognition of the emotional pain experienced by clients and empathetic responses to their expressed distress. The nurse must

NURSING CARE PLAN

Post-Trauma Response

NURSING ASSESSMENT DATA

Subjective: "I can't think about anything except the explosion." "I get so anxious I can't do anything right." "I keep feeling like it is all my fault it happened." "Whenever I think about it, I can't breathe and my heart beats fast." "I have difficulty sleeping, because I have nightmares that wake me up." "I just don't seem to care about my job or anyone else now." "I get so angry and upset, but I keep it bottled up inside." Wife reports preoccupation is interfering with work and relationships at home. *Objective:* tense facial muscles, wringing of hands, pacing; *DSM-IV diagnosis:* Post-traumatic stress disorder.

NANDA Diagnosis: Post-trauma response related to experience of surviving explosion at workplace 6 months ago

Outcomes	Interventions	Rationale	Evaluation
Short term	• Develop nurse-client relationship; see NIC interventions for anxiety reduction, calming technique, cognitive restructuring, coping, and sleep enhancement	• Nurse-client relationship fosters self-acceptance and self-esteem.	**Short term**
1. Will accurately perform relaxation exercises *within 1 week.*			1, 2. Met in 1 week
2. Will participate in social activity with family *within 1 week.*		• There is evidence that the identified NIC interventions for support-system enhancement are effective.	3, 4, 5. Met in 2 weeks
3. Will relate increased amount of sleep *within 2 weeks.*	• Use contracting for desired behaviors	• Contracting is a basic concept in behavioral therapy.	**Long term**
4. Will express relief from feeling responsible for explosion *within 2 weeks.*	• Teach client relaxation exercises and guided imagery and encourage use at first symptoms of anxiety and before attempting to sleep	• Relaxation and guided imagery exercises provide the control that decreases anxiety.	1. Partially met in 1 month; experiencing ability to meet expected demands at work; however, still reports occasional episodes feeling stress related to event during breaks
5. Will report a decrease in somatic symptoms (pacing, wringing of hands, tense muscles, palpitations) *within 2 weeks.*	• Assist client in identifying support group and begin discussing traumatic experience	• Allows client to know that others understand and accept feelings; provides support and opportunity to reduce impact of event by talking about it.	2. Met in 1 month
Long term *Within 1 month:*	• Use cognitive restructuring techniques to assist client in gaining a realistic appraisal of role in the event	• Assist client in gaining a realistic appraisal of role in the event and to identify realistic life goals.	3. Partially met; sleeps three nights without awaking because of nightmares; review relaxation and other sleep-enhancing techniques and continue for 2 weeks
1. Will report ability to concentrate at job.	• Assist client in identifing source of angry feelings and developing constructive coping methods for expressing anger	• Angry feelings cannot be worked through until source is identified. Healthful coping methods are necessary to function at optimal levels of ADLS.	4. Partially met; reports awareness that anger was directed primarily at self; recognizes when angry with others and has had success with dealing directly with anger; has not been consistent with implementation; review and role-play; continue for 4 weeks
2. Will report improved relationships with family.			
3. Will sleep five of seven nights without waking.			
4. Will report relief of feelings of anger.	• Work with family to teach about disorder and identify methods of assisting client	• Involves family in client's treatment and strengthens support systems.	5. Met in 1 month
5. Will verbalize realistic future plans.			

INTERDISCIPLINARY TREATMENT PLAN

Critical Pathway: Anxiety 300.OX; Panic 300.OX, PTSD 309-89

Patient Name: _____ Case Manager: _____ Physician: _____ Medical Record #: _____
Admit date: _____ Expected LOS: _____ UR days certified: _____ Discharge Date: _____ Actual LOS: _____

Day/Date:	0–8 Hours	8–24 Hours	Day 2	Day 3	Day 4	Day 5
ASSESSMENTS AND EVALUATIONS	Nursing Nutritional screen Admit note Precautions	H & P, Social HX, RT/TA; Dr: Initial TX Plan/Admit Note, AIMS Assess sleep patterns	Precaution Evaluation	Psych Eval done Social Hx on chart Precaution Evaluation Assess for level of care	Assess for readiness for discharge	Assess for goals achieved
PROCEDURES	Lab ordered-Admit profile UA, UDS, UCG, EKG, Other:	Lab done: UA, UDS, UCG, EKG, Other:	Lab results checked Abnormals called to Dr.	Follow-up for abnormal lab results		
CONSULTS	IT ordered Y/N FT ordered Y/N GT ordered Y/N Psych Testing Order Y/N	GT started Psych Testing done	Schedule MTP meeting	IT started, FT started Psych Testing Results Home Contract		
TREATMENT PLANNING	NI: Axis III	RT/TA started	RT/TA started School started (youth)	Master TX Plan Updated RT/TA entry	MTP reflects psych testing results	Assess client support network
INTERVENTIONS	Assess Suicidal/Aggressive potential	Communicate in calm nonthreatening manner	Low stimuli; identification of causative factors	Explore anxiety triggers	Help develop and rehearse problem-solving skills	Encourage independent decision making
MEDICATIONS	Meds ordered, Informed Consent		Drug interaction checked by Pharmacist/Dr. signs informed consent	Antianxiety meds as short term intervention only	Meds evaluated/readjusted	Discharge instructions for medication self-admin
LEVEL TEACHING	Level ordered Patient Rights Orient to Unit	Orient to Program	Reevaluate Medication Teaching Stress Reduction; Goals	Reevaluate for PHP Meds reinforced; Positive coping mechanism	Reevaluate for D/C Decision making; Relaxation techniques	Reevaluate Promote self-reliance and diversional activities
NUTRITION/DIET CONTINUUM OF CARE	Diet Ordered: Initial D/C Plans	Chart daily intake Outcome survey	Chart daily intake Evaluate support system	Weight, chart intake D/C Plan update/revise	Chart daily intake After Care Plan written	Diet D/C instruction Outcome survey
PATIENT OUTCOMES	Controls self-harm/aggr.	Patient feels more secure	Anxiety levels decreased	Anxiety cycle interrupted	Uses problem solving skill	Promote cntl/self-worth

NOTE: (Variances included on the second page of the pathway) which is not shown; PsychPaths™ © 1994 Strategic Clinical Systems, Granbury, Texas.

The Nursing Process

keep in mind at all times the feelings of horror experienced by clients with PTSD. Statements such as, "That must have been very hard for you," although therapeutic once a working relationship is established, may be perceived as a belittlement of the clients' intense feelings and/or an implication that the pain was in the past rather than continuing into the present. Clients tend to feel understood and accepted when nurses are attentive listeners and communicate interest in the following ways:

- Help clients describe their experiences
- Clarify perceptions of what clients disclose
- Provide feedback that promotes clients' self-care
- Remain nonjudgmental about client's shameful or horrific perceived experiences

Nurses provide information to clients about the development and persistence of their post-traumatic symptoms and about the strategies that are useful in managing and resolving their problems. The nurse may find that teaching exercises and methods to reduce sleep disturbances can meet some short-term goals of providing immediate relief from feelings of tiredness that result with recurrent nightmares and insomnia.

Cognitive coping resources are balanced with those invested in emotional regulation. Clients are helped to refocus their attention toward identifying and then proceeding with behavioral changes that promote a healthy lifestyle. The nurse assists with identification and support of adaptive cognitive coping skills. The client will require assistance with establishing appropriate, achievable goals. Participation in problem solving is used to decrease clients' preoccupation with symptoms.

There are some indications that individuals with PTSD may increase the severity of the distress through irrational thinking and internal attributions for the traumatic event (Ellis, 1994; Leung, 1994). The nurse assists clients to challenge ideas about the event and substitute more realistic thoughts and expectations of themselves. For example, individuals who suffer guilt for not having rescued others should be helped to learn new thoughts and to question the assumptions that they "should" have assisted others. Assisting clients to recognize the realistic limits of their control over the stressful event is essential. Increased use of cognitive coping resources such as logical thinking facilitates a client's sense of being in control and fosters hope that problems can be solved.

Preoccupation with symptoms decreases as clients are better able to manage their emotions and thoughts and solve problems. Interventions that help clients explore the traumatic experience in detail and think about how they influence thoughts, feelings, and behavior provide opportunities to explore the positive and negative aspects. Involvement in this process facilitates the integration of the traumatic experience. The understanding achieved through logical analysis also helps clients assign meaning to the event and begin the process of letting go of their preoccupation with it. Many clients will find that developing rituals or ceremonies specific to themselves can facilitate their letting go of the trauma.

Grieving process

Another major focus of nursing care, often implemented through counseling, is helping the client grieve. The inability to experience the grieving process has been suggested as a factor in the persistence of post-traumatic symptoms. Loss is inherent to traumatic events. Even if victims survive without tangible loss, there are intangible losses such as the sense of safety and the threat of loss. Survivors have lost loved ones, friends, or property. When these losses are not acknowledged by others, the survivors are left to grieve without the needed support. The symptoms of the grieving process and the quests associated with mourning are found among survivors of catastrophic events (see Chapter 36). The implementation of the interventions associated with support system enhancement presented in Box 24-3 are important in assisting with the grieving process.

Emotional regulation

Clients need an opportunity to begin identifying the relationships between current symptoms and the traumatic events. Box 24-4 lists the principles of emotional regulation. The nurse should assist with making these connections as they become clear. The nurse should be aware of helping the client discuss the losses that have occurred and the changes that have resulted from the trauma. There should be an opportunity to evaluate past behaviors in relation to the actual situation not the situation as they or others think they "should" have acted. The nurse needs to assist the client with recognizing and labeling feelings and finding ways to safely express them. The client may need to learn adaptive coping strategies for handling the feelings of anger and resentment that evolve. Techniques to manage anger have been helpful in treating PTSD (Gerlock, 1994). It may be necessary to set limits with some clients who experience anger and rage. Redirecting energy toward physical activities may help.

Talking in detail about a traumatic event and exploring the experience appear to be beneficial when done immediately after the crisis and for a short time thereafter. When in-depth supportive debriefing does not occur, clients may be left with residual problems or experience a delayed reaction. Focusing on assisting clients to develop and use interpersonal social skills can be helpful

The Nursing Process

Box 24-3

Support System Enhancement

DEFINITION

Facilitation of support to patient by family, friends, and community

ACTIVITIES

Assess psychological response to situation and availability of support system

Determine adequacy of existing social networks

Identify degree of family support

Identify degree of family financial support

Determine support systems currently used

Determine barriers to using support systems

Monitor current family situation

Encourage the patient to participate in social and community activities

Encourage relationships with persons who have common interests and goals

Refer to a self-help group, as appropriate

Assess community resource adequacy to identify strengths and weaknesses

Refer to a community-based promotion/prevention/ treatment/rehabilitation program, as appropriate

Provide services in a caring and supportive manner

Involve family/significant others/friends in the care and planning

Explain to concerned others how they can help

Reprinted with permission from McCloskey J.C., & Bulechek, G.M. (Eds). (1996). Nursing interventions classification (NIC), (2nd ed.). St. Louis: Mosby.

Box 24-4

Principles of Emotional Regulation

- Accept feelings
- Accept symptoms
- Identify resources and activities
- Realize psychologically painful situations
- Accept reality
- Foster optimistic attitude
- Avoid blaming others
- Accept help and support
- Resume activities of daily living (ADLs)

From Lundin, T. (1994). The treatment of acute trauma: Post-traumatic stress disorder prevention. Psychiatric Clinics of North America, 17, 385-391.

Box 24-5

Principles of Milieu Therapy

- Treat the symptoms that caused the hospitalization
- Protect the client and others from physical harm; some clients with PTSD exhibit delusions and hallucinations that may be destructive to the client and the milieu
- Dissociation is one of the major symptoms of PTSD; encourage the client to become involved in the therapeutic milieu
- For clients who are hypervigilant, provide an environment that is quiet and free of noise and multiple activities
- Set limits and boundaries regarding the client's behavior

in integrating the experience through talking about and sharing it with others. Participating in support groups provides opportunities to discuss the experience and find solutions for problems and symptoms.

Clients require help in integrating the trauma experience into their lives. They may need to share some experiences with the nurse. The nurse must be prepared to listen and assist clients in attaching meaning to their experiences, accepting what has occurred, and getting on with their lives. There needs to be some degree of closure and resolution. Being able to resolve some experiences can allow individuals to move forward more comfortably.

Milieu Therapy

The nurse has an important role in the management of the milieu for clients hospitalized for PTSD. (For an overall discussion on milieu management see Chapter 19).

Box 24-5 lists some important considerations in the milieu management for clients with PTSD.

Self-Care Activities

Nursing interventions that may help clients manage their symptoms of chronic anxiety include physical activity that alters brain chemistry and mood. The nurse can help clients establish a schedule of walking, jogging, or swimming. Weightlifting may also be suggested as a means of releasing tension and improving mental concentration. Nurses can also help clients cope with acute emotional states by encouraging participation in activities they enjoy. Clients who derive pleasure and relaxation from playing a musical instrument, painting, sculpting, or writing may use these activities as therapeutic self-interventions. The nurse teaches clients how to use relaxation and deep-breathing exercises and guided imagery to manage their stress and

The Nursing Process

anxiety. The therapeutic relationship provides support to clients as they learn how to use these strategies and control the impact of their emotional status on coping.

Empowerment

Powerlessness is an important aspect of a post-traumatic response. Nurses help clients search for and use strategies for empowering themselves. Initially, clients may benefit from keeping a journal in which they document descriptions of situations, thoughts, and feelings associated with the occurrence of flashbacks, intrusive thoughts, nightmares, and problems. Nurses collaborate with clients in the examination of the journal for how thoughts and feelings facilitate or reinforce triggering circumstances. Exploration of these thoughts and feelings is then used to help clients identify and use strategies for detoxifying situations that trigger and perpetuate their post-traumatic responses. Teaching new coping strategies and cognitive skills can also increase the sense of control clients experience.

Family intervention

Whenever one member of a family experiences PTSD, all members experience trauma (Brende & Goldsmith, 1991). The family should be included in treatment. After the initial period, family members need information to assist health care providers in identifying signs and symptoms that indicate that the individual is having residual problems and to seek assistance as quickly as possible. Psychoeducational strategies can facilitate the family's ability to provide the safety and support the individual with PTSD needs.

Psychobiological Interventions

Although no specific medication has been proven effective to treat PTSD as a disease, medication is used to control the excessive autonomic arousal that creates barriers to life and treatment goals. By managing symptoms clients are able to put greater distance between themselves and the event, to put the event behind them, and to gain greater control over physiological and psychological factors. Six goals for pharmacotherapy in PTSD are listed in Box 24-6. Distinguishing between acute and chronic PTSD affects both the selection and the duration of drug therapy. Box 24-7 summarizes the mnemonic BICEPS used to represent the treatment principles in acute PTSD.

When there is a comorbid diagnosis, health care providers should carefully consider which pharmacological agents to use, factoring in the PTSD symptoms to be treated. Even in clients without comorbidity, polypharmacy may be required for optimal results, because pharmacological agents tend to be used for spe-

Box 24-6

Goals for Pharmacotherapy in Post-Traumatic Stress Disorder

- Reduce intrusive symptoms
- Improve avoidance symptoms
- Reduce tonic hyperarousal
- Relieve depression, anhedonia
- Improve impulse regulation
- Control acute dissociative and psychotic features

Box 24-7

Treatment Principles in Acute Post-Traumatic Stress Disorder

Treatment can be described as BICEPS:
Brief
Immediate
Centrally administered (coordinated)
Expectation of return to normal functioning
Proximally given
Superficial (i.e., no attempt should be made to explore deep, unresolved conflicts)

cific groups of symptoms. Studies indicate that tricyclic antidepressants (TCAs), monoamine oxidase inhibitors (MAOIs), and the new serotonergic agents such as selective serotonin reuptake inhibitors (SSRIs) are useful in the treatment of symptoms associated with PTSD. The MAOI phenelzine (Nardil) is used to relieve the intrusive symptoms; however, the side effects of this drug, along with the dietary restrictions and contraindication to use alcohol, precludes its use for many clients experiencing trauma, especially those with substance abuse comorbidity. The addiction potential and the possibility of disinhibition with resultant impulsive or hostile behavior with clients using clonazepam should be considered. Also, depressive symptoms have been associated with benzodiazepine pharmacotherapy. The nurse should be aware of the individual's likelihood for abuse and also consider the possibility of disinhibition with the resultant impulsive or hostile behavior with clients on benzodiazepine.

Antipsychotic agents are not used in the treatment of PTSD. Although clients may exhibit symptoms such as hallucinations, these are often dissociative and can be managed by other techniques such as anger management. However, some clinicians do use neuroleptics for

The Nursing Process

TEACHING POINTS

Clients With Post-Traumatic Stress Disorder

Teach the client, family, and/or significant others the following:

1. Symptomatology, progression, and treatment of PTSD

2. Relationship of the symptoms to the traumatic event

3. Information about the development and persistence of their PTSD symptoms

4. Traumatic event needs to be discussed and feelings explored

5. Hypervigilance, sleep disturbances, guilt, and other reactions are normal responses to a catastrophic situation

6. Techniques and strategies to cope with the symptoms of PTSD

7. Avoid the use of alcohol and other drugs to alleviate feelings of distress

8. If acute symptoms of anxiety following exposure to a trauma do not subside within 4 weeks, help should be sought

brief periods in low doses to treat suspiciousness and paranoia (although there is currently no support for this from research findings). The comorbid association between PTSD and borderline personality may also indicate the need for a neuroleptic. Electroconvulsive therapy may occasionally be used to treat severe depression in clients with PTSD.

The response to pharmacotherapy of PTSD is relatively slow. It may take 8 weeks or longer for the beneficial effects of drug therapy to become evident, and longer treatment may further maximize gains. Other considerations in medication adherence include cost of the medicine, frequency of dosing, and assessment of personal benefit. Medication adherence is an important factor in recovery but can be compromised by side effects.

Anticholinergic side effects of TCAs may hinder medication adherence and may impair the attainment of therapeutic levels. Other problems that occur with tricyclics are orthostatic hypotension, weight gain, and excessive sedation. Sexual dysfunction may be an important factor in compliance with the tricyclic, serotonergic, and MAOI antidepressants. Dietary and alcohol restriction with the MAOIs may also affect adherence. See Chapter 15 for further information on specific side effects and Chapter 16 for techniques to enhance adherence to medications. Conservative tapering of medications is advisable in this population. It should not be done while the client is exploring deep unresolved conflicts in a continued therapeutic process.

Health Teaching

Health teaching for clients with PTSD may encompass a variety of areas. The major goal of health teaching is to teach clients strategies to reduce their PTSD symptoms. Teaching Points for clients with PTSD are presented above. See Chapter 16 for additional health teaching/psychoeducation suggestions. The Research Highlight on p. 452 discusses anger management as cognitive/behavioral strategy.

Case Management

The most important management of PTSD in the community is the control of client symptoms and the safety of the client. Nursing assessments contribute to the multidisciplinary data base used in the development of a comprehensive care plan. Nurses monitor, evaluate, and document clients' responses to therapies and progress and participate in multidisciplinary team treatment planning.

Health Promotion and Health Maintenance

At present it is not known whether PTSD can be prevented. Efforts directed toward prevention should include managing the immediate and acute stress responses. Debriefing and defusing, through open discussion of the traumatic event, the meaning the situation has for the individual, and the responses to the event, are ways of reducing stress. Pharmacological methods may also be required to manage the acute phase of anxiety and stress (see Chapter 15). Long-term studies in which individuals are identified immediately after suffering a catastrophe are needed to determine whether PTSD can be prevented through early management.

RESEARCH HIGHLIGHT

Gerlock A. A. (1994). Veterans' responses to anger management intervention. *Issues in Mental Health Nursing.* 15, 393-408.

Summary

The purposes of this retrospective quasi-experimental study was to determine whether there is a relationship between specific confounding variables and veterans' anger scores both before and after an anger management class and whether there was a change in anger scores following the class.

The sample consisted of 51 male veterans who attended classes on anger management in cohorts of 6 to 12 persons. The cohort groups attended class sessions for 8 weeks. The classes used a cognitive-behavioral approach to anger management. Each class included didactic segments on physiological, behavioral, and cognitive cues to the anger response; early learning experiences with anger; anger triggers and what makes one vulnerable to anger; short-term anger payoffs versus longer term consequences; other feelings; and steps at solving abusive anger problems. The final 2 weeks of classes consisted of sharing outcomes, identifying anger themes, and establishing daily anger management plans.

Both state and trait anger scores dropped significantly following the classes. Major themes identified by the participants included childhood trauma, being a victim of physical violence, and witnessing domestic violence. Veterans with a history of childhood trauma had higher final trait-anger scores. An overwhelming number of subjects reported either a past or present drug and/or alcohol problem.

A cognitive-behavioral approach to anger management was effective in reducing anger in this study. Further study is needed to determine whether these effects remain over time.

Implications for Nursing Practice

Based on the conclusions of this and related studies, it is important for psychiatric nurses who work with clients with PTSD to do the following:

1. Explore their own thoughts and feelings about anger
2. Assess for anger in trauma survivors
3. Provide clients with PTSD with information about anger arousal
4. Assist individuals who survive trauma to relate past experiences to current feelings and responses
5. Be aware that clients with PTSD who also have substance abuse problems may be helped in programs that treat substance abuse
6. Suggest that clients with PTSD keep journals or anger logs to assist them in viewing their experiences objectively and to serve as evidence of one method of their abilities to be in control

Hypnosis, eye movement desensitization, and imaginal flooding are examples of techniques most often employed by other disciplines to decrease anxiety, detoxify traumatic memories, and resolve flashbacks, intrusive thoughts, and sleep disturbances (Leung, 1994: Lundin, 1994). Nursing interventions should be directed toward helping clients understand what is involved in these therapies and formulate questions for their therapists when they have concerns, providing support for their participation, and supporting their decisions related to plan of care and treatment choices. Nurses in advanced practice may function as therapists with clients and consultants with health care professionals.

COMMUNITY RESOURCES

Department of Veterans Affairs
Call for regional office
(800)827-1000
National Alliance for the Mentally Ill
200 North Glebe Road, Suite 1015
Arlington, VA 22203-3754
(800)950-6264
National Institute of Mental Health
for list of publications
5600 Fishers Lane
Rockville, MD 20857

National Mental Health Association
1201 Prince Street
Alexandria, VA 22314-2971
Society for Traumatic Stress Studies
435 North Michigan Avenue, Suite 171
Chicago, IL 60611-4067
Phone: (312)644-0828
Fax: (312)644-8557

THE CONSUMER'S VOICE

Post-Traumatic Stress Disorder

Will Brady

This disorder (if I can call it that) has affected my life in many ways. Sometimes a sudden shift in my emotional state may occur, which is perplexing at times, since I am not always aware of what triggers have caused the response. It can be a simple reminder of my own past trauma, perhaps a violent scene on television or in a film. Other times, I sit through such things without any problem at all. This unpredictability in and of itself is hard to deal with. If I knew, for example, that every time I watched a film about child abuse that some emotional or other disturbance would resurface, it could be easily avoided. The problem is that one cannot always be aware of triggers for this problem. Some things are obvious, others are discoverable, and still others are vague and elusive.

I sometimes have difficulty sleeping, or become distrustful of others. There is sometimes a persistent premonition as if I were expecting some unpleasant event to weave through my average day. It is a difficult problem, but for the most part I am able to lead a productive life.

One event that stays in my mind occurred when I took a job as a client advocate in an inpatient psychiatric facility. When I was introduced to my co-workers in a large meeting, one of the employees called out, "I think it is important that everyone knows he used to be a client." This not only was hurtful in that the intent was to present me in a negative light, but it also robbed me of the opportunity to share that information myself. My status as an ex-patient is not something that I choose to keep hidden in general, but I found this experience to be stigmatizing. It also drummed up some old and negative feelings from early traumatic experiences.

I have been abusive to myself in the past and involved myself in abusive relationships. Sometimes I think that so much of my mental energy has been devoted to overcoming the initial trauma and recognizing triggers for preventing its recurrence that I have not properly learned to protect myself in other ways. Although I can react and see with clarity a necessary course of action in a crisis, I am not so in tune with more subtle and interpersonal interactions that are not threatening on the surface, such as abusive partners in a relationship.

To cope with my symptoms when things get difficult, I do a variety of things, some of which may seem contradictory but actually are not. When necessary, I isolate myself. I often find that a long walk in the woods is calming. I keep a journal, writing my thoughts in it, keeping track of events, and using it as a memory enhancer. One of the coping mechanisms I use is to view this "disorder" for what it truly is—a complex and powerful aspect of myself. It is that part of me that afforded me protection during a time of stress and abuse when I was overpowered by circumstances and events in my environment. It is that part of me that allowed me to survive rather than be destroyed by overwhelming forces.

I channel my anger into productive activities like splitting firewood, mountain climbing, or other exercise. I have tried to turn negative habits into positive outlets for my emotions, like reliving my own past experience through my artwork. My work as a client advocate often serves as an outlet for a lot of energy and, from time to time, I see myself as I once was through my interactions with clients. This is helpful and also keeps me motivated to help others.

Allowing time for me to heal and giving myself enough physical and emotional distance from the initial perpetrator of my trauma has been helpful. I have a small group of dependable friends with whom I can discuss things. They are a cornerstone of support in my life, but trying to increase my own self-reliance as a devlopmental experience is also important. Striking an overall balance is key to recovery from trauma for me. This allows me to recognize myself as an individual, and the friends that make up my support system allow me to recognize myself as a part of a community or perhaps a surrogate family of my own making.

I'm skeptical about what "help" the caring professions have been able to provide. My own experience has been that, more often than not, efforts by caregivers have often made things worse for me. Sometimes the desire to help is there on the part of professionals, but often the therapeutic process seems to be about making the professional feel that she or he is being helpful. There are, no doubt, supportive professionals who may be helpful, but in my personal experience I have rarely come into contact with them.

The expectation that clients in the inpatient setting will share the most intimate parts of their lives with any professional caregiver is unrealistic. Rapport must be developed not with the symptoms, but the individual. Meaningful sharing can come only after this. I suggest that some part of the clinical record document the client's interpretation of events. I believe that including the client's experience of things is relevant and will go a long way toward building trust and a therapeutic alliance.

The Nursing Process

 CRITICAL THINKING QUESTIONS

Bob was admitted to the hospital after he had an explosive outburst and threw furniture around his living room. Bob is 32 years old, has been married for 3 years, and has a 1-year-old daughter. Bob is a member of the volunteer rescue squad in his community that responded to the crash site of a commercial aircraft in which 120 persons were killed. Only 10 persons survived. Bob's wife reported that he had nightmares and trouble sleeping since the crash. He is more aloof and withdrawn from friends and family.

1. What are your feelings about listening to Bob's experiences at the crash site?
2. What would be essential to establish before he would feel comfortable talking with you?
3. What would be important to discuss with his wife, and how can she best be involved in his care?
4. What are helpful methods to assist Bob to understand and control his feelings of anger?
5. What are possible feelings that Bob is experiencing but keeping covered?
6. Identify at least three nursing diagnoses and interventions that may be applied to Bob.
7. What information does Bob need to manage successfully at home?

Evaluation

The outcomes stated earlier in this chapter are individualized for each client and must be evaluated on an ongoing basis. Long-term evaluation helps determine if the long-term therapeutic work of people with post-traumatic stress response meets the following:

- Memories of the traumatic event are confronted and a meaning attached to it that facilitate healing.
- They are able to listen to feedback on their disclosure of the traumatic experience and associated feelings and accept the empathy and help provided by the listener.
- They are able to give up the victim role and control their thoughts, feelings, and behaviors, demonstrating a healthy self-concept and lifestyle.

KEY POINTS

- Events and circumstances that involve actual or potential death or serious injury to the self or others can create intense fear, helplessness, or horror, which are the stressors that contribute to a post-traumatic stress response.
- Events and circumstances that increase a person's vulnerability to the development of post-traumatic stress symptoms include war, rape, crime-related events, natural disasters, technological disasters, childhood sexual abuse, severe and disabling physical injuries, and living with someone who is abusive.
- Covictims are people also at risk for developing a post-traumatic stress response because of their exposure to catastrophes as eyewitnesses, rescuers, or caregivers or their relationship to victims.
- A post-traumatic stress response develops in people who, before exposure to the catastrophe, were healthy and did not necessarily have premorbid psychological problems. The traumatic nature of a catastrophe is the source of the post-traumatic stress response.
- Some people have personal vulnerabilities that increase the severity and persistence of post-traumatic stress symptoms.
- Comorbid psychiatric disorders may occur with post-traumatic stress disorder (PTSD).
- Symptoms of post-traumatic stress that are problematic for the victims include hypervigilance and arousal, guilt, dissociation (depersonalization, psychogenic amnesia and fugue, and flashbacks), and avoidance of triggers.
- Symptoms of PTSD are similar across cultural groups; however, the strategies for assessment and intervention are diverse and need to be based on culture.
- Intervention outcomes usually focus on the client's ability to give up the victim role and control thoughts, feelings, and behaviors, demonstrating a healthy self-concept and lifestyle.

REFERENCES

American Psychiatric Association (1980). *Diagnostic and Statistical Manual of Mental Disorders, third edition.* Washington, DC: Author.

American Psychiatric Association (1994). *Diagnostic and statistical manual of mental disorders, fourth edition.* Washington, DC: Author.

Blanchard, et al. (1991). Changes in plasma norepine phrine to combat related stimuli among Vietnam veterans with post-traumatic stress disorder. *Journal of Nervous and Mental Disease, 179*(6), 371-379.

Blank, A.S. (1994). Clinical detection, diagnosis, and differential diagnosis of post-traumatic stress disorder. *Psychiatric Clinics of North America, 17,* 351-383.

Boudenyne, P.A., & Hyer, L. (1990). Physiological responses to combat memories and preliminary treatment outcomes in Vietnam veterans post-traumatic stress disorder patients treatment with direct therapeutic exposure. *Behavior Therapy, 21*(1), 63-87.

Bremner, J., Southwick, S., Brett, E., & Fontana, A. (1992). Dissociation and posttraumatic stress disorder in Vietnam combat veterans. *American Journal of Psychiatry, 149,* 328-332.

Brende, J., & Goldsmith, R. (1991). Post-traumatic stress disorder in families. *Journal of Contemporary Psychotherapy, 21,* 115-124.

Brown, P., & Wolfe, J. (1994). Substance abuse and post-traumatic stress disorder comorbidity. *Drug and Alcohol Dependence 35*(1), 51-59.

Butler, P.D., et al. (1990). Corticotropin-releasing factor produces fear-enhancing and behavioral activating effects following infusion into the locus coeruleus. *Journal of Neuroscience, 10:*176-183.

Buydens-Branchey, L., (1990). Duration and intensity of combat exposure and post-traumatic stress disorder in Vietnam veterans. *Journal of Nervous and Mental Diseases, 178*(9), 582-587.

Dinan, T.G., et al. (1990). A pilot study of a neuroendocrine test battery in posttraumatic stress disorder. *Biological Psychiatry, 23:*665-672.

Ellis, A. (1994). Post-traumatic stress disorder (PTSD): A rational emotive behavioral theory. *Journal of Rational Emotive and Cognitive Behavior Therapy, 12*(1), 3-25.

Emotional trauma haunts Korean POWs, (1991). *Science News, 139*(5), 68.

Gerlock, A.A. (1994). Veterans' responses to anger management intervention. *Issues in Mental Health Nursing, 15,* 393-408.

Goodwin, J.M., Cheeves, K., & Connell, K. (1990). Borderline and other severe symptoms in adult survivors of incestous abuse. *Psychiatric Annals, 20*(1), 22-32.

Green, B.L., Lindy, J.D., Grace, M.C., Gleser, G.C., Leonard, A.C., Karol, M., & Winget, C. (1990). Buffalo Creek survivors in the second decade: Stability of symptoms. *American Journal of Orthopsychiatry, 60*(1), 43-53.

Keane, T., & Wolfe, J. (1990). Comorbidity in post-traumatic stress disorder: An analysis of community and clinical studies. *Journal of Applied Social Psychology, 20,* 1776-1788.

Kolb, L.C. (1993). The psychobiology of PTSD: Perspectives and reflections on the past, present, and future. *Journal of Traumatic Stress, 6*(3), 293-307.

Koopman, C., Classen, C., Cardena, E., & Spiegel, D. (1995). When disaster strikes, acute stress disorder may follow. *Journal of Traumatic Stress, 8*(1), 29-46.

Kramer, T., Lindy, J., Green, B., & Grace, M. (1994). The comorbidity of post-traumatic stress disorder and suicidality in Vietnam veterans. *Suicide and Life-Threatening Behavior, 24*(1), 58-67.

Lazarus, R.S. & Folkman, S. (1984). *Stress, appraisal, and coping.* New York: Springer.

Leung, J. (1994). Treatment of post-traumatic stress disorder with hypnosis. *Australian Journal of Clinical and Experimental Hypnosis, 22,* 87-96.

Litz, B., Keane, T., Fisher, L., & Marx, B. (1992). Physical health complaints in combat-related post-traumatic stress disorder: A preliminary report. *Journal of Traumatic Stress, 5,* 131-141.

Machell, D.F. (1993). Combat post-traumatic stress disorder, alcoholism, and the police officer. *Journal of Alcohol and Drug Education, 38,* 23-32.

McGaugh, J.L., et al. (1990). *Brain organization and memory: Cells, systems, and circuits.*

Moss, M., Frank, E., & Anderson, B. (1990). The effects of marital status and partner support on rape trauma. *American Journal of Orthopsychiatry, 60*(3), 379-390.

Opp, R., & Samson, A.V. (1989). Taxonomy of guilt for combat veterans. *Professional Psychology, Research and Practice, 20*(3), 159-165.

Orr, S.P. (1990). Psychophysiologic studies of post traumatic stress disorder. In E.L. Giller (Ed.). *Biological assessment and treatment of post traumatic stress disorder.* Washington, DC: American Psychiatric Press.

Pitman, R.K., et al. (1990). Naloxone-reversible analgesic response to combat-related stimuli in post traumatic stress disorder. *Archives of General Psychiatry, 47:*541-544.

Post-traumatic Stress: Part I (1991), *The Harvard Mental Health Letter, 7*(8) 17-20.

Schwarz, E., & Perry, B. (1994). The post-traumatic response in children and adolescents. *Psychiatric Clinics of North America, 17,* 311-326.

Shaley, A., et al. (1990). Post-traumatic stress disorder: Somatic comorbidity and effort tolerance. *Psychosomatics, 31*(2), 197-203.

Shives, L.R. (1994). *Basic concepts of psychiatric-mental health nursing,* (3rd ed.). Philadelphia: J.B. Lippincott.

Spector, J., & Huthwaite, M. (1993). Eye-movement desensitisation to overcome post-traumatic stress disorder. *British Journal of Psychiatry, 163,* 106-108.

Squire, L.R., & Zola-Morgan, S. (1991). The medial temporal lobe memory system. *Science, 253:*2380-2386.

Tomb, D.A. (1994). The phenomenology of post-traumatic stress disorder. *Psychiatric Clinics of North America, 17,* 237-250.

Ullman, S. (1994). Adult trauma survivors and post-traumatic stress sequelae: An analysis of reexperiencing, avoidance, and arousal criteria. *Journal of Traumatic Stress, 8,* 179-188.

Walker, G. (1990). Crisis-care in critical incident debriefing. *Death Studies, 14*(2), 121-133.

Weiss, D., Marmar, C., & Schlenger, W. (1992). The prevalence of lifetime and partial post-traumatic stress disorder in Vietnam theater veterans. *Journal of Traumatic Stress, 5,* 365-376.

Yates, J., & Nasby, W. (1993). Dissociation, affect, and network models of memory: An integrative proposal. *Journal of Traumatic Stress, 6,* 305-326.

Chapter 25

Impulse-Control Disorders

Pam Price-Hoskins

LEARNING OUTCOMES

After studying and applying the concepts of this chapter, the learner will be able to:
- Describe the tension and alienation of persons with impulse-control disorders.
- Apply appropriate theoretical frameworks to specific impulse problems.
- Determine antecedents and correlates of aggressive behavior.
- Intervene with persons displaying impulsive behavior.
- Refer persons with impulse problems to appropriate community resources for long-term support and treatment.

KEY TERMS

Antecedents	Explosive lifestyle	Pyromania
Assault	Explosiveness	Remorse
Compulsivity	Fight-or-flight syndrome	Restraint
Consequences	Impulsivity	Seclusion
Constant observation	Kleptomania	Seizure equivalents
Contingencies	Limit setting	Self-monitoring
Contracting	Paraphilias	Time-out
De-escalation	Pathological gambling	Trichotillomania
Escalation		

The news abounds with reports of impulsivity: on the Internet, on television, in newspapers. The impulsivity and aggression content has increased in magazines and books. Gun control continues to be a national social and health issue. The breakdown of societal taboos against violence is occurring, even as there are more laws and greater attempts to stop the epidemic.

Impulsivity can be a pathological disorder, a symptom, or a personality trait. There are two kinds of impulsivity: functional and dysfunctional. Functional impulsivity results from excitement and is accompanied by outgoingness, verve, and ebullience. It is often perceived as a personality trait. Dysfunctional impulsivity results in destructive behavior and may be either a symptom or a pathological disorder.

Destructive impulsivity is a public health epidemic, requiring millions of dollars to identify, control, and eradicate. Unfortunately, immunization is an unlikely solution. The roots are probably not biological but rather social, and the solutions must be found in the societal arena.

The financial burden associated with impulsivity is difficult to estimate but may be as high as $80 billion in direct and indirect costs. However, the upsurge of violence in society is not related to mental illness. Much of the aggression is the result of a coercive interactive lifestyle (Morrison, 1994) and not a mental disorder. Only about 5% of all persons with mental illnesses are destructively impulsive or physically aggressive.

However, the percentage of clients with impulse-control disorders is increasing in inpatient units because danger to oneself or others (threat of violence) or inability to care for oneself are the only criteria for admission to inpatient treatment. In the not-too-distant future the large majority of inpatients will be impulsive and aggressive, and nurses will be required to manage both individual and unit-level impulsivity and aggression. Even then, the amount of violence occurring in inpatient psychiatric units will be considerably less than that occurring in homes and on the streets.

The purpose of this chapter is to provide a theoretical and intervention framework for the practice of nursing with clients who have impulse-control disorders. Because some aggression is a result of impulse disorders, aggression is addressed in this chapter as well.

EPIDEMIOLOGY

Risk factors for aggression and impulsivity include personal history of aggression and impulsivity, family history, head injury, and temporal lobe seizure disorder. Factors such as socioeconomic status and poverty are associated with aggression and impulsivity but the association is unclear (Brill, 1993). Persons of every age group, socioeconomic status, culture, and gender may be aggressive and impulsive. No groups are left untouched by these behaviors.

Men and women are equally likely to be aggressive. However, women are more likely to be aggressive at home with family members and friends, whereas men tend to be more aggressive in public places with strangers (Newhill, Mulvey, and Lidz, 1995) (see the Cultural Highlights box on p. 458).

Once aggression has been used successfully, it becomes increasingly more difficult to give it up as a pattern of interaction with others. Besides becoming a "habit" that is perceived as out of the client's control, its ability to deliver immediate results is powerfully reinforcing. Hence the history of violence itself is the greatest predictor of future violence.

THEORETICAL FRAMEWORK

Theoretical correlates of impulsivity and aggression include biological and psychosocial explanations. Psychosocial correlates have had strong proponents until the past decade. Research into biological factors has greatly improved knowledge about these troublesome behaviors. Ultimately, the biological and psychosocial correlates will be intimately woven together for a thorough understanding of impulsivity and aggression.

Biological Correlates

Two biological correlates are primarily involved in the determination of behavior and are highly related to impulsivity and aggression. They include the following:

- Brain structures, particularly the limbic system, frontal and prefrontal cortex, and temporal lobes
- Neurotransmitters, particularly the monoamines: serotonin (5HT), dopamine, and gamma-aminobutyric acid (GABA)

Head injury

Head injuries may result from birth trauma, accidents, or physical abuse. Head injuries may result in permanent change to personality and emotional expression. Injuries or lesions in the limbic structures, temporal lobes, and frontal lobes are associated with aggression. Damage to the prefrontal lobes of the cerebral cortex often results in behavioral disinhibition and overt criminality (Garza-Trevino, 1994).

Seizures

Only temporal lobe epilepsy (TLE) and multiinfarct dementias occurring in the temporal lobes are highly

CULTURAL HIGHLIGHTS

Women and Anger

Theory

There are two kinds of anger: trait anger and state anger. *Trait anger* is the ongoing general tendency to be angry. High trait anger is seen in persons who react with anger to more situations with a higher level of intensity than those with low trait anger. Both systolic and diastolic blood pressure are related to trait anger. *State anger* is the tendency to respond to particular situations with anger.

Anger is expressed in four ways: anger-in, or suppression; anger-out, or explosiveness and aggression; anger-discuss, or talking about anger; and anger-symptoms, or converting anger to somatic expression. Both anger-in and anger-out are harmful to individuals and to relationships. Anger symptoms are harmful to the individual, because the person remains unaware of the anger and its toll. Only anger-discuss is considered healthy.

Ventilation of anger does not necessarily diminish anger or produce relief. Ventilation, that is, forceful release of anger, is different than anger-discuss, in which words and reflection are used to defuse the anger.

Application to Women

1. There is no evidence to support myths such as women's propensity to suppress anger and married women's inclination to suppress anger.

2. Married women are less likely than unmarried women to hold in their anger.

3. Women with high school educations have more anger-in and anger symptoms than women who are college graduates.

4. When women are divided into three occupational groups (high group: private practitioners, executives, and entrepreneurs; medium group; nurses, teachers, and other human service workers; low group: clerical workers, secretaries, and homemakers), the low category uses more anger-in; the medium group has the highest scores on trait and state anger.

5. Women with adult children are more likely to suppress anger; mothers with elementary school children scored highest on anger-out, Trait anger is highest in women with preadult children.

6. As age increases, women tend to have less anger-out and fewer unhealthy thoughts but more anger-in.

7. Anger symptoms are highest in women in their forties and early fifties, which is also thought to be the most stressful life stage for women.

8. Women with more emotional symptoms, such as nervousness and irritability, often seen during perimenopause, score significantly higher in anger symptoms than women who have only physical complaints such as hot flashes and night sweats. This may indicate that menopause intensifies but does not cause psychological distress.

9. Women with psychiatric histories do not differ from medical and nonclinical groups on trait anger.

10. Women with psychiatric histories are significantly more stressed than are the medical and the nonclinical groups.

11. No statistically significant differences on any of the factors of anger exist between African-American and caucasian women.

12. Chinese-American women score higher on trait anger and anger-out than African-American and caucasian women. Primary targets of the anger were husbands.

13. Anger-prone women are likely to think that situations are unfair and have been deliberately provoked.

14. There is an inverse relationship between anger-discuss and anger-in.

Adapted from Thomas, S.P. (1993). Anger and its manifestations in women. In S.P. Thomas (ed.), Women and anger. *New York: Springer.*

related to aggression; however, neither are considered a cause of aggression (Harper-Jacques and Reimer, 1992).

There are two kinds of aggression associated with seizures: (1) a nonspecific, nondirected aggression that occurs during the ictal (physically visible) phase of a seizure and is purely defensive in nature, and (2) postictal aggression, which is specific and directed. The client is confused and agitated at that point and is prone to misinterpretation of environmental stimuli such as taking vital signs.

Neurotransmitter dysfunction

Research consistently suggests the role of the serotonergic system in aggression, probably the S_2 receptors in the prefrontal areas of the cerebral cortex (Barratt, 1993). Neurotransmitters can malfunction through a surplus or a deficit of a neurotransmitter at the front end (neuron) or the back end (receptor) of the synaptic cleft (see Chapter 13). Depending on the neurotransmitter and the site of the dysfunction, a client may be (1) hyperaroused and prone to impulsivity and aggression or (2) very difficult to stimulate and prone to slow reactions and poor ability to defend self.

Perception and interpretation

A third area for dysfunction is the interaction between the cortical (cognitive) functions and the limbic (emotional) functions. The interaction between these two aspects of the brain is called "the emotional circuit" (Harper-Jacques and Reimer, 1992) and is where meaning is assigned to particular perceptions. If the limbic and/or the cortical areas, or the emotional circuit, is dysfunctional, the meaning attributed to an event may be out of synchronization with the meaning assigned by persons in the environment. This explains why staff members sometimes do not know why a client becomes upset; the client's brain dysfunction creates the misinterpretation.

Psychosocial Correlates

Psychosocial explanations of impulsivity and aggression include psychodynamic theories, and family/community socialization. Biological correlates and psychosocial correlates are often found together in individual clients.

Psychodynamic theories

Psychodynamic theories, or theories about causality arising from within the minds and emotions of individuals, have some empirical support. Ego deficit theory, projection, and anxiety are psychodynamic theories outlined here.

Ego Deficit Theory   Ego deficit theory is a common psychodynamic explanation of impulsivity and aggression. Theoretically, the ego does not have the support needed to develop a strong sense of reality, to test reality, or to develop adequate problem-solving and decision-making skills. Research indicates that early insecure attachment correlates with aggression in later childhood (Constantino, 1995).

Projection   Clients who are impulsive and whose impulses are converted to aggression usually define themselves as victims who are protecting themselves from aggression or provocation (Crowner et al., 1995).

Anxiety   The events that trigger impulsivity and aggression are usually anxiety-laden. Anxiety may lead to the *fight-or-flight syndrome, the limitation of a person's choices to just two: to fight (become physically or verbally aggressive) or to run away* (see Chapter 10). Anxiety is a whole-person experience with a strong biological basis. Anxiety creates an abundance of neurotransmitters, leading to hyperarousal and hypervigilance (see Chapters 13 and 14). If circumstances are such that the person cannot run away either by leaving or by saving face, aggression is often the only perceived choice. Persons who become aggressive under these conditions feel justified in their actions, believing they had no choice.

Family and community socialization

Although family and community norms do not constitute a theory, extensive data support the role of families and communities in the socialization of their members into beliefs and behaviors about aggression. Families and communities define appropriate behavior and socialize their members to those norms. Some families and communities teach, "Do unto others as you would have them do unto you." Others teach, "Do unto others before they do it unto you." Children learn impulsiveness from a child-rearing style characterized by alternating patterns of apathy and abuse (L'Abate, 1994). For example, one afternoon the children yelling and throwing food brings a disinterested glance from their mother, who is watching television. That evening, yelling and throwing food brings on rage and beatings for all three children. Children growing up in violent culture are bewildered by tenderness or kindness. As adolescents, they may interpret tenderness and kindness as weakness and an invitation to take advantage of another person. Some persons have been treated with respect so rarely that they do not know how to act appropriately in response.

When violence is accepted by adults, even a nonviolent child may become violent as that child becomes an adolescent. Violent boys tend to regard themselves as healthy, whereas violent girls do not. A girl who is comfortable with her violence is likely to be seriously disturbed. If a child is violent, the violence may be outgrown. If a teen is violent beyond the age of 13, the pattern is likely to continue into adulthood (Marohn, 1992).

Morrison (1994) has culled from several studies an emerging personality type that is aggressive; it is characterized by power and control. This is a person whose aggression is neither an impulse-control disorder nor biologically based. This is a person who chooses violence as a way to interact with the environment. Socialization into this style may occur in many ways, such as through membership in a gang, watching others who are able to get their needs met through this style, and reinforcements when this style is used. (See Chapter 16 for information on learning theory.)

The Nursing Process

Assessment

Common clinical profiles assist health care professionals in understanding how clients with impulse disorders may present themselves. Screening tools and assessment questions are also found in this section.

Clinical Profiles

The most common clinical behaviors exhibited by persons with impulsivity and aggression are explosiveness, escalation, impulsivity, compulsivity, remorse, kleptomania, pyromania, pathological gambling, trichotillomania, and paraphilias. Each of these is explored.

Explosiveness

Explosiveness *is a sudden, rapid, violent release of energy that is used for or has destructive potential.* If the client has a history of temporal lobe epilepsy (TLE), multiinfarct dementias, Alzheimer's disease, or Korsakoff syndrome, there may be little warning before an explosive episode occurs. A detailed history may reveal antecedents such as excessive sensory stimulation or an abrupt, unannounced change that is perceived as threatening. This information may assist the nurse to anticipate and prevent explosive episodes.

There are two kinds of explosiveness associated with seizures. A nonspecific, nondirected aggression that occurs during the ictal phase of a seizure is purely defensive in nature. Postictal aggression may occur due to a misinterpretation of environmental stimuli and is more likely to cause harm. A third kind of explosiveness is attacks made by clients who do not have epilepsy but who have **seizure equivalents,** *disorganized discharges of energy leading to unprovoked fights.*

Temporal lobe epilepsy may be misdiagnosed as rage reaction. Here the client does not show any physical manifestation of an epileptic seizure but rather has a history of getting into vicious fights with little or no provocation. These clients may complain of a sense of "inner pressure" before the fight and often do not remember what occurred during the fight. Such persons have difficulty relating to others and often abuse alcohol, perhaps in an attempt to self-medicate. To complicate matters, the fights are usually viewed by significant others as a consequence of the alcohol; therefore the temporal lobe epilepsy may remain undiagnosed.

Organic brain conditions such as Alzheimer's disease or Korsakoff syndrome in the advanced stages may pre-cipitate aggressive episodes. However, because persons with organic brain conditions have deterioration in all aspects of personality, the aggression is often unfocused, unintentional, and not dangerous.

Another form of explosiveness occurs in clients with **explosive lifestyle,** *a long-standing life pattern of impulsively acting on rageful, frustrated, and hateful impulses because of an inability to think before acting.* Such a person experiences guilt or remorse after an aggressive act and may say things like, "I don't know what came over me," or "I saw red and the next thing I knew, I was punching him."

Escalation

Clients' behaviors may take a pattern of **escalation,** *increasing intensity of anger, hostility, and verbal and nonverbal agitation and aggression.* Escalation occurs on a continuum from verbal statements with angry affect to physical aggression against a person and/or the environment.

Verbal aggression is indicated by forceful words and tone of voice that reinforce the forceful message. For a client who does not usually curse, cursing may indicate that the client is exceptionally angry and is being verbally aggressive. Escalation from verbal aggression would include more body language: red face, distended neck and face veins, hands clenching and unclenching, and leaning forward or moving closer to a person or an object. Further escalation entails large motor activity such as pacing, swinging arms, or pounding one hand into another. The client's voice may become much louder; the client may not be able to address the issue logically any longer but may only be able to threaten. A client may escalate rapidly, over a period of minutes, or slowly, over 2 or 3 days. Escalation may be caused by feelings that the client does not know how to express or are too strong to verbalize.

If not interrupted, either by the client or by the staff or family, the escalation may end in assault. **Assault is** *defined as client-initiated physical contact of a forceful nature* and includes hitting, kicking, slapping, biting, choking, or throwing an object with physical contact (Crowner et al., 1995).

Impulsivity

Impulsivity *is defined as thoughtless action, planlessness, intolerance for routine and rules, restlessness, impatience, and incautiousness* (Eysenck and Eysenck,

The Nursing Process

1978). Impulsive persons quickly convert anger to aggression (Lancee, et al., 1995), whereas persons with lower impulsivity do not easily convert anger into aggression. It is important to identify whether the impulsive client is psychotic or nonpsychotic; this information helps the nurse plan for safety and intervention. Psychotic clients direct aggression at others; staff members respond with fear and anxiety, rapid action, and control of client behavior with seclusion and restraint. Nonpsychotic clients direct aggression toward self or property; staff members respond by engaging in conversation to control self-destructive behavior.

It is also important to assess whether behavior is truly impulsive, or whether it is calculated and planned. Behavior may also be compulsive or driven in such a way that the client perceives there is no choice but to act. Impulsive and compulsive behaviors are considered symptoms of illness, but they do not exonerate the client from responsibility for those behaviors (Harris and Morrison, 1995).

Compulsivity

Compulsivity is an irrational drive to act impulsively and sometimes repetitively. Compulsivity is often an attempt to control impulsivity and aggression. Some compulsions are somewhat socially acceptable, such as workaholism and compulsive exercise. Others are destructive to society, as well as to the individual and the family, such as alcoholism, drug addiction, and compulsive risk taking that endangers life. In the future, a cause or causes, probably biological, will be found to underlie all compulsive and impulsive mechanisms (Yager, 1989).

Remorse

Remorse is sorrow and guilt for one's behavior and a desire to make amends. Remorse rarely occurs when clients perceive that the action was necessary to defend themselves from bodily harm, when clients do not remember and do not believe they committed the act (as during the ictal phase of a seizure), or when intimidation was the purpose of the behavior. However, clients often feel remorseful when they remember the act, accept responsibility for their behavior, and recognize the harm caused. Staff members prefer clients to feel remorseful and often interpret the behavior as "bad" if remorse does not occur. Staff members label behavior as "sick," however, if remorse does occur. Staff members respond more empathetically and helpfully to clients with sick behavior than with bad behavior.

Kleptomania

Kleptomania is an impulse disorder characterized by a compulsion to steal, especially in the absence of economic necessity or personal desire. Kleptomania is exceedingly rare and occurs in only about 5% of the persons caught shoplifting. The buildup of tension immediately before the compulsion to steal is characteristic as is the sense of relief and pleasure immediately after. The items stolen are hardly ever used; they are given away, returned surreptitiously, or hidden.

Pyromania

Pyromania is an impulse disorder characterized by an uncontrollable impulse to start fires. There may be a biochemical connection to fire starting, in that low levels of monoamine metabolite levels and 5-hydroxyindoleacetic acid (5-HIAA) have been found in samples of cerebrospinal fluid drawn from fire starters (Vikkunen et al., 1987). However, the psychodynamic theories still predominate. Pyromania may be an expression of frustration and rage, a show of power, a sexual perversion, or a cry for help. Fire starting may be an issue in the treatment setting because it presents a safety hazard.

Pathological gambling

Pathological gambling is an impulse disorder characterized by preoccupation with gambling, spending more money or gambling longer than intended, restlessness and irritability if unable to gamble, a need to increase the amount and time spent gambling, and an inability to stop gambling in spite of enormous personal consequences. The characteristics are strikingly similar to the signs of substance-related disorders (see Chapter 27). Although many persons gamble, only about 2% to 3% of the population (around 2 to 3 million persons) demonstrate pathological gambling.

Trichotillomania

Trichotillomania is an impulse-control disorder characterized by pulling out one's hair, resulting in noticeable hair loss. The impulse cannot be resisted despite the consequences, is immediately preceded by increasing tension, and is followed by relief. Most often, the scalp is the source of the hair, though eyebrows, eyelashes, beards, and pubic hair may also be plucked. This form of self-mutilation may have a physiological basis, since persons with mental retardation and Tourette's disorder have increasingly been identified with the disorder. It could be a form of disinhibition or brain dysfunction.

Paraphilias

In addition to the above-mentioned disorders related to impulsivity, there are *sexual disorders, called **paraphilias,** in which impulsivity is a major symptom.* These disorders are treated on an outpatient basis or in forensic units and usually are not directly treated by nurses.

TABLE 25-1

Paraphilias

DISORDER	DEFINITION	DISTINGUISHING CHARACTERISTICS
Transvestic fetishism	Recurrent or persistent cross-dressing in the clothes of the opposite sex for release of tension or for sexual pleasure	Some transvestites are transsexuals, whereas some are homosexuals, cross-dressing to attract other homosexuals. Intense frustration is experienced when there is interference with cross-dressing. Cross-dressing is generally used for the purpose of sexual excitement.
Zoophilia (Bestiality)	The act of deriving sexual pleasure from animals	Sexual activity with animals is the exclusive method of achieving sexual pleasure.
Pedophilia (Child molesting)	The act of obtaining sexual pleasure by molesting a child in the prepuberty stage of development	Pedophiles are often male and in their late thirties or early forties. The offender is often familiar to the child and may be a relative, friend, or acquaintance. The child is generally at least 10 years younger than the offender who may be oriented toward children of the same or opposite gender.
Exhibitionism	The act of deriving erotic pleasure from briefly exposing the genitals to a surprised victim	The act generally occurs in a public place. Pleasure stems from seeing the shocked reaction of the viewer. Masturbation sometimes accompanies the act of exposure. Victims are generally female children or adults.
Voyeurism	The act of deriving sexual pleasure through viewing sex organs or sex acts of an unsuspecting victim	The voyeur's primary sex activity is viewing the sexual behavior of others. Generally occurs in early adulthood and is a chronic condition.
Sexual masochism	The act of deriving sexual pleasure and gratification by experiencing physical or mental pain and humiliation	The masochist desires to be dominated in the sexual relationship and is excited by the idea of being the recipient of pain. It involves being humiliated, bound, beaten, or otherwise made to suffer.
Sexual sadism	The act of receiving sexual pleasure and erotic gratification through infliction of physical or psychological pain on another	The sadist achieves orgasm from sadistic acts even when other sexual outlets are available. The desire to dominate is a primary dynamic. Generally, it involves a nonconsenting partner but may sometimes involve a consenting partner. Rape may be committed by persons with this disorder.

TABLE 25-2

Tools used to measure aggression

TOOL	DESCRIPTION
IVE Inventory (Eysenck and Eysenck, 1978)	Measures impulsiveness, venturesomeness, and empathy, with validity and reliability established by the authors; tool is commonly used with clients with mental illness
Overt Aggression Scale (Yudofsky et al., 1986)	Measures aggression in four areas: verbal aggression and physical aggression against self, objects, and other people
Past Feelings and Acts of Violence Scale (quoted in Botsis et al., 1994)	Measures feelings and actions that clients have exhibited in the past

The Nursing Process

Names, definitions, and characteristics of selected paraphilias are found in Table 25-1.

Screening Tools

Other disciplines rely on selected tools to measure impulsivity. Some of these tools are listed in Table 25-2.

Assessment Questions

Assessment questions focus on three areas: *(1) the events and issues occurring before the impulsivity and aggression, referred to as* **antecedents;** *(2) the events and issues occurring during the behavior, known as* **contingencies;** *and (3) the events and issues occurring after the behavior, called* **consequences,** both positive and negative, that are directly linked with the behavior.

The assessment questions themselves may escalate anxiety. The nurse should remain sensitive to the client's verbal and nonverbal behavior, with the first priority being to develop a positive relationship with the client. Intruding into physical or psychological space is anxiety-provoking and should be avoided.

Focus on antecedents

Predictors of violence include the following (Gallop, McCay, and Esplen, 1992):

- History of violence
- Client verbal aggression
- Anxiety
- Substance abuse
- Severity of pathology
- Acute stage of illness

Both impulsivity and aggression are usually preceded by anxiety, internally or externally generated. Understanding the client's history of impulsivity and aggression may assist the nurse in preventing, managing, and helping the client to regain control. Table 25-3 gives an example of an interview for assessing the client's history of aggression.

Focus on contingencies

Contingencies, or situational factors, include internal provocations and external events. Assaults linked to some interpersonal element are in some way provoked. Contingencies of aggression identified through research (Durivage, 1989; Gallop, McCay, and Esplen, 1992; Katz and Kirkland, 1990) include the following:

- Medication administration
- Shift or staff change in inpatient units or treatment programs

- Low level of interaction between staff and clients
- Inconsistent limit setting and social expectations
- Lack of a predictable schedule
- Staff role ambiguity
- Low staff morale
- Lack of a competent, committed authority figure
- Manipulative, fearful staff interactions with clients
- Rigid intolerance
- Authoritarian style

Using the assessment of the client, the nurse identifies factors in the client's history that may be repeated in the treatment environment and for which interventions need to be planned. For instance, the client assessed in Table 25-3 has difficulty with male authority figures. Avoiding assignment of male staff members to this client would decrease the opportunity for power struggles. When limits need to be set or the client confronted, a female may be the more appropriate choice for the intervention. Conflicts with the client's male psychiatrist and consulting neurologist should be expected; staff should plan to assist the client during interviews with them and assist the client to look back over power struggles and help him separate his old history from his current interactions.

Focus on consequences

Consequences may actually reinforce impulsive or aggressive behavior. When unreasonable requests and demands get met because of the impulsiveness or aggressiveness, the behavior is rewarded, and clients are encouraged to use the same style again. Consequences may be social or natural. Natural consequences automatically follow the action, such as pain after an injury or a sense of power when someone is intimidated. Social consequences are those controlled by persons and organizations in society, such as prison after a guilty verdict for rape or alienation from family after an aggressive outburst. In psychiatric treatment, some consequences are natural and should be interrupted only with great forethought and for very good reasons. However, social consequences in a treatment environment are very important as a deterrent for impulsive and aggressive behavior. These are controlled by staff, must fit the inappropriate behavior, and must be implemented consistently.

Focus on escalating tension

Unless head-injured, very few clients become explosive without warning. Most become increasingly and visibly more agitated and verbally louder and more demanding. Assessing the escalation of tension and intervening to

The Nursing Process

TABLE 25-3

Example of an initial interview with an aggressive client

SAMPLE QUESTIONS	POSSIBLE ANSWERS (C: CLIENT; F: FAMILY)
Have you ever had a head injury? Please tell me all the times you remember.	C: Well, starting when I was little I was in lots of accidents, and I probably hurt my head some. I fell out of a tree once and had stitches in my head. I wrecked my bike and my motorcycle. When I was 18, I spent the night in the hospital with a concussion. And I got my ears boxed a few times when I was a kid.
	F: Since we've been married, Bill has had three car accidents. He had dizziness and ringing in his ears all three times but was too hardheaded to get a checkup. He still has bad headaches.
Have you ever had a seizure or a fit?	C: I have blackouts sometimes.
	F: Sometimes he just stops in midsentence and stares off into space for a minute, then comes back around and picks up where he left off.
Who lived with you as you were growing up?	C: Mom, Grandad, and Grandma at first. Then with Mom and Mark; I guess he was like a stepdad.
Was your home generally happy?	C: No way! They were mad about something night and day. Mind you, I deserved most of the beatings. Mom even deserved some of what she got-from Grandpa and from Mark.
	F: And now he's the same way with the kids and me. We had some hard slaps when I was growing up but nothing like he dishes out.
How badly were you hurt?	C: Lots of black eyes, a few broken ribs, cigarette butts flipped at my head just for the fun of it, but I deserved some of it. I had a smart mouth; I just couldn't help it, though. I just had to stand up to him. I felt like I'd die if I didn't.
You thought he might kill you?	C: No, not really. I thought I'd die inside if I didn't stand up for Mom and me.
	F: But he can't stand to see his son do the same thing for me.
	C: That's different, Sarah. Don't talk like that to the nurse. That's our business!
Do you feel picked on sometimes?	C: All the time. Since Mark, I guess I just find people to pick on me. Bosses, especially. They want slobbering servants to lick their shoes. I usually just walk out on a job, I get so fed up.
	F: Yeah, and the last two places he trashed as he was leaving. I think they didn't file charges because they were afraid he'd hurt them.
	C: I might have, too. But I felt a lot better after I made them pay for the way they treated me.
Let's change the subject here. Are you comfortable enough to talk about what goes on in your home?	C: What are you going to ask?
I'm going to ask about how much you yell, how loud you sound to your wife and kids, and how physically aggressive you get.	C: I don't want to answer any more questions. I want to stop now.

The Nursing Process

prevent aggression and impulsivity is the nurse's primary goal. The myth that all assaults can be predicted and that competent staff will prevent them must be confronted (Poster and Ryan, 1994). Although staff can do much to assess, prevent, mitigate against, and stop assaults, clients must be held accountable for their own behaviors.

Focus on the nurse's self-assessment

When a nurse is faced with an impulsive, aggressive, and/or disruptive client, several feelings are common: fear, anger and revenge, masochistic acceptance, entrapment, exploitation, demoralization, helplessness, and cynicism (Daum, 1994). Feelings facilitate action, and the nurse has an ethical responsibility to act therapeutically with the client. Therefore the nurse has an ethical responsibility to assess and manage thoughts and feelings that would hinder a therapeutic relationship. A self-assessment is helpful in managing thoughts and feelings. See Box 25-1 for examples of self-assessment questions.

BOX 25-1

The Nurse's Self-Assessment

How do I usually respond to impulsivity in others? Do I become more controlling? Irritated? Anxious? Helpless? Get impulsive myself?

How do I respond to verbal aggression in others? Verbal aggression toward me? Threatened physical aggression toward me? Toward persons I love or feel responsible for? Physical aggression toward property? My property? Property of great value?

What am I afraid of? Am I afraid to set limits or confront the client? In what ways are my feelings affecting my relationship with the client? In what ways are my feelings influencing my performance of the nursing role?

Does the client remind me of someone I know? Are my feelings more strongly related to the client or to the person I know (transference)?

If this client acts out, am I comfortable that I can handle my own behavior? Maintain control of the environment, including other clients? How would I assist the client to regain control?

Do I think this person deserves to be punished for past behavior? For the behavior toward me? Toward other clients or staff? Which of my actions are punishing rather than therapeutic?

Nursing Diagnosis

Impulsive and aggressive behaviors may be placed either in the first or the second part of the nursing diagnosis (see Chapter 5). Examples of aggression and impulsivity that could be either in the first or the second part of the diagnosis are found in Box 25-2.

The *Diagnostic and Statistical Manual of Mental Disorders, Fourth Edition* (DSM-IV) defines impulsivity and aggression as symptoms of several other disorders such as schizophrenia, panic disorder, PTSD, and substance-related disorders. A classification of impulse disorders, not elsewhere classified, is shown in Box 25-3.

BOX 25-2

Nursing Diagnoses of Aggression and Impulsivity

INEFFECTIVE INDIVIDUAL COPING (RUNNING AWAY) IS THE:

First part of diagnosis
Outcome is to remain in the area and to draw in journal.

Second part of diagnosis
Interventions include placing precautions on elopement; removing shoes and access to coat; having staff member sit next to client when client is most likely to bolt and assist with management of anxiety; allowing client to exhibit signs of restlessness, such as twisting in chair, tapping foot, and swinging leg during group; and asking other clients to ignore the behaviors.

IMPAIRED SOCIAL INTERACTION (VERBAL AGGRESSION) IS THE:

First part of diagnosis
Outcome is to use an "I" statement when expressing anger.

Second part of diagnosis
Interventions include monitoring signs of increasing tension and unwillingness to talk; asking the client at regular intervals to rate tension and validate whether it is building, remaining the same, or diminishing; developing a game plan with clients for going to their rooms if they begin to yell or speak angrily, with the understanding that a staff member will accompany clients so they can have their say.

The Nursing Process

DSM-IV Impulse-Control Disorders Not Elsewhere Classified

Intermittent explosive disorder
Kleptomania
Pyromania
Pathological gambling
Trichotillomania
Impulse-control disorder NOS (not otherwise specified)

Reprinted with permission from American Psychiatric Association. (1994). Diagnostic and statistical manual of mental disorders, fourth edition. *Washington, DC: Author.*

Outcome Identification

In general, outcome criteria for resolution of aggressive and impulsive behaviors include the following:

- *Decrease in destructive behavior*—Because aggression and impulsivity are chronic conditions and must be managed over a lifetime, one of the goals is to decrease the intensity and number of destructive episodes, while concomitantly decreasing the actual amount of destruction, personally, in relationships, and toward property. As clients begin to manage their aggression and impulsivity, small gains are important and need to be celebrated.
- *Change in the consequences of impulsive behavior*—For persons who have managed increasing tension through impulsivity, the greatest consequence and reward is the relief that follows the behavior. It is powerfully reinforcing because the tension becomes unbearable if it is not discharged. However, the client's personal reward system can be altered. For example, when Jonette beats her children because of her own tension buildup, the consequence is battered, frightened, psychologically scarred children. She momentarily feels better, but the guilt and remorse and the loss of her relationship with her children are grave consequences. Jonette must learn to value the health of and relationships with her children more than she values discharging her personal tension in this destructive manner. It takes a change in her personal value system to allow work on this long-term goal.
- *Increase in coping skills for impulsivity and aggression*—The client's perceptions of and reactions to stressors are more important than the stressful

event itself (Botsis et al., 1994). Therefore an important long-term goal for clients with aggressive and impulsive behavior is to develop coping skills.
- *Improvement in self-monitoring*—One of the major methods of self-management is *self-monitoring or becoming aware of the triggers, thoughts, and feelings that contribute to building tension.* Assisting the client to identify those triggers, thoughts, and feelings, and developing the discipline to wait to act while making time to think about alternatives is a long-term goal but well worth the effort. Managing environmental and internal stimuli is a large part of self-monitoring.

Planning

Planning tools used with clients who are impulsive and aggressive consist of nursing care plans, interdisciplinary treatment plans, and treatment protocols. The examples presented here are tools developed for use in individual institutions or are research-based.

Nursing Care Plan

Nursing care plans for clients who are aggressive and impulsive are developed depending on clients' abilities to consistently, cognitively engage in their own treatments. A nursing care plan for a client with psychosis is found on p. 467.

Interdisciplinary Treatment Plan

Consistency in responding to impulsivity and aggression is powerful for rewarding positive behavior and reinforcing consequences of negative behavior. The multidisciplinary team has more difficulty responding consistently to aggression and impulsivity than to almost any other behavior. The desire to build and maintain rapport can interfere with a team member's willingness to follow through consistently with team decisions. The fear of the client acting out when other team members are not around may prevent a nurse from setting limits and following through on consequences. Because the behavior is provocative and reminds staff members of their own personal issues (transference) and vulnerabilities, they have their own ideas about what is best for the client and tend to want to implement their own plans. It is in the client's best interest for the entire team to agree on a plan and then follow through consistently without undermining the integrity of the plan in any way. An interdisciplinary treatment plan for responding to intermittent explosive disorder is found on p. 468.

NURSING CARE PLAN

Aggressive, Psychotic Client

NURSING ASSESSMENT DATA

Subjective: About 3 hours after admission to a psychiatric inpatient unit for inability to care for self, client was sitting in corner of day room. *Objective:* Feet drawn up in chair, rocking, crying, and muttering incoherently; high-pitched cough, as if choking on a small object; hollers out, "I want water." When no one came toward her immediately, she jumped up, turned over the card table with a jigsaw puzzle, and started throwing everything at hand that she could pick up; *DSM-IV diagnonis:* Psychosis NOS.

NANDA Diagnosis: Risk for violence related to ineffective individual coping

Outcomes	Interventions	Rationale	Evaluation
Short term 1. Will not hurt self or others *while in inpatient treatment.* 2. Will not destroy property *while in inpatient treatment.* **Long term** 1. Will maintain relationships with significant others with no physical aggression toward self or others *within 3 weeks.*	• Immediately take a glass of water to client. "Here is the water you asked for, Denise." • Ask client to help you clean up the mess or to unpack her belongings in her room. • Inform Denise that yelling and throwing things are not good ways to get her needs met and that next time she will be escorted to seclusion. Do this when there is a quiet time without onlookers. • Assign a staff member to observe client closely but from a distance. If client shows signs of escalating, ask client to go to room. If client refuses, escort client to room or to seclusion room. Obtain an order for seclusion. • Start neuroleptic medication as soon as possible. Do a baseline AIMS test for tardive dyskinesia, and baseline lying and standing blood pressure before first dose. • Maintain high expectations for participation and behavior control but low demand for compliance until client is clinically improved.	• Meeting needs and stated requests rewards clear request; gives Denise a chance to stop aggression without losing face. • Gives client choices, both of which are acceptable and need to be done. • Communicating the expectations in a clear, concise way lowers anxiety; doing so in private and when client is calm is respectful and more likely to be heard. • Clients usually show signs of increasing escalation. However, being too close to client may invade personal space and increase client's anxiety. Civil liberties may be violated only with a physician's assessment and collaboration with the nurse. • Psychosis is a brain disorder, and aggression when psychotic is instinctive vs. deliberate. The sooner a chemical balance is attained, the sooner client can be expected to take responsibility for her behavior. Baseline data establish a comparison standard. • She is easily overstimulated and can help make determinations about tolerance level of stimulation and activity.	**Short term** 1. Met 2. Two salad bowls were broken in the first 24 hours of hospitalization. **Long term** 1. Met

▇▇ **INTERDISCIPLINARY TREATMENT PLAN**

Critical Pathway: Intermittent Explosive Disorder

Patient Name: _____   Case Manager: _____   Medical Record #: _____
Admit date: _____   Expected LOS: _____   UR days certified: _____   Physician: _____   Actual LOS: _____
Discharge Date: _____

Day/Date:	0–8 Hours	8–24 Hours	Day 2	Day 3	Day 4	Day 5
ASSESSMENTS AND EVALUATIONS	Nursing Nutritional screen Admit note Precautions	H & P, Social HX, RT/TA; Dr: Initial TX Plan/Admit Note, Pred. Eval. AIMS Scale	Precaution Evaluation Document sleep patterns; note body language & facial expression as anger indicators.	Psych Eval done Social Hx on chart Assess for and discourage manipulative behavior	Assess for readiness for discharge	Assess for goals achieved Include patient and family in process
PROCEDURES	Lab ordered-Admit profile UA, UDS, UCG, EKG, Other:	Lab done: UA, UDS, UCG, EKG Other:	Lab results checked Abnormals called to Dr. Consider EEG	Follow-up for abnormal lab results	Check CBC for immunosupression if Tegretol is used	
CONSULTS	IT ordered Y/N FT ordered Y/N GT ordered Y/N Psych Testing Order Y/N	GT started Psych Testing done	Schedule MTP meeting Invite family	IT started, FT started Psych Testing Results Home Contract		Explore community resources as applicable ie, Tough Love.
TREATMENT PLANNING	NI: Axis III		RT/TA started School started (youth)	Master TX Plan Updated; RT/TA entry, family informed		Give copy of area meeting places and times
INTERVENTIONS	Assess Self-Harm Aggression potential	Convey calm non-threatening attitude.	Structure Milieu (encourage patient to i.d. anger triggers)	Identify strengths and accomplishments	Help develop and rehearse problem-solving skills	Assess client support network
MEDICATIONS	Meds ordered, Informed Consent signed by pt. and/or guardian.	Med teaching for client and family give written info. (Re: side affects & expected outcomes.)	Drug interaction checked by Pharmacist/Dr. signs informed consent	Meds evaluated/ readjusted Teaching reinforced	Develop system to remember meds and have pt. rehearse	Discharge instructions for medication self-admin for family administration.
LEVEL TEACHING	Level ordered Patient Rights Orient to unit and program	Boundaries maintenance and impulse control.	Re-evaluate level Consistent limit setting with logical consequences	Re-evaluate level Delayed gratification Positive coping mechanisms	Re-evaluate level Decision making; Anger control.	Re-evaluate for PHP Promote self-reliance & diversional activities
NUTRITION/DIET CONTINUUM OF CARE	Diet Ordered: Initial D/C Plans	Chart daily intake Outcome survey	Chart daily intake Placement search	Weight, chart intake D/C Plan update/ revise	Chart daily intake After Care Plan written	Discharge instruction Outcome survey
PATIENT OUTCOMES	Controls self-harm/ Aggression	Anxiety decrease	Expresses anger appropriately	Makes + self statements	Uses problem solving skill	Broaden support system

PsychPaths™ © *Strategic Clinical Systems, Granbury, TX.*

The Nursing Process

Treatment Intervention Protocols

Several intervention protocols have been developed to save time in writing the same interventions repeatedly, and to give the nurse time to individualize the interventions. Intervention protocols relevant to clients who are aggressive and impulsive are anger-control assistance and appropriate stimulation of the neurobiological system.

Anger-control assistance

Anger-control assistance is helpful for clients who are impulsive or whose anxiety or tension easily converts to aggression. A nursing intervention classification has been developed (Box 25-4) for anger-control assistance.

Stimulation of the neurobiological system

Overstimulation of the neurobiological system occurs when there is damage to the structures of the brain, or the neurotransmitters are over- or under functioning. The reticular-activating system may also not be able to screen out irrelevant stimuli, bombarding the client with too much information too quickly. Teaching methods to help clients to modulate stimulation include the following:

- Help client to learn self-monitoring of inner pressure or overstimulation
- Instruct client to leave any activity during which the inner pressure begins
- Keep environmental stimuli at moderate levels (e.g., room temperature at 70 degrees, room lighting at 70 to 100 watts, voices at conversation level)
- Repair all irritating electrical light aberrations (e.g., buzzing, flickering, clanking)
- Have client wear headphones with tapes or music when noise level is loud or annoying
- Encourage client to avoid overstimulating or chaotic places and events, such as fairs, horse races, and bars

Box 25-4

Anger-Control Assistance

DEFINITION

Facilitation of the expression of anger in an adaptive non-violent manner

ACTIVITIES

Establish basic trust and rapport with patient

Use a calm, reassuring approach

Determine appropriate behavioral expectations for expression of anger, given patient's level of cognitive and physical functioning

Limit access to frustrating situations until patient is able to express anger in an adaptive manner

Encourage patient to seek assistance of nursing staff or responsible others during periods of increasing tension

Monitor potential for inappropriate aggression and intervene before its expression

Prevent physical harm if anger is directed at self or others (e.g., restrain and remove potential weapons)

Provide physical outlets for expression of anger or tension (e.g., punching bag, sports, clay, and writing in a journal)

Provide reassurance to patient that nursing staff will intervene to prevent patient from losing control

Use external controls (e.g., physical or manual restraint, time outs, and seclusion) as needed, to calm patient who is expressing anger in a maladaptive manner

Provide feedback on behavior to help patient identify anger

Assist patient in identifying the source of anger

Identify the function that anger, frustration, and rage serve for the patient

Identify consequences of inappropriate expression of anger

Assist patient in planning strategies to prevent the inappropriate expression of anger

Identify with patient the benefits of expressing anger in an adaptive, nonviolent manner

Establish expectation that patient can control his/her behavior

Instruct on use of calming measures (e.g., time outs and deep breaths)

Assist in developing appropriate methods of expressing anger to others (e.g., assertiveness and use of feeling statements)

Provide role models who express anger appropriately

Support patient in implementing anger control strategies and in the appropriate expression of anger

Provide reinforcement for appropriate expression of anger

Reprinted with permission from McCloskey, J.C. & Bulechek, G.M. (Eds.) (1996). Nursing interventions classification (NIC). (2nd ed.). St. Louis: Mosby.

The Nursing Process

Implementation

Although all nursing roles are enacted with clients with impulsive and aggressive disorders, several will be highlighted to emphasize factors to consider with this population. The roles to be explored are counseling, milieu management of aggression, psychobiological interventions, health teaching, and health promotion and maintenance.

Counseling

Standards of care for the development of rapport with clients with aggressive and impulsive disorders are found in Box 25-5. Cognitive-behavioral therapy has efficacy with persons with disorders of impulse. In fact, it is considered an essential adjunct to medication treatment if lasting change is to occur (L'Abate et al., 1992). Management of impulsiveness is usually the goal of therapy because impulsiveness appears to be a chronic condition (Butz and Austin, 1993).

Groups are useful with anger management. The group focuses on dysfunctional thoughts, decatastrophizing, identifying the worst-case scenarios and their aftermaths, assisting clients to think before acting, preparing for provocation, role playing, role reversal, and relaxation training to induce a sense of self-control (Anderson-Malico, 1994). Relaxation training without the tools for management of anger has not been effective in decreasing anger and aggression (Novacco, 1979) (see Chapter 14). In contrast, 12-step groups for impulsive behaviors such as alcohol and drug abuse have been "extraordinarily useful" in curbing impulsively destructive behaviors (McCown and VandenBos, 1994).

Contracting

***Contracting** is the development of a written agreement between a client and the nurse or treatment team in which the client's specific behaviors and their consequences are delineated.* A reward contract may say something such as, "If I do not yell at my roommate in the next 24 hours, I will earn two movie passes." A consequence contract may say something such as, "If I talk loudly out of anger, I will not work out on the weights that same day." The contract should consist of the following:

- What the client wants to change
- The specific new behaviors to be practiced
- The consequences for exhibiting the unhealthy behavior
- The rewards for practicing the new behavior

BOX 25-5

Establishing Rapport With an Aggressive Client

DEFINITION

Establishment of a relationship of mutual trust, built on certain guidelines to which both parties agree

ACTIVITIES

- Create an alliance with clients around the problems as they define them (see Chapter 9).
- Maintain a physical distance from the clients that they determine to be comfortable (see Chapters 6 and 8).
- Do not move toward clients who are exhibiting increasing agitation.
- Do not reach out or touch clients who are escalating.
- Consistently approach clients from the front and side, getting their attention before moving into their personal space.
- Maintain a balance between a focus on preventing aggression and a focus on the client as a person.
- Discuss with clients behaviors that are indicative of escalating aggression—*before* they are exhibited; tell clients the consequences of various behaviors.

- Assist clients to attend to the initial symptoms of aggressive behavior.
- Help clients identify appropriate ways to discharge and ventilate tension, such as jogging, weight lifting, guitar playing, relaxation exercises, clay modeling, and painting.
- Work toward having clients communicate when they need assistance from staff in controlling their own behavior.
- Discuss with the team the appropriateness of demonstrating to clients holding techniques, restraint, or seclusion; demonstration decreases a client's fear of the unknown and may facilitate an alliance with clients who are afraid of being punished for losing control.
- Express a concern for and an interest about the client's perceptions and problems.
- Set limits on inappropriate behaviors. "We will not allow you to hurt yourself or others."

The Nursing Process

Conflict management

Management of conflict is necessary because conflict causes anxiety, which is experienced as inner tension. Aggression and impulsiveness are used to manage the inner tension. Adults usually learn to manage conflict as a replacement of the impulsiveness and aggression characteristic of children. Conflict management is a strategy that clients can use to manage impulsiveness and aggression.

Conflict occurs because people want two different outcomes or actions that are, on the surface at least, mutually exclusive. For instance, John wants to leave the day hospital environment to pick up his food stamps. Staff members do not want John to leave because they believe he is avoiding some of the causes of his anxiety. There are three outcome options (Fisher, Ury, & Patton, 1991):

- Win-win, in which both parties get some part of their stated goals and feel all right about the compromises and/or creative solutions developed to get to a satisfactory solution
- Win-lose, in which one party gets what is wanted and the other gets nothing of what is wanted
- Lose-lose, in which all negotiations break down and neither party gets anything wanted

Applying this to John, a win-win solution would be for him to pick up the food stamps after the process group. A win-lose solution would be for the staff to insist that John stay for the group and not address John's stated need to pick up his food stamps. A lose-lose solution would be for John to walk out of the program and refuse to come back; he gets his food stamps, but he and the staff lose the opportunities afforded in continuing therapy. Even a win-lose solution is ultimately a lose-lose situation; when one party loses, there is a compulsion to get even, to win and make the other party lose.

Milieu Therapy

A useful strategy for aggressive and impulsive clients is environmental manipulation. The goal is to provide a predictable, stable social structure. Stability helps clients to participate in the unit milieu and to maintain control of their own behavior. Even something as simple as transfer to a different unit may precipitate aggression. There are several guidelines for managing the environment.

First, furnishing the unit with safety in mind can decrease the likelihood of damage to persons and property. Second, when someone with aggressive potential is on the unit, staff members need to be visible and available. If a client is to be given upsetting information, other staff members need to know when the client is to be told, and

contingency plans developed. Third, when a client is escalating, other clients, staff, and objects need to be moved away from the area. This serves two purposes: (1) increased safety for everybody if the client loses control, and (2) decreased opportunity for other clients to become anxious and thus precipitate aggressive or impulsive actions in some of them. Fourth, assist the client to a quiet, nonstimulating room and turn down lights and music to decrease the amount of stimulation bombarding the client.

De-escalation

Some techniques to use for ***de-escalation,*** *or defusing a potentially aggressive situation,* include the following:

- Avoiding power struggles (allow clients to win struggles for control without giving in to unrealistic demands)
- Giving clients what they define as important if at all possible
- Teaching clients verbal skills of negotiation and collaboration
- Encouraging client involvement in decision making
- Showing respect when clients act independently
- Instituting consequences for violent or threatening behavior

Limit setting

Limit setting *is clarifying appropriate, expected behavior in light of potential or actual inappropriate behaviors.* Inappropriate client behaviors include verbal abuse of staff and other clients, manipulative and exploitive behavior, threats, sexual and physical aggression, and inappropriate familiarity. Setting firm limits on unacceptable and inappropriate behaviors in a nondefensive manner is part of the nursing role. Research on styles of limit setting indicates that the nurse's approach to limit setting makes a difference in the client's response (see Research Highlight on p. 472).

Retaliation although at times tempting, is inappropriate, unprofessional, and unethical. The alternative is to develop a treatment plan in conjunction with the treatment team that addresses the aggressive or impulsive behavior and to follow that treatment plan. Box 25-6 provides interventions for limit setting.

Time-out

Time-out *is a strategy for behavior control in which clients, on prompting from staff or family, voluntarily remove themselves from the environment.* Time-out decreases the potential for client and staff or family injury,

The Nursing Process

RESEARCH HIGHLIGHT

Lancee, W.J., Gallop, R., McCay, E., & Toner, B. (1995). The relationship between nurses' limit-setting styles and anger in psychiatric inpatients. *Psychiatric Services, 46* (6), 609-613.

Summary

The purpose of the study was to explore the influence of nurses' limit-setting styles on inpatient psychiatric clients' anger.

The dependent, or outcome, variable was state anger. The independent variables measured were limit-setting style, psychiatric diagnosis, and impulsivity. The six limit-setting styles tested* included the following:

1. Belittlement ("You act like a child, you get treated like a child.")

2. Platitudes ("We practice the Golden Rule here; treat others as you want to be treated.")

3. Solution without options ("OK, you need time away from each other right now.")

4. Solution with options ("OK, because you need time away from each other right now, do you two want to go to your own rooms or someplace else while you cool off?")

5. Affective involvement without options ("Uh oh, looks like you two have gotten on each others' nerves.")

6. Affective involvement with options ("Uh oh, things feel tense. Is now a good time to talk, or shall we meet back here together after some cool-off time?")

The subjects were 56 psychiatric inpatients who agreed to respond to four role-play situations that commonly occur between clients and nurses on an inpatient unit. The clients acted out their responses. The Spielberger Scale was used to measure the amount of anger generated in each scenario.

The amount of impulsivity was directly related to the amount of anger generated, no matter what the limit-setting style or diagnosis. The limit-setting styles were found to be directly related to anger, with belittling correlated with the highest anger scores, affective involvement with options correlated with the lowest anger scores. Schizophrenia was correlated with the least amount of anger. Diagnosis was not statistically related to impulsivity.

The amount of anger generated with limit setting may be influenced by the nurse's limit-setting style.

Implications for Nursing Practice

1. Belittling is an ineffective style used to set limits, almost always generates considerable anger, and may actually precipitate aggression.

2. Affective involvement, or establishing rapport and relationship, is correlated with the least amount of anger, though anger is still generated.

3. Offering options is an effective strategy, whether with or without affective involvement.

4. The most effective strategy across all diagnoses and across levels of impulsivity is affective involvement with options.

5. The nurse's interaction style is not the only factor, but is certainly one factor, in the amount of anger and aggression expressed by psychiatric inpatients.

The phrases were not used in the study, but illustrated the limit-setting styles.

increases the client's control of and responsibility for own behavior, and is less intrusive than seclusion or restraint.

If the client is unable to choose time-out or cannot control behavior within a reasonable period of time, seclusion or restraint is the next most restrictive step. Involuntary time-out is not a legal entity. The client either chooses voluntarily to use a quiet space, or is involuntarily forced into seclusion or restraints. Open door, closed door, and locked door are variables that do not legally enter into the definition. The only variable is the client's choice.

The Nursing Process

BOX 25-6

Limit Setting

DEFINITION

Establishing the parameters of desirable and acceptable patient behavior

ACTIVITIES

Discuss concerns with patient about behavior

Identify (with patient input, when appropriate) undesirable patient behavior

Discuss with patient, when appropriate, what is desirable behavior in a given situation or setting

Establish reasonable expectations for patient behavior, based on the situation and the patient

Establish consequences (with patient input, when appropriate) for occurrence/nonoccurrence of desired behaviors

Communicate the established behavioral expectations and consequences to the patient in language that is easily understood and nonpunitive

Communicate established behavioral expectations and consequences with other staff who are caring for patient

Refrain from arguing or bargaining about the established behavioral expectations and consequences with the patient

Assist patient, when necessary and appropriate, to show the desired behaviors

Monitor patient for occurrence/nonoccurrence of the desired behaviors

Modify behavioral expectations and consequences, as needed, to accommodate reasonable changes in the patient's situation

Initiate the established consequences for the occurrence/nonoccurrence of the desired behaviors

Decrease limit setting, as patient behavior approximates the desired behaviors

Reprinted with permission from McCloskey, J.C., & Bulechek, G.M. (Eds.). (1996). Nursing interventions classification (NIC). (2nd ed.). St. Louis: Mosby.

Seclusion and restraint

Seclusion is any involuntary confinement of a person alone in a room that the person is physically prevented from leaving. Restraint is any method of physically restricting a person's freedom of movement, physical activity, or normal access to the body.

Whenever seclusion and/or restraints are used, the client is also placed on constant observation status. *Constant observation is continuous one-on-one monitoring of a client to ensure the safety and well-being of the client and others.* Some ways to increase the therapeutic potential of restraints include the following:

• Planning with client what will happen if client loses control, including seclusion or restraint

• Planning with client to intervene in escalation before restraint becomes necessary, including contracting

• Discussing alternatives to restraint if loss of control occurs

• Asking client if face up or face down is a better position if restraint is necessary

• After a restraint episode is discontinued, debriefing with client feelings, thoughts, and understanding about why restraint was used and clarify any misinformation

• Informing and continuing to inform client before and during a restraint procedure about why it is being done and what client behavior is required to discontinue the procedure

Guidelines for the use of seclusion and restraint are found in Box 25-7 and include monitoring and documentation requirements. Many of the guidelines for seclusion and restraint are determined by the state courts; one held in Alabama in 1992 may change some of the current national standards (Recent court ruling..., 1992).

Reintroduction into the milieu

When someone loses control and becomes verbally or physically aggressive, the relationships the client has with staff members and other clients have been violated. In relationships, persons are expected to behave courteously and thus be worthy of trust. The persons in the community who feel that trust has been broken, whether clients or staff, need an opportunity to reestablish the relationship. Usually a one-to-one visit between the client and staff provides an opportunity to talk through the event and the feelings and perceptions and to establish a connectedness again. A clinical example follows:

Cletus S., a 17 year old, had "adopted" 15-year-old Stony while they were both hospitalized on the adolescent unit.

The Nursing Process

BOX 25-7

Guidelines for the Use of Seclusion and Restraint

CLINICAL INDICATIONS AND CONTRAINDICATIONS

- To safely contain a client who is exhibiting out-of-control behavior
- To prevent a client from injuring self or others (according to the 1992 Alabama ruling, this is the only indication for restraint)
- To prevent serious disruption of the therapeutic environment or the likelihood of significant property damage
- To intervene proactively as part of a comprehensive treatment plan with specific goals and assessment parameters
  Seclusion and restraint may **never** be used in the following circumstances:
- As punishment (i.e., staff members are angry because client repeatedly ignores reasonable requests)
- For the convenience of staff (i.e., during change of shift report or short staffing)
- As a substitute for individualized treatment (staff members indicate they do not have time to stay with client while parents are visiting, so client is placed in seclusion)

PROTOCOLS

- An as-needed order is never permitted.
- A physician or registered nurse authorized by the physician may make the decision to initiate seclusion and/or restraint based on the client's current behavior. The physician must be notified as soon as possible but no later than 1 hour after restrictions are initiated.
- Each order to restrain or seclude must include an expiration time, and under no circumstance can the time be greater than 24 hours. (In Alabama the restriction is a maximum of 8 hours.) A physician must make a clinical assessment of the client and sign the order within 24 hours. (In Alabama a physician must see the client in person within 4 hours, preferably within 1 hour.)

- The client must be treated in a manner that demonstrates respect, maximizes comfort, minimizes pain, and precludes harm. Staff rights to dignity, modesty, respect, comfort, and freedom from pain are also a consideration during the initiation of seclusion and restraint.

ASSESSMENT AND DOCUMENTATION

- Clients in seclusion and/or restraints must be assessed at regular intervals, usually every 15 minutes, and their behavior documented.
- Clients in restraints must have circulation of the limbs checked every 15 minutes. For poor circulation, range-of-motion exercise is completed, and for chafing, padding is added to the restraint. The intervention is documented.
- Documentation must occur hourly that the client has been offered the opportunity to drink water and to void or defecate; intake and output should be accurately recorded. If the client can maintain control, a toilet, rather than a urinal or bedpan, may be used.
- Documentation must occur three times a day and in the evening that meals or snacks have been offered and how much was eaten.
- At least every 24 hours, the client has the right to wash, brush teeth, comb hair, put on deodorant, and so forth. Sometimes the activities can wait until the client is out of seclusion or restraint, but at no time can the client's physical hygiene be neglected for an indefinite period.
- An administrative record of all clients in seclusion or restraint and the lengths of time of the restrictions is to be kept and reviewed monthly. The record is used to improve quality, review utilization of resources, and detect patterns of the use of seclusion and restraint. The goal is to entirely eliminate the use of seclusion and restraint.

Stony lost control yesterday and used a ping-pong paddle to damage some of the items in the day room. He had permitted Cletus to get close, to talk with him, and to take the paddle. Cletus had purposely distracted Stony so that the security officers could get hold of Stony to take him to seclusion. After the event, Cletus felt guilty about betraying Stony, did not know how Stony felt about him, and was concerned about how things would be between them when Stony came back into the community. The nurse for these two clients discussed their need to reestablish their relationship. She set up a meeting between them in Stony's seclusion room. The door remained open and the nurse remained

near enough to intervene, if needed. The young men talked and shared and reestablished the relationship that had been important to both.

Reestablishment of rapport, both for staff and for clients, first requires acknowledgement of one's own thoughts and feelings about the aggressing client. For instance, the primary nurse for Stony might have said to peers, "I've tried so hard to be comfortable around Stony. Now I'm faced with overwhelming fear, and I'm furious with him. I don't know whether I can continue to work with him." Second, communicate perceptions, thoughts,

The Nursing Process

and feelings related to the aggression incident. It is helpful for clients to say their thoughts and feelings, as in a community meeting. Staff may communicate to peers in a staff or debriefing meeting. The energy built up by anger and fear can be expressed, making it easier to communicate those same thoughts, and feelings with caring and concern to the aggressing client. The client needs an opportunity to listen and to express thoughts and perceptions too.

Staff consistency

Although staff consistency probably is not as instrumental in aggression management as often believed, it is an important factor in creating a healthy milieu. Staff consistency is facilitated when the following occurs:

- There are very few rules, and all are aimed at implementing treatment concepts such as safety and respect
- The concepts are emphasized repeatedly, and exceptions to rules and policies are made as long as they do not violate the concepts
- The rules facilitate adjustment to the outside world and not primarily to the treatment milieu

Clients test rules. The more rules a treatment environment has, the more testing that occurs. Staff members have a difficult time being both rule implementers and therapeutic staff persons if the rules become the predominant method of interaction between staff and clients.

Staff training and peer review

Staff experience aggressive and impulsive feelings, as well as clients. Maintaining control over the feelings and acting constructively are good methods of role-modeling for clients, who are aware of the rush of feelings in others, as well as in themselves. Staff training is essential to help maintain control of one's behavior. Techniques for the prevention of aggression can be taught to professionals, family members, peace officers, and other members of society who come into contact with aggressive persons. The Community Resources box on p. 476 provides some training resources.

Staff discussion of interactions with clients can take place in individual sessions or in small groups. The goal of the discussion is to allow the staff member to examine personal behaviors, feelings, and thoughts in a safe, nonjudgmental atmosphere with someone who can assist with those issues. The persons who assist can be any licensed team members with advanced degrees. However, they cannot be someone who evaluates or is in a position to reward or punish the staff member.

Peer review requires mature staff members who are fair, honest, and caring toward one another but who do not have personal relationships away from work. This is necessary because giving and receiving feedback may be perceived as threatening to relationships; some staff members are unwilling to threaten a personal relationship by being honest with professional feedback. The goal is to examine one's own and another's behavior objectively and fairly and to share those observations with another. Peer review gives staff members an opportunity to learn from feedback and to develop additional expertise.

Psychobiological Interventions

Beta-blockers (propranolol is the most common and the most effective) have been used quite successfully for decreasing violent outbursts in clients with organic bases for rage. Though the exact mechanism of the effect is not known, there is a belief that there is "a final common pathway mediating aggression of any origin," because the medication treats aggression arising from such a wide variety of disorders. The four most likely explanations include the following (Haspel, 1995):

- Helping the prefrontal cortex provide appropriate inhibitory functions that were injured by some accident or lesion
- Decreasing the stimulation caused by excess production of neurotransmitters; beta-blockers block beta-adrenergic receptors
- Blocking the central nervous system stimulation that triggers the locus ceruleus and its projections
- A combination of the three above and the affinity of beta-blockers to displace 5-HT from its receptors; these effects apparently reduce both predatory and impulsive aggression (Haspel, 1995)

Because of the link to the serotonergic system, the use of SSRIs (selective serotonergic reuptake inhibitors) and MAOIs (monoamine oxidase inhibitors) are also common (see Chapter 15). These may be prescribed for children and for adults.

Another medication currently in clinical trials for aggression is clozapine (Ratney et al., 1993), particularly with treatment-resistant, severely aggressive persons with subaverage intelligence. Clinical anecdotes document dramatic decreases in aggression with these clients (Bellus, Stewart, and Kost, 1995). Medication Tips on p. 477 provide some guidelines for giving medications to clients who are aggressive and impulsive.

The Nursing Process

COMMUNITY RESOURCES

Aggression Management Program
Developed by the Hospital of the University of
Pennsylvania, Philadelphia (Martin, 1995).

**CAPE (Controlling Aggressive Patients
Effectively)**
P.O. Box 53277
Oklahoma City, OK 73152-3277
(405)522-0007

CPI (National Crisis Prevention Institute, Inc.)
3315-KN 124th Street
Brookfield, WI 53005
(414)783-5787

Mandt Training
One- and two-day programs for staff in nursing homes,
hospitals, emergency departments, and facilities for
clients with mental disorders.
P.O. Box 831790
Richardson, Texas 75083-1790
(214)669-1362

REB Security Training, Inc.
Two-day program for security officers and others in
managing and controlling aggression.
P.O. Box 697
Avon, CT 06001
(203)677-5936

Wickersty and Associates, Inc.
Offers programs on controlling aggression in
hospitals.
P.O. Box 646
Bladensburg, MD 20710-0646
(800)966-3866.

SUGGESTED READINGS

Gertz, B. (1980). Training for prevention of assaultive
behavior in a psychiatric setting. *Hospital and Community Psychiatry, 31,* 628-630.

Lehmann, L.S. et. al. (1983). Training personnel in the
prevention and management of violent behavior.
Hospital and Community Psychiatry, 34, 40-43.

Sacramento Management of Assaultive Behavior Task
Force. (May 1, 1987). *Management of assaultive behavior.* Sacramento: California Department of Mental Health.

Thackrey, M. (1987). *Therapeutics for aggression: Psy-
chological/physical crisis intervention.* New York:
Human Sciences Press. (Documents a 4-hour course
on management of crises.)

Health Teaching

Because production of the monoamines are diet related
(as are the use of monoamine inhibitors), clients may
be taught healthy eating habits specifically to assist
with neurotransmitter development. Vitamins needed
are niacin and thiamine, both found in whole-grain
breads, enriched cereals, pork, liver, and legumes
(Harper-Jacques and Reimer, 1992). Plenty of sleep and
modulating stimuli are also helpful in decreasing impulsivity and aggression. Avoiding excessive stimuli is a
good way for clients to manage irritability and impulsiveness.

Although communication skills are not likely to decrease the amount of aggression in an adult's life, the
same is not true for adolescents. Adolescents often have
a difficult time verbalizing their feelings and separating
thoughts, feelings, and actions. Communication skills are
useful to adolescents in reducing aggression that comes
from the frustration of being unable to communicate or
not being heard (Marohn, 1992).

Conflict resolution and negotiation skills are also useful, as mentioned earlier. See Teaching Points on p. 478
for ideas on teaching these skills.

Health Promotion and Health Maintenance

Several health promotion and maintenance strategies for
clients with impulsiveness and aggression have been
mentioned throughout this chapter. There are two others to examine more closely: prevention of aggression
and relationship interventions.

The Nursing Process

 MEDICATION TIPS

Impulsive and Aggressive Clients

1. Nurses should tell clients the truth about medications and the behaviors they are designed to help.

2. The nurse should determine, each time medication is given, that clients know what they are receiving, the dosage, and the therapeutic effect; the nurse should seek an evaluation of the medication each time the client receives it. Aggressive and impulsive clients may resist taking psychotropic medications and may have difficulty with compliance once they are self-medicating. Evaluation helps clients to internalize the need for medication.

3. The nurse should make sure clients actually take medication. Often, aggressive clients will check their medications because they do not trust the real motivation behind the nurse or the physician giving the medication to them. Liquid medication may be necessary. If crushing medication is a viable option, the nurse should check with the pharmacist to see if the medication can be crushed without losing any of its therapeutic effects.

4. Giving as-needed intramuscular medications is usually a hazardous job because clients who are in the midst of uncontrolled behavior receive them. To decrease hazards to both clients and staff the nurse should do the following:

   a. If the order permits discretion, the nurse should offer clients the option of PO or IM medications. The nurse should ignore any verbal escalation if clients agree to take medication by mouth.

   b. The nurse should have medication ready. The nurse should not make client or staff wait before medication is given.

   c. If client refuses to take medication, the nurse should not give it unless there are court papers on the chart to pursue legal detention of client for danger to self or others (see Chapter 3).

   d. If an IM injection is necessary, there should be enough staff to hold clients, should they become aggressive.

   e. If possible, the nurse should give injections in a quiet place, out of the view of other clients. Often, others will perceive staff as intimidating or abusing the client and will themselves become more anxious and possibly impulsive and aggressive.

   f. The nurse should wear gloves and take the syringe to the room in a small box. The nurse should place the syringe in the box as soon as the injection is given. Do not recap the needle. The box offers a safe way to travel through the hall and among staff and clients without creating a hazard for the nurse or others. The uncapped needle and syringe should be disposed in the nearest hazard control box, usually in the medication room.

   g. Clients should be told that medications should begin to help in about 10 minutes. The nurse should check back in about 10 minutes and ask clients their evaluations of the effects of the medications. This dialogue encourages the client to participate in planning and implementing care.

Prevention of aggression

Prevention of aggression has been suggested in several areas:

- Aggressive prenatal programs for mothers who abuse alcohol and drugs

- Parenting classes that emphasize personal responsibility for one's behavior
- Problem-solving skills taught in schools (Touchet, Shure & McCown, 1993)
- Decrease in exposure to violence, victimization, and trauma (Herman, Perry, and Vander Kolk, 1989)

The Nursing Process

TEACHING POINTS

Conflict Management Strategies for Clients Who Are Aggressive

The following strategies can be both taught and role-modeled as staff members work with clients.

1. Acknowledge that a conflict exists.

2. Both parties must decide if the conflict needs to be resolved. Sometimes a conflict exists but does not affect the parties' abilities to continue the relationship. For instance, the nurse may think that curfew time for night treatment clients should be 8 pm, and the clients coming in may prefer 10 pm on the weekends. The conflict does not matter if neither party has the authority to alter the time.

3. If the conflict gets in the way of trust, and the parties have the authority to resolve it (or at least to make a mutually determined recommendation) the following principles are helpful:

   a. The goal is a solution that both parties would support. This is a win-win solution and quite often, neither party has thought of the solution before negotiations begin; this solution is a synergistic creation of honest, forthright, respectful listening and problem solving.

   b. Nurses should assume that they can learn a lot by listening to the other person. If nurses believe that changing their minds means losing face or losing ground, they are in a win-lose or a lose-lose posture. This is not helpful. Nurses can change their minds and approach the negotiations again.

   c. Nurses should find out what the other party really wants. For instance, a group of adolescents on an inpatient unit may say they want to stay up to watch the news on television. By unit rule the lights are out by 10 PM. The adolescents really want 30 additional minutes of phone time and it would be nice to watch the news as well. The staff really wants to finish charting before 10 PM. Until the real interests of the two sides are out in the open, there is no way to reach one of several creative alternatives available to these two groups.

   d. Nurses should maintain respectful, honest, assertive communication. They should confront disrespectful, dishonest, aggressive, or passive communication by indicating that it jeopardizes a win-win solution to the issue.

   e. If the meeting has reached an impasse, or if the client or staff can only discuss for a limited amount of time, another time to meet with new ideas and suggestions should be arranged. If no new ideas are forthcoming, the side with no new ideas should be asked whether they want to continue to look for a more satisfactory solution than the one with which they are currently living.

Compiled from Fisher, R., Ury, W., & Patton, B. (1991). Getting to yes: Negotiating agreement without giving in. *New York: Simon and Schuster and Houghton Mifflin Company.*

- Enhancement of parent-child attachment experiences
- Provision of opportunities for alternative relationships with caring adult figures

Relationship interventions

Aggression occurs because of environmental provocation. Aggression may occur either when the aggressor knows and is angry with another person or does not know or perceive the other person as human. Both of these conditions may occur because of mental illness,

such as paranoia or dissociative identity disorder. However, they often occur with persons who have no mental illness.

To humanize relationships for aggressive people may be a challenge. To effectively intervene with a client, nurses find ways to "give in without giving up," that is, declining or giving up a power struggle while not giving in to unreasonable demands (Harris and Morrison, 1995). Getting to know somebody makes aggression against them more difficult. Staying in touch with the humanness of an enraged person is another challenge.

The Nursing Process

THE CONSUMER'S VOICE

Impulse-Control Disorder

Anonymous

Having an impulse-control disorder is like having a time bomb ticking inside of you all the time. You never know when the fuse is going to ignite and explode without having a chance to snuff it out and not hurt anybody. It's like a red haze sweeps over me, and I can't think clearly or feel anything other than rage. I have to get rid of it, and my instinct is to do that by striking out. I am ashamed of the fact that in doing so I have physically and emotionally hurt members of my family. In my rage, I have said and done horrible things to my wife and children. I have told them they were stupid (and much worse). I have thrown full plates of food because the potatoes were mashed, not baked, or the chicken was broiled, not fried. My family has told me, and I can tell, that they feel like they are walking on eggshells all the time. They never know when the eggs will crack—sometimes for no apparent reason—and another reign of terror will begin. Unfortunately for all of us, no one ever really confronted me about my explosiveness. They just ran for cover, waiting for the storm to be over, hoping no one got hurt in the crossfire.

So until recently (and I am now 51) I never realized that I had a problem. I thought this was the way all "real" men acted. After all, my father beat me and my brothers with a strap on a regular basis and verbally reamed us out regularly. It was only after my first wife finally divorced me, and I broke the collarbone of my second wife's 8-year-old son and she pressed charges that the court forced me to go to a treatment program for persons with impulse-control problems.

I thank God every day for this program. I'm only sorry that I wasn't forced to go to something like this before I did so much damage to my family and, I'm sure, others as well. The most important thing the doctors, nurses, and social workers do is treat me with patience and respect, even though I've done such awful things. They use behavioral strategies to help me recognize and deal with my anger and explosiveness before it gets out of control. If one approach doesn't work, they come up with another one.

I'm not cured; I may never be, but I'm a lot better now. I am talking about my feelings rather than acting on them, for the first time in my life. The support group I attend, where other people understand and accept me, is very important to me. My wife and her kids are also hanging in there with me. We are going to family therapy together, which means a whole lot to me. I live one day at a time and pray for the strength to be in charge of myself.

Evaluation

Evaluation of outcomes established with the client and communicated in the client's treatment plan completes the nursing process and forms the assessment for a revision of the plan. Besides outcomes evaluation, staff examines the relative success of interventions used, with input from the client and family or significant others.

When interventions have been successful and goals accomplished, it is possible for clients to manage their own aggressions and impulsiveness with some occasional coaching by significant others. Relationships are improved and work and school are less disrupted by poor judgment and unacceptable behavior. The client is less alienated from others and has an opportunity to make constructive contributions to family and society.

KEY POINTS

- Clients with impulsive and aggressive behaviors are often alienated from friends and family, have a difficult time establishing and maintaining relationships, and feel that their emotions and behavior are out of control.
- Theoretical explanations for impulsive and aggressive behaviors are primarily biological in nature, although some kinds of aggression and impulsivity have psychodynamic, family, and social causes or reinforcers.
- Behaviors common to impulsivity and aggression are explosiveness, escalation, and remorse. Impulse control disorders include intermittent explosive disorder, kleptomania, pyromania, pathological

CRITICAL THINKING QUESTIONS

Jim J. was brought to your hospital in handcuffs from the city jail where he had spent 3 days for assault. His family had arranged for admission to the day treatment program with insurance certification for 5 days of treatment. Jim is 23 years old and has a history of impulsive aggression, theft, and drug use. As you approach Jim, the police officers, and four arriving family members, Jim stands up very straight, takes a step toward you, and says in a low, threatening tone, "You think *you* are going to help me? I could wrap one hand around your throat."

1. What is your first impresssion of Jim? What are your thoughts, feelings, and actions toward him? What are your thoughts, feelings, and actions toward yourself?
2. Describe three possible responses to Jim, each designed to be therapeutic. Give a rationale for each.
3. What are the five most essential pieces of information you need about Jim? How would each contribute to the assessment you need to develop a plan of care for Jim?
4. How long would you want to leave Jim in handcuffs? Why? How would you work with him to get the handcuffs removed? What therapeutic purposes would release from the restraint serve, if accomplished within 15 minutes of arrival to the facility?
5. In what ways would you work with Jim and the other patients in the day program to minimize intimidation and eliminate aggression? Whose assistance, among your multidisciplinary team members, would you need?

gambling, and trichotillomania. Sexual disorders are characterized by impulsivity and are called paraphilias.
- The most common antecedent for aggression is history of aggression. The most common contingency is a relationship issue in which the client has felt provoked. The release of tension for both impulsive and aggressive clients is often the greatest consequence and reinforces the behavior. Other consequences are destructiveness to the client, to relationships, and to property.
- Nurses can best manage their own aggressive and impulsive feelings by doing self-assessments when they experience inner pressure, anxiety, anger, or

fear. In addition, formal staff training shows how to manage oneself.
- Positive outcomes for clients with aggressive and impulsive disorders include a decrease in destructive behavior, increase in management skills for impulsivity and aggression, and improvement in self-monitoring.
- Some common standards of care used with clients who are impulsive and aggressive are anger control assistance and management of the stimulation of the neurobiological system.
- Nursing roles that have special applications with clients who are aggressive and impulsive are counseling, milieu management, psychobiological interventions, health teaching, and health promotion and maintenance.
- The use of seclusion and restraints have many legal requirements, because these interventions interfere with the client's constitutional right to freedom.

REFERENCES

American Psychiatric Association (1994). *Diagnostic and statistical manual of mental disorders, fourth edition.* Washington, DC: Author.

Anderson-Malico, R. (1994). Anger management using cognitive group therapy. *Perspectives in Psychiatric Care, 30* (3), 17-20.

Barratt, E. (1993). Impulsivity: Integrating cognitive, behavioral, biological, and environmental data. In W. McCown, J. Johnson, & M. Shure (Eds.), *The impulsive client: Theory, research, and treatment.* Washington, DC: Author.

Bellus, S.B., Stewart, D., & Kost, P.P. (1995). Clozapine in aggression: Letter to the editor. *Psychiatric Services, 46* (2), 187.

Botsis, A.J., Soldatos, C.R., Liossi, A., Kokkevi, A., & Stefanis, C.N. (1994). Suicide and violence risk: I. Relationship to coping styles. *Acta Psychiatrica Scandanavia, 89,* 92-96.

Brill, N.Q. (1993). *America's psychic malignancy.* Springfield, IL: CC Thomas.

Butz, M., & Austin, S. (1993). Management of the adult impulsive client: Identification, timing, and methods of treatment. In W. McCown, J. Johnson, & M. Shure, (Eds.), *The impulsive client: Theory, research, and treatment.* Washington, DC: American Psychological Association.

Constantino, J.N. (1995). Early relationships and the development of aggression in children. *Harvard Review of Psychiatry, 2* (5), 259-273.

Crowner, M., Peric, G., Stepcic, F., & Ventura, F. (1995). Psychiatric patients' explanations for assaults. *Psychiatric Services, 46* (6), 614-615.

Daum, A.L. (1994). The disruptive antisocial patient: Management strategies. *Nursing Management, 25* (8), 46-51.

Durivage, A. (1989). Assaultive behavior: Before it happens. *Canadian Journal of Psychiatry, 34,* 393-397.

Eysenck, S.B.G., & Eysenck, H.J. (1978). Impulsiveness and venturesomeness: Their position in a dimensional system of personality description. *Psychological Reports, 43*, 1247-1255.

Fisher, R., Ury, W., & Patton, B. (1991). *Getting to yes: Negotiating agreement without giving in.* New York: Simon and Shuster and Houghton Mifflin Company.

Gallop, R., McCay, E., & Esplen, M.J. (1992). The conceptualization of impulsivity for psychiatric nursing practice. *Archives of Psychiatric Nursing, 6* (6), 366-373.

Garza-Trevino, E.S. (1994). Neurobiological factors in aggressive behavior. *Hospital and Community Psychiatry, 45* (7), 690-699.

Harper-Jacques, S., & Reimer, M. (1992). Aggressive behavior and the brain: A different perspective for the mental health nurse. *Archives of Psychiatric Nursing, 6* (5), 313-320.

Harris, D., & Morrison, E.F. (1995). Managing violence without coercion. *Archives of Psychiatric Nursing, 9,* (4), 203-210.

Haspel, T. (1995). Beta-blockers and the treatment of aggression. *Harvard Review of Psychiatry, 2* (5), 274-281.

Herman, J., Perry, I.O., & Van der Kolk, B. (1989). Childhood trauma in borderline personality disorder. *American Journal of Psychiatry, 146*, 490-495.

Katz, P., & Kirkland, F.R. (1990). Violence and social structure on mental hospital wards. *Psychiatry, 53*, 262-277.

L'Abate, L. (1994). *A theory of personality development.* New York: Wiley & Sons.

L'Abate, L., Farrar, J., & Serritella, D. (1992). *Handbook of differential treatments for addiction.* Needham Heights, MA: Allyn and Bacon.

Lancee, W.J., Gallop, R., McCay, E., & Toner, B. (1995). The relationship between nurses' limit-setting styles and anger in psychiatric inpatients. *Psychiatric Services, 46* (6), 609-613.

Marohn, R. (1992). Management of the assaultive adolescent. *Hospital and Community Psychiatry, 43* (6), 622-624.

Martin, K.H. (1995). Improving staff safety through an aggression management program. *Archives of Psychiatric Nursing, 9* (4), 211-215.

Morrison, E.F. (1994). The evolution of a concept: Aggression and violence in psychiatric settings. *Archives of Psychiatric Nursing, 8* (4), 245-253.

Newhill, C.E., Mulvey, E.P., & Lidz, C.W. (1995). Characteristics of violence in the community by female patients seen in a psychiatric emergency service. *Psychiatric Services, 46* (8), 785-789.

Novacco, R. (1979). Cognitive regulation of anger and stress. In P. Kendall, & S. Hollan (Eds.). *Cognitive-behavioral interventions: Theory, research, and procedures.* New York: Academic Press.

Poster, E.C., & Ryan, J. (1994). A multiregional study of nurses' beliefs and attitudes about work safety and patient assault. *Hospital and Community Psychiatry, 45* (11), 1104-1108.

Ratney, J.J. et. al. (1993). The effects of clozapine on severely aggressive psychiatric inpatients in a state hospital. *Journal of Clinical Psychiatry, 54*, 219-233.

Recent court ruling in Alabama's Wyatt case modifies 20-year-old patient care standards. (1992). *Hospital and Community Psychiatry, 43* (8), 851-852.

Thomas, S.P. (Ed.). (1993). *Women and anger.* New York: Springer.

Touchet, M., Shure, M., & McCown, W. (1993). Interpersonal cognitive problem solving as prevention and treatment of impulsive behaviors. In W. McCown, J. Johnson, & M. Shure (Eds.), *The impulsive client: Theory, research, and treatment.* Washington, DC: American Psychological Association.

Vikkunen, M., Nuutila, A., Goodwin, F.K., & Linnoila, M. (1987). Cerebrospinal fluid monoamine metabolite levels in male arsonists. *Archives of General Psychiatry, 44*, 241.

Yager, J. (1989). Clinical manifestations of psychiatric disorders. In H.I. Kaplan & B.J. Sadock (Eds.). *Comprehensive textbook of psychiatry* (5th ed.). Baltimore: Williams and Wilkins.

VIDEO RESOURCES

Psychiatric Emergencies
Pamela E. Marcus
Module 3: Violence, Aggression, Suicide, and Posttraumatic Stress Disorder

Chapter 26

Personality Disorders

Norine J. Kerr

LEARNING OUTCOMES

After studying and applying the concepts of this chapter, the learner will be able to:

- Discuss the epidemiology and risk factors of personality disorders.
- Differentiate among relevant theories that attempt to explain the biological, sociocultural, and psychodynamic correlates of personality disorders.
- Discuss the essential biopsychosocial symptoms and characteristics of personality disorders.
- Apply the nursing process to the care of clients diagnosed with personality disorders.
- Use current theories about personality disorders to formulate relevant nursing diagnoses and realistic outcome criteria for individuals diagnosed with personality disorders.
- Discuss the relationship between nursing care plans for two common nursing diagnoses used with clients with personality disorders (PDs) and interdisciplinary treatment plans for PD.
- Evaluate established nursing care plans for the nursing diagnoses personal identity disturbance and potential for violence.

KEY TERMS

Activities of daily living (ADLs)	Hypersexual behavior	Projection
Affect	Idealization	Reality testing
Devaluation	Impulse control	Relatedness
Distorted self-perception	Judgment	Splitting
Dysphoria	Mood	Stimulus filter/stimulus barrier
Ego-dystonic	Object constancy	Thought processes
Ego-syntonic	Poor impulse control	Unhealthy manipulation
Healthy self-perception		

In the past, health care professionals and even the public referred to people with personality disorders (PD) as sociopaths, psychopaths, deviants, perverts, or antisocial people. The negative connotations of these terms contribute to the stigma of PD as a mental health disorder. Even today, some health care professionals who were educated many years ago and who do not work in the field of psychiatric-mental health might describe clients who have personality disorders as people who act out in society and have "no feelings toward others" and no "conscience" or sense of guilt. Some clients with the diagnosis of PD do reflect these descriptors. However, today people with PD are considered to have "presenting problems" that reflect dysfunctional behavioral patterns, rather than the overt psychotic symptoms seen in acute schizophrenia. Their behaviors reflect problems with impulse control, judgment, reality testing, self-perception, mood, and activities of daily living (ADLs) and lead to recurring patterns of ineffective social, vocational, sexual, and interpersonal functioning (Kerr, 1990). In other words, their overall dysfunctional behavioral patterns are pervasive, inflexible, and generally do not fit with the norm of the person's culture. Often, their distressing and "unlikable" behavior is apparent in adolescence or early adulthood (American Psychiatric Association [APA], 1994).

The purpose of this chapter is to help the learner understand PDs so that individuals with these disorders can receive the emotional support needed to cope and to change. When certain patterns of thinking and behaving create recurrent problems in a person's life, as seen in alcohol and drug abuse, relationship difficulties, chronic depression, and school or work failures, a PD may be involved. PDs involve the very structure of the client's character (ego), so treatment usually is long-term and changes are slow to occur. Clients with this diagnosis may require hospitalization during periods of crisis, although their basic problems are of a more long-standing nature.

EPIDEMIOLOGY

Accurate statistics on people who meet the diagnostic criteria (APA, 1994) of PD are difficult to determine. A great deal of stigma is attached to these diagnoses, and reimbursement for Axis II diagnoses is a related issue. (Axis II refers to a category of the *Diagnostic and Statistical Manual of Mental Disorders, Fourth Edition,* [DSM-IV] multiaxial assessment system. Axis II is used to report PDs and mental retardation.) It is suspected that many people with PD are never clinically diagnosed, since many are in the mainstream of society experiencing difficulties in life in general and in work and personal relationships specifically. However, their difficulties are rarely to the degree that hospitalization of any length is required. Therefore many people with PD never seek treatment, nor do they come to the attention of health care professionals. Thus they remain uncounted and add to the difficulty of determining exact statistics on this mental disorder.

Clients with PDs who demonstrate a high potential for violence most commonly draw attention from nurses. According to the data available, 5% to 15% of the adult population has some form of PD. They tend to come from younger age groups and often, socially impaired environments (e.g., urban areas with a high incidence of transient persons, lower socioeconomic neighborhoods, and prisons). Regardless of the parents' social class, clients diagnosed with PD tend to have lower incomes. In areas with high social disintegration, the rate of PD is three times as great as in more organized environments. Researchers believe these data support the hypothesis that personality disorders can be influenced by social support and personal change (Kaplan and Sadock, 1995). The significance of this disorder is emphasized by the following statistics (Soloff et al., 1994): 9% to 28% of persons who complete suicide are diagnosed with PD; about one third of adolescents and young adults who complete suicide have a PD. Clients who have attempted suicide represent up to 55% of those diagnosed with PD; borderline PD represents the most common diagnosis. The DSM-IV (APA, 1994) groups the various PDs as follows:

- Cluster A: eccentric
- Cluster B: erratic
- Cluster C: fearful

Clustering helps to group recurring patterns of behavior with certain PDs. The incidence of PDs is often presented according to these clusters.

Cluster A, Eccentric: Paranoid, Schizoid, and Schizotypal

The incidence of the Cluster A PDs is somewhat difficult to establish since these individuals seldom seek assistance, given their withdrawn and distrustful nature. Paranoid PD is more common in men than women by about 7 to 5 (Perry and Vaillant, 1989), an estimated 0.5% to 2.5% of the population (Kaplan, Sadock, and Grebb, 1994). Prevalence of schizoid personality disorder in the general population has been estimated at 7.5% (Kaplan, Sadock, and Grebb, 1994), and it is more commonly diagnosed in men. According to one study, schizotypal PD occurs in 3% of the population (Millon, 1987). Research indicates that one significant risk factor for PD is a genetic predisposition to the disorder. Individuals who have a first-degree relative with schizophrenia are at risk (see discussion related to biological correlates on p. 484).

Cluster B, Erratic: Antisocial, Borderline, Histrionic, and Narcissistic

The incidence for the Cluster B PDs is also difficult to establish, although many of these individuals can be found in prisons. Prevalence estimates of antisocial PD in the United States range from 3% in men to less than 1% in women (APA, 1994). Borderline PD (BPD) occurs in about 1% to 2% of the population and is more common in women than men (Kaplan, Sadock, and Grebb, 1994). Attempted and completed suicides are high in BPD. Risk factors for BPD are presented in the assessment section of this chapter. Prevalence of histrionic PD is thought to be about 2% to 3% of the population and is twice as common in women (Perry and Vaillant, 1989). Anecdotal reports suggest that narcissistic PD ranges from 2% to 16% in the psychiatric population and less than 1% of the general population. It is more common among men than women (Perry and Vaillant, 1989).

Cluster C, Fearful: Avoidant, Dependent, Obsessive-Compulsive, Not Otherwise Specified

The incidence for Cluster C PDs is equally difficult to determine. According to Kaplan, Sadock, and Grebb (1994), avoidant PD (APD) is common, affecting about 1% to 10% of the population, yet specific gender ratio statistics are not available. Perry and Vaillant (1989) cite one study in which 2.5% of the sample was diagnosed with dependent PD (DPD). More common in women than men, DPD was seen most often in the youngest children of families. The specific statistical prevalence of obsessive-compulsive PD is unknown (Kaplan, Sadock, and Grebb, 1994); it is diagnosed more often in men who are the oldest children (Townsend, 1993). Passive-aggressive PD (PAPD) and depressive PD are now listed in the DSM-IV as PDs not otherwise specified (NOS) and are categorized under Cluster C. There is little or no prevalence data on PAPD, and due to the newness of DPD as a category, no epidemiological data are available. It is suspected that because depressive disorders are so prevalent in the general population, DPD is also fairly common.

THEORETICAL FRAMEWORK

There is no single theoretical explanation for the development and persistence of the dysfunctional behavioral patterns of PD. There are theories that account for some but not all symptoms experienced by these individuals. These include biological, sociocultural, and psychodynamic correlates. These three theoretical frameworks have general acceptance in the psychiatric-mental health field. Each will be explored in this chapter and applied to nursing.

Biological Correlates

Genetic/hereditary

Preliminary work in genetic and biological domains suggest a link to the development of PDs. Such evidence indicates that a psychobiological perspective would be useful in the diagnosis and treatment of personality disorders (Siever and Davis, 1991). Research indicates that familial associations and inheritable PD characteristics have been noted in Cluster A personality disorders. Studies suggest that clients who have a family history of psychiatric disorders such as alcoholism, drug addiction, or schizophrenia have a genetic predisposition to PDs that fit Cluster A. For example, schizotypal PD is seen more often in individuals with first-degree biological relatives who have been diagnosed with schizophrenia than in individuals of the general population. Cluster B personality disorders are considered to have a genetic predisposition as evident in studies that show a higher incidence in identical twins than fraternal twins (APA, 1994; Perry and Vaillant, 1989; Siever and Davis, 1991).

Brain chemistry

Several studies indicate that there is a disturbance or imbalance in the dopamine and serotonin neurotransmitters of persons with schizotypal PD (Siever, 1992). The question in relation to PDs might be: Do individuals develop PDs because they have different brain chemistry or because there are psychosocial forces at work? The role of psychobiological intervention will be discussed further in the implementation section of this chapter.

Studies report that the rapid eye movement (REM) latency is shorter in people with major depressive disorder, in addition to being shorter and more varied in people with BPD. It is proposed that the reduction in REM latency is related to the activity of the muscarinic agonist arecoline and may contribute to affective instability, the classic symptom of BPD (Siever and Davis, 1991).

Autonomic nervous system

High anxiety levels have been noted in clients with the Cluster C PDs. Examples of high anxiety can be seen in clients diagnosed with avoidant personality disorder. For example, the client with avoidant PD "avoids" developing a relationship for fear of rejection and the related anxiety of such rejection. Persons diagnosed with NOS passive-aggressive PD decrease their anxiety by avoiding the direct expression of anger. They do this by procrastinating about something that may evoke confrontation and anger.

Although the biological correlate of this anxiety/inhibition theory is not well-studied, there are some findings that support that clients with PD experience this type of pathological anxiety. For example, these anxiety-inhibited individuals are found to have increased cortical and sympathetic arousal (Siever and Davis, 1991). Signs of depression are noted in Cluster C obsessive-compulsive PDs. The fact that obsessive-compulsive symptoms have been helped greatly with drugs, including antidepressants, also suggests a biological component.

Another view of the relationship between the autonomic nervous system and PD focuses on the hypothalamus. One of the purposes of the hypothalamus is to integrate sympathetic and parasympathetic activities (Guyton and Hall, 1995). According to Kerberg (1993), pain activates the "punishing center" of the hypothalamus. For example, infants whose orientation to the world is based on "hurting" tend to cope by using greater amounts of aggression. It is this excessive aggression that powers the development of borderline, passive-aggressive, histrionic, and narcissistic personality disorders (Kernberg, 1993).

Hormonal

Aggressive tendencies have been found in persons with increased levels of androgens (i.e., substances that stimulate or produce male characteristics, as the male hormone). Studies suggest that impulsive behaviors may be linked with increased levels of estrone, 17-estradiol, and testosterone (Raine and Mednick, 1989). Other studies have reported higher levels of noradrenergic metabolites in gamblers and volunteer subjects demonstrating sensation-seeking behaviors (Siever and Davis, 1991).

Most studies recommend further research on biological correlates to fully understand the development of PD. Some of the discussion on the biological correlates suggests that sociocultural and psychodynamic factors also play a role in the development of PD. Discussion of sociocultural explanations of PD also suggest that psychodynamics are a factor.

Sociocultural Correlates

Personality is shaped by the values, beliefs, attitudes, and norms manifested by the culture in which a person lives. Cultural and ethnic groups pass their values on to their members. Other societal influences, such as high levels of crime and violence, contradict American values about closeness and trust. Rising crime rates generate fear and insecurity that make people reluctant to risk closeness or contact with strangers or new acquaintances. People are more cautious in deciding who they can trust, which promotes suspiciousness that can be easily reinforced by experience. Some urban residents, particularly the elderly, become prisoners in their homes because of fear and associated involuntary social withdrawal.

The current phenomenon of the immediate gratification of the "me" generation is influenced and magnified by the media. Environmental theorists suggest that this contributes to the overall problems of impulse control as well as the pattern of poor impulse control in those diagnosed with PD.

Within society's varied ethnic and cultural groups, families play a role in passing down their culture to family members. Chapter 12 emphasized that within the family structure, individuals develop ways of communicating with each other and society. For example, through family interactions, an individual learns about relationships, ways of handling aggression, and physical and personal space management.

Townsend (1993) suggests that clients from Cluster A: paranoid PD have often been subjected to parental antagonism, serving as scapegoats for displaced parental aggression. The childhoods of schizoid individuals have been described as bleak, cold, unempathetic, and devoid of nurturance and support. The family dynamics of the individual with a schizotypal personality disorder may be characterized by parental indifference, impassivity, or formality. Closeness feels neither natural nor comfortable, and social skills are not developed. Eventually, the person begins to tune out reality. At the same time, clients diagnosed with Cluster B antisocial type personalities are seen to come from a chaotic home environment (Perry and Vaillant, 1989) in which the intermittent appearance of impulsive parents does more harm than good. At the same time, certain family dynamics have been proposed to account for clients diagnosed with Cluster C PDs such as obsessive-compulsive and passive-aggressive PD. The prominent feature of families of children who later develop obsessive-compulsive disorder (OCD) was overcontrol (Antoni, et al., 1987). Parents expected their children to live up to impossible standards and then condemned them when they failed. Such children then become driven to avoid punishment and to find safety in conforming to the external rules and regulations in their lives. Antoni, et al. (1987) cites contradictory parental attitudes and inconsistent training methods as major factors in the development of PAPD. Such children may receive the kindness and support they crave, or they may be the recipients of hostility and rejection at any moment without provocation.

The social nature of the family and the various everyday living interactions of a family environment play significant roles in the way people feel about themselves, as well as in how they act with family members and others in society. As discussed in Chapter 12, the family often plays a significant role in the development of psychopathology, and personality disorders prove no exception. These sociocultural factors are intertwined with the psychodynamic correlates of PD.

Psychodynamic Correlates

A widely held explanation for why PDs develop is offered by ego developmental and object-relations theorists. For instance, Mahler, Pine, and Bergman (1975) believe that many clients who develop PDs encounter difficulties at the separation-individuation stage of development (18 months to 3 years). This phase parallels the development of the child's capacity to walk and, therefore to physically separate from the mother. Normally, children at this stage feel expansive and elated, as they realize their potential for gaining control over their bodies and environment (see Chapter 7). Their exuberant quest for mastery leads them away from mother, causing physical separation.

Children supported in their moves away will grow secure in the maternal attachment and not be afraid of abandonment. Under "good enough" conditions, **object constancy** is obtained, *which means the child can evoke a stable and consistent mental image of the mother to derive comfort when she is not physically present.* For this reason, children can tolerate their short departures from mothers' sight without undue anxiety.

In general, the psychodynamic view contends that inadequate parenting results in individuals who do not complete developmental tasks related to autonomy and separation/individuation. Children experience inadequate parenting in an environment that is indifferent, cold, and emotionally deficient. This results in impaired object constancy and leaves them particularly vulnerable to separations and losses later in life. Issues and conflicts surrounding abandonment, dependency, control, and/or authority permeate clients with PD.

From the psychodynamic view, symptoms of PD emerge from ego developmental deficiencies or impairment. Another way of understanding these symptoms is to examine ego competencies. By understanding ego competencies, the psychiatric nurse can target interventions that assist clients to move beyond their blocked development and develop ego competencies needed to lead a satisfying life. Ego or coping competencies most relevant to PD include the following (Bellak, 1973):

- *Impulse control involves the ability to delay urges to take action in an attempt to contain rising anxiety.* Individuals with PDs tend to have **poor impulse control;** *they use action, rather than reflection, to manage painful internal states.* Such acting out is done in an attempt to obscure emotional pain through action. When certain feelings, thoughts, and/or impulses become dimly perceptible, clients take action to dispel them. This habitual response of "escape through action" becomes clients' primary pattern of attempting to cope. In addition, their incapacity to tolerate internal discomfort leaves them with little capacity for reflection or introspection, at least initially. Poor impulse control may be evident in self-destructive behaviors, such as cutting oneself, overspending, engaging

in high-risk sexual behaviors, or abusing drugs or alcohol; for clients with PD who are **ego-syntonic** *these behaviors are viewed as an acceptable part of their personality,* rather than **ego-dystonic** or *inconsistent with their personality.* These clients commonly use chemicals to alter their mood or state of consciousness in an effort to act out.

- **Mood** *refers to a pervasive dynamic emotion,* and **affect** *refers to responses to changing states of emotion* (APA, 1994). Ideally, persons can modulate affect, so their moods are neither excessively low nor high. Depression is common in PDs, often having the characteristics of "abandonment depression," first described by Masterson in 1976. To *abandon* means to withdraw protection, support, or help from another or to break a close association coupled with feeling a complete lack of interest in the fate of the person given up. To abandon means that one person actively withdraws something that is needed by another. Understandably, feelings of abandonment create a variety of dysphoric feelings and responses. **Dysphoria** *is a disorder of affect characterized by depression and anguish.* It is this magnitude of loss that characterizes abandonment depression, with rage, guilt, fear, passivity, and feelings of emptiness all coexisting with the profound sense of loss.

- **Judgment** *refers to the ability to compare probable consequences of choices based on actions.* Ideally, persons use what they have learned in prior situations to avoid future negative consequences. The ability to think, anticipate, and effectively problem solve is impaired when a person is ruled by impulses. Clients with PD show poor judgment when they continue to engage in self-defeating behaviors in spite of predictable harm to themselves.

- **Reality testing** *involves objectively evaluating the outside world and distinguishing between inner and outer sources of stimuli, as well as processing and interpreting sensory data without distortion.* Clients with paranoid personality disorders might perceive a casual comment as harsh criticism, in which case, their poor reality testing is their excessive use of "projection." **Projection** *is a psychological defense mechanism in which feelings, thoughts, or impulses, which originate from within the self, are perceived as originating from outside the self.* That is, clients may not perceive that their interpretation of the above casual comment as negative criticism originates from within themselves, from their own hard criticism or self-appraisal rather than from the person saying it. A person's ability to accurately process what is happening within oneself, and in the external environment are impaired to the extent that the person uses projection as a defense.

• *Healthy self-perception* *involves being able to hold a stable, realistic sense of self that is free from both self-hate and self-glorification. A distorted self-perception is derived, in part, when* "good" *and* "bad" *aspects of self and others cannot be integrated.* This is known as **splitting,** *in which opposing emotional feelings, such as love and hate, are actively separated from each other. For example, the self or others are seen as "all good or all bad."* This defense mechanism precludes awareness of self or others as whole beings, with both good and bad features. Instead, the positive aspects of self and others are exaggerated through **idealization** (*to envision as perfect*), and the negative aspects of self and others are exaggerated through devaluation (to degrade one's worth).

• **Relatedness** *refers to the quality and degree of one's interpersonal interaction.* Clients with PDs often relate to others in rigid and inflexible ways, making it difficult to establish intimate relationships. For example, clients with dependent PD exhibit the interpersonal style of clinging, often behaving in a helpless, dependent, and regressive manner (moving toward). Clients who use a distancing mode avoid contact with persons, either by devaluing others or withdrawing from them. Schizoid clients just try to avoid contact altogether. Other clients interact in ways designed to push nurses away (moving against others). A client with APD or BPD may tell the nurse, in response to attempts to listen or empathize, that the approaches being used are simplistic, useless, and probably harmful. The problem occurs when one interpersonal style is adhered to rigidly, despite whether the consequences are positive or negative.

• **Thought processes** *refer to the ability of a person to think logically, make judgments, and express ideas in ordered, logical ways* (see Chapter 8). Although clients with PD usually express themselves in ways that reflect ordered and logical thinking, their attention, concentration, and retention are often impaired. The client's thinking may be excessively concrete or diffuse, and either may cause the person's speech to lack a clear focus, or it may be excessively constricted and guarded. When experiencing turmoil or conflict, these clients may not comprehend what others are saying. The intrusion of urgent thoughts and fantasy can cause disruptions in communication. Conceptual thinking suffers to the degree that logical thought processes are impaired (see Chapter 29). Clients with PD usually show no sign of delusions or other forms of thought disorders.

• **Activities of daily living (ADLs).** *Competence in ADLs requires a person to use the full range of ego skills to carry out basic needs related to ADL skills of dress, hygiene, and nutrition.* Difficulties with ADL skills vary in each subcategory of PD, although most clients have some degree of difficulty in maintaining a healthy lifestyle. Lack of hygiene may result in body odor, tooth decay, and multiple health problems. Grooming may be poor, creating an unkempt, disorganized, or bizarre appearance. Many clients with PDs do not manage their nutritional needs adequately, resulting in either deficient or excessive food intake. Often, they have no set routine of daily activities, which creates disturbances in their activity levels, such as excessive sleep, chronic inactivity, hypomanic behavior, and insomnia.

• **Stimulus filter/stimulus barrier** *refers to a person's physiological capacity to screen and regulate incoming sensory stimuli.* Clients who have difficulty filtering sensory stimuli experience a diffuse excitability, which makes them feel like "jumping out of their skin." An excessive response to noise and light may occur, resulting in agitated restlessness. The person's attention span is often poor because of being absorbed with the experience of overstimulation. In spite of hypersensitivity and excitability, such clients may seek even more stimuli.

The *Nursing Process*

Assessment

Clinical Profiles

Table 26-1 lists the three clusters used by the DSM-IV (APA, 1994) to organize the various types of PDs. Clinical profiles of each of the PDs are also summarized in this table; they are mood, self-image, behavior, relatedness/interpersonal style, cognitive mode, and primary ego defense mechanism are included for each personality disorder subcategory. The majority of clients diagnosed with PD are treated in community settings and do not require hospitalization. Hospitalization is necessary when clients with PD demonstrate a high risk for self harm/mutilation (e.g., suicide threats or gestures) or clients experience PDs connected with a major Axis I diagnosis such as schizophrenia or major depression. Clients usually have presenting symptoms in acute crisis situations.

As illustrated in Table 26-1, the predominant characteristics related to the above areas determine the cluster and subsequent subcategory of each PD. These four areas are explained in the six characteristics indicated in this table: mood, self-image, behavior, relatedness, cognitive mode, and defense mechanism. The enduring pattern is characterized by the following:

- It is inflexible and pervasive across a broad range of personal and social situations
- It leads to clinically significant distress or impairment in social, occupational, sexual, and other important areas of functioning
- It is stable and of long duration, and its onset can be traced back to at least adolescence or early adulthood
- It is not better accounted for as a manifestation or consequence of another mental disease
- It is not a result of the direct physiological effects of a substance (e.g., illicit drugs or medication, or a general medical condition).

Assessment Tools

The nurse is usually aware of the client's particular PD diagnosis. In addition to conducting a complete nursing health assessment, the nurse or other health care professionals often use focused assessment tools. It is important for the nurse completing the comprehensive assessment to compare the directly assessed data with other indirect sources of data, as well as review the data presented in Table 26-1.

To measure ego strengths and deficits in clients with PDs, focused assessment tools, in addition to comprehensive assessment tools, are needed. One focused assessment tool designed specifically for this purpose is Ego Mental Competency (EMC) (Kerr, 1990). This instrument allows the nurse to identify the most acute ego deficits and the areas of greatest ego strengths so that ego competencies can be mobilized to deal with identified problems. The Ego Mental Capacity (EMC) is a focused assessment tool used for persons diagnosed with PD. An example of a question from the EMC used to assess impulse control is "How often do you think before you act in situations like that?" (Kerr, 1990). The answer to this question, as well as others from the EMC and the comprehensive assessment, derive the necessary data for the formulation of one or even several nursing diagnoses.

The Personality Disorder Rating Scale is another instrument used to determine clients' degree of difficulty with everyday life. This tool assesses depressed mood; anger-hostility; sense of self; interpersonal aspects; and level of anxiety, appetite, sleep, and energy (Salzman et al., 1995). It can be used to determine baselines for clients to measure outcomes during and after treatment. It is now believed that PDs can be diagnosed in adolescents (Johnson et al., 1995). It is important that qualified healthcare professionals use valid and reliable instruments, whether they are checklist tools, structured interview guides, or a combination of both, as part of the assessment process.

As previously stated, clients with PDs are admitted to a psychiatric unit when they get into some kind of crisis, for example, self-mutilation, suicidal feelings, and others. Other clients who are admitted have an Axis I diagnosis of schizophrenia, major depression, or substance abuse, as well as an Axis II diagnosis of PD. The PD symptoms may be overshadowed until the more acute phase of the illness begins to resolve. Because personality characteristics are learned very early in life, or may even be inherited, treatment aimed at character change takes years. Most treatment situations, resulting from current managed care policies, are short-term and crisis-centered, and are aimed at strengthening coping competencies. Both strategies are appropriate and can be used effectively in combination.

Text continued on p. 495.

TABLE 26-1 DSM-IV personality disorders

MAJOR CHARACTERISTICS, SIGNS, AND SYMPTOMS OF CLUSTER A: ECCENTRIC

TYPES	MOOD	SELF-IMAGE	BEHAVIOR	RELATEDNESS	COGNITIVE MODE	DEFENSE MECHANISM
Cluster A						
Paranoid	**IRASCIBLE:** Displays a cold, sullen, churlish, and humorless demeanor; attempts to appear unemotional and objective, but is edgy, envious, jealous, quick to react angrily or take personal offense	**INVIOLABLE:** Has persistent ideas of self-importance and self-reference; entirely innocuous actions and events are experienced as personally derogatory and scurrilous; is pridefully independent and highly insular; experiences intense fears of losing identity, status, and powers of self-determination	**DEFENSIVE:** Is vigilantly alert to anticipate and ward off expected derogation and deception; is tenacious and firmly resistant to sources of external influence and control	**PROVOCATIVE:** Displays a quarrelsome, fractious, and abrasive attitude; precipitates exasperation and anger by a testing of loyalties and a searching preoccupation with hidden motives	**SUSPICIOUS:** Is skeptical, cynical, and mistrustful of the motives of others, construing innocuous events as signifying hidden or conspiratorial intent; reveals tendency to magnify tangential or minor social difficulties into proofs of duplicity, malice, and treachery	**PROJECTION:** Actively disowns undesirable personal traits and motives and attributes them to others; remains blind to one's own unattractive behaviors and characteristics, yet is overalert to and hypercritical of similar features in others
Schizoid	**FLAT:** Is emotionally impassive, exhibiting an intrinsic unfeeling, cold, and stark quality; reports weak affectionate or erotic needs; rarely displays warm or intense feelings; apparently unable to experience pleasure, sadness, or anger in any depth	**COMPLACENT:** Reveals minimal introspection and awareness of self; seems impervious to the emotional and personal implications of everyday social life	**LETHARGIC:** Appears to be in a state of fatigue, low energy, and lack of vitality; is sluggish, displaying deficits in activation, expressiveness, and spontaneity	**ALOOF:** Seems indifferent and remote, rarely responsive to the actions or feelings of others, possessing minimal "human" interests; fades into the background; is unobtrusive; has few close relationships; prefers a peripheral role in social, work, and family settings	**IMPOVERISHED:** Seems deficient across broad spheres of knowledge; evidences vague and obscure thought processes that are below intellectual level; communication is easily derailed; sequence of thought is conveyed through a circuitous logic	**INTELLECTUALIZATION:** Describes interpersonal and affective experiences in a matter-of-fact, abstract, impersonal, or mechanical manner; pays primary attention to formal aspects of social and emotional events

Continued.

TABLE 26-1—cont'd

DSM-IV personality disorders

	MAJOR CHARACTERISTICS, SIGNS, AND SYMPTOMS OF CLUSTER A: ECCENTRIC—cont'd				
TYPES	**MOOD**	**SELF-IMAGE**	**BEHAVIOR**	**RELATEDNESS**	**COGNITIVE MODE**	**DEFENSE MECHANISM**
Schizotypal	**DISTRAUGHT:** Reports being apprehensive and ill-at-ease, particularly in social situations; is agitated and anxiously watchful and distrustful of others and wary of their motives; manifests drab, apathetic, sluggish, joyless, and spiritless appearance; reveals marked deficiencies in face-to-face rapport and emotional expression	**ESTRANGED:** Possesses permeable ego-boundaries and struggles with recurrent social perplexities and experiences of depersonalization, derealization, and dissociation; sees self as forlorn, with repetitive thoughts of life's emptiness and meaninglessness	**ABERRANT:** Exhibits socially gauche habits and peculiar mannerisms; is perceived by others as eccentric and disposed to behave in an unobtrusively odd, aloof, curious, or bizarre manner	**SECRETIVE:** Prefers privacy and isolation with few, highly tentative attachments and personal obligations; has drifted over time into increasingly peripheral vocational roles and clandestine social activities	**AUTISTIC:** Mixes social communication with personal irrelevancies, circumstantial speech, ideas of reverence, and metaphorical asides; is ruminative; appears self-absorbed and lost in daydreams with occasional magical thinking, obscure suspicions, and a blurring of fantasy and reality	**UNDOING:** Bizarre mannerisms and idiosyncratic thoughts appear to represent a retraction or reversal of previous acts or ideas that have stirred feelings of anxiety, conflict, or guilt; ritualistic or "magical" behaviors serve to repent for or nullify assumed misdeeds or "evil" thoughts

	MAJOR CHARACTERISTICS, SIGNS, AND SYMPTOMS OF CLUSTER B: ERRATIC				
Cluster B						
Antisocial	**CALLOUS:** Is insensitive, unempathetic, and cold-blooded, which are expressed in wide-ranging deficits in social charitableness, human compassion, or personal remorse; exhibits a course of incivility, as well as an offensive, if not ruthless, indifference to the welfare of others	**AUTONOMOUS:** Sees self as unfettered by the restrictions of social customs and the restraints of personal loyalties; values the image and enjoys the sense of being free, unencumbered, and unconfined by persons, places, obligations, or routines	**IMPULSIVE:** Is impetuous and irrepressible, acting hastily and spontaneously in a restless, spur-of-the-moment manner; is short-sighted, incautious, and imprudent, failing to plan ahead or to consider alternatives; is not likely to heed consequences	**IRRESPONSIBLE:** Is untrustworthy and unreliable, failing to meet or intentionally or negating personal obligations of a marital, parental, employment, or financial nature; actively violates established social codes through duplicitous or illegal behaviors	**DEVIANT:** Construes events and relationships in accord with socially unorthodox beliefs and morals; is disdainful of traditional ideals and contemptuous of conventional values	**ACTING OUT:** Rarely constrained inner tensions that might accrue by postponing the expression of offensive thoughts and malevolent actions, socially repugnant impulses are not sublimated, but are discharged directly in precipitous ways, usually without guilt

TABLE 26-1—cont'd

DSM-IV personality disorders

MAJOR CHARACTERISTICS, SIGNS, AND SYMPTOMS OF CLUSTER B: ERRATIC—*cont'd*

TYPES	MOOD	SELF-IMAGE	BEHAVIOR	RELATEDNESS	COGNITIVE MODE	DEFENSE MECHANISM
Borderline	LABILE: Mood has either marked shifts from normality to depression to excitement or has extended periods of dejection and apathy, interspersed with brief spells of anger, anxiety, or euphoria	UNCERTAIN: Experiences the confusions of an immature, nebulous, or wavering sense of identity; seeks to redeem actions with expression of contrition and self-punitive behaviors	PRECIPITATE: Displays a desultory energy level with sudden, unexpected, and impulsive outbursts; abrupt, endogenous shifts in drive state and in inhibitory control places activation equilibrium in constant jeopardy	PARADOXICAL: Although needing attention and affection, is unpredictably contrary, manipulative, and volatile, frequently eliciting rejection rather than support; reacts to fears of separation and isolation in angry, mercurial, and often self-damaging ways	CAPRICIOUS: Experiences rapidly changing, fluctuating, and antithetical perceptions of thoughts concerning passing events; contradictory reactions are evoked in others, creating, in turn, conflicting and confusing social feedback	REGRESSION: Retreats under stress to developmentally earlier levels of anxiety tolerance, impulse control, and social adaptation; among adolescents, is unable to cope with adult demands and conflicts, as evident in immature, if not increasingly infantile, behaviors
Histrionic	FICKLE: Displays short-lived dramatic and superficial emotions; is overreactive, impetuous, and exhibits tendencies to be easily enthused and as easily angered or bored	SOCIABILITY: Views self as gregarious, stimulating, and charming; enjoys the image of attracting acquaintances and pursuing a busy and pleasure-oriented social life	AFFECTED: Is overreactive, stimulus-seeking, and intolerant of inactivity, resulting in impulsive, unreflected, and theatrical responsiveness; describes penchant for momentary excitements, fleeting adventures, and short-sighted hedonism	FLIRTATIOUS: Actively solicits praise and manipulates others to gain needed reassurance, attention, and approval; is demanding, self-dramatizing, vain, and seductively exhibitionistic	FLIGHTY: Avoids introspective thought and is overly attentive to superficial and fleeting external events; integrates experience poorly, resulting in scattered learning and thoughtless judgments	DISSOCIATION: Regularly alters self-presentations to create a succession of socially attractive but changing facades; engages in self-distracting activities to avoid reflecting on and integrating unpleasant thoughts and emotions

Continued.

TABLE 26-1—cont'd
DSM-IV personality disorders

TYPES	MOOD	SELF-IMAGE	BEHAVIOR	RELATEDNESS	COGNITIVE MODE	DEFENSE MECHANISM
	MAJOR CHARACTERISTICS, SIGNS, AND SYMPTOMS OF CLUSTER B: ERRATIC—cont'd					
Narcissistic	LIGHT: Manifests a general air of nonchalance and imperturbability; appears coolly unimpressionable or buoyantly optimistic, except when narcissistic confidence is shaken, at which time either rage, shame, or emptiness is briefly displayed	ADMIRABLE: Confidently exhibits self, acting in a self-assured manner and displaying achievements; has a sense of high self-worth, despite being seen by others as egotistic, inconsiderate, and arrogant	ARROGANT: Flouts conventional rules of shared social living, viewing them as naive or inapplicable to oneself; reveals a careless disregard for personal integrity and an indifference to the rights of others	EXPLOITIVE: Feels entitled; is unempathic; expects special favors without assuming reciprocal responsibilities; shamelessly takes others for granted and uses them to enhance self and indulge desires	EXPANSIVE: Has an undisciplined imagination and exhibits a preoccupation with immature fantasies of success, beauty, or love; is minimally constrained by objective reality; takes liberties with facts and often lies to redeem self-illusions	RATIONALIZATION: Is self-deceptive in devising plausible reasons to justify self-centered and socially inconsiderate behaviors; offers alibis to place oneself in the best possible light, despite evident shortcomings or failures
	MAJOR CHARACTERISTICS, SIGNS, AND SYMPTOMS OF CLUSTER C: FEARFUL					
Cluster C Avoidant	ANGUISHED: Describes constant and confusing undercurrents of tension, sadness, and anger; vacillates between desire for affection, fear of rebuff, and numbness of feeling	ALIENATED: Sees oneself as socially isolated and rejected by others; devalues self-achievements; reports feelings of aloneness and emptiness, if not depersonalization	GUARDED: Warily scans environment for potential threats; overreacts to innocuous events and anxiously judges them to signify personal ridicule and threat	AVERSIVE: Reports extensive history of social pan-anxiety and distrust; seeks acceptance but maintains distance and privacy to avoid humiliation and derogation	DISTRACTED: Is preoccupied and bothered by disruptive and often perplexing inner thoughts; the upsurge from within oneself of irrelevant and digressive ideation upsets thought continuity and interferes with social communication	FANTASY: Depends excessively on imagination to achieve need gratification and conflict resolution; withdraws into reveries as a means of safely discharging affectionate as well as aggressive impulses

TABLE 26-1—cont'd

DSM-IV personality disorders

MAJOR CHARACTERISTICS, SIGNS, AND SYMPTOMS OF CLUSTER C: FEARFUL—cont'd

TYPES	MOOD	SELF-IMAGE	BEHAVIOR	RELATEDNESS	COGNITIVE MODE	DEFENSE MECHANISM
Dependent	**PACIFIC:** Is characteristically warm, tender, and noncompetitive; timidly avoids social tension and interpersonal conflicts	**INEPT:** Views self as weak, fragile, and inadequate; exhibits lack of self-confidence by belittling own aptitudes and competencies	**INCOMPETENT:** Ill-equipped to assume mature and independent roles; is docile and passive, lacking functional competencies, avoiding self-assertion, and withdrawing from adult responsibilities	**SUBMISSIVE:** Subordinates needs to stronger, nurturing figure, without whom feels anxiously helpless; is compliant, conciliatory, placating, and self-sacrificing	**NAIVE:** Is easily persuaded, unsuspicious, and gullible; reveals a Pollyanna attitude toward interpersonal difficulties; watering down objective problems and smoothing over troubling events	**INTROJECTION:** Is firmly devoted to another; wanting to believe an inseparable bond exists between them; submits any independent views in favor of others to preclude conflicts and threats to the relationship
Obsessive-compulsive	**SOLEMN:** Is unrelaxed, tense, joyless, and grim; restrains warm feelings and keeps most emotions under tight control	**CONSCIENTIOUS:** Sees self as industrious, reliable, meticulous, and efficient; fearful of error or misjudgment and hence overvalues aspects of oneself that exhibit discipline, perfection, prudence, and loyalty	**DISCIPLINED:** Maintains a regulated, repetitively structured, and highly organized life pattern; is perfectionistic, insisting that subordinates adhere to personally established rules and methods	**RESPECTFUL:** Exhibits unusual adherence to social conventions and proprieties; prefers polite, formal, and correct personal relationships	**CONSTRICTED:** Constructs world in terms of rules, regulations, time schedules, and social hierarchies; is unimaginative, indecisive, and notably upset by unfamiliar or novel ideas and customs	**REACTION-FORMATION:** Repeatedly presents positive thoughts and socially commendable behaviors that are diametrically opposite to the deeper, contrary, and forbidden feelings within; displays reasonableness and maturity when faced with circumstances that evoke anger or dismay in others

Continued.

TABLE 26-1—cont'd

DSM-IV personality disorders

MAJOR CHARACTERISTICS, SIGNS, AND SYMPTOMS OF CLUSTER C: FEARFUL—cont'd

TYPES	MOOD	SELF-IMAGE	BEHAVIOR	RELATEDNESS	COGNITIVE MODE	DEFENSE MECHANISM
Personality Disorder Not Otherwise Specified, for example, Passive-Aggressive (Negativistic)	HOSTILE: Has an excitable and pugnacious temper that flares readily into contentious argument and physical belligerence; is mean-spirited and fractious; is willing to do harm, even persecute others, to get one's way	COMPETITIVE: Is proud to characterize self as assertively independent, vigorously energetic, and realistically hard-headed; values aspects of oneself that present tough, power-oriented image	FEARLESS: Is unflinching, recklessly daring, thick-skinned, and seemingly undeterred by pain; is attracted to challenge, risk, and harm, as well as undaunted by danger and punishment	INTIMIDATING: Reveals satisfaction in competing with, dominating, and humiliating others; regularly expresses verbally abusive and derisive social commentary; exhibits vicious, if not physically brutal, behavior	DOGMATIC: Is strongly opinionated and closed-minded, as well as unbending and obstinate in holding to one's preconceptions; exhibits broad-ranging authoritarianism, social intolerance, and prejudice	ISOLATION: Can be cold-blooded and remarkably detached from the impact of one's destructive acts; views objects of violation impersonally, as symbols of devalued groups devoid of human sensibilities

The Nursing Process

Nursing Diagnosis

The nurse's diagnostic thinking process during assessment assists the nurse in deriving accurate nursing diagnosis(es) for the client with PD. Although the nurse always considers indirect data, such as the established DSM-IV diagnosis, the most important data is the client's direct assessment data and the comparison of this data with established defining characteristics for the NANDA nursing diagnosis under consideration. Although length of stay for clients with Personality Disorder continues to decrease, the diagnosis of BPD (Cluster C) represents those most often treated in the inpatient setting (Miller, Eisner, and Allport, 1994).

Assessment occurs throughout treatment, because clients replay their dysfunctional patterns of interaction within the treatment milieu. On the basis of these assessments, one or several diagnoses and related goals or outcome identification statements are formulated and revised throughout an episode of care. The nursing care plan indicating a common nursing diagnosis used for these clients and a related plan of care is presented on p. 496. Additional nursing diagnoses common for clients with personality disorders are presented in Box 26-1.

Outcome Identification

To have a positive impact on clients with PD, outcome identification must be realistic and measurable. To accomplish this aspect of the nursing process, data related to the specific ways in which clients attempt to defend against internal pain and aggression and the effects these attempts have on their lives are crucial in establishing short- and long-term goals.

Outcomes for clients with PD require some change in their behavior. Many of the characteristics of selected PDs illustrate the difficulty they present in establishing realistic and measurable goals for the client with PD. For example, the client with narcissistic PD portrays a confident self-image of, "I am the greatest; I don't need to change." The client with paranoid PD projects the issues as everyone else's fault, so "Why do I have to change?" Also, the client with borderline PD has such marked mood shifts that a discussion of established goals is met with a response such as, "I never agreed to that!"

The enduring patterns shown by clients with dysfunctional behavior PD combined with short hospital stays for acute crisis, make establishing timelines difficult. Evaluating long-term goals is difficult during inpatient hospitalization as well as in the community setting. Although this situation is further compounded by clients' nonadherence to treatment plans (Koenigsberg, 1994; Springer and Silk, 1996), the issue of adherence to treatment may be a realistic measurable long-term goal for clients with PD. As study continues on the validity of diagnosing Personality Disorder in adolescents, it is hoped that early diagnosis and treatment will contribute to more realistic outcome identification, client adherence to treatment regimens, and better outcomes, especially the meeting of long-term goals (Johnson et al., 1995).

Planning

Planning refers to the establishment of a standardized nursing care plan and its relationship to the interdisciplinary treatment plan. A nursing care plan for a client with a personality disorder is presented on p. 496. It is based on the nursing diagnosis "risk for violence," a common nursing diagnosis used by nurses who work with clients diagnosed with PD who come for treatment in a variety of settings.

Nurses do not work in a vacuum. The other mental health care team members share the same goal—that of helping the client to function at the most optimal level possible. Interdisciplinary treatment for hospitalized clients with PD usually consists of contracts, prevention of regression, medications, and various forms of therapy. Activity therapists have much to offer clients in their quest for health, as do the social worker, psychiatrist, psychologist, and supportive personnel. Nursing staff members bring to the team the unique perspective of the psychiatric-mental health nurse (ANA, 1994). This means that for nurses to carry out their standards of care, their

---

Box 26-1

Common Nursing Diagnoses for Clients With Personality Disorders

- Risk for violence: directed at others, related to excessive internal aggression, as evident in frequent fights, and one term in prison for assault
- Self-esteem disturbance, related to lack of self-assertive skills, as evident in extreme passivity in interpersonal relationships and verbalized sense of inadequacy
- Noncompliance with milieu structure related to self-concept disorder, as evident in verbal assertions of being special and exempt from rules and expectations
- Personal identity disturbance, related to failure to achieve object constancy, as evident in self-destructive response to recent separation from therapist (3 weeks)

Risk for Violence

NURSING ASSESSMENT DATA

Subjective: states, "I have been angry for as long as I can remember. I started fighting in kindergarten because fighting made me feel better." *Objective:* Several scars on face and arms; threatened two clients on the unit; communicates in a hostile, intimidating style; *DSM-IV diagnosis:* bipolar personality disorder.

NANDA Diagnosis: Risk for violence: directed toward others, related to poor impulse control and modulation of affect

Outcomes	Interventions	Rationale	Evaluation
Short term	• Determine that client understands unit policies, structure, expectations, and requirements for privileges.	• Establishes boundaries so that the significance of deviations can be immediately processed.	**Short term**
1. Will contract for nonviolence on the unit *on admission*			1. Met; on admission
2. Will practice the verbal skills necessary to put anger into words *within 3 days*	• Develop a contract with the client in which there is an agreement to nonviolence.	• Contracting, a basic principle of cognitive therapy, signals volitional agreement to not act destructively.	2. Partially met; verbal outburst accompanied by door slamming on two occasions; rediscussed goal with client
3. Will stabilize in mood and daily functioning in *1 week*		• Contracting provides clarity that consequences do and will occur; intent is to engage client's reality ego.	3. Not met; still having mood swings; discuss with team
4. Will sublimate aggressive energy into constructive outlets *within 24 hours*	• Pose questions that help the client to reflect on internal feelings and thoughts.	• Being able to put into words, rather than actions, internal feelings will help client to think before acting, thereby enhancing coping skills.	4. Partially met; has been walking 2 miles daily; see #2 above
Long term			**Long term**
1. Will understand the source of violent feelings during the safety of the therapeutic relationship *within 12 months*	• If the client engages in destructive behavior and cannot respond to "talking it out," immediately interrupt the behavior by whatever appropriate means is available, e.g., quiet or seclusion rooms, physical restraints, or medication.	• Assuming the ego function of impulse control for the client prevents destructive behavior and provides the possibility the client will learn to internalize this function.	1. Not met; too soon to evaluate
2. Will use appropriate community resources on own, particularly groups, for further support in finding more effective ways to cope *within 6 months*	• When using external controls, explain the rationale for doing so and continue to talk with the client.	• Once the show of force begins, the client can get lost in the shuffle; talking to the client *during* the incident conveys some degree of respect in the worst of circumstances.	2. Partially met; accepted referral for anger control group
	• Help the client identify triggers that prompt aggressive outbursts and the significance of the triggering event.	• To assist the client in developing insight about behaviors.	
	• Assign or refer client to an anger control group; refer to the NIC anger control assistance interventions in Box 26-2.	• Anger protocols indicate to the client that there are other options for dealing with anger.	
	• Educate client about community resources available to help constructively channel destructive impulses.	• Allows the client to understand that other sources of support are available.	

INTERDISCIPLINARY TREATMENT PLAN

Outpatient Clinical Pathway: Personality Disorder

Patient Name: _____   Sex: _____   Age: _____   Clinician: _____   Physician: _____
Diagnosis: _____   DSM IV: _____   ICD-9: _____   Referral Source: _____
Payor Source: _____   Current Medications: _____
Chief Complaint in patient's words: _____

	Pre-Treatment	Beginning Phase (Sessions 1-4) First Week	Middle Phase (Sessions 5-8)	End Phase (Sessions 8-12)	Follow Through
Assessment	☐ Why has pt called; what is crisis ☐ What does pt want to accomplish ☐ Assess Risk Potential ☐ Suicidality ☐ Homicidality ☐ Substance Abuse ☐ Psychosis/mania	☐ Confirm DX by DSM-IV ☐ Ethnic, cultural, social ☐ Personality patterns ☐ Functional style ☐ Current stressors ☐ Risk factors & suicidality ☐ Resources/support ☐ Evaluate for RX (for co-morbid symptoms-anxiety, depression, substance abuse)	☐ Response to RX for co-morbid disorders ☐ Risk factors & suicidality ☐ Psychosocial stressors & adaptive responses ☐ Pt's view of self/others, thinking, experiencing of emotions & relationships ☐ Pt/family/significant other involvement in therapy	☐ Response to RX ☐ Evaluate RX compliance ☐ Assess if pt has more productive coping methods ☐ Level of independent functioning ☐ Potential for regression	☐ Contact to find out what has changed ☐ Contact to find out how pt has progressed ☐ Or, have pt call in with progress report
Treatment Interventions	☐ If risk, refer to inpatient ☐ Refer to non-therapy services (legal, vocational, financial, spiritual) if needed ☐ Set appointment for pt to come in today	☐ Refer to physician for RX medical exam, & DX tests ☐ Complete Medical Exam ☐ Consider diagnostic tests (EEG, Drug Screen) ☐ RX informed consent ☐ Focus: Crisis Stabilization ☐ Mutually contracted treatment plan: clear limits, expectations, consequences ☐ Emphasize active participation & compliance	☐ Stimulate helpful awareness how personality type interferes with functioning, relationships ☐ Support pt's attempts to be involved in therapy ☐ Focus: Expectations for Mature Behavioral Change ☐ Evaluate & Revise Treatment Plan ☐ Refer to group therapy	☐ Update Treatment Plan include support groups ☐ Finalize AfterCare Plan ☐ Refer to support group & community resources ☐ Focus: Pt's Style for Specific Problem Solving Issues ☐ Let pt know therapist is available PRN with set limits ☐ Express genuine interest in how things turn out for pt	☐ Provide intermittent short-term therapy as needed ☐ Evaluate effectiveness of AfterCare Plan ☐ Provide additional community resources, as needed
Treatment Evaluation & Patient Outcomes	☐ Long-term TX goal: Personality change-new methods of interacting ☐ Short term TX goal: Crisis stabilization ☐ Pt Outcome: Does not harm self or others	☐ Pt has absence of suicidal homicidal ideation/risk ☐ Pt provides ideas about what needs to be changed ☐ Pt returns to same/better level of functioning than before crisis w/o catastrophe	☐ Pt recognizes responsibility for self ☐ Pt able to identify precipitating factors to crisis & how to avoid them	☐ Pt establishes & maintains an interpersonal relationship without evidence of manipulation or exploitation ☐ Pt demonstrates use of constructive coping skills	☐ Pt/family participating in follow-up care & community treatment ☐ Pt continues to work on therapy on his/her own to maintain wellness.

Criteria listed above is only a guideline and is not intended to be a standard of care. PsychPaths™ © Strategic Clinical Systems, Granbury, Texas.

The Nursing Process

Box 26-2

Anger Control Assistance

DEFINITION

Facilitation of the expression of anger in an adaptive nonviolent manner

ACTIVITIES

Establish basic trust and rapport with patient

Use a calm, reassuring approach

Determine appropriate behavioral expectations for expression of anger, given patient's level of cognitive and physical functioning

Limit access to frustrating situations until patient is able to express anger in an adaptive manner

Encourage patient to seek assistance of nursing staff or responsible others during periods of increasing tension

Monitor potential for inappropriate aggression and intervene before its expression

Prevent physical harm if anger is directed at self or others (e.g., restrain and remove potential weapons)

Provide physical outlets for expression of anger or tension (e.g., punching bag, sports, clay, and writing in a journal)

Provide reassurance to patient that nursing staff will intervene to prevent patient from losing control

Use external controls (e.g., physical or manual restraint, time outs, and seclusion) as needed, to calm patient who is expressing anger in a maladaptive manner

Provide feedback on behavior to help patient identify anger

Assist patient in identifying the source of anger

Identify the function that anger, frustration, and rage serve for the patient

Identify consequences of inappropriate expression of anger

Assist patient in planning strategies to prevent the inappropriate expression of anger

Identify with patient the benefits of expressing anger in an adaptive, nonviolent manner

Establish expectation that patient can control his/her behavior

Instruct on use of calming measures (e.g., time outs and deep breaths)

Assist in developing appropriate methods of expressing anger to others (e.g., assertiveness and use of feeling statements)

Provide role models who express anger appropriately

Support patient in implementing anger control strategies and in the appropriate expression of anger

Provide reinforcement for appropriate expression of anger

Reprinted with permission from McCloskey J.C., & Bulechek G.M. (Ed.) (1996). Nursing interventions classification (NIC), *(2nd ed.).* St. Louis: Mosby.

own assessments and plans must be integrated into the total plan of care.

Because of the relative infrequency of inpatient treatment of clients with PD, interdisciplinary treatment plans for inpatient treatment of PDs are not currently available.

An interdisciplinary treatment plan, referred to as a clinical pathway and designed for the nonhospitalized client with PD is presented on p. 497. It indicates what outcomes are expected after 6 to 12 treatment sessions. The hope is that the client with PD will seek treatment before going into a full blown crisis, which is the usual reason for hospitalization. Regardless of whether a client with PD is being treated on an inpatient or outpatient basis, or whether a formal written interdisciplinary treatment plan is available, the nurse implements the nursing care plan in concert with the intentions of the interdisciplinary treatment team. Inherent in every nursing or interdisciplinary care plan is the agreement among staff that the plan will be carried out consistently

by all members of the team. Staff who have a plan before a crisis develops will respond more smoothly in the actual crisis. Consistency is critical to the successful outcome of a planned response for crisis-provoked behavior.

Implementation

Consistency in implementing treatment approaches among the nursing staff and interdisciplinary team is paramount when working with clients with PDs, and it is the essential component of milieu management. Clients with PDs are especially able to discern the issues around which staff members, particularly across disciplines, are not in agreement. Staff members are vulnerable to polarization in these issues and must manage their own disagreements and resolve them satisfactorily. The entire team must also insist that clients continue to focus on their own issues, instead of staff and unit issues. Violent and hypersexual behavior creates anxiety in all staff as

The Nursing Process

does other characteristics indicated in Table 26-1. Most of these characteristics can cause a great deal of anxiety for nurses and other team members. For example, the quarrelsome attitude of the client with paranoid PD or the angry impulsive outbursts of the client with BPD cause anxiety in the staff. Nurses should anticipate their anxiety. The important strategy is to assess it and reduce it. Anxiety is contagious. The object is to not transfer anxiety back to an already anxious client or others in the milieu. A nurse's anxiety can affect the establishment of a therapeutic nurse-client relationship (Peplau, 1963). A variety of nursing interventions can be implemented with clients diagnosed with PDs (Box 26-2). The nursing interventions reflect the desired outcomes and are usually indicative of the predominant defining characteristics assessed by the nurse as well as the treatment setting.

Counseling

Counseling is essential for clients with PDs. For counseling efforts to be successful, the nurse must understand the specific constellations of personality characteristics that help create the client's difficulties, as well as demonstrate mutual respect and openness. The client with a schizoid personality may need the nurse's help to share feelings about surgery, while a client with a histrionic personality may need help containing emotions. Only by understanding the particular constellation of feelings, beliefs, and behaviors of each kind of personality disorder can the nurse tailor counseling strategies to meet the unique needs of each client.

Clients with PDs are encountered in all areas of nursing, extending far beyond the walls of psychiatric institutions. Counseling is conducted by psychiatric nurses who are prepared at the basic and advanced levels. Most often, the entry level nurse performs counseling within the framework of a nurse-client relationship (see Chapter 9) or formal and informal groups (see Chapter 11). Counseling in the form of family therapy (see Chapter 12) is most often performed by the advanced practice nurse.

The nurse should carefully monitor the evolution of the nurse-client relationship to ensure that a dependence on the nurse is not developing. Effective counseling skills with such clients make the difference in whether a "difficult" client or family situation in a medical/surgical or clinical setting is managed successfully by the nurse.

Depending on the setting, nurses functioning within the basic scope of psychiatric nursing may be involved with various types of groups (see Chapter 11) of clients with PD. Group therapy can be quite effective with these clients; the elements of universality and belongingness are especially important. Group therapists must have expertise in setting appropriate limits while still maintaining an atmosphere where self-exploration is the norm. A few empirical studies have demonstrated that short-term supportive group therapy has better client outcomes for short-term hospitalization than psychoanalytic therapy; however, there are conflicting findings (Springer and Silk, 1996).

Behavioral approaches

An example of a behavioral approach used with clients with PD is solution-focused therapy. Specific goals are made by the client. The nurse helps clients find the "solutions" needed to accomplish the goals. Therapy is discontinued once goals have been achieved, unless new goals are formulated. The success of the therapy is measured only within the context of whether goals are met. Basic level nurses use many principles of behavioral therapy when counseling clients within the nurse-client relationship. This kind of therapy is often well-received by clients with OCD and can be effective with other Personality Disorders as well.

Cognitive therapy

Because rigid and faulty thinking are so prevalent in clients with PDs, cognitive therapy is also useful. In cognitive therapy, it is assumed that one's thoughts generate feelings and that by changing thoughts, feelings can be changed (Ellis, 1994). Various kinds of irrational thought patterns are brought to the client's attention (e.g., inappropriate generalization) so these processes can be eliminated. Although nurses functioning at the basic level may use principles of cognitive therapy in counseling sessions, cognitive therapy is usually conducted by the advanced practice nurse.

Milieu Therapy

The aim of milieu management is the creation of an optimal environment for growth and change. Most experts agree that a milieu is therapeutic to the degree that clients are involved with each other. Thus the unit is structured for high client-client contact, as well as for high client-staff interaction. Nurses direct their efforts at creating a milieu in which norms of honesty, openness, curiosity, respect, and self-reflection predominate.

As clients act out their dysfunctional patterns in the present, feedback is given about how and why such patterns adversely affect their best interests. For example, clients with avoidant and dependent PD can discover how their fear of rejection cripples their interpersonal

The Nursing Process

effectiveness and can learn to practice assertiveness skills. The use of **unhealthy manipulation** of staff by these clients is expected. *This refers to the use of manipulation as the primary and sometimes only method for getting one's needs met, usually by treating others as objects through dehumanizing acts and exclusion of the needs of anyone else* (Chitty and Maynard, 1986). This type of maladaptive manipulation may be directed to an individual or to the milieu in general. A prime example is seen in the seducer role used by many clients diagnosed with APD. Here the client demonstrates **hypersexual** or *intense sexual behaviors*. The person may wear very sexually suggestive clothes, flirt with a particular nurse, only focus on sexual topics, try to kiss staff or other clients, touch others on the unit in sexual areas, or get in bed with another client. The behavior makes all in the milieu uncomfortable, and the end result is that it keeps the clients more isolated. Clients with APD and BPD will undoubtedly violate some structure that elicits the need for limit setting. Ideally over time, confrontations and limit setting by the nurse and staff lead to greater client self-awareness and insight.

A review of Table 26-1 highlights a number of the dysfunctional behavioral characteristics of clients with PD, for example, the impulsive behavior of the antisocial client who fails to plan ahead, is late for a group meeting, and is angry that the group did not wait. The unexpected and impulsive outbursts of the client with BPD often disrupt the status quo of a unit activity. In general, the client with PD tends to disrupt the environment, whether it is a hospital unit, partial hospitalization program, or even a group therapy session in a community mental health agency.

It is important for the nurse to not stereotype clients with PD. Rather, the nurse and team must handle unacceptable behaviors in a consistent manner. Most situations require some type of consistent limit setting in relation to client violence (physical, sexual, or verbal) toward self or others, cheating/lying, or other type of unhealthy manipulation of staff or clients. Each occurrence can be an opportunity for client growth and development. Consistency and sensitivity of the staff are paramount when using limit setting within the context of milieu management or the nurse-client relationship.

The nurse, as a key member of the team, is often responsible for establishing, implementing, and evaluating a limit-setting protocol for negative behaviors with staff input. A limit-setting protocol should include the following:

- Specific boundaries so that the significance of deviations can be immediately processed

- Contracting, a basic principle of cognitive therapy, to ascertain volitional agreement from the client to not act destructively (see Chapters 9 and 26)
- Specific information regarding the consequences that will occur if rules are not followed, in an attempt to engage client in social realities
- Options for dealing with anger and other physically violent or hypersexual behaviors; this should be indicated verbally to the client as well as in writing, for example, "being able to put into words, rather than actions, your (client's) feelings will help you think before acting, it will help you develop more useful and socially acceptable coping skills, and will help you be less impulsive"
- At the beginning of each shift, a member of the staff is designated to be the "communicator" during the implmentation of limit-setting protocol; the designated person has the specific role of talking with the client once the protocol is initiated; this role is particularly important for dealing with violent behavior; sometime once the show of force begins, the client can get lost in the shuffle; talking to the client during the incident conveys some degree of respect in the worst of circumstances

It cannot be stressed enough how important it is that the staff is consistent in setting limits on all negative behaviors. Often situations escalate to a crisis level when limit setting is inconsistent. Another helpful strategy is to have staff members review the general limit-setting protocol as well as rehearse it with a focus on various behaviors that disrupt the milieu setting. Such strategies help staff to respond in a firm, sensitive, consistent manner from the smallest infraction of the milieu's rules to the most threatening, unsafe violent act.

Self-Care Activities

Some clients with PDs need help with ADLs. The nurse may assist the client with ADLs in terms of hygiene/grooming, nutrition, and/or rest. In some cases this involves assistance with leisure-time activities. Clients with social-skills deficits often can benefit from social-skills training and education. Nurses can implement these activities either one-on-one or in group situations.

Psychobiological Interventions

Psychobiological intervention is usually prescribed in combination with some other form of therapy. Despite new approaches in both types of interventions, the

The Nursing Process

client with PD, especially BPD, remains difficult to treat. Almost all classes of psychiatric drugs have been tried with these clients (Koenigsberg, 1994). Some of the positive results of psychiatric drugs support the theories discussed in the biological correlates section presented earlier in this chapter.

Because depression is so pervasive in clients with PD, antidepressants such as MAOIs and even lithium have proven helpful in providing symptomatic relief. When their depression is well-controlled, clients have more energy to work on their issues, and the tendency to resort to alcohol and drugs to self-medicate may be diminished.

Neuroleptics are indicated in clients with schizotypal PD when psychotic-like symptoms are present in periods of decompensation (Siever and Davis, 1991). Thiothixene (Navane) has been shown to be useful with schizotypal clients in decreasing levels of illusions, ideas of reference, obsessive-compulsive symptoms, and phobic disorders (Perry and Vaillant, 1989). Both the anticonvulsant drug carbamazepine (Tegretol) classified as a mood stabilizer, and the MAOI drug tranylcypromine (Parnate) have been associated with a decrease in impulsive, self-destructive behaviors. Haloperidol (Haldol) and Navane have decreased paranoid thinking, anxiety, and hostility in some clients while violent episodes found in antisocial clients have been helped with the use of lithium carbonate and propanolol (Inderol).

Fluoxetine (Prozac) may reduce anger and related impulsive behaviors and borderline traits (Salzman et al., 1995; Siever and Davis, 1991). Kramer's (1993) *Listening to Prozac,* claims that low doses of Prozac given to nonclinically ill persons with depression results in profound character changes in these individuals. Labeling these individuals "rejection sensitive," Kramer describes them as "prickly" in reaction, expecting the worst, perceiving rejection where none was intended, defensive in attitude, and fearful in nature (characteristics commonly seen in client's with PD's). Within weeks of starting Prozac they became more open, less sensitive, more social and outgoing, and less fearful. Kramer reasons that these individuals, although not clinically depressed, were "wired differently" from early trauma responses, which caused sympathetic arousal, adrenal hyperactivity, and neurochemical imbalance. Early trauma responses cause these reactions, he claims, making certain individuals more susceptible to later stresses. Apparently, emotional experiences of rejection and abandonment, in particular, do predispose certain people to subclinical serotonin/norepinephrine depletion.

Although these medications in the borderline population seem to decrease selected target symptoms, for example, depression, to a manageable level, they have little or no effect on the personality patterns of this group. Furthermore, nonadherence to psychotherapy and pharmacology remains high (Koenigsberg, 1994). As with any client receiving medications, clients with PD need to be taught about their medications and side effects, especially clients in the community setting (see Chapter 15 for further information).

Health Teaching

Health teaching, especially from a psychoeducational framework, can be effective in helping clients with PD achieve more satisfying, productive, and healthier patterns of living. In fact, clients with PD tend to be especially open to the major goal of learning about their own illnesses (see Chapter 16). When clients with BPD hear about the concepts of splitting, abandonment depression, and acting out, they resonate with the material. They begin to have hope that they are not alone and that with work and effort they can grow beyond their current difficulties. An important aspect of health teaching is for nurses to become comfortable talking with clients regarding their illnesses (see the Community Resources box on p. 502).

Case Management

The case management interventions are based on a comprehensive approach. The interdisciplinary treatment plan on p. 497 illustrates this important approach.

Health Promotion and Health Maintenance

Clients with PDs are at risk for other disorders. Hence, health promotion and disease prevention interventions are aimed at identifying and diagnosing those clients at risk for PDs.

Evaluation

Although the plan of care, specifically the identified outcomes, is assessed continuously, evaluation is a formal process in which the nurse assesses whether identified outcomes are achieved in the specified timeline. Given the long-term nature of PD, it can be particularly difficult to evaluate the outcomes of treatment. The nursing care plan presented on p. 496 indicates that the nurse should evaluate outcomes and should document progress toward these goals. The Research Highlight on p. 502 reflects the long-term nature of PDs.

The Nursing Process

COMMUNITY RESOURCES

Because of the high incidence of comorbidity between PDs and depression, the following organizations are recommended as resources for individuals with PDs.

Depression After Delivery
P.O. Box 1282
Morrisville, PA 19067

National Alliance for the Mentally Ill (NAMI)
200 North Glebe Road, Suite 1015
Arlington, VA 22203-3754
(800)950-6264

National Depressive and Manic Depressive Association
730 North Franklin, Suite 501
Chicago, IL 60610
(312)642-0049

National Foundation for Depressive Illness
P.O. Box 2257
New York, NY 10116
(212)370-7190

RESEARCH HIGHLIGHT

Gunderson, J., et al. (1993). Stages of change in dynamic psychotherapy with borderline patients: Clinical and research implications. *Journal of Psychotherapy Practice and Research, 2*(1), 64-71.

Summary
The phases during the course of long-term therapy for five successfully treated clients with BPD were analyzed. Baseline functioning (socially dysfunctional) was determined using DSM-III criteria for the BPD subjects and compared with baseline after 4 years of therapy.

Phase 1, first year of therapy, was characterized by clients engaging in a broad range of acting-out behaviors. Phase 2, second year, was marked by diminished severity of clients' self-destructive actions. Four clients found part-time and/or low-level employment, involving nondemanding, routine tasks. Phase 3, acting out greatly diminished as the clients gained emerging trust in the fact that the therapists cared about them, but this was accompanied by intensified hostility as limits were set within the therapeutic relationship. Phase 4 and 5 were characterized by an increased expression of a range of affects, both within and outside of therapy. Social role performance included more self-responsibility and career ambitions, and friendships were developed.

Certain changes in clients with borderline personality disorders during long-term therapy can be expected. If years of therapy have failed to yield progression into Phase 2, the nurse therapist should seek supervision and expect assistance during long-term therapy.

Implications for Nursing Practice
- Understand that change is not only possible for these clients, but follows a particular and predictable course
- Use more supportive approaches during the beginning phase of treatment and more exploratory approaches later in treatment
- Focus interventions on assisting clients to manage their impulses, understanding that impulse control often is a reliable measure of change in the early years
- Assist family members to maintain more realistic performance expectations
- Assist these clients to become involved with some sort of social support, understanding that initially such involvement will be intermittent and conflictual
- Although the course of therapy will certainly vary from client to client, seek supervision or assistance if the therapy is not resulting in outlined changes within a reasonable time.

The Nursing Process

THE CONSUMER'S VOICE

Borderline Personality Disorder

Marc Jacques

What perspective can I offer you, you who are but a distant concept to me and me to you. I will start by telling you that I most often want to be someone or something else, for I am never satisfied with who I am, even though I possess great skill and talent. Like a child trying to catch a soap bubble so are jobs and friends to my ever-changing identity. I often remember the losses and feel deep sorrow. In the constant endings of my friendships I have spread seeds of my intense anger and often harvest violent consequences at times least expected. Many tell me I always look angry, which makes me so. For years I have watched my close relationships dissolve in front of my tearful eyes, so to protect myself, I say sour grapes and then accuse abandonment. In loneliness I strive for affection and acceptance, but my judgements are polluted by my pain of past failures. Many times I self-medicated with street drugs to try to feel better, but that too was a black hole. My stress has caused me to hear God gig-gle and Lucifer laugh, although I believe neither exist. It is no wonder depression and low self-esteem dog my path. In my desperate times I have tried to kill myself but like a poor marksman I just cannot hit the bull's eye. Even in my attempts at death I have felt that I could do nothing right.

Through education, I have worked hard uncovering myself from the sands of despair so tirelessly trying to bury me. It has been a process of discovery and I have forged success and a will to live from the knowledge and hope of recovery, an idea once alien to my treatments. I have come to know that medication without hope and support is a cruel and lonely prison. I strongly believe I have become stable mostly because of the understanding that I could do so. To those who read this, it is my sincerest hope that you understand and learn that the concept of recovery will make the greatest difference to the greatest number of people.

KEY POINTS

- Many individuals with PDs remain undiagnosed and are not often hospitalized.
- Clients with PD struggle with ego deficits and lack of separateness and individuality.
- The splitting defense mechanism, normal in early childhood but pathologic if relied on past puberty, accounts for much of the difficulty with staff and peers in treatment settings.
- Clients with PDs can only be fully understood when biological variables are considered. Recent research developments in the neurobiological field have revealed a number of findings related to the role of genetics, hereditary, brain chemistry, the autonomic nervous system, the hypothalamus, and the hormonal system.
- The specific areas to assess are impulse control, mood, judgment, reality testing, self-perception, object relations, thought processes, mastery of ADLs, and stimulus filter/stimulus barrier.

- In terms of separation-individuation, the goal of nursing care is to help clients develop a sense of self and to take responsibility for their own thoughts, feelings, and actions.
- In terms of ego function, the goal of nursing care is to help clients develop strength in the areas of ego deficit; this is done by modeling healthy behavior through strengthening weak ego functions.
- PD is considered an Axis II diagnosis, and clients are usually not hospitalized unless they are a threat to themselves (e.g., suicidal) or to others or if the PD occurs with a major Axis I disorder such as schizophrenia, substance abuse, or mood disorder.
- Long-term therapy may bring about desired behavioral changes, but the enduring patterns are major obstacles to desired outcomes.
- Currently a combination of short-term therapy and psychopharmacology are desirable approaches and can be successful if the client adheres to the treatment plan.

CRITICAL THINKING QUESTIONS

Janet, 22, was admitted to a local psychiatric hospital after calling a suicide hotline and threatening to kill herself. The hotline traced the call and alerted the police, who picked her up at home and brought her to the hospital. Janet had been in therapy at a local mental health clinic for 2 years because of depression and feelings of "emptiness." Her problems had escalated about 3 months before admission, at which time she began to complain that the therapy was not helping. This was in stark contrast to prior assertions that the therapy was "the only thing holding my life together."

At the same time, Janet began to sleep late and miss work. In the evenings she "partied" heavily with alcohol and marijuana, and became sexually involved with a variety of men. She also withdrew from usual social activities and refused to associate with her family. Her hostility toward her therapist, Dr. B., became pronounced; she complained especially about his "critical attitude" toward her. She was sleeping poorly and having horrifying nightmares. She would call Dr. B. in the middle of the night when she had nightmares, but then she would miss her regularly scheduled appointments.

When admitted to the unit, Janet isolated herself from both staff and other clients. When approached by staff, she could become quite caustic and was quickly able to elicit a defensive response in staff. An exception was seen in her response to an older female mental health technician, with whom she seemed to feel quite comfortable.

After several days on the unit, Janet's behavior shifted dramatically. Her withdrawn behavior gave way to a demanding, aggressive interpersonal style. She complained about being placed on unit confinement, stating that she had never intended to kill herself. She was particularly derisive toward evening staff, who had enforced the unit "rule" that clients be in their rooms by 11 PM She claimed in the community meetings that such rules reflected the "gestapo" mentality of staff. Soon, other clients began to stay up past the appointed time.

Staff members became increasingly polarized in their feelings toward Janet. Some felt she was "nothing but a spoiled brat," needing only to learn that "she was no better than anyone else." Other staff believed she was being treated too harshly. As staff members' trust in one another eroded, Janet seemed to grow increasingly cheerful.

1. In what ways does Janet demonstrate the typical behavior patterns and ego deficits seen in BPD?
2. What is the nature of Janet's self perception?
3. Which behaviors demonstrate her tendency to use action as a means to deal with painful, internal states?
4. In what sense does Janet act entitled? (*Entitlement* involves the belief that one has a rightful claim to special privileges, when in fact, one does not.)
5. Would you consider this client to have a sociopathic disorder? Why or why not?
6. In what ways are Janet's symptoms related to her relationship with Dr. B.?

- Consistency in implementing the established plan of care is important, especially in relating to limit setting for negative client behaviors.
- Evaluating client outcomes is difficult with clients with PDs, given enduring patterns of behavior, decreased lengths of hospital stay, and lack of adherence to treatment.

REFERENCES

American Nurses Association (ANA). (1994). *A statement on psychiatric-mental health clinical nursing practice and standards of psychiatric-mental health clinical nursing practice.* Washington, DC: Author.

American Journal of Nursing (AJN). (1965). Anxiety recognition and intervention. *American Journal of Nursing, 65*(9), 129-152.

American Psychiatric Association. (1994). *Diagnostic and statistical manual of mental disorders,* 4th ed. Washington, DC: Author.

Antoni, M., Levine, J., Tischer, P., Green, C., & Millon, T. (1987). Refining personality assessments by combining MCMI highpoint profiles and MMPI codes, Part V: MMPI code 78/87. *Journal of Personality Assessment, 51*(9), 375-387.

Bellak, L. (1973). *Ego functions in schizophrenics, neurotics, and normals: A systemic study of conceptual diagnostic and therapeutic aspects.* New York: John Wiley & Sons.

Chitty, K. K., & Maynard, C. K. (1986). Managing manipulation. *Journal of Psychosocial Nursing and Mental Health Services, 24*(6), 8-13.

Ellis, J. A., & Spanos, N. P. (1994). Cognitive-behavioral interventions for children's distress during bone marrow aspirations and lumbar punctures: a critical review. *Journal of Pain & Symptom Management, 9*(2), 96-108.

Gunderson, J., Waldinger, R., Sabo, A., & Najavito, L. (1993). Stages of change in dynamic psychotherapy with borderline patients. *Journal of Psychotherapy Practice and Research, 2*(1), 64-70.

Guyton, A., & Hall, J. E. (1995). *Textbook of medical physiology* (9th ed.). Philadelphia: Saunders.

Johnson, B. A., Brent, D. A., Connolly, J., Bridge, J., Matta, J., Constantine, D., Rather, C., & White, T. (1995). Familial aggregation of adolescent personality disorders. *Journal of American Academy Child Adolescent Psychiatry, 34,* 798-804.

Kaplan, H., & Sadock, B. (1995). *Comprehensive textbook of psychiatry* (6th ed.). Baltimore, MD: Williams and Wilkins.

Kaplan, H.I., Sadock, B. J., & Grebb, J.A. (1994). *Kaplan and Sadock's synopsis of psychiatric behavioral sciences clinical psychiatry* (7th ed.). Baltimore: Williams & Wilkins.

Keltner, N. (1992). Culture as a variable in drug therapy. *Perspectives in Psychiatric Care, 28*(1), 33-36.

Kernberg, O. (1993). The psychopathology of hatred. In R. Glick & S. Roose (Eds.), *Rage, power, and aggression: The role of affect in motivation, development, and adaptation, vol. 2* (pp. 61-79). New Haven, CT: Yale University Press.

Kerr, N. (1990). Ego competency: A framework for formulating the nursing care plan. *Perspectives in Psychiatric Care, 26*(1), 13-24.

Koenigsberg, H. W. (1994). The combination of psychotherapy and pharmacotherapy in the treatment of borderline patients. *Journal of Psychotherapy Practice and Research, 3*(2), 93-107.

Kramer, P. D. (1993). *Listening to Prozac.* New York: Viking.

Mahler, M. S., Pine, F., & Bergman, A. (1975). *The psychological birth of the human infant.* New York: Basic Books.

McCloskey, J. C., & Bulechek, G. M. (Eds.) (1996). *Nursing interventions classification (NIC): Iowa intervention project (2nd ed.),* St. Louis: Mosby.

Miller, C.R., Eisner, W., Allport, C. (1994). Creative coping: A cognitive-behavioral treatment program for borderline personality disorder. *Archives of Psychiatric Nursing, 8,* 280-285.

Peplau, H. (1963). A working definition of anxiety. In S. F. Burd & M. A. Marshall (Eds.), *Some clinical approaches to psychiatric nursing* (pp. 323-327). New York: Macmillan.

Perry, J., & Vaillant, G. (1989). Personality disorders. In H. Kaplan & B. Sadock (Eds.), *Comprehensive textbook of psychiatry* (vol. 2) (5th ed.). Baltimore: Williams & Wilkins.

Raine, A., & Mednick, S. (1989). Biosocial longitudinal research into antisocial behavior. *Review in Epidemiology, 37,* 515-524.

Salzman, C., Wolfson, A. N., Schatzberg, A., Looper, J., Henke, R., Albanese, M., Schwartz, J., & Miyawaki, E. (1995). Effect of fluoxetine on anger in symptomatic volunteers with borderline personality disorder. *Journal of Clinical Psychopharmacology, 15*(1), 23-29.

Siever, L. J. (1992). Schizophrenia spectrum personality disorder. In A. Tasman, & M. B. Riba (Eds.), *American psychiatric press review of psychiatry, vol I,* Washington, DC: American Psychiatric Press.

Siever, L.J., & Davis, K.L. (1991). A psychobiological perspective on the personality disorders. *American Journal of Psychiatry, 148*(12), 1647-1657.

Soloff, P.H., Lis, J.A., Kelly, T., Cornelius, J., & Ulrich, R. (1994). Risk factors for suicidal behavior in borderline personality disorder. *American Journal of Psychiatry, 151,* 1316-1323.

Springer, T., & Silk, K.R. (1996). A review of inpatient group therapy for borderline personality disorder. *Harvard Review of Psychiatry, 3*(5), 268-278.

Townsend, M. (1993). *Psychiatric mental health nursing: Concepts of care.* Philadelphia: JA. Davis.

Wester, J. (1991). Rethinking inpatient treatment of borderline clients. *Perspectives in Psychiatric Care, 27*(2), 17-20.

Chapter 27

Substance-Related Disorders

Madeline A. Naegle

LEARNING OUTCOMES

After studying and applying the concepts of this chapter, the learner will be able to:

- Formulate a self-assessment for health risks related to alcohol and other drug use.
- Assess the dysfunctional behavior patterns of clients with alcohol and other drug problems.
- Describe the effects of common drugs of abuse.
- Define concepts related to abuse and dependence.
- Formulate nursing care plans for clients with drug and alcohol problems.
- Discuss the implications of dual diagnoses in planning nursing care.
- Discuss the relationship substance of use and abuse to the health and health care of individuals.

KEY TERMS

Abstinence	Denial	Manipulation
Abuse	Detoxification	Physiological dependence
Addiction	Dual diagnoses	Polysubstance abuse
Avoidance	Enabling	Process addiction
Binge drinking	Euphoria	Psychological dependence
Blackout	Formal intervention	Recovery
Codependence	Gateway drug	Relapse
Craving	Grandiosity	Tolerance
Cross dependence	Impulsiveness	Wernicke-Korsakoff syndrome
Cross tolerance	Intoxication	Withdrawal delerium

ubstance abuse and addiction are major problems in society today. Every segment of society, regardless of race, gender, or age is affected. Mood-altering substances can be traced in history to earliest societies. Some substances that are used grow naturally, whereas others are manufactured illicitly or even legitimately in laboratories. They may be smoked, inhaled, ingested, or injected and used for social, religious, or self-medicating purposes. Because dependence affects all spheres of an individual's life and disturbs the whole person, it is considered a wholistic disease.

Substance abuse and dependence were first described as disease processes in the 1960s with the introduction of Jellinek's work on alcoholism. Dependence on alcohol and other drugs is now generally accepted and is classified in the American Psychiatric Association's *Diagnostic and Statistical Manual of Mental Disorders, fourth edition,* (DSM-IV) as a psychiatric disorder (APA, 1994).

In today's society, the substances that are abused include caffeine, nicotine, alcohol, steroids, stimulants, depressants, heroin, and cocaine. Persons do not usually think of caffeine found in coffee, tea, or sodas, or the nicotine found in tobacco as mood-altering substances. They also fail to consider the mood and behavioral changes that alcohol produces and do not consider it a drug, although its potential for inducing dependence is high. Because alcohol, caffeine, and nicotine are legal and easily obtained, their mood-altering capacities are not usually emphasized. *The abuse of more than one substance at a time is referred to as* **polysubstance abuse.**

Not all abuse or dependence involves a substance. In recent years it has become evident that activities such as overeating, excessive computer use, and gambling, which result from strong compulsion and are repetitive, are behaviorally similar to dependence or addiction. Some researchers classify these activities as "process addictions," and the persons who engage in them respond to treatment approaches that are similar to those used with persons who are dependent on substances. Gambling is an example of a process addiction.

The widespread distribution of substances, coupled with limited treatment for drug and alcohol dependence, guarantee that nurses employed in all settings will encounter clients with drug and/or alcohol problems. In addition, nurses are affected by the alcoholism or drug dependence of family members or friends.

In addition to learning to care for others with substance-related disorders, nurses need to recognize their own vulnerabilities to abuse of alcohol, tobacco, caffeine, and other drugs. Since 1981, professional nursing organizations have sought to educate their members about the incompatability of practicing nursing while experiencing problems with alcohol and other drugs. Although nurses have about the same rates of substance abuse and dependence as the general public, they are at special risk, because drugs are readily available in the work-place and health care professionals are inclined to self-medicate. Substance abuse and dependence by nurses and the efforts being used to prevent and decrease their prevalence are also discussed in this chapter.

This chapter provides basic knowledge and information about the skills that are necessary for health promotion, treatment, and rehabilitative intervention for substance-related disorders. Table 27-1 defines terms commonly associated with substance abuse and dependence, and gives examples of each. Each term will be further discussed in this chapter.

EPIDEMIOLOGY

Substance abuse ranks high among serious health problems. Although illicit drug use and alcohol consumption have declined gradually since 1979, the widespread use of and dependence on these substances continue among a significant number of individuals. Nicotine, now classified by the Food and Drug Administration (FDA) as an addictive substance, is linked to more deaths annually than the human immunodeficiency virus/acquired immunodeficiency syndrome (HIV/AIDS), cancer, and other substances combined. Seventy percent of Americans drink alcohol at least once per year, and alcohol use and abuse are factors in the injuries, deaths, and social problems of many citizens.

The costs of substance abuse to society are high. Lives are lost, and loss of work productivity costs millions of dollars each year. Alcohol is a factor in 40% of all motor vehicle accidents, and alcohol and other drugs are often implicated in boating or athletic accidents (National Institute of Drug Abuse [NIDA], 1994). Costs include not only lives lost but also medical care, long-term services to the disabled, and increased insurance rates. Health care expenditures for clients who use alcohol, drugs, and nicotine are estimated to be greater than $166 billion annually (Substance Abuse and Mental Health Services Administration, 1994). The link between violence and alcohol and other drugs is well-documented. Alcohol is a factor in vandalism on college campuses, date rape, sexual assault, and domestic violence. Under the influence of alcohol, young adults are more likely to engage in unsafe sexual practices (Noell, et al, 1993), and parents are more likely to abuse their children.

The epidemiology of drug and alcohol abuse and dependence is not as well-documented as that for other less stigmatized and more commonly recognized diseases. Major national surveys are conducted to identify the prevalence of problems, but drug users are often reluctant to participate or tend to underreport use. In addition, although it is estimated that 15.3 million individuals have a problem with alcohol and many millions of

TABLE 27-1

Terms common to substance-related disorders

TERM	DEFINITION	EXAMPLE
Abstinence	*Intentional nonuse of psychoactive substances*	There is no social or other consumption of alcohol.
Abuse	*A maladaptive pattern of substance use manifested by recurrent and significant adverse consequences*	A women uses excessive amounts of amphetamines to maximize work output or to lose weight.
Addiction	*Compulsive use of a psychoactive substance or repetition of compulsive behavior; characterized by tolerance, psychological dependence, and withdrawal*	There is use of large amounts of alcohol despite interpersonal and social problems related to use.
Blackout	*A brief amnestic period during which the individual is conscious and appears to be functioning normally*	An individual cannot recall conversations or events of the previous evening during which he or she was drinking heavily.
Codependence	*Dysfunctional behavior patterns characterized by excessive focus on the emotional, social, and physical needs of another*	An individual fails to retain sufficient funds for one's own needs while supporting another financially.
Craving	*A nearly irresistible urge to obtain and use a psychoactive drug*	The individual experiences an intense longing to obtain a substance or engage in an activity.
Cross dependence	*A state that results when an individual addicted to one drug develops biochemical changes that support addiction to another drug*	The individual dependent on morphine manifests dependence on methadone.
Cross tolerance	*The development of tolerance to other drugs by the continued exposure to a particular drug*	The repeated use of sedative hypnotics may result in a high tolerance for alcohol.
Denial	*A defense mechanism manifested in a failure to recognize or acknowledge realistic facts or events*	There is denial that smoking two packs of cigarettes per day has negative implications for health.
Detoxification	*The medically supervised decrease in drug dosage while maintaining physiological stability*	A provider gradually decreases benzodiazepines to the point of discontinuation.
Drug misuse	*Use of a drug for purposes other than those for which it was intended*	The individuals ingest antihistamines to induce sleep.
Dual addiction	*Simultaneous addiction to two psychoactive drugs*	The individual is dependent on alcohol and cocaine.
Dual diagnosis	*The coexistence of a major psychiatric disorder and a substance related disorder*	There is a use of marijuana to lessen secondary symptoms, such as hallucinations, of schizophrenia.
Enabling	*Behaviors by others that result in a friend's or family member's continued use or abuse of a drug*	Individual maintains a lifestyle that includes regular drinking despite a spouse's abuse of alcohol.
Intoxication	*A reversible substance-specific syndrome due to recent ingestion of or exposure to a substance*	Individual experiences pressured speech, rapid activity, and psychomotor disturbance following cocaine ingestion.

TABLE 27-1—cont'd

Terms common to substance: related disorders

TERM	DEFINITION	EXAMPLE
Process addiction	*Strong compulsions that result in repetitive activities with negative social, emotional, and legal consequences*	A person regularly spends the entire weekly household budget on lottery tickets.
Psychological dependence	*Subjective experience of a need for a drug to experience "normal" functioning*	The user feels "driven" to obtain and consume a drug or to engage in a particular behavior.
Physiological dependence	*A cluster of cognitive, behavioral, and physiological symptoms linked to a pattern of repeated self-administration resulting in tolerance, withdrawal, and compulsive drug taking*	The individual dependant on heroin uses large amounts of the drug and continues to use it to avoid uncomfortable symptoms that occur when use ceases.
Recovery	*Abstinence and healing obtained as a function of a drugfree lifestyle*	"Recovery" implies that life is meaningful, rewarding, and manageable without the use of drugs.
Relapse	*A temporary lapse into addictive behaviors*	The individual may experience a "binge" of excessive use over a number of days or up to 2 weeks.
Tolerance	*The need for greatly increased amounts of the substance to achieve intoxication or the "desired effect"*	The individual must now snort 2 gm of cocaine because the effect of the drug is not the same euphoria previously attained when taking 1 gm.
Withdrawal	*A substance-specific syndrome that follows the cessation of or reduction in intake of a psychoactive drug on which an individual is physiologically dependent*	On sudden cessation of triazolam (Halcion) an individual develops symptoms of insomnia and disorientation.

others are affected by a family member's problems with drugs and alcohol (NIDA, 1993), few of these individuals ever enter treatment. They do, however, seek medical treatment for other illnesses and are treated for the long-term effects of alcoholism, such as pancreatitis, hypertension, or kidney failure.

Risk Factors

Certain factors place some individuals at greater risk than others for the development of abuse and dependence. "At-risk" suggests that biological, psychological, or environmental conditions may predispose a person to the development of a drug and/or alcohol problem. Risk factors include the following.

- The heavy use of alcohol and other drugs or the presence of abuse or dependence by family members
- The presence of psychological conflict, which a person may attempt to resolve through drug use
- Genetic predisposition, which is derived from biological factors
- Inborn tolerance, which may result in excessive alcohol or other drug intake

Other psychological factors that predict risk for alcohol and drug abuse have been noted (NIDA, 1994) and include the following:

- Failure in school
- Rebelliousness and alienation
- Early antisocial behavior
- Need for immediate gratification
- Lack of empathy
- Frequent lying
- Insensitivity to punishment
- Peer pressure and choice of peers who use drugs
- Siblings who use drugs
- Inadequate parental direction and discipline

Community and cultural factors also play a role in determining risk for alcohol and other drug abuse. Communities with high levels of mobility, crime, and delinquency, as well as high population density, are high-risk environments and experience higher rates of dependence among their residents. Poverty and deprivation are also significant risk factors (NIDA, 1993).

Substance-related disorders do not respect age. Fetal exposure to alcohol puts unborn children at risk and may lead to fetal alcohol syndrome. Young children, adolescents, and older adults are all at risk. Chapters 33, 34, and 35 discuss the substance-related issues of these populations.

As the most powerful unit of socialization, the family transmits cultural beliefs, myths, and values about drug use. Likewise, peers and media personalities deliver messages about drug use, drug-using lifestyles, and through advertising, the desirability of drugs as a means of achieving relaxation.

Alcoholic beverages have been produced by civilizations since the beginning of time. Among cultural groups, there are wide variations in alcohol and drug use (see the Cultural Highlights box below). The types of beverages have varied globally by region, and the use of wines and spirits are subject to cultural traditions of families. Some groups have used wine strictly for celebratory purposes, others for religious rituals, and some for sustenance.

Many cultural groups do not consider alcohol a drug, although few would deny its psychoactive properties. When wine is produced at home and consumed daily at meals, little attention is paid to its addictive potential or to the consideration of potential links between health problems and its consumption. The result is that among many groups, especially those of Mediterranean descent, a double standard exists for alcohol and for other drugs. Illicit drugs are considered dangerous and unhealthy, but alcohol is accepted and not considered threatening to the individual, family, or society.

THEORETICAL FRAMEWORK

Increasingly, clinicians and researchers are acknowledging that many variables contribute to the development of drug dependence. These variables are neither predictable nor the outcome of singular causes. The disease model provides a context from which to consider interacting variables, which include biochemical and genetic predisposition, family history, social and environmental influences, temperament and character, and developmental resilience. Just as the interaction of some or all of these variables may cause dependence, they may also explain why some individuals do not develop symptoms.

Several models are discussed here, current perspectives hold that no one theoretical framework adequately explains substance abuse or dependence and that several biopsychosocial factors and multiple socioenvironmental influences are involved.

Disease Model

Substance dependence meets the criteria for a disease for the following reasons:

- It can be diagnosed.
- It is a primary disorder.

CULTURAL HIGHLIGHTS

- In a 1991 survey of preadolescents in a Mediterranean culture, more than 35% of responding youths (n = 252) reported drinking beer and wine for the first time between the ages of 10 and 11, as compared with American youth, in which the average age of first nonreligious consumption of alcohol is 12 (NIDA, 1994).
- The incidence of cocaine-related emergency department episodes among African-American males steadily increased 10.1% between 1985 and 1992. Reported incidence for African-American females for the same period increased 5.2% (National Center for Health Statistics, 1994.)
- Various Hispanic ethnic groups differ widely in their drinking behaviors. For example, Cuban Americans have lower rates of alcohol and drug abuse than either Mexican Americans or Puerto Ricans (NIDA, 1987).

- In Mexican-American populations, the Curandero (folk healer) uses a combination of counseling and herbs such as *babo de San Ignacio* (which causes nausea and vomiting when consumed) to treat alcoholism (Trotter, 1979).
- "Stories" by Native Americans that relate the Alcoholics Anonymous (AA) experience and translate the Twelve Steps of AA in language acceptable to Native American heritage are used in the treatment of Native Americans who identify with the traditional culture (AA, 1989).
- Ceremonies that use tribal rituals of cleansing (sweat house) and ritual prayers intended to restore harmony between an individual and the universe are incorporated into treatment of drug abuse and alcoholism by Native Americans (AA, 1989).

• It is the cause of other medical and psychiatric problems.
• It is predictable and progressive in its course.
• It is treatable.

The similarity between dependence and other diseases is evidenced by both psychological and physiological factors. Individuals who are addicted to substances are genetically predisposed to addiction and have chemically altered brain function. Psychologically they are obsessed with the use of the drug for its pleasurable qualities and exhibit evidence of compulsive, self-defeating drug-use patterns. Dependence on certain drugs is analogous to having allergy. The person with an allergy is not held responsible for the allergy and is not expected to control the untoward response to the allergen, but rather is expected to exhibit the usual responses to it. The vulnerable individual is also expected to avoid the allergen so as not to experience a negative consequence. Applying this analogy to substance dependence supports a nonblaming attitude and acknowledges that maintaining abstinence and managing the disease are the responsibilities of the client.

Accepting a lack of control over the substance and the need to abstain from its use are cornerstones of successful treatment. Control is accepted and expected to be in the hands of some power greater than oneself. Recovery consists first of abstinence, then physical, emotional, and spiritual healing. Complete recovery is not considered possible; hence the term "recovering."

Jellinek (1960) is credited with articulating the disease model of alcoholism. The current model, revised from Jellinek's early work, incorporates the following:

• There is a unique entity that can be identified as alcoholism.
• Persons with alcoholism and prealcoholism are essentially different from those who do not have the disease.
• Persons with alcoholism may sometimes experience an irresistible physical craving for alcohol or a strong psychological compulsion to drink.
• Persons with alcoholism gradually develop loss of control over drinking and possibly even the ability to stop drinking.
• Alcoholism is a progressive disease that develops through a distinct series of phases as long as the person continues to ingest alcohol.
• Alcoholism is a permanent and irreversible condition.

Biological Correlates

Biochemical explanations of dependence include theories about neurochemical action, craving and reward mechanisms in the brain, and genetic predisposition to abuse of alcohol or other substances.

Neurotransmitters

The neurotransmitter model holds that drugs work by inhibiting, stimulating, or changing the release or action of neurotransmitters in the brain. Neurotransmitters implicated in dependence include serotonin, dopamine, norepinephrine, and acetylcholine. During normal neurotransmitter action, presynaptic cells release neurotransmitters into the synaptic cleft, where they exert specific effects on postsynaptic target neurons or receptor sites. Normal neurotransmitter action ends when there is *reuptake* into presynaptic cells or a breakdown of the neurotransmitters by enzymes (see Color Plate).

Cocaine, amphetamines, and other stimulants produce an excitatory or stimulant response by increasing the production of dopamine, serotonin, norepinephrine, and acetylcholine. Hyperstimulation in the central nervous system (CNS) results in psychological effects such as heightened energy, increased tolerance to pain, and improved intellectual performance. *Tolerance* develops, *requiring increased amounts of the drug to create the desired effect.* Increased amounts of the drug result in an overabundance of neurotransmitters with consequent development of additional receptor sites. If a decrease in drugs occurs, neurotransmitter levels decrease, causing understimulation of the CNS. Craving for the drug or withdrawal symptoms may then follow.

Craving

The term *craving was initially used to describe the strong overpowering urge for opiates experienced by opiate-dependent clients experiencing acute withdrawal. It currently describes the desire to use certain abused substances at any time.* The craving response involves the reward centers of the brain, genetic influences on neurotransmission, and biochemical changes caused by alcohol or other drugs themselves.

Blum and Payne (1991) propose a three-phase model to explain craving: setup, substitution, and destruction. *Setup* refers to the genetic predisposition an individual has to dependence. Genetically predisposed individuals are believed to have a reduced supply of enkepalins or a reduced ability to release these neurotransmitters in the hypothalamus. A predisposed individual may have an increased number of opioid receptors and reduced dopamine receptors in the nucleus accumbens (the reward center of the brain). Feelings of well-being are therefore reduced. The "setup" is that alcohol and other drugs cause dopamine release, reversing the deficit and leading to strong feelings of well-being.

Once alcohol "rewards" the brain receptors, *substitution* occurs. Alcohol and other drugs are substituted and cause a release of dopamine, temporarily offsetting the genetic dopamine deficiency. The *destructive* phase involves increased intake of the substance to achieve the desired CNS effects (tolerance). Damage to the reward center results in intensified craving. The process is a cyclical "trap." Furthermore, the chronic use of a drug to satisfy craving slows the rate of neurotransmitter production and release, resulting in withdrawal symptoms or tolerance.

The subjective experience of craving alcohol, cocaine opiates, or nicotine plays a significant role in relapse in individuals who have stopped using a substance but feel powerless to resist its lure. The mechanisms involved in craving also account for withdrawal symptoms that occur when a substance is abruptly discontinued.

Normally, excessive amounts of neurotransmitters are "recycled" into the presynaptive neurons in a process called *reuptake* (see Chapter 13). Some drugs block reuptake, prolonging stimulation of the central nervous system. Cocaine blocks reuptake of serotonin and dopamine, increasing the amount of excitatory neurotransmitters. *An exaggerated feeling of well-being* or *euphoria* associated with cocaine results. Alcohol, barbiturates, and benzodiazepines block the reuptake of the modulator neurotransmitter, gamma-aminobutyric acid (GABA), and enhance binding at receptor sites. The calming and sedative effects of alcohol, benzodiazepines, and barbiturates are the results. Hallucinogenic drugs such as LSD and PCP reduce the supply of serotonin and GABA in the synaptic cleft. This reduction permits excessive dopamine and acetylcholine activity, which results in hallucinations, delusions, and paranoia.

Genetics

The current belief is that there is a genetic or familial predisposition to dependence, and the substance of choice may vary from generation to generation. Outcomes of family, twin, and adoption studies, as well as molecular genetic research, suggest that genetically determined traits, not a specific gene, determine the type of dependence an individual may develop. In this view, the individual enters life with a certain genetically determined "protection" or "predisposition" to dependence. It is hoped that the conclusive identification of biological genetic markers will contribute to the early identification of the disease, diagnostic specificity of subtypes, and the matching of interventions to specific subtypes. Researchers believe that genetic disturbance results in neurotransmitter imbalance.

Although much of the research has involved dependence on alcohol, abuse of and dependence on other drugs are being explored. The extremely complex nature of symptoms of dependence contributes to the recognition that there is no single gene that determines whether or not a person develops the disease. In fact, researchers believe that the genetic predisposition to alcohol is polygenetic and that the genes related to alcoholism (alcogens) may interact and exert influence across symptoms or subtypes (Crabbe and Goldman, 1992). The subtypes most commonly used today are Type I and Type II, which may be loosely characterized as distinguishing alcoholism *without* and *with* antisocial personality traits (Cloninger, Bohman, and Sigrardson, 1981).

Physiological outcomes

Substances of abuse act primarily on the CNS, but they also manifest effects on vital signs, the respiratory system, psychomotor behavior, and other biological systems. The body regards any drug as a poison. How a drug affects an individual depends on the individual's size, age, and health as well as the mode of entry of the drug and the dose of the substance. Table 27-2 lists common drugs of abuse and describes their behavioral effects, sites of action, and duration of effects.

All drugs of abuse have the potential for lethal effects by enhancing suicidal ideation or by causing toxicity and/or overdose. Likewise, abrupt withdrawal may cause life-threatening symptoms. Because not all clients acknowledge their abuse or dependence, nurses must recognize the physical signs of problematic alcohol and other drug use. Complaints of early morning vomiting, chronic diarrhea, gastritis, anorexia, and vague undiagnosed abdominal pain are common gastrointestinal (GI) complaints of individuals who ingest substances (Kinney, 1996). Hypertension and dysrhythmia are common cardiovascular symptoms. Unexplained trauma, sleep complaints, and sexual dysfunction are other symptoms that should alert the nurse to further assess the individual for alcohol and other drug use. Prolonged or chronic use has the potential to cause serious impact on body systems. Box 27-1 lists the consequences of chronic use of alcohol. In drug-dependent individuals, physical signs include poor hygiene, dental carries, vein scarring, abscesses, and erosion of the nasal septum.

Family Correlates

Alcoholism has been called a family disease, meaning that dependence on alcohol serves to maintain homeostasis in the family. Alcohol or drug abuse by an adolescent may be a means of preserving the parents' marriage. Dependence may also develop as a sequel to abuse or neglect in a dysfunctional family in which the child fails to develop a healthy sense of self. Others believe that the use of substances is a learned coping behavior fostered within the family.

Bowen (1978) discussed substances as part of the triangulation process in families (see Chapter 12). He viewed use of a substance as a means of avoiding problems within the marriage and family. Energy and emotion

TABLE 27-2

Common mood-altering drugs

DRUG NAME	EFFECTS	SITE OF ACTION	LENGTH OF EFFECT
Hallucinogens			
Mushroom (psilocybin)	Altered body image	Central nervous system (CNS)	Onset: 40 to 60 min.
LSD (lysergic acid diethylamide)	Euphoria		Duration: 6 to 12 hr.
Mescaline (from the peyote cactus)	Sharpened perceptions		
DOM (dimethoxymethylam-phetamine)	Somatic effects: dizziness, tremors, weakness, nausea		
STP (no chemical name)	Psychosis-like symptoms		
MDA, Ecstasy (methylene dioxyamphetamine)	Emotional swings		
	Suspiciousness		
	Bizarre behavior		
	Increased blood pressure		
	Increased temperature		
	Objective signs: dilated pupils, flushing, tremors		
Cannabinoids			
Marijuana	Failure of judgment and memory	CNS	Dependent on route of administration
Hashish	Mild intoxication	Cardiovascular system	Dose dependent
	Euphoria		
	Relaxation	Respiratory system	Onset: 20 to 30 min.
	Sexual arousal		Duration: 3 to 7 hr.
	Panic states		
	Visual hallucinations		
	Objective signs: reddened eyes, dry mouth, incoordination		
	Heart rate increases to 140/min.		
Opiates: Semisynthetic and Synthetic Analgesics			
Codeine	Analgesia (therapeutic)	Nervous tissue	Onset: 20 to 30 min.
Morphine	Euphoria	CNS (opiate receptors)	Duration: 4 to 8 hr.
Heroin	Escape		
Dilaudid	Reduction in sexual and aggressive drives	Respiratory system	
Methadone			
Demerol	Respiratory depression		
Darvon	Sedation, sleepiness		
Designer drugs	**Objective signs:** hypertension, pupillary constriction, constipation		

TABLE 27-2—cont'd

Common mood-altering drugs

DRUG NAME	EFFECTS	SITE OF ACTION	LENGTH OF EFFECT
Sedative-Hypnotics and Anxiolytics			
Barbiturates	Drowsiness, sedation	CNS	Dependent on route of administration
Seconal	Euphoria	Cardiovascular system	Dose dependent
Nembutal	Escape, loss of aggressive and sexual drives	Respiratory system	Onset: 30 to 40 min.
Amytal	Emotional lability		Duration: 4 to 5 hr.
Tuinol	Poor judgment		
Barbiturate-like (quaaludes)			
Benzodiazapines (Librium, Valium)	**Objective signs:** blood pressure decreased 10-30 mmHg; slightly decreased temperature; decreased urinary output; decreased pulse and respirations		
Buspirone (BuSpar)			
Stimulants			
Amphetamine, Methaphetamine, Dexedrine, Benzadrine	Euphoria, grandiosity	CNS	Onset: route-related 10 to 30 min.
Ritalin	Stimulation, energy, anxiety	Peripheral nervous system	Duration: drug related
Preludin	Relief of fatigue	Cardiovascular system	
	Depression		
Cocaine	Wakefulness		
Crack	Suppression of appetite		
	Aggressive feelings, paranoia		
	Objective signs: sweating, dilated pupils, increased blood pressure, rapid heart and respiratory rates, tremors, seizures		
Phencyclidines			
PCP (phencyclidine) (Angel dust)	Detachment from surroundings	CNS	Rapid onset: 2 to 3 min. up to 45 min.
	Decreased sensory awareness		Duration: drug- and dose-related
	Illusions of superhuman strength		
	Acute intoxication		
	Objective signs: flushing, fever, sweating, coma, agitation, confusion, hallucinations, paranoia, violence		
Inhalants			
Benzene (paint thinner, cleaning fluid, glue)	Euphoria	Cardiac effect	Onset: immediate
Nitrites	Giddiness, headache, fatigue, drowsiness	CNS	Duration: 20 to 45 min.
Nitrous oxide	**Objective signs:** dysrythmias, damage to kidneys, liver abnormalities		

TABLE 27-2—cont'd

Common mood-altering drugs

DRUG NAME	EFFECTS	SITE OF ACTION	LENGTH OF EFFECT
Alcohol			
Alcohol	Relaxation, sedation, release of inhibitions	CNS	Onset: 20 min. to 1 hr.
Beer		Respiratory system	Duration: dose related
Wine	**Objective signs:** incoordination, nausea, vomiting, slurred speech		
Xanthines			
Caffeine	Stimulation	CNS	Onset: 10 to 30 min.
	Restlessness		Duration: 3 to 7 hr.
	Anxiety		
	Objective signs: decreased heart and respiratory rates, diarrhea, gastric disorder, insomnia, tremors		
Nicotine			
Cigarettes	Stimulation	CNS	Onset: immediate
Smokeless tobacco	Enhanced performance	Respiratory system	Duration: 5 to 15 min.
		Cardiovascular system	
		Endocrine system	

are invested in a third, outside "substance." The result is that the person using alcohol or another drug is distanced from the partner, negating any possibility for intimacy in the marital relationship. Children also remain in a distant position in the triangle.

Psychodynamic Correlates

Psychodynamic theories have historical value, and psychological issues are important factors for clients in maintaining recovery. They evolve from analytical and self-psychological models. The analytical view identifies drug use as a symptom of unmet current or developmental needs; a symptom of unconscious, unresolved dependency needs; a symptom of unconscious self-destructive drives; or the craving for ecstatic experience. In analytical terms, drug use provides "secondary gain," that is, the individual is able to gratify some need not otherwise recognized, expressed, or met.

The self-psychology model also addresses the psychological needs of the individual and proposes that drug-taking serves an ego-enhancing function. It was once thought that drugs were used to "medicate" distressful states such as depression, self-esteem disturbances, im-

Box 27-1

Physiological Consequences of Chronic Alcohol or Drug Use

- Cardiovascular effects: hypertension, stroke, cardiac enlargement, anemias, and blood dyscrasias
- Gastrointestinal (GI) problems: esophagitis, gastritis, cancers of the GI tract, hemorrhage, pancreatitis, hepatitis, and cirrhosis of the liver
- Skin problems: acne rosacea, dermatitis, telangiectasia, spider angioma, and palmar erythema
- Malnutrition and nutritional diseases
- Neurological problems: peripheral neuropathy
- Korsakoff's syndrome
- Sexual dysfunction
- Blood dyscrasias: thrombocytopenia and leukopenia

pulsivity, or acute or chronic dysphoria (low-level emotion). Uncomfortable moods such as rage, shame, and loneliness were sedated. Feelings of unworthiness, weakness, or depression were changed by stimulants, thereby defending the individual against these feelings.

Another theory proposes that clients become fixated at the oral stage of development in infancy. Ingestion of substances is seen as a way of fulfilling past unmet oral needs.

Psychodynamic theories are no longer widely accepted as explanations of substance-related disorders, but rather they explain psychological variables that may contribute or prevent the development of symptoms.

Behavioral Correlates

Behaviorists describe drug and alcohol problems as learned maladaptive behaviors or habits developed in response to external stimuli, such as involvement in a drug subculture or exposure to heavy alcohol use by adults. The underlying causes of the behavior are less important than the immediate rewards experienced by the user, such as escape, avoidance of negative feelings, indirect expression of anger, and rebellion. Continued use of substances results in reinforcement—either positive or negative—of the behavior and its social, physiological, and psychological consequences.

A drug may initially appear to facilitate the individual's functioning. For example, when alcohol diminishes shyness and creates social ease, the user experiences positive feedback that reinforces a pattern of use. Drugs such as alcohol and heroin result in the continued need for reinforcement by the drug effects rather than an experienced need to learn positive coping skills. Environmental stimuli may become "triggers" or signals that elicit craving, or the desire to use.

Dysfunctional patterns of behavior have also been associated with substance dependence. Dependent individuals often use manipulation, that is, they *attempt to meet their own needs at the expense of others.* Insensitivity to others can result from an insensitivity to oneself as a person. *Grandiosity is the irrational thought that one is entitled to special treatment and that everyone should know of the entitlement.* Grandiosity is often an effect of stimulant use, may be a personality characteristic independent of drug use, and often is a behavior that must be addressed in early recovery.

The defense mechanism of denial is considered a key behavioral symptom of individuals with addictive symptoms. *Denial is manifested in statements and behaviors that indicate that the individual does not acknowledge, see, or experience concern about the consequences and scope of excessive drug use.* Denial exists to some degree in the thinking of all persons with drug and alcohol abuse and dependence problems.

*Behaviors by others that serve to perpetuate the addictive or dependent behavior are termed **enabling.*** Family and friends may unwittingly reinforce drug-using behaviors by becoming *codependent.* ***Codependence** is considered by many to be a learned dysfunctional behavior pattern characterized by an extreme emotional, social, or physical focus on another person, without regard to personal needs or realistic social expectations.* Codependent individuals inadvertently reinforce the use of alcohol or drugs by supplying the substance or means for its purchase, attempting to control intake, or providing excuses for socially deviant behaviors such as excessive spending or failure to appear at work.

The *Nursing Process*

Assessment
Clinical Profile

Alcohol-related disorders
Alcohol is a natural substance formed by the fermentation of sugar by yeast spores. It is the most widely abused drug in the United States. Since alcohol content varies by type of beverage, a "standard drink" measure is used to determine the amount of alcohol consumed by an individual. Fig. 27-1 lists standard drink equivalents for beer, wine, and distilled spirits.

Physiological effects of alcohol use Alcohol is absorbed directly from the stomach and exerts system depression and physiological effects throughout the body almost immediately. In low doses, alcohol produces relaxation, loss of inhibitions, loss of concentration, drowsiness, slurred speech, and sleep.

Chronic use results in multisystem problems. Chronic use of alcohol may result in ***Wernicke-Korsakoff syndrome.*** Wernicke's encephalopathy, also called Wernicke's syndrome *is a form of dementia and results from thi-*

The Nursing Process

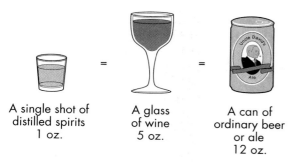

A single shot of distilled spirits 1 oz.

=

A glass of wine 5 oz.

=

A can of ordinary beer or ale 12 oz.

Fig. 27-1 Standard drink equivalents.

TABLE 27-3

Correlation between blood-alcohol level and behavioral/motor impairment	
RISING BLOOD-ALCOHOL LEVEL*	**EXPECTED EFFECTS**
20–99	Impaired coordination, euphoria
100–199	Ataxia, decreased mentation, poor judgment, labile mood
200–299	Marked ataxia and slurred speech, poor judgment, labile mood, nausea and vomiting
300–399	Respiratory failure, coma, death

*mg/100 mL blood (mg % or mg/100 mL)

amine deficiency. *Symptoms include paralysis of ocular muscles, diplopia (double vision), ataxia (muscular incoordination), somnolence, and stupor.* Korsakoff psychosis is *characterized by confusion and short-term memory loss, and confabulation. It usually accompanies Wernicke encephalopathy.* Thiamine arrests and reverses the syndrome in some cases. However, if thiamine replacement therapy is not initiated, death may occur.

Chronic alcohol use may cause cirrhosis of the liver. Cirrhosis involves the widespread destruction of functional liver cells that are replaced with fibrous nonfunctioning (scar) tissue. Complications of cirrhosis include portal hypertension, ascites, esophageal varices, and hepatic encephalopathy. Complications of cirrhosis are life-threatening and require aggressive treatment. Any future ingestion of alcohol by clients who have cirrhosis and/or its complications may result in death.

Blood-alcohol level The amount of alcohol in the bloodstream is measured by the blood-alcohol level (BAL). This level has limited clinical usefulness because of the rapid elimination rate of alcohol. Table 27-3 lists blood-alcohol levels and their expected behavioral effects.

The DSM-IV lists several disorders that are related to problematic use of alcohol. Those discussed here include the following: alcohol intoxication, alcohol abuse, alcohol dependence, and alcohol withdrawal

Alcohol intoxication *Intoxication with a substance refers to the development of a reversible substance-specific syndrome resulting from the ingestion of or exposure to a substance.* Persons who are intoxicated are often "drunk." Signs and symptoms of alcohol intoxication include the following:

- Changes in mood
- Belligerence or aggressive behavior
- Poor psychomotor coordination
- Impaired memory

- Impaired judgment
- Impaired social functioning
- Blackouts
- Physical signs including nystagmus
- Blood-alcohol level of 100-200mg/100mL
- Bradycardia
- Diaphoresis

Jeffrey is an 18-year-old college freshman who entered a large urban university after completing high school in his hometown in rural New Jersey. During the fall fraternity pledging period, Jeffrey, a strong student who is active in campus government affairs, tried hard liquor for the first time. He changed from his reserved self to being more gregarious, telling jokes, and making overtures to women.

Soon his speech became slurred and he made a belligerent remark to one of his close friends, who suggested to Jeffrey that perhaps he could not "hold his liquor." In response, Jeffrey swung a punch in his friend's direction, but because he was so poorly coordinated, Jeffrey missed his mark. When he passed out on a chair, his date and a friend roused him enough to get him home and to bed. That next day, Jeffrey did not remember trying to strike his friend.

Alcohol abuse Alcohol abuse is a common and often undiagnosed pattern of excessive alcohol consumption. Excessive consumption must occur for at least a 12-month period to be considered abuse. The symptoms of alcohol abuse include the following:

- Tolerance to the effects of alcohol
- Problematic consumption

The Nursing Process

- Maladaptive drinking patterns
- Problems in fulfilling role obligations
- Social isolation
- Denial
- Unpredictable drinking behavior
- Changes in eating and stress management activities
- Frequent relapses to heavy consumption

Other patterns that occur in relation to abuse include phases of intermittent *episodic* heavy consumption balanced with phases of abstinence or light drinking. These alternating periods can last for weeks or months. Individuals may also engage in binge drinking. **Binge drinking** *is a pattern of regular, heavy drinking limited to specific periods of time, such as weekends or vacations.* Sudden termination of such heavy consumption may result in withdrawal or alcohol hallucinosis, but only if the individual becomes physiologically dependent during the period of binging.

Box 27-2 describes the DSM-IV criteria for substance abuse. These criteria may be applied to the abuse of any substance.

Alcohol dependence   Alcohol dependence is a more severe disturbance than alcohol abuse and is characterized by loss of control over the use of alcohol, a pattern of compulsive use, and the expenditure of substantial periods of time and energy in the consumption of alcohol. Dependence may be only psychological or may include both physiological and psychological components. Box 27-3 describes the DSM-IV criteria for substance dependence. These criteria are applied to clients who are dependent on alcohol or other substances.

Alcohol withdrawal   When alcohol or any drug of abuse is terminated abruptly by a person who is physiologically dependent, a specific pattern of signs and symptoms emerge. Onset of symptoms begins within 6 to 12 hours following the cessation of or reduction in prolonged heavy alcohol use. Symptoms of alcohol withdrawal include the following:

- Nausea and vomiting
- Course tremors of hands, tongue, and eyelids
- Malaise and weakness
- Sweating
- Elevated temperature
- Anxiety
- Depressed mood and irritability
- Headache
- Insomnia

If untreated, withdrawal may progress to alcohol **withdrawal delirium,** *which is characterized by seizures, transient hallucinations and illusions, severe agitation, elevated vital signs, severe nausea and vomiting, and marked autonomic hyperactivity.* Onset of delirium occurs on the second or third day following cessation of alcohol ingestion and can be avoided with medical intervention that includes intravenous (IV) fluids and gradually reduced doses of medications (sedative-hypnotics). Untreated delirium may result in death. See Chapter 31 for a full discussion of delirium.

Stimulant drugs

CNS stimulants that are often abused include cocaine, amphetamines, nonamphetamine stimulants, caffeine, and

Box 27-2

DSM-IV Criteria for Substance Abuse

A. A maladaptive pattern of substance use leading to clinically significant impairment or distress, as manifested by one (or more) of the following, occurring within a 12-month period:
   (1) Recurrent substance use resulting in a failure to fulfill major role obligations at work, school, or home (e.g., repeated absences or poor work performance related to substance use, substance-related absences, suspensions, or expulsions from school; neglect of children or household)
   (2) Recurrent substance use in situations in which it is physically hazardous (e.g., driving an automobile or operating a machine when impaired by substance use)
   (3) Recurrent substance-related legal problems (e.g., arrests for substance-related disorderly conduct)
   (4) Continued substance use despite having persistent or recurrent social or interpersonal problems caused or exacerbated by the effects of the substance (e.g., arguments with spouse about consequences of intoxication, physical fights)
B. The symptoms have never met the criteria for substance dependence for this class of substance.

From American Psychiatric Association. (1994). Diagnostic and statistical manual of psychiatric disorders, fourth edition. *Washington, DC: Author.*

The Nursing Process

nicotine. Cocaine is the most potent and is derived from the leaves of the coca plant, while caffeine and nicotine are the most prevalent and widely used stimulants.

Cocaine, amphetamines, and nonamphetamine stimulants exert their influence by augmenting or potentiating the excitatory neurotransmitters epinephrine, norepinephrine, and dopamine. They are known as psychomotor stimulants. On the street, amphetamines are known as *bennies, splash, speed, crystal, and black beauties.* Diet pills are called *uppers,* and cocaine is referred to as *coke, blow, snow, lady, and flake. Crack* is the form of cocaine that is smoked or inhaled.

Caffeine is a common ingredient in coffee, tea, colas, and chocolate. Nicotine is the primary psychoactive ingredient in tobacco products. Caffeine and nicotine are generally cellular stimulants and exert their actions directly, increasing rates of cellular metabolism.

Physiological effects of cocaine Cocaine stimulates the CNS and is abused recreationally because of its pleasurable effects. Persons who abuse cocaine may "binge"

on high doses of the drug on an episodic basis followed by a 2- to-3–day recuperation known as a "crash." Or they may be chronic daily users of smaller doses that increase over time as their tolerance increases. Cocaine helps individuals to feel more powerful, more confident, and more decisive.

Intoxication with cocaine increases the myocardial demand for oxygen, resulting in an increased heart rate. When vasoconstriction occurs, myocardial infarction, ventricular fibrillation, and sudden death may occur. When inhaled, cocaine can cause pulmonary hemorrhage, bronchitis, or pneumonia. Chronic cocaine snorting causes nasal rhinitis. Cocaine exerts a powerful aphrodisiac effect, which may be one reason for relapse or continued use of the substance.

Cocaine abuse Cocaine abuse is a maladaptive pattern of cocaine use manifested by recurrent and significant adverse consequences, including legal difficulties that may result from possession and use of the drug. Signs and symptoms of cocaine abuse include denial

---

Box 27-3

DSM-IV Criteria for Substance Dependence

A maladaptive pattern of substance use, leading to clinically significant impairment or distress, as manifested by three (or more) of the following, occurring at any time in the same 12-month period:

(1) Tolerance, as defined by either of the following:
   (a) A need for markedly increased amounts of the substance to achieve intoxication or desired effect
   (b) Markedly diminished effect with continued use of the same amount of the substance

(2) Withdrawal, as manifested by either of the following:
   (a) The characteristic withdrawal syndrome for the substance (refer to Criteria A and B of the criteria sets for Withdrawal from the specific substances)
   (b) The same (or a closely related) substance is taken to relieve or avoid withdrawal symptoms

(3) The substance is often taken in larger amounts or over a longer period than was intended

(4) There is a persistent desire or unsuccessful efforts to cut down or control substance use

(5) A great deal of time is spent in activities necessary to obtain the substance (e.g., visiting multiple doctors or driving long distances), use the substance (e.g., chain-smoking), or recover from its effects

(6) Important social, occupational, or recreational activities are given up or reduced because of substance use

(7) The substance use is continued despite knowledge of having a persistent or recurrent physical or psychological problem that is likely to have been caused or exacerbated by the substance (e.g., current cocaine use despite recognition of cocaine-induced depression or continued drinking despite recognition that an ulcer was made worse by alcohol consumption)

SPECIFY IF:

With physiological dependence: evidence of tolerance or withdrawal (i.e., either Item 1 or 2 is present)
Without physiological dependence: no evidence of tolerance or withdrawal (i.e., neither Item 1 nor 2 is present)

COURSE SPECIFIERS (SEE P. 527):

Early Full Remission
Early Partial Remission
Sustained Full Remission
Sustained Partial Remission
On Agonist Therapy
In a Controlled Environment

From American Psychiatric Association. (1994). Diagnostic and Statistical Manual of Psychiatric Disorders, fourth edition. Washington, DC: Author.

The Nursing Process

and avoidance, maladaptive behavioral changes, episodes of problematic use, feelings of euphoria, enhanced self-confidence, neglect of responsibilities, interpersonal problems and conflicts, legal risks and infractions, periodic heavy use alternating with abstinence, and negative physical signs including anorexia and weight loss. The following example illustrates cocaine abuse.

> Frank W., a 45-year-old lawyer, is seeking treatment because of marital problems. He reports that problems in his marriage began 3 years ago when he began to feel attracted to another woman and became disinterested in sex with his wife. At that time, he introduced his wife to cocaine sniffing, an activity which he had enjoyed in his twenties, but from which he had refrained since he married. Sniffing cocaine for brief periods at the end of a social evening seemed to enhance sexual interest for both of them. After that, Frank began using cocaine at the office one evening in the middle of the week. More recently, he has been sniffing cocaine every weekday evening and on weekends. The resulting decrease in available income, a 10-pound weight loss, and agitation, were noticed by his wife, and she accused him of using cocaine and concealing it from her. He is seeking assistance, although he is exceedingly ambivalent about his drug use and denies that it is a problem.

Cocaine intoxication Cocaine and its solid form "crack," which is smoked, induce rapid euphoric responses, the onset of which varies according to the mode of ingestion (smoking, snorting, injecting). Signs and symptoms of cocaine intoxication are both behavioral and psychological. Signs and symptoms of cocaine intoxication are a "high" feeling, euphoria, enhanced vigor, gregariousness, restlessness, hypervigilance, anxiety, alertness, grandiosity, psychomotor agitation, cardiac dysrhythmias, dilated pupils, and impaired social and occupational functioning. The following clinical situation illustrates some of the consequences of cocaine intoxication.

> Kathy C. is a 24-year-old graphic designer who works for a large advertising firm in San Francisco. Last week she was arrested for the first time and spent the evening in jail before her boyfriend could post bail and remove her from custody. When he arrived, she explained that she and several colleagues had "celebrated" a recently acquired contract and had ended up sniffing cocaine. Realizing that she was late, she left while still intoxicated and was involved in a minor traffic accident. During the ensuing scuffle, she used profane language and shoved a police officer at the scene.

Opioid drugs

Opioids are narcotic analgesics that suppress the CNS and exert both sedative and analgesic effects. They are used therapeutically to relieve pain, control diarrhea, and relieve coughing. Opioids are derived from the juice of unripe seed capsules of poppy plants. Morphine is the primary active ingredient of opium. Heroin is the common street form of the drug. Opioid (known on the street as "black," "poppy," "tar," or "big O"), morphine (known as "Miss Emma," "white stuff," or "M"), and codeine (known as "terp," "romo," and "robo") are also popular opiod drugs of abuse.

Opioids desensitize users to both psychological and physiological pain and induce a sense of euphoria. Individuals quickly develop dependence on, as well as profound tolerance to, opioids. Strict controls exist about the accessibility of opioids, and therefore use of these drugs is illicit and illegal. Despite this, heroin is readily available in the United States and is used experimentally and regularly by about 3% of the population. Demerol, a synthetic opioid, is the main drug, after alcohol, to which health care professionals become addicted. It quickly induces physiological dependence.

Opioid intoxication Opioid, or heroin, intoxication consists of clinically significant maladaptive behavior or psychological changes that develop during or shortly after use of an opioid such as heroin. Initially the individual is euphoric and relaxed and has pinpoint pupils. If an overdose occurs, anoxia ensues and pupils dilate, followed by signs of impending coma. Signs and symptoms of opioid intoxication are initial euphoria and relaxation, pupillary constriction, apathy, impaired judgment, dysphoria, slurred speech, impairment in attention or memory, depressed respirations and other vital signs, confusion and/or disorientation, and drowsiness or coma. Clients who abuse heroin are at greater risk to develop AIDS (Naegle, 1994).

Marijuana use

A 1993 household survey by the National Institute of Drug Abuse (NIDA, 1994) found that 9% of the population had smoked marijuana in the past year. Marijuana is second only to alcohol as the most widely abused drug. Marijuana is composed of the dried leaves, stems, and flowers of the cannibis plant, and hashish, which is more potent, is a resin derived from the flowering tops of the plant. Marijuana is usually smoked in loosely rolled cigarettes or in pipes. It is known on the street as "weed," "pot," "stick," "grass," "Mary Jane," and "hay." Hashish is known as "hash," "ganga," or "charas."

The drug derived from the plant depresses the central nervous system. Increased doses produce sedation, hypnosis, and anesthesia. It also produces euphoria, anxiety, grandiosity, hypervigilance, impaired judgment, tachycardia, elevated blood pressure, pupillary dilation, nausea,

The Nursing Process

vomiting, and perspiration or chills. Intoxication occurs immediately and lasts for about 3 hours.

The recreational use of marijuana is controversial. There is evidence that it is a ***gateway drug,*** *that is, that it may lead to abuse of more potent substances.* It has been used to treat the pain, nausea, and vomiting associated with chemotherapy. However the long-term efficacy of the drug has not been established. The following clinical example illustrates why its use is a concern.

Timmy is a 14-year-old who began hanging out with older teens who smoked pot. He recently tried it with no ill effect and has progressed to almost daily use. His school grades have dropped, he is increasingly irritable at home, and he has dropped his association with most of his peers. He has become socially isolated. Last Saturday night, 1 month after he began to smoke pot, Timmy was admitted to the emergency room and treated for cocaine intoxication. During a follow-up interview with an addiction counselor and his parents, he revealed that he had been shoplifting to support his pot addiction. He claims that the incident with cocaine was his first.

Prescription drugs

Prescription drugs are among the most abused substances. The problem is rarely addressed, in part because actual prevalence is unknown. Prescription drugs are sold on the street, but most often, they are obtained with prescriptions from physicians or other providers. Prescribers may be ignorant about the potential abuse of prescription drugs, may rationalize excessive consumption of prescription drugs by clients, or may overuse drugs with clients rather than treat or refer them for non-pharmacological interventions.

Sedative-hypnotic agents and anxiolytic drugs are the most common prescription drugs that cause physiological and psychological dependence. These drugs are CNS depressants that cause behavioral depression, which ranges on a continuum from therapeutic relief from anxiety, sedation, sleep, and anesthesia to physiological dependence to, and in large enough doses, death. Signs and symptoms of dependence on prescription drugs in the anxiolytic (benzodiazepine) class include tolerance, impaired judgment, drug-seeking behaviors, compulsive use, and self-medicating behaviors. The following example illustrates progressive dependence that is characteristic of individuals who are dependent on prescription drugs.

Nancy M. is a 33-year-old secretary in a large, well-known law firm. She was prescribed chlordiazepoxide (Librium) when she injured her back skiing 5 years ago. At the time, she used it occasionally after straining the existing injury or when feeling particularly nervous. She progressed to taking it regularly and doubled the dose (10 mg.) after bad days at

the office. Three months ago, she complained to her physician that the medication was no longer relieving her back pain. When he was reluctant to renew the prescription, she became tearful and expressed the fear that she could not function without the medication. He prescribed Xanax (2 mg.) but warned her that the medication was addictive and to curtail daily use.

One week after beginning the medication, Nancy pronounced that it was "not helping" and increased her daily use to 4 mg. When she was unable to renew her prescription with her physician, she located another physician who began prescribing medication for her. She currently sees five different prescribers who give her medication. At present, she is taking four to five times the daily therapeutic dose.

Dual diagnoses

In recent years there has been a significant increase in the number of individuals with diagnoses of major mental and/or emotional disorders who also abuse or are dependent on drugs. Between 15%–43% of clients in the mental health care system have co-occurrence of a major mental disorder and a substance-related disorder. Actual prevalence of comorbidity or dual diagnoses is obscured, because statistics do not reflect combined data from psychiatric and substance abuse treatment centers. In addition, "dual diagnoses" are often not established because of traditional patterns of identifying primary and secondary diagnoses. The result is that one of the disorders receives insufficient attention, and care is fragmented.

The mental disorders are related to substance use disorders in the following ways:

- They may precede the substance abuse or dependence, placing the individual "at-risk."
- They may influence and exacerbate the course of the abuse or dependence.
- They may emerge as a consequence of substance abuse.
- They may become linked over time with the symptoms of dependence.

Clients who have coexisting mental and substance-related disorders have many needs. They require frequent inpatient hospitalizations and appear to have lower recovery rates than clients with only a diagnosis of substance-related abuse disorders. Furthermore, the use of alcohol, illicit drugs, and illicitly obtained prescription drugs aggravates and/or precipitates recurrence of dysfuctional symptoms and can even induce related delirium, dementia, or other organic disorders.

These clients respond best to treatment in an environment that treats the mental disorder; that includes interpersonal stimulation, which is low in intensity and not

The Nursing Process

too demanding; that links clients with Twelve-Step programs; and that promotes abstinence.

The following clinical example illustrates the complexity of symptoms in a client who has dual diagnoses of alcohol dependence and major depression.

Mr. Y. is a 66-year-old retired bartender who has had two past hospitalizations following suicide attempts. He is admitted for alcohol detoxification by his son who says he found him unconscious at home. Mr. Y. says he had been on a 2-week "bender," and family members report he has always been a heavy drinker.

Following detoxification, Mr. Y. expresses having feelings of boredom and hopelessness since his retirement. He does not share with staff his previous episodes of suicidal behavior. While on a pass to attend an Alcoholics Anonymous (AA) meeting, he attempts suicide with "pills" he had hidden in his car.

RESEARCH HIGHLIGHT

Kearney, M.H., Murphy, S., Irwin, K., & Rosenbaum, M. (1995). Salvaging self: A grounded theory of pregnancy on crack cocaine. *Nursing Research, 44* (4), 2-7.

Summary

The purpose of this qualitative nursing study was to develop a grounded theory to encompass the main issues and problems faced by pregnant women who use crack cocaine and the actions they take in response to pregnancy.

The 60 women recruited for the study were active drug users who used cocaine or crack on the average of once weekly. A snowball sampling technique was used to obtain participants, and each was compensated $40; individuals who provided referrals were compensated $20. Data were gathered in audiotaped interviews that lasted 1 hour, and data were organized along the lines of inquiry based on women's narratives. Summary and field notes were also used. Grounded theory analysis included (1) preliminary data categorization, (2) substantive coding, and (3) theoretical coding.

The basic problem of pregnancy in the context of crack cocaine use was threatened selfhood. The action taken was a process of "salvaging self."

The process of "salvaging self" emerged as the women attempted to redirect their lives and make the best of an already damaged pregnancy experience. Salvaging included a focus on the self as an individual. The salvaging process was initiated at different times during the women's pregnancies and consisted of two phases: facing the situation and evading harm." "Facing the situation" was a phase of judging the pregnancy situation and weighing options. Judgments were made about three categories of meaning: value, hope, and risk. "Evading harm" included initiating actions based on judgments, which fell into the categories of harm reduction and stigma management.

The women in the study were seeking to salvage their own lives for the sake of their infants' well-being. Values of pregnancy and motherhood were conventional in contrast to the world of drugs and prevailing impoverished and crisis-filled lifestyles. Self-protection parallels other observations of women's responses to threats in the forms of pregnancy, drug addiction, and sexual preference.

Implication for Nursing Practice

The nurse should do the following in managing pregnant clients who are addicted to substances:

- Explore the links between stereotyping by health care providers and the threats to the self-esteem of pregnant women who are addicted.
- Understand the psychological processes that accompany changes to self-concept throughout pregnancy.
- Affirm the value of the pregnant woman as a whole person, separate from the developing fetus.
- Develop strategies that create a foundation for a trusting relationship with women who are addicted and of childbearing age.
- Discuss guidelines for nurses in the development of care plans for women who are addicted using prenatal and drug treatment facilities.
- List actions that can be included in health teaching to reduce risks to pregnant women and their fetuses.
- Discuss the ethical implications of questioning women about illicit drug use and the confidential management of such information.

The Nursing Process

Special populations
Substance abuse occurs regardless of age, socioeconomic status, or profession. Children are born to addicted women, adolescents report excessive alcohol use, and the elderly are the largest consumers (and misusers) of over-the-counter (OTC) medications. Furthermore, professionals, including physicians and nurses, are also among those with substance use problems.

Pregnant women who abuse substances Cocaine, alcohol, marijuana, heroine, nicotine, amphetamines, and tobacco are substances abused by pregnant women. It is estimated that 6% to 8% of pregnant women have serious problems with alcohol. Illicit drug use among pregnant women ranges from 4% to 32% (Redding and Selleck, 1993). The psychosocial profile of pregnant women who abuse substances includes the following:

- Chaotic family history
- History of trauma and loss
- Unstable lifestyle
- Poor parental role models
- Few positive social supports
- Poor self-esteem
- Guilt, shame, and anxiety about abuse or dependence
- Noncompliance with prenatal care or absence of any prenatal care
- Legal or school problems

Infants born to women who are addicted to cocaine and/or opiates are themselves physiologically addicted to the substance and experience withdrawal symptoms at birth. Furthermore, many are born with other disabilities. Some of the issues and problems facing women who are addicted to cocaine are found in the Research Highlight on p. 522.

Women who are heavy smokers may bear infants of low birth weight. Fetal alcohol syndrome (FAS) occurs in children of women who consumed alcohol during pregnancy; the effects are dose-related. The characteristics and facial dysmorphology of children with fetal alcohol syndrome are depicted in Fig. 27-2.

Impaired professionals Substance abuse among nurses has received increasing attention in recent years. In 1984, The American Nurses' Association (ANA) reported that approximately 5% of nurses were alcohol-dependent and 8% to 10% abused alcohol and/or other drugs. (ANA, 1984). Recent studies indicate that the prevalence of alcohol and other drug problems in nurses is similar to that of other groups of women in American society.

Recognizing that a peer is impaired by substance abuse is difficult and is most often met with denial or hostility if that individual is confronted. Clues that indicate that a nurse's performance may be impaired by a substance are found in Box 27-4. Nurses who suspect a peer of diverting drugs or of abusing substances should

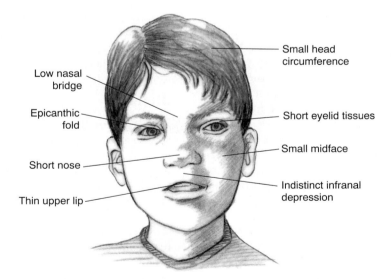

Fig. 27-2 Characteristics of children with fetal alcohol syndrome (FAS). Children with FAS often exhibit the following characteristics: pre- and postnatal growth retardation, developmental delays, intellectual impairment, neurological abnormalities, and characteristic facial dysmorphology.

The Nursing Process

Box 27-4

Clues to Possible Substance Abuse in Nurses

- Decline in appearance and performance
- Mood swings
- Memory lapses
- Frequent absence from floor
- Excess time spent in restroom
- Working extra shifts
- Increased incidents/accidents when nurse is on duty
- Increased number of clients who report unrelieved pain or insomnia
- Inaccurate drug counts
- Increased vial breakage and drug wastage

Box 27-5

CAGE

CAGE Screening Tool

C Have you ever felt you ought to **cut down** on your drinking?

A Have people **annoyed** you by criticizing your drinking?

G Have you ever felt bad or **guilty** about your drinking?

E Have you ever had a drink first thing in the morning—an **eye opener**—to steady your nerves or get rid of a hangover?

NOTE: *More than one positive response indicates a probable drinking problem.*

From Ewing, J.A. (1984). Detecting alcoholism: The CAGE questionnaire. Journal of American Medical Association, 252 *(14),* 1905-1907.

document their observations and report their findings to appropriate nurse managers.

State boards of nursing are responsible for determining if a nurse's substance abuse or dependency jeopardizes public safety. Some may refuse to grant or to reinstate a suspended license. Others collaborate with expert panels to ascertain if a nurse's substance abuse poses a threat to public safety and to refer the nurse for treatment. Collaborating state boards and nursing associations may institute or cooperate to monitor substance use when a nurse is in the recovery process. The National Student Nurses Association has developed guidelines that are similar to those of its parent organization.

Some form of peer assistance program currently exists in most states to help nurses who are impaired by substances or psychiatric illness. Peer assistance programs aim to assist impaired nurses to recognize their problems, obtain treatment, and establish or regain accountability for professional practice. Typically the nurse with an impairment problem makes a contract for recovery that details treatment requirements, monitoring guidelines, frequency and length of peer support contracts, and the personal and professional consequences of relapse. The following clinical example demonstrates symptoms of impaired performance by a student nurse.

Jillian is in the last semester of her nursing education. She has been an academic honor student and has excelled clinically until this semester. Jillian occasionally uses OTC stimulants when studying for examinations. She is a popular student and began drinking socially with her peers two semesters ago. She has smoked tobacco since her senior year in high school.

Recently her friends have noticed memory lapses and mood swings. Her clinical instructor observed that she leaves the floor often and spends long periods of time in the restroom.

The head nurse on the unit where Jillian is a student informed her instructor that there has been an increased number of complaints about pain from clients in Jillian's care, despite documented administration of analgesics to them. Jillian's instructor carefully observed and documented incidents of drug diversion and unusual behavior. She confronted Jillian and referred her to the peer assistance program. Jillian agreed to a treatment program and monitoring. She will not be permitted to sit for her state board examination until she has had 2 drug-free years monitored by the peer assistance treatment program in her state.

Screening

Screening for the use of substances is an essential first step in assessment in any setting and is incorporated into general history taking. Screening identifies a client's potential problem with alcohol or other drugs. Interviewing, observation, and inspection provide the data for screening and assessment about the nature and extent of an individual's involvement with a drug (Box 27-5). Assessment is a dynamic and ongoing process. Making positive contact with the client and establishing rapport are the first priorities. The overriding goals of assessment include the following:

- Determine whether a drug and/or alcohol problem exists

The Nursing Process

TABLE 27-4

Screening tools

TOOL/TEST	PURPOSE	FORMAT
CAGE (Ewing, 1984)	Assesses immediate or recent past use of alcohol	Four questions; positive responses indicate probable drinking problem (Box 27-5)
TWEAK (Russell, Martier, and Sokal, 1991)	Assesses immediate or recent past use of alcohol during pregnancy	Seven-point scale; responses indicate severity of drinking problem
AUDIT (Saunders et al., 1995)	Assesses quantity and frequency of alcohol use over past year	Ten-item test; a score of 8 or more indicates need for further in-depth assessment
Brief MAST (Pokorny, Miller, division Kaplan, 1972)	Assesses for use of alcohol; no time frame; longer administration time	Twenty-item test; yes/no answers; standardized scores that indicate severity of drinking
T-ACE (Sokol, Martier, and Ager, 1989)	Detects high-risk drinking behavior in pregnant women	Four items; positive answers indicate probable risk for problematic alcohol use
CHARM (Sumnicht, 1991)	Assesses risk of problematic substance use in elderly	Five questions; responses indicate intent of use by elderly; positive responses indicate degree of medically hazardous use in older adults
Trauma Scale (Skinner et al., 1986)	Assesses history of trauma and related drinking beginning with eighteenth birthday	Five items; one positive answer indicates probable drinking problem (Box 27-6)
DAST (Skinner, 1982)	Assesses drug abuse in all age groups	Twenty-eight items; a score of 5 or more posi-

- Determine the level and severity of the problem
- Motivate the client to change problematic behavior
- Enhance or create motivation for treatment

The nurse assesses use of substances to detect patterns that place the individual at risk for negative health consequences and illness. The extent of the assessment varies with the setting in which the nurse is providing care. In the primary care setting, for example, nurses evaluate and treat clients who are in early, middle, and late or chronic states of substance abuse or dependence. The nurse first screens and assesses for potential problems using history taking and brief screening instruments. Several screening instruments have been developed. Table 27-4 lists selected tests along with their purposes and brief synopses of their formats.

If screening indicates that the client has a problem with alcohol or other drugs, further evaluation is needed. Fig. 27-3 illustrates a decision tree for screening clients in primary care settings (NIAAA, 1990). The

Trauma Scale in Box 27-6 is part of the decision-tree screening and produces data about the relationship of trauma to substance-using behavior. It is brief (five questions) and touches on physical injury, habits of driving under the influence, the influence of drugs or alcohol on behavior, and residual effects of injury that influence mental status.

Focused Assessment

Follow-up interviews complete the assessment, whether in a primary care or an acute treatment setting. In addition to setting the tone for a therapeutic alliance, assessment interviews with clients who abuse substances provide opportunities to review findings and explain their meanings and health implications. They are also used to discuss clients' interests in and readiness for referral and treatment. Table 27-5 lists focused assessment questions intended to obtain information about the target behaviors of individuals with an alcohol or other drug problem, as well as examples of client responses.

The Nursing Process

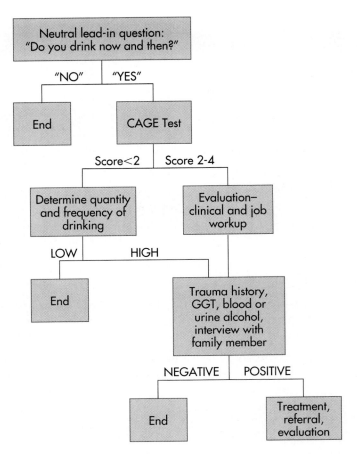

Fig. 27-3 Decision tree for primary care screening. High consumption is defined as 60 to 80 gm of absolute ethanol per day. Significant trauma history would be indicated by a score of 2 or higher on the five-item trauma scale (see Box 27-6). (From National Institute on Alcohol Abuse and Alcoholism [NIAAA]. [1990]. *Seventh Special Report to the U.S. Congress on Alcohol and Health.* Publication Number [ADM] 281-88-0002, p. 197. Washington DC: Department of Health and Human Services.)

Blood and Urine Tests

In addition to information obtained during screening and follow-up assessment interviews, blood and urine tests are performed to validate and/or expand interview findings. Among the blood tests ordered are blood-alcohol levels, hepatic screening tests, glucose, hemoglobin and hematocrit levels, and HIV screening.

Urine toxicology screens are widely used as a method of screening for illicit substance use. They should be administered randomly and more than once to reduce false positives. False positives may occur with certain foods (e.g., poppy seeds) and medications (e.g., decongestants). Nurses should be aware that some substance use may not be detectable in urine screens or may only be detectable for a short time. Cocaine and LSD last as little

as 12 hours, while benzodiazepines can last up to 24 to 48 hours after the last dose. Inhalants are not detectable in urine at all.

Nursing Diagnosis

Dysfunction related to psychoactive drug use exists on a continuum from use to dependence. The DSM-IV (APA, 1994) describes substance-related disorders for 10 classes of drugs and polysubstance use (see Table 27-2). The major diagnoses fall into categories of abuse, dependence, intoxication, and withdrawal for each group. The DSM-IV also addresses disorders induced by the use or misuse of substances, such as sleep and mood disorders. The diagnostic category polysubstance-related

The Nursing Process

Box 27-6

Trauma Scale Screening Tool

Five Questions About History of Trauma Since Eighteenth Birthday:

1. Have you had any fractures or dislocations of your bones or joints?
2. Have you ever been injured in a traffic accident?
3. Have you ever injured your head?
4. Have you ever been in an assault or fight (excluding sports)?
5. Have you ever been injured while drinking?

NOTE: *More than one positive response would indicate a probable drinking problem.*

From Skinner, H.A., Holt, R., Schuller, J., & Roy, J. (1986). Identification of alcohol abuse using laboratory tests and a history of trauma. Annals of Internal Medicine, 101, *847-851.*

disorder refers to the repeated use over a 12-month period of at least three groups of substances (not including caffeine and nicotine). The course of substance dependence is further defined in the DSM-IV by six descriptions that specify the duration of type of remission. Course specifiers for substance dependence include the following:

- Early full remission
- Early partial remission
- Sustained full remission
- Sustained partial remission
- On agonist therapy
- In a controlled environment

Nursing diagnoses are established following assessment for substance-related health manifestations. Table 27-6 lists selected nursing diagnoses used in relation to substance abuse and dependence and examples of possible defining characteristics. NANDA diagnoses have been adopted by the ANA in its publication, *Standards of Addiction Nursing* (1988) (see Appendix B).

Outcome Identification

Treatment outcomes of the client with a substance-related disorder vary with the phase and severity of abuse or dependence. Other important factors are the characteristics of the individual and the drug on which the individual is dependent. The need for inpatient hospitalization, for example, is determined by the individual's ability to refrain from using the drug, and the health

risks that unmonitored withdrawal from the drug may cause. Inpatient hospitalization also provides an opportunity for clients to put distance between themselves and the drug supply. This applies similarly to the individual who cannot refrain from gambling, smoking, or compulsive sexual activity.

Goals of inpatient hospitalization include providing clients with basic understanding of the effects of drug use and dependent behavior on physical and mental health, helping them begin the steps toward lifestyle change, and introducing them to Twelve-Step self-help groups. Hospitalization for detoxification or medically supervised withdrawal requires a minimum stay of 10 days to 2 weeks, depending on contributing factors such as the number of drugs the client is using, contributing medical conditions, age of the client, emergent conditions such as organic mental changes, completeness of discharge plans, managed care dictates, and the availability of community resources to support aftercare.

Aftercare includes a variety of treatment modalities, but minimal expectations include involvement in ongoing counseling or a psychotherapeutic relationship and participation in a self-help group such as Narcotics Anonymous (NA) or Alcoholics Anonymous (AA). Aftercare may also include living in a halfway house or attending a day center (Sullivan, 1995).

Controlled drinking may be the appropriate goal for some. Individuals who have recovered from a state of alcohol abuse or early addiction without formal intervention may be able to drink moderately. *Total abstinence,* while a difficult goal, is however required for most individuals. Achieving and maintaining total abstinence, including a gratifying life in sobriety, requires the development of new coping mechanisms, social support including economic stability, and a level of mastery that permits some control over the circumstances of one's life. Recovery is a lifetime process, and most individuals who have experienced success in sobriety consider that their efforts must be ongoing.

Planning

Planning care for individuals with substance-related disorders is a complex process. Approximately 6% of psychiatric clients have drug and alcohol problems that meet criteria for abuse or dependence. Even when persons with these problems do not have a diagnosed psychiatric illness, their mental health is clearly changed by drug use.

Researchers suggest that implementing treatment and reaching positive outcomes are best achieved if both client and nurse understand the client's readiness

The Nursing Process

TABLE 27-5

Focused assessment: abuse of a psychoactive substance

NURSING ASSESSMENT	TARGET BEHAVIORS	EXAMPLES: CLIENT RESPONSES
Client Interview		
Tell me about your drinking? What other drugs do you use?	Drugs used	"I drink socially." "What do you mean by drugs?"
When do you use them (every day, weekly, monthly, weekends)?	Frequency: regular use, binging	"Sometimes I'll start drinking on Fridays—before I know it, it's Monday."
How do you use the drug (snorting, drinking, injection)?	Route of administration	"Somebody usually passes around a joint."
How much, on average, would you take at a time?	Identifying maladaptive patterns: amount in grams, ounces, joints, cubes	"We *breath it up*—we wouldn't inject," "A couple of tokes," "A few glasses of wine."
Where do you use?	In social setting only? Alone? Part of the drug subculture (shooting galleries, clubs)?	"Some of us just get together when one of us gets some good stuff."
Assess Motivation for Use		
What would you say the drug does for you?	Interpersonal, psychological, or cognitive rewards of use as perceived by the client	"XTC just makes me feel loving toward everyone."
What are the "benefits" you experience when you use (euphoria, escape)? What is good for you about your use? What does the drug do for you?	The function the drug serves for the user	"One or two drinks and I'm really mellow." "I'm really on task when I snort."
Have you had legal, marital, or financial difficulties recently?	Interpersonal, legal, or monetary problems as consequent to drug/alcohol use	"Got laid off work last week." "I'm broke."
Do you think such problems could be related to your using drugs? Do you ever think you may be drinking too frequently?	Other events linked with excessive use: illness, assault, domestic violence, child abuse charges, DWI, debts	"Naw, I never use all that much." (Denial of links between drugs and impaired performance.)
Evaluate Evidence and/or Severity of Problem		
Has your wife (son, friend, employer) ever expressed concern over your use of drugs and/or alcohol?	Changes noted by others; often these are linked to use	"Sometimes my mom gets all bent out of shape about my drinking. She's kind of a teetotaler."
Do you sometimes feel you are not in control of your need to use or the amount you use?	Loss of control over drinking and/or drug use; rules about when and how much to drink (suggests fears over controlling use)	"Well, I guess I drink more than last year, but then again, I am making more money."
How do you try to control use?	Efforts to control use; switching beverages, limiting contact with other users, etc.	"I can handle that amount if I am not depressed or just needing a place to sleep."
How long have you had trouble with use or restricting the amount you use? How long have you been trying to cut down?	Duration of problem; loss of control over use	"I have been shooting up pretty steadily since Christmas." "My dad died, etc."

The Nursing Process

TABLE 27-6

Selected nursing diagnoses common to addiction nursing practice

NURSING DIAGNOSIS	EXAMPLES OF DEFINING CHARACTERISTICS
Sensory-perceptual alterations	Fluctuation in mental status, confusion, disorientation, blackouts, hallucinations ataxia, history of flashbacks, history of seizures, intolerance to activity, diminished self-esteem, discomfort, homeless lifestyle, practice of unsafe sex, severe withdrawal syndrome
Altered nutrition: less than body requirements	Report of inadequate dietary intake; change in appetite and dental caries
Thought process, altered	Mood swings, restlessness, impairment of recent memory, lack of insight, dementia
Noncompliance	Continuing pattern of addiction, verbalization of noncompliance, inability to set goals
Communication, impaired verbal	Inability to express feelings, slurring of speech, inappropriate speech patterns
Spiritual distress	Distress in human spirit caused by guilt, shame, grief, self-blame, lack of meaning in life
Powerlessness	Passivity, a perceptual experience of loss of control, inappropriate efforts to assert control over self
Social interaction, impaired	Actual, secondary to intoxication; relationships changed by substance use
Sexual dysfunction	Problems of inorgasmia and erectile dysfunction as a result of drug abuse
Violence, risk for: self-directed	Self-destructive acts initiated while under the influence of a drug
Violence, risk for: directed at others	Marital conflicts, assault, sexual assault, rape, or child abuse associated with substance abuse

to change problematic behaviors. Individuals with substance-related disorders have been observed to pass through the following preliminary stages before such change is initiated:

- *Precontemplation,* in which clients have no intention to change behavior in the foreseeable future, often because they are unaware of problems
- *Contemplation,* in which clients are aware of the problem and are seriously thinking about doing something about it
- *Preparation,* in which clients combine intention and begin to change their behaviors
- *Action,* in which changes in behavior, experience, or environment begins
- *Maintenance,* in which clients work to prevent relapse and consolidate the benefits of action (Prochaska, DiClemente, and Norcross, 1992).

Life factors as well as feelings can influence an individual's readiness or motivation to change. Negative consequences of abuse, such as HIV-positive status, arrest for a driving while intoxicated (DWI) charge, or loss of professional licensure can influence change. Desires or aspirations, such as the wish to have a child, may increase motivation. Loss of income, serious threats to self-esteem, the expectations of significant others, changes in health status, and dramatic life events may also be motivators. Finally, the extent to which the individual notices and acknowledges cognitive impairment, mood changes, or spiritual distress can also provide motivation.

Planning for nursing care occurs on individual and interdisciplinary treatment team levels. A nursing care plan for an inpatient client with dual diagnoses of marijuana abuse and borderline personality disorder is presented on p. 530.

A sample critical pathway reflecting interdisciplinary treatment team planning for a client with substance abuse with an expected length of inpatient hospitalization of 7 to 14 days is presented on p. 531. This pathway suggests a 7- to 14–day length of stay, whereas the current norm generally allows reimbursement for 3 days of inpatient alcohol detoxification and 7 days of inpatient drug withdrawal.

Dual Diagnoses

Nursing Assessment Data

Subjective: Confusion, auditory hallucinations, apprehension, agitation. Client states:"I smoked a little marijuana on my weekend pass." *Objective:* Response to internal stimuli, including fantasy and auditory hallucinations; inappropriate laughing; pacing; and mumbling incoherently; *DSM-IV Diagnoses:* Cannabis abuse and borderline personality disorder.

NANDA diagnosis: Sensory-perceptual alteration, auditory, related to substance use (smoking marijuana)

Outcomes	Interventions	Rationale	Evaluation
Short term 1. Will differentiate external reality from internal process *within 12 hours.* 2. Will exhibit appropriate affect *within 12 hours.* 3. Will verbalize an understanding of effects of drug abuse on personality organization *within 7 days.*	• Orient client to unit • Acknowledge client's internal processes • Administer as needed medication • Provide symptom management following drug use • Use NIC drug withdrawal interventions protocol • Observe for adverse reactions to withdrawal protocol (see Box 27-8)	• Important to reenforce reality and nature of client's setting • Biological means can be used to increase cognitive organization and prevent adverse reactions to withdrawal	**Short term** 1. Met in 3 hours. 2. Not met. Drug effect persists. Continue supportive listening and reality orientation. 3. Not met. Client continues to exhibit resistance. Unwilling to participate in problem planning at present. Reassess plan.
Long term 1. Will accept that psychoactive drugs aggravate personality disorder. 2. Will seek healthy alternatives to cope with feelings.	• Acknowledge client's laughter, but do not respond • Acknowledge that laughter is not about a shared reality • Facilitate interaction when client has difficulty with communication • Assist client to identify the problem or situation that causes distress • Require client to attend problem-solving group next day • Discourage decision making when client is under influence of drug • Support self-acceptance • Encourage client to evaluate behavior • Provide factual information regarding diagnosis and treatment • Assist client with developing healthy modes of coping such as relaxation techniques • Appraise and discuss with client alternative responses • Encourage client's gradual mastery of uncomfortable feeling states	• Responsive communication and active listening validates appropriate affect. • Group attendance will educate client on how drug use impairs problem-solving skills. • It is necessary that client is able to fully attend to information obtained in group. • Acceptance, encouragement, and reinforcement of links between behavior and comfort states lessens denial. • Relaxation and other coping techniques are healthy alternative behaviors to drug use. • Knowledge of and mastery of feelings are behavioral relapse prevention strategies.	**Long-term** 1. Not met. Client continues to test limits. Reinforce limit setting. 2. Not met. Client refuses participation in coping strategies session. Reassess plan.

::::: INTERDISCIPLINARY TREATMENT PLAN

Critical Pathway: Substance Abuse

Initiation: _____   Substance Abuse

Date: _____   Diagnosis: _____

DRG#: _____

AVG LOS: <u>7, 14 Days</u>

ACTUAL LOS: _____

	Day 1	Day 2-5	Day 6-12 (14 Day CP only)	DAY 6-7 (7 Day) Day 13-14 (14 Day)
Medical Interventions	PA Intro, H&P, MSE, Review old records. Order Approp. Protocol, Diet, Act. level. Order other meds/tests/consults as indic. Educate re: detox process. Initiate TX plan.	Address medical complications. Review labs, tests, consults. Complete TX plan. Evaluate Dx/condition. Order/adjust meds as needed. Monitor detox progress. Psych Eval if indicated.	Continue w/med mgmt. & eval. ID med w/aftercare needs & refer as needed. Consent form & educate re: Antabuse or HIV test, if indicated. Educate re: disease aspects. Review/update TX plan. Cont. Psych Eval if indicated.	Complete medical, psych aftercare plan, D/C summaries to referring MD, Clinics, Med. D/C Summary. D/C instruction plan. D/C order. Prescriptions.
Nursing Interventions	PN Intro. Nsg. Assess MSE, check family/SO involvmt. Initiate approp., protocol,TX plan. Seizure/fall prec. if indic. Monitor/enc. po intake, assist w/ ADL's PRN, wt., UA for drug screen. Orient pt to unit/prog. & Pt. "buddy". Protocol/detox education, ID other Educ. needs. ID D/C Planning. Risk Factors. Manage pts. off unit w/staff.	Continue w/protocol.Assess/assist involvmt. In milieu & Family/SO visits. Monitor sleep, appetite, mental status, Update TX plan. Assist ADL's PRN. UA on @2nd Day, PN session w/PL. Give recovery assignment(s) w/AT. Educate pt/family re: disease, meds, coping. Manage pts. off unit w/staff.	Assess/assist involvmt in milieu.Assess family/SO visits. MSE. Review/Update TX plan/aftercare plan.VS qd. PN session. Review assignment(s) w/pt. & AT. Off unit w/staff. Continue w/ education days 2-5. Manage pts. off unit w/staff.	Nsg D/C summary. Review Nsg TX goals VS qd. Review D/C plans & assess understanding of education (day 2-13). Call PP/FH for pt. transfer report, if indicated. PN/Pt termination session. Manage pts. off unit w/staff.
Social Work Interventions	Social Work Introduction; emergency intervention PRN.	D/C Plan/Aftercare consultation PRN. ID D/C Risk factors. Assist w/ psycho-social complications. TX plan.	Counseling w/ family/SO PRN. Community referrals as indic. Family educ. Review/update TX plan.	Finalize referral/aftercare process. SW D/C summary.
Addiction Therapist	AT Introduction; Emergency Intervention PRN.	Counseling session. Complete Psycho-social & coord. completion of TX plan w/in 72 hrs.Initiate & coord. F/U plan. Early Recovery Educ. Give Recovery Assignment(s) w/PN.	Review/Update TX plan. Refer for aftercare. Continue counseling. Continue w/ education (day 2-5) Review assignment(s) w/ pt. & PN.	Addiction Therapist D/C Summary. Counseling session to terminate therapy. Complete/review/document aftercare plan.
Psychology Interventions	Conduct cognitive & Beh. Eval. PRN.; Emergency Intervention PRN.	Provide consult. to TX team in Psychol/Beh. aspects of TX plan.	Admin. Psych testing if indic. Review findings w/pt. & team. Rev/update TX plan.	Make recommended re: continued psychological assess. & intervention following D/C.
Key Patient Outcomes	Pt. will begin to safely detox from Substance(s) w/in protocol parameters.	Pt. will safely detox from Substance(s) (w/in 3-5 days)	Pt. will partic. in 100% of classes/grps @ _____. Pt. will practice coping skills @ _____. Pt. will ID relapse triggers @ _____. Pt. will sleep .5 hrs/night @ _____. Pt. will positively contribute w/in milieu. @ _____.	Pt. will ID plan to cope w/ relapse triggers @ _____. Pt. will verbalize understanding of disease process & meds, if indicated @ _____. Pt. will state F/U plan @ _____. Pt. will ID one present feeling re: current situation @ _____.

Key: *7 day CP Circle = Variance; Date = Progress Note re: specific evaluation/intervention/goal. (Variances are included on the second page of the pathway, which is not shown.)*
PsychPaths™ © 1994 Strategic Clinical Systems, Granbury, Texas.

The Nursing Process

Implementation

Intervention with clients to prevent the onset of substance-related disorders and to treat early, middle, and late stages of substance-use problems include counseling, milieu management, self-care, psychobiological strategies, health teaching, case management, health promotion, and health maintenance. Nurses working with clients with substance-related disorders follow the *Standards of Addictions Nursing Practice*.

Counseling

Counseling provides clients who have substance-related disorders reality-oriented support with problem solving, decision making, and emotional and psychological functioning as they learn to cope without the use of psychoactive drugs.

Individual counseling strategies

Psychotherapy cannot be effective if judgment and cognition are impaired by drug effects. Therefore it is not initiated until the client is sober and drug-free. The length of time needed is determined by the amount of drug the individual has been consuming and the frequency of consumption. The individual who has been consuming at least 1 pint of distilled spirits daily for several months, for example, requires a period of abstinence sufficient to clear the brain of residual alcohol.

A contract to cease or decrease drug use should then be made between the client and nurse. Accepting a contract, even though the client may "lapse" or "slip," is an indicator of the client's desire to terminate and control drug use. Counseling focuses on dysfunctional behaviors.

Denial is the hallmark symptom of individuals who are addicted. Individuals often need help in accepting the existence of a problem and letting go of the denial that the behavior or substance use causes problems in interpersonal relations, work, or other areas of life. Because denial of the negative consequences of substance abuse is so strong, building motivation is an important outcome for early intervention.

One means of increasing motivation and decreasing denial is the *formal "intervention." Family members, employers, friends, and colleagues who have been affected by the client's substance use make lists of how the client's substance use has impacted their lives. These are presented to the client with the guidance of an experienced addiction counselor.* When clients recognize the impact of their substance use on others, they become motivated to engage in treatment.

It is important that the nurse not confront the client's denial directly, but listen to the client carefully and with respect. The nurse should then point out discrepancies in the client's statements or observed contradictions in reports, or the reality of certain events (e.g., "You tell me that your cocaine use was not interfering with your work, and yet you mentioned yesterday that you had been laid off.").

As the client discusses symptoms and/or signs of abuse or dependence, the nurse labels the behaviors with terms that describe the symptom, such as "unsuccessful efforts at cutting back" and "lack of control over intake." With other members of the team with whom the client has contact, the nurse makes plans that address the connections between drug use or abuse and the client's problems in current or past life circumstances. This might include discussions that link health problems with drug use. For example, compromised respirations are linked to chain smoking, or liver disease is linked to excessive alcohol use.

Counseling efforts address other dysfunctional behaviors associated with abuse and dependence. These behaviors include manipulation, impulsiveness, avoidance, grandiosity, and anger.

Manipulation is getting one's needs met at the expense of another person. Insensitivity to others comes from insensitivity to oneself as a person. Therapeutic responses to clients who manipulate include the following:

- Treat clients with dignity and respect
- Use assertive communication
- Hold firmly to reasonable limits
- Expect that all rules apply to all clients with consistent consequences

Ultimately, manipulative patterns subside as clients begin to recognize themselves as persons worthy of dignity and respect. They no longer have to "steal" time, energy, or attention. They can ask directly for what they need.

Impulsiveness is a tendency to act suddenly without thought or conscious decision making. Impulsiveness is a method of discharging the discomfort of anxiety before actually experiencing it. Therapeutic responses to impulsiveness include the following:

- Respond to demands by delaying the response for a reasonable time
- Expect the client to explain the thinking behind the act or demand
- Treat impulsive acts with grave concern for their consequences
- Expect clients who have made impulsive decisions to seek feedback from their peer groups, family members, and staff and to objectively weigh that feedback

The Nursing Process

Avoidance *is a pattern of escaping from others through physical and emotional distancing.* Avoidance of relationships is common for newly recovering persons. They do not have well-developed social skills and have often spent years during which relationships were modified by substances instead of respect, self-disclosure, honesty, and intimacy. Self-disclosure is frightening to those clients, because the self has been systematically destroyed by substances. Learning who one is and developing one's values and beliefs, likes and dislikes must occur before one has a self to give to another in an intimate way.

Avoiding feelings also occurs, because feelings have not been acknowledged and the skills needed to respond to feelings have not been developed. There is often the irrational belief that one has to do something about feelings—one's own as well as others'. Therapeutic responses to avoidance include the following:

- Invite clients to join in safe activities such as board games or team endeavors
- Ask experienced clients to model for newly diagnosed clients the process of acknowledging feelings and tolerating the internal pain
- Clarify the boundaries of the therapeutic relationship between client and nurse and adhere to those boundaries at all times, even beyond treatment

Grandiosity *is the irrational thought that one is entitled to special treatment and that everyone should know of the entitlement.* Members of Twelve-Step groups call this characteristic "terminal uniqueness." They tend to tease and chide one another humorously about believing they are the only ones who ever experienced the worst, the best, or the only anything. Therapeutic responses to grandiose behavior include the following:

- Help client identify the similarities between self and others
- Empathize with the feelings of fear and inferiority
- Reflect feelings when the client acts or talks in a grandiose manner
- Tell clients that recovery depends on honest feedback from peers and that it is in their best interest to develop positive relationships

Anger is a common emotional response in persons with substance dependence who are beginning the recovery process. Persons with substance-related disorders are angry about many things: having the disease, the consequences of the disease, having to give up the chemical and all it did for them, having to start life over, wasted time, lost relationships, poor judgment, and the experiences they had when they used the substance.

For clients with substance-related disorders, learning to own and experience anger internally is fundamental to dealing with anger in a healthy way. Putting one's body response and thoughts into words, deciding what one can control, and acting only after due deliberation are lifetime processes for those who have an ingrained dysfunctional response to anger. Therapeutic responses to dysfunctional anger include the following:

- Set limits on verbal and physical abuse.
- Suggest that clients find a quiet place and take time-out if they think they might lose control of their behavior.
- Ask clients to describe how they are feeling inside ("I feel hot in my face, and the shirt is itching on my forearms." "I have a huge knot the size of a fist and hard as a rock on my left side.")
- Process the events that preceded the anger to gain insight into the cause of the anger.
- Help clients distance from other persons' actions, words, and feelings and not be affected by them.

Family counseling

Family counseling focuses on the effects of drinking or drug use on the family system. Stopping substance abuse, defining the nature and boundaries of the family system, stabilizing the family, and assisting with the development of new coping skills are primary goals of family treatment when drugs have been a central organizing principle for the family. Education about drugs and their effects on personal functioning and relationships serves to enlighten family members about the implications of drug use and may prevent the development of later problems.

Efforts to address dysfunctional family patterns or negative environmental influences should be part of the plan of care. Examples of this include substance abuse by family members other than the identified client, patterns of interaction that include inflexible and inappropriate roles, and problems of domestic violence and sexual abuse.

Family traditions or transgenerational patterns may reinforce the very behaviors that the substance abuser must change. Unless family behaviors are addressed, it is unlikely that the client alone can disengage from the dysfunctional traditions of the family system.

Support groups

There are many groups modeled on the Twelve-Step approach of AA to support clients with substance-related disorders and their families. Table 27-7 lists several self-help groups, the populations they serve, and the purposes of each. Many anonymous groups have a strong spiritual component and require that clients acknowl-

The Nursing Process

TABLE 27-7

Self-help groups

GROUP	POPULATION SERVED	PURPOSE
Alcoholics Anonymous (AA) 475 Riverside Drive New York, NY 10163 (212) 870-3400	Individuals who desire to stop drinking	AA is a voluntary anonymous worldwide fellowship. Members seek sobriety, freedom from alcohol through the practice of the Twelve Steps, and the development of a drugfree lifestyle.
Narcotics Anonymous (NA) P.O. Box 9999 Van Nuys, CA 91409 (818) 780-3951	Individuals who desire to refrain from the use of narcotics	NA is a voluntary anonymous fellowship. Members seek a drugfree lifestyle through the practice of the Twelve Steps, including insights into personal, spiritual, and social concerns.
Al-Anon P.O. Box 862, Midtown Station New York, NY 10018 (212) 302-7240	Friends and relatives of individuals with drinking problems	Through a Twelve-Step fellowship, relatives and friends work toward a sense of distance, objectivity, and personal sanity as they deal with those who have drinking problems.
Nar Anon P.O. Box 2562 Palos Verdes, CA 90274 (213) 547-5800	Friends and relatives of individuals who are addicted to narcotics	To recover from behaviors associated with drug addiction. Goals include self-care, self-development, spiritual growth, and detachment from the person who is addicted.
Ala Teen P.O. Box 862, Midtown Station New York, NY 10018 (212) 302-7240	Adolescents and young persons whose lives have been affected by the addiction of someone close to them	Develop perspectives on personal life, self-related responsibilities, and a spiritual and emotional cognitive being.
Children of Alcoholic Parents (CAPs) 1225 E. 11 Mile Rd. Royal Oak, MI 48067 (810) 541-4013	Adult children of alcoholics and otherwise dysfunctional families	Gain insight into personal behaviors developed in response to life with a dysfunctional parent/family.
Families Anonymous P.O. Box 3475 Culver City, CA 90231-3475 (310) 313-5800	For persons whose lives have been affected by the use of mind-altering substances and related behavior of a relative or friend.	Gain insight into personal behavior and an understanding of addiction.
Gamblers Anonymous P.O. Box 17173 Los Angeles, CA 90010 (213) 386-8789	Compulsive gamblers	This is a voluntary, anonymous fellowship in which members seek recovery from compulsive, repetitive behaviors in games of chance.
Smokenders 4455 E. Camelback Rd. Ste. D-155 Phoenix, AZ 85018 (602) 840-7414	Individuals wishing to stop smoking	A structured support group that helps individuals stop or reduce smoking habits.

The Nursing Process

Box 27-7

The Twelve Steps of Alcoholics Anonymous

1. We admitted we were powerless over alcohol—that our lives have become unmanageable.
2. Came to believe that a Power greater than ourselves could restore us to sanity.
3. Made a decision to turn our will and our lives over to the care of God as we understood Him.
4. Made a searching and fearless moral inventory of ourselves.
5. Admitted to God, to ourselves, and to another human being the exact nature of our wrongs.
6. Were entirely ready to have God remove all these defects of character.
7. Humbly asked Him to remove our shortcomings.

8. Made a list of all persons we had harmed and became willing to make amends to them all.
9. Made direct amends to such people wherever possible, except when to do so would injure them or others.
10. Continued to take personal inventory, and when we were wrong promptly admitted it.
11. Sought through prayer and meditation to improve our conscious contact with God as we understood Him, praying only for our knowledge of His will for us and the power to carry that out.
12. Having had a spiritual awakening as the result of these steps, we tried to carry this message to alcoholics and to practice these principles in all our affairs.

NOTE: *The Twelve Steps are reprinted with permission of Alcoholics Anonymous World Services, Inc. Permission to reprint this material does not mean that AA has reviewed or approved the contents of this publication. AA is a program of recovery from alcoholism only— use of the Twelve Steps in connection with programs and activities that are patterned after AA, but that address other problems, does not imply otherwise.*

edge that they are powerless, their lives are unmanageable, and they have a need for God, however they have come to know Him. Box 27-7 lists the Twelve Steps of AA.

Milieu Therapy

Substance abuse treatment takes place in a variety of settings. Acute inpatient treatment takes place in specialized detoxification units, in a general hospital for medical problems or withdrawal symptoms, at long-term rehabilitation centers, or in therapeutic communities. Table 27-8 lists selected settings for care, describes them, and gives the purposes of each.

A therapeutic milieu for clients with substance abuse problems is similar to a therapeutic milieu of a psychiatric setting. Safety is a key priority, including the safety provided by skilled nurses when clients experience withdrawal or other conditions and are in uncomfortable physical states. Similarly, expectations about the management of antisocial, self-destructive, and aggressive behavior must be clear. The milieu is "therapeutic" inasmuch as it provides opportunities for "corrective experiences" in social interaction and encourages learning how to manage feelings. For individuals with substance-related disorders, this means learning to tolerate frustrations and the intense craving for the drug in ways that are constructive and ultimately prevent retreat into an intoxicated state.

Self-Care Activities

Self-care is an important component in preventing the development of substance abuse problems, achieving successful initiation and completion of treatment, and preventing relapse. For most individuals who have been diagnosed with abuse or dependence, any drug use initiates a rapid return to addiction.

Recovery requires that clients address old, drug-dependent coping mechanisms and old feelings of discomfort that supported their drug use. Relapse prevention enables the individual to see life circumstances, feelings, and negative relationships as manageable without the use of drugs. Relapse prevention includes the anticipation and discussion of social, environmental, and family patterns that evoke a desire to engage in the process addiction or to use a substance. Repeated "rehearsal" of ways to address anticipated situations can counteract some of the negative feelings that support a return to dysfunctional behavior.

One easy and common reminder of risk is the term *HALT.* HALT refers to the universally understood conditions of **h**unger, **a**nger, **l**oneliness, and **t**iredness, states that often trigger the temptation to get a "quick fix" with food, sex, alcohol, or some other drug to feel better. Clients are taught self-care to avoid these conditions. Social support, manifested in encouragement, listening, love, and companionship of family, friends, and colleagues, decreases loneliness, provides positive feedback, and affirms that one is a likeable, worthy person.

The Nursing Process

TABLE 27-8

Treatment settings

SETTING	DESCRIPTION	PURPOSE
Inpatient hospitalization	A 2-to-4–week hospitalization in a unit of a general hospital, residential treatment center, or psychiatric hospital; milieu provides "corrective" emotional experiences	Provides safety; restricts access to the drug; provides monitoring of self-destructive behaviors
Detoxification	Supervised medical regimen to withdraw the client from drugs that have induced psychological and physiological dependence	Monitoring negative psychological and physiological effects of drug withdrawal by gradually decreasing medication ingested and treating responses
Rehabilitation	Long-term hospitals that address all phases of treatment; halfway houses that provide a sheltered and emotionally and financially supportive environment with peers	Provide transition from highly structured medically modeled settings to independent community life and outpatient treatment with support of Twelve-Step programs; vocational counseling is key to return to work
Therapeutic community	Group living situations based on hierarchical community structure and governance; heavy use of psycho-education, peer group influence, disciplined drug-free lifestyles; examples include Phoenix House, Day Top Village	Assist individual in self-examination, behavioral change, and social adjustment without use of drugs

Nurses, like their clients, need to focus on caring for themselves. Because of demanding academic and professional lives, and the altruistic tradition of nursing, nurses and nursing students often place the needs of others before their own, to their own detriment. Research suggests that nurses recovering from substance abuse and psychiatric illness are at risk for insufficient development of self-care activities. For example, Hutchinson (1988), in her work on recovering nurses, indicates that one's own identity is replaced by the professional role. The nurse as a *person* is overshadowed by the nurse as a *professional.* This interferes with the nurse's development and maintenance of recreational activities, appropriate exercise regimens, social life, and family obligations.

Some nurses attempt to relieve their professional stress by using alcohol and other drugs, which leads to abuse and dependence. Similarly, while there is much evidence on the detrimental effects of smoking on health, nurses continue to be the largest group of smokers among health care providers. Physicians, attorneys, and others for whom professional identity leads to the neglect of personal physical and mental health needs are equally vulnerable.

The support of colleagues (peer support) is a key element to the recovery of health care professionals who have substance abuse and mental disorders. State and na-

tional nursing associations, for example, have organized "help lines" to respond to family and individual inquiries, offer peer counseling, and make referrals for nurses who are concerned about their drug use and/or mental health or who have been treated for such problems. In the workplace, employee assistance programs also provide brief counseling and referral in a confidential manner.

Skill-development teaching is an important component of self-care development. Deficits in life skills are thought to contribute to drug abuse vulnerability. Among the skills that may be developed are vocational/employment, job search strategies, social skills, assertiveness training, and relaxation/stress management strategies.

Psychobiological Interventions

Pharmacological intervention

Pharmacological interventions for the treatment of substance-related disorders are limited at the present time. However, as the biochemical functions involved in abuse and dependence are more clearly understood, effective treatments should develop. Table 27-9 lists commonly used pharmacological treatment approaches. Medication tips related to drugs used in the treatment of abuse and dependence are listed in the box on p. 537.

The Nursing Process

TABLE 27-9

Pharmacological interventions

INTERVENTION	DEFINITION
Agonist substitution	Treatment with a medication that has pharmacological actions similar to the abused drug; methadone treatment of heroin addiction and nicotine chewing gum treatment of tobacco dependence are examples
Maintenance	Chronic treatment at a stabilized dosage; methadone maintenance is an example
Detoxification	Short-term treatment with progressively decreasing dosages to suppress withdrawal signs and symptoms following cessation of drug of abuse
Antagonist treatment	Treatment with a medication that blocks the pharmacological effects of abused substance (e.g., naltrexone HCl [ReVia]; naloxone [Narcan])
Symptomatic treatment	Treatment with a medication whose pharmacological mechanism of action is not related to that of the abused drug but whose effects might alter some of the symptoms of drug abuse, i.e., benzodiazapine, hypnotic/tranquilizer
Aversion treatment	Use of a pharmacological agent to deter craving; use of antabuse for drinking is an example

 MEDICATION TIPS

Methadone

- The standard dosage of Methadone may have to be adjusted to reach optimal effect.
- Methadone should never be stopped suddenly; the dose must be tapered downward.
- Combining other psychiatric medications with Methadone should be done only with close monitoring.
- Combining alcohol, illicit drugs, and Methadone can produce adverse and possibly life-threatening responses.

Nicotine Transdermal Patches (Habitrol, Nicoderm, Prostep)

- Patches combined with community programs such as "Smokenders" and support groups such as Nicotine Anonymous are most effective.
- "Triggers" (feelings, situations, stressful events) that increase craving need to be identified.
- A program of diet and exercise initiated in early abstinence and while on the patch can deter weight gain.

Disulfiram (Antabuse)

- The client must be committed to abstinence; otherwise daily ingestion of the drug will compromise well-being.
- Alcohol must not be used in food preparation.
- Products that contain alcohol, such as mouthwash and over-the-counter medications, must be avoided.
- If alcohol is consumed after taking Antabuse, the client must seek medical consultation immediately.

Naltrexone HCL (ReVia)

- ReVia must never be combined with opioids.
- ReVia is contraindicated for clients with liver disease.
- The client must be drugfree for 7 to 10 days before administration.
- The client should participate in supportive treatment while taking the drug.
- The client should report withdrawal-like or hepatic symptoms immediately and stop taking the drug.

Disulfiram (Antabuse) has traditionally been used as a form of aversive treatment. Taken orally in doses of 250 mg to 500 mg., it blocks the oxidation of alcohol at the acetaldehyde stage and results in a highly unpleasant reaction to the beverage. Because this reaction can include hypotension, nausea, and vomiting, clients are carefully screened and should be committed to not ingesting alcohol. Informed consent is required.

Agonist substitution, that is the use of a medication with pharmacological effects similar to the drug of dependence, is also used. This approach includes the use of benzodiazepines in medically supervised withdrawal

The Nursing Process

from alcohol, the use of nicotine (Nicoderm or Habitrol) patches for individuals trying to stop smoking, and the use of nicotine (Nicorette) gum.

Methadone maintenance is a type of agonist substitution. The use of methadone (Dolophine), usually in a maintenance dose of around 75 mg., is based on the premise that certain individuals no longer produce sufficient endorphins for a feeling of well-being, resulting in drug-seeking behavior and its inappropriate mental, social, and legal consequences. Methadone "normalizes" the chemical state of these individuals, who are then more responsive to counseling, vocational training, and the development of lifestyles that are more productive and socially gratifying. Methadone maintenance programs are increasingly focused on concomitant provision of supportive counseling, group work, Twelve-Step programs, and access to comprehensive health care.

On recovery from drug dependence, clients may manifest symptoms separate from the psychoactive effects of the drug of addiction and require symptomatic treatment. Some common examples of this are the onset of depression following treatment for cocaine dependence and the appearance of anxiety reactions in clients treated for alcoholism. Carefully monitored use of antidepressant and anxiolytic drugs may be warranted.

Antagonist treatment refers to the use of medication that blocks the pharmacological effects of the abused drug. The most common antagonist is naltrexone HCl (ReVia), an opioid reception antagonist that works by blocking both craving and the pleasure of getting high. It has been used in the past to treat meperidine (Demerol) dependence and to counteract the effects of heroin and other opioid substances, and more recently to treat alcohol dependence. Clients must not have used opioids within the past 7 to 10 days. A naloxone HCl (Narcan) challenge test should be negative before treatment, and urine screening should be used to verify absence of opioids. The drug should not be given until the client is free of withdrawal symptoms. Naltrexone HCl is an adjunct to treatment and should only be prescribed to clients in recovery, relapse prevention, or Twelve-Step programs.

Withdrawal protocols

Withdrawal occurs when an individual who has become physiologically dependent on alcohol and/or other drugs stops using the drug. Detoxification and withdrawal are potentially life-threatening and require careful biophysiological monitoring. The withdrawal protocol and the duration of the process are dependent on the type and amount of drug. A careful history of daily use should be obtained and verified. Drugs whose actions are similar to the drug of dependence are used in progressively decreasing doses. For alcohol withdrawal, benzodiazepines

---

Box 27-8

Substance Use Treatment

Alcohol Withdrawal

DEFINITION

Care of the patient experiencing sudden cessation of alcohol consumption

ACTIVITIES

Withdraw the drug gradually during detoxification
Create a low-stimulation environment for detoxification
Monitor vital signs during withdrawal
Monitor for delirium tremens
Administer anticonvulsants or sedatives, as appropriate
Medicate to relieve physical discomfort, as needed
Approach abusive patient behavior in a neutral manner
Address hallucinations in a therapeutic manner
Maintain adequate nutrition and fluid intake
Administer vitamin therapy, as appropriate
Monitor for covert alcohol consumption during detoxification
Listen to patient's concerns about alcohol withdrawal
Provide emotional support to patient/family, as appropriate
Provide verbal reassurance, as appropriate
Provide reality orientation, as appropriate
Reassure patient that depression and fatigue commonly occur during withdrawal

Reprinted with permission from McCloskey, J.C., & Bulechek, G.M. (1996). Nursing interventions classification (NIC), *(2nd ed.), St. Louis: Mosby.*

---

such as diazepam (Valium) in doses decreasing from 20 to 30 mg daily are used. Box 27-8 lists nursing interventions for a client in alcohol withdrawal. Box 27-9 lists care for a client experiencing drug detoxification.

Health Teaching

Health teaching involves using substance-related facts and research findings to educate individuals, families, and communities. Health teaching facilitates clients' understanding of health and the relationship of substance use to health maintenance.

Health teaching is an important part of treatment. Education begins once withdrawal from the substance is complete and the client is cognitively able to process information. Preventive education includes disseminating information to young schoolchildren, adolescents, and parents about drug and alcohol use. High-risk populations such as pregnant women and the elderly should

The Nursing Process

Box 27-9

Substance Use Treatment

Drug Withdrawal

DEFINITION

Care of a patient experiencing drug detoxification

ACTIVITIES

Provide symptom management during the detoxification period

Determine history of substance use

Discuss with patient the role that drugs play in his/her life

Assist the patient to recognize that drugs provide a sense of assertiveness, heightened self-esteem, and frustration tolerance

Assist the patient to identify other means of relieving frustrations and increasing self-esteem

Monitor for paranoia and hesitancy to trust others during the detoxification period

Encourage self-disclosure

Monitor for body image distortions and anorexia

Provide adequate nutrition

Monitor for hypertension and tachycardia

Monitor for depression and/or suicidal tendencies

Medicate to relieve symptoms during withdrawal, as appropriate

Encourage exercise to stimulate the release of endorphins

Encourage involvement in a support group such as Narcotics Anonymous

Facilitate family support

Reprinted with permission from McCloskey, J.C., & Bulechek, G.M. (1996). Nursing interventions classification (NIC), *(2nd ed.) St. Louis: Mosby.*

Box 27-10

Federal Educational, Research, and Service Resources

National Clearinghouse for Alcohol and Drug Information (NCADI)
P.O. Box 2345
Rockville, MD 20847-2345
(800)729-6686

Center for Substance Abuse Prevention (CSAP)
5600 Fishers Lane
Rockwall II, Room 9D 10
Rockville, MD 20857
(301)443-0365

Center for Substance Abuse Treatment (CSAT)
5600 Fishers Lane
RW II, Suite 618
Rockville, MD 20857
(301)443-2467

National Institute of Alcohol Abuse and Alcoholism (NIAAA)
Willco Building, Suite 409
6000 Executive Blvd.
Bethesda, MD 20892-7003
(301)443-3860

National Institute for Drug Abuse (NIDA)
5600 Fishers Lane
Rockville, MD 20857
(301)443-1124

also be targeted. Content should include information about the health implications of drinking alcohol and using OTC, illicit, and prescription drugs. It should also contain facts and figures supported by research findings. Factors that predispose individuals to the development of drug-related problems, such as a family history of drug and alcohol dependence and family traditions of heavy consumption, should also be included when educating children, adolescents, and adults. Findings related to disease, such as the development of cancers of the head and neck in persons who smoke pipes and persons who use smokeless tobacco, the prevalence of lung cancer in persons who smoke, and problems related to drinking and driving, are supported by research and should be included in public health education. Similarly, information

to support abstinence by pregnant women should be incorporated into routine health care; but most certainly it needs to be part of health teaching for clients in recovery. Such links between drug use and potential consequences should be in a matter-of-fact, nonthreatening manner, and clients should be assisted to make their own decisions about drug use. Box 27-10 lists federal agencies that are funded to provide information that assists nurses in their role as health educators. Teaching Points that can be shared with a client who is diagnosed with marijuana abuse are listed on p. 540.

Case Management

Case management of clients with substance-related disorders is a complex process that should involve not only the client but also family and significant others, employers, and legal authorities. Case management begins in the hospital with detoxification and early intervention. Services needed by clients with substance-related disorders

The Nursing Process

TEACHING POINTS

Client With a Diagnosis of Marijuana Abuse

The nurse should teach the client, family, and/or significant others the following:

- Persons who become psychologically dependent on one drug are predisposed to dependence on other drugs and alcohol.
- Once an intention to recover is made, there are often "slips" or returns to use in the early weeks of recovery.
- Persons trying to recover from drug use are most vulnerable to "slips" when they are around persons and places and experience feelings and events linked with previous drug use. The recovering person needs the support of family and friends to make new associations and develop new leisure activities.
- Persons have the most success in recovery when involved in self-help groups. These groups offer members who are

learning to recover the opportunity to share experiences, provide tips on dealing with uncomfortable feelings, and provide emotional support, 24 hours per day.
- Others involved with the individual who is abusing drugs need to guard against making that person's recovery the focus of their relationship. Do not try to control the individual's access to or use of a drug. Responsibility for recovery must be assumed by the individual who is abusing drugs.
- Persons often have to attempt recovery several times before a drug-free life is firmly in place or drug use is no longer a prominent part of their lives. Renewed efforts should never be demeaned or discouraged.

Box 27-11

Substance Use Prevention

DEFINITION

Prevention of an alcoholic or drug use lifestyle

ACTIVITIES

Assist patient to tolerate increased levels of stress, as appropriate

Prepare patient for difficult or painful events

Reduce irritating or frustrating environmental stress

Reduce social isolation, as appropriate

Support measures to regulate the sale and distribution of alcohol to minors

Lobby for increased drinking age

Recommend responsible changes in the alcohol and drug curricula for primary grades

Conduct programs in schools on the avoidance of drugs and alcohol as recreational activities

Encourage responsible decision making about lifestyle choices

Recommend media campaigns on substance use issues in the community

Instruct parents in the importance of example in substance use

Instruct parents and teachers in the identification of signs and symptoms of addiction

Assist patient to identify substitute tension-reducing strategies

Support or organize community groups to reduce injuries associated with alcohol, such as SADD and MADD

Survey students in grades 1 to 12 on the use of alcohol and drugs and alcohol-related behaviors

Instruct parents to support school policy that prohibits drug and alcohol consumption at extracurricular activities

Assist in the organization of post-activities for teenagers for such functions as prom and homecoming

Facilitate coordination of efforts between various community groups concerned with substance use

Reprinted with permission from McCloskey, J.C., & Bulechek, G.M. (1996). Nursing interventions classification (NIC), *(2nd ed.). St. Louis: Mosby.*

---

include medical care, counseling, peer support, self-help group support, behavioral reconditioning, skill and vocational development such as job-finding skills, social skills, assertiveness skills, stress management skills, and other types of long-term treatment.

Because dependence is a chronic illness, services should be linked to stages of recovery. The client's financial resources and the current health care climate, which limits insurance coverage for clients who are addicted and dependent on drugs, should be considered.

The Nursing Process

THE CONSUMER'S VOICE

Substance-Related Disorder: Dual Diagnoses

Michael Lonergan

I am a 32-year-old man. During much of my life I have experienced a great deal of turmoil. At age 20 I was diagnosed with general psychosis and substance abuse. My first experience with psychiatric nurses was in an emergency room. I came in high on opium, intoxicated with whiskey, and psychotic as hell. My family was present but unaware of my needs. The nurses and doctors quickly sedated me and treated my presentation and psychosis with perphanazine (Trilafon).

Did my family and professionals know who I really was? Did they treat my disorder with my consent and involve me in my treatment? What about my addiction? These issues were not adequately addressed. As a result, the last 12 years have been filled with quite interesting experiences. I feel I have just recently come into my own; by this I mean I have gained responsibility for myself and left a world in which I was reacted to and treated with medications and therapy in response to my presentation.

Most of my experience with psychiatric nurses has been in emergency rooms, hospitals, and partial hospital settings. I was treated by professionals for my mental health issues but not my substance abuse. Looking back I wish I had been detoxed from my substance abuse prior to receiving treatment for my psychosis and mental illness. I might then have escaped some of my experiences as a mental health client, such as coping with a disability, living in poverty, and being treated as incompetent when viewed according to my behaviors and not who I was.

The most stigmatizing and discriminating experience I had was constantly being informed by professionals that I shouldn't do too much because I might get sick again. Surprisingly, my refuge came from my affiliation with Alcoholics Anonymous. I lived the Twelve Steps of AA and endured the mental health world. It was the persons in AA who encouraged me to go on with my life, become educated, become employable, and be involved in all of my affairs.

I initially survived the discrepancies between my mental health treatment and Twelve-Step affiliation, because I was able to separate the two. Professionals helped me separate AA from mental illness, because my treatment was separate. At the time I felt this separation was a good thing, but looking back I could have used support and the opportunity to integrate both issues to help me connect a little bit easier than I did.

Today I have a masters degree in mental health administration and work for the state of Connecticut as a Coordinator of Consumer Services in a Department of Mental Health and Addiction Services district office. I want to share with psychiatric nurses that I personally recognize the validity of their profession and its necessity in the treatment of substance-related disorders. They can help me and others with substance-related disorders by doing the following:

- Detoxing a substance abuse client before psychiatric treatment begins
- Emphasizing and supporting the development of natural supports and community integration for a substance-related disorder
- Always encouraging the person to go on with life, once stable

Health Promotion and Health Maintenance

Psychiatric-mental health nurses employ strategies and interventions to promote and maintain mental health and prevent mental illness (ANA, 1994). The prevalence of substance abuse and dependence disorders suggests the need for nurses to become involved in activities aimed at preventing illicit use or misuse of substances. Box 27-11 lists nursing interventions aimed at preventing substance use.

Individuals who show early signs of developing drug use problems, that is *"hazardous" drinking* (consumption of 14 drinks per week or 5 drinks on each occasion) need to be counseled about the risks of excessive drinking patterns (Saunders et al., 1993). Giving feedback to clients that links alcohol consumption with health or the interpretation of test findings such as an elevated GGT indicating liver damage can motivate the client to decrease the amount of alcohol consumed.

The Nursing Process

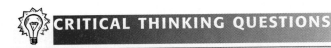

CRITICAL THINKING QUESTIONS

Alice G. was referred to the emergency department by her general practitioner who has been treating her excessive weight gain with Preludin. Ms. G., 35 years old, is 5'3" and weighs 170 lbs. She has no history of psychiatric illness. As the nurse gathers data for a brief history, she notes that Ms. G. is poorly groomed, is diaphoretic, and has elevated blood pressure and dilated pupils. She keeps asking to be excused to urinate. When the nurse requests that she try to sit still to finish the interview, Ms. G. responds irritably, "Why are you trying to make this more difficult for me? Can't you see that I am a nervous person?" She then becomes apologetic and tearful and states, "I am just so afraid of this place."

1. How might the nurse feel about this client?
2. How do attitudes about medications and drugs influence your assessment of clients?
3. What are common attitudes about obese women?
4. What are common attitudes about the need and ability for clients to control their use of substances?
5. What nursing interventions would be most effective in increasing the client's physical comfort and reassuring her about the safety of the treatment setting?
6. What tests should be performed to determine Ms. G.'s level of substance use?
7. What are the outcomes of Preludin overdose?
8. What medications should be given to counteract behavioral agitation in response to Ms. G.'s symptoms?
9. What referrals should be planned for Ms. G. following hospitalization?

Many health care professionals believe that recovering from dependence and compulsive dysfunctional behaviors is a lifelong process and is best supported by Twelve-Step self-help groups that provide peer fellowship aimed at maintaining abstinence.

Substance abuse and dependence takes its toll on the physical health status of clients. The nurse's role in the care of this situation includes the following:

• Help the client connect substance use to physical consequences
• Encourage the client to seek regular primary health care and dental care

• Teach clients to manage chronic health problems that do not resolve after detoxification
• Implement protocols for medical treatment of the problems while the client is in treatment

Evaluation

Outcomes evaluation for clients with substance-related disorders is an essential part of their nursing care. All phases of treatment need careful documentation. Nursing research in particular is needed to determine the effectiveness of intervention aimed at maintaining sobriety and preventing relapse (Gerace, Hughes, and Spunt, 1995).

KEY POINTS

• Use, abuse, and dependence on substances occur in most cultures worldwide and are linked to social and legal problems, as well as physical and mental health problems.
• The causes of the disorders of abuse and dependence on psychoactive drugs result from the interaction of biological, social, cultural, and psychological states and traits.
• Disorders related to drug use can be prevented through changes in social and cultural traditions and by health teaching about the risks and potential negative outcomes of drug use.
• Nurses incorporate knowledge about drug use, abuse, and dependence in all roles implemented in general practice as well as in the specialties of psychiatric-mental health and addictions nursing.
• Nursing care in acute and chronic states of substance-related disorders is systematic, client-oriented, and outcome-directed.
• The successful treatment of abuse and dependence is determined by the extent to which comprehensive care addresses the physical, emotional, social, and spiritual realms of the client's life affected by drug use.
• Self-assessment and an understanding of personal characteristics that predispose them to substance use, abuse, and dependence is essential for nurses.

REFERENCES

Alcoholics Anonymous. (1989). *AA for Native Americans* (Pamphlet #P21-406). New York: General Services Board, Alcoholics Anonymous.

American Nurses' Association. (1984). *Addictions and psychological dysfunction in nursing.* New York: Author.

American Nurses' Association. (1988). *Standards of addiction nursing practice with selected diagnoses and criteria.* Kansas City, MO: Author.

American Psychiatric Association (1994). *Diagnostic and statistical manual of psychiatric disorders,* (4th ed.). Washington, DC: Author.

Bailey, S.L. (1992). Adolescents' multisubstance use patterns: The role of heavy alcohol and cigarette use. *American Journal of Public Health, 82*(9), 1220-1224.

Barry, K.L., & Fleming, M.F. (1993). The alcohol use disorders identification test (AUDIT) and the SMAST-13: Predictive validity in a rural primary care sample. *Alcohol & Alcoholism, 28*(1):33-42.

Blum, K., & Payne, J.E. (1991). *Alcohol and the addicted brain.* New York: Macmillan.

Bowen, M. (1978). *Family therapy and clinical practice.* New York: Aronson.

Clement, J.A., Williams, E.B., & Waters, C. (1993). The client with substance abuse/mental illness: Mandate for collaboration. *Archives of Psychiatric Nursing, 74*(4), 189-196.

Cloninger, C.R., Bohman, M., & Sigvardson, S. (1981). Inheritance of alcohol abuse: Cross-fostering analysis of adopted men. *Archives of General Psychiatry, 38*(8), 861-868.

Crabbe, J.C., & Goldman, D. (1992). Alcoholism: A complex genetic disease. *Alcohol Health and Research World, 16*(4), 297-303.

Ewing, J.A. (1984). Detecting alcoholism: The CAGE questionnaire. *Journal of American Medical Association, 252*(14), 1905-1907.

Gerace, L.M., Hughes, T.L., & Spunt, J. (1995). Improving nurses' responses toward substance-nursing patients: A clinical evaluation project. *Archives of Psychiatric Nursing, 9*(5), 286-294.

Hutchinson, S. (1988). Chemically dependent nurses: The trajectory toward self-annihilation. *Nursing Research, 35*(40), 196-201.

Jellinek, E.M. (1960). *The disease concept of alcoholism.* New Haven, CT: College and University Press.

Kearney, M.H., Murphy, S., Irwin, K., & Rosenbaum, M. (1995). Salvaging self: A grounded theory of pregnancy on crack cocaine. *Nursing Research, 44*(4), 2-7.

Kinney, J. (1996). *Clinical manual of substance abuse (2nd ed.).* St. Louis: Mosby.

Naegle, M. (1994). Drug use and HIV: Health care provider perspectives. *Journal of the Association of Nurses in AIDS Care.* May-June, 39-46.

National Center for Health Statistics (1994). *Health, USS, 1993.* Hyattsville, MD: Public Health Service.

National Institute of Drug Abuse. (1987). *Finding from the Hispanic Health and Nutrition Examination Survey: Use of selected drugs among Hispanic: Mexican Americans, Puerto Ricans, Cuban Americans.* Rockville, MD: Author.

National Institute of Drug Abuse. (1993). *National survey results on drug use.* From *Monitoring the future study, 1975-1992. Vol. I: secondary school students* (NIH publication no. 93-9597). Rockville, MD: Author.

National Institute of Drug Abuse. (1994). *The national household survey on drug abuse: Population estimates, 1993.* Rockville, MD: Author.

Pokorny, A.D., Miller, B.A., & Kaplan, H.B. (1972). The brief MAST: A shortened version of the Michigan Alcoholism Screening Test. *American Journal of Psychiatry, 129*(3), 3342-345.

Prochaska, J., DiClemente, C.C., & Norcross, J.C. (1992). In search of how people change: Application of addictive behaviors. *American Psychologist, 47*(9), 1102-1111.

Redding, B., & Selleck, C. (1993). Perinatal substance abuse: Assessment and management of the pregnant woman and her children. *Nurse Practitioner Forum, 4*(4), 216-223.

Russell, M., et al., (1991). Screening for pregnancy risk drinking: TWEAKING the tests. Research Institute on Alcoholism. *Buffalo Alcohol, 15,* 368.

Saunders, J.B., Aasland, O.G., Babor, J.F., De la Fuente, J.R., & Grant, M. (1993). Development of the Alcohol Use Disorder Identification Test (AUDIT): WHO Collaborative Project on early detection of persons with harmful alcohol consumption. *Addiction, 88*(6), 791-804.

Skinner, H.A. (1982). The drug abuse screening test. *Addiction Behavior, 7*(4)363-371.

Skinner, H.A., Holt, R., Schuller, J., & Roy, J. (1986). Identification of alcohol abuse using laboratory tests and a history of trauma. *Annals of Internal Medicine, 101,* 847-851.

Sokol, R.J., Martier, S.S., & Ager, J.W. (1989). T-ACF questions: Practical pregnancy detection or risk drinking. *American Journal of Obstetrics and Gynecology, 160,* 863-868.

Substance Abuse and Mental Health Services Administration (SAMHSA). (1994). *The economic costs of alcohol and drug abuse and mental illness.* BKD54. Rockville, MD: Author.

Sullivan, E. (1995). *Nursing care of clients with substance abuse.* St. Louis: Mosby.

Sumnicht, G. (1991). *Sailing white horses: Adventures with older substance abusers.* Madison, WI: Prevention and Intervention Center for Alcohol and Other Drug Abuse.

Trotter, R.T. (1979). Evidence of an ethno-medical form of aversion therapy on the United States-Mexico border. *Journal of Ethnopharmacology, 1*(3), 279-284.

VIDEO RESOURCES

Case Studies in Emergency Nursing Video Series:
Dealing with the Intoxicated/Impaired Patient
Psychiatric Emergencies Video Series:
Module 2: Intoxification, Abreactions, Side Effects
Mosby's Psychiatric Nursing Video Series:
Volume 4: Substance Abuse
Mosby's Nursing Care of Clients with Substance Abuse Video Series:
Substance Abuse in the Hospital
Substance Abuse in Perinatal Care
Substance Abuse in Families, Children, and Adolescents
Substance Abuse in the Community
Substance Abuse in Chemical Dependency Treatment Centers
Dual Diagnoses

Chapter 28

Eating Disorders

Melissa Hedinger Cottrell
Anita Leach McMahon

LEARNING OUTCOMES

After studying and applying the concepts of this chapter, the learner will be able to:

- Describe the significant dysfunctional behaviors of clients with anorexia nervosa, bulimia nervosa, and binge eating disorders.
- Explain the continuum of eating regulation responses.
- List the target behaviors of clients with restricting and bingeing type eating patterns.
- Identify the medical complications of eating disorders.
- Identify biopsychosocial risk factors in the development of eating disorders.
- Describe the criteria that indicate a need for hospitalization of a client with an eating disorder.
- Apply the nursing process to the care of clients with eating disorders.
- Outline nursing management strategies used in the care of clients with eating disorders.

KEY TERMS

Anorexia nervosa	Cognitive restructuring	Obesity
Antecedent	Consequence	Purging
Binge eating	Contracting	Response
Binge eating disorder	Cue	Substitution
Body image	Drive	Visualization
Bulimia nervosa	Morbid obesity	

One of life's major challenges is to find a way to nourish the body and also remain within sociocultural expectations related to thinness and beauty. Early in life, a child's family is responsible for the child's dietary intake. As children mature, their abilities to regulate their food intake may be altered by multiple factors that potentially trigger dysfunctional eating patterns. The inability to regulate healthy eating patterns by over- or under-eating interferes with biological, psychological, and sociocultural integrity.

Anorexia nervosa, bulimia nervosa, binge eating, and some types of obesity are disorders that involve the dysfunctional eating behavioral patterns of overconsumption or underconsumption of food. *Anorexia nervosa* has been recognized as a mental disorder for more than 100 years. *This eating disorder is characterized by an intense drive for thinness, severe dieting efforts, and extreme weight loss leading to emaciation and possible death. Bulimia nervosa is an eating disorder characterized by the excessive intake of calories, referred to as binge eating, within a specific period of time. Binge eating is then followed by the purging activities of self-induced vomiting, laxative abuse, diuretic abuse, and/or compulsive exercise to avoid weight gain. Purging is the act of expelling an agent from the body.*

Binge eating disorder (BED) has been included in the *Diagnostic and Statistical Manual of Mental Disorders, Fourth Edition, (DSM-IV)* as a potential future classification. *It is characterized by the symptoms of bulimia and impaired control behaviors such as eating rapidly, eating large amounts of food until feeling uncomfortably full, eating alone and when not hungry, and feeling embarrassment, disgust, guilt or depression after overeating* (Trumpey, 1996).

Obesity is one of the most common health problems in the United States. *Obesity is defined as a body weight of 20% above ideal body weight. Morbid obesity is a term used to classify weight that is 100% above ideal body weight.*

The continuum of self-destructive eating behaviors displayed by clients is explored in this chapter (Box 28-1). Emphasis is placed on the psychobiological causation of eating disorders. Predisposing medical issues and behavioral dynamics of clients with anorexia, bulimia and binge eating disorder (BED), as well as clients who are obese will be reviewed. The primary purpose of this chapter is to prepare learners to assist clients in the management of symptoms associated with anorexia nervosa, bulimia nervosa, BED, and obesity.

EPIDEMIOLOGY

Eating disorders, although related, have distinct epidemiological features. The secret nature of associated dys-

---

Box 28-1

Continuum of Learned Eating Regulation Responses

Functional   Dysfunctional

1   2   3   4   5   6

1. Intake of daily balanced meals with an appropriate caloric range
   Maintenance of appropriate body weight according to height and age
   Positive image relating to nourishing body for health purposes
2. Occasional increased or decreased caloric intake.
3. Overeating or fasting as a result of external and/or internal stressors.
4. Frequent episodes of compulsive overeating, purging, and/or restriction of caloric intake
5. History of compulsive overeating, purging, and/or dieting that leads to the inability to identify feelings of hunger and/or satiety
6. Restriction of food intake daily
   Anorexia
   Binge eating followed by purging
   Compulsive overeating

---

functional behaviors, as well as the cultural taboos that label such behavior as deviant, make accurate reporting of data difficult. The following is an epidemiological profile for individuals with anorexia:

- Ninety-five percent are female.
- Age of onset is generally early in adolescence, although some women show symptoms in their early 30s.
- Research studies report a range of incidence from 1 in every 100 to 1 in every 800 females between the ages of 12 and 18.
- Mortality is reported to be between 5% and 18%.

Approximately 66% of the male population and 59% of the female population are considered obese. Mortality for individuals who are obese is statistically higher than for individuals with normal weight. Some studies have found that for those individuals whose obesity has persisted for more than 5 years, treatment is most likely ineffective (Halmi, 1994). Recent studies suggest that 20% to 40% of clients who are obese have significant problems with binge eating (Pheln, 1990). Although binge eating is found in normal-weight individuals, existing statistical data seem to suggest that it is more prevalent in persons who are obese.

Available epidemiological data about clients with bulimia nervosa are as follows:

- They may be either male or female. Some studies report a 1:1 ratio between men and women who have bulimia.
- Onset of bulimia most likely occurs in adolescence or early adulthood.
- Statistics about mortality are unavailable.
- Bulimia nervosa is generally found in 1% to 2% of the adolescent and young-adult population.
- Approximately 90% of all clients with bulimia are female.

Recent studies show an increase in male athletes who purge to meet their specific target weights (wrestlers and gymnasts). It is not uncommon for individuals with anorexia nervosa to also develop bulimia nervosa. Approximately one third of persons with bulimia nervosa have previously had anorexia. Between 6% and 10% of clients with bulimia die of physiological complications or suicide (Sansone and Dennis, 1994).

Sexual abuse has been observed in 30% to 50% of all adult women diagnosed with an eating disorder. The theory suggests that a female with anorexia starves to obtain an impish, childlike body to free herself from further sexual exploitation. Clients with bulimia purge, or vomit, to throw up or cleanse themselves from forced sexual experiences (Waller, 1992).

THEORETICAL FRAMEWORK

Over the years many theorists have attempted to explain the origins of eating disorders. Presently the prevailing research indicates strong biological explanations for the disease and a belief in a genetic predisposition to the development of symptoms. Familial, psychodynamic, cognitive, behavioral, and environmental explanations further enhance our understanding of clients with eating disorders.

Biological Correlates

The biological regulation of appetite and eating behavior is an extremely complex process that involves multiple body systems. The premise that the hypothalamus contains the appetite regulation center is of particular interest for those who work with clients with eating disorders. Neurotransmitters, neuromodulators, particularly enzymes and hormones, contribute to the bodies control of feeling and satiety. Serotonin in particular is implicated as an inhibitor of food intake and acts as a *satiety agent,* that is, it signals that hunger is satisfied and the person can stop eating. Excessive cortisol signals the hypothalamus, resulting in loss of appetite with subsequent weight loss (Kaye and Weltzin, 1991).

Other hypotheses suggest eating disorders may be variants of mood disorders or possibly caused by decreased endogenous opioid activity. Both anorexia nervosa and bulimia nervosa are associated with pervasive endocrine dysfunction including amenorrhea (absence of menses) and thyroid disorders. Early studies of anorexia illustrate abnormal pituitary-ovary regulation, with luteinizing hormone (LH) reverting to an immature prepubescent pattern. Findings seem to indicate that endocrine disturbances may parallel or reflect mood, appetite, and behavior and may indeed play a role in the cause of anorexia nervosa and bulimia nervosa (Halmi, 1994).

Carbohydrates such as sugar play a large part in BED and obesity. Sugar triggers the craving mechanism. Beta-endorphins, stimulated by increased sugar intake, act to stimulate more binge eating.

Anorexia nervosa is a disorder that makes conflicting demands on the food-intake system. Body weight drops, which creates a need for nutrients, while simultaneously, a number of factors also act to inhibit eating. Factors that have been found to regulate food intake and play a part in cause of symptoms of anorexia nervosa include osmotic pressure changes, blood pressure, body temperature, gastric emptying rate, food palatability, learned food aversions, and zinc availability.

Genetic Correlates

Eating disorders tend to run in families. Relatives of an individual with anorexia nervosa or bulimia nervosa are more likely than the general population to develop an eating disorder. Twin studies are less conclusive, but in general, a high "concordance" rate for anorexia nervosa in identical twins suggests either a genetic predisposition or environmental/familial influence in the development of eating disorders.

For more than a century, researchers have known that body weight is hereditary. Studies have shown that if one parent is obese, the child has a 50% chance of being obese. If both parents are obese, the child has an 80% chance of obesity (Skunkard and Meyer, 1993). Current studies on obesity are beginning to validate the influence of genetic coding on individuals' weights and sizes.

Cognitive-Behavioral Correlates

Behaviorists believe that eating disorders stem from learned maladaptive behaviors. Emphasis is placed on observable behavioral events, related antecedents, and consequences and responses that result from the behavior. Most health professionals view dieting as the one single antecedent that proceeds maladaptive eating behaviors.

Learning theory is based on the basic concepts of drive, cue, response, and reward. A ***drive is an internal*** *or external stimulus that motivates individuals to take action.* For example, they believe primary drives such as hunger are biological, but secondary drives such as binge eating are learned responses to anxiety.

A *cue is an internal and/or external response signal that, if noticed, predicts when, where, and what response will occur.* Persons may notice, for example, that they feel anxious. A *response is an activity such as thinking, feeling, or behaving that is a reaction learned through frequent rewarded experiences.* A response is what a person does as a result of a cue. For example, an individual may respond to the feeling of anxiety (cue) by eating. The reward or consequence is the reinforcement a person receives as a result of the learned response. In this example the decrease in anxiety is the reward. A decrease in anxiety is thought to be the major reinforcement for eating disorders.

Antecedents are the behaviors, feelings, moods, or events that trigger an individual's behaviors—in this case, eating. For example, the U.S. culture has created an active daily lifestyle. An occasionally skipped meal may serve a "brief functional purpose." Binge eating or fasting because of external and/or internal stressors may then quickly lead to dysfunctional eating responses. These persons may begin to use food for purposes other than nutrition, such as to assist in satisfying unmet social and/or psychological needs.

Consequences are the results of behaviors. For eating disorders, they range from self-starvation to morbid obesity. Box 28-1 illustrates a continuum of learned eating regulation responses. Frequent episodes of compulsive overeating, purging, and/or restriction of caloric intake, and indications of dysfunctional eating responses provide immediate gratification, thus improving mood or satisfying needs. The person's inability to regulate eating habits leads to alterations in the biological, psychological, social, and cultural behaviors of individuals.

Another premise of the behavioral theorists involves two kinds of conflict. The *avoidance-avoidance conflict* occurs when one must choose between two undesirable alternatives. For example, a person with anorexia may want to avoid gaining weight and at the same time may want to avoid ill health. The *approach-avoidance conflict* occurs when the person has ambivalent feelings toward the same object. The individual wishes simultaneously to approach and to avoid the object. For example, a person who is obese may want to lose weight but does not want to decrease intake.

Psychodynamic Correlates

According to many theorists and researchers who study eating disorders, Hilde Bruch has had the greatest impact on the psychoanalytical treatment of clients with eating disorders. Before the time of Bruch, anorexia nervosa was generally seen as a "form of conversion hysteria," and the refusal to eat symbolized "the repudiation of sexuality, especially fantasies surrounding oral impregnation" (Swift, 1991). Bruch emphasizes pre-oedipal development, observing that anorexia clients display major deficits in the sense of self-identity and autonomy. In her view, anorexia demonstrates underlying powerlessness (Bruch, 1978). Several other psychological and personality factors have been associated with the development of eating disorders (Box 28-2).

Familial Correlates

Family environment is thought to have a major influence in the development of eating disorders. Of historical note is the fact that Minuchin and his colleagues (1978) were among the first to label anorexia nervosa as a "psychosomatic illness" and list the dynamics present in families of clients with anorexia. They included enmeshment, rigidity, overprotectiveness, and conflict avoidance. These theories help explain family dynamics and assist family therapists who intervene with clients and their families.

It is believed that the child with anorexia is overprotected by parents who are generally hypervigilant, particularly of basic needs. The mother is generally the overprotective and domineering parent and may be particularly concerned about the nutritional needs of her child. However, fathers of children with anorexia have been identified as passive and withdrawn. Fathers play a special role by helping girls move from childhood to adulthood. The father of a child with anorexia may distance himself from his daughter, setting up the situation in which as a young lady, the daughter attempts to reverse the biological process and become "Daddy's little girl" once more.

Boundaries within and around the family are rigid. The child with anorexia takes a "peacemaker" or go-between role with parents and may unwittingly become

---

Box 28-2

Psychological and Personality Factors Associated With the Development of Eating Disorders

High need for achievement and perfectionism
Significant adolescent turmoil
Impaired self-concept or body image
Struggles with identity formation
Mood instability
Social phobia
Poor impulse control
Low self-esteem
Intolerance or overcontrol of emotions

involved in spousal conflict. The child aims to not embarrass the family and remains quiet about or denies any domestic discord. Children with anorexia depend on parental assessment of their behaviors and are loyal at all costs to family values; consequently, they become "good little girls" or "good little boys" at the cost of their autonomy.

With the onset of adolescence, conflict develops between peer involvement and family loyalty. This is generally the time that symptoms of eating disorders begin. The onset of anorexia is often linked to stressful events involving loss, separation, or change in the family. The severity of symptoms is thought to be related to the degree of family enmeshment and rigidity and to the length of time the child has been involved in the parental conflict. Because of learned conflict-avoidance patterns and the closed system boundaries, the family unites to "protect" the child with anorexia, thus rewarding the symptoms. According to family theories, the body and weight loss of the person with anorexia become the property of the whole family. Weight and food become the family's central concern.

Research about the background and family history of individuals who eventually develop bulimia or develop BED is sparse. Recent data suggest that factors such as chronic illness, the presence of obsessive-compulsive disorders (OCDs), phobias, parental divorce, and a death in the family dominate the family histories in more than 50% of studies of individuals with bulimia. (Pheln, 1990). Other data indicate a high correlation between addictive drinking behavior of parents and development of bulimic symptoms in their children. Married women with bulimia tend to experience role difficulty and are more dependent and passive than individuals who do not have bulimia (Waller, 1992).

According to Stunkard and Meyer (1990) and other researchers studying obesity, there is not a specific family prototype for the development of obesity in children unless it is genetically predestined. However, in early studies, Bruch (1970) noted that clients who were obese came from homes where food rights were used as control mechanisms, such as when to eat, what to eat, and how much to eat. She found that parents would give or withhold food for multiple reasons that did not relate to the child's hunger. Food could be given as a sign of love or used to pacify in a cold, unfeeling household. Children were rarely allowed to decide for themselves if they were hungry. She believed the end result was that they developed into adults who were unable to recognize hunger and other body sensations.

Environmental Correlates

Sociocultural pressures play an important role in the development of eating disorders. Although men also have eating disorders, their body shapes and sizes are not often used to measure masculinity. Most women, however, carry cultural ideals of "appropriate body shapes." Society continues to pass on the underlying message through the media that "life is exciting but only for those who fit the cultural stereotype of the perfect woman" (Fontaine, 1991). The increase of mass media in the twentieth century has been an important factor in identifying "acceptable" body shapes. Visual and print media serve as primary stimuli for encouraging thinness, which adds fuel to women's obsession with weight and the glamorization of thinness.

The *Nursing Process*

Assessment

Clinical Profile

Anorexia nervosa

Anorexia nervosa is an eating disorder of life-threatening proportion, characterized by a relentless pursuit of thinness, intense fear of becoming fat, and delusional disturbance of **body image,** *the subjective view one has of one's physical appearance.* It has been referred to as self-starvation. Box 28-3 identifies behaviors, feelings, and conditions characteristic of anorexia nervosa.

Physical signs and symptoms, psychosocial patterns, behaviors, family dynamics, and cultural influences must be considered in any description of clients with anorexia. The weight loss associated with anorexia nervosa may produce life-threatening cardiac dysrhythmias. Death from resulting malnutrition has been reported for 10% to 15% of these clients.

A wide variety of physical signs and symptoms occur, including hypothermia, cold intolerance (accompanied by cyanosis and numbness of extremities), bradycardia, hypotension, electrolyte imbalance, sleep disturbances, and skin changes. Peripheral edema is common. Teeth and gums often show signs of deterioration as a result of frequent self-induced vomiting.

The Nursing Process

Box 28-3

Characteristics Associated With Anorexia Nervosa

Drastic reduction in food intake
Preoccupation with foods to prevent weight gain
Phobia for foods that produce weight gain
Self-induced vomiting
Amenorrhea for at least three consecutive menstrual periods
Frequent self-administered enemas
Body-image distortion (feels fat), despite excessive thinness
Emaciated appearance
Denial of weight loss and thinness
Denial of self as sexual being
Fear of sexual maturity
Pattern of excessive exercise
Frequent use of repression and regression as defense mechanisms
Strained family relationships
Feelings of powerlessness
Narrow range of interests
Disturbed self-concept
Perfectionism
Overachievement
Depression

Gastric complications include gastritis, lowered acid secretion, and delayed emptying of the stomach with subsequent acute dilation and possible rupture. The pumping chambers in the heart become weakened, and the cardiac output is decreased. Estrogen deficiency leads to amenorrhea. Other endocrine disorders are often not diagnosed. Lowered testosterone production in men causes impotence. Decreased sexual energy is common to both genders. Altered function of pituitary, thyroid, and adrenal hormones with resulting signs and symptoms also occurs. An increased incidence of osteoporosis has been observed in some clients. Peripheral nerve paralysis results from nerve compression caused by lack of body cushioning (Kaplan, Sadock, and Grebb, 1994).

During the initial stages of anorexia nervosa, the individual's behavior may be difficult to distinguish from a "normal dieter." Persons attempting to lose weight avoid foods such as fats, proteins, sweets, and breads. Unlike normal dieters, an individual with anorexia nervosa continues food restriction after others have achieved a "normal" body weight. The client with anorexia begins to learn to eat less and daily may eat only a few bites of food.

Clients with anorexia nervosa also display unusual responses to eating or to eating situations. Instead of looking forward to being with others at meals, they find excuses for eating alone. Behavioral changes may also include an increasing preoccupation with the body. Clients begin monitoring the body changes that result from their weight loss (visibility of the ribs, decreased size of the abdomen, and loss of body fat). As the disorder progresses, dieting is the primary factor of life and becomes the center of all thoughts, feelings, and actions. Weight loss is the measure of personal success, self-esteem, and control.

Persons with anorexia tend to be perfectionists with highly compulsive traits. As children they were described as "the model child," "passive," "over-obedient," and "introverted." They are the overachievers who enjoy pleasing others (especially parents or those in authority) to the exclusion of their own needs. They feel helpless, hopeless, and isolated and constantly struggle for control. Their superior "goodness" serves as a defense against a profound sense of inadequacy and ineffectiveness (Conrad, Sloan, and Jedwabny, 1992).

It has been suggested that clients with anorexia have problems developing self-identity. Clients may be nonassertive, may avoid taking risks, and may depend on family members to make personal decisions for them. Although they may excel academically, their lack of self-esteem leads to feelings of boredom, helplessness, and personal ineffectiveness. Normal peer relationships are not developed, and interactions are usually limited to one person at a time and remain on a superficial level. Often clients with anorexia are depressed.

Physiological complications of anorexia nervosa

As a general rule, medical complications in anorexia nervosa are primarily results of a starvation-induced hypometabolic state. In an attempt to adapt and survive, the body shifts into a hypometabolic state to conserve resources. The thyroid slows metabolism and the output of hormones. Body temperature decreases, causing sensitivity to cold. The client's heart rate and blood pressure decrease, resulting in light-headedness, and reflexes become sluggish. The client's skin becomes dry, and hair loss is common. Nonessential physiological functions such as menstruation cease.

As the disease progresses and starvation intensifies, the body feeds itself on the remains of body fat and protein. The client's body muscle mass decreases, and in the latter stages of starvation the heart muscle becomes rigid, less contractile, and less efficient. Cardiac conduction abnormalities develop, resulting in dysrhythmias and death.

The Nursing Process

Laboratory findings in clients with anorexia reveal anemia, decreased white blood cell and platelet levels, elevated beta-carotene levels (which produce yellow skin color with no known explanation), and elevated cholesterol levels. Vomiting, laxative abuse, and diuretic abuse are methods clients use to lose weight. Medical complications of maladaptive weight loss methods are found in Table 28-1. If these complications are not treated, death may occur. Mortality rates resulting from complications of anorexia nervosa vary between 5% to 8% (Sansone and Dennis, 1994). Criteria from the DSM-IV for clients with anorexia nervosa (Box 28-4) reflect the body image and denial issues of these clients.

Bulimia nervosa

Bulimia nervosa is an eating disorder commonly referred to as the *binge-purge syndrome*. It is characterized by episodic rapid consumption of large amounts of food in a short time (usually less than 2 hours). Termination of the eating episode results from abdominal pain, sleep, social interruption, or self-induced vomiting.

Clients with bulimia generally consume high-caloric, easily ingested food and do so in secret. They may make repeated attempts to lose weight employing any of the following measures: severely restricted diets, strenuous exer-

Box 28-4

DSM-IV Criteria for Anorexia Nervosa

- Refusal to maintain body weight at or above a minimally normal weight for age and height (loss of 15% or greater average body weight)
- Intensive fear of weight gain or becoming fat, although client is currently underweight
- Disturbance in body image
- Denial of seriousness of current low body weight
- Absence of menarche

RESTRICTING TYPE

Client does not regularly engage in binge-eating, self-induced vomiting, or purging behaviors (use of laxatives, diuretics, or enemas).

BINGE-EATING/PURGING TYPE

During anorexic phase, client engages in binge-eating or purging behavior.

From American Psychological Association. (1994). Diagnostic and statistical manual of mental disorders, fourth edition. *Washington, DC: Author.*

TABLE 28-1

Possible medical complications of commonly used weight-loss methods

VOMITING	LAXATIVE ABUSE	DIURETIC ABUSE
Parotid gland enlargement (neck area	Nonspecific abdominal complaints (cramping, constipation)	Hypokalemia (low potassium)
Erosion of tooth enamel and increased cavities	Sluggish bowel functioning ("cathartic colon")	Fatigue; diminished reflexes; if severe, possible cardiac dysrhythmia; if chronic, serious kidney damage
Tears in esophagus	Malabsorption of fat, protein, and calcium	Fluid loss; dehydration, light-headedness, thirst
Chronic esophagitis		
Chronic sore throats	Electrolyte imbalance	Electrolyte imbalance
Difficulty swallowing	Dehydration	
Stomach cramps		
Digestive problems		
Anemia		
Electrolyte imbalance		

The Nursing Process

cise, self-induced vomiting, frequent enemas and use of cathartics, amphetamines, and/or diuretics. They experience weight fluctuations greater than 10 pounds in 1 day as a direct result of binge eating and bodily fluid shifts.

Unlike persons with anorexia whose emaciated appearance is often the hallmark of the disorder, most bulimics are of approximately normal weight and appear to be "physically well." However, heart disease, hypertension, and diabetes are common in clients with bulimia.

As in anorexia nervosa, the onset of bulimia nervosa is usually preceded by dieting. Episodes of prolonged and severe caloric restriction lead to binge episodes followed by some form of self-induced compensatory behaviors to avoid weight gain. Clients with bulimia generally center their self-value and worth on their shape, size, and weight. As the illness progresses, the client generally experiences increased feelings of isolation and self-deprecation.

Clients with bulimia generally begin purging to rid their bodies of calories consumed during a binge. There is often an increase of symptoms during times of stress. Binge-purge cycles may vary in frequency from occasional to multiple times per day. As the disorder progresses, a lifestyle is developed to facilitate the binge-purge process. This lifestyle is accompanied by feelings of isolation, self-deprecating thoughts, labile and/or depressed moods, and low self-esteem.

Clients with bulimia fully recognize their abnormal eating patterns. A great amount of time and energy is spent planning and carrying out binge-purge episodes. Binge eating eventually becomes a "soothing" way to cope with a variety of unpleasant feelings such as frustration, anger, fear, boredom, and loneliness. Abuse of alcohol, street drugs, and amphetamines to maintain weight may be characteristic of some clients with bulimia. A higher incidence of both stealing and poor interpersonal relationships has been reported in some studies (Palmer, 1990).

Somatic preoccupation, guilt about secretive eating behavior, indecision, and lack of motivation are other hallmarks of clients with bulimia. Self-mutilative behaviors, suicidal thoughts, mood swings, and suicide attempts are common.

The depression found in clients with bulimia is often associated with the family theme of loss: loss of competence and self-esteem, resulting in low levels of differentiation; loss of respect for parental authority, loss of shared goals; or loss of friend or loved one through death, illness, or distance.

Medical complications that develop in bulimia nervosa are generally results of binging or the subsequent compensatory behaviors that result from vomiting, laxative abuse, or diuretic abuse. Binging may result in abdominal distention, bloating, and pain.

Self-induced vomiting can result in multiple medical complications. During vomiting, the acid gastric contents of the stomach can erode tooth enamel. Vomiting may also result in salivary gland enlargement (the parotid and/or submandibular glands). Vomitus may also cause extensive upper-gastrointestinal (GI) tract irritation. This irritation can cause sore throat, difficulty swallowing, and indigestion.

Clients who abuse syrup of ipecac to induce vomiting are at increased risk for severe GI difficulties. Forceful vomiting may create a tear in the mucosa of the GI tract (blood in vomitus). Prolonged vomiting can cause the loss of potassium and can result in altered cardiac functions. Low potassium levels can precipitate cardiac dysrhythmias (Sansone and Dennis, 1994).

In women with bulimia, the menstrual cycle may be present, irregular, or absent. Stomach ulcers and rectal bleeding with hemorrhaging may occur and are the primary causes of death in clients with bulimia. Electrolyte imbalance—the result of diuretic and/or laxative abuse—is common and may be life-threatening. Box 28-5 identifies the DSM-IV criteria for bulimia nervosa.

Box 28-5

DSM-IV Criteria for Bulimia Nervosa

- Recurrent episodes of binge eating characterized by eating a large amount of food in a specific period of time
- Loss of control during the eating episode (inability to stop eating or control amount of food intake)
- Recurrent inappropriate actions to avoid weight gain, such as self-induced vomiting, laxative abuse, misuse of diuretics, enemas, or other medications
- Fasting after food binges for extended periods of time
- Controlling weight through excessive exercise
- Self-esteem controlled by body shape and weight

PURGING TYPE

During bulimic episode, client regularly self-induces vomiting and abuses laxatives, diuretics, or enemas

NONPURGING TYPE

During bulimic episode, client fasts or uses excessive exercise to compensate for extensive food intake

From American Psychological Association. (1994). Diagnostic and statistical manual of mental disorders, fourth edition. Washington, DC: Author.

The Nursing Process

Obesity

Obesity is identified as a serious health problem, although it is not classified as an eating disorder in DSM-IV (APA, 1994). Obesity is defined as 20% above ideal body height/weight index. Morbid obesity is classified as 100% above ideal body height/weight index.

Multiple theories have been proposed to explain the etiologic factors of obesity. Many believe that genetics, and neurobiological and endocrine structures contribute to appetite, eating behaviors, fat distribution, and body size. Multiple medical complications are associated with obesity and include hypertension, gall bladder disease, cardiovascular disease, diabetes, and trauma to weight-bearing joints. Clients generally are dissatisfied with their body shape and size, and also have low self-esteem. Many report childhood sexual abuse.

Binge eating disorder

Many individuals who are obese are compulsive overeaters. BED is the uncontrolled craving for and ingestion of food that stops when an individual either vomits or falls asleep. It is believed that the triggers for compulsive overeating are the result of a decrease in energy utilization. This decrease of energy is completely independent of the fuel or stored body fat an individual has. Macronutrient regulation and identification of how neuropeptides influence food cravings are currently being researched. Binge eating may initially be a response to external or internal stressors, which quickly leads to dysfunctional eating responses. Individuals begin to use food to meet social and/or psychological needs. Individuals with a history of binge eating beyond a period of 3 to 6 months eventually exhibit an inability to identify when feelings of hunger and satiety begin (APA Working Group, 1993). Box 28-6 lists suggested criteria for making a diagnosis of BED.

Persons who are binge eaters generally lack interest in exercise programs and prefer passive, observer activities. Often they feel helpless and hopeless about their abilities to lose weight. They use excessive eating behavior or binging to substitute for feelings such as anger, guilt, boredom, inadequacy, ambivalence, loneliness, or unattractiveness. For some, overeating may be a way of expressing hostility, showing rebellion against authority, reducing anxiety, or it may be an attempt at independence.

Focused Assessment

The assessment process used for a person who has or is suspected of having an eating disorder involves observation of the client's behavior, the interview process, and

Box 28-6

Criteria for Binge Eating Disorder

- Recurrent episodes of binge eating at least twice per week for 3 months
- No use of extreme measures to lose weight
- Awareness that eating patterns are abnormal
- Fear of not being able to stop eating voluntarily
- Depressed mood and self-deprecating thoughts following eating binges
- No evidence of body image disturbance other than body size dissatisfaction
- Overeating episodes not related to anorexia, bulimia, or physical disorder
- Consumption of high-calorie, easily ingested food during binge
- Secretive eating during binge
- Repeated efforts to diet in an effort to lose weight
- Negative affect, which often starts the binge eating
- Frequent weight fluctuations of greater than 10 lbs. caused by alternating binging and dieting

validation of information with significant others. A complete health assessment that includes inspection of gums and mouth should be performed. Because affective disorders are prevalent among clients with anorexia, bulimia, and BED, information about mood changes, suicide potential, and family history of affective disorders should be included in the data base. Information about family functioning is also essential. Questions that should be asked by the nurse to obtain an accurate data base are found in Table 28-2.

Nursing Diagnosis

Caring for clients with eating disorders requires the nurse to make clinical judgments about the clients' needs. For the hospitalized client with anorexia or bulimia, a diagnosis most often focus on the binge-and-purge eating patterns, the life-threatening seriousness of their nutritional state (overweight or underweight), and their delusional body image.

At present, behavioral syndromes for anorexia nervosa and bulimia nervosa are reported in DSM-IV (see Boxes 28-4 and 28-5). When psychological factors are a component of the etiology of a particular client with obesity, another diagnostic descriptor is used: psychological factors affecting physical condition. In an effort to refine terminology used to differentiate the binge-purge syndrome from bingeing behavior alone, the DSM-IV

The Nursing Process

TABLE 28-2

Focused assessment of clients with eating disorders

ASSESSMENT TOPIC	QUESTIONS
History of eating disorder	What difficulties are you currently experiencing with food?
	What is your current weight and height?
	What was your highest weight and when?
	What was your lowest weight and when?
	How old were you when you first noticed eating problems?
	What circumstances occurred prior to your eating problems?
	Do you have a history of binging episodes?
	Do you have a history of purging episodes?
	How many binge-purge episodes do you experience daily?
	Is there a pattern to your binge-purge cycles?
Preoccupation with food	How often do you think about food in a 24-hour period?
	Describe some of your thoughts.
Vomiting	How frequent are vomiting episodes?
	Are they self-induced?
	Do you use syrup of ipecac?
Laxative and diuretics use	How often do you use laxatives or diuretics?
	Is ther a particular pattern of use?
	What type do you use?
	How much do you use?
	How long have you been using laxatives or diuretics?
Abuse of amphetamines/over-the-counter stimulants	How often do you use stimulants?
	What type do you use?
	How much do you use?
	How long have you been using diet pills?
Exercise pattern	Describe the fequency and type of exercise you do.
	(Is there evidence of hyperactivity/hypoactivity?)
Body weight distortion	How do you feel about your size?
	(How does perception correspond to observed reality?)
Menstrual history	Is amenorrhea or irregular menses present?
	How long have your periods been irregular?
Sleep patterns	How much do you sleep?

The Nursing Process

TABLE 28-2—cont'd

Focused assessment of clients with eating disorders

ASSESSMENT TOPIC	QUESTIONS
	Do you eat at night?
	Do you binge at night?
Sexuality	Have you ever been sexually abused?
	Are you sexually active?
	(Is sexual activity appropriate to age and lifestyle?)
Addictive behaviors	Have you ever stolen anything?
	Do you gamble?
	How much and what kind of alcohol do you consume and where do you consume it?
	Do you smoke marijuana?
	Do you use illicit drugs?
Maladaptive social functioning	Describe problems at work or school.
	Tell me about your friends.
	How long have you had the friendships?
Related disorders	Are you depressed?
	Have you ever thought about suicide or attempted suicide?
	Is there a history of family depression?
	(Is a personality disorder evident?)
Family functioning	Describe a typical family mealtime.
	Which of your family members are overweight? Which are too thin?
	Does anyone in your family eat too much? Too little?

(1994) has included BED, which is commonly called compulsive overeating, as a diagnostic area needing further exploration.

Whenever an eating disorder is the diagnosis, comorbidity is considered, since several factors increase an individual's risk for eating disorders. First- and second-degree relatives of individuals with anorexia nervosa and bulimia nervosa have an increased incidence of depression, obsessive-compulsive disorder (OCD), bipolar disorders, and substance abuse problems (Sansone and Dennis, 1994). Approximately 20% of clients with anorexia and 40% of clients with bulimia meet the DSM-IV criteria for major depression. It is hypothesized that clients with an affective illness are more vulnerable to the development of an eating disorder once they begin dieting. OCD traits are observed and documented in the population of clients with eating disorders. This correlates specifically with the client's obsessive drive for thinness at all costs. Substance abuse has also been identified in one third of all clients with bulimia. One hypothesis states that alcohol and/or other substance use may be a coping response to isolation and dysphoria. Axis II diagnoses—the personality disorders—are also prevalent among clients with eating disorders. See Table 28-3 for DSM-IV diagnostic categories and selected North American Nursing Diagnosis Association (NANDA) nursing diagnoses with corresponding examples of assessment data.

The Nursing Process

TABLE 28-3

Corresponding DSM-IV and NANDA diagnoses and assessment data

DSM-IV DIAGNOSIS	NANDA DIAGNOSIS	ASSESSMENT DATA
Anorexia nervosa, restricting type	Nutrition altered: less than body requirements related to fear of weight gain and starvation behavior	Refusal to maintain body weight for age and height
	Powerlessness related to lack of control over food avoidance	Intense fear of becoming fat, although underweight
	Anxiety related to fear of weight gain as evidenced by rituals associated with food intake	
Anorexia nervosa, binge eating/purging type	Self-multilation, risk for, related to excessive exercise and/or self-induced vomiting	Binge eating and/or purging behavior during anorexic episode
Bulimia nervosa, purging type	Self-mutilation, risk for, related to feeling of inadequacy as evidenced by medical complications/injuries due to excessive exercise and/or self-induced vomiting	Reoccurring episodes of binge eating in specific periods of time (1-2 hours)
	Powerlessness related to perceived lack of control over eating behaviors and/or binging-purging	Recurrent compensatory behaviors to avoid weight gain (purging and laxative and/or diuretic abuse)
	Body image disturbance related to fear of weight gain as evidenced by rituals associated with food intake and purging	Self-evaluation is based solely on body size
Bulimia nervosa, non-purging type	Nutrition altered: more than body requirements related to excessive intake of calories as evidenced by being above ideal body weight	Reoccurring episodes of binge eating in a specific period of time
	Body image disturbance related to fear of weight gain as evidenced by rituals associated with food intake	Self-evaluation is based solely on body size
Binge eating disorder	Nutrition altered: more than body requirements related to excessive food intake, being 20% above ideal body weight, and decreased physical mobility	Eating excessive food high in caloric value over specific period of time

Outcome Identification

There are several outcomes desired for clients with anorexia nervosa and bulimia nervosa and for those with binge eating disorder. During hospitalization, priority should be given to achieving a state of nutritional balance that is adequate to sustain life and prevent serious physiological sequelae. Long-term outcomes should be concerned with asserting control over one's life, incorporating a realistic view of one's body, and developing trusting interpersonal relationships. Examples of outcomes related to eating disorders are presented in Box 28-7.

Planning

Nursing care provided to clients with eating disorders occurs in various settings and is part of an interdisciplinary effort. Client's biological status is always a primary concern. Outpatient treatment allows clients the greatest opportunity to self-regulate their eating patterns while

The Nursing Process

Box 28-7

Outcomes for Clients With Eating Disorders

ANOREXIA NERVOSA

Janie will comply with dietary regimen without deviance for 2 weeks.

Janie will gain 2 pounds weekly until ideographic weight is achieved.

Janie will set a reasonable weight for herself and when weight is obtained, she will identify how she will remain at the desired weight.

BULIMIA NERVOSA

Marsha will spend time with a member of her family or a friend following meals.

Marsha will verbalize her feelings and use persons as opposed to food when she is anxious.

BINGE EATING DISORDER

Alan will initially reduce episodes of compulsive eating from two times weekly to twice monthly.

Alan will attend Overeaters Anonymous meetings three times weekly.

---

establishing autonomy. This level of care also assists clients to manage their financial resources sparingly.

Acute inpatient care provides clients the opportunity to be monitored 24 hours per day and is necessary when physiological symptoms are life-threatening. The client's intake and output can also be closely observed. A nursing care plan for a client with anorexia being treated in an outpatient setting is presented on p. 557. A nursing care plan for a client with bulimia requiring hospitalization for binge-purge behaviors is found on p. 558.

The client with chronic anorexia provides a multitude of challenges for the interdisciplinary treatment team. A clinical pathway representing an interdisciplinary treatment plan for a client with anorexia being treated in an acute care setting is presented on p. 559.

Implementation
Counseling

Counseling interventions for clients with eating disorders are initially aimed at formation of therapeutic nurse-client relationships. Individuals who seek help for eating disorders generally do so because significant others have urged them to obtain assistance. When they seek help on

their own, they are generally highly ambivalent and do not know how to accept assistance in restructuring their eating patterns. Clients at the beginning of hospitalization may be angry. This anger is often expressed as hostility toward the nurse; clients deny the need for help despite deep wishes for nurturance.

Once trust is established in the relationship, the client may begin the working phase, let down defenses, and reveal feelings of depression and neediness. Therapeutic responses during this phase should include active listening and "feeding rituals." Each contact with the client should be structured into two parts: listening and supportively reflecting the client's feelings and experiences. This procedure enables the client to gain a sense of identity and to express feelings of sadness and loneliness. It is during this stage that clients begin to realize the extent of their illnesses. The binging and purging symptoms may be under control, but the client's recovery is just beginning. During this phase, clients are generally unable to ask for help but are most receptive to nurturance.

Clients who in the past have been sexually abused should be referred to advance practice colleagues who specialize in treating the effects of trauma and/or abuse. The body-image distortion of the client with an eating disorder is one of the most difficult aspects of the illness. Nurses should be encouraged to assist clients in distinguishing between body-image distortion (size and shape) and dissatisfaction of specific body parts and areas. Box 28-8 on p. 560 lists body-image enhancement interventions.

Cognitive-behavioral management

Cognitive-behavioral interventions are extremely effective in the treatment of clients with eating disorders. Techniques include substitution, visualization, contracting, cognitive restructuring, and assertiveness training.

Substitution *Substitution is a successful behavioral technique that involves substituting dysfunctional eating behaviors with healthful alternative behaviors.* Behavioral antecedents (those cues associated with dysfunctional eating patterns) need to be determined. Clients should first be asked to recall and then keep a careful log of activities, binge eating episodes, and purging behaviors (e.g., vomiting and laxative abuse). They should also be instructed to describe feelings, thoughts, fears, stressful situations, or boredom and to note times and sequences of all activities. Using the log, nurses can assist clients to identify behavioral cues or antecedents associated with the onset of dysfunctional eating behaviors. Alternative responses can then be planned and substituted for the destructive eating behavior. For example,

The Nursing Process

NURSING CARE PLAN

Client With Anorexia Nervosa

NURSING ASSESSMENT DATA

Subjective: Client states, "I look so fat," despite that she is 30 lbs. under ideal weight. *Objective:* Client refused to intake specific foods high in caloric value-refusal to maintain adequate weight for age and height. Past history of treatment in an eating disorder program. Current stabilization of fluids and electrolytes. *DSM-IV diagnosis:* Anorexia nervosa

NANDA Diagnosis: Body image disturbance related to fear of weight gain

Outcomes	Interventions	Rationale	Evaluation
Short term 1. Will continue to maintain adequate body weight *weekly*. 2. Will verbalize fears of food in *weekly* therapy sessions. 3. Will perform relaxation techniques prior to meals *daily*. 4. Will maintain *daily* foods and feeling journal. **Long term** ***Within 1 month:*** 1. Will maintain stabilized body weight without loss. 2. Will act on ability to increase high-risk food intake.	• See NIC interventions for anxiety reduction and coping enhancement. • Weigh client at specific intervals. • Reward client for weight gain. • Monitor client's daily calories consumed. • Instruct client on how to increase caloric intake. • Teach client relaxation techniques. • Discuss with client and family perceptions or factors interfering with client's ability to eat.	• There is consensus and research data to support specific NIC interventions. • Clients with eating disorders need assistance with feelings of anxiety and in learning enhanced coping skills. • Assists in facilitating client's weight gain. • Reduces client's anxiety and facilitates improved self-esteem. • Anorexia nervosa affects the entire family. Families have rigid boundaries, are enmeshed, and its members have low levels of self-differentiation.	**Short term** 1. Met weekly. If client fails to meet weekly goal, revise. Collaborate with multidisciplinary team. 2. Met weekly. Client capable of identifying fear of foods. 3. Met daily. 4. Met daily. **Long term** 1. Partially met. Client has increased protein and fat intake by 10%. Continue to monitor. 2. Partially met. Client had gained 16 lbs. 6 weeks after discharge. Continue to monitor.

when feeling lonely, a client is taught first to recognize and "own" the loneliness, then to avoid eating, and finally to substitute it with, for instance, telephoning a friend.

Visualization *Visualization is a way of programming changes in behavior through the use of positive and creative mental images.* Visualization has been effective for clients seeking weight control and other forms of self-improvement; for reducing stress, anxiety, and shyness; and for healing and controlling pain. For clients with eating disorders who also have thought disorders, affective disorders, or borderline personality dis-

order (i.e., dual diagnoses), these interventions are not appropriate.

Relaxation is the first step in the process. The client can then be "guided" to mentally visualize or create specific scenes or images using all the senses. For example, a person may be encouraged to create a mental image of what it is like to feel hungry (e.g., an empty jar or a hollow tree). The client should then be guided to change the image to one of fullness or satisfaction. The empty jar is filled with flowers, and the hollow tree provides a home for wild birds. Audiocassettes can be used so that clients may practice the exercise independently at the

The Nursing Process

NURSING CARE PLAN

Client With Bulimia

NURSING ASSESSMENT DATA

Subjective: Client states she feels like she is out of control during an eating episode. *Objective:* Recurrent episodes of binge eating characterized by eating large amounts of food in a specific period of time. Recurrent inappropriate actions to avoid weight gain (i.e., self-induced vomiting, laxative abuse, enemas, or excessive exercise. *DSM-IV diagnosis:* Bulimia nervosa

NANDA Diagnosis: Nutrition, altered: less than body requirements related to dysfunctional eating patterns

Outcomes	Interventions	Rationale	Evaluation
Short term 1. Will identify safe amount of food an individual may keep down *daily* without purging. 2. Will regain fluid and electrolyte balance *in 2 weeks.* 3. Will expand acceptable foods by increasing two phobic foods *per week.* **Long term** 1. Will decrease time spent focusing on calculating calories and/or obsessing on physical appearance. 2. Will abstain from purging behavior.	• Provide nutritional consultation to client. • Provide emotional support to client while experiencing feelings of fullness, bloating, and delayed gastric emptying. • Monitor client's fluids and electrolyte status. • Teach client to replace caloric anxiety with staff support and coaching. Use cue cards with rational statements (e.g., "Just because I feel fat doesn't mean I'm fat. Food is necessary to fuel my body.").	• Collaboration with client facilitates client's control. • Clients experience a fluid shift after discontinuing use of purging process. • Clients who purge experience potassium and carbon dioxide imbalance, creating cardiac complications. • Cognitive restructuring is supported by research as the most effective psychosocial treatment for bulimia.	**Short term** 1. Met daily. 2. Met in 2 weeks. 3. Not met. Evaluate plan with interdisciplinary team. **Long term** 1. Partially met. In 1 month client experiences less obsessing but still calculates fat intake. 2. Fully met. Client and family report no further purging behaviors.

recommended frequency of two to three times a day for 20 minutes.

Contracting *Contracting is a set of rules, reinforcements, and consequences agreed on by the nurse and client.* It should include a list of prohibited and permitted behaviors and the reward or reinforcement for contract fulfillment as negotiated between the client and the treatment team. Bed rest is an often-used negative reinforcement, whereas watching television, visits outside the unit, and visitors to the unit are positive reinforcements. Items generally negotiated in the contract with clients with anorexia or bulimia are noted in Box 28-8.

During the contract negotiation process, client independence should be fostered, and attempts should be made to distinguish client's motivation from expectations of others. Contracts should be generally based on behavioral protocols established by the treatment team and on the most recent research findings. Protocols reward appropriate behaviors, generally in a prescribed progressive manner.

Cognitive restructuring Cognitions or beliefs an individual has about eating behavior and body weight should be examined for irrational elements. *Cognitive restructuring involves exploring these irrational be-*

INTERDISCIPLINARY TREATMENT PLAN

Clinical Pathway: Anorexia Nervosa

Patient Name:
Date of Admission:

Average LOS: 21 days
Actual LOS:
Number of Authorized Days:

	Days 1-2	Days 3-9	Days 10-16	Days 17-21
Physician Actions	Assess in holistic manner, admission orders provide restriction orders as needed, order lab and EKG, collaborate with dietician to initiate refeeding goal	Review lab, past medical records, facilitate completion of master treatment plan, identify appropriate level of patient activity, identify if use of psychotrophic medications is indicated, repeat labs as needed.	Update treatment plan with team, review level of physical activity, monitor medication intake and rule out side effects, initiate discharge planning, repeat labs as needed.	Discharge plans and follow-up confirmed mediation titrated, outpatient caloric intake and activity level established
Nursing Actions	Holistic admitting assessment; monitor intake; orient to unit; vital signs and weight	Monitor intake and output, vital signs as ordered, document weight and core body temperature daily, observe for excessive exercise or hoarding of food, encourage verbalization of fear related to food intake, provide support at mealtime while establishing firm limits on expected food intake, monitor patient activity.	Continue to monitor patient activity, vital signs as ordered, continue to weigh as needed, observe for increased signs of anxiety as weight increases; continue to encourage interaction with peers in hospital unit.	Continue to monitor weight increase and patient activity level, reinforce needs for after care and provide list of community support groups
Psychology Actions	Introduction to primary therapist	Initiate evaluation of coping mechanisms of a family system facilitated by eating disorder; initiate cognitive restructuring.	Assess function eating disorder provides family system, encourage to verbalize feelings of anger, frustration as opposed to silent self-destructive behavior (ie. starvation), facilitate adaptation of effective coping mechanisms.	Family and/or individual couples therapy for parents is useful in assisting age-appropriate separation and symptom alleviation.
Dietary Actions	Identify caloric intake prior to admission; assess client food likes and dislikes

Patient verbalizes commitment to attempt recovery agreeing to assigned dietary intake. | Assess patient's current dietary intake and revise caloric intake if clinically indicated.

Attends 100% of meals, meets nutritional goals as established by patient and treatment team as indicated to facilitate food intake, verbalize feelings of anxiety/fear | Continue to assess dietary intake and increase caloric intake as clinically indicated.

Continue to attend 100% of meals, meets 100% of established nutritional goals. Continue to identify risk foods and weight points that trigger anxiety. | Collaborate with team in creating "ideal" discharge caloric intake, assist in identifying 3-5 day meal plan with grocery list and client's ability to "handle" food.

Commits to eating 100% of discharge meal plan, makes 2 personal meals their last week of treatment, identify anxiety relating to personal preparation of food. Verbalize fear of maintaining discharge body weight. |

Courtesy Laureate Psychiatric Clinic and Hospital Eating Disorders Program, Tulsa, Oklahoma.

The Nursing Process

Box 28-8

Body Image Enhancement

DEFINITION

Improving a patient's conscious and unconscious perceptions and attitudes toward his/her body

ACTIVITIES

Determine patient's body image expectations, based on developmental stage

Use anticipatory guidance to prepare patient for changes in body image that are predictable

Determine whether perceived dislike for certain physical characteristics creates a dysfunctional social paralysis for teenagers and other high-risk groups

Assist patient to discuss changes caused by illness or surgery, as appropriate

Help patient determine the extent of actual changes in the body or its level of functioning

Determine whether a recent physical change has been incorporated into patient's body image

Assist patient to separate physical appearance from feelings of personal worth, as appropriate

Assist to determine the influence of a peer group on the patient's perception of present body image

Assist patient to discuss changes caused by puberty, as appropriate

Assist patient to discuss changes caused by a normal pregnancy, as appropriate

Assist patient to discuss changes caused by aging, as appropriate

Teach the patient the normal changes in the body associated with various stages of aging, as appropriate

Assist the patient to discuss stressors affecting body image due to congenital condition, injury, disease, or surgery

Identify the significance of the patient's culture, religion, race, gender, and age on body image

Monitor frequency of statements of self-criticism

Monitor whether patient can look at the changed body part

Monitor for statements that identify body image perceptions concerned with body shape and body weight

Use self-picture drawing as a mechanism for evaluating a child's body image perceptions

Instruct children about the functions of the various body parts, as appropriate

Determine patient's and family's perceptions of the alteration in body image versus reality

Identify coping strategies used by parents in response to changes in child's appearance

Determine how child responds to parents' reactions, as appropriate

Teach parents the importance of their responses to the child's body changes and future adjustment, as appropriate

Determine whether a change in body image has contributed to increased social isolation

Assist patient in identifying parts of body that have positive perceptions associated with them

Identify means of reducing the impact of any disfigurement through clothing, wigs, or cosmetics, as appropriate

Assist patients to identify actions that will enhance appearance

Assist the hospitalized patient to apply cosmetics before seeing visitors, as appropriate

Facilitate contact with individuals with similar changes in body image

Identify support groups available to patient

Assist client at risk for anorexia or bulimia to develop more realistic body image expectations

Use self-disclosure exercises with groups of teenagers or others distraught over normal physical attributes

Reprinted with permission from McCloskey J.C., & Bulechek G.M. (Eds.). (1996). Nursing interventions classification (NIC), *(2nd ed.) St. Louis: Mosby.*

liefs and substituting more realistic, rational ones. For example, a client with bulimia can be taught that there are no "forbidden foods" but rather excessive quantities of them. Distortions of reality can be "relabeled" and corrected with cognitive confrontation. The distortion that all fats are forbidden can be directly confronted with specific facts relating to the body's need for and use of fats.

Positive and negative reinforcement Positive and negative reinforcement involves rewarding desirable behaviors and punishing undesirable ones. Positive reinforcement is the application of a rewarding consequence following the display of a specific behavior. Negative reinforcement is the removal of an adverse condition following the display of a specific behavior. Positive rein-

The Nursing Process

Box 28-9

Sample Contract for Clients With Eating Disorders

- The client must eat prescribed meal plan.
- Meals are to be eaten with staff, who record intake.
- The client has 1 hour to eat each meal.
- Initially the client may not attend exercise groups and is required to stay on the unit.
- The nurse may limit activity on the unit, as needed.
- The nurse may restrict the client to the day room when restriction is warranted because of contract violations.
- The client is restricted from the kitchen and bathroom use is monitored for 2 hours following meals.
- The client is weighed as ordered at the same time, in the same clothing, and with the same scale prior to morning voiding. Client can record own weight, if indicated.
- If client refuses to eat required portions, the client is restricted to the day room until the next meal is eaten.
- A meal equals at least three substantial servings (i.e., a substantial dinner includes one portion each of carbohydrate, protein, and vegetable).
- For underweight clients, no weight below the highest achieved weight (in hospital); for overweight clients no weight gain above the lowest achieved in the hospital. Weight loss or weight gain results in reevaluation of the client's commitment to treatment.
- When on bed rest or confined to the day room, client may not have visitors.

The contract is explained to the client and signed by both client and nurse. It is renegotiated as client needs and progress indicates.

forcement may involve permitting a client increased activity periods when he or she gains weight. Negative reinforcement may permit the nurse to restrict activity if the client loses weight. Positive and negative reinforcement interventions should be carefully planned by the multidisciplinary team and negotiated in the form of a therapeutic contract.

Assertiveness training Persons with eating disorders have major issues with control and therefore have difficulty with self-identity and assertiveness. Some assertiveness techniques that can be taught to clients include the following:

- Accept apologies
- Give and accept compliments
- Give and receive criticism
- Say "no" rather than do what others want

Clients should be given multiple opportunities to assert their feelings related to treatment and to learn to use their voices rather than bingeing or purging to express personal feelings.

Nutritional counseling

Because of designing complex eating plans, a registered dietitian is generally caring for clients with eating disorders a member of the interdisciplinary treatment team. The nurse may intervene by reinforcing the dietitian's nutritional counseling and carrying out orders to implement dietary recommendations. In general, nutritional counseling is an essential role of the nurse. The Research Highlight on p. 562 emphasizes the necessity of counseling young women about adequate nutritional intake.

Group counseling

Groups for clients with eating disorders focus on the dysfunctional behaviors and underlying dynamics. They aim to decrease clients' feelings of isolation and provide peer encouragement to clients who wish to change dysfunctional eating patterns. Support groups provide clients with opportunities to increase their social network and reshape perceptions of self and the environment. Clients learn solutions to their problems through sharing with others in similar situations.

Overeaters Anonymous (OA) is a Twelve-Step program that supports individuals with weight problems. This is an appropriate intervention because of the codependent dynamics present in some clients who experience eating disorders. Local chapters of the National Eating Disorders Association also provide support group intervention for clients and their families.

Family counseling

Family intervention for clients with eating disorders is multidimensional and includes psychoeducation as well as supportive and insight-oriented family therapy. The psychoeducational approach includes teaching the family about the dynamics of the illness, individual behaviors and reasons for them, and interactive family dynamics. Education allows family members to gain cognitive insight into what is happening within the family system. The goal of family counseling should be to facilitate the development of adaptive coping behaviors. The nurse's role is to refer families for therapy sessions or family support groups.

Milieu Therapy

In inpatient settings nurses are usually in charge of maintaining the therapeutic milieu. Nursing responsibilities

The Nursing Process

RESEARCH HIGHLIGHT

Portsmouth, K., Henderson, K., Graham, N., Price, R., Cole, J., & Allen, J. (1994). Dietary calcium intake in 18-year-old women: Comparison with recommended daily intake and dietary energy intake. *Journal of Advanced Nursing, 9*(20), 1073-1078.

Summary

The purpose of this study was to ascertain if young Australian women consumed adequate calcium during an important time in their lives. Subjects consisted of 113, 18-year-old university students in Western Australia who were asked to complete a health questionnaire developed specifically for this study. The average daily intake of calcium and the number of kilojoules* consumed were calculated using a 4-day record kept by all subjects. Subjects were instructed not to alter their normal dietary habits during the research period.

Diet records were analyzed for calcium and energy intakes using the diet software package. The average amounts of calcium and energy consumed per day for individual subjects were then calculated. Pearson's correlation coefficient was used to determine the relationship between the variables. An Alpha level of 0.05 was accepted for significance.

The mean calcium intake for the group of 18-year-olds was 734 mg/day. Of the group, 68% had a calcium intake below the 800 mg RDA. Thirty-two percent of the population had mean energy intakes below 6,300k. Chronic caloric/energy restriction was reported by the majority of subjects as a means to limit weight gain.

Implications for Clinical Practice

- Nurses should be aware that many young women have inadequate dietary calcium intakes.
- The amount of dairy products that hold calcium are generally high in caloric value, which increases fat and protein.
- Young women are reluctant to increase the calcium in their diet due to increased calories.
- Nurses may advise clients with insufficient calcium intake to elevate dietary calcium levels by increasing foods such as low-fat dairy products (skim milk, low-fat cheese, and yogurt), salmon, tofu, and broccoli.
- As the adolescent population ages it will be at increased risk for osteoporosis.

*Kilojoules are a measure of caloric intake.

include maintaining client safety and keeping the unit free of abusive substances such as diet pills, diuretics, laxatives and syrup of ipecac. Nurses are also responsible for enforcing the contracts established for clients by the team (see Box 28-9).

Self-Care Activities

Management of clients with eating disorders requires multiple interventions that involve self-care activities. Physical parameters such as vital signs, electrolytes, weight, intake and output, and caloric intake should be monitored and recorded. Accompanying the client to the bathroom to prevent vomiting and observing for signs of laxative abuse is another nursing responsibility. Providing for physical activity as needed and permitting clients

to choose appropriate exercise protocols facilities the client's self-esteem.

Exercise may be used by the client with anorexia or bulimia as a means to lose weight and alter body size. Exercise should not be allowed until the client is physically stable. Clients should be encouraged to limit all physical activity until weight gain occurs. Clients who are obese should be encouraged to begin exercise slowly after being authorized to exercise by their physicians. Beginning an exercise program with pool activities is generally best for these clients.

Psychobiological Interventions

Many clients with anorexia restrict their medications because they perceive them as foreign substances that

The Nursing Process

cause weight gain. Clients who display multiple obsessive-compulsive disorder (OCD) traits, however, may benefit from treatment with medications such as fluoxetine (Prozac) and clomipramine (Anafranil) and should be encouraged to adhere to taking them when they are prescribed.

Clients with bulimia have experienced some positive responses to treatment with antidepressant medications. Imipramine (Tofranil), desipramine (Norpramin), trazadone (Desyrel), and fluoxetine have been shown to be effective in reducing bulimic symptoms. More research is needed about the efficacy of psychopharmalogical treatment.

For clients with eating disorders, staff members should treat food as medication. Food is prescribed and recorded as such. Medication Tips related to eating disorders are listed below.

Health Teaching

A key intervention in the management of clients with eating disorders is education about and management of their symptoms. Once the client's physical state is stable, education should generally be the first intervention used. Meal planning and nutritional instruction can begin immediately for clients with bulimia and clients who are binge eating.

Clients with anorexia begin an educational program after they have achieved their goal weight. The purpose of waiting before discussing management with clients who have anorexia is related to their obsessive preoccupation with food and their persistent drive to maintain a state of thinness when self-starvation behaviors may be life threatening. The initial focus of education for a client with anorexia should be on the life-threatening seriousness of dysfunctional eating behaviors. Control of intake

should be prescribed, much like medication would be. The primary goal is to facilitate an increase in the client's weight.

Clients with eating disorders should be taught alternative and healthy eating patterns. The Teaching Points below indicates ways in which the preparation and eating of food may be modified to achieve desired goals.

Case Management

Effective intervention with clients with eating disorders requires collaborative efforts by the client, nurse, family, and others who participate in their care. The physical problems of the client need to be managed by the physician or nurse practitioner. Social workers and nurses with advanced preparation should work together to help resolve the complex family issues of these clients. A dietitian may be involved in the meal planning process and a physical therapist helps exercise programs. Inpatient behavioral modification programs are planned by the interdisciplinary team and implemented by the nursing

TEACHING POINTS

Healthy Eating Patterns

The nurse should teach the client, family, and significant others the following:
- Shop for food after eating.
- Buy and prepare smaller (for clients who are obese) or larger (for clients with anorexia) quantities of food.
- List favorite and least favorite foods. Compare and determine caloric value of each.
- Eat in a specific spot on the unit (or at home).
- Do not eat while doing other activities, such as reading or watching television.
- Decrease (for clients who are obese) or increase (for clients with anorexia) high-calorie foods
- Use smaller (for clients who are obese) or larger (for clients with anorexia) plates to make portions look larger or smaller.
- Eat slowly and chew thoroughly.
- Put utensils down and wait 15 seconds between bites.
- Plan snacks that need to be chewed to satisfy oral needs (carrots, apples, celery).
- Drink sips of water at the table and at prescribed times.
- Determine nonfood-related rewards such as attending a movie or going shopping.

MEDICATION TIPS

Clients With Eating Disorders

- Clients should avoid laxatives, diuretics, and diet pills.
- Client should consult health care provider before taking over-the-counter medications.
- Client should inform health care provider about eating disorder whenever medication is prescribed.
- Antidepressant medication has been helpful to some clients with eating disorders.

The Nursing Process

staff or behavior specialist who has the 24-hour responsibility for a client's behavior.

Contracts are negotiated with clients and involve the collaboration with everyone involved in the client's care. Consistency is key to the success or failure of behavioral protocols that facilitate the client's timely movement from one level of care to another.

Health Promotion and Health Maintenance

Promoting optimum health of clients is a key component of health promotion. Support groups for individuals with eating disorders exist for this purpose. A list of national organizations that offer information to clients with bulimia and anorexia is found in the Community Resources box below. These national organizations provide information about the location of support groups and also list various treatment facilities and licensed therapists who specialize in treating clients with eating disorders. Educating the public about the dangers of unsupervised dieting and alerting parents and school officials about the symptoms of anorexia and bulimia are key preventive goals of nurses.

Evaluation

Clients with maladaptive eating patterns provide a variety of challenges to nursing personnel. Dealing with internal psychological conflict while encouraging nourishment of the body is a mutual challenge of client and nurse. Effectiveness of treatment can be evaluated in the following areas:

- Has the client initiated/progressed toward more adaptive eating patterns?
- Have biological and psychological needs been addressed and corrected?
- Have associated social and cultural problems been resolved?
- Has a relapse prevention plan been developed?

Nursing care should be modified as needed. The chronic nature of eating disorders often requires that clients participate in long-term maintenance treatment programs, which include ongoing outpatient treatment, medication management, and participation in a support group or other twelve-step organization such as Overeaters Anonymous.

KEY POINTS

- The client with anorexia nervosa engages in relentless pursuit of thinness, intensely fears becoming fat, and has a delusional disturbance of body image.
- Individuals with anorexia nervosa have the potential to literally starve themselves to death and must be treated as dangers to themselves.
- Bulimia nervosa is an eating disorder commonly referred to as *binge-purge syndrome*. It is characterized by episodic rapid consumption of large amounts of food in a short time. Termination of an

 COMMUNITY RESOURCES

American Anorexia and Bulimia Association
293 Central Park West, Suite 1R
New York, New York 10024
(212) 501-8351

Anorexia Nervosa and Bulimia Resource Center
111 Majorca Avenue
Coral Gables, Florida 33134
(305) 448-8325

Eating Disorders Awareness and Prevention
603 Stewart Street, Suite 803
Seattle, WA 98101-1229
(206) 382-3587

National Association of Anorexia Nervosa and Associated Disorders (ANAD)
P.O. Box 7
Highland Park, IL 60035
(847) 831-3438

National Eating Disorders Organization (NEDO)
(formerly National Anorexic Aid Society)
6655 South Yale Avenue
Tulsa, OK 74136
(918) 481-4044

Overeaters Anonymous (OA)
6075 Zenith Court, Northeast
Rio Rancho, New Mexico 87124-6424
(505) 891-2664

The Nursing Process

THE CONSUMER'S VOICE

Eating Disorders

Gabrielle Kitchener

To me, having anorexia is like having a police guard around me at all times admonishing me not to eat. Even though I now know the guard is only in my head, it was and still is at times as real to me as if a guard were actually standing beside me. Although thoughts about the fear of being fat are unwanted and just pop into my head, they can take over and become my life goal and purpose if I do not fight them.

When I was 11 years old I did not have much insight. I allowed the guard in my head to take over, so much so that I spent 2 years in Connecticut Valley Hospital trying to obey this guard who would not allow me to eat. During much of that time I let others make decisions for me, because I wanted someone to "save me." I couldn't understand why someone couldn't just wave a magic wand and cure me. It was only when I realized that I was the one who held the key to unlocking myself from the guard that I started making decisions and eating for myself.

Although I am no longer actively anorectic, I still fight the negative thoughts daily. I try to eat in a relaxed, supportive environment with other persons rather than alone. This way I am not alone with my thoughts, and I can focus on the social as well as nutritional aspects of eating. When I eat alone, I eat more junk food, and I think about calories. Also when I am alone I think about being sinful and evil, without worth. I try to be with others, listen to music, or write to get away from these negative thoughts. My friends help me by providing support and encouragement. My faith also helps me, offering me hope during my darkest times. Music and writing help me. Sitting in my rocking chair while listening to music is soothing. Writing poetry or writing down my thoughts is an outlet for my pent-up emotions. I enjoy going on religious retreats, which help me find peace and refocus—away from daily stressors.

Anorexia has had a profound impact on my life, both positively and negatively. It has caused me to have health problems, increased my susceptibility to suicidal thoughts, and perhaps contributed to the early onset of a muscle disease I now have. When I was a teenager, it affected my social life, because I was preoccupied with the problem and isolated myself. I was stigmatized by my family and friends. My parents' friends asked why I hadn't "gotten over it" yet. My friend's mother wouldn't allow me to socialize with my friend once she found out I had an eating disorder, because my friend might "catch it." Having anorexia has also influenced me positively, because it has given me greater insight into the problems of other people and a special sensitivity to others with eating disorders. I have greater empathy for people with any mental health problem because of our similar experiences.

The mental health care delivery system helped me only when I was given choices and was involved in goal setting and planning for my own treatment. I was helped especially by a counselor at a supervised apartment I lived in. The counselor would sit down in the evenings with me and just talk—about my worries, my fears, and my hopes. I ate better when eating was not tied to a behavioral program. Seclusion and withholding of my belongings did not help me, and I wouldn't recommend it for others with eating disorders.

Force feeding (i.e., tube feeding) should only be used as a lifesaving measure. It should not be used as a means of control. It is important to feed the spirit as well as the body. A person with anorexia (don't label me an *anorectic*) is not a dog who is being conditioned to respond to a Pavlovian bell. Don't judge; remember that the person is in pain and always needs compassion as well as firmness and guidance.

eating episode takes place when abdominal pain, sleep, social interruption, excessive exercise, or self-induced vomiting occurs. Laxatives and/or diuretics may also be used to purge.
• Binge eating disorder (BED) is characterized by symptoms of bulimia and impaired control behav-

iors such as eating rapidly, eating large amounts until uncomfortably full, eating alone, eating when not hungry, and feeling disgust or guilt after overeating.
• Clients who have parents who are obese have a genetic predisposition to obesity.

CRITICAL THINKING QUESTIONS

Ann P. was brought to the psychiatric unit for an evaluation. According to Ann's husband, "she just quit eating about 1 year ago." Ann reports struggling with body image issues since she was a teenager. Upon completion of the nursing interview, Ann's husband becomes angry and states, "None of this would have happened if she would just eat."

1. What is your first impression of Ann?
2. What is your first impression of Ann's husband?
3. How do you feel about your own body shape and size?
4. What information do you need to gather to effectively assess Ann?
5. In what ways would you work with Ann to encourage and support her to increase her food intake?
6. Should Ann's activity level be restricted, and if so, how?
7. What information should Ann's husband be given about eating disorders?

• Family dynamics encourage clients to sacrifice self in an attempt to stabilize the family system.
• The majority of clients with eating disorders are female.
• Sociocultural factors influence the manner in which women perceive their bodies. Many young women believe "thinness will make me happy."
• Behavioral techniques such as positive and negative reinforcement, guided imagery, substitution, and cognitive restructuring help clients who binge and purge or eat compulsively to control their eating disorders.
• Eating disorders are sometimes treated with pharmacological agents such as selective serotonin reuptake inhibitors.

REFERENCES

APA Working Group on Eating Disorders. (1993). American Psychiatric Association practice guidelines: Practice guidelines for eating disorders. *American Journal of Psychiatry, 150,* 207.

American Psychiatric Association. (1994). *Diagnostic and statistical manual of mental disorders, fourth edition,* Washington, DC: Author.

Bruch, H. (1970). Psychotherapy in primary anorexia nervosa. *Journal of Mental and Nervous Diseases, 150,* 51-66.

Bruch, H. (1978). *The golden cage.* Cambridge, MA: Harvard University Press.

Conrad N., Sloan S., & Jedwabny J. (1992). Resolving the control struggle on an eating disorders unit, *Perspectives in Psychiatric Care, 28,* 13.

Holmi, K.A. (1994). Eating disorders: Anorexia nervosa, bulimia nervosa, and obesity. In RE Hales, S.C. Yudofsky & J.A. Talbott (Eds.). *Textbook of Psychiatry* (2nd ed). Washington D.C. American Psychiatric Press.

Kaplan, H.I., Sadock, B.J. & Grebb, J.A. (1994). *Synopsis of Psychiatry* (7th Ed.) Baltimore: Williams and Wilkins.

Fontaine, K.L. (1991). The conspiracy of culture: women's issues in body size. *Nursing Clinics of North America, 26,* 669.

Kaye, W., & Weltzin, T. (1991). Neurochemistry of bulimia nervosa. *Journal of Clinical Psychiatry, 52,* 21-28.

Kaye, W., & Weltzin, T. (1991). Serotonin activity in anorexia and bulimia nervosa: Relationship to the modulation of feeding and mood. *Journal of Clinical Psychiatry, 52,* 41-48.

Koepp, W., Schildbach, S., Schmager, C., & Rohner, R. (1993). Borderline diagnosis and substance abuse in female patients with eating disorders. *International Journal of Eating Disorders, 14*(1), 107-110.

Minuchin, S., Rosman, B., & Baker, L. (1978). *Psychosomatic families: Anorexia nervosa in context.* Cambridge, MA: Harvard University Press.

McCloskey, J.C., & Bulechek, G.M. (1996) *Nursing interventions classification (NIC)* (2nd ed.). St. Louis: Mosby.

Palmer, T. (1990). Anorexia nervosa, bulimia nervosa: Causal theories and treatment. *Nurse Practitioner, 15,* 12-21.

Pheln, K.W. (1990). Anorexia nervosa and bulimia: Incidence and diagnosis. *Nurse Practitioner, 15*(4) 22-25, 28, 31.

Sansone, R., & Dennis, A. (1994). *Overview of eating disorders.* Columbus, Ohio: National Anorexic Aid Society.

Stunkard, A.J., & Meyer, J.M. (1993) *Genetics and human obesity: Theory and therapy* (2nd ed). New York: Raven Press.

Swift, W.J. (1991). Bruch revisited: The role of interpretation of transference and resistance in the psychotherapy of eating disorders. In C. Johnson (Ed.). *Psychodynamic treatment of anorexia and bulimia.* New York: Guilford Press.

Trimpey, L. (1996). *Taming the feast beast: How to recognize the voice of fatness and end your struggle with food forever.* New York: Delacort.

Waller, G. (1992). Sexual abuse and bulimic symptoms in eating disorders: Do family interaction and self-esteem explain the links? *International Journal of Eating Disorders 12*(3), 235-240.

Wolfe, Barbara E. (June, 1995). Dimensions of response to antidepressant agents in bulimia nervosa: A review. *Archives of Psychiatric Nursing, IX,*(3), 111-121.

Chapter 29

Schizophrenia and Other Psychotic Disorders

Mary Walker

LEARNING OUTCOMES

After studying and applying the concepts of this chapter, the learner will be able to:

- Summarize biological and psychosocial correlates of schizophrenia.
- Explain differences between Type I and Type II schizophrenia.
- Describe cognitive, perceptual, affective, behavioral, and social changes seen in persons with schizophrenia.
- Discuss epidemiological factors related to schizophrenia.
- Discuss assessment tools used in the evaluation of schizophrenia.
- Develop a nursing care plan for a client with schizophrenia.
- Describe interventions related to counseling, milieu therapy, self care, psychobiology and health teaching.
- Explain the value of using case management and an interdisciplinary approach with persons who have schizophrenia.
- Use preventive interventions for at-risk populations.

KEY TERMS

Cognition	Fixed delusion	Positive symptoms
Delusion	Hallucination	Psychosis
Delusional system	Illusion	Thought broadcasting
Depersonalization	Labile	Thought insertion
Derealization	Negative symptoms	Type I schizophrenia
Ego boundary	Paranoia	Type II schizophrenia
Expressed emotion	Perception	Water intoxication

chizophrenia and other psychotic disorders have been described for hundreds of years. These disorders have carried with them a burden of fear, stigma, and superstition that contribute to their devastating effects.

Schizophrenia is the major illness in a group of disorders having psychotic features. These features are characterized by loss of ego boundaries and impairment in reality testing. This could include the presence of hallucinations or delusions. Clients with these disorders often exhibit disorganized thinking (as noted by abnormal speech patterns) and grossly disorganized behavior.

Globally, the occurrence rates of schizophrenia are similar, affecting about 1% of the population. Thus 1 to 2 million people in the United States have the disorder. Some of these individuals experience intermittent symptoms; others will follow a severe and persistent course. The estimated cost of schizophrenia to society was estimated at $48.2 billion in 1983, and it is projected to reach $55 billion by 2007 (Murphy and Moller, 1993). In addition, the personal and family costs of the illness cannot be calculated.

The purpose of this chapter is to generate insight into the world of a person with psychoses and to explore the role of the nurse in caring for the client with schizophrenia in hospital- and community-based settings. In addition, this chapter outlines the nursing process for individuals, families, and the community that transcends specific treatment settings.

EPIDEMIOLOGY

To put schizophrenia in perspective, it is useful to look at statistical data that describe this phenomenon. Schizophrenia is an illness with a fairly stable prevalence over the past 50 years. Rates of this disorder are higher for those with first-degree relatives who have schizophrenia. The onset of schizophrenia is at 15 to 45 years of age, but most commonly is first seen in a person's late teens or early twenties. The average age of onset is 19 years (Keith and Regier, 1991), although women tend to develop symptoms of the illness 3 to 4 years later than men (Betemps and Ragiel, 1994).

The course of the illness varies. Of those with schizophrenia, 25% to 33% have unrelenting symptoms from the first episode, and in 50%, these symptoms appear intermittently. In other individuals, there is one psychotic break, and then no symptoms are seen thereafter (Keith and Regier, 1991). In addition, persons with schizophrenia have higher mortality and suicide rates. One in ten will succeed with suicide attempts in the first 10 years of the illness (Betemps and Ragiel, 1994). Interestingly, persons with schizophrenia have abnormally low rates of rheumatoid arthritis but are at higher risk for heart disease (Aksu and Myers, 1994). Some risk factors for the development of schizophrenia are listed in Box 29-1.

Box 29-1

Risk Factors for Schizophrenia

- Close relative with schizotypal personality disorder
- Close relative with schizophrenia
- Winter/spring birthdate
- Second trimester prenatal influenza infection
- 15 to 45 years of age
- Early history of attentional deficits

Although schizophrenia is seen in all parts of the world, symptoms are remarkably similar across different cultural groups. Efforts are under way by the World Health Organization (WHO) to standardize diagnostic criteria for schizophrenia. Studies conducted to date have indicated that schizophrenia can be diagnosed reliably in various settings, since core symptoms are so much alike (Karno and Jenkins, 1993). For example, in most cultural groups studied, predominant symptoms were a sense that the person's thoughts were being taken away, read by an alien agency or broadcast. Often, people with schizophrenia across cultural groups used identical comments to describe the distress of auditory hallucinations (Betemps and Ragiel, 1994). If particular cultural beliefs are misinterpreted as delusions or "odd thinking" an illness may be diagnosed in error.

There are, however, mental illnesses specific to a particular cultural group, which may resemble psychotic symptoms. Evidence exists of overdiagnosis and misdiagnosis of schizophrenia among African-American and other ethnic groups, so providers must be astute in exploring symptoms (Campinha-Bacote, 1994). Diagnosticians may incorrectly label a person with schizophrenia if a culturally sensitive assessment has not first been completed.

Another striking finding noted is that the course of schizophrenia seems to be milder and more benign in developing countries than in countries such as the United States. Since many other cultures tend to have low amounts of "expressed emotion" such as criticism, hostility and overinvolvement in family settings, it has been postulated that this may be why individuals with schizophrenia may fare better in these cultures (Karno and Jenkins, 1993). Some other considerations and examples of cultural factors are found in the Cultural Highlights box on p. 569.

THEORETICAL FRAMEWORK

Biological Correlates

The current predominant biological research conducted to explain symptoms of schizophrenia can be grouped into two general approaches, neurophysiological and neuroanatomical.

CULTURAL HIGHLIGHTS

Assessment
- Clients from different cultures may exhibit varying symptoms. For example, in persons from developed countries depression is less often associated with schizophrenia (Ragiel, 1994).
- They may also exhibit paranoid or other delusions related to powerful agencies in their culture such as demons or spirits versus the government.

Diagnosis
- Cultural context of the symptoms must be reviewed by the health care team. For example, the delusion that illness or death may come to an individual through a supernatural force may reflect the culture bound syndrome of "voodoo illness" in some African-American and Black Caribbean cultures (Campinha-Bacote, 1994).

Intervention
- Close monitoring of side effects should be done with the person's heritage in mind. Extrapyramidal symptoms (EPSs) may be seen at lower effective doses in Asian Americans. (Campinha-Bacote, 1994)
- Family involvement in care should be sensitive to cultural issues. Explore sensitive family issues gently but completely in Asian-American families; they may communicate in a less direct manner than the dominant American culture (Frye D'Avanzo, 1994). This could also be misconstrued as a speech or language disorder in the client.
- Some cultural groups such as those of Hispanic descent emphasize inclusion of the extended family in treatment plans. Efforts should be made to include family members,

Neurophysiological factors

Metabolic activity One neurophysiological correlate of illness is related to the metabolic activity of the brain.

By the use of positron emission tomography (PET) scanning and single photon emission computed tomography (SPECT), researchers are able to measure regional cerebral blood flow. PET scans also measure the metabolic rate of glucose in areas of the brain. Many studies have shown that individuals with schizophrenia have decreased blood flow and decreased glucose metabolism notably in the frontal areas of the brain *(hypofrontality)* as seen in Color Plate 8. Neuropsychological testing of cognitive functions also tends to confirm this finding. Frontal lobes govern planning, abstract thinking, and social judgement so one can surmise that this deficit is seen behaviorally as an inability to act in socially acceptable ways (Grinspoon, 1992). An example of this would be a client who begins to travel across the country without any personal possessions, money, or possibly the exact location of the destination. Short-term memory may also be diminished as a result of hypofrontality (Keefe and Harvey, 1994).

In addition, abnormalities of temporal lobe functioning have also been reported from electroencephalogram (EEG) studies. Hallucinations have been associated with accelerated glucose metabolism in the left temporal lobe. There is also evidence of generalized cortical and subcortical dysfunction, which could account for the varying symptom presentations in this disorder (Waddington, 1993).

Neurotransmitter theory The neurotransmitter theory model proposes that symptoms of schizophrenia are related to dysfunction in one of four neurotransmitter systems: dopamine, serotonin, norepinephrine, and gamma-aminobutyric acid (GABA) systems of the brain (Csernansky and Newcomer, 1994). Of these, the dopamine system has been the most extensively studied. The major problem is an excess of dopamine in certain brain areas in people with schizophrenia.

Despite the amount of research into this area, however, there is still a poor understanding of the specific relationship between dopamine dysfunction and subsequent deficits (Cohen and Servan-Schreiber, 1993). It is postulated that one or perhaps a combination of the following accounts for symptoms:

- Overall increase in dopamine levels: It has been found that antipsychotic medication works primarily by lowering dopamine level.
- There could be an increased number or sensitivity of the dopamine receptor sites in the brain.
- There could be a decrease in the number of presynaptic dopamine receptors or autoreceptors. These autoreceptors inhibit dopamine synthesis so that too few would have the net effect of keeping dopamine levels higher.
- It is possible that there is a lowered amount of a naturally occurring dopamine antagonist in the brain. GABA, for example, may prevent the creation of dopamine, so if GABA is too low, increased dopamine may result (Thompson, 1990).
- Five dopamine receptor subtypes are as follows:
  - D_1 receptors have no known direct role in producing psychotic symptoms, but have been found to influence D_2 functioning.
  - D_2 receptors are located in the limbic and motor neuron centers. Overactivation may be responsible

for "positive" psychotic symptoms such as hallucinations, paranoia, and delusions. Color Plate 5 in the Chapter 13 color insert presents images depicting the location of the D_1 and D_2 receptors.

- D_3 receptor stimulation may be linked with "negative" symptoms such as blunted affect, emotional withdrawal, and apathy.
- D_4 receptors are located in neuron centers that influence regulation of stress-related dopamine activities and thought processes and possibly are associated with "positive" symptoms as D_2 receptors.
- D_5 receptors are found only in limbic regions and may be related to behavior. (Seemen, 1995)

The serotonin and norepinephrine systems have been less intensely studied, but it is thought that these may act to modulate systems within the limbic areas (Csernansky and Newcomer, 1994). Interest in the serotonin system has been aroused recently with the discovery that some of the newer antipsychotic medications such as clozapine (Clozaril) have an affinity for serotonin 5-HT_2 receptors. These medications seem to target both "positive" and "negative" symptoms such as hallucinations and avolition (Hultunen, 1995).

Information processing The way people with schizophrenia process information is also thought to reflect an abnormality in neurophysiology. Specifically, individuals with schizophrenia are less able to perceive, attend to, and retain information received from the environment (Gold and Harvey, 1993). Clients with schizophrenia seem to have generalized deficits as well as specific abnormalities.

In the left hemisphere of the brain, dysfunction has been examined in terms of overactivation and consequent temporal abnormalities. The result is seen as a delay in processing incoming sensory information. For example, a client may take longer to respond to questions. Antipsychotic medication is believed to help speed up this process.

Attentional impairments are noted to include deficits in the ability to sustain attention to relevant information while at the same time to ignore extraneous information (Siever et al., 1993). Consequently, all incoming information seems important, and it is difficult to focus on a task without being distracted.

Memory Memory is a cognitive process that is also affected by schizophrenia. Specifically, clients show impairment in verbal and visual memory suggesting bilateral hemispheric abnormalities. Storage of images to the short-term memory is slower, and a lowered number of neurons in the prefrontal cortex may also affect memory. This could be seen as a decrease in stored memory and decreased retrieval of stored information into conscious awareness (Freeman and Karson, 1993).

Finally, an interesting neurophysiological phenomena has been noted among people with schizophrenia, schizotypal personality disorder, and relatives of people with schizophrenia. When confronted with a slowly moving target such as a pendulum, clients exhibit impairment in tracking the movement smoothly with their eyes. This has been linked to frontal brain dysfunction, but the exact mechanism of this is not known (Siever et al., 1993).

Neuroanatomical factors

In addition to altered physiology, there are specific and measurable abnormalities in the actual structure of the brain, which have been determined with the advent of scanning techniques and other physiological tests. Computed tomography (CT) and magnetic resonance imaging (MRI) scanning have elucidated striking differences between the brains of persons with schizophrenia and normal brains. The five areas of abnormality that will be examined are as follows:

1. *Decreased cerebral and cranial size.* This has also been viewed as "cortical atrophy." However, some researchers believe that smaller cerebral and cranial sizes are results of faulty development of the brain rather than a shrinking of established brain mass (Nasrallah, 1993).
2. *Lowered numbers of cortical neurons.* This phenomena is seen more distinctly in the frontal lobes (Freeman and Karson, 1993). Negative symptoms of schizophrenia are believed to be a result of frontal lobe dysfunction, although it is not known whether this accounts for these symptoms.
3. *Decreased volume of other brain areas.* Persons with schizophrenia tend to have a smaller volume of limbic temporal lobe structures, especially in the hippocampus region (Nasrallah, 1993). Diminution of the substantia nigra and putamen exists in some studies. Color Plate 8 in the Chapter 15 color insert depicts areas of decreased brain volume.
4. *Ventricular abnormalities.* Considerable evidence supports a phenomena of cerebral ventricle enlargement especially of the third and lateral ventricles. Also seen is an increased prominence of cortical sulci and fissures (Cannon and Marco, 1994). Asymmetries of ventricular enlargement have been noted in the temporal horns on the left side as compared with the right. Asymmetries of the Sylvan fissures, which are normally larger in the left hemisphere, are smaller. These abnormalities are created by faulty development of the brain from genetic or other early factors (Crow, 1995). Fig. 29-1 presents MRI scans depicting ventricle

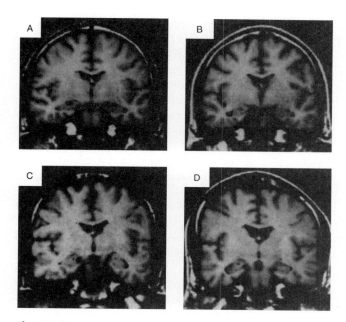

Fig. 29-1   Magnetic resonance imaging (MRI) scans of two sets of monozygotic twins. One twin in each set was diagnosed with schizophrenia (*B* and *D*). *B* and *D* show subtle enlargement of the lateral ventricles in the affected twins as compared with the unaffected twins (*A* and *C*). (From Suddath, R.L. et al. (1990). Anatomical abnormalities in the brains of monozygotic twins discordant for schizophrenia. *The New England Journal of Medicine, 322*(12) 789-794.)

enlargement in twins with schizophrenia versus the size of ventricles in unaffected twins.

5. *Thalamic changes.* Reduced volume has been found in the thalamic nuclei in several studies (Freeman and Karson, 1993). This has been of interest to researchers because many symptoms of schizophrenia can be explained by abnormalities in this area of the brain (Andraeson, 1995).

Genetic Correlates

One of the earliest observations of persons with schizophrenia was that the illness aggregates (clusters) in families. The risk for schizophrenia in a first-degree relative of a person with schizophrenia is 9.7 times greater than the general population (Kendler and Diehl, 1993). From studying twins, it has also been found that a monozygotic twin has a nearly 50% rate of developing schizophrenia if the sibling is schizophrenic (Kaplan, Sadock, and Grebb, 1994).

In addition, findings from studies of children with schizophrenia in their families but who were adopted indicate that these children have a higher risk of developing schizophrenia themselves. This, of course, lends sup-

port to a model of schizophrenia that implicates genetic transmission. However, recent adoption studies show that among troubled families, there is an increased risk of schizophrenia, which is consistent with the idea that the illness may occur when genetically susceptible persons experience stressful environments (Kendler and Diehl, 1993).

Psychosocial Correlates

Historically, in the absence of specific biological causes, it was believed that psychosocial factors were primarily responsible for the development of psychosis. Psychodynamic and family theories were espoused to explain the etiologic factors of a psychotic illness. These theories are no longer accepted today as viable explanations for the occurrence of schizophrenia.

Familial Correlates

Specific aspects of family life have been studied that seem to be linked to relapse in schizophrenia. One of these is the quantity and quality of expressed emotion in the family. *Expressed emotion, or EE, is a concept that refers to three main communication and behavioral factors in family relationships: criticism, hostility, and overinvolvement.* Families may be classified as having high or low EE based on the Camberwell Family Interview (CFI) (Gamble, 1994). Those families with high EE tend to be either highly overinvolved, hostile, or critical, whereas families with low EE tend to be more warm, understanding, and tolerant. If a person with schizophrenia lives in a family situation with high EE, that person has a higher probability of relapse than does a person living in a low EE setting (Karno and Jenkins, 1993). However, these factors are not identified as causing schizophrenia but could exacerbate symptoms of an underlying biological dysfunction. Expression of emotion is not necessarily a static concept though, and may fluctuate during time. This may represent a reciprocal relationship between the family and the client's illness process (Stirling et al., 1993).

Sociocultural Correlates

Evidence for the biological bases of schizophrenia is strong, but biological theories do not completely explain why some individuals have an earlier onset or have a serious and persistent course. To integrate understanding of the biological and environmental influences on schizophrenia, the stress vulnerability model of schizophrenia has been proposed. This model postulates that certain individuals have genetic or earlier-acquired impairments that make them vulnerable to developing psychosis when exposed to stress (Gardner and Thompson,

1992). The stress vulnerability model proposes that certain people have a permanent vulnerability to develop schizophrenia (O'Connor, 1991).

According to this perspective, the onset or relapses of psychotic symptoms results from interactions among personal vulnerabilities, (especially psychosocial), and personal and environmental protectors (O'Connor, 1991).

Thus the nurse should be careful not to assume a judgmental attitude toward clients and "blame" them for relapse (see the Research Highlight below). Minimizing stress and maximizing the protective factors should theoretically lessen occurrence and severity of psychotic episodes. Examples of stressors that could be minimized or eliminated might include:

- Living in a hostile, critical environment
- Numerous environmental changes
- Job pressures
- Poor social skills
- Low self-esteem
- Poverty
- Lack of good health habits
- Stigmatization

Protective factors that could be encouraged include:

- Engaging the client in a positive support system such as a support group
- Family education on creating a low EE family atmosphere
- Social skills training
- Focus on a client's strengths in addition to his/her challenges.
- Advocacy for supportive employment

A phenomena called "downward economic drift" occurs in many persons with schizophrenia and often places them in a low socioeconomic status (Dohrenwend et al., 1992). This lack of resources then compromises the individuals ability to obtain optimal services and in fact, 30% receive their treatment from a general medical physician or nonmental health human service provider (Betemps and Ragiel, 1994).

Another view states that this illness is a cultural creation of modern Western civilization because it was first defined in a Western cultural context. Foucault (1973) and Szasz (1974) believe that the concept of "madness" with which schizophrenia is very much intertwined, is a culturally produced definition that is neither universally valid nor defined as a medical disease. Szasz supports the position that psychiatric diagnoses are stigmatizing labels and that one is ill only if one feels ill. He believes that people should not be labeled and treated as ill simply because they demonstrate behavior that has traditionally and culturally been labeled as ill. Although this idea has its followers, the concept is not universally accepted. However, there are several grass-roots organizations such as the National Alliance of Mentally Ill (NAMI), who agree that labels of mental illness are stigmatizing and more focus should be placed on these disorders as neurobiological diseases rather than as subjective illnesses.

RESEARCH HIGHLIGHT

Fetter, M.S., & Lowery, B.J. (1992). Psychiatric rehospitalization of the severely mentally ill: Patient and staff perspectives. *Nursing Research, 41* (5), 301-305.

Summary
The purpose of this study was to examine client and staff beliefs about what caused client relapse and what impact that belief had on clients. Clients were interviewed separately and asked to list a cause of why they were rehospitalized. Results indicated how clients thought that internal and uncontrollable aspects of their illnesses were the cause of readmission. Staff members also tended to attribute problems to something internal in the client; however, they were more likely to see the cause as inadequate effort, something under the client's control.

Implications for Nursing Practice
- If clients believe that readmission to the hospital is uncontrollable, it may be necessary to intervene so that a self-fulfilling prophecy or a fatalistic view of the future does not occur.
- Nurses must guard against a judgmental attitude toward clients. Even with the best effort, on the client's part, relapse may not always be avoidable.

The *Nursing Process*

Nurses encounter clients with schizophrenia and their families in a variety of settings. A client who is acutely disturbed may be admitted to a short-term, acute-care inpatient setting for stabilization that provides a foundation for psychiatric rehabilitation, or a long-term residential setting for extended symptom management and rehabilitation. The client may receive treatment in a halfway house, day-treatment center, community rehabilitation program, outpatient clinic, or the home, all of which contribute to maximizing the client's highest level of functioning and integration within a family and community setting.

Assessment

Clinical Profile

Psychosis is a term used as a defining characteristic for a number of neurobiological disorders including schizophrenia. The term *psychosis* has many definitions, none of which are universally agreed upon. In its most limited sense, *psychosis* refers to the experience of positive symptoms such as hallucinations or delusions with an absence of insight about their dysfunctional nature (American Psychiatric Association [APA], 1994). In a broader sense, it also includes other positive symptoms such as disorganized speech and behavior (or catatonia) and negative symptoms (Box 29-2). Psychosis can also be considered on a severity continuum, from a brief psychotic disorder to schizophrenia, which in its most severe form is a persistent, lifelong disorder (Box 29-3). Table 29-1 highlights major features of schizophrenia and related disorders (APA, 1994). Box 29-4 identifies subtypes of schizophrenia.

Positive and negative symptoms

The symptomology of schizophrenia is often grouped into two categories, positive and negative symptoms.

This does not refer to the relative desirability of the symptoms. *Positive symptoms* refer to an excessive amount or gross distortion of normal function. *Negative symptoms* denote a lessening or complete loss of normal functions (see Box 29-2).

Positive symptoms are often reduced by the administration of traditional antipsychotic medication. Some of the newer antipsychotic medications such as clozapine (Clonaril) and risperidone (Risperdal) have been effective in lessening negative symptoms as well.

BOX 29-2

Positive and Negative Symptoms of Schizophrenia

POSITIVE SYMPTOMS

Hallucinations
Delusions
Disorganized speech
Looseness of associations
Bizarre behavior

NEGATIVE SYMPTOMS

Poverty of speech (Alogia)
Affective blunting
Anhedonia
Social withdrawal
Apathy
Avolition
Poor grooming
Attentional impairment

BOX 29-3

Continuum of Increasing Severity of Psychotic Disorders

LESS SEVERE		MORE SEVERE	
Brief psychotic disorder	Schizophreniform disorder	Substance-induced psychosis	Schizoaffective disorder
Delusional disorder		Psychosis related to a	Schizophrenia
Shared psychotic disorder		medical condition	

The Nursing Process

TABLE 29-1

Major features of schizophrenia and related disorders

DSM-IV DIAGNOSIS	MAJOR FEATURES
Brief psychotic disorder	Presence of one or more of the following: • Delusions • Hallucinations • Disorganized speech • Grossly disorganized or catatonic behavior Symptoms that are culturally sanctioned should not be included. The duration of an episode is at least 1 day, but less than one month with an eventual full return to premorbid functioning. The pressure or absence of stressors should be noted as should postpartum onset (within 4 weeks after delivery).
Delusional disorder	Nonbizarre delusions of at least 1 month's duration that might include situations that occur in real life such as being followed, poisoned, infected or deceived. Person has not met criteria for schizophrenia. Apart from the impact of the delusion, functioning is not markedly impaired and behavior is not odd or bizarre.
Shared psychotic disorder (folie à deux)	A delusion develops in a person in the context of a close relationship with another person(s) who has an already established delusion. The content of the delusions are similar.
Schizophreniform disorder	Meets criteria for schizophrenia, but an episode of the disorder lasts at least 1 month but less than 6 months. Good prognostic features are evident with two or more of the following: • Onset of psychotic symptoms within four weeks of the first noticeable change in usual behavior or functioning • Confusion present at height of psychotic episode • Absence of flat or blunted affect • Good premorbid social and occupational functioning
Substance-induced psychotic disorder	Prominent hallucinations or delusions that have developed during, or within a month, of substance intoxication or withdrawal or are related to medication use.
Psychotic disorder due to a general medical condition	Presence of prominent hallucinations or delusions that do not occur exclusively during the course of a delirium, nor are accounted for by another mental disorder. Evidence from the history, physical, or laboratory findings that the symptoms are a direct result of a medical condition.
Schizoaffective disorder	An uninterrupted period of illness which, at some time, includes either a major depressive episode, a manic episode, or a mixed episode concurrent with the symptoms of schizophrenia. During the same period, there are hallucinations or delusions for at least 2 weeks without accompanying mood symptoms. Symptoms of a mood disturbance are present for a significant portion of the illness.

The Nursing Process

TABLE 29-1—cont'd

Major features of schizophrenia and related disorders

DSM-IV DIAGNOSIS	MAJOR FEATURES
Schizophrenia	At least two of the following, each present for a significant period of time during a 1 month period: • Delusions • Hallucinations • Disorganized speech • Grossly disorganized or catatonic behavior • Negative symptoms Also present for a significant period of time since the onset of disturbance is one or more major areas of dysfunction in work, interpersonal relations or self-care that is markedly below the level achieved before onset. Continuous signs of the disturbance persist for at least 6 months.

BOX 29-4

Subtypes of Schizophrenia

PARANOID SCHIZOPHRENIA

• Tends to occur in later life and is characterized by suspiciousness and delusions of persecution and grandeur

DISORGANIZED SCHIZOPHRENIA

• Characterized by a flat or incongruous affect
• Bizarre mannerisms and social isolation occur
• The onset of this type of schizophrenia occurs early in life and tends to be chronic.

CATATONIC SCHIZOPHRENIA

• Noted by periods of behavior that fluctuate between a complete stupor and mutism, and psychomotor agitation accompanied by almost constant talking and shouting

UNDIFFERENTIATED SCHIZOPHRENIA

• A category used when clients' symptoms are mixed and cannot fit into a clearly defined category

RESIDUAL SCHIZOPHRENIA

• Characterized by at least one episode of psychosis but currently no psychotic features are present
• Some symptoms such as social isolation and other behavioral and cognitive changes may still persist.

Negative symptoms can be further classified into primary and secondary symptoms. The primary symptoms are those considered to be resulting from core neural defects. Secondary negative symptoms are caused by the following individually or in combination:

• Extrapyramidal side effects of medication (e.g., emotional blunting)
• Demoralization, depression from the presence of the illness or medication side effects
• Effects of chronic institutionalization such as lack of stimulation leading to apathy and withdrawal
• Withdrawal as a result of psychotic symptoms themselves such as auditory hallucinations telling a person to hide (Andraeson, 1995)

A preponderance of negative rather than positive symptoms in a client seems to correlate with a poorer course and prognosis (Aksu and Myers, 1994).

Because of this relatively distinct grouping of symptoms and variable response to antipsychotic medication, two subtypes of schizophrenia, Type I and Type II, have been proposed (Andraeson, 1985). *Type I schizophrenia is characterized by more positive symptoms,* whereas *Type II schizophrenia refers to clients who exhibit more negative symptoms.* Type I, or positive schizophrenia, may have an acute onset, and the course of the prognosis is more optimistic. Antipsychotic medications typically are helpful in ameliorating these symptoms which suggests an underlying defect in the dopamine system (Andraeson, 1985).

The Nursing Process

TABLE 29-2
Altered thought and language patterns in schizophrenia

PATTERN	DEFINITION	EXAMPLE
Thought Patterns		
Autistic thinking	• Elementary and concrete form of thinking • May be private and highly symbolic • May be incoherent to others	Susan used to write out pages of "scientific" jargon, which she claimed explained the process of space flight to the planet Pluto.
Magical thinking	• Belief that one's thoughts control situations, persons, or events	Mike states that he can determine which song will be played next on the radio by thinking about that song.
Concrete thinking	• Lack of the ability to form abstract thoughts	A nurse used an example of a job interview while explaining how to cope with stress. The client commented on how the interviewee got to the job interview instead of focusing on the more abstract concept of coping with any stressor.
Looseness of association (asyndetic speech)	• Thoughts seem fragmented • One idea is not clearly connected to the next idea	James states to the nurse, "You should have let me operate on you. Are you my mother? I can go eat lunch now."
Overinclusiveness	• Addition of many irrelevent items in speech • May be a result of impaired reticular activating system, which would normally inhibit overstimulation (Kaplan & Sadock, 1994)	Bill answers the nurse's request for her address and then goes on to talk about the city and state in which she lives as well.
Language Patterns		
Neologism	"New word" devised that has special meaning only to the client	"Raffity" was a word used by Sylvia to mean someone she could not trust.
Echolalia	Repetition of words or phrases heard from another person	After the nurse asked Julie to take her medication, Julie repeated, "Medication medication, medication."
Verbigeration	Purposeless repetition of words or phrases	For many days, Randy repeated "NASA goes to the moon. NASA goes to the moon."
Metonymic speech	Use of words with similar meanings interchangeably	Joan may say "please pass the spoon," when the intended message is "Please pass the fork."
Clang association	Repetition of words or phrases that are similar in sound but in no other way	A client might say, "I want to go on an outing to the park, lark, dark, bark."
Word salad	Form of speech in which words or phrases are connected meaninglessly	Paul might say, "Baby, throw ocean blue."
Stilted language	An overly and inappropriately formal communication pattern, usually written, which seems artificial and intellectual	Edith might say, "Good morning, Judy. It is an exceptionally bright and glorious day, and I will attempt to be fastidious in my appreciation of it."
Pressured speech	Speaking as if words are being forced out quickly (reflects the client's racing	"I need my medication. Please give it to me because it was due 10 minutes ago, and I feel very anxious and up-

The Nursing Process

TABLE 29-2—cont'd

Altered thought and language patterns in schizophrenia

PATTERN	DEFINITION	EXAMPLE
Poverty of speech	Diminished amount of speech	Michael responded to interview questions by answering in short phrases such as, "Maybe," and "I don't know," and others.
Poverty of content of speech	Adequate amount of speech but lacking in substantial information	Christine said she "wanted to go on an overnight pass because it was time."
Mutism	Absence of verbal speech	Susan sat in the corner of the dayroom sucking her thumb (also reflecting regression) and would not respond verbally to any attempts at communication.

Type II schizophrenia is thought to have a more insidious onset with chronic dysfunction such as those associated with negative symptoms. Brain imaging techniques have noted a higher incidence in structural brain defects with these persons (Andraeson, 1985). Type II schizophrenia is also helped by the newer "novel" antipsychotic medications. These drugs affect the serotonin as well as dopamine systems, which suggests serotonin involvement in the creation of negative symptoms (Jibson and Tandon, 1996).

Although with a mental illness changes occur in every area of a person's life, clients with schizophrenia exhibit marked changes in their cognition, perception, affect, behavior, and socialization. Each of these will be reviewed in depth, and clinical examples will be provided to illustrate a lifelike picture of the client's experience.

Cognitive impairment

The term *cognition refers to mental or thinking processes. It involves purposefully obtaining, storing, and retrieving information and knowledge; this is the use of intellect, reason, and judgment.* One of the major characteristics of schizophrenia is the disruption of usual ways of thinking.

The person with schizophrenia deviates from logical thought patterns that characterize adult thinking and returns to earlier, more elementary thought patterns. This results in the inability to produce complex thoughts and coherent sentences. It is presumably a result of problems in neurotransmitter function that accelerates, delays, or blocks information processing or transmission. Impairment also includes problems with memory, thought and language patterns, thought content, and difficulty with decision making.

Persons with schizophrenia have serious problems in processing information normally. In particular, this can be seen as poor concentration, distractibility, and an inability to maintain attention to the task at hand. A common nursing request is for a client to take a shower. If the client does not do this, it may be viewed as "noncompliance" when, in fact, the act of taking a shower is a series of steps that a person with alterations in information processing may not be able to sequence. The client may not even be able to communicate to the nurse why he or she is unable to take a shower.

This has implications for nursing interventions. For example, psychoeducational groups may have limited success if they are not short, well-focused, and actively engaging the client. It may be difficult for the client to maintain concentration even with the best of intentions to do so.

Memory deficit is also a cognitive change seen in schizophrenia. This is exhibited by the person having problems retrieving information already learned or by the person with an impairment in encoding items into short- or long-term memory. When their symptoms are being managed well by antipsychotic medication, some clients do not remember what is was like to be ill. In some cases, they stop taking medication because they are not able to connect getting better and staying better with taking medication. This noncompliance therefore represents more than simply oppositional or unmotivated behavior; it relates directly to memory dysfunction.

Cognitive impairment is also reflected in the thought and language of the client. Thought patterns, of course, cannot be directly observed, so this is evaluated by observing the client's form of speech. This is often characterized by odd or unusual language patterns, which are summarized in Table 29-2.

The Nursing Process

TABLE 29-3

Types of delusions and examples

DELUSION	DEFINITION	EXAMPLE
Ideas of reference	A person believes certain events, situations, or interactions are directly related to himself/herself.	Dick, a 40-year-old man, telephones the police to inform them that he sees two people standing in front of his house who must be talking about him.
Delusions of persecution	A person believes he or she is being harassed, threatened, or persecuted by some powerful force. A person may be driven to act in drastic ways by such persecutory thoughts.	Monica, a 35-year-old unemployed bookkeeper, has always led an isolated life with few friends or recreational interests. She worked for a large corporation where the clerical staff was about to become unionized. Monica became convinced that the supervisors were harassing the employees, including her, because they had voted to become union members. She believed that she was being singled out and harassed by her supervisor who was giving her the heaviest and most difficult workload of all the bookkeepers.
Delusions of grandeur	A person attaches special significance to his or her position in relation to others or the universe, or has an exaggerated sense of self-importance that has no basis in reality.	Jane, a 45-year-old unmarried woman, walked around carrying a bundle swaddled in a baby blanket. She said it contained the baby Jesus and that she was his mother, Mary. She refused to put the bundle down because she thought other persons, envious of her special position, were trying to kidnap her baby.
Somatic delusions	A person believes that his or her body is changing or responding in an unusual way that has no basis in reality.	Joe, age 50, had gallbladder surgery in a general hospital. Following the surgery, he began to complain to his family that he was convinced other vital organs had also been removed at the time of surgery. He claimed that his stomach had been removed, which he viewed as punishment for not taking his physician's advice about losing weight.

Thought content is often impaired as well, in the form of *delusions. These are strongly held beliefs that are not validated in reality, and ones that the client has not always held.* One client experienced a delusion that she had been assigned to perform maneuvers with the U.S. National Guard in an empty lot in her neighborhood. *When delusions are elaborate and detailed,* they are known as a *delusional system.* This client believed that she had received her orders for the maneuvers from persons on television and could name specific jobs to which she had been assigned. *When the beliefs are unshakable and contradictory information does not refute the delusions for the person, it is termed a fixed delusion.* When the client was told that the National Guard does not use private citizens to assist them, she stated that it was a special community project authorized by the governor. She refused to accept information that contradicted the delusion. *Some clients believe that another person can place thoughts into their minds, known as **thought insertion** even to the point of controlling them. Other clients may believe they can send their thoughts into other's minds. This is known as **thought broadcasting.** Table 29-3 presents types of delusions with examples.

A person with schizophrenia also has an impairment of decision making abilities. This actually represents deficits in several functions such as lack of insight, problem-solving skills and an inability to initiate tasks. At times, this is seen as an inability to use "common sense" or to use general knowledge that others take for granted. For example, the nurse might tell a client that his or her next appointment is at 10 o'clock next Friday, and unless

The Nursing Process

clarified, the client might assume 10 PM rather than the more obvious 10 AM time.

Some clients may have problems understanding the value and use of money. They may go shopping and purchase a lot of merchandise, then be surprised when they appear at the check-out counter because the items cost more than the 20 $1 bills they have in their pocket. These persons may think that because they have many bills that it means they have much value.

Perceptual changes

Another problematic area for clients with schizophrenia is their difficulty in perceiving reality accurately. The term *perception refers to the response of sensory receptors to external stimuli such as pictures or sounds.* Perception not only involves the ability of the client to receive stimuli through the appropriate receptor but also to be able to integrate, interpret, and respond to them appropriately. Perception involves the following three-step process:

1. The ability to receive sensory input through sight, hearing, taste, touch, and smell
2. The ability to attend to the stimulus that concurs with reality
3. The ability to respond and act appropriately to the information

For example, persons normally can see, smell, and hear a fire, and they must also be able to understand what is a fire. Then, persons must be able to protect themselves from being burned. Clients with disturbances in perception may have difficulty receiving the correct sensory stimulus or may have trouble understanding how others would respond to it. For example, if a fire alarm sounds, it may be misperceived as an alarm clock and a client may therefore not seek safety.

Illusions and hallucinations　Persons misperceive stimuli in two ways—through illusions and hallucinations. An *illusion is a misperception of real objects in the environment. It tends to occur when lighting is poor and one object is mistaken for another.* When a person first awakens or is in a darkened room, a table in the room may look like a crouching figure. Normally, this misperception is corrected quickly when a light is turned on or when the person touches the object and recognizes it. In schizophrenia, these misperceptions may not be readily corrected even with more information. The illusions may persist and become confusing to the client. These misperceptions may be transient or may become integrated as a part of the client's reality.

Hallucinations and changes in body feelings are two of the most noted perceptual changes experienced by clients with schizophrenia. A *hallucination is a sensation or image that occurs without external stimulus.* Hallucinations may be auditory, visual, olfactory, gustatory, or tactile. The most common types of hallucinations are auditory and visual. Tactile, olfactory, and gustatory hallucinations are usually associated with organic conditions such as withdrawal from drugs or alcohol. Types of hallucinations with examples are listed in Table 29-4.

Sense of self　Another area of altered perception is related to sense of self. *Ego boundary refers to a person's sense of self as a distinct individual, separate from others and the environment.* A sense of boundary develops to demarcate self from everything else. For example, Joe believes that when a nurse places her hand on his arm, his body becomes a part of the nurse's body. Body image is a person's perception of the physical aspects of his body, both internally and externally. In schizophrenia, clients may have such diffuse ego boundaries that they may not know where they end and the external environment begins.

Depersonalization occurs when there is a feeling of unreality about the self. Clients may feel as if they are fused to part of the environment, or may feel dead or in a trance. One client wore no shoes because he did not know where his body ended and the floor began. He needed to have contact with the floor with his bare feet to determine his position. Loss of ego boundaries may also be experienced by people taking lysergic acid diethylamide (LSD) or other hallucinogenic drugs.

Schizophrenia sometimes produces *an unreal quality in the person such that the environment seems to be in an altered state. This is known as derealization. Persons may feel as if they do not know where they are, or they may be having a sense of déjà vu in which the environment may look familiar but appears dreamlike.*

Affective changes

Affect is the way emotions or feelings are experienced and exhibited. The hypothalamus and other brain structures, notably the amygdala, hippocampus, and higher cortical areas, are involved with normal emotional process of emotion to occur.

Emotions can be hyperexpressed, hypoexpressed, or expressed in an incongruent manner. Clients with schizophrenia most often have hypoexpression of emotions that is frustrating to them because people think they have no emotion. One client related that he often tries to smile but his face does not work. However, many

The Nursing Process

TABLE 29-4

Types of hallucinations and examples

TYPE	DEFINITION	EXAMPLE
Auditory	Voices or sounds that do not relate to objective reality are heard by the client but not by others.	A client heard music that was not heard by others.
Command	A type of auditory hallucination is heard in which voices demand that the person perform some action, often aggressive, toward self or others.	Randy heard a screaming voice insisting that he mutilate his arms with needles.
Olfactory	Odors are smelled that appear to be coming from specific or unknown places.	Julie states she smells onions no matter where she goes.
Gustatory	Tastes are experienced that have no basis in reality.	Randy states that, whenever he is in a room full of people, he develops a burning sensation in his tongue.
Tactile	Strange body sensations are felt that may or may not be part of a delusional system. At times tactile hallucinations involve misperceptions about body parts. This type of hallucination is common in alcohol toxicity.	A client in alcohol withdrawal feels as if insects are crawling inside his body.
Visual	Objects not present in reality are seen.	Sylvia thinks she sees a door close out of the corner of her eye when in fact, it remains open.

clients report no longer even experiencing feelings internally.

These clients may also lack the ability to identify and label their emotions. When asked how they feel about a situation, they may respond by saying, "I don't know." This may be based on an impaired capacity to recognize and name what they are experiencing rather than avoidance or resistance. The affective changes noted in clients with schizophrenia are detailed in Table 29-5.

Another associated symptom of schizophrenia is the potential for aggressive behavior. Although persons with schizophrenia do not commit more acts of violence than the general public (Torrey, 1994), there may be an increased risk for impulsive and/or aggressive behavior if a client is receiving command hallucinations to harm others or is exhibiting paranoia. The client should be asked if they have intentions to hurt themselves or others, and this should be followed up with more specific questions with regard to plan, method, and target.

Depression is also an associated affective symptom of schizophrenia. One source states that a secondary depression may develop in about 25% of clients after an acute exacerbation of their illness (Aksu and Myers, 1994). Symptoms of depression may be easily confounded with symptoms of schizophrenia such as altered sleeping and eating patterns, anhedonia, affective flattening, alogia and avolition. Antipsychotic medications can also create a drug-induced akinesia that may mimic depression. The nurse should be alert to the possibility of depression in assessment activities.

Behavioral changes

There are characteristic behavioral or motor activity changes seen in the client with schizophrenia. Table 29-6 explains some of the major changes seen in this realm.

When persons have been taking antipsychotic medication for a long time, a characteristic set of movements may develop. These movements are not characteristic of schizophrenia but are directly related to drug therapy. This set of behavioral symptoms is known as *tardive dyskinesia (TD)*. These symptoms might be exhibited as facial grimacing or odd tongue movements. See Chapter 15 for a more thorough explanation of TD.

In addition, physical appearance is likely to change when the client with schizophrenia is acutely psychotic. Clients may dress in bizarre combinations of clothes such as a bathing suit with an overcoat, or they may wear the same clothes every day, unlaundered. Appearance may deteriorate, especially related to negative symptoms. This might include disheveled, and dirty

The Nursing Process

TABLE 29-5

Affective changes of schizophrenia and examples

AFFECTIVE CHANGE	DEFINITION	EXAMPLE
Inappropriate affect	Expression of feeling incongruous to the situation and not consistent with cultural expectations	Client smiles as he relates the death of his mother.
Blunted affect	Emotional response is appropriate to the situation but not as strong as one would expect	Client shows mild irritation in a situation where others would be very angry.
Flat affect	No emotional expression; face is blank, masklike	Client relates having a good time on a recreational trip but shows no facial or verbal expression of pleasure.
Anhedonia	Loss of the sense of pleasure	Client reports that bowling was once enjoyable but now is not interested in any recreational sport.
Overreaction	Increased emotional sensitivity and responses from expected cultural norms	A client with schizophrenia exhibits a rage reaction when her mother refuses to allow her to watch an X-rated videotape in their home.
Mood lability	Emotions that fluctuate rapidly	Client is quietly sitting and conversing with the nurse about a superficial topic then quickly begins to laugh hysterically and cry uncontrollably.
Ambivalence	Experience of having two opposite feelings at the same time; these feelings make the person want to do two opposite things at once	Client states he is committed to treatment in the inpatient program, but several minutes later he demands to leave, complaining he is being held against his will.
Aggressive behavior	Actual or intended harming of another	Instructed by voices to do so, the client picked up a trash can and threw it at her sister.
Depression	Psychiatric condition characterized by low mood, altered sleeping and eating patterns, anhedonia, and avolition	The client has reported loss of appetite and he states he feels that life is not worth living since he has developed schizophrenia.

clothes, sloppy, unkempt appearance, and lack of personal hygiene. These symptoms are often the first clue to family members that something is amiss and may signal a potential or impending relapse. Related behavioral changes may include lack of persistence in work or school activities.

Social changes

The person with schizophrenia not only must deal with all the affective, perceptual, cognitive, and behavioral changes, but also often experiences a low level of social functioning and self-care. Social problems for clients may be a direct or indirect result of the schizophrenia. Direct social changes occur when the biological symptoms of

the disorder prevent the person from socializing and forming relationships within accepted norms, or when the brain deteriorates to a point of having no motivation. Behaviors directly contributing to social changes include the inability to communicate coherently, loss of drive and interest, deterioration of social skills, personal hygiene, and mistrust. In addition, direct social changes may be influenced by the clients poorly formed ego and body boundaries, and an inability to filter stimuli.

Indirect effects are those that occur as a secondary process to the biological symptoms. These include low self-esteem, poor academic and vocational performance in comparison to peers, dependency, and stigmatization from others.

The Nursing Process

TABLE 29-6

Behavioral changes and examples in schizophrenia

BEHAVIORAL CHANGE	DEFINITION	EXAMPLE
Catatonia	Alteration in motor behavior, either seen as an absence of most movement or extreme agitated excitability	Nancy sat in the unit lounge for hours curled up in a fetal position.
Waxy flexibility	Condition where a client remains in any body position in which they are placed This was more commonly seen before the advent of psychotropic medications.	Samuel kept his arm in a position suspended over his head until it was physically lowered by the nurse.
Automatism	Client performs motor functions with a slow, rigid quality	When asked to take his medication, Jesse obeyed in a programmed, robotlike manner.
Negativism	Extreme oppositional stance to all requests The client may, in fact, perform the opposite of what is asked. This may be a reaction to internal versus external cues.	When asked to take his medication, Ned screamed at the nurse and threw the medicine on the floor.
Stereotypy	Repetitive patterns of movement that may or may not imitate others behavior	Candace nodded her head and rubbed her arms with her hands repeatedly.
Echopraxia	Imitation of body position to look like another person This may be related to a clients attempting to mimic "normalcy." It may also be related to a client's difficulty with body boundaries.	Laura smiled and crossed her arms when she noticed the nurse doing this.
Avolition	Condition in which a person is not motivated to performs tasks This is related to neurotransmitter changes.	Fred's mother believes he is lazy because he is not able to get out of bed until noon.

When brain changes (possibly in the frontal area) occur so that the client exhibits a lack of drive and motivation, this can also have social consequences. It takes a certain amount of energy to initiate activities with others and follow through with social or vocational commitments. If a person is experiencing a preponderance of negative symptoms, he or she may lack the energy to nurture relationships.

Social skills such as appropriate behavior in public may also be altered by generalized brain changes. A client, for example, may masturbate in public or speak intimately with strangers. This may also be a reflection of poorly formed ego and body boundaries. Clients may not have a good sense of when it is appropriate to discuss personal matters with others or how close to stand next to others when conversing. Clients may talk to themselves in response to hallucinations. They may also exhibit poor grooming. Most persons are frightened and repelled by this behavior, which may be reflected in avoidance or even in some cases of aggression toward the client.

Another brain change that decreases socialization is a tendency of some clients to feel suspicious and untrusting. This may be related to changes in perceptions. Trust with clients is developed by providing consistent interactions over a period of days or weeks. At the extreme, clients may exhibit *paranoia which refers to an exaggerated suspiciousness*. This condition may be manifested by the client's feeling that everyone is against him

The Nursing Process

or her, or that powerful agencies are plotting to inflict harm. Such clients may believe that their food is poisoned or that staff members are going to kill them. Some remain watchful and are terrified of any lapse in their vigilance.

Clients who have difficulty with perceptions and relationships or who tend to isolate themselves may have difficulty finding employment or maintaining a stable job. This can be made worse by cognitive and other behavioral changes. Without adequate income, many clients become homeless and may become dependent on social services. These clients then become some of the thousands of homeless mentally ill viewed as "street people."

Clients may also exhibit dependency. This is an overreliance on others to meet physical or emotional needs. Overreliance may have become a part of the client's life style related to a learned helplessness. However, persons with persistent mental disorders have greater dependence needs when the disorder is not properly controlled.

Persons with schizophrenia may have an impairment of the reticular activating system, which means they are easily overstimulated and need to separate themselves from people and noise to decrease the stimuli. The above factors make it difficult to establish relationships, provide for adequate self-care, and find and maintain employment.

Comorbidity of Schizophrenia and Substance Abuse

One of the most challenging problems in the assessment and treatment of clients with schizophrenia is their concurrent use of illicit drugs and alcohol. Although drug abuse has been found to have decreased among students, drug use has probably been on the increase among those persons with schizophrenia (Selzer and Lieberman, 1993). Clients with schizophrenia may be attempting to self-medicate troubling symptoms of the illness or side effects of antipsychotic medication. Of the clients with schizophrenia, 48% receive a diagnosis of drug abuse or dependence and this group has a poorer prognosis (Aksu and Myers, 1994). When there is a chemical dependency and a major mental illness present, it is referred to as a *dual diagnosis,* or "mentally ill, chemical abusing and addicted" (MICAA) (see Chapter 27).

Psychosis Related to Medical Conditions

Psychosis can also be present as a result of certain medical conditions. A wide variety of these conditions may produce psychotic symptoms. For example, hallucinations and delusions have, in some cases, been associated with temporal lobe epilepsy (APA, 1994). Alcohol and certain drugs may also mimic signs of psychosis. The nurse should initially maintain a high level of suspicion with clients who have the presenting symptoms of psychosis. A careful general history should be taken with all clients, as well as performance of physical assessment to aid in correct determination of interventions.

Another factor worth noting is that clients with schizophrenia have been known to have a decreased sensitivity to pain (Dworkin, 1994). Medical symptoms in general tend to be underreported, and persons with schizophrenia may exhibit physical illness through behavior changes rather than verbal complaints (Krach, 1993). This phenomena may have serious implications if life-threatening disorders minimized by the client are not attended to.

Focused Assessment

A comprehensive assessment is outlined in Chapter 5. Although the focus of this assessment is on clients who are acutely disturbed, the principles and content of an assessment are the same regardless of the setting. In practice, clients' present symptoms become apparent in a wide variety of settings to seek assistance. The assessment of persons with schizophrenia includes collection of data about the person, the family, and the accommodated changes in the cognitive, perceptual affective, behavioral, and social spheres of experience. Table 29-7 is a sample focused assessment for the client with schizophrenia, the family and the environment.

The ability to gather data may be limited by the client's presenting symptoms and behavior, which need to be assessed individually. In addition, family members may not be present or available. Consequently, the initial assessment process may extend over time until the client is sufficiently responsive or other reliable informants are available.

Because the client who is acutely disturbed is often frightened by the idea of being interviewed, the nurse tries to ensure that the environment is as calm as possible. Distracting stimuli should be avoided. Lighting should be well-lit and not shadowy. Privacy is needed, but not to the extent that the client feels anxious and threatened by it. Sufficient personal space is to be allowed so that the client's boundaries, which may be fragmented or diffuse at this time, are not invaded.

The nurse introduces himself or herself, addresses the client by name, speaks in a clear way, uses understandable language, clarifies questions, and uses restatement to ensure understanding of the client's response. Prolonged eye contact may be threatening to the client. The nurse's

The Nursing Process

TABLE 29-7

Focused assessment of a person with schizophrenia

Joe H. is a 30 year old African American who has come to be assessed by the nurse for an acute exacerbation of paranoid schizophrenia. He was brought to the community mental health center by his mother and sister with whom he has been living. The mental health center nurse has also been contacted by the client's case manager to see if the client needed to be hospitalized.

Assessment Data

Mental Status Examination

Joe's appearance is disheveled. His hair is dirty and he is wearing layers of clothes although the temperature outside is mild. He appears to be older than his stated age. His attitude toward the nurse is guarded. During the interview, his eyes continually scan the room, and he stands and paces occasionally. Joe's speech is rapid and seems pressured. His thoughts are only tangentially connected. He describes delusions of persecution where government investigators are slowly trying to poison him because he is aware of an extraterrestrial and U.S. government plot to take over the world.

The client states his mood is anxious. Affect appears fearful and angry at times. Joe is oriented to time, place, person, and date. Memory is intact, and the client is able to name the last five presidents of the United States. Joe is able to copy a simple clock figure; however, when asked to explain the proverb, "People in glass houses should not throw stones," he answered, "Because it might break their house"—a concrete answer to an abstract question.

Joe's insight into his symptoms is poor, as well as his judgment, since he wants to go to the Federal Building and talk with the head of the Federal Bureau of Investigation (FBI), "so I can tell him to stop harassing me."

History

Joe's first psychotic break came at age 20 when he was in college studying to be an electrical engineer. He has had two relapses since then. He lives with his mother and sister and has never lived alone. He has held no permanent employment and has only a few acquaintances.

Social Data

Currently, his only social outlet is attending church once a week with his family. He stopped doing this 1 month ago, when he began to believe that certain church members were part of the plot to take over the world. However, the family cites their church as a source of strength and support.

Family Data

Both the mother and sister comment to the nurse, "We love Joe, but he is threatening us at home and beginning to believe we are in on the 'plot.' We don't know if we can manage him at home any more." Typical family members' responses to the client are frustration and verbal expressions of criticism and anger.

QUESTIONS/OBSERVATIONS	POSSIBLE ANSWERS
Assessment of the Person Experiencing Psychosis	
"What problems have you been having lately?"	"I haven't been thinking straight. I'm really nervous. Where are the guards? Are you taking me to jail now?"
"You are at the mental health center. What was it that led up to your coming here?"	"I don't know. I've had trouble with my family. Did they report me? Is that why my case manager picked me up?"
Observe for cognitive changes such as concrete thinking, delusions, magical thinking, or autistic communication.	The nurse notices the lack of ability to sort out facts, make sense of the circumstances.
Observe for symptoms such as hallucinations, somatization, or depersonalization.	"Oh, it's nothing. Can you hear it? That buzzing sometimes drives me crazy. I can ignore it, though."
"You seem to be listening to something. Could you tell me about it?"	"Do you hear that voice? No, of course not. I don't hear it either."
Observe for congruency of thought and affect. Observe for negative symptoms such as flat affect.	Shakes head vigorously. Client smiled and giggled while talking.
Observe for unusual gestures, posture, gait, tone of voice, mannerisms, suspiciousness; note physical appearance.	Client was unshaven and smelled strongly of body odor and urine; clothes were soiled. After shaking head vigor-

The Nursing Process

TABLE 29-7—cont'd

Focused assessment of a person with schizophrenia

QUESTIONS/OBSERVATIONS	POSSIBLE ANSWERS
	ously, client continued to glance around the room, sitting on hands, rocking back and forth.
"Tell me about using alcohol or other drugs."	"I drink sometimes. When I feel like I'm going to explode, I get drunk or smoke a couple of joints. You going to tell the cops?"
"When you are at your best, what is your life like for you?"	"I hear those sounds sometimes, but I just ignore them. I go to a day-treatment center four days a week."
"How have you been able to manage at home not being able to think straight?	(Silence)
"What makes you feel tense? What do you do when you're tense?"	"I feel really upset when my sister yells at me. All she does is tell me how worthless I am. When she does that, I usually go to my bedroom and listen to music with my headphones."
"When have you had emotional problems before?"	"Other people think I have problems. I've been locked up three times before, but they were the ones with the problems."
"How long have you had schizophrenia?"	"Oh, I don't remember."
"Can you tell me about any previous relapses you have had?"	"I'm not having a relapse. Don't you understand that the world is coming to an end?"
Assessment of the Family	
"Tell me about your family." "Who are you closest to?" "Who do you live with?"	"Mom, Miriam, and Dude—he's a Pomeranian. I live with all of them."
"What was it like growing up in your family?"	"Okay. I guess like everybody else's. Some fighting, some laughing. Everybody was very serious. I was the only one who laughed. They thought I was strange."
"What is your relationship like with your mom?"	"She is a nice person. Probably shouldn't have had kids. She is too serious to like children."
"Did anybody in your family ever have mental illness?"	"I don't know. I was adopted when I was 2 years old. They said my real mother couldn't take care of me anymore."
"What kinds of activities is each person responsible for?"	"Mom cooks and cleans and works at a department store. Miriam studies. Dude and I play."
Note avoidance of issues or events, or short, incomplete answers. "Is there anything that is difficult to talk about in your family?"	"Everything. I don't know. It's pretty tense at our house. We talk about me looking for a job. Mom cries a lot. I don't know."
Observe for evidence of divergent opinions or thoughts. "Are individual decisions respected?"	"We disagree about everything. I want to get a job and go to college and get an apartment. Mom wants me to take a bath. Her goal for me is to have clean underwear. Miriam could not care less."
"How have the client's changes affected you as a family?"	MOTHER: "He's such a fine boy. I just wonder if I did everything I could. What do you think, Nurse?"

The Nursing Process

TABLE 29-7—cont'd

Focused assessment of a person with schizophrenia

QUESTIONS/OBSERVATIONS	POSSIBLE ANSWERS
	MIRIAM: "I'm tired of him getting all the attention. Nothing I do counts."
Assessment of the Environment	
"Tell me about your education."	"I graduated from high school and got through half a semester of college."
"How well do you get along with other people when you work?"	"I've been a grocery clerk. I sold ties in a store and did odd jobs and deliveries. I kinda like to work. But the people start treating me strange. I don't like them talking about me. I quit them all."
"Where do you live?"	"I live at 234 Capon Street, upstairs and to the left."
"Are you a member of any particular, cultural, religious, or ethnic group?"	"I am an African American."
"What are that group's beliefs about your symptoms?"	"They all think that if I tried harder, I could get over this. Then sometimes they think that, because I'm adopted, I might never get over it."
"Tell me about your friends. How long do your friendships tend to last? How do you make friends?	"Friends come and go. Only family stays, they say. I don't know. It's hard for me to get close to people. Maybe there's something wrong with me."
"What community services are you aware of or are you currently using?'	"I swim at the YMCA. I like swimming. I feel strong in my arms, but I don't lift weights. I don't want to be dangerous, just strong. I get medication here at the Community Mental Health Center. Sometimes I see the doctor here. Mary Smith is my case manager."
"Tell me about your extended family. Who gives you support?"	"I have a wonderful grandfather. He takes me to lunch every week. He listens to me, helps me figure out things. He encourages me to do things other guys do. I love the heck out of him."
"What do you do in your spare time?"	"I draw. I watch TV. I stay up late and watch TV, then sleep late in the morning, until noon most days."

Physical Assessment Data

1. Laboratory data
   Complete Blood Count (CBC) - within normal limits
   Blood chemistry - within normal limits
   CT scan - shows slightly enlarged 3rd and lateral brain ventricles
   Electroencephalogram (EEG) - within normal limits

2. Abnormal Involuntary Movement Scale (AIMS)
   Negative for tardive dyskenesia (TD) at this time

3. Past presence of neuroleptic malignant syndrome
   Family and client report no presence.

4. Current vital signs and physical examination are within normal limits.

5. Past medication taken—Family reports that the client had been taking haloperidol (Haldol) until 2 years ago when it "made his face feel stiff."

6. Current medicine prescribed - Thiothixene but client reports he has discontinued taking it in the last 2 months because, "I am fine, I don't need any medication."

The Nursing Process

attitude and feeling will be reflected in the approach to the client. A calm, unhurried, and competent manner may go a long way toward helping the client respond to the fullest extent possible. The most important goal of the initial interview is to help the client develop a sense of trust with the nurse and to gather baseline information to begin care planning and initiate discharge planning.

Assessment Scales

There are a variety of structured methods that can assist nurses in obtaining assessment data about a client. As part of the initial interview, it is helpful to conduct a mental status examination. This is a standardized method of obtaining information about a client's thoughts, feelings, and gross cognitive functioning at the present time. The elements of a mental status examination are developed in Chapter 5.

The nurse can use numerous other scales that aid in initial or ongoing assessment of a client's progress or functioning. These are listed in Table 29-8 with a brief description of each scale.

It is very challenging for the nurse to interview a client who is experiencing an acute psychotic episode. In this situation, the nurse should attempt to obtain only the most important information pertaining to the client and defer other elements of the assessment to a later time.

Significant others may be able to provide crucial information such as a history of physical problems, a brief history of the illness, circumstances surrounding this admission, medications prescribed, allergies and usage of illicit drugs and alcohol. This quick assessment can then be expanded in a day or so after the client becomes more stable. At this time, the nurse can conduct a more thorough interview. The client may feel more trusting of the nurse at this time as well and may be more open in his or her responses.

A nurse working in an outpatient setting may also spread assessment out over time. Possibly, more extensive neuropsychological testing will be done and records and treatment plans from other facilities, if applicable, will be obtained to create a long-term rehabilitation plan.

Nursing Diagnosis

The nursing diagnosis is formulated from the assessment and includes identification of the client's strengths and problems. Other disciplines use a symptom-based diagnostic system which is contained in the *Diagnostic and Statistical Manual, Fourth Edition (DSM-IV)* (APA,

TABLE 29-8

Assessment scales measuring aspects of schizophrenia

INSTRUMENT	DESCRIPTION
Extrapyramidal Symptoms Rating Scale (ESRS)	Measures presence of extrapyramidal motor behavior
Abnormal Involuntary Movement Scale (AIMS)	Easily used tool to track changes in motor symptoms, which may be indicative of TD
Global Assessment Scale (GAS)	Assesses functional status as well as symptoms and may be used over time to measure changes (O'Connor and Eggert, 1994)
Positive & Negative Symptom Scale (PANS)	Useful for determining extent of positive and negative symptoms of schizophrenia
Brief Psychiatric Rating Scale	Well-validated tool of 16 items that measures separate symptom areas as well as giving a total pathology score (Acorn, 1993)
Moller-Murphy Symptom Management Scale (MM-SMAT)	Can be used by clinicians as well as clients and families to provide a systematic method of identifying and coping with symptoms of schizophrenia (Murphy and Moller, 1993)

1994). Table 29-9 represents a comparison between DSM-IV diagnostic criteria and nursing diagnoses.

Nursing diagnoses change as the client changes. As the nurse observes and interacts with the client and the client's condition changes, patterns of additional problems and strengths emerge. Initial problems may be modified or resolved as the client's level of integration changes.

Outcome Identification

The overall goal of working with clients with schizophrenia is to promote the highest level of wellness as de-

The Nursing Process

TABLE 29-9

Comparison of DSM-IV diagnostic criteria with selected NANDA nursing diagnoses

NANDA DIAGNOSES*	DSM-IV DIAGNOSES†
Altered thought processes related to increased anxiety	Paranoid schizophrenia
Risk for other-directed violence related to auditory command hallucinations and persecutory and grandiose delusions	
Social isolation related to bizarre behavior	Disorganized schizophrenia
Altered health maintenance related to lack of knowledge in basic health practices and participation in high-risk behaviors	
Compromised ineffective family coping related to lack of knowledge of effective communication/management patterns with client and lack of knowledge of resources	Catatonic schizophrenia
Impaired social interaction related to skills deficit in communicating with others	

*From North American Nursing Diagnosis Association. (1994). NANDA nursing diagnoses: definitions & classification, 1995-1996. St. Louis: Mosby.
†Reprinted with permission from American Psychiatric Association (1994). Diagnostic and statistical manual of mental disorders, fourth edition. Washington, DC: Author.

fined by the client in relation to work, school, social relationships, and self-care. This outcome is achieved through:

- Symptom monitoring
- Relapse prevention
- Early intervention

The foundation for positive outcomes actually begins during the assessment phase. This information gives guidance to the nurse to formulate accurate nursing diagnoses which, in turn, guide goal and outcome development. For example, on assessment, the nurse may discover that the client continues to have auditory hallucinations, but the voices are faint and the client can easily block them out with distractions. Another piece of data suggests that clients stay in their homes because they do not know how to appropriately socialize with others. Although the nursing diagnosis of "altered thought process" may be appropriate to address the first symptom, the client may instead have more interest in learning how to initiate relationships. "Impaired verbal communication" may then be a better focus for a nursing diagnosis with the corresponding goal of improving social communication.

Another consideration for outcome development is that schizophrenia is a chronic illness, and there is a high probability (up to 50%) of recurrence of psychotic symptoms. Outcomes therefore should be realistic to avoid discouragement for both the nurse and the client. Both persons need to be aware that some outcomes may take a long time to accomplish.

And above all, outcomes need to be developed with the active participation of the client if at all possible. The goals must be consistent with the client's ability to tolerate anxiety, since learning and change are anxiety-provoking experiences. Mutually developed, realistic outcomes can work as a tool to foster the client's self-esteem as each goal met strengthens the client's confidence that the illness can be managed.

When considering goals with clients, the nurse and client should first develop short-term goals that can be accomplished within several days during a hospital stay. These outcomes focus on decreasing danger to self or others and management of acute symptoms. Simultaneously, the nurse must be planning long-range goals with the client, which are geared to psychiatric rehabilitation, community reintegration, and optimization of mental health. These outcomes are usually accomplished after the client is living in the community.

Communication among service providers throughout the client's care is crucial to ensure that outcomes are attained. A continuous integrated and "seamless" flow of treatment between inpatient and outpatient settings will help assure quality outcomes for a client.

Planning

The short-term goal of treatment planning is to assist the client with schizophrenia to make the transition from an unstable to a stable level of wellness. Long-term treatment goals and plans involve assisting the client to actualize his or her potential, which includes facilitating a satisfactory quality of life as defined by that person (Murphy and Moller, 1996). This requires an approach

The Nursing Process

that is consumer- and family-focused; their input is integral to effective treatment planning.

A nursing care plan for a client with schizophrenia is presented on p. 590. An interdisciplinary treatment plan in the form of a clinical pathway for inpatient treatment of a schizophrenic episode is presented on p. 591.

Implementation
Counseling

Supportive-educative counseling

Nurses are in a pivotal role to provide support and intervention to decrease positive and negative symptoms of schizophrenia. The symptoms with which nurses assist clients are anxiety, mistrust, managing hallucinations and delusions, communication with one who is experiencing loose associations, and managing social withdrawal.

Anxiety Anxiety occurs because a person feels threatened or because of biochemical dysfunction. In either situation, a prime consideration is alleviating or decreasing the anxiety. The nurse can help clients with this by:

- Maintaining a calm presence with them during acute phases.
- Encouraging clients to put feelings into words or talk about the experience. This will help "ground" the client. The client should feel safer and not abandoned.
- Exploring with the client the meaning of the experience in terms of identifying the threat.
- Discussing why the client may be experiencing anxiety at this time.
- Helping the client identify negative or erroneous self messages that could contribute to the feelings.

For example if a client feels anxious when saying to himself or herself, "I shouldn't have made that mistake on my ceramic project; I'm a worthless person," the nurse can help the client rephrase the negative (and faulty) self-talk into, "I made a small mistake on this project but that's okay; I'm just learning how to do ceramics." This technique, called cognitive restructuring, often modulates the anxious feeling (see Chapter 30).

Mistrust Nurses find that clients with schizophrenia display profound mistrust of self, others, and the world around them. Biological theories state that mistrust is caused by a person's inability to interpret environmental cues realistically. General approaches to dealing with a suspicious person highlight reliability and consistency in all interactions. Trust develops gradually, and clues to its presence are openness of thoughts and feelings, as well

as seeking out contact with the nurse. When structuring the nurse-client relationship, the nurse should:

- Be specific about the times and places of meetings. Clients with altered perceptions may misinterpret ambiguous messages.
- Address the duration of the relationship whenever possible. It is helpful for clients to understand time boundaries with the nurse.
- Follow through with the schedule. This demonstrates consistency and reliability. Even if a client appears indifferent, it may represent a facade and subsequently take weeks to regain the client's trust even when an unavoidable or unexplained absence occurs.
- If the client is in the hospital, schedule several short periods of time with the client and space them throughout the shift. Mistrustful clients may be unable to tolerate prolonged interpersonal contact without becoming anxious about anticipated social discomfort. They may also feel threatened by verbal intrusion with premature personal questions before trust is established.
- To reduce a client's anxiety during meetings or conferences in which clients are involved, all people should be introduced and the goals of the meeting stated.
- It is helpful for the nurse to assign one or two staff members to work consistently with a client who has difficulty trusting others, so that the client does not have to expend energy forming relationships with many different people.
- Other team members should also be aware of the care plan so that their approaches to the client are consistent with that of the direct caregiver's to promote the client's trust in all staff members.

Mistrustful clients are also acutely sensitive to the genuineness of others and aware of inauthentic behaviors.

Honesty is also a component of genuineness. It demonstrates to the client that the nurse can be trusted. The client should be assured of confidentiality. Questions about care should be answered. Clients have a right to be informed about their treatment, to be involved in planning their care, and to know the rationale for any treatment.

Clients often anticipate impending separations such as vacations and job changes, and terminate the relationship before the separation occurs. Changes in schedule and anticipated absences should be discussed in advance so that opportunities for fantasy about abandonment are minimized.

NURSING CARE PLAN

Medication Nonadherence

NURSING ASSESSMENT DATA

Joe H. is a 30-year-old African-American who has come to the inpatient unit of Hillside Hospital after being judged a threat to others by staff at the community mental health center. *Subjective data:* Client states, "I am not taking medicine. It is poison." He relates an FBI/CIA plot against him, threatening to hurt family members because they are part of the plot. He asks the nurse, "Are you with the FBI?" *Objective data:* Guarded attitude, disheveled appearance; affect anxious, pacing. Height 6'1", weight 160 lbs. Additional assessment data received from the community mental health nurse (see Table 29-7); *DSM-IV diagnosis:* paranoid schizophrenia.

NANDA Diagnosis: Altered thought processes related to medication nonadherence

Outcomes	Interventions	Rationale	Evaluation
Short term ***Within 3 days*** 1. Will verbalize a decrease in anxiety as measured on an anxiety scale from 1 (low) to 10 (high). 2. Will verbalize no threats to staff or family. 3. Will question delusional beliefs. **Long term** ***Within 1 month*** 1. Will list at least 3 benefits of taking medication as prescribed. 2. Will state he views FBI/CIA plot as fake. 3. Family will report client is grooming self and eating at least 2 meals per day.	• Refer to Interdisciplinary Treatment Plan clinical pathway on p. 591. • RN to meet with client 5 minutes every 2 hours during day and evening shift without demands • RN case manager will initiate stepwise progression of challenging delusional beliefs regarding medicine • All staff give full explanations of team actions especially regarding medications • RN should question delusions but focus on conversation about how medication noncompliance has impacted his functioning • After 3 days, refer client for small group medication management module • Observe client closely to ensure that he is swallowing medication • Monitor response to medication and observe for side effects • Discuss management strategies for specific side effects and what interventions to use at home	• Standardized plan of care promotes optional treatment continuity • Short, frequent meetings with client will promote trust • Some research indicates that delusional beliefs can be modified with a series of graded challenges with a trusted provider • Minimizes misinterpretation • Disputing delusional belief in the absence of a trusting relationship may entrench delusions • Focus on "here and now" group topics facilitates problem solving that is associated with effective medication self-management; small versus large groups are less threatening for paranoid clients • If client believes medication is poison, he may try to "cheek" or not swallow medication • Teaching/monitoring medications is an essential nursing responsibility • A sufficient knowledge base provides the foundation for self-responsibility	**Short term** 1. Met in 3 days 2. Partially met (client not verbalizing threats to staff) in 3 days 3. Met in 3 days **Long term** 1. Met in 1 month 2. Partially met—in one month client still believes there could be an FBI/CIA plot, but does not think it directly involves him, nor are family or church involved in plot 3. Met in 1 month

INTERDISCIPLINARY TREATMENT PLAN

Clinical Pathway

Initiation:_____   Diagnosis: <u>SCHIZOPHRENIA</u>   DRG: <u>430</u>_____

Date:_____   AVG LOS:_____   Actual LOS:_____

	Day 1	**Day 2-6**	**Day 7-11**	**Day 12-16**
Medical Interventions	H&P, MSE: thought process & content, misperceptions, SI/HI. Eval. for Sub Abuse. Order labs, EKG 40+. Admission orders. Drug Screen. Restrict for 24 hrs.	Complete Treatment Plan. Establish antipsychotic dose. Assess for Changes in MSE. Review labs & old record. Re-eval. restriction.	Update Treatment Plan. Monitor symptoms, meds, & side effects. Continue Group/Individual therapy. Initiate D/C plans for F/U.	Discharge Instruction Form. Discharge orders. Prescriptions & F/U appt. Terminate therapy.
Nursing Interventions	Admission Assessment Documentation. Assess for command hall., paranoid del., thought of self harm. Monitor intake. Orient to ward, schedule & give ITP. Vital signs & wt.	Assess adaptation to ward. Provide structured environment. < stimulation, > contact with reality. Intro to sm. grp. act. Monitor hall., del., thoughts of harm (SI, HI), level of anxiety, response to meds. Assist with grooming. Educate pt/family illness/meds.	Continue monitor (see previous). Evai. participation in reality oriented act. Eval. independence in ADL's. Eval. med/illness teaching.	Continue monitor/eval. (see previous) Complete D/C summary. AMI referral. Reinforce need for continued aftercare & meds.
Social Work Interventions	Emergency Intervention	Assessment by 3rd workday. Identify living situation, financial status & support systems. Initiate D/C planning	Continue counseling pt/family. Review with pt/family available support systems.	Coordinate pass with caregiver to eval. reintegration into community. Terminate counseling. Make out-patient appts.
Psychology Interventions		Initiate Psych Testing	Review findings	
Recreation Therapy Interventions	Initial contact	Initial RT Assessment completed. Introduce pt. to Socialization grp.	Begin/continue leisure/discharge plan. Eval. reality orientation/relatedness.	Complete Leisure Discharge plan(s). Terminate therapy.
Key Patient Outcomes	Pt. verbalizes feelings of safety @_____	Visible during meals @_____ Attends ward/team activities @_____ Maintains control i.e., @_____ Identifies current meds @_____	Visible on ward 50% of time @_____ Independent ADL's @_____ Improved personal hygiene @_____	< &/or cessation of sxs of altered thought process/content, misperception, self harm @_____ Cessation of agitation @_____ Improved judgment @_____ Improved relatedness @_____ F/U & meds @_____

Patient Identification
Key: *Circle-Variance*
#-Date-Progress Note re: specific evaluation/intervention goal
@-Achievement date
(Variances are contained on a second page, which is not included.)
Courtesy VA Medical Center, Baltimore, Maryland

The Nursing Process

Testing is another aspect of mistrust. Testing refers to the client's attempt to determine the nurse's interest, caring, and sincerity. Clients may test the nurse by engaging in socially unacceptable behavior. Clients need to find out that nurses will not be put off by attempts to drive them away. As clients accept the nurse's sincerity, testing behavior diminishes.

The nurse can also help mistrustful clients learn how to expand feelings of trust from the nurse to others. Nurses can help clients identify behaviors that are characteristic of trusting and trustworthy people. The client who has a reliable set of criteria to follow regarding trustworthiness will feel more secure about initiating and partaking in relationships.

Managing hallucinations   One of the most common and troubling symptoms of schizophrenia is the experience of hallucination. There are four levels of intensity of auditory hallucinations: comforting, condemning, controlling, and conquering.

As hallucinations become stronger, they often become more verbally demeaning to the client. The "voices" may also demand that the client comply with certain actions. These are termed *command hallucinations.* Command hallucinations may be particularly dangerous, since they often involve demands that the client harm self or others (Moller, 1990).

Medications are administered that specifically target hallucinations, but there are also behavioral techniques. Such techniques include thought stopping (e.g., saying "stop and go away"), or distraction strategies such as watching television, talking with someone, or listening to music with headphones, which will also tend to decrease their frequency and strength (Buccher et al., 1996). Specific interventions for hallucination management are presented in Box 29-5.

Research has shown that as interpersonal and self-care skills improve, hallucinations decrease. Clients with schizophrenia who participate in active recreational programs also show decreased psychosis (Corrigan and Storzbach, 1993). Auditory hallucinations may also be diminished if clients are taught to engage in humming during the hallucination. This is thought to interfere with subvocal muscular activity associated with a hallucinations (Green and Kinsbourne, 1990).

Managing delusions   According to Keith and Regier (1991), the most common symptom of schizophrenia is the presence of bizarre delusions. Thus the nurse often assists clients in dealing with this symptom. Because this is considered another positive symptom of schizophrenia, antipsychotic medication is also helpful in decreasing delusions.

In addition, nurses can address delusions with psychosocial interventions. A danger in directly attempting to change the client's mind is that the delusion may, in fact, be even more strongly held. However, a study is under way that indicates that if a graded, collaborative, nonconfrontational approach is used with clients who have delusions, these ideas may become less firmly held and some ideas rejected completely. This entails the following:

- Do not directly challenge the validity of the delusion.
- First attempting to modify the beliefs that are the least strongly held by asking clients to just *consider* alternative interpretations of the situation
- Examine evidence for their beliefs with them and point out how that could be seen a different way
- Encourage the client to voice arguments against their own beliefs (Chadwick and Lowe, 1990)

These techniques are only effective in the context of a trusting relationship and must not be carried out in a highly confrontational manner. Some clients never relinquish their delusions but may be able to function if the delusion remains nonthreatening and if they can learn not to talk about it except with people who are tolerant of them.

Looseness of associations   Communicating with a client who has schizophrenia can be a challenging process if that person exhibits altered thought processes reflected in disturbed speech and language. The nurse should attempt to understand the client's experience and help the client see the interest the nurse has in communication. This helps prevent a mutual withdrawal where difficulty in communication leads the client and nurse to stop working on a relationship. The nurse should be looking for meaning behind the loose association and should comment directly on that aspect of speech. When clients speak in tangential patterns that seem unfocused, nurses may have to gently interrupt the person to get them to return to the topic. Sometimes the nurse comments on the underlying feeling that the speech seems to evoke.

For example, one client was restricted from independently smoking cigarettes because he was at-risk for burning himself. His reply to the nurse was, "I am commander of this camp and you aren't going to get your paycheck." The nurse stated, "It must be frustrating and leave you with a powerless feeling to be given this restriction." These simple techniques and genuine commitment to engaging the client communicates caring and facilitates further communication.

The Nursing Process

BOX 29-5

Hallucination Management

DEFINITION

Promoting the safety, comfort, and reality orientation of a patient experiencing hallucinations

ACTIVITIES

Establish a trusting, interpersonal relationship with the patient

Monitor and regulate the level of activity and stimulation in the environment

Maintain a safe environment

Provide appropriate level of surveillance/supervision to monitor patient

Record patient behaviors that indicate hallucinations

Maintain a consistent routine

Assign consistent caregivers on a daily basis

Promote clear and open communication

Provide patient with opportunities to discuss hallucinations

Encourage patient to express feelings appropriately

Refocus patient to topic, if patient's communication is inappropriate to circumstances

Monitor hallucinations for presence of content that is violent or self-harmful

Encourage patient to develop control/responsibility over own behavior, if ability allows

Encourage patient to discuss feelings and impulses, rather than acting on them

Encourage patient to validate hallucinations with trusted others (e.g., reality testing)

Point out, if asked, that you are not experiencing the same stimuli

Avoid arguing with patient about the validity of the hallucinations

Focus discussion upon the underlying feelings, rather than the content of the hallucinations (e.g., "It appears as if you are feeling frightened")

Provide antipsychotic and antianxiety medications on a routine and PRN basis

Provide medication teaching to patient and significant others

Monitor patient for medication side effects and desired therapeutic effects

Provide for safety and comfort of patient and others when patient is unable to control behavior (e.g., limit setting, area restriction, physical restraint, and seclusion)

Discontinue or decrease medications (after consulting with prescribing caregiver) that may be causing hallucinations

Provide illness teaching to patient/significant others if hallucinations are illness based (e.g., delirium, schizophrenia, and depression)

Educate family and significant others about ways to deal with patient who is experiencing hallucinations

Monitor self-care ability

Assist with self-care, as needed

Monitor physical status of patient (e.g., body weight, hydration, and soles of feet in patient who paces)

Provide for adequate rest and nutrition

Involve patient in reality-based activities that may distract from the hallucinations (e.g., listening to music)

Reprinted with permission from McCloskey, J.C., & Bulechek, G.M. (Ed.). (1996). Nursing interventions classification (NIC), *(2nd ed.). St. Louis: Mosby.*

Social withdrawal Clients with schizophrenia exhibit isolation from others as a result of mistrust, altered reality testing, and lack of social skills. Clients who are withdrawn often respond slowly to nursing interactions. They usually need consistent, repeated approaches by nurses. Such clients may be mute and immobile or reclusive. Intervention includes establishment of interpersonal contact, facilitation of communication and of social participation.

Communication with withdrawn clients requires much patience from the nurse. To sit in silence with a mute person can be uncomfortable if one is more accustomed to verbal clients. The nurse may be tempted to fill the silence with trivia or aimless chatter and may

also communicate discomfort by fidgeting. The nurse facilitates communication with the client by doing the following:

- The nurse should determine the client's concerns and use this information to stimulate interest and client participation.
- The nurse should avoid filling up silences by talking about self, which conveys lack of interest in the client. Continuous talking by the nurse also conveys that the client is not expected to verbalize.
- The nurse should ask open-ended questions and pause to provide opportunities for the client to respond.

The Nursing Process

- The nurse should avoid direct questions that may be perceived as intimidating or not respectful of the client's privacy.
- The nurse should tend to the client's nonverbal communication. A completely silent client may communicate a great deal through body movements, gestures, and posture. Clients who are withdrawn may indicate their nonverbal participation in an interaction through establishment of direct eye contact, particularly when it has previously been avoided. Relaxation or alertness in body posture may be a first sign of comfort with the nurse.
- The nurse should use nonverbal methods of communicating. Some direct eye contact with the client conveys interest, concern, and caring. Leaning toward the client but maintaining a comfortable distance communicates that the nurse's attention is focused on the client. Touch should be used judiciously with the client until after assessment of response to touch has been done.
- The nurse should provide physical care is an important way of conveying concern. Reading magazines, eating, playing games, and taking walks are ways of promoting relatedness in a less demanding way because there is no requirement for verbalization in those activities. However, opportunities for talking may evolve out of experiences both the nurse and the client enjoy.

The client should play a key role in setting the pace for development of closeness. The one-on-one relationship provides the foundation for intervention with the withdrawn client. However, the nurse also strives to help the client gradually develop social relationships with a variety of other people. As nurse and client become more comfortable with each other, the nurse may gradually include others in social situations.

Psychotherapy

Nurses with specialized training, may provide individual therapy, group conduct therapeutic groups and implement family intervention for clients in inpatient or outpatient settings. These treatment modalities are modified somewhat for clients with schizophrenia but many basic principles remain the same.

Individual therapy When working with clients who have schizophrenia, a supportive, pragmatic focus is useful. This may include collaborative problem solving; management of specific symptoms; and assisting the client with social and personal functioning, spiritual needs, and

vocational adjustment. Educational interventions may be promoted by modeling healthy behaviors, or role playing communication or social skills with the client. A most therapeutic intervention noted by a majority of clients is positive feedback and a focus on what the client is doing well, rather than a focus solely on shortcomings (Beeber, 1995).

Cognitive therapy is also a tool nurses use in individual therapy to develop more resilience to stress and develop strategies to deal with problems (Gardner and Thompson, 1992). For example, a client might be encouraged to check out perceptions of others in socially approved ways instead of not voicing suspicious thoughts.

Therapeutic groups Group therapy has become more scrutinized in the past several years because it is seen as an economical modality and provides socialization opportunities for clients. A wide variety of group therapies can be beneficial to clients with schizophrenia. Overall, the therapeutic factors that can be accomplished in groups include the following:

- Instillation of hope
- Opportunity for catharsis of feelings
- Sense of belongingness in a cohesive group
- Interpersonal interaction and learning
- Self-understanding
- Universality or the sense of not being alone with one's problem
- Guidance from others
- Opportunity to reenact and reframe past family problems
- Identification as a member of a group (Yalom, 1985)

For clients with schizophrenia, six types of therapy groups are are most commonly employed: medication maintenance, social skills training, educational, interpersonal, and self-help. In all these groups, outcomes are better if the therapist takes an active role and the process is highly structured and supportive (Kahn and Kahn, 1992). Ambiguity should be kept to a minimum as clients may misinterpret less than clear expectations. Interventions should be direct and concrete and should match abilities of the client. The length of the sessions should match attention span and tolerance for stimulation. A 30-to-45–minute session may be most appropriate. Making the session a pleasant, positive experience for the clients is of prime importance. Many clients may have had negative social experiences in the past and may be very anxious about a group setting. The nurse should also strive to keep conflict or expressed negative

The Nursing Process

emotion in these groups to a minimum to keep anxiety low among clients.

Family interventions Interventions with family members should be incorporated whenever possible for clients with schizophrenia. Since schizophrenia tends to run a persistent course, clients often reside with family members and rely on them as a major source of support. The nurse may be asked to provide crisis intervention in the home or long-term guidance and education to promote positive coping patterns and to help prevent relapse.

One of the most consistently stated needs by caregivers is for information about the client's illness and practical interventions for coping with symptoms of the illness (Pfeiffer and Mostek, 1991). One modality that can be used effectively is to conduct multiple family groups where several families come together to provide support and receive practical information. These groups can also teach coping skills such as relaxation, recreation, and assertiveness to family members. They can also provide validation of family members' feelings and problematic situations.

A key intervention in working with families is to provide education about communicating feelings. Since high expressions of emotion in the family tends to increase the risk of relapse in clients, the nurse should recommend interactions that are warm, understanding, and tolerant instead of overinvolved, hostile, or critical (Gamble et al., 1994).

Specifically, it should be emphasized to family members that:

- They are in no way being blamed for the client's illness or relapse
- "Normal" families may criticize each other, but clients with schizophrenia are especially sensitive to any critical comments
- They should decrease any negative personal comments about the client to *below* what would be considered average for other families
- Involvement with the client should be concerned, yet matter-of-fact
- Extensively monitoring many aspects of the client's life such as behavior, dress, personal hygiene, and others, can increase stress for the client and can possibly increase the possibility of relapse

Finally, interventions for families should have as a goal, strengthening of support systems, both formal and informal. The National Alliance for the Mentally Ill (NAMI),

Schizophrenics Anonymous, and Recovery, Inc., are examples of organizations that provide support and resources for families and clients (see the Community Resources box below).

Milieu Therapy

Safety

An important consideration when working with clients who have schizophrenia is the maintenance of safety in the environment. Positive symptoms of a client, such as command hallucinations or delusions of persecution may compel a client to take risks or commit aggressive acts. One client interpreted literally the biblical passage, "If your eye causes you to sin, pluck it out, and if your hand causes you to sin, cut it off." By not

 COMMUNITY RESOURCES

Persons With Schizophrenia

National Alliance for the Mentally Ill (NAMI)
200 North Glebe Road, Suite 1015
Arlington, VA 22203-3754
(703) 524-7600 or toll free (800) 950-6264

National Association of Psychiatric Survivors (NAPS)
P.O. Box 618
Sioux Falls, SD 57101-0618
(605) 334-4067

National Empowerment Center
130 Parker Street
Lawrence, MA 01843

National Mental Health Consumers Association
P.O. Box 1166
Madison, WI 53701

Recovery, Inc.
802 North Dearborn Street
Chicago, IL 60610
(312) 337-5661

Schizophrenics Anonymous
1209 California Road
Eastchester, NY 10709
(914) 337-2252

The Nursing Process

comprehending the abstract concept of this passage, the client cut out his eye and amputated his hand, which caused his death through hypovolemic shock. The nurse should assist the client in complying with taking antipsychotic medications, since these affect the positive symptoms.

Memory problems, related to possible hippocampal dysfunction, may create unsafe situations if clients do not remember locations of important items such as clinic phone numbers or appointment dates. The nurse may need to work with the client to create a concrete system of managing this problem. For example, the client could always have a particular drawer in which important papers are kept.

Negative symptoms such as anergia might precipitate a dangerous situation if a client did not react quickly enough in an emergency. Reviewing basic safety precautions for the client's residence is an important nursing function.

Poor judgment, possibly related to frontal lobe dysfunction, may lead clients into high-risk sexual encounters or threatening environments. Specific guidelines about how to reduce risk for human immunodeficiency virus (HIV) infection, for example, are necessary. Clients should be strongly encouraged not to use alcohol and drugs, since they will impair judgment further.

Safety is accomplished structurally in the health care facility by unit policies and/or outpatient policies delineating safety measures. In the home, it involves conducting an assessment for general physical safety. Another safety consideration is a contingency plan for action if a relapse occurs. A plan could be contracting with a client. For example, the client may agree to contact the registered nurse case manager if auditory hallucinations become commanding or aggressive. On an inpatient unit, physical containment of a client may be necessary with the use of mechanical restraints for a short time if the client is an immediate danger to self or others. This should always be accompanied by the one-to-one presence of staff with the client, a thorough explanation of what is being done, and behaviors the client needs to exhibit to be released from restraints. Application of physical restraints is a collaborative effort requiring physicians order and always used as a last resort.

Productive activities

One goal of treatment is usually the repatterning of a dysfunctional lifestyle by engaging the client in a daily structure of activities that can be integrated as a permanent part of the client's life. This is needed because if there are prominent negative symptoms mediated by hypofrontal-

ity, the client may show social withdrawal, apathy, and loss of initiative. These symptoms may preclude a sense of meaning and purpose in life.

It is also useful to engage clients in purposeful activity to detract from the positive symptoms of auditory hallucinations. A structured activity program must be developed with client goals in mind, not simply to fill time for the client. Even basic expectations of getting up in the morning, grooming, and eating breakfast help clients establish a normal routine and transfer the schedule to job or ongoing therapy expectations. Some activities may be directly related to employment such as being involved in a sheltered workshop or participating in volunteer work. Other activities may be geared toward managing a job interview or increasing attention span, which might have indirect effects on vocation.

Some programs are provided to assist clients in managing leisure time. Formal recreational outings or simply engaging the client in a game of cards are two activities where clients can learn new ways to use free time.

Nurses can also provide opportunities for clients to sharpen skills of daily living. Banking, shopping, meal preparation, child care, and housework are all areas that are important for functioning. Practical education in these areas individually or in groups can assist clients in being more independent. For more detailed interventions on psychiatric rehabilitation, see Chapter 38.

Living arrangements

There is no one optimal residence for clients who have schizophrenia. Some persons marry, hold jobs and live with little assistance. Others may require some supervision for medication and activities of daily living (ADLs). These people may prefer to live in group homes or board and care homes. A halfway house is a form of transitional living for when a client may not be ready to live independently but instead needs more time or assistance to increase functional abilities.

Many clients rely on close relatives for housing, especially parents and siblings, and others require an intensive level of care that is provided by nursing homes or long-term hospitalization. Unfortunately, many persons with schizophrenia are homeless.

The nurse is a key member of the interdisciplinary team who decides with the client and family the most appropriate living arrangements for furthering the client's long-term goals. One consideration is the relative degree of brain dysfunction that the client is experiencing. For example, if the client has many positive symptoms and only moderately controlled psychosis a higher level of care and structure will be needed. Perhaps a brief inpatient stay for stabilization may be appropriate. If a

The Nursing Process

client has predominant negative symptoms, a community-based case management program would be more suitable.

Special programs are available that attempt to slowly integrate clients into a job and socialize them. These programs (often called "Job Clubs") first work with a client to determine the type of work for which he or she is best suited. They may begin training clients by having them perform work at the clubhouse or with a staff member at another job site. The goal is for the client to experience a job in a "safe" setting where training or education can be extended if necessary and the client can feel successful. Since culture in the United States values productivity, engaging in meaningful work can be an important component in a client's self-esteem. Nurses are in a good position to advocate for vocational rehabilitation for those clients who are appropriate.

Social skills training

Another significant milieu intervention that the nurse can implement is a program of social skills training. Formal training modules are available to assist clients in learning conversation skills, assertiveness, and social cues. This is especially helpful for those clients who have negative symptoms such as social isolation, poverty of speech, and attentional impairment. All staff should take responsibility for modeling appropriate social skills as well as positively reinforcing any attempts clients make in their social interactions. The nurse may need to actually teach the client appropriate ways of beginning a conversation or maintaining a relationship because these basic skills may never have been learned. The nurse may need to role play situations with the client for optimal integration of these skills. See also Chapter 38.

Self-Care Activities

Hygiene and grooming

As noted earlier, persons with schizophrenia have deficits in information processing and cognitive functioning. This may result in clients not adequately providing self-care. The nurse needs to assess the self-care problem (e.g., are delusions about poisoned water evident?) and design interventions that address the specific self-care problem. For example, Ralph F. had memory dysfunction that required him and the home care nurse to create a system of reminders to always brush his teeth after his morning coffee, wash his clothes on the day of his favorite television program, and change his clothes on calendar days marked with red dots.

Sleep

Many people with schizophrenia have altered sleep patterns. This may be because of psychotic symptoms or neurochemical changes in the brain. Altered sleep patterns are specifically seen in reductions in REM or the dream stage of sleep (Freeman and Karson, 1993). The nurse should assess typical patterns and work with the client to promote a healthy pattern of rest and sleep. General sleep hygiene principles should be initiated such as maintaining a regular time to go to bed and awaken, discouragement of daytime napping, elimination of caffeine from the diet, and the practice of physical relaxation techniques. Moderate exercise during the day or afternoon also encourages sleep.

If the client is having difficulty staying awake during the day because of sleepiness associated with medication, the nurse should explore with the physician the possibility of giving the bulk of the medication in the evening or adjusting the dosage.

Nutrition

Eating habits should always be assessed by the nurse to determine adequacy of daily nutrition. Some clients may have delusions about food or their ability to digest it. Other clients may not take time to eat or may not know how to prepare balanced meals. Other clients may consume large amounts of fat and salt in the form of easy-to-obtain "fast food."

If clients are suspicious, they may prefer to eat foods brought from home or food in sealed packages. For clients with low attention spans, high-quality snacks throughout the day may be a better alternative than three sit-down meals. Teaching clients about excess fats, sugars, and salt in their diets can empower them to make healthier choices for "fast food."

Caffeine consumption may be significant, especially among psychiatric clients (Byrne et al., 1991). Caffeine estimates should always be assessed because its use can interfere with antipsychotic medication and can contribute to sleep disturbances and mood irritability. Nurses should encourage decaffeinated alternatives and teach clients to expect a period of withdrawal after caffeine is stopped.

Exercise

Research shows a link between physical activity and emotional well-being. Persons with schizophrenia tend to have poor fitness levels in comparison to clients who have other psychotic conditions (Sheehan, 1991).

Regular exercise can produce notable benefits besides the obvious physical conditioning. Since clients with schizophrenia tend to have a poor body image and

The Nursing Process

boundaries, basic fitness exercises with some exploratory type gymnastic movements can assist the client to acquire a better self-image. In addition, the use of noncontact team sports may provide a mechanism for antisocial clients to interact nonverbally (Sheehan, 1991).

Health needs

A high incidence of unrecognized medical illness exists among clients with psychiatric disorders (Byrne et al., 1991). This may be related to decreased pain perception, lack of knowledge about disease processes, or the belief that physical complaints are "delusional." The nurse should give information to the client and family about health resources and encourage periodic physical and dental examinations. Clients should be taught routine breast or testicular examinations and given straightforward information about protection from sexually transmitted diseases. Any complaints of physical illness should be carefully explored.

The use of tobacco is also prevalent among clients with mental illnesses and may be related to self-medication of anxiety or decreased Parkinsonian side effects of antipsychotic medication, since nicotine is thought to decrease some medication levels (Selzer and Lieberman, 1993). Smoking cessation should be strongly encouraged and expected. Resources to assist clients to stop smoking, such as a nicotine patch, are readily available.

Psychobiological Interventions

During an acute inpatient phase, a key role for the nurse is to monitor the effectiveness of medications prescribed and note any adverse side effects that might require adjustment of the medication.

Antipsychotic medication is the mainstay of treatment for those with psychosis. Different classes of these medications may be prescribed until target symptoms of psychosis are reduced or eliminated and side effects are minimal. Novel combinations of medication may be used, as well, to alleviate concomitant symptoms. For example, a client may be prescribed an antipsychotic as well as an antidepressant medication if the client is experiencing significant depression.

Alprazolam (Xanax) is an antianxiety medication also used occasionally in addition to an antipsychotic because it is believed to augment the neuroleptic's effect in reducing negative symptoms such as blunted affect.

Carbamazepine (Tegretol), an antiseizure medication, can be also used, in conjunction with the antipsychotic medication. It is thought to lessen positive symptoms and aggressiveness if these are prominent (Keefe and Harvey, 1994).

Education about medication is important, because clients have a right to know what they are being prescribed and what are the effects of the medication. The nurse can inform the client that without medication, the relapse rate is 60% to 70% within the first year of diagnosis. If medication is taken, the relapse rate is 40% and then drops to 15% when there is a combination of medication, group education, and support.

Clients often have difficulty taking their medication regularly. This is related to a number of psychobiological brain changes. Among the positive symptoms, clients who experience paranoid delusions may believe that their medication is poisonous. Disorganized thinking may mitigate against taking medication because clients may have good intentions but may become distracted from the goal. Memory dysfunction might create a situation where they forget a scheduled dose.

Negative symptoms may also preclude clients from taking medication consistently. If a client is experiencing amotivation, he or she may be apathetic toward a regular medication regimen. Poor insight may create a situation where the client does not feel ill, and therefore feels no need to take any medication. In addition, if a client is experiencing social problems such as homelessness or inadequate income, there may be problems even acquiring and storing medication. Teaching should focus on increasing acceptance of taking the medication, since nonadherence is a significant and common problem.

A basic medication education program should review:

- What the medication is, including trade and generic names
- When and how often it is to be taken
- How it works/what symptoms it affects
- What are the side effects and how to deal with them, such as taking the bulk of the dosage in the evening if sedation is a problem and if the prescribing provider concurs (see the Medication Tips on p. 599)
- Any special considerations such as if they are able to drive or operate heavy machinery
- Potential interactions with other drugs, alcohol, or food
- Who to contact if there are problems or questions about medication at home

Neuroleptic malignant syndrome

Neuroleptic malignant syndrome (NMS) is a serious side effect of neuroleptic or antipsychotic medication. Although it is rare, affecting only 1% to 2% of clients on med-

The Nursing Process

MEDICATION TIPS

Antipsychotic Medications

- Drowsiness may occur at the initiation of therapy. Until you know how the medication is affecting the client, advise him or her to be careful with activities such as operating machinery or driving.
- Dizziness can occur especially after awakening in the morning. Tell client to rise slowly when getting out of bed.
- Dry mouth may be experienced. Clients should drink some water or eat sugar-free mints to help. (Observe for water intoxication.) Constipation may occur. Clients should eat fiber-rich foods, drink fluids, and exercise to help avoid this.
- Sunburns are more of a possibility when taking this medication. Clients should use sunscreen whenever they are exposed to the sun.
- Liquid forms of antipsychotic medication are not absorbed as well when caffeine is consumed 30 minutes before or after taking the medicine (Gaumer, 1992).

- Clients should not take antipsychotic medication within 1 hour of taking antacids or diarrheal medication, since the antipsychotic medicine tends not to be absorbed as readily (Gaumer, 1992).
- Tell clients never to share medication with another.
- Tell clients to develop a system for remembering to take their medications, such as compartmentalized pill boxes or pairing medication times with other regular activities.
- Clients should determine with their physicians what to do if doses are missed.
- Tell clients: DO NOT STOP TAKING MEDICATION EVEN IF YOU ARE FEELING WELL.

ication, it can cause serious neurological damage, and death rates may range from 14% to 30% (Blair and Dauner, 1993). See Chapter 15 for an in-depth discussion of NMS.

Tardive dyskinesia

One of the most serious and irreversible side effects of antipsychotic medication is tardive dyskinesia (TD). This condition is characterized by abnormal involuntary muscle movements that may affect the face or extremities. Any person that takes antipsychotic medication is at-risk for TD but those over age 50 seem to be at higher risk. Those who have taken antipsychotic medication for a number of years and have an affective component to their illness are more prone to TD.

There is no specific treatment for this side effect. Antipsychotic medication is discontinued as soon as any symptom of TD is observed. When this protocol is followed, clients may have up to a 50% chance that TD will diminish. In other clients, the side effect remains permanently (Gaumer, 1992). The nurse's responsibility is to educate clients about the possibility of tardive dyskinesia and to conduct periodic assessments using tools such as the AIMS test (see Chapter 15).

Water intoxication

Another nursing consideration to be kept in mind when working with clients with psychotic disorders is the possibility of polydipsia leading to water intoxication. Polydipsia refers to an excessive intake of fluid. *Water*

intoxication is the ingestion of water or fluid in excess of the body's ability to excrete it (Henley et al., 1992). Water intoxication can also be measured by laboratory data as a serum sodium concentration of 120 mEq/L or less. This can produce agitation, confusion, altered consciousness levels, convulsions and in some cases, death (Bugle et al., 1992). This condition can occur in as many as 18% of clients with serious neurobiological disorders at some point in the course of illness (Davidhizar, 1991) and can be a challenging behavior for clients to try to change. Nursing interventions may involve the following:

- Systematically control and monitor intake and output. This can be a challenge because clients can be singleminded in obtaining fluids.
- Engage the client in a structured environment (e.g., groups, recreation, etc.). This is helpful to divert clients attention away from obtaining fluid.
- Weigh the client twice daily and put in place a system of behavioral management if the client gains more than an agreed on amount reflecting excessive water consumption.
- Encourage the client to chew gum or eat ice chips.
- Educate the client about the effects of water intoxication.
- Enlist the client's collaboration in decreasing water intake instead of setting up a power struggle against the client. One creative nurse gave a set of yellow plastic paint chips to a client with an indwelling

The Nursing Process

urinary catheter. The client knew that he had to stop drinking water when the urine in his bag matched an agreed on color of paint chip corresponding to an unsafe urine concentration.

Health Teaching

Psychoeducation about coping with symptoms of schizophrenia is one of the most vital functions for nurses working in acute or long term community settings. One aspect of teaching should include basic education of clients and family about schizophrenia; symptoms, course, prognosis, treatment, and support resources; and symptom management.

Finally, a program of systematic symptom monitoring is an important part of health teaching. By identifying early signs of relapse, the client and family are empowered to take steps to prevent rehospitalization or lessen exacerbation of illness (O'Connor, 1991). See the Teaching Points presented below.

Case Management

Clients with schizophrenia are high users of physical and mental health services. They are often faced with a bewildering array of services and providers, each of whom provides only a portion of the client's needs. Also, clients with neurobiological disorders have symptoms such as social isolation and altered information processing, which make it even more difficult for clients to access and use treatment services (see Chapter 17).

For these and other reasons, many practice settings use a case management approach to care, having one nurse take responsibility for the coordination of all care received by a client and family. The case manager serves as a link between inpatient and community-based staff to ensure that the client's care continues uninterrupted. Needed services are also ensured, since the case manager has extensive knowledge of community resources and how to access them.

The case manager is typically involved in the client's discharge planning from inpatient care. This role also involves contacting the client in the community to work with him or her with the goal of minimizing relapse. For example, a case manager may meet with the client and inpatient treatment team before a client is discharged. The case manager then, when the client is at home, may encourage the client to take prescribed medication (see Chapters 17 and 38).

Health Promotion and Health Maintenance

Although the nurse may not be able to prevent the development of schizophrenia, he or she can work to promote the highest level of wellness possible for individuals. A nurse not only has a role with individual clients and families, but may have as a "client" the community at large. Interventions in this area include targeting at-risk populations. For example, low-income or homeless people with schizophrenia need interventions to increase their quality of life and use of health care services. Teaching coping strategies and providing practical assistance

TEACHING POINTS

Client With Schizophrenia

Teach the client, family and/or significant others the following:

- The neurobiological etiologic factors and interrelationship of the role of stress
- That there is a 70% relapse rate if medications are not taken on a regular basis and a 30% relapse rate if medication regimen is followed (studies indicate that relapse is less likely to occur if the family involvement is warm and supportive of the client)
- To identify the early warning signs of relapse (e.g., feeling tense, difficulty concentrating, trouble sleeping, increased withdrawal, increased bizarre/magical thinking, increased suspiciousness) that come *before* frank (obvious) psychotic symptoms

- To report the early warning signs of relapse and/or medication side effects to their primary health care professional
- To not use substances that can exacerbate a psychotic relapse (e.g., marijuana, alcohol, psychomotor stimulants like amphetamines, crack, or cocaine)
- To identify and access sources of ongoing support in dealing with the client (see the Community Resources box on p. 595)
- The development of problem-solving skills related to environmental stress of ADLs
- The importance of keeping the home environment a low expressed emotion versus a high expressed emotion and why
- Manage delusions or hallucinations

The Nursing Process

Schizophrenia

Anonymous

I have schizophrenia. I was diagnosed in 1988, a year after my father committed suicide. My doctor said the trauma from his suicide caused my schizophrenia.

In the beginning, I heard voices and didn't understand what was happening to me. I drank alcohol to escape from the voices, but I would just get drunk. I stayed awake many nights, unable to sleep because I was afraid of what the voices said. Imagine hearing someone talk to you and not being able to see them. The voices teased me, made fun of me, and scared me. I lost my apartment and everything I owned. I was flunking out of college, and I spent all of the inheritance I had received from my father. Finally I was hospitalized. I spent 2 months in the hospital and was put on medication.

About a year and a half after my hospitalization the voices went away. I was very happy. I have coped with my illness by taking my medication, eating well, and getting enough sleep. I make sure to structure my day and to not isolate myself. I also go to therapy and talk about what is bothering me to learn how to cope with difficult situations.

I have been discriminated against because of this diagnosis. In 1993, I had a job at a restaurant, and my boss knew I was a member of a psychosocial club called Primetime, a place where the psychiatrically disabled get jobs, socialize, and train for work. The direc-

tor of Primetime helped me get the job at the restaurant. The restaurant owner wouldn't let me wait tables even though I had experience, so I bussed tables and didn't get any tips from the other waitresses for helping them. None of the other waitresses were friendly. They all hung out together and ignored me.

The mental health care delivery system has helped me through therapy and work. Going to therapy once a week allows me to discuss what is bothering me and helps relieve stress. Having a therapist who believed I could hold down a job and reach my goals helped me. Being on medication has helped control my symptoms and helped me cope. My current job has helped in my recovery. Through it, I have gained more self-esteem and learned a lot.

To cope with schizophrenia it is important to take the necessary medication, go to therapy, get enough sleep, and eat well. Work with the doctors and therapists, and tell them what is going on and how you feel. It is also important to stay away from street drugs and alcohol. A suggestion I have for professionals who work with people who have schizophrenia is to listen to what they say, have patience, and educate them about the illness. This will help them understand what they have and how to deal with it so that they can recognize the symptoms and have a better quality of life.

with ADLs are preventive interventions that can be incorporated into various programs for this population. Design and implementation of community programs are more effective if consumers and professionals participate in the process. See Chapters 18 and 38 for in-depth discussions of health promotion and maintenance interventions for this client population.

Advocacy and political action on behalf of persons with mental illness are also parts of the health promotion role of nurses. Some nurses run for governmental office or act as consultants to public officials on health care. Others join with consumer groups to help educate the

public about mental illness. Supporting legislation to protect rights of individuals with major mental illnesses can be accomplished by keeping informed of upcoming legislation on a state and federal level.

Evaluation

The last phase of the nursing process is an analysis of interventions and outcomes to determine to what extent goals have been achieved. Since goals are formulated to be measurable, this should be a straightforward process. If nurse and client agree that goals have been achieved,

The Nursing Process

the nurse might choose to continue interventions at a less intense level but may strive to maintain outcomes reached. If goals have not been met, the nurse needs to determine whether the interventions were actually addressing the cause of the problem. New interventions may be attempted then, before modifying objectives. Evaluation may then become the first step of a new nursing process cycle.

CRITICAL THINKING QUESTIONS

Melissa T. is a 22-year-old college senior who has been admitted to the acute psychiatric unit of University Hospital. She was accompanied by her parents who live 100 miles away.

Melissa had been brought to the hospital by campus police who had found her in the student union screaming at the television to stop "telling me to hurt myself." She admits to prior illicit drug use but a preliminary urinalysis did not show the presence of any drugs at this time. Her appearance is somewhat disheveled, but she is calm and appears confused. Her affect is flat, but she states that her mood is good. Melissa is not oriented to time, date, or place; however, she does know her name and she knows who are her parents. She says, "I keep hearing someone telling me to kill myself; it must have come from the television." She shows poor judgment and insight in wanting to leave the hospital because "there is nothing wrong with me." According to her parents, Melissa has not exhibited any bizarre behavior in the past. Physical examination and vital signs are within normal limits.

1. What are additional nursing assessment tools that would aid in the evaluation of Melissa? What results might you expect?
2. What are three nursing diagnoses that would be important for this client? In what order would you prioritize them? Give your rationale.
3. In what ways does this client fit a "typical profile" of a client with schizophrenia? In what ways does she not?
4. What interventions would you implement to maintain the safety of Melissa and others?
5. Explain how you would involve Melissa's family in her treatment plan?
6. What discharge plans might you project for Melissa?

KEY POINTS

- Schizophrenia is a neurobiological disorder that is one of a group of disorders having psychotic features.
- Schizophrenia affects about 1% of the worldwide population.
- Although the cause of schizophrenia has not been established, the illness is correlated with neurotransmitter dysregulation, altered information processing, hemispheric dysfunction, and neuroanatomical abnormalities
- Genetic studies indicate that there is a higher incidence of schizophrenia among first-degree relatives.
- Persons with schizophrenia have higher incidence of relapse if they are living in families with a high level of expressed emotion.
- The stress-vulnerability model of schizophrenia is one theory postulating that some individuals are born with a tendency to develop schizophrenia when exposed to sufficient stress.
- Initial assessment of an acutely psychotic client should focus on establishing trust and gathering the most critically needed data.
- Positive symptoms of schizophrenia refer to those behaviors or experiences that are increased or grossly distorted from the norm.
- Negative symptoms refer to conditions reflecting a lessening or loss of normal functions.
- Type I schizophrenia is associated with "positive" symptoms such as hallucinations and elusions.
- Type II schizophrenia has a preponderance of "negative" symptoms such as social isolation and low motivation.
- Symptoms on schizophrenia include cognitive dysfunction, changes in perception, affective, behavioral, and social changes.
- Tardive dyskinesia and neuroleptic malignant syndrome are two serious side effects of antipsychotics.

REFERENCES

Acorn, S. (1993). Use of the Brief Psychiatric Rating Scale by nurses. *Journal of Psychosocial Nursing, 31*(5), 9-12.

Aksu, E.M., & Myers, H.E. (1994). Schizophrenia: Pathophysiology and treatment aspects. *Journal of American Academy of Physicians Assistants, 7,* 175-82.

Altshuler, L. (1991). Neuroanatomy in Schizophrenia and Affective Disorder. *Journal of the California Alliance for the Mentally Ill, 2*(4), 27-30.

American Psychiatric Association (1994). *Diagnostic and statistical manual of mental disorders, fourth edition.* Washington, DC: Author.

Andraeson, N.C. (1984). *The broken brain.* New York: Harper and Row.

Andraeson, N.C. (1985). Positive vs. negative schizophrenia: A critical evaluation. *Schizophrenia Bulletin, 11*(3), 380-389.

Andraeson, N.C. (Winter, 1994). NARSAD Research Newsletter. In *Alliance for the Mentally Ill of Iowa Newsletter,*

Andraeson, N. (1995). *Negative symptoms in schizophrenia* (videotape). ProCom Div Wheeler Communications Group, Inc.

Bateson, G., Jackson, D.D., Haley, J., & Weakland, J. (1956). Toward a theory of schizophrenia. *Behavioral Science, 1,* 251-64.

Beeber, L.S. (1995). The one-to-one relationship in psychiatric nursing: The next generation. *Psychiatric nursing 1946-1994: A report on the state of the art.* St. Louis: Mosby.

Betemps, E.J., & Ragiel, C. (1994). Psychiatric epidemiology: Facts and myths on mental health and illness. *Journal of Psychosocial Nursing, 32*(5), 23-28.

Blair, D.T., & Dauner, A. (1993). Neuroleptic malignant syndrome: Liability in nursing practice. *Journal of Psychosocial Nursing, 31*(2), 5-17.

Bowen, M. (1978). A family concept of schizophrenia. In M. Bowen (Ed.), *Family Therapy in Clinical Practice.* New York: Aronson.

Buccheri, R. Trygstad, L., Kanas, N., Waldron, B. & Dowling, M. (1996). Auditory hallucinations in schizophrenia. *Journal of Psychosocial Nursing, 34:2,* 12-25.

Bugle, C., Andrew, S., & Heath, J. (1992). Early detection of water intoxication. *Journal of Psychosocial Nursing, 30*(11), 31-34.

Byrne, C., Isaacs, S., & Voorberg, N. (1991). Assessment of the physical health needs of people with chronic mental illness: One focus for health promotion. *Canada's Mental Health, 3,* 7-12.

Campinha-Bacote, J. (1994). Transcultural psychiatric nursing: Diagnostic and treatment issues. *Journal of Psychosocial Nursing, 32*(8), 41-46.

Cannon, T.D., & Marco, E. (1994). Structural brain abnormalities as indicators of vulnerability to schizophrenia. *Schizophrenia Bulletin, 20*(1), 89-102.

Chadwick, P.D.J., & Lowe, C.F. (1990). Measurement and modification of delusional beliefs. *Journal of Consulting and Clinical Psychology, 58*(2), 225-232.

Cohen, J.D., & Servan-Schreiber, D. (1993). A theory of dopamine function and its role in cognitive deficits in schizophrenia. *Schizophrenia Bulletin, 19*(1), 85-104.

Corrigan, P.W., & Storzbach, D.M. (1993). Behavioral interventions for alleviating psychotic symptoms. *Hospital and Community Psychiaty, 44*(4), 341-347.

Crow, T.J. (1995). The meaning of the morphological changes in the brain in schizophrenia. *Current Approaches to Psychosis, 4,* 8-9.

Csernansky, J.G., & Newcomer, J.W. (1994). Are there neurochemical indicators of risk for schizophrenia? *Schizophrenia Bulletin, 20*(1), 75-88.

Davidhizar, R. (1991). Understanding water intoxication. *Advancing Clinical Care, May-June,* 16-19.

Dohrenwend, B.P., Levav, I., Shrout, P.E., Schwartz, S., Naveh, G., Link, B.G., Skodol, A.E., & Stueve, A. (1992). Socioeconomic status and psychiatric disorders: The causation-selection issue. *Science, 255,* 946-952.

Drake, R.E., Alterman, A.I., & Rosenberg, S.R. (1993). Detection of substance use disorders in severely mentally ill patients. *Community Mental Health Journal, 29*(2), 175-192.

Dworkin, R.H. (1994). Pain insensitivity in schizophrenia: A neglected phenomenon and some implications. *Schizophrenia Bulletin, 20*(2), 235-248.

Fetter, M.S., & Lowery, B. (1992). Psychiatric rehospitalization of te severely mentally ill: Patient and staff perspectives. *Nursing Research, 41*(5), 301-305.

Foucault, M. (1973). *Madness and civilization.* New York: Vintage.

Freeman, T., & Karson, C.N. (1993). The neuropathology of schizophrenia. *Psychiatric Clinics of North America, 16*(20), 281-293.

Frye, B., & D'Avanzo, C. (1994). Cultural themes in family stress and violence among Cambodian refugee women in the inner city. *Advances in Nursing Science, 16*(3), 64-77.

Gamble, C., Midence, K., & Leff, J. (1994). The effects of family work training on mental health nurse's attitude to and knowledge of schizophrenia: A replication. *Journal of Advanced Nursing, 19,* 893-896.

Gardner, B., & Thompson, S. (1992). The use of cognitive behavioural therapy with people with schizophrenia. *Journal of Clinical Nursing, 1,* 283-288.

Gaumer, C.B. (1992). *Menninger clinic medication manual.* Menninger Clinic, Topeka, Kansas.

Gold, J.M., & Harvey, P.D. (1993). Cognitive deficits in schizophrenia. *Psychiatric Clinics of North America, 16*(2), 295-312.

Gold, J., Randolph, C., Carpenter, C., Goldbert, T., & Weinberger, D. (1992). The performance of patients with schizophrenia on the Wechsler Memory Scale-Revised. *The Clinical Neuropsychologist, 6*(4), 367-373.

Green, M.F., & Kinsbourne, M. (1990). Subvocal activity and auditory hallucinations: Clues for behavioral treatments? *Schizophrenia Bulletin, 16*(4), 617-625.

Grinspoon, L. (1992). *The Harvard Mental Health Letter, 8,* 11.

Haier, R. (1990). Research Update in Schizophrenia. *The Journal of the California Alliance for the Mentally Ill, 1,* 12.

Henley, J., Fagan-Pryor, E., & Haber, L. (1992). Nursing program to meet the challenge of caring for patients with water intoxication. *Issues in Mental Health Nursing, 13,* 59-67.

Huttunen, M. (1995). The expanding role of serotonin-dopamine antagonists in psychoses treatment. *Current Approaches to Psychoses: Diagnosis and Management, 4,* 2-3.

Jansen, E. (1994). A self psychological approach to treating the mentally ill, chemically abusing and addicted (MICAA) patient. *Archives of Psychiatric Nursing, 8*(6), 381-389.

Jibson, N.D., & Tandon, R. (1996). A summary of research findings on the new antipsychotic drugs. *Psychiatric Nursing Forum, 2,* 1-7.

Kahn, E.M., & Kahn, E.W. (1992). Group treatment assignment for outpatients with schizophrenia: Integrating recent clinical and research findings. *Community Mental Health Journal, 28*(6), 539-550.

Kaplan, H.I., & Sadock, B.J. (Eds.). (1994). *Comprehensive textbook of psychiatry (6th ed.).* Baltimore: Williams & Wilkins.

Karno, M., & Jenkins, J.H. (1993). Cross-cultural issues in the course and treatment of schizophrenia. *Psychiatric Clinics of North America, 16*(2), 339-350.

Keefe, R., & Harvey, P. (1994). *Understanding schizophrenia.* The Free Press, N.Y.

Keith, S.J., Regier, D.A., & Rae, D.S. (1991). Schizophrenic disorders in L. N. Robins & D.A. Regier (Eds.), *Psychiatric disorders in america.* New York: The Free Press.

Kendler, K.S., & Diehl, S.R. (1993). The genetics of schizophrenia: A current genetic-epidemiologic perspective. *Schizophrenia Bulletin, 19*(2), 261-285.

Kim, M.J., McFarland, G.K., & McLane, A. (Eds.). (1993). *pocket guide to nursing diagnosis (5th ed).* St. Louis: Mosby.

Krach, P. (1993). Nursing implications: Functional status of older persons with schizophrenia. *Journal of Gerontological Nursing, 19*(8), 21-27.

Krach, P., & Yang, J. (1992). Functional status of older persons with chronic mental illness living in a home setting. *Archives of Psychiatric Nursing, 6*(2), 90-97.

Mednick, S.A., Huttunen, M.O., & Machon, R. (1994). Prenatal influenza infections and adult schizophrenia. *Schizophrenia Bulletin, 20*(2), 263-267.

Moller, M. (1989). *Understanding and communicating with the person who is hallucinating.* (Videotape). Omaha, NE. NurSeminars, Inc.

Murphy, M.F., & Moller, M.D. (1993). Relapse management in neurobiological disorders: The Moller-Murphy symptom management assessment tool. *Archives of Psychiatric Nursing, 7*(4), 226-235.

Nasrallah, H.A. (1993). Neurodevelopmental pathogenesis of schizophrenia. *Psychiatric Clinics of North America, 16*(2), 269-280.

O'Connor, F. (1991). Symptom monitoring for relapse prevention in schizophrenia. *Archives of Psychiatric Nursing, 5*(4), 193-201.

Pallast, E.G.M., Jongbloet, P.H., Straatman, H.M., & Zielhuis, G.A. (1994). Excess seasonality of births among patients with schizophrenia and seasonal ovopathy. *Schizophrenia Bulletin, 20*(2), 269-276.

Pfeiffer, E.J., & Motek, M. (1991). Services for families of people with mental illness. *Hospital and Community Psychiatry, 42*(3), 262-264.

Pincus, J. & Tucker, G. (1985). *Behavioral neurology.* Oxford, UK: Oxford University Press, Oxfold, U.K.

Prescott, C.A., & Gottesman, I.I. (1993). Genetically mediated vulnerability to schizophrenia. *Psychiatric Clinics of North America, 16*(2), 245-267.

Seeman, P. (1995). Dopamine receptors as new targets for novel drugs. *Current Approaches to Psychosis: Diagnosis & Management, 4,* 2-3.

Selzer, J.A. & Lieberman, J.A., (1993). Schizophrenia and substance abuse. *Psychiatric Clinics of North America, 16*(2), 217-144.

Sheehan, M. (1991). Sports therapy in mental illness. *Nursing Standard, 20*(6), 33-37.

Siever, L.J., Kalus, O.F., & Keefe, S.E. (1993). The boundaries of schizophrenia. *Psychiatric Clinics of North America, 16*(2), 217-244.

Stirling, J., Tantam, D., Thomas, P., Newby, D., Montague, L., Ring, N., & Rowe, S. (1993). Expressed emotion and schizophrenia: The ontogeny of EE during an 189 month follow up. *Psychological Medicine, 23,* 771-778.

Szasz, T. (1974). *The myth of mental illness.* New York: Harper & Row.

Thompson, L.W. (1990). The dopamine hypothesis of schizophrenia. *Perspectives in Psychiatric Care, 26*(3), 18-23.

Tieaskie, L. (1992). NMS: Rare and dangerous drug reaction. *American Journal of Nursing, Feb,* 67-70.

Torrey, E.F. (1994). Violent behavior by individuals with serious mental illness. *Hospital and Community Psychiatry, 45*(7), 653-661.

Waddington, J. (1993). Neurodynamics of abnormalities in cerebral metabolism and structure in schizophrenia. *Schizophrenia Bulletin, 19*(1), 55-69.

Yalom, I. (1985). *The theory and practice of group psychotherapy.* Basic Books: New York.

Chapter 30

Mood Disorders

Judith Haber

LEARNING OUTCOMES

After studying and applying the concepts of this chapter, the learner will be able to:
- Discuss the epidemiological risk factors related to the development of depression, bipolar disorder, and suicide
- Discuss biological and psychosocial correlates of mood disorders
- Differentiate between cognitive, affective, behavioral, and physiological changes associated with depression and mania
- Identify focused assessment criteria and assessment instruments for depressed, manic, and suicidal clients
- Develop a nursing care plan for a client with depression, mania, or who is suicidal
- Discuss nursing interventions related to counseling, milieu management, self-care, psychobiology, and health teaching for clients with mood disorder.
- Explain the value of using case management and an interdisciplinary approach with mood disorders
- Describe health promotion and preventive interventions for populations at risk for mood disorders
- Discuss outcome indicators to use when evaluating the effectiveness of nursing intervention for clients with mood disorders
- Select self-care strategies that nurses can use to maintain a realistic perspective and therapeutic effectiveness

KEY TERMS

Affect
Anniversary reaction
Cognitive distortions
Completed suicide
Delayed grief reaction
Double depression
Electroconvulsive therapy (ECT)
Grief
Hypomania

Lethality
Levels of intention
Mood
Nodal events
Phototherapy
Postpartum blues
Postpartum depression
Postpartum psychosis
Rapid cycling

Seasonal affective disorder (SAD)
Social role strain
Suicide attempts
Suicide intent
Suicidal ideation
Suicidal gestures
Suicidal threats
Tunnel vision

All people experience a wide range of moods and an equally large repetoire of emotional responses as a dimension of human existence. *Mood refers to a sustained internal emotional state associated with characteristic emotions and feelings that are reflected in a person's personality and influence how that person functions.* In contrast, **affect** *refers to the external expression of current emotional content* (Kaplan, Sadock, and Grebb 1994).

For centuries, extremes in mood have fascinated artists, scientists, writers, and philosophers who have attempted to link extremes of mood with positive attributes such as genius, creativity, productivity, and charisma, but also with negative attributes such as madness, despair, grandiosity, and destructiveness. Indeed, some of society's most respected celebrities—Vincent Van Gogh, the artist; Sylvia Plath, the writer; Frederic Neitzsche, the philospher; Jerry Garcia, the rock star; and Abraham Lincoln, the politician—represent famous people whose lives were affected, both positively and negatively, by a mood disorder.

Mood disorders are the most common, yet challenging of the neurobiological conditions encountered by psychiatric mental-health nurses, affecting at least 10 to 15 million Americans at any given time. It is estimated that of the 30,000 annual suicides in the United States, approximately 16,000 are associated with depressive disorders. Generally, mood disorders involve a single or recurring depressive (unipolar) and/or manic (bipolar) episodes. They also occur as dimensions of other non-mood conditions including eating, personality, panic, and obsessive-compulsive disorders (OCDs), as well as drug or alcohol intoxication or withdrawal. People, not uncommonly, experience mood disorders, especially depression, associated with physical health problems such as diabetes, cancer, human immunodeficiency virus/acquired immunodeficiency syndrome (AIDS), chronic fatigue syndrome (CFS), fibromyalgia, multiple sclerosis (MS), and cerebrovascular accident (CVA), or as consequences of the use of selected prescription medications. For others, backaches, headaches, and other somatic complaints are the manifestations of depression that go undiagnosed or untreated about 50% of the time because they masquerade as physical health problems that are not connected to depression. All too often, symptoms of depression are inappropriately dismissed as understandable responses to stress, weakness of character, or an attempt to get attention. As such, mood disorders are mental health problems commonly encountered in mental health as well as primary and specialty care settings.

Despite the fact that mood disorders cause as much suffering and economic loss to persons and their families as heart disease, cancer, and other chronic physical illnesses, fewer than half of individuals with major mood disorders receive treatment. In some cases they do not seek treatment because of social stigma and a sense of hopelessness, or they are not correctly diagnosed by primary care providers because many physical health problems have similar symptoms (insomnia, weight loss, fatigue) that make recognition of mood disorders more difficult.

Differentiating persons who are experiencing normal mood fluctuations from those with depressive or bipolar (manic-depressive) disorders for which treatment is appropriate presents an ongoing challenge to mental health professionals. Psychiatric nurses encounter clients with mood disorders, ranging from mild to severe, in a variety of inpatient and outpatient settings. The purpose of this chapter is to examine depressive and bipolar disorders, including suicide, develop an understanding of the biopsychosocial theories that explain mood disorders, and learn how to intervene effectively with clients experiencing these conditions.

EPIDEMIOLOGY

It is estimated that one in four persons will experience some type of mood disorder during his or her lifetime. Major depressive disorder is the most common mood disorder, with a lifetime prevalence of approximately 15%. Depression may range from mild and moderate states to severe states with or without psychotic features. Psychotic depression, however, is relatively uncommon, accounting for less than 10% of all depressions.

Major depression is estimated to occur two times more often in women than men. Although a specific genetic transmission pattern has not been identified, major depression is 1.5 to 3 times more common among first-degree relatives of persons with this disorder than among the general population (Kaplan, Sadock, and Grebb, 1994; American Psychiatric Association [APA], 1994). Major depression appears to have a recurring pattern. Of persons having a single episode of major depression 50% to 60% can be expected to have a second episode. Persons who have had a second episode have a 70% chance of having a third episode. Untreated, most episodes of major depression last 6 to 24 months. The prevalence rates for major depressive disorder appear unrelated to ethnicity, education, income, or marital status.

Although depression can occur at any age, the most common age of adult onset for men and women is between ages 25 and 44. The age of highest risk is the 18-to-44 age group, particularly those ages 18 to 24. In fact, there has been a progressive increase in acute and recurring depression for each cohort of persons born during successive decades of the twentieth century. Studies of depression also reveal an earlier age of onset of depression among younger cohorts, suggesting that the rate of depressive disorders may be rising in successively younger age groups (Bourdon et al., 1992).

Box 30-1 identifies risk factors associated with suicide. The National Institute of Mental Health Epidemiologic Catchment Area Study (ECA) assessed the lifetime prevalence of suicide attempts. Findings indicated that in people with no lifetime history of any psychiatric disorder, the suicide rate is 1%. Among people with a lifetime history of major depressive disorder, the rate of suicide is 18% (Bourdon et al., 1992). Of the 30,000 annual suicides, 16,000 in the United States annually are associated with depressive disorders. The relationship between depression and death is significantly stronger in men. Data also suggest that suicide is occurring more often in those over 60, particularly white single men, and those under 24 (Mellick, Buckwalter, and Stolley, 1992). Family members and loved ones are also considered victims of suicide. Multiply the 16,000 suicides annually that are related to depressive disorders by as few as four family members or close friends for each, and the result is 64,000 persons who have suffered unusual and traumatic grief and whose lives will forever be affected by their loss (Box 30-1).

Bipolar I mood disorder is less common than major depressive disorder, with a lifetime prevalence of about 1%, similar to the figure for schizophrenia. Because bipolar I disorder tends to have a recurring pattern, the cost of this neurobiological disorder to the 1 to 3 million people affected, their families, and society is significant. More than 90% of people who have a single manic episode, will have future episodes. Roughly 60% to 70% of manic episodes occur immediately before or after a major depressive episode, with each person having a unique cyclical pattern. The number of lifetime episodes (both manic and depressive) tends to be higher for bipolar I disorder compared with major depressive disorder. The interval between episodes tends to decrease as the person ages.

THEORETICAL FRAMEWORK

Theories related to explaining the development of mood disorders, including depression, bipolar disorder, and suicide are numerous but can be logically grouped in relation to biological, psychosocial, and familial theories. Some of these theories conflict with one another, some are supported by research, but some are not, and certainly not all of them are applicable to any one person. Rather, they represent the range of major theories that propose to explain the occurrence of specific mood disorders.

Biological Correlates

Common biological theories focus on neurotransmitter, neuroendocrine, circadian rhythm, kindling and behavioral sensitization, and genetic hypotheses.

Neurotransmitter hypothesis

Several neurotransmitters, including three biogenic amines—epinephrine, norepinephrine, and serotonin—as well as acetylcholine, dopamine, and gamma-aminobutyric acid (GABA), are proposed to be involved in the pathophysiologic factors of mood disorders. The receptor-sensitivity hypothesis suggests that alterations in neurotransmitter or neuroreceptor sensitivity in the central nervous system (CNS) may be related to the development of depression and/or manic-depressive disorder.

One hypothesis focuses on a possible overactivity of the norepinephrine (NE) autoreceptor. Autoreceptors function as the neuron's own feedback system and tell the neuron when enough neurotransmitter has been released into the synapse. This hypothesis proposes that instead of regulating the normal release of NE in the synapse, an overactive autoreceptor inhibits normal amounts of NE from entering the synapse. Since antidepressant medications also affect the NE receptor cells after several weeks on this kind of medication regimen, this might explain the several-week lag time for onset of therapeutic effectiveness. It may take longer to change the NE receptors than it does to increase the amount of NE in the synapse. From another perspective, the antidepressant effect may be caused by an upregulation or increase of the NE receptor cells of the postsynaptic membrane which allows more NE to be received (Lowery, 1996; Montano, 1994).

BOX 30-1

Risk Factors Related to Suicide

Family history of suicide
Family history of substance abuse
Prior suicide attempts
History of mood disorder
Depression
Psychosis (hallucinations, delusions)
Substance abuse (use of or withdrawal from)
General medical illnesses
Organic brain disorders (delerium, dementia)
Personality disorders
Impulse control disorders
Anxiety
Stress (acute or chronic)
Isolation
Loss of a significant other
Loss of self-esteem
Loss of social and economic resources
Guilt
Ambivalence
Gender and age (caucasian males over age 60)

Serotonin (5-HT), another neurotransmitter, is also involved in mood disorders. Studies have found that concentrations of serotonin are low in mood disorders. Low concentrations of serotonin metabolites have been found in the cerebrospinal fluid of some suicidal clients. One of the newest classes of antidepressants, the selective serotonin reuptake inhibitors (SSRIs), act almost exclusively on the serotonin system, supporting a key role for serotonin in mood disorders. Although current SSRIs act primarily through the blockade of serotonin reuptake, thereby causing more of it to be available to bind to the receptors of the postsynaptic neuron, future generations of antidepressants may have other effects on the serotonin system. The identification of multiple serotonin receptor subtypes suggests that other mechanisms including antagonism of the $5-HT_2$ receptor and agonism of the $5-HT_{1A}$ receptor, may be examples of other effects of antidepressants on the serotonin system (Hayes, 1995).

Acetylcholine, another biogenic amine, has also been targeted for involvement in mood disorders. It has been proposed that too little acetylcholine can cause depression and too much norepinephrine can cause mania, suggesting that an imbalance between these two neurotransmitters contributes to the cause of mood disorders. Dopamine, usually associated with the biological basis of schizophrenia, exerts an influence similar to acetylcholine. Low levels of dopamine are associated with depression, whereas increased levels, particularly in combination with the NE system, are associated with mania.

GABA, an inhibitory neurotransmitter from the amino acid family, has been identified as a modulator of other neurotransmitter systems. GABA has a wide range of effects, is present in 30% of nervous synapses, and increased GABA activity has been found to paradoxically have an antidepressant and antimanic effect (Hayes, 1995; Kaplan, Sadock, and Grebb, 1994). Thus GABA may be another neurotransmitter that plays an important role in the cause of mood disorders. Finally, the peptide neurotransmitters, the newest classification of neurotransmitters to be discovered, are also highlighted as regulators of other neurotransmitters. Although their mechanism of action is not well-understood, they are often found together in the same neuron as other neurotransmitters involved in mood disorders such as 5-HT, NE, and GABA. Specific peptides such as endogenous opioids, found to coexist with 5-HT and NE, are thought to be involved with stress, pain, and mood. Substance P, thought to coexist with acetylcholine and NE, is primarily found in sensory neurons (Devane, 1994; Hayes, 1995).

Dietary influences on the production and metabolism of neurotransmitters are also being studied. Dietary amino acids such as tryptophan, tyrosine, and choline are precursors of neurotransmitters. Dietary additives as well as naturally occurring chemicals may influence the development of depression and mania. Salicylates, caffeine, sugar, and preservatives may interact with neurotransmitters to influence brain function (McEnany, 1990; Wurtman, 1988).

It is obvious that there is no single neurotransmitter implicated in the development of either major depression, bipolar disorder, or suicidal behavior. Rather, the dysregulation hypothesis proposes that there is a generalized dysregulation of the mechanisms that regulate neurotransmission activities at the synapse. Support for this perspective is derived from evidence that neurotransmitter systems interact with each other; the activity of one affects and modulates the activities of the others. Moreover, medications used to treat mood disorders are targeted to specific neurotransmitters and appear to restore more effective neurotransmitter regulation. In general, decreased activity within the 5-HT-NE neurotransmitter system is associated with depression and increased activity of the NE-dopamine system is associated with mania (Goodwin and Jamison, 1990; Hayes, 1995; McEnany, 1990).

Neuroendocrine hypothesis

A correlation between hormonal activity and mood disorders has been considered for many years. Among the symptoms of depression that suggest endocrine changes are decreased appetite, weight loss, insomnia, changes in libido, gastrointestinal (GI) disorders, and mood changes. Mood changes have also been associated with endocrine disorders such as Cushing's disease, hyper- and hypothyroidism, autoimmune thyroiditis, and estrogen therapy. Recently, new biochemical assay techniques have detected alterations in hormone activity concurrent with depression.

Most neuroendocrine research in mood disorders suggests the disinhibition of the hypothalamic-pituitary-adrenal (HPA) axis and the hypothalamic-pituitary-thyroid (HPT) axis. Cortico-releasing factor (CRF), a hypothalamic peptide, stimulates the release of adrenocorticotropic hormone (ACTH) from the anterior pituitary. ACTH causes the adrenal cortex to secrete cortisol which in turn regulates the further release of CRF from the hypothalamus. The entire HPA axis has a circadian rhythm; most of the cortisol released from the adrenal glands comes in periodic bursts during the early morning hours. In people who do not have mood disorders, cortisol levels are relatively flat from late afternoon until 3 or 4 AM, when they begin to increase and spike at regular intervals, until about noon, when they gradually begin to level off again. In contrast, clients with physiological evidence of depression have been shown to have erratic cortisol spikes over a 24-hour period. The regulation of CRF is complex and involves neurotransmitters associated with mood disorders, especially depression, including serotonin, norepinephrine, and acetylcholine. Hyperactivity of the HPA axis and hypersecretion of cortisol in depressed clients has been extensively documented. The cortisol levels seem to return to normal as the depression subsides and, as such, appears to be related to the depression itself rather than to stress or mere hyperactivity (Jefferson and Greist, 1994).

Dysregulation of the HPT axis may also be associated with mood disorders. A consistent finding has been that about one third of all clients with major depression, who have an otherwise normal HPT axis, have a blunted release of thyroid-stimulating hormone (TSH) in response to an infusion of thyroid-releasing hormone (TRH). However, the value of this finding is limited by data which indicate that this same abnormality is also reported for other psychiatric diagnoses. Recent research has focused on the possibility that a subset of depressed clients have an unrecognized autoimmune disorder that affects their thyroid glands. Findings suggest that 10% of clients with mood disorders, particularly bipolar I disorder, have detectable concentrations of antithyroid antibodies. Another potential association is between hypothyroidism and the development of a rapid cycling course in clients with bipolar I disorder. Although the exact mechanism for its efficacy is unclear, clients with rapid cycling bipolar I disorder have been treated effectively with thyroid hormone (Kaplan Sadock, and Grebb, 1994; McEnany, 1990).

Three tests may prove effective in diagnosing mood disorders, and provide biological markers differentiating unipolar from bipolar depression and mania from schizophrenia:

- The *corticotropin-releasing factor (CRF) stimulation test* evaluates the pituitary's ability to respond to corticotropin-releasing hormone (CRH) and secrete sufficient amounts of ACTH to induce normal adrenal activity.
- The *thyroid-releasing hormone (TRH) infusion test* assesses the pituitary's ability to secrete sufficient amounts of thyroid-stimulating hormones (TSH) to produce normal thyroid activity.
- The *dexamethasone suppression test (DST)* is based on the observation that in clients with biological evidence of depression, late afternoon cortisol levels are not suppressed after a single dose of dexamethasone.

Biological rhythms

Characteristic rhythms seem to be related to all body processes. Although alterations in body rhythms have not been found to cause mood disorders, their relevance in terms of cyclical recurrence, seasonality, and circadian rhythms is at the forefront of psychobiological research.

Mood disorders are characterized by episodes that are recurrent, often occurring and remitting spontaneously. Two subtypes of mood disorders are typically cyclical in nature, bipolar disorder (especially rapid cycling bipolar I disorder) and depressive disorder with seasonal pattern (often referred to as *seasonal affective disorder [SAD]*) (Betrus and Elmore, 1991; McEnany, 1996a). In the case of bipolar disorder, cycles may be days, weeks, months, or even years. Cycles related to seasonal affective disorder occur annually at the same time each year as people react to environmental changes such as temperature, light, or latitude. The sleep cycle is linked to the timing of circadian rhythms and to alterations in the brain's ability to follow environmental cues such as light and darkness, or disturbances in the intensity of circadian rhythms such as those caused by sleep disturbances, temperature changes, mood cycling, and cortisol and thyrotropin abnormalities (see Chapter 13).

Persons who are depressed or experiencing manic episodes have certain characteristic changes in biological rhythms and physiology. For example, clients with depression commonly report circadian rhythm disturbances related to sleep such as difficulty falling asleep, and awakening in the middle of the night and early morning. Persons having manic episodes, however, identify circadian rhythm disturbances related to hyposomnia.

Mania has been associated with circadian rhythms in three ways: phase shifting, loss of patterning, and disorders of amplitude (Restak, 1989). All-night sleep studies of clients with depression demonstrate that sleep problems associated with depression are related to the timing of rapid eye movement (REM) sleep. Findings indicate that REM sleep begins too early in the night and lasts too long, up to twice as long as the first REM period in persons who are not depressed. Consistent with this finding, the sleep electroencephlograms (EEGs) of persons with depression are abnormal, with 90% of these individuals experiencing shortened REM latency. Normally, when people fall asleep, the fifth stage of sleep (REM or dream sleep) occurs in 60 to 90 minutes. In clients with depression it occurs in 5 to 30 minutes, thus indicating that there is sleep dysregulation in these clients. The outcome of this circadian rhythm disturbance is that persons with depression spend less time in the more refreshing slow wave stages of sleep, particularly stages 3 and 4, and more time in REM sleep. This finding may explain why persons with depression complain of feeling tired and unrefreshed after a full night's sleep. There is also a decrease in the total sleep time, an increased percentage of dream time, an increased number of spontaneous middle-of-the-night awakenings, and difficulty falling asleep (Kaplan, Sadock, & Grebb 1994; McEnany, 1996b).

Changes in the pattern of melatonin secretion in people with SAD may be responsible for the seasonal mood variation of this population. Low levels of the neurotransmitter melatonin (a further synthesis of serotonin secreted by the pineal gland) are associated with light and pigmentation of the skin. The pineal gland translates basic information about the environment (e.g., light, temperature) into neuroendocrine functions through the synthesis and release of melatonin. The synthesis and release of melatonin occurs within a circadian rhythm that is dependent on light (suppresses melatonin) and darkness (releases melatonin) for its completion. Stress, through a complex neuroendocrine mechanism, can inhibit melatonin synthesis (McEnany, 1996b; Restak, 1989). The fact that light suppresses melatonin output provides the rationale for using phototherapy with people who have SAD. This intervention applies a full spectrum of light to persons with SAD to influence melatonin output and relieve symptoms in a nonpharmacological manner.

Kindling

According to the kindling hypothesis, early episodes of mood disorders require precipitating events, which act as subthreshold electrical stimuli. However, later episodes may occur spontaneously because the person has been sensitized by stable, low doses of the stimulation over time. Repeated exposure to precipitating events may result in more frequent occurrence of mood disorder episodes. This pattern is consistent with the clinical picture that is observed in persons with depression and bipolar disorder. Early episodes of depression and/or mania may be precipitated by external psychosocial stressors in vulnerable persons, but later episodes may occur in the absence of any observable external stressor. In addition, both depression and bipolar disorder may be characterized by a recurrent pattern, one that occurs with greater frequency and intensity over time (Kaplan, Sadock, and Grebb, 1994; McEnany, 1990; Montano, 1994).

Consistent with the limbic kindling hypothesis are reports of EEG changes or dysrhythmias in persons with mood disorders. Symptoms such as irritability; periodic, uncontrollable mood shifts with depression or euphoria; preseizure auras; poor response of psychotic symptoms to antipsychotic medications; and hyposexuality may be mood-related symptoms of complex partial seizures (ictal equivalents). In addition, reports of increased prevalence of EEG abnormalities in both clients who are manic and those who are depressed are increasingly common, without such clients displaying any overt evidence of seizure activity. However, repeated daily subthreshold (subictal) seizure activity may be a major factor in the symptoms of mood disorders, particularly bipolar disorder (Kessler et al., 1989). For example, persons with rapid cycling bipolar disorder may show bitemporal paroxysmal sharp waves on the EEG without any overt evidence of epilepsy.

Further support for the role of limbic kindling in mood disorders is that the neurotransmitters most closely associated with mood disorders, NE, 5-HT, and GABA, inhibit kindling. In addition, major treatments for bipolar disorder are consistent with the kindling hypothesis. For example, lithium blocks behavioral sensitization, carbamezapine (an anticonvulsant) blocks kindling, and valproic acid (another anticonvulsant) inhibits the metabolism of GABA while simultaneously activating GABA synthesis, yielding an overall effect of increased GABA availability (McEnany, 1990). Post (1989) also observed that valproic acid/valproate (Depakene) seems to be particularly effective in clients who fail to respond to medications such as lithium, especially those with the rapid cycling form of bipolar disorder.

Genetic hypothesis

Genetic data strongly suggest that a significant factor in the development of a mood disorder is genetics. However, the pattern of genetic inheritance is complex, but best illustrated by the findings of family, adoption, twin, and linkage studies. Moreover, there is a stronger genetic component for the transmission of bipolar I disorder than for the transmission of major depressive disorder.

Family studies Family studies have repeatedly found that the first-degree relatives of subjects with bipolar I disorder are 8 to 18 times more likely to have bipolar I disorder than are the first-degree relatives of control subjects. They are also 2 to 10 times more likely to have major depressive disorder. In a similar way, first-degree relatives of subjects with major depressive disorders are 1.5 to 2.5 times more likely to have bipolar I disorder than are the control subjects and two to three times more likely to have major depressive disorder. The findings of family studies illustrate that the likelihood of having a mood disorder decreases as the degree of relationship widens. For example, a cousin is less likely to be affected than is a brother or sister (Kaplan, Sadock, and Grebb, 1994).

Adoption and twin studies The findings of adoption studies also support the genetic basis for the inheritance of mood disorders. The data indicate that the biological children of affected parents are at greater risk for a mood disorder, even if they are raised in nonaffected adoptive families (Jefferson and Greist, 1994). Twin studies have found that the concordance rate for bipolar I disorder in monozygotic twins is 33% to 90% and about 50% for major depressive disorder. In contrast the concordance rates for dizygotic twins are about 5% to 25% for bipolar I disorder and 10% to 25% for major depressive disorder (Kaplan, Sadock, and Grebb, 1994).

Linkage studies   No genetic linkage has been consistently associated with mood disorders. Associations between mood disorders, particularly bipolar I disorder, have been reported for chromosomes 5 and 11, as well as the X chromosome. The D_1 receptor gene is located on chromosome 5, whereas the gene for tyrosine hydroxylase, the rate-limiting enzyme for catecholamine synthesis, is located on chromosome 11. Linkage has also been suggested between bipolar I disorder and a region on the X chromosome. However, this finding has not been consistently replicated (Kaplan, Sadock, and Grebb, 1994).

The most reasonable explanation of the genetic studies is that the particular genes identified in the positive studies may be involved in the genetic inheritance of mood disorders in the families studies but may not be involved in the genetic inheritance of mood disorders in other families. Although a pattern of genetic inheritance is associated with mood disorders, a distinct genetic mechanism is not apparent at the time.

Psychosocial Correlates

Psychodynamic theory

The object loss theory of depression is associated with traumatic separation of a person from significant objects of attachment. Contemporary object loss theory identifies two important issues related to loss: (1) loss during childhood as a predisposing factor for adult depression and (2) separation in adult life as a precipitating stressor for depression. Children ordinarily form a bond with the mother figure by 6 months of age. If the bond is severed, the child experiences separation anxiety and profound grief related to loss of the loved object. The loss experienced during these early years and the subsequent mourning process are thought to influence personality development and predispose such persons to respond dysfunctionally to losses that occur in later life (Bowlby, 1980). Interestingly, psychodynamic theorists understand manic-depressive cycles as a reflection of a failure in childhood to establish loving object relationships (Klein, 1975).

The object loss theory remains an unvalidated hypothesis, however, as to whether persons who have sustained loss of a significant object in childhood are sensitized to losses in adult life and as a result of early losses, become depressed significantly more often than those without such experiences. Although studies indicate that as a group, persons with depression have sustained more parental loss than control groups, including normal or other diagnostic groups, this factor alone is not sufficiently universal to account for all forms of depression. Furthermore, there is even debate about the beneficial or immunizing effects of having coped successfully with an early loss in the development of resilience (Wagnild and Young, 1990).

Another psychodynamic perspective about mood disorders views depression as a turning inward of anger that is not directed at the appropriate object and is accompanied by feelings of guilt. This process is initiated by loss of an object toward whom the person feels both love and hate (ambivalence) and is unable to express anger because it is considered inappropriate or irrational. In addition, the person may have developed a life-long pattern of containing feelings, especially those that are viewed negatively. Angry feelings are then directed inward. Freud (1953) believed that the self-destructive act of suicide could be regarded as a strike against the hated and loved object as well as against the self. Klein (1975) has regarded mania as a set of defensive operations designed to idealize others, deny any aggression or destructiveness toward others, and restore relationships with lost love objects. There is no empirical support for this theoretical perspective. In fact, external redirection of anger has not not always led to clinical improvement in depression or bipolar disorder.

Cognitive theory

The cognitive theory of depression developed by Beck (1979) is based on the premise that individuals experience depression because of cognitive misinterpretations that involve distorted thinking. Beck proposes that depression is a cognitive problem that is based on a negative evaluation of self, the world, and the future (cognitive triad). In contrast to other theories, this theory proposes that negative thoughts are of primary importance and negative feelings (sadness, hopelessness, worthlessness, guilt, and other emotions) are of secondary importance. Cognitive theorists suggest that in the course of development certain learned experiences sensitize persons, making them vulnerable to depression. The values, acquired beliefs, and assumptions made *(silent assumptions)* are often irrational but do influence thoughts and ultimately feelings in a negative manner so that these individuals and their world are perceived as a glass half-empty rather than as one half-full. Such persons also make *logical errors,* which consist of faulty information processing and errors in thinking that maintain the person's belief in the validity of their negative thoughts, despite the presence of contradictory evidence. They acquire a tendency to think rigidly, making *extreme, absolute judgments known as **cognitive distortions*** (Table 30-1). According to cognitive theory, the person who is predisposed to depression will use mechanisms such as cognitive distortions to explain an adverse event as a personal shortcoming.

TABLE 30-1

Cognitive distortions

COGNITIVE DISTORTION/DEFINITION	EXAMPLE
ALL-OR-NOTHING THINKING—Seeing things in terms of black-or-white categories; this kind of dichotomous thinking leaves no room for interpreting experience in shades of gray	Because Steve did not complete every aspect of a project perfectly, on time, and without stress, he thinks that he is a failure.
OVERGENERALIZATION—Make a broad generalized conclusion based on a single incident or piece of evidence	At a party, Nancy went up to a woman she had met at church a few months ago and reintroduced herself. The woman chatted briefly and then excused herself to talk to someone else. Nancy immediately assumed that nobody at the party was interested in what she had to say.
MENTAL FILTER—Picking out a single negative detail and dwelling on it exclusively so that the whole situation is perceived negatively	Jack, an architect, who was uncomfortable with criticism was praised for the quality of his recent detailed blueprints but was asked by his boss if he could get the next job out a little quicker. He went home depressed, having decided that his employer thought he was dawdling.
DISQUALIFYING THE POSITIVE—Rejecting positive experiences by finding a way to discount them	Jane has been experiencing less tension and stress at department meetings, but tells herself that this change is only because there is less turmoil going on at work this month.
JUMPING TO CONCLUSIONS—Arbitrarily jumping to a negative conclusion that is not justified by the facts of the situation	Phillip finds out that Jessica, a former girlfriend, has just broken up with the man she has been dating. When she agrees to go out with him, he concludes that she is (1) angry at her boyfriend and knows he will find out, (2) depressed and on the rebound, or (3) afraid of being alone again.
CATASTROPHIZING—Exaggerating the importance of an event, response, or part that one plays in a situation	Allison is convinced that the recent headaches she has been having suggest that she must have a brain tumor.
SHOULD STATEMENTS—Operate from a list of inflexible rules about how self and others should act	Seth believed that he should never feel angry, jealous, or hurt. He should always feel happy and serene.
LABELING AND MISLABELING—Attaching a negative label to self or another, instead of describing an error	Jasmine who dropped and spilled a new bottle of perfume, proceeded to label herself as a "complete klutz" who never does anything without screwing up.
PERSONALIZATION—Seeing self as the cause of an external event for which the person is not primarily responsible	Gene, a father of two, blames himself when he sees any sadness in his children.

The outlook of clients with depression is dominated by pessimism. They anticipate future adversities and experience them as though they are happening in the present or have already occurred. Table 30-2 shows that predictions tend to be influenced by cognitive distortions so that they are overgeneralized and extreme. Since they view the future as an extension of the present, clients with depression expect their perceived failure to continue indefinitely. Essentially, pessimism dominates their activities, wishes, and future expectations (Beck, 1979).

When persons with depression are not in a depressed mood or are only mildly depressed, they are capable of realistic self-evaluation, basically able to discern both strengths and weaknesses. If depression does occur, often following one or more life stressors, the negative cognitive perceptions occur. As depression becomes more severe, negative thinking increasingly replaces objective thinking; each experience is interpreted as further evidence of failure (tunnel vision). Consequently, a person will view self as inadequate, defective, or deprived. The world is viewed as making exorbitant demands or as pre-

TABLE 30-2

Cognitive, affective, behavioral, and physiological changes associated with depression

PHYSIOLOGICAL	COGNITIVE	AFFECTIVE	BEHAVIORAL
Amenorrhea	Ambivalence	Anger	Aggressiveness
Changes in appetite and weight (anorexia and weight loss, overeating and weight gain)	Confusion	Anxiety	Agitation
	Inability to concentrate	Apathy	Alcoholism
	Indecisiveness	Bitterness	Changes in activity level
Dizziness	Loss of interest and motivation	Dejection	Drug addiction
Gastrointestinal upset:		Despair	Flat affect
• Constipation	Obsessional thoughts	Despondency	Intolerance
• Indigestion	Pessimism		Irritability
• Nausea		Fatigue	
• Vomiting	Self-blame	Gloom	Lack of spontaneity:
Lethargy	Self-destructive thoughts	Guilt	• Robotlike movements
Pain:	Self-doubt	Helplessness	• Unchanging facial expression
• Backache	Suicidal thoughts	Hopelessness	Poor personal hygiene
• Chest pain	Thoughts slow	Ineffectiveness	Poverty of speech:
• Headache	Uncertainty	Isolation	• Marked decrease in amount of speech
Sexual changes:		Joyless	• Long pauses
• Decreased sexual desire		Loneliness	• Low monotone vocal pitch
• Decreased responsiveness		Low self-esteem	Psychomotor retardation:
• Impotence		Overwhelmed	• Slowing of movement and speech
Sleep disturbances:		Powerless	Social withdrawal and/or isolation
• Difficulty falling asleep (initial insomnia)		Sadness	Suicidal gestures and attempts:
• Waking up during the night (middle insomnia)		Worthlessness	• Repeated car accidents
• Early morning awakening (terminal insomnia)			• Self-inflicted lacerations or abrasions
• Hypersomnia (excessive sleeping)			• Food bingeing, purging, or starvation
Weakness			

senting impossible obstacles to overcome. Hypersensitive to loss and defeat, it is anticipated that current difficulties or suffering will continue indefinitely. The person is oblivious to experiences of success or pleasure. Not surprisingly, anger is difficult to acknowledge because the person with depression feels responsible for and deserving of insults, failures, rejections, and other life problems. Low self-esteem is experienced along with apathy, indifference, and inactivity, which is often observed as withdrawal and passivity. The physical symptoms of depression, such as low energy, may also be explained by the person's pessimistic view of the future, leading to the "psychomotor inhibition" typically seen with depressed clients.

At the severe end of the depression continuum, suicidal thoughts, wishes, and actions can be regarded as an extreme expression of the wish to escape the everpresent suffering and feelings of failure. Feelings of hopelessness, with no chance of improvement, the person with depression sees suicide as a logical solution. It promises to end their misery and relieve their family of a burden, and the person begins to believe that everyone would be better off if he or she was dead. Tunnel vision only fuels the inability to perceive or think about more positive life-affirming solutions.

Research studies provide considerable support for the cognitive theory of depression, thereby providing an empirically supported theoretical foundation for understanding the depressed person's thought patterns and for structuring nursing intervention. In fact, the Agency for Health Care Policy Research (AHCPR) (USDHHS, 1994) *Guidelines for the Detection and Treatment of Depression in Primary Care* identify cognitive therapy as one of the brief therapy models yielding effective outcomes for the treatment of depression.

Hopelessness Model

The hopelessness model of depression is derived from the learned helplessness theory first proposed by Seligman (1975). Originally based on experiments with laboratory animals, studies with humans led to the assumption that learned helplessness was a model of depression. The major concept of this model is when persons believe they have no control over situations or are unable to reduce suffering or obtain praise because they are depressed.

More recently, Abramson, Metalsky, and Alloy (1989) have constructed a more complex model, derived from attribution theory, called the hopelessness theory of depression. It represents a reformulation of the original learned helplessness theory of depression. This model suggests that inferred negative consequences and negative characteristics about self contribute to the formation of hopelessness and, in turn to the symptoms of hopelessness depression. The chain begins with the perceived occurrence of negative life events that serve as "occasion setters" for persons to become hopeless. Because not all people become hopeless and depressed when confronted with negative life events, Abramson, Metalsky, and Alloy (1989) proposed three types of inferences that influence whether a person will become hopeless and, in turn, depressed when dealing with negative life events:

- Inferences about why the event occurred
- Inferences about the consequences that will result from the occurrence of the event
- Inferences about the self, given that the event occurred

When negative life events are attributable to stable versus unstable causes and global versus specific causes, and are viewed as important, hopelessness is likely to oc-cur. Inferred negative consequences are most likely to lead to hopelessness when the consequence is viewed as important, not able to be remedied, unlikely to change, and affecting many areas of life. When inferred characteristics about the self (e.g., self-worth, abilities, personality, or desirability) are negative, hopelessness and depression may ensue. This is particularly likely when a person believes that such characteristics are not changeable and that they will interfere with important outcomes in many areas of life.

The three kinds of inferences may not be equally important in contributing to whether a person becomes hopeless and, in turn, becomes depressed. However, the likelihood of generalized hopelessness increases with the extent to which a person expects that highly desired outcomes will not occur. In contrast, circumscribed pessimism occurs when persons exhibit the negative outcome/hopelessness expectation about only a limited area and, as a result, have less severe symptoms of depression (Abramson, Metalsky, and Alloy, 1989).

The hopelessness model is now strikingly similar to Beck's cognitive model of depression previously described. The hopelessness model is also proposed as a sufficient, but not necessary, cause of depression. Other physiological and psychological factors can also produce symptoms of depression. Finally, research studies investigating the relationship between the hopelessness model and depression are still being empirically validated.

Behavioral Model

Social learning theory (Bandura, 1977) provides the primary behavioral model related to depression. This model proposes that psychologic functioning, including depression, is understood in terms of continuous reciprocal interaction between personal factors. These factors include cognitive processes, behavioral factors, and environmental factors all operating as interdependent factors that influence one another. The extent to which these factors, singly or in combination, influence a person differs in various settings and for different behaviors.

This theory views individuals as capable of exercising considerable control over their own behaviors. Persons are active participants in selecting, organizing, and transforming incoming stimuli. In this context, they are not powerless objects controlled by their environment who merely react to external influences, nor are they totally free to do whatever they choose. Rather, individuals and their environment have a mutual influence on each other.

Reinforcement is a central concept of the behavioral model and important to understanding the behavioral view of depression. Social learning theory recognizes that there is a broad range of reinforcers (positive and negative) for any given behavior. Person-environment interactions with positive outcomes provide positive reinforcement. As a result the person feels good, which strengthens the person's behavior, and increases the likelihood that it will occur more often in the future. In contrast, little or no rewarding interaction with the environment will be regarded as a negative outcome, causing the person to feel sad or blue. Depressed people are thought to have person-environment interactions that elicit too many negative or too few positive outcomes. A key assumption of this model is that a low rate of positive reinforcement is integral with the development of depression (Jarrett and Rush, 1996).

Keeping the person-environment influence in mind, two likely reinforcement situations may occur: (1) the person may not initiate appropriate behaviors that yield positive reinforcement and (2) the environment, including persons in the environment, may not provide positive reinforcement.

These two situations are not uncommon since persons with depression have been identified as individuals lacking social skills needed to interact effectively. Similarly, others find the thought patterns and behavior of persons with depression to be negative, offensive, pessimistic, and they try to avoid them. The net result is often a situation of mutual withdrawal. When experiences commonly thought to be positively reinforcing events (e.g., success at work or school) are perceived to be absent, depression is likely to occur. Depression also occurs when certain negative life events (e.g. marital discord and verbal or physical abuse) are experienced (Segal and VanderVoort, 1993).

The behavioral model emphasizes an interactional perspective, one that highlights an active rather than a passive view of persons, and which addresses the importance of the person-environment relationship. From this perspective, the goal of intervention is to assist the person with depression to increase the quality and quantity of positively reinforcing interactions and to decrease those that are negative reinforcers. Empirical support for the efficacy of the behavioral model in the treatment of depression is evident. This is operationalized in treatment approaches such as social skills training, activity scheduling (Lewinsohn et al., 1984), problem solving, and self-control therapy (Palmer-Erbs, 1996).

Stress model

The stress response can, as discussed in Chapter 14, include mood disturbances. Stressors that may result in mood disturbances include social role strain, loss, and life events.

Social role theory   Social role stressors, most notably social role strain, have emerged as factors related to the development of depression. This is particularly relevant in light of the predominance of depression among women and the increasing interest in gender socialization processes and women's changing societal role (Ruble et al., 1993; Warren, 1994; Weissman et al., 1993).

The term *social role strain refers to aspects of a role that are considered problematic or undesirable.* The findings of Glazenbrook and Munjas' (1986) classic study on the relationship between role strain and depression demonstrated a significant relationship between those variables in women. Role strain in marriage emerges as a major stressor related to depression for men and women. In a classic study, Gove (1972) studied the rates of mental illness among married men and women. He found higher rates of mental illness for married women, whereas single, divorced, and widowed women had lower rates than men. Gove concluded that marriage has a protective effect for men, but not for women.

Another stressor attributed to the differential rates of depression in men and women may be the role strain inherent in both marriage and parenting. The literature on dual-career families indicates that a working woman often has to combine and juggle the roles of worker, spouse, and parent, documenting the additive nature of the roles and responsibilities that contribute to role strain and overload (Beeber, 1996; Carter and McGoldrick, 1989). Since the majority of adult women can expect to spend most of their adult life working and more than half of today's working women have children, the importance of having a supportive partner cannot be underestimated. Although a causal relationship between social role-strain and depression has not been established, the presence of significant role-related stressors in a person's life suggests a vulnerability to depression among specific target populations.

Loss   Loss may be real or imagined. It may involve loss of a person, object, physical functioning, self-esteem, status, or prestige. Because of their symbolic meaning, many losses appear to be more important than the observer would consider appropriate, as in the following example:

> Laura lost a locket given to her by her grandmother before her death. This was a momento she wore every day. The chain must have broken and the locket must have dropped without Laura realizing it until that evening when she was changing into her nightgown. Laura had no idea when or how this loss had occurred. Having been very close to her grandmother, she was devastated by the loss, her only tangible connection to this special relative.

Even seemingly positive or pleasurable events such as a job promotion, graduation from school, marriage, or a geographic move can generate feelings of sadness and loss of old friends and colleagues, independence, security, neighborhood associations, and memories of the past. Of paramount importance in estimating the magnitude of the loss is the person's perception of the actual and symbolic significance of the event. The stronger the kinship or sense of attachment, the security needs met by this person or object, the dependence-independence bonds, and the intensity of ambivalence, the more intense the sense of loss is likely to be.

Adults throughout the life cycle are constantly experiencing losses. Since losses are stressors that usually represent something negative—a deprivation—persons are challenged to find meaning in these losses and use this understanding to achieve personal integration and recovery (Cotton, 1990). The normal mourning process facilitates the resolution of uncomplicated grief reactions or simple bereavement associated with loss. Denial, anger, anxiety, pain, despair, acceptance, and hope are some of the characteristic emotions persons experience as they navigate the turbulent waters of the mourning process. Typically, this process is not smooth; rather, it is characterized by turmoil, pain, regression, and potential problems. Individuals often wonder if it is normal to feel this way. They worry that the "depression-like feelings" they are having are not sadness and "the blues" associated with mourning, but "real depression." They wonder if they will ever see light at the end of the tunnel.

When a loss occurs through death, certain factors influence mourning outcomes including: the age of the person, preparation for bereavement (anticipated or unanticipated death), previous warnings, preventability of the loss, and expression of feelings (McGoldrick and Walsh, 1991).

Although the loss of a loved one is a major stressor, most people resolve this loss through uncomplicated grief reactions and bereavement and do not experience pathological grief or depression. The acute grief reaction is usually resolved within 6 to 8 weeks, even though complete healing and recovery will take at least 1 full year. Nurses should be aware of specific internal and external factors, as highlighted in Box 30-2 which inhibit mourning (Cotton, 1990). Although not all people who experience loss will develop depression, loss and separation are stressors that may precipitate depression for targeted populations at risk (Rahe, 1979; McGoldrick, 1991).

Life events   *Life events of an important nature* often called **nodal events** have been implicated as a predisposing influence in the development of depression (Miller, 1988). Research findings suggest that on average, persons with depression reported almost three times as many important life events during the 6 months before the onset of clinical depression than did control subjects (McGoldrick, 1991; Rahe, 1979). Life events perceived as undesirable and potential precipitants of depression include loss of self-esteem, interpersonal discord, socially undesirable occurrences, and major disruptions of life patterns. In general, those nodal events regarded as exit events (subtractions and losses) are more likely than entrance events (additions and introductions) to be followed by exacerbation of psychiatric symptoms (especially depression), physical health changes, and impairment in social functioning (Rahe, 1979). Certainly,

the concept of nodal events overlaps with the concept of loss discussed in the previous section.

Nodal events such as separation, divorce, marital conflict, and childhood physical and sexual abuse are examples of exit and entrance events that can precipitate or accompany depression. When multiple nodal events occur with a brief period, stress escalates dramatically, as does the likelihood of depression and other stress-related symptoms. Moreover, **anniversary reactions** (*affective responses around the anniversary of a nodal event such as a death, divorce, or illness that occurred in the family*) can take the form of appropriate reminiscent sadness; depression; suicidal thoughts, gestures, or attempts; and other stress-related symptoms.

From the many theories discussed in an effort to provide a comprehensive perspective about mood disorders, it is evident that no single theory sufficiently explains the nature or development of a mood disorder. Each theory contributes to an understanding of mood disorders; many of them overlap and interrelate. Recent research also highlights multiple causes for mood disorders. A holistic perspective on mood disorders reflects the interaction of biologic and psychosocial theories that combine to contribute to the development of depressive and bipolar disorders.

BOX 30-2

Factors Inhibiting the Resolution of Loss Through Mourning

EXTERNAL FACTORS

- Immersion of the mourner in practical, necessary tasks that accompany the loss (e.g., funeral arrangements, search for immediate employment, or resolving estate business) that divert or distract the person from dealing with the emotional issues related to the loss
- Lack of support from the person or family's support system inhibits the mourner's expression of grief in all its forms (e.g., anger, guilt, sadness, regret, or anxiety) and blocks their opportunity to reminisce about and review the lost relationship
- Indiscriminate use of tranquilizers and antidepressants that suppress normal expression of grief and may ultimately lead to more complex depressive reactions

INTERNAL FACTORS

- Suppression of crying and/or anger because they are deemed "socially unacceptable" or viewed as evidence of "weakness" or "mental illness"
- Belief that the quality and quantity of emotions associated with the loss is so unique it cannot be communicated
- The mourner's lack of understanding about the impact of previous losses and their response to such events

The *Nursing Process*

Clients with mood disorders and their significant others are encountered by nurses in a variety of settings. Severely depressed and manic clients who are a danger to self or others and/or who have psychotic features may be admitted to inpatient psychiatric units for treatment stabilization. Such clients may have other nonmood, co-occurring psychiatric disorders such as alcohol or drug abuse, borderline personality disorder, eating disorder, panic disorder, or obsessive-compulsive disorder. Both depression and bipolar disorder tend to be recurring mental health problems, a factor that emphasizes the importance of maximizing the client's highest level of functioning, family integration, and community participation (USDHHS, 1993; Gitlin et al., 1995). Increasingly, the majority of clients with mood disorders are treated in community-based mental health settings including: day-treatment, dual diagnosis, home care, case management, or group homes; halfway houses; community mental health centers; and private practice.

Assessment

Since all people experience a wide range of moods and a large repertoire of emotional responses, nurses are challenged to determine when a person's mood represents (1) normal emotional responsiveness, (2) a healthy functional response that shows attempts to overcome the stress of loss associated with grief and mourning, or (3) a dysfunctional response characterized by its intensity, pervasiveness, persistence, and the extent to which it interferes with a person's usual biopsychosocial functioning.

Mood disorders involve disturbances in physiological, cognitive, affective, and behavioral regulation as identified in Tables 30-2 and 30-3. Major affective disorders are classified into two subgroups, depressive and bipolar disorders, depending on whether depression is the only evident mood disorder or both depressive and manic episodes occur over time. These two disorders, as well as suicide, are the foci of the nursing process section of this chapter.

Clinical Profile

Grief reactions
Grief, the normal subjective response to loss of a loved person through death or separation, also occurs following the loss of a valued object, cherished possession,

prized ideal, or a job; or loss of security, status, or self-esteem. The feelings of grief associated with loss are universal. Often, the feelings are so intense, they temporarily bring normal daily activities to a standstill. Interestingly, persons going through the mourning process often report symptoms that are indistinguishable from depression, yet under these circumstances they and others accept these feelings as normal. Their pain, stress, suffering, and impairment of functioning can last for days, weeks, or months, but are resolved eventually through the mourning process. Grief responses can be uncomplicated and functional, running a time-limited consistent course that is modified by factors listed in Box 30-2.

In contrast, ***delayed grief reactions*** *represent dysfunctional responses to loss, implying that something has prevented mourning from running its normal course.* Two types of dysfunctional grief reactions have been identified in the classic work of Lindemann (1944), the delayed reaction and the distorted reaction. Depression is one type of a distorted grief reaction.

Evidence of a delay in the work of mourning or a delayed grief reaction is often indicated by a persistent lack of expressed emotion following a loss. Absence of emotional expressiveness may not be evident at the beginning of the mourning process, it may diminish or halt once it has started, or it may do both. Expression of grief can be delayed for weeks, months, or even years. The underlying emotions do not go away, they may be triggered by deliberate attempts to recall and emotionally re-experience the loss. They may also occur spontaneously through accidental or coincidental recall of the original loss and its related emotions that are triggered by some current event, including anniversary reactions, as in the following example:

> When Ann's 18-month-old son Alex died from Tay-Sachs disease, she did not completely grieve the loss of this child. Already pregnant with a second child, her husband urged Ann to "put this loss behind her," since a "normal" baby would arrive in 4 months. However, each year the grieving response recurred on the anniversary of Alex's death.

Depression
Major depressive disorder, (sometimes called unipolar depression), is characterized by one or recurrent episodes of major depression without episodes of mania or hypomania (low-level mania). Major depression may range

The Nursing Process

TABLE 30-3

Physiological, cognitive, affective, and behavioral changes associated with mania

PHYSIOLOGICAL	COGNITIVE	AFFECTIVE	BEHAVIORAL
Dehydration	Denial of realistic danger	Confident	Aggressiveness
Lack of need for sleep	Distractibility	Elation	Argumentativeness
Lack of adequate nutrition	Exalted opinion of self	Euphoria	Excessive spending of money
Weight loss	Flight of ideas	Expansiveness	Grandiose acts
	Grandiosity	Extroverted	Heightened sexual drive and activity
	Illusions	Free of worry	Hyperactivity
	Lack of judgment	Happiness	Impulsive
	Loose association	Humorous	Increased motor activity
	Short attention span	Intolerant of criticism	Intrusive
		Labile mood	Irresponsibility
		Lively	Irritability
		Suspicious	Manipulative
		Uninhibited	Meddling
			Poor personal hygiene and grooming
			Provocativeness
			Verbosity

from mild to moderate states to severe states with or without psychotic features. Depressive disorders should not be confused with the sad or depressed mood that normally accompanies specific life events, particularly losses or disappointments that generate grief responses. A sad or depressed mood is only one of many signs and symptoms of a clinical depression, as highlighted in Table 30-4.

The physiological, cognitive, affective, and behavioral patterns of depression presented in Table 30-2 vary from person to person. This list shows the array of possible changes associated with major depression. Not all persons experience all of them. In fact the presenting symptoms are unique for each person and sometimes contradictory. In one individual, sadness and slowness may predominate; in another, agitation or anger may be prominent. Whatever the pattern, a key assessment consideration is that the client experiences his or her current condition as a "change" (i.e., they seem unlike themselves) in functioning that persists for at least 2 weeks and leads them to seek help.

Depressed mood is the most common manifestation of depression. Often, persons do not describe themselves as "depressed," but as sad, blue, downcast, down in the dumps, or unable to enjoy life. Although each of these adjectives describes the unhappiness associated with depression, none of them captures the intensity and pervasiveness of the depressed mood state. Tearfulness and crying are also common; yet some persons with depression do not cry, describing themselves as "beyond tears." Anxiety is another affect that accompanies depression, a pervasive feeling of worry and fear connected

The Nursing Process

TABLE 30-4

Focused assessment for mood disorders

ASSESSMENT CATEGORY AND RELATED QUESTIONS	POSSIBLE ANSWER: CLIENT WITH DEPRESSION	POSSIBLE ANSWER: CLIENT (OR *FAMILY*) WITH BIPOLAR DISORDER
Family history		
Tell me about anyone in the family who has been depressed or has had extreme mood swings (highs and/or lows).	C: My mother periodically had severe depression. She was in and out of hospitals from the time I began high school.	C: Granny was higher than a kite off and on. I don't have that problem, I just enjoy life! F: His grandma had mood swings all of her adult life. They began coming closer together as she got older; she died in a mental institution
How was she treated for it?	C: She had shock treatments several times. She was a zombie for awhile, but they helped, sometimes for several years.	C: Granny, Granny, they just kicked her in the fanny!
Client's History of Mood Disorders (Number, Type of Episodes, Severity of Episode, Cycle Length, Psychotic Features)		
Tell me about any previous depressive (lows) or manic (highs) episodes you have had; if you start from the first time this happened, describe a typical episode.	C: I've never been in the hospital before. Usually, I feel like a gray cloud, now I feel like an ugly, useless black cloud.	C: It happens not often enough. Being singled out from the rest really puts me over the crest. F: He's been having these mood swings for about the last 6 years. They started when we got married and always occur in the spring. I can see him getting higher and higher, wanting to party, travel, spend. I have to take the checkbook and credit cards away or we would be bankrupt. He's so clever; he finds ways to charge things where we have no accounts, then I have to deal with the telephone complaints. Once he's hospitalized and medicated, he comes down and is ready to go home.
Responsiveness to Previous and/or Current Treatment (e.g. TCAs, SSRIs, MAOIs, Lithium, or Other Mood Stabilizers or ECT)		
What treatments have you taken condition? How effective have they been?	C: I was on antidepressants once for a few months. I felt better and stopped taking them.	C: Drugs! I hate drugs! They rob your zest for life! F: He's taken lithium for 4 years on and off. He doesn't like the hand tremors. About 3 months after he stops taking it, he starts acting strange, and we start all over again.

Continued.

The Nursing Process

TABLE 30-4—cont'd

Focused assessment for mood disorders

ASSESSMENT CATEGORY AND RELATED QUESTIONS	POSSIBLE ANSWER: CLIENT WITH DEPRESSION	POSSIBLE ANSWER: CLIENT (OR *FAMILY*) WITH BIPOLAR DISORDER
Mood Changes		
How would you describe your usual mood? How does your current mood differ from your usual mood?	C: I think I'm always a little depressed, but nothing like my mother was. But I do worry that I'll end up like her.	C: I feel great! I'm floating on cloud nine! Who could be happier, but cross me, and you're finished!"
How much pleasure are you getting from things you normally like to do?	C: No pleasure in anything; not family, friends, work, nothing.

Sometimes I'm a real happy-go-lucky person, lots of friends, creative at my job, love to vacation. Now, I feel like I'm on an island with no bridges . . . . | C: I'm a very busy person—I have places to go, things to do, and people to see. Gotta go, no more time to waste! |
Cognitive Changes		
Tell me about your ability to concentrate. How much difficulty do you have focusing on or completing a task or job? Tell me what it's like for you to try to put your thoughts together.	C: I can't do anything. I'll be standing at the sink and wonder why I am standing there . . .	C: Not only can I concentrate, I'm working on a special project for the President, yes, the President. That's all I can say, it's top secret!
How do you feel about the future?	C: Bad things keep happening; it's going to get worse . . .	C: When I look into my crystal ball, I see nothing but bright crystals. Not bad, not bad!!!
Have you had any thoughts of harming yourself? If so, can you describe them for me?	C: I'd like to go to sleep and not wake up—no more problems	C: Don't get me pissed off, or you'll really have to worry about me being a cut up!
Have you ever thought of killing yourself as a way out of this (if answer is yes, do suicide assessment in Table 30-6)?	C: I just don't want to wake up.	C: I told you, bug off!
Behavioral Changes		
How much time have you been spending with friends lately? To what extent is this different from your usual social habits or activity level?	C: I haven't even been going to work, just dragging myself out at some point in the day is a struggle. Then I just sit there, I have nothing to say.	F: He hasn't slowed down. He has made long distance calls to I don't know where, He made airline reservations for Rome; I cancelled them just in time. He's negotiating to buy a new business and a big new house. He only went to work to quit. He thinks they don't appreciate him enough. I can't get him to lie down, slow down, nothing—I'm exhausted and he still has energy to spare.

The Nursing Process

TABLE 30-4—cont'd

Focused assessment for mood disorders

ASSESSMENT CATEGORY AND RELATED QUESTIONS	POSSIBLE ANSWER: CLIENT WITH DEPRESSION	POSSIBLE ANSWER: *CLIENT (OR FAMILY)* WITH BIPOLAR DISORDER
Have any changes occurred in your lifestyle in the last 6 months or year? If so, describe them to me. Tell me about anybody important to you who has been sick or died in the past year? How has this affected you?	C: My dad died last year. I have to take care of my brother Ronnie who had polio; he lived with my dad. Our youngest daughter just left her husband, What else could go wrong? A lot I suppose . . .	C: My mother died, the old witch, I was glad to see her go, always meddling, meddling!
What kind of financial or legal problems are you facing?	C: None, just the usual day-to-day struggle.	C: None! And . . . that's none of your darn business!
To what extent has your use of alcohol or drugs changed over the past year? If there have been changes, describe their effect on you.	C: I wish I liked to drink, maybe it would help. My primary care provider gave me tranquilizers; I only took one. It only made me feel like more of a zombie.	F: The best I can tell he has signed legally binding contracts for a total of $250,000. If we can't get out of those contracts, we're bankrupt. I can't go through this again . . .
Physical Changes		C: A little nip now and again just makes me feel perfect, yes perkier instead of murkier!
Have there been changes in your sleep patterns? Appetite? Weight? Interest in sex? Anxiety level? If there have been changes, please describe them to me.	C: My only escape is sleep, all I want to do is sleep, but I can't fall asleep or stay asleep. I toss and turn and wake up feeling exhausted. I've lost 15 lbs. in the last month…sex, no I don't think so…I feel like a blob, but sometimes I feel like my heart is going to burst out of my chest.	C: Eat, who has time to eat? I told you I'm a busy person. I don't need sleep, I need a typist; can you type? The President is sending a messenger for the first draft of my project.

with agitation. Depression or anxiety may exhibit diurnal variation; certain times of the day (morning or evening) are either better or worse.

Sometimes persons will seek medical care for somatic problems without associating them with the physiological, cognitive, affective, or behavioral changes of depression. Such complaints might include gastrointestinal distress, headaches, back pain, insomnia, palpitations, dizziness, appetite changes, fatigue, and changes in sex drive. Individuals often focus on "physical" health problems rather than "psychiatric" problems, because it is more socially acceptable to have abdominal distress or a backache than the profound sadness, loss of concentration, or feeling of emptiness associated with depres-

sion. They also have a concrete explanation for why their "get-up-and-go got up and left them." This is particularly true in cultural groups for whom mental health problems represent a source of shame, loss of face, or weakness of character, as illustrated in the Cultural Highlights box on p. 622.

To differentiate appropriate diagnostic cues about depression versus physical health problems, nurses, especially those working in primary care settings, should be attentive to the spectrum of somatic symptoms that the client describes, while paying equal attention to issues related to mood and cognition. In addition, nurses should be able to distinguish between mood disorders such as major depression or manic episodes, and mood

The Nursing Process

CULTURAL HIGHLIGHTS

Mood Disorders

Assessment

In some cultures, depression may be experienced or expressed in somatic terms rather than with sadness or guilt. Complaints of "nerves" and headaches (Latino or Mediterranean cultures), problems of the heart (Middle Eastern cultures), or being "heartbroken" (among the Hopi Indians) may provide cues that express the depressive experience (Hulme, 1996; Lipson, 1992; Muecke and Sassi, 1992).

Diagnosis

Among Mexican cultures, "susto" is a culture-bound folk illness that mimics depression. When a Mexican-American client and/or family member describes their relative as having "susto," the nurse and other members of the mental health team should consider traditional, as well as culture-specific, assessment data in determining whether diagnosis of psychopathologic factors such as major depression is appropriate (Campinha-Bacote, 1994).

Intervention

1. Mexican-American families may be more responsive to the inclusion of a folk healer called *curandero* in the treatment plan, a person they view as the appropriate healer for "susto" (Campinha-Bacote, 1994).

2. Monitoring side effects of antidepressants is especially important with Hispanic clients who appear to have a higher toxic effect of tricyclic antidepressants (Lawson, 1986).

3. African Americans are more susceptible to tricyclic antidepressant (TCA) delirium than caucasians. For a given dose of TCA, African Americans have higher blood levels and faster therapeutic response (Strickland et al., 1991)

4. The therapeutic ranges of lithium for clients who are manic in Japan and Taiwan were reported to be 0.4 to 0.8 mEq/L, as compared with 0.6 to 1.2 mEq/L in the United States (Lin, et al., 1986).

5. Participation in outpatient mental health programs by African-American clients may be maximized in referrals that are made to church-affiliated versus hospital or mental health center programs (Campinha-Bacote, 1992).

---

disorders related to medical conditions and/or those that are substance-induced.

There are several subgroups of major depressive disorder—psychotic, melancholic, atypical, seasonal, and postpartum—that nurses need to understand and with which they need to be familiar. Two subgroups, depression with seasonal pattern and depression with postpartum onset, are presented in greater detail.

Depression with seasonal pattern *Depression with seasonal pattern is referred to as **seasonal affective disorder (SAD)**. SAD is associated with a recurring seasonal pattern, usually related to the shortened daylight of fall and winter and that disappears in spring and summer* (APA, 1994a). Apparently, humans' internal biological clock slows down in winter and speeds up in spring and summer. Of the population living in temperate zones, 25% normally experience some degree of

change in mood or weight in response to the onset of winter (Bushnell and DeForge, 1994).

This depressive disorder is characterized by lethargy and fatigue, "afternoon slumps," hypersomnia, irritability, anxiety, social withdrawal, and increased appetite, including carbohydrate craving and weight gain (Bushnell and DeForge, 1994; Glod, 1991). Research findings suggest that SAD results from a seasonal disturbance in circadian rhythms caused by the absence of appropriately intense and timed light cues, coupled with dysregulation of melatonin metabolism. It is hypothesized that serotonin decreases as melatonin increases, resulting in depressed activity and depressed mood. High carbohydrate levels also increase serotonin. The carbohydrate-craving phenomenon observed in adult clients with SAD may be an effort by those persons to relieve or self-regulate depressive symptoms (Krauchi, Wirz-Justice, and Graw, 1990).

The Nursing Process

Depression with postpartum onset Postpartum mood variations are a normal postdelivery occurrence. *Postpartum blues* are experienced by 50% to 70% of women. *Transient in nature, these episodes occur within 1 to 5 days postpartum, last 1 to 10 days, and resolve spontaneously* (Ugarriza, 1995). *Characterized by malaise, fatigue, crying, mood instability, anxiety, and mild confusion, the syndrome is generally mild and brief.* Treatment consists of education, reassurance, and time to resolve this normal response.

Postpartum psychosis is a relatively rare syndrome, occurring in only 1 or 2 of every 1000 postpartum women, *typically begins two or three days after delivery.* Women are at-risk for developing postpartum psychosis for the first 30 days following delivery. *Postpartum psychosis consists of either depressive or manic disorders;* the *Diagnostic and Statistical Manual of Mental Disorders, Fourth Edition* (DSM-IV) lists it as an atypical psychosis (APA, 1994a). *Characteristically, the mother has difficulty caring for the infant, appears confused, and complains of poor memory, although performing normally in memory tests.* Tearfulness, feelings of worthlessness, psychomotor retardation, and appetite and sleep disturbances are seen in women with postpartum psychosis. An inordinate concern about the baby's health, guilt about lack of love, and delusions about the infant's being dead or defective may also be present. The mother may deny having given birth and acknowledge hearing voices that command her to hurt the baby (Beck, 1992; Ugarriza, 1995). Although serious, postpartum psychosis can be treated effectively. However, the recurrence rate following subsequent pregnancies is 30% to 51% and many clients subsequently develop bipolar disorder (Ugarizza, 1995).

Postpartum depression develops anywhere from 2 weeks to 12 months after delivery with most cases occurring within 6 months. The risk of postpartum depression is 10% to 15%; the rate is higher for women with a psychiatric history. In contrast to postpartum psychosis, *postpartum depression has an insidious onset* (Affonso, 1992). *The symptoms are far more severe than those of the "blues" and are capable of generating debilitating problems for the woman such as intense feelings of inadequacy, inability to cope, social withdrawal, weight gain, loss of normal interests, and multiple somatic complaints* (Beck, 1992, 1995; Ugarizza, 1995).

Dysthymic disorder

Dysthymic disorder, another depressive disorder, is characterized by a chronically moderately depressed mood and other symptoms that are similar to but milder than major depression. Persons with dysthymia describe their mood as sad or "down in the dumps" most of the day and on more days than not for at least 2 years (APA, 1994a). When in a depressed mood, at least two of the following symptoms are present: poor appetite or overeating, insomnia or hypersomnia, low energy or fatigue, low self-esteem, poor concentration or difficulty making decisions, and feelings of hopelessness. Eric K., a client with dysthymic disorder, describes his self-criticism and lack of confidence in his ability to accomplish tasks as "a way of life," part of the fabric of his self-image for as long as he can remember. Persons with dysthymic disorder sometimes have what is called **double depression,** that is, *they develop a major depressive episode on top of the moderate depression that appears to be ever-present.* Eric K. differentiates between dysthymia and major depression by describing the "gray cloud" versus the "black cloud" experience.

Bipolar disorder

Bipolar disorders are mood disorders in which there is at least one or more manic or hypomanic episodes, with or without a history of a major depressive episode (APA, 1994a). Bipolar disorders are characterized by mood swings from profound depression to extreme euphoria (mania), with intervening periods of normal mood (euthymia). The frequency, duration, and severity of manic and/or depressive episodes varies and is unique to each individual. For example, the interval between episodes (recurrences) can be years, months, weeks, or even hours. *When four or more mood episodes (either manic, depressive, or both) occur within the same year, a **rapid cycling** specifier is designated* (APA, 1994a). Box 30-3 identifies types of bipolar disorders. Although bipolar disorder occurs less often than depressive disorders, it is estimated that approximately 2 million Americans have bipolar disorder. Of those who have an initial manic episode, 75% will have more than one episode, and almost all those with manic episodes will have depressive episodes.

Physiological, cognitive, affective, and behavioral changes associated with the manic phase of bipolar disorder are listed in Table 30-3. *A somewhat milder clinical portrait called **hypomania** is not severe enough to cause marked impairment in social or occupational functioning, does not include psychotic features, nor does it require hospitalization.*

During a manic episode, the mood is elevated, expansive, or irritable. Motor activity is excessive and frenzied, the person takes on too many activities, exhibits pressured speech, distractibility, hypersexuality, and inflated self-esteem; exercises poor judgment; is unable to an-

The Nursing Process

BOX 30-3

Types of Bipolar Disorders

BIPOLAR I DISORDER

Bipolar I disorder is the diagnosis given to a person who is experiencing, or has experienced, one or more manic episodes or a mixed episode (client exhibits rapidly alternating moods, sadness, irritability, or euphoria, accompanied by symptoms associated with depression and mania). The client may also have experienced episodes of depression.

BIPOLAR II DISORDER

Bipolar II disorder is characterized by recurrent episodes of major depression with the episodic occurrence of hypomania. The person has never experienced an episode that meets the full criteria for a manic or mixed episode.

CYCLOTHYMIC DISORDER

A chronic mood disturbance of at least 2 years duration, involving numerous episodes of hypomania and depressed mood of insufficient severity or duration to meet the criteria for either bipolar I or bipolar II disorder.

ticipate consequences of actions; and has flight of ideas. Psychotic features, including delusions (usually grandiose or paranoid) and command hallucinations, may be present, which give rise to a risk for self-injury, suicide, and danger to the client's safety.

When the mood is elevated or euphoric, it is often infectious. Clients present a happy-go-lucky, confident picture. Clients who are manic report feeling happy, unconcerned, carefree, and devoid of problems. However, their mood has no connection to the reality of the situation or the feelings of others. In fact, some clients have extraordinarily grandiose delusions about their power, influence, and importance. Their self-esteem is inflated, they are self-confident, and their ego knows no bounds. They often involve themselves in grandiose, but seemingly senseless and risky ventures that often fail and create enormous financial hardship for colleagues, friends, or family members. Yet they have no guilt or remorse about the havoc they create. In fact they seem to court danger, while denying its presence.

As their mood escalates, their boundless energy, scheming, manipulation, and inability to predict consequences often result in excessive spending, substance abuse, heightened sexual drive, promiscuity, and misdemeanors. In contrast, the client's mood may be irritable

or hostile, particularly when plans are thwarted. They can be argumentative and provocative and "turn on you," seemingly at the drop of a hat. Clients in manic states also exhibit behaviors such as mood lability with rapid shifts from elated to depressed moods and may alternately laugh and cry within minutes of each other.

Because of the hyperactivity of a client who is manic, characteristic physical changes include inadequate nutrition related to lack of time to eat and serious weight loss related to insomnia and overactivity. When clients are in extreme manic states, dehydration may become a life-threatening problem that requires immediate attention.

As the mood state becomes increasingly expansive, speech is often disturbed; clients are overtalkative, and logical speech is replaced by confusing, loud, and rapid language. Speech may become full of irrelevancies, and plays on words are common to the extent that looseness of associations and flight of ideas are evident. There is marked impairment in occupational functioning, typical social activities, or relationships with others and may require hospitalization to prevent harm to self or others, particularly when there are psychotic features.

Suicide

Although suicide and suicide potential occur in a number of psychiatric disorders including major depression, bipolar disorder, schizophrenia, dementia, substance abuse, dissociative identity, and personality disorders, the highest incidence of suicide potential and fatal acts occurs in persons experiencing major depression. The suicide rate for depression is three times greater than suicide related to any other psychobiological disorder. Suicidal behavior is usually considered to include suicide gestures, suicide attempts, and completed suicide.

Suicidal ideation is defined as the presence of thoughts or contemplation about suicide. However, there is no self-destructive action related to these thoughts. Similarly, suicide gestures represent acts of self-injury, the goal of which is inflicting hurt and receiving attention rather than actual self-destruction. Many persons, as well as health professionals, often underestimate the significance of suicide gestures such as taking 10 aspirin or acetaminophen (Tylenol), lacerating the wrists or throat with a nail file or a soda can tab top, and driving at breakneck speeds. Often considered an attention-getting device rather than an early warning sign or cry for help, suicide gestures may be erroneously disregarded. All suicidal behavior should be taken seriously, whatever the intent, and deserves the serious attention of health professionals.

Suicide threats are indirect or direct statements that hint, suggest, or declare the intent to end one's life

The Nursing Process

and usually occur before overt suicidal activity takes place. For example, the suicidal person's verbal message might say, "I'm such a burden, you'd all be better off without me" or, "You'd take care of my family, wouldn't you?" Taken in the context of recent life stressors such as chronic unemployment, debilitating illness, school failure, or major depression, such statements take on credibility. For example, Martin, age 50, has been unemployed for 3 years. He finds himself thinking repeatedly, "I expected to have no problem locating another job based on my computer skills, but now I am convinced that I'll never get another job. My severance, unemployment, and savings are all gone . . . all I have left is my life insurance . . . I'm worth more dead than alive." This example also illustrates the fact that cognitive functioning of suicidal people is often characterized by *a rigid style of perceiving and reacting that makes it difficult for them to formulate alternative approaches or solutions to problems* (Rickelman and Houfek, 1995). *This pattern is sometimes called* **tunnel vision** *and is predominantly pessimistic in nature.*

Individuals also communicate suicide threats nonverbally; they give away prized possessions, make out wills, or make funeral arrangements. Sometimes they systematically withdraw from social activities and friendships until they are totally isolated.

Suicide threats often symbolize the ambivalence associated with ending one's life. On one hand, it represents the flickering hope that someone will recognize the danger and rescue the person from self-destructive impulses. On the other, it represents the hopelessness that things will never change for the better or that anyone cares enough to prevent the person from self-harm.

Suicide attempts *include those self-directed actions taken by a person that are intended to result in death if not interrupted.* **Suicide intent** *is the seriousness or intensity of the wish of a person to end his or her life.* The **level of intention** *is associated with the development of and specificity of the suicide plan, including method, time, and place* (Buchanan, 1991). Suicide is intentional when a person takes or plans to take a direct, conscious part in self-destructive behavior (e.g., taking one's life by hanging). Suicide is subintentional when a person plays an indirect role in ending their life. Subintentional behavior may be a way of fulfilling conscious and unconscious wishes (e.g., some vehicular accidents may be suicides; driving too fast on dangerous roads may result in a fatal accident that is the equivalent of suicide; or chronic alcohol abuse) (Adams, 1992).

All suicide attempts should be taken seriously! However, assessment emphasis should be placed on the lethality of the method threatened or attempted. **Lethality,** *the risk of danger or death,* is positively correlated with any plan that is straightforward, easy to carry out, and has little or no margin of error. The difference between planning to put a gun to one's head and pulling the trigger versus planning to take an overdose of pills is obvious. There is little margin of error with the gun, one gun being about as lethal as another. The margin for error with pills can be large or small; it depends on (among other things), the type of pills, the number of pills, and the possibility of reflex vomiting while the pills are being swallowed. Bizarre plans may be evidence of psychosis, but this may also be true of many simple, highly lethal plans that are dictated by hallucinatory voices (command hallucinations). For example, a young man who was rescued from the edge of a high roof said that he had been instructed by "an angel of the Lord" to "rise up to meet God." In general, clients who are psychotic are a high-risk group because of their impulsivity and distorted thought processes. However, any client, psychotic or otherwise, who displays a high level of impulsivity is at increased risk for self-destructive behavior and suicide.

The availability of means is crucial for even the simplest suicide plan to succeed. For a person who has a gun but no bullets, there is still an important barrier between life and death and, perhaps, a ray of hope. For a person who has a loaded gun in his dresser drawer, which he plans to use as soon as his wife leaves for work, there is little ambivalence about attempting suicide.

Completed suicide *results from self-directed actions that result in death.* It may take place after suicidal threats, gestures, or attempts have been missed or ignored, or the functional use of coping mechanisms fail. However, some people do not provide easily identifiable warning signs. An important dimension of assessment includes determining how and to what extent the client's patterns of daily living have recently changed. For example, changes in sleep, eating, hygiene, work, and social habits are often indicators of severe dysfunction. Assessment of recent stressors are also critical factors that precipitate suicidal action. Nurses should consider the impact of a job loss; geographic move; threat of incarceration; family or marital problems that create feelings of estrangement, alienation, or hopelessness; loss of a loved one through death, divorce, or separation; or an anniversary reaction to that loss. Nurses also need to be alert to clients whose severe depression suddenly shows significant improvement. This may mean that the client has made a decision to commit suicide, their ambivalence has been resolved and they feel relieved because a solution to their hopeless dilemma has been reached.

Completed suicides generate many feelings in the survivors (the significant others) that are difficult to com-

The Nursing Process

municate. Their pain cannot be communicated to their dead loved one; it is difficult to share with each other or the outside world. Anger, family disintegration, and stigmatization have been identified as significant forms of pain (Derni and Howell, 1991). One sister stated, "My feelings about my brother's suicide was and still is a lot of anger toward him for being such a jerk . . . it was such a selfish act, it just fit with the way he had been from the time I had known him." A sense of family disintegration is particularly expressed by those who have lost a parent. A son remarked, "I not only lost my father, but anything that resembled family life." The sense of being stigmatized by neighbors, friends, and other members of the community is highlighted by a daughter who stated, "I stopped going to church, which I hoped would help me heal, because I would see members of the congregation whispering about us during the church service and avoiding us during the social hour afterwards. I felt like a leper." These kinds of experiences can lead to unresolved or delayed grief reactions and depression.

Focused Assessment

Clinical interview
Focused assessment of clients with mood disorders includes focused data collection about (1) individual and family history of depression or bipolar disorder, (2) mood changes, (3) cognitive changes including suicidal ideation, (4) behavioral and social changes, and (5) physical changes. The mental status examination is always included in the comprehensive assessment of the client with mood disorders. Assessment data are collected from the client, family members, and significant others in the client's support system. Nonclient data sources become particularly important when the client is severely depressed or having a manic episode. Table 30-4, pp. 618-621, presents assessment categories, focused assessment questions, and possible client answers that nurses can use when interviewing clients with depressive and bipolar disorders.

Physical assessment
Physical assessment is an essential part of the comprehensive client assessment. Physical health problems and related medications need to be identified to establish a data base that enables providers to differentiate depression as a primary mood disorder from depression as a co-ocurring disorder of alcohol, drug intoxication, or withdrawal. Various nonpsychiatric medical conditions and use of related prescription and nonprescription medications can be associated with mood disorders, especially

depression. (AHCPR, 1993). Laboratory tests listed in Table 30-5 may be used in the assessment process.

Assessment scales
Standardized provider-completed or client self-rating scales listed in Table 30-5 are also used to assess the presence or severity of depression or bipolar disorder. These scales should be used in combination with the clinical interview, laboratory tests, and a physical examination.

Suicide assessment
A suicide assessment includes evaluation of the risk that a client will engage in self-destructive behavior. Table 30-6 provides guidelines for assessment of clients who present a constellation of risk factors related to suicide. High lethality and high intention indicate a need for continued observation in a safe setting such as an inpatient unit. Assessment of suicidal risk is an ongoing process that continues for at least 3 months following a depressive episode (Cardell and Horton-Deutsch, 1994).

Nursing Diagnosis

Nursing diagnoses need to reflect the broad range of biopsychosocial problems demonstrated by depressed, bipolar, and/or suicidal clients. The congruence of North American Nursing Diagnosis Association (NANDA) nursing diagnoses and DSM-IV medical diagnoses that are derived from the same assessment data base are presented in Table 30-7 for depressed and/or suicidal clients and clients with bipolar disorder.

When a client is depressed or a client is suicidal, depressed or not, priority NANDA nursing diagnoses reflect documentation about potential for injury, suicide, overall safety, physical health and self-care patterns, and alterations in thought processes, self-concept, and social interaction. For the client in a manic state, additional priority nursing diagnoses most often focus on potential for injury, impaired physical health and health habits, as well as impulsivity, manipulation, and intrusion into the living space of other clients and staff.

Outcome Identification

Establishing realistic outcome criteria with clients who have mood disorders is particularly important. Overall goals include (1) reduction and removal of symptoms, (2) restoration of the client's occupational and psychosocial functioning, (3) improvement in the client's quality of life, and (4) decreasing the likelihood of relapse and recurrence.

The Nursing Process

TABLE 30-5

Assessment screening tools for clients with mood disorders

PURPOSE	ASSESSMENT SCALE
Depressive symptoms or severity of depression	Schedule for Affective Disorders and Schizophrenia (SADS) (Endicott and Spitzer, 1978) (provider-completed interview guide or change version)
	Beck Depression Inventory (BDI) (Beck et al., 1961) (self-report)
	Zung Self-Rating Depression Scale (Zung, 1965) (self-report)
	Hamilton Rating Scale for Depression (HRS-D) (Hamilton, 1968) provider-completed interview guide
	Center for Epidemiologic Studies Depression Scale (CES-D) (Radloff, 1977) self-report
	Montgomery-Asberg Depression Rating Scale (MADRS) (Montgomery and Asberg, 1979) (self-report)
Laboratory tests	TRH stimulation test and CRH stimulation test (both differentiate unipolar from bipolar disorders and mania from schizophrenia)
	DST (provides evidence of biologically based depression)
	Sleep and waking EEGs
	Thyroid function tests
Geriatric depression	Geriatric Depression Scale (Yesavage et al., 1983) (self-report)
Suicide	Hopelessness Scale (Beck et al. 1974) (provider-rated)
	Suicide Assessment Scale (Hoff, 1989)
Biological or rhythm alterations (sleep, appetite, eating, mood, menstrual)	Personal journal detailing patterns for 1 to 2 weeks
Bipolar disorder	Symptom Checklist 90 (SCL-90) (Derogatis, 1977) Minnesota Multiphasic Personality Inventory (MMPI)
	Young Mania Scale (Young, et al., 1978)
	Manic State Scale

Maintaining the client's safety needs to ensure survival is always the first priority for clients with mood disorders as well as those with other mental health problems. To illustrate this point, see the nursing care plan and related outcomes in Chapter 25 on p. 467 for the nursing diagnosis risk for violence, which is also applicable for suicidal clients who have depressive or bipolar disorder. Nevertheless, some criteria that may be used for measurement of outcomes for clients with depression are as follows:

• Exhibits no evidence of self-harm

• Sets realistic goals for self
• Attempts new activities and interacts appropriately with others
• Focuses attention and concentrates when reading or problem-solving
• Identifies strengths, as well as weaknesses
• Eats a well-balanced diet to prevent weight loss and maintain nutritional status
• Bathes, washes, and combs hair, and dresses in clean clothing without assistance

TABLE 30-6

Assessment of risk for suicide

ASSESSMENT FACTOR	LOW RISK (1 POINT)	MODERATE RISK (2 POINTS)	HIGH RISK (3 POINTS)
Suicidal ideation	No current suicidal thoughts	Intermittent or fleeting suicidal thoughts	Constant suicidal thoughts
Prior suicide attempts	No previous attempts	Past attempts of low lethality	Past attempts of high lethality
Suicide plan	No plan	Has plan without access to planned method	Has carefully thought out plan with actual or potential access to method
Lethality of plan	Low lethality of plan (e.g., superficial scratching)	Moderate lethality (e.g., swallowing 20 aspirin; reckless driving)	High lethality of plan (e.g., hanging, gun, jumping, carbon monoxide)
Current morbid thoughts (e.g., preoccupation with death, reunion fantasies)	Rarely	Intermittent	Constantly
No Harm Contract	Reliably signs No Harm Contract	Signs No Harm Contract, but is ambivalent	Unwilling or Unable to Sign No Harm Contract
Current alcohol and/or drug use	Infrequently to excess	Frequently to excess	Continual abuse
Behavioral symptoms: • Anxiety • Hopelessness • Helplessness • Anger/rage • Guilt/shame • Impulsivity • Isolation	None to two symptoms present	Three to four symptoms present	Five to seven symptoms present
Support systems	Several friends, coworkers, and relatives available	Few or only one friend, coworker, or relative available	None available
Coping mechanisms	Generally constructive	Some are constructive	Predominantly destructive

Total score _____

RN signature _____

Date and time _____

Scoring directions

1. Assess each assessment factor.
2. Circle one descriptor for each assessment factor that *best* describes the client.
3. Assign appropriate points (1, 2, or 3) to each factor.
4. Add the points for each assessment factor to arrive at a total score.

Scoring key

10-13 = No precautions

14-19 = Moderate risk precautions (15-min checks)

20 or above = High risk precautions (1:1 constant observation) above

Adapted from Hatten, C.I., & Valente, S.M. (1984). Suicide assessment and intervention (2nd ed.). *Norwalk, CT: Appleton-Century Crofts.*

The Nursing Process

TABLE 30-7

Comparison on DSM-IV diagnostic criteria for major depression and related NANDA nursing diagnoses

DSM-IV CRITERIA*	NANDA DIAGNOSES†
Major Depression	
At least five of the following symptoms (including one of the first two) must be present most of the day, nearly every day, for at least 2 weeks:	
Depressed mood	Hopelessness
Loss of interest or pleasure	Coping, ineffective individual; social interaction: impaired
Weight loss or gain	Nutrition, altered: more than/less than body requirements
Insomnia or hypersomnia	Sleep pattern disturbance
Psychomotor retardation or agitation	Mobility, impaired physical
Fatigue or loss of energy	Fatigue; self-care deficit (specify)
Feelings of worthlessness or excessive guilt	Self-esteem, disturbance in
Impaired concentration or indecisiveness	Thought processes, alteration In
Thoughts of death or suicide	Violence, risk for: self-directed
Mania	
Three or more of the following symptoms must be present to a significant degree for at least one week:	
Inflated self-esteem or grandiosity	Self-esteem, disturbance in
Decreased need for sleep	Sleep pattern disturbance
Pressured speech	Communication, impaired verbal
Flight of ideas	Thought processes, altered
Distractibility	Thought processes, altered
Increase in goal-directed activity or psychomotor agitation	Social interaction: impaired; self-care deficit (specify) mobility, impaired physical
Excessive involvement in pleasurable activities that are likely to yield negative consequences	Coping, ineffective individual

*Reprinted with permission from American Psychiatric Association. (1994). Diagnostic and statistical manual of mental disorders, fourth edition. Washington, DC: Author.
†From North American Nursing Diagnosis Association. (1994). NANDA nursing diagnoses: Definitions and classification, 1995-1996. St. Louis: Mosby.

- Sleeps 5 to 8 hours per night and verbalizes feeling well-rested

The following criteria may be used for measuring outcomes for the client who is manic:

- Demonstrates no evidence of harm to self or others
- Verbalizes understanding of recurrent nature of bipolar disorder

- Verbalizes that hallucinatory and delusional activity has stopped
- Does not manipulate others for gratification of own needs
- Accepts limits established by staff and accepts responsibility for own behavior
- Interacts appropriately with others (without dominating or monopolizing)

The Nursing Process

- Verbalizes a more realistic self-concept
- Sleeps 5 to 8 hours per night without medication
- Eats a well-balanced diet to prevent weight loss and maintain nutritional status
- Showers, washes, combs hair, and dresses appropriately

Planning

Planning care for clients with mood disorders is a multidisciplinary effort. For psychiatric nurses, as well as for other team members, priorities in planning care include symptom reduction, restoration of the client's functional status, improvement in his or her quality of life, and prevention of relapse and recurrence of future episodes. To accomplish this, treatment consists of three phases: acute, continuation, and maintenance (USDHHS, 1993).

The objective of the *acute* treatment phase is to reduce or eliminate the symptoms of the mood disorder and restore occupational and psychosocial functioning. This phase usually lasts 6 to 12 weeks and if clients are symptom-free at the end of that time, they are then in remission. A portion of the acute treatment phase may take place in an inpatient setting such as the hospital, particularly if the client is at risk for harming self or others. A nursing care plan related to cognitive restructuring, which is an intervention with demonstrated effectiveness for clients with depressive disorders, is presented on p. 631. This care plan is particularly effective during the acute treatment phase and can be used in both inpatient and outpatient settings. A critical pathway that illustrates an example of an inpatient interdisciplinary treatment plan for clients with major depressive disorder appears in Chapter 17. A critical pathway illustrating an example of an inpatient interdisciplinary treatment plan for clients with bipolar disorder is presented on p. 632. Other portions of the acute treatment phase occur in partial hospital and outpatient settings.

The objective of *continuation* treatment is to prevent relapse, which is a return of the current depressive or manic episode. Since mood disorders tend to recur, continuing treatment is essential in relapse prevention. Nurses need to remember that the risk of relapse is highest during the first 4 to 6 months after recovery. Therefore continuation treatment of mood disorders should last for 4 to 9 months after return to symptom-free status. This treatment phase takes place in outpatient settings.

The objective of *maintenance* treatment is to prevent the recurrence, or return, of a new episode of the mood disorder. This approach is commonly accepted for bipolar disorder, but is relatively new for depressive disorders. Research findings indicate that clients who have had three or more episodes of major depression have a 90% chance of having another episode (National Institute of Mental Health [NIMH], 1985). Therefore they are considered to be appropriate candidates for continuation treatment that prevents new episodes or lengthens the time interval between episodes (USDHHS, 1993). The appropriate length of maintenance treatment may vary from 1 year to a lifetime, depending on the client's history and other factors. This treatment phase also takes place in outpatient settings.

Effective planning must consider the phases of treatment for mood disorders. Nurses should discuss the three phases with the client and family or significant others so that they understand the treatment trajectory and have realistic expectations about it. In so doing they can knowledgeably join in with formulating and adhering to the treatment plan.

Implementation

Counseling

Nurses begin working with clients who are depressed, suicidal, and/or manic by establishing a therapeutic relationship (see Chapter 9). Therapeutic use of self and communication skills are the nurse's major intervention strategies for operationalizing the counseling implementation standard.

Therapeutic use of self

When nurses work with clients who are depressed, their approach should be warm and accepting. They should demonstrate empathy, honesty, and hope. It is not easy to provide warm, compassionate care to someone who is unresponsive, helpless, and hopeless or agitated and demanding. Nurses may even feel angry or resentful of the client's helplessness and hopelessness, believing that the client has "much to be grateful for" and should be able to "get a grip" on their depression. Nurses should avoid being overly enthusiastic and giving false reassurance. Patience, belief in the potential of each person to grow and change, and hope are needed. When this is communicated to the client both verbally and nonverbally, the client may begin to respond.

On the other hand, when nurses work with clients experiencing manic episodes, their approach should be warm but firm. Clients who are manic can be disruptive; they commonly dominate group meetings or individual counseling or therapy sessions with talkativeness, short attention span, flight of ideas, lack of insight, rapid mood swings, and hyperactivity. Although they may appear to participate in the nurse-client relationship, their commu-

Cognitive Restructuring

NURSING ASSESSMENT DATA

Subjective: Cynthia states, "Under the best circumstances I am not an optimistic, outgoing, and confident person; this cancer has put me over the edge. I see gloom and doom everywhere." *Objective:* Cynthia, a 47 year old woman, diagnosed with lung cancer 8 months ago, has had symptoms of major depression (psychomotor agitation, loss of pleasure, sad pessimistic mood, worthlessness, and guilt) since completing chemotherapy and radiation 2 months ago. Following a suicide attempt, she was hopitalized for 5 days of treatment stabilization and is now admitted to the day treatment program of the same hospital. She is taking Pamelor 100 mg. qd. hs and Xanax .25 mg. tid. *DSM-IV diagnosis:* major depression, single episode.

NANDA Diagnosis: Coping, ineffective individual related to cognitive distortions

Outcomes	Interventions	Rationale	Evaluation
Short term *Within 3 days* 1. Will identify cognitive distortions that reinforce negative self-perceptions. 2. Will label painful feelings associated with cognitive distortions. *Within 1 week* 3. Will identify stressors that trigger cognitive distortions and related emotions. **Long term** 1. Will analyze beliefs that contribute to negative assumptions and interpretations of stressful events *within 2 weeks.* 2. Will replace faulty or inaccurate interpretations (cognitive distortions) with more realistic interpretations of stressful situations and positive self-perceptions *within 1 month.*	• Establish nurse-client relationship-trust • See Box 30-4 • Explain how beliefs influence cognitive assumptions about situations and interactions that lead to faulty interpretations about self, situations, and interactions, as well as distressing emotions and behavior • Assist client in exploring connections between thoughts, feelings, and behavior • Ask client to identify cognitive distortions that illustrate how he or she processes information, particularly in stressful situations • Assist client in examining the validity of cognitive thought patterns • Teach client how to use a Cognitive Distortion Log to increase awareness of stressful events, faulty interpretations, and related emotions through documentation • Explore and test more realistic interpretations of self, situations, and interactions • Teach client how to use Cognitive Distortion Log to replace faulty interpretations with more realistic interpretations and related emotions • Assist client in developing effective coping skills that increase self-help competence (see Chapter 14)	• Increases client willingness to problem-solve • Practice guidelines provide a research-based standard for nursing intervention • Core beliefs about self and others are highly charged, emotional, very rigid, and very low in awareness • Thoughts often mediate affect and behavior • Negatively biased cognition is a core process in depression • Collaborative questioning facilitates reality testing, development of alternative perspectives, and problem solving • Self-monitoring precedes ability to change • Facilitates more rational responses about self, the environment, and the future • Self-monitoring progress in reframing negative cognitions and related emotions • Effective coping skills increase positive self-perception; reduce stress and related anxious and depressed feelings	**Short-term** 1. Met *in 3 days* 2. Not met *in 3 days (met in 5 days)* 3. Met *in 1 week* **Long term** 1. Met *in 2 weeks* 2. Partially met *in 1 month*

⊞ INTERDISCIPLINARY TREATMENT PLAN

Critical Pathway: Bipolar Manic 296.4x, depressed 296.5x, mixed 296.6x, cyclothmia 301.13

Patient Name _____ Case Manager _____ Physician: _____ Medical Record # _____

Admit date: _____ Expected LOS: _____ UR days certified: _____ Discharge Date: _____ Actual LOS: _____

Day/Date:	0-8 Hours	8-24 Hours	Day 2	Day 3	Day 4	Day 5
ASSESSMENTS & EVALUATIONS	Nursing Assessment Nutritional screening, wt Admit note, Precautions	H & P, Social HX, RT/TA; Dr. Initial TX Plan/Admit Note, Assess Sleep patterns, AIMS	Precaution Evaluation Observe for audio/visual hallucinations	Psych Eval done Social Hx done Precaution Evaluation	Assess readiness for discharge	Assess for goals achieved
PROCEDURES	Lab ord.; Adm. prof., UA, UDS, UCG, EKG, Other:	Lab done: UA, UDS, UCG, EKG, Lithium level	Lab results checked Abnormals called to Dr.	Physician progress note r/t abnormal lab values	Note baseline renal functions.	Consider serum Lithium, tegretol, Valproic acid Psych Testing results
CONSULTS	IT ordered Y/N FT ordered Y/N GT ordered Y/N	GT started, limit group size Psych Testing Order Y/N	Schedule MTP meeting	IT started, FT started Psych Testing Done Home Contract		Psych Testing results
TREATMENT PLANNING	NI: _____ Axis III	Structured schedule promotes pt. security	RT/TA started School started	Master TX Plan Update/Revise, RT/TA		Consider level of care change
INTERVENTIONS	Assess safety needs monitor anxiety stimulus	Decrease stimuli during manic phase	Reality orientation	Reinforce control over social behaviors	Assess client support network	Focus on strength and accomplishments
MEDICATIONS	Meds ordered, Inf. Con.		Drug interaction ✓'d, Dr. signs inf. Consent	Meds side-effects evaluated	Observe/document response to Rx,	Discharge instructions for medication self-admin
LEVEL	Level ordered		Re-evaluate	Re-evaluate	Re-evaluate consider PHP	Re-evaluate
TEACHING	Patient Rights Orient to Unit	Orient to Program	Sx. of lithium toxicity, fluid balance	Lithium takes 1-2 weeks to alleviate mania	Symptoms of recurrent illness	Teach family S/S of Rx. non-compliance
NUTRITION/DIET	Type: _____	Diet adequate in sodium	I&O, 2500-3000 ml/day	I&O, encourage fluids	Chart daily intake	Dischg. dietary instr.
CARE CONTINUUM	Initial D/C Plans	Outcome Survey	Placement Search	Discharge Plan updated/rev	After care plan written	Outcome Survey, follow-up appts. set
PATIENT OUTCOMES	Controls violent impulses	Aggitation dec., sleep 6-8 hrs.	Aggressive response to hallucinations prevented	Increased self-esteem	Broaden support group	Foster self-reliance

*PsychPaths™ ©Copyright 1994, All Rights Reserved. Strategic Clinical Systems, Inc., Granbury, Texas.
(Variances are contained on a second page, which is not shown.)*

The Nursing Process

nication is often superficial, a strategy used to resist genuine involvement in the therapeutic process.

Clients who are manic are also experts at sensing a vulnerable area in another person or in a group. They use this sensitivity to manipulate and exploit others, which in turn alienates others and provokes angry defensive responses from clients and staff alike. These strategies are diversionary maneuvers used to avoid examining their own problems. Nurses are, perhaps, particularly susceptible to these feelings because of their caregiver role and have the most frequent contact with the client who is manic. Feedback, constructive confrontation, limit-setting, simple explanations, and concise, truthful answers to questions and statements are often used intervention strategies. For the nurse working with manic clients, peer or team support or supervision is an essential component of maintaining an objective perspective.

Facilitating expression of feelings

Nurses use counseling intervention strategies to facilitate the expression of feelings in clients with depression. These clients have difficulty identifying and expressing feelings, especially anger, guilt, worthlessness, sadness, hopelessness, and anxiety. They tend to view such feelings as unacceptable. Awareness of such feelings tends to frighten them and reinforce their already low self-esteem. Clients who are suicidal often feel embarassed at being unable to cope with their problems, thinking that their feelings are not worthy of any attention.

Nurses demonstrate acceptance of the client's thoughts and feelings through active listening and use therapeutic communication strategies such as empathy, facilitative questions and statements, feedback, and confrontation to promote the expression of feelings in clients with depression. If the nurse distances from or overtly rejects the client and his or her feelings, the client's belief that it is not safe to express oneself is reinforced. Similarly, it is particularly important not to try to talk clients out of their sadness by being inappropriately cheerful and optimistic or by offering false reassurance. Comments such as, "Don't be upset . . . everything will be fine," invalidate the client's experience. Realistic reassurance occurs when the nurse acknowledges the client's pain and despair but expresses hope by reinforcing that depression is a self-limiting disorder and that although recovery is slow, the future will be better.

Helping a client become aware of aggressive feelings will be successful when it is done slowly, tentatively, and with genuine patience. Providing feedback is one way to start. Feedback should always be framed in a tentative way to decrease resistance: "I notice that when you talk about your husband, you get a certain look on your face. I may be wrong about this, but it looks to me like a feeling of irritation. What were you aware of feeling just now as we were talking?" This is different from saying, "When you talk about your husband you are obviously angry." The second response is disrespectful, imparts a sense of threat, and creates anxiety for a person who has difficulty expressing feelings. The first response is respectful of the client's individuality, leaving the person free to consider the possibility or reject it. Often the first response will be an automatic denial such as, "Of course I'm not angry with my husband." The nurse then retreats for the moment, but over time and with repeated interventions, the client may become trusting enough to view the expression of feelings with more comfort.

Once a client is willing to share concerns about negative emotions, the nurse must understand the full range of emotions before selecting an intervention. For example, nurses cannot simply assure clients that anger is acceptable. Aggressive feelings may contain elements of destructive impulses that are harmful to self or others. Appropriate anger is indeed healthy, but a client may be harboring hate, vindictiveness, and wishes for revenge. If these feelings are labeled okay, the client may feel that they have been given permission to act on them, which may be frightening. The client, feeling the nurse does not understand, may retreat into isolation and secrecy.

When nurses accept a client's anger, despair, guilt, or anxiety without criticism, that person is encouraged to feel that awareness of and expression of such feelings need not be destructive or a sign of weakness. Increased emotional responsiveness may at first be frightening to clients for whom depression has been a flight from painful emotions, particularly anger. Facilitating expression of feelings by calm acceptance leads clients out of their depression; as emotional responsiveness returns, so does a reasonable basis for hope. Many clients experiencing both depressive and manic states have problems expressing anger and need to learn assertive behavior (see Chapter 14).

Facilitating self-esteem

Clients who are depressed and suicidal often feel worthless and of little value to self or others. Feelings of guilt, usually an exaggerated sense of responsibility for some wrongdoing, only reinforce those feelings of low self-esteem. Improvement of a client's self-esteem begins when the nurse does the following:

1. Schedules specific time to spend with the client that ensures privacy and communicates the client's importance as an individual

The Nursing Process

2. Demonstrates acceptance of clients even if they are negative and pessimistic, thereby promoting feelings of self-worth

3. Focuses on strengths and accomplishments and minimizes failures

4. Promotes attendance at therapy and activity groups that offer structured opportunities for success that are not time-consuming or difficult and that reinforce feelings of success and competence

5. Promotes independence and self-responsibility by collaborating on goals and problem-solving strategies

6. Assists the client to identify which parts of self the client wants to change and which parts of self maintain low self-esteem

7. Provides positive reinforcement for successes but not so much that it is inconsistent with the client's negative view of self

8. Encourages the client to recognize areas of change

9. Teaches the client assertiveness skills (see Chapter 14)

10. Involves the client in social skills training to restructure old and shape new social behaviors through contracting, rehearsal, and role playing

Cognitive restructuring

Cognitive interventions are directed at (1) increasing the client's self-esteem, (2) increasing the client's sense of control over goals and behaviors and, (3) modifying the client's negative thoughts and expectations. As illustrated in Box 30-4, cognitive interventions examine how beliefs influence cognitive assumptions about situations and interactions that lead to faulty interpretations about self, situations, and interactions, as well as distressing emotions and behavior. The outcome of cognitive restructuring interventions is a more realistic evaluation of situations and interactions that increases the client's optimism, self-esteem, and self-confidence (Young and Klosko, 1993). Research findings indicate that cognitive interventions may be more effective with acute rather than recurrent major depressive disorder (Thase et al., 1994).

Clients with depression often define their problems negatively. This is because their thinking is dominated by negative ideas; they do not perceive their behavior and their interpretation of events as possible causes of depression. They often assume a passive, victim stance and wait for someone or something to lift their mood. As a result, clients will, despite successful performances, take a pessimistic or hopeless view of outcomes and

their part in achieving them and continue to have low self-esteem.

The nurse begins by encouraging the client to explore his or her thoughts and feelings. The nurse accepts the client's perceptions, but need not accept the client's conclusions. Negative thinking is often an automatic process of which the client is unaware. Use of the cognitive distortions listed in Table 30-1 is often a helpful tool to aid clients in increasing their awareness of typical negative thinking patterns. The nurse can help the client explore the extent to which negative thoughts occur. Once aware of the frequency of this pattern, the client can be taught how to substitute a realistic thought for an automatic negative one that generally represents a misperception, irrational belief, or cognitive distortion. For example, a client who states, "I have been and always will be a coward," might be instructed to substitute a more realistic thought such as, "My fears vary from time to time and from situation to situation." Clients are also encouraged

---

BOX 30-4

Cognitive Restructuring

DEFINITION
Challenging a patient to alter distorted thought patterns and view self and the world more realistically

ACTIVITIES
Help the patient accept the fact that self-statements mediate emotional arousal

Help patient understand that the inability to attain desirable behaviors frequently results from irrational self-statements

Point out styles of dysfunctional thinking (e.g., polarized thinking, overgeneralization, magnification, and personalization)

Assist patient in labeling the painful emotion (e.g., anger, anxiety, and hopelessness) that he/she is feeling

Assist patient in identifying the perceived stressors (e.g., situations, events, and interactions with other people) that contributed to stress

Assist patient to identify own faulty interpretations about the perceived stressors

Assist patient to replace faulty interpretations with more reality-based interpretations of stressful situations, events, and interactions

Reprinted with permission from McCloskey J.C. and Bulechek G.M. (Eds). (1996). Nursing interventions classification (NIC) (2nd ed.). St. Louis: Mosby.

The Nursing Process

to test the validity of their ideas. For example, a client states, "Nobody wants to talk to me at a party; I'm a social misfit." The client contracts to initiate or respond to conversation with three people at the next party he attends and then evaluate if his negative idea about his social desirability is valid. Table 14-5 on p. 257 is also a helpful tool for clients to use when reappraising beliefs that provide the basis for cognitive distortions.

Concurrently, the client can be encouraged to increase positive thinking by evaluating personal assets, strengths, accomplishments, and opportunities. Clients should also be helped to move from unrealistic to realistic goals, as well as decreasing the importance of unattainable goals. These interventions decrease stress and depressive feelings and increase the client's self-understanding and self-esteem (Young and Klosko, 1993; Jarrett and Rush, 1994).

Group interventions
Whether the group focus is group therapy, social skills training, or psychoeducation, involvement in therapeutic groups provides multiple benefits to clients with mood disorders and their significant others (Maynard, 1993; Pollack, 1993).

Group therapy   Group therapy for clients with major depression provides a vehicle for expression of feelings of hopelessness and ambivalence. Knowledge that others have similar feelings coupled with empathy and support from group members:

- Decreases guilt
- Facilitates learning about their own behavior patterns and the effect of them on others based on feedback from group members
- Decreases sense of loneliness and isolation by learning that other people have similar problems, which reduces powerlessness and hopelessness
- Increases self-understanding and control over their own lives
- Increases social support through group relatedness
- Develops skills in coping with stress from listening to other group members
- Provides a sounding board for realistically modifying their perceptions and expectations of self and others
- Facilitates development of more satisfying relationships.

Pollack (1993) reports that clients with bipolar disorder positively evaluate group therapy sessions that include only clients with that diagnosis. Respondents of this study indicated that they liked communicating with

people who could relate to how they were feeling, they valued the information received about the disorder and the medications to treat it, and they benefited from hearing about other members experiences, such as how they were coping. The self-management of bipolar disorder group model also described by Pollack (1995a) is designed to increase client accountability through a combined approach integrating educational, group dynamic, and psychotherapeutic characteristics.

Social skills groups   Nursing intervention through the use of group social skills training provides a strategy for shaping social skills that improves effectiveness in social interactions. Socialization has a modifying effect on depression by providing an experience incompatible with social withdrawal. It also promotes increased self-esteem through the positive reinforcers of approval, acceptance, recognition, and support.

Nurses use behavioral principles to facilitate the sequential learning of effective social skills when they collaborate with clients to:

- Assess the client's social skills and interests through observation and by encouraging description of behaviors interfering with social interaction
- Identify gaps in the client's social skill repetoire
- Instruct the client about corrective social behaviors
- Role model effective social skills
- Role play and rehearse problematic social situations and interactions
- Provide feedback and positive reinforcement when effective social skills are used
- Encourage the client to test new skills in actual or other social situations and interactions
- Discuss generalizing the use of newly developed skills in other aspects of the client's life

To facilitate the application or generalization of social skills, nurses work with clients to identify career, recreational, religious, cultural, and personal interests. Community resources such as self-help groups (see the Community Resources box on p. 636), organizations, special interest groups, and clubs (e.g., women's groups, single parents groups, biking clubs, church groups, professional organizations, and neighborhood associations) all provide socialization opportunities. Clients with depression, in particular, often need significant encouragement and support when working on the development of social skills.

Postvention on the psychiatric unit following suicide   When a client commits suicide during or following hospitalization, postvention groups, which focus

The Nursing Process

COMMUNITY RESOURCES

American Association of Suicidology
2459 South Ash
Denver, CO 80222
(303)692-0985

Depression After Delivery
P.O. Box 1282
Morrisville, PA 19067
(215)295-3994

National Alliance for the Mentally Ill (NAMI)
200 North Glebe Road, Suite 1015
Arlington, VA 22203-3754
(800)950-6264

National Depressive and Manic-Depressive Association
730 North Franklin, Suite 501
Chicago, IL 60610
(312)642-0049

National Foundation for Depressive Illness
P.O. Box 2257
New York, NY 10116
(212)370-7190

Suicide Prevention Center, Inc.
184 Salem Avenue
Dayton, OH 45406
(513)297-4777

National Institutes of Health (NIH)
National Institute of Mental Health (NIMH)
Information Resources and Inquiries Branch
5600 Fishers Lane, Room 7C-02
Rockville, MD 20857
(301)443-4513
(800)421-4211 (Depression/awareness, recognition and treatment information)

NIMH Mood Disorder Publications

1. *Depressive illnesses: Treatments bring new hope* (NIH Publication No. 93-3612)

2. *Bipolar disorder* (NIH Publication No. 93-3679)

3. *Lithium* (NIH Publication No. 93-3476)

4. *Plain talk about depression* (NIH Publication No. 93-3561)

5. *Helping the depressed person get treatment* (NIH ADM Publication No. 90-1675)

6. *La depresion: Existen tratamientos eficaces (Depression: Effective treatments are available)* (SP-1703)

on the survivors, the staff, and other hospitalized clients on the inpatient unit are useful to begin resolving the trauma of a completed suicide. When clients kill themselves despite preventive measures, staff members and other clients often have an intense reaction that includes anger, guilt, helplessness, and hopelessness. Clients on the unit may also demonstrate self-destructive behavior or even carry out their own suicides. Staff members tend to go through a process of grieving in addition to experiencing guilt, failure, and helplessness (Cooper, 1995).

It is usually helpful to assemble staff members and clients in groups so that they can share and express their feelings of loss. Such feelings may include other clients' anger and fear for their own safety. Surviving clients (e.g. family members) may identify with the person who has committed suicide; they may be afraid that they, too, will succumb to their own self-destructive impulses and that

staff members will be unable to prevent this. The professionals have the responsibility of supporting and protecting clients as well as working through their own feelings.

Family interventions

Families of clients with depression experience frustration and anger when making an effort to express love and care that is seemingly not appreciated, as illustrated in the Research Highlight on p. 637. Guilt over feelings of frustration and anger adds to the burden. The family needs to know that the person with depression often responds negatively to expressions of love, feeling needful yet undeserving or demanding yet unable to receive. A person with depression may try to respond in a reciprocal, loving way but may be unable to do so. Family members thus feel drained and rejected. Although most depressive symptoms decrease following treatment, fam-

The Nursing Process

RESEARCH HIGHLIGHT

Badger TA. (1996). Family members' experience living with members with depression. *Western Journal of Nursing Research.* 18:2, 149-171.

Summary

Families of relatives with depression experience difficulties with communication, marital adjustment, expressed emotion, problem solving, and family functioning. Not surprisingly, depression has its most negative impact on families during acute depressive episodes. The purpose of this qualitative study was to describe family members' experiences in living with a member with depression.

Findings suggest that this process can be described as family transformations. In the first stage of this process, acknowledging the stranger within, family members described observing the metamorphosis of the person and other family members, finding socially acceptable explanations, living two lives, searching for reasons and solutions, and hoping for what was. In the second stage—fighting the battle—family members alternated between the strategies of holding their ground, moving forward to counteract the metamorphosis, and working the system to get help for the family member who was ill. In the third stage, family members described gaining a new perspective, identified preserving oneself, refocusing on others, redesigning the relationship, and becoming hopeful as strategies used in this final stage. Family members are significantly affected by having a family member with depression.

Implications for Nursing Practice

Based on the conclusion of this study, it is important for psychiatric-mental health nurses to:

- Assist families to develop nonstigmatizing explanations of their relatives behavior
- Reinforce family's lack of blame for their relative's depression
- Include relatives in care planning and intervention to decrease isolation and increase a knowledgeable approach
- Provide an opportunity to express feelings about having a family member with depression
- Assist family members in identifying community resources and support systems to decrease stress and caregiver burden
- Encourage family members to identify strategies for redistributing family role responsibilities

ilies consistently continue to experience difficulties during remission (Badger, 1996).

It is important that nurses conduct family meetings or family therapy sessions with families of clients who are depressed to determine the extent to which relatives or friends in the client's support system reinforce or support the client's depression. When persons become depressed, they often receive a lot of attention from others who interact with them in a helpful, caring, nurturing, or annoyed manner. However, when a person behaves in a nondepressed manner, minimal attention is given. This interaction pattern reinforces dysfunctional depressed ways of acting. Therefore one goal of family therapy is to have family members positively reinforce nondepressed behavior and ignore dysfunctional depressive behaviors.

Family intervention is also needed with significant others of clients with bipolar disorder. Family members need support in coping with the recurrent nature of bipolar disorder, particularly the mood highs and lows, the related behavioral changes, and their impact on the family. During the depressed phase of the cycle, the family interventions discussed above are helpful. When the manic phase occurs, family member are often frustrated by and angry about their family member's often hostile, impulsive, acting-out behavior. Because judgement is impaired and grandiosity abounds, the effect on the family of indiscriminate spending, commitment to foolish business ventures, promiscuity, and alcohol or drug abuse can be profound. Family therapy helps members learn about bipolar disorder, its treatment, and symptom management strategies such as limit setting, and relapse prevention. It also helps families deal with the marital conflict that is often evident (APA, 1994a).

When a family member commits suicide, intervention with the family is extremely important (Anderson, 1991). Grief following the loss of a loved one by natural causes generally involves a temporary healing process, but grief following a suicide is a self-perpetuating agony of loss from death, rejection, and disillusionment.

Often the social or religious rituals and amenities through which bereaved families receive comfort and

The Nursing Process

support from friends who share their loss are lacking when a suicide is involved. The family feeling shame and/or guilt and fearing censure from others may not observe mourning rituals such as a wake, shiva, or funeral service. It is not uncommon for friends, and even relatives, to feel that they do not know what to do for the family, or even what to say. As a result, they often do nothing. This reinforces the family's sense of isolation and confirms and perpetuates their guilt.

Children are particularly vulnerable to the death of a parent by suicide. Behavioral problems such as nightmares, bedwetting, clinging, and a decline in school performance are sometimes related to a family's tendency to try to keep from the child the facts of the parent's death, generally by making up an explanation that is supposedly less traumatic. Children often know the truth anyway; they are perceptive and may also be the recipient of thoughtless remarks made by family friends, teachers, or friends. However, children are often denied the opportunity to deal with the fact of suicide because of the family's closed communication system.

Nurses who can listen, accept, and support the family are a valuable family resource. One mother, following the suicide of her 20-year-old son, described the pain, "Like ocean waves crashing on you. You're covered with the salty wet tears. You just want the undertow to take you. How can you listen to me? But thank you for not abandoning me."

Referral to community bereavement groups for adults, children, or the entire surviving family is beneficial. Sometimes feeling the pain is too great to share with a group; it takes time for family members to feel ready to attend self-help group meetings.

MIlieu Therapy

Interventions related to milieu therapy include monitoring safety needs, limit setting, management of environmental stimuli, and structuring time and activities.

Monitoring safety needs

Nursing intervention related to preventing self-harm is a priority action. A decision about the level of suicide risk is made when the initial assessment is completed (see Table 30-6). Associated with that decision is one about the level of observation, precautions to be taken, and limits on activity and freedom of movement. This information is reviewed with the client, reinforcing the rationale for maintaining a safe environment.

Sometimes a client commits to and signs a "No Harm Contract" in which the client agrees not to inflict self-harm for a specified period. The client also agrees to

give others any possibly lethal objects such as guns or knives and to contact the provider should he or she be tempted to act on self-destructive impulses. Family and supportive others should also be included in the contracting process; they are important allies in managing a suicidal client. When suicidal clients are treated on an outpatient basis:

1. Both client, family, and provider need names and telephone numbers to cover any emergencies
2. The clients should be supervised at all times by family, friends, or health care personnel and should never be left alone
3. The nurse should monitor all medications the client is taking
4. The client should only have a few days' supply of medications to avoid risk of overdose

Other clients (including those who do not agree to contracting) may require involuntary commitment to a secure hospital unit if they are a danger to self and/or others. When clients have expressed suicidal thoughts or made suicidal gestures or attempts, the outcome is for the client to feel safe, in control of, and responsible for his or her behavior related to safety.

Clients in the emergency room, on a medical or surgical unit or critical care unit for serious complications following an attempt or on the psychiatric unit require one-on-one observation and nursing care. This means that the client is in full view *at all times,* including when in the bathroom. Clients who are confused delerious, self-mutilating, or psychotic with active command hallucinations are at high risk and also require one-on-one observation.

Other interventions include removing possessions that represent a danger to the client's safety, such as razors, pocket knives, scissors, metal nail files, shoelaces, belts, jewelry, and medications. Locking the doors to the unit, posting suicide precaution notices, and communicating the suicide observation status of each client at risk (at change of shift report) are other specific interventions.

A period of maximum observation is not merely "standing guard" but provides an opportunity to begin returning control to the client, to establish rapport, to communicate expectations related to safety, and to begin establishing a therapeutic alliance. As the risk of suicide decreases, constant one-on-one observation may be reduced to 15-minute, half hour, or hourly checks. Sometimes clients sign an observation form and make verbal reports at 15-minute intervals. This approach helps clients take responsibility for their own safety.

The level of observation is reviewed by the health care team every 24 hours. Changes in client behavior

The Nursing Process

such as a sudden lifting of depression, escalating command hallucinations or impulsivity, or reemergence of self-mutilating behavior are carefully documented and communicated immediately to team members.

Clients who are impulsive and/or who do not respond to verbal limit setting may require chemical or physical restraints. One-on-one nursing care is required, and the rationale related to use of restraints for safety is explained to the client. Seclusion and restraints are *only* used when all other behavioral safety approaches have been ineffective. They are discontinued as the impulsive behavior decreases (see Chapter 25).

Decreasing environmental stimuli
Management of environmental stimuli is particularly important for manic clients who have difficulty filtering stimuli, which only increases their distractability and hyperactivity. Environmental stimuli can be decreased by soft lighting, low noise level, and simple room decorations. There should be as few people as possible in the client's environment. The client may need to be removed from the general unit milieu, which may be too stimulating, and spend time in a quiet room. Seclusion also may be used to provide a low stimulus environment and/or to manage threatening or aggressive behavior. The nurse provides input to the team about the client's tolerance for external stimuli. For example, initially the manic client may be unable to tolerate highly structured, confining group activities. Therefore choice of activities should consider the client's low threshold for excitability and distractability. Examples of activities that are effective are walks, housekeeping chores, painting, dance, or movement therapy. Firm, clearly stated instructions will facilitate transitions from one activity to another.

Limit setting
Limit setting is often a major milieu management issue with clients who are manic. Demanding, disruptive, hostile, aggressive, and manipulative behavior is characteristic of clients in the manic phase of bipolar disorder. For example, many of their verbalizations are sarcastic, belittling, or confrontational. They become loud and verbally abusive at the slightest delay or frustration. They may refuse to make their bed, pick up their clothing, or carry out assigned responsibilities on the unit. Staff may be asked repeatedly for special favors such as buying small items from outside or to make exceptions to the unit rules. They may try to relate to staff more as friends than as professionals, often using a "divide and conquer" approach (e.g., asking a special favor of one staff member after it has been refused by another).

Other clients and staff may treat these clients with caution and try not to upset them because they are afraid that they will become physically aggressive. Their disruptive behavior may consume all of the staff's time and energy, leaving other clients to fend for themselves. The client's grandiose beliefs are reinforced if the entire treatment program is disrupted by his or her inappropriate behavior.

Clients with depression may also need limits set on their nonparticipatory behavior and demands to be satisfied. Nursing interventions related to limit setting include the following:

- Staff on all shifts must agree on constructive limits and a unified, consistent approach to limit setting. They should be written down, posted conspicuously, and followed through consistently. Frequent staff meetings should be held to reduce faulty communication.
- Expectations should be established for personal responsibility and behavior such as adhering to program policies, cleaning rooms, or no body contact with other clients or staff.
- Consequences of not meeting expectations should be defined.
- Positive feedback (reinforcement) for appropriate behavior should be provided.
- Limits should be set on demanding, manipulative, hostile, or aggressive behavior. Nurses should encourage other clients to carry out agreed limits. Pressure applied by peers is sometimes more effective than pressure applied by staff.
- Corrective feedback should be given in an objective manner that communicates the impact of the behavior on others.
- Reinforcement of negative behavior should be avoided, and ignored or minimally responded to.
- Nurses should refrain from defensive personal responses to criticism, profanity, or physical attack.
- The data (versus judgments) about the behavior should be documented.
- After an episode is over, the client should be given an opportunity to discuss thoughts and feelings experienced before, during, and after the episode.
- Alternative coping strategies should be explored

Since an overall objective of nursing care is to help clients increase their self-control, limit setting is carried out with this goal in mind. Nurses help clients learn to monitor their own behavior, evaluate its impact on others, and choose coping strategies that capitalize on the person's strengths.

The Nursing Process

Promoting physical activity

Clients with mood disorders are encouraged to participate in physical activity. Physical activity releases energy, produces feelings of well-being, generates feelings of control, and produces feelings of accomplishment. Physical activity is one component of milieu therapy and can be done individually or in groups.

Walking, jogging, swimming, bicycling, and aerobics are popular exercises that have a positive effect on the client's overall feeling of well-being, self-esteem, and accomplishment. Movement therapy, dance therapy, sports, and calesthenics are also satisfying forms of physical activity that promote release of tension and nonverbal expression of feelings. Clients are encouraged to participate in activities that were formerly reinforcing even if they do not want to do them. Clients may progress from solitary involvement to group involvement in physical and other activities.

As clients progress, recreational needs become important. Planning renewal of an activity previously enjoyed—an outing, a movie, dinner out, a social gathering, or playing a sport or a game—also provides clients with a legitimate sense of accomplishment.

Self-Care Activities

Physical well-being may be forgotten in both depression and mania and clients may be incapable of self-care activities. Clients who are depressed often have significant changes in physiologic functioning related to nutrition and sleep, as well as self-care deficits related to hygiene and grooming. The more severe the depression, the more important the physical care. Nurses may need to monitor the diet, record intake and output, and weigh clients daily who have no appetite and have lost weight. Monitoring laboratory values such as sodium, potassium, urine, specific gravity, and acetone provides objective data about changes in hydration and nutritional status. Staying with the client during meals, arranging for preferred foods, and encouraging frequent small meals may be helpful. Sometimes clients increase their caloric intake when food becomes a way of coping with anxiety. This is more common in clients who are mildly or moderately depressed, but can contribute to reinforcement of low self-esteem. In this situation, nurses can, when the person is receptive, work with the client on weight management strategies.

Sleep disturbances are common. Typically, clients may have difficulty falling asleep (initial insomnia), may incur early morning awakening (terminal insomnia), or may wake during the night and have difficulty returning to sleep (middle insomnia). Clients are discouraged from sleeping during the day to promote more restful sleep at night. Antidepressant medications are usually administered at night so that clients get the maximum sedative effect at night, thereby promoting uninterrupted sleep, and so that they are not drowsy during the day. However, the SSRI antidepressants (e.g., paroxetine [Paxil], Fluoxetine [Prozac], and sertraline [Zoloft]) are taken in the morning to prevent insomnia. Clients may require prescribed sedative medication at bedtime to promote sleep until a normal sleep pattern is restored. Nurses can help clients with relaxation techniques, warm baths, or backrubs to soft music to promote relaxation. Limiting caffeine, especially late in the day, eating regularly, and staying active during waking hours may also promote more normal sleep patterns.

Neglect of hygiene and grooming is common and is related to psychomotor retardation, loss of energy, diminished interest, and low self-esteem. Nurses may have to assist them with bathing or dressing. They should do this matter-of-factly, explaining that help is being offered because the client is unable to do it independently right now. However, nurses should not maintain or reinforce the client's helplessness or dependency longer than is necessary and should always encourage clients to care for themselves whenever possible. Cleanliness and interest in appearance should be noticed and positively reinforced. Sometimes nurses rush the client or do a task themselves to save time; this does not facilitate the client's recovery and should be avoided.

Clients who are manic primarily need protection from themselves. They may be too busy to eat, drink, shower, change clothes, or sleep. Eating problems should be handled in the same way as with clients who are depressed. In addition, high-calorie foods that can be eaten without utensils and drinks that can be consumed easily while standing or moving are suggested. These clients sleep little, so a quiet environment, sedation, and opportunities for frequent short naps will promote restoration of a regular sleep pattern as will other sleep-promoting strategies used with clients who are depressed. Clients who are manic may also need assistance in selecting clothes and carrying out hygiene activities. Clients need to be provided with flexible opportunities to shower and change. Loose, comfortable clothing is preferable. Setting limits and using a firm approach may be necessary because of the hyperactivity and lack of judgement of the client who is manic.

Psychobiological Interventions

Pharmacological interventions

Antidepressant medications are considered to be a treatment of choice for clients with major depression. They

The Nursing Process

are administered to elevate the mood and alleviate other cognitive, affective, behavioral, and physiological changes associated with major depression. At this time no single antidepressant medication is clearly more effective than another (USDHHS, 1993). As discussed in Chapter 15, there are three types of antidepressant drugs commonly used tricyclics, nontricyclics, and monamine oxidase inhibitors (MAOIs).

Despite their recognized effectiveness, antidepressant medications have their limitations. Foremost is the fact that there is a lag time of 2 to 6 weeks before the therapeutic effect begins. Also important is the fact that they have side effects that can influence the client's willingness to continue taking them for extended periods. For example, a fairly common side effect of selected antidepressants is problems with sexual function. That side effect decreases the client's motivation to adhere to their antidepressant medication regimen. This highlights the importance of the nurse's role in client education; the nurse's ability to teach the client how to manage side effects in ways that minimize distress can often make the difference in the client's ability to commit to the medication protocol. Medication Tips for clients taking antidepressants can be found on p. 642.

Another problem with antidepressants is their toxicity. Tricyclics are lethal when high doses are taken, which makes them particularly dangerous for clients who need them most, suicidal clients. Finally, not all clients benefit from antidepressants and it is difficult to predict who will respond to which drug. Sometimes it takes several trials using different antidepressants or a combination of antidepressants and other psychoactive medications to achieve a therapeutic effect (Nemeroff, 1994).

For clients with acute manic episodes, hypomania, and bipolar disorder, mood stabilizers are thought to be the drug of choice. Since it takes 1 to 2 weeks for mood stabilizers to achieve a therapeutic effect, an antipsychotic medication may also be used during the first few days or weeks of an acute manic episode to manage severe behavioral excitement and acute psychotic symptoms. The overall objectives of psychopharmacological management are to produce a remission of symptoms and prevent recurrence of future episodes.

Other disorders with an affective component such as schizoaffective disorder, recurrent unipolar depressive disorder, catatonia, and alcoholism are sometimes effectively treated with mood stabilizers, especially when they are cyclical in nature. Mood stabilizers have also been reported effective in treating nonaffective disorders such as temporal lobe epilepsy, eating disorders, borderline personality disorder, and aggressive conduct disorder As discussed in detail in Chapter 15, lithium, carbamazepine (Tegretol), and valproate (Depakene) are commonly used mood stabilizers (Keltner and Folks, 1991). Because of the potential for lithium toxicity as well as unpleasant and/or dangerous side effects of mood stabilizers in general, nursing interventions include pretreatment health history and physical, monitoring of lithium levels and blood counts, management of lithium toxicity, and client education (see the Medication Tips on p. 642).

Lithium is a toxic medication with a narrow range of therapeutic effectiveness (0.5-1.5 mEq/ml). Blood levels are drawn regularly on an outpatient basis because a high blood concentration can be lethal. Clients need to know that if they have vomiting or diarrhea, they need to refrain from taking lithium that day.

Many clients dislike taking mood stabilizers because although they dislike the "lows" of depression, they do not want to give up the "highs" of mania. For example, Bobby L. said that he quit taking his medication because he hates "feeling dead." He said that when he's on a manic high, he feels alive, important, and creative. The lithium, as he sees it, robs him of energy, vitality, and a sense of importance. As a result clients may refuse to take it, hide it in their hands or clothes ("palm it"), refuse to swallow it ("cheek it"), or discard it.

Education about the disorder and its recurrent nature as well strategies for managing the specific side effects the client finds objectionable, helps the client to internalize the importance of taking the medication regularly. As indicated in the Cultural Highlights on p. 622 nurses must also be aware of cultural variations when considering appropriate doses, monitoring client responses to, and observing for side and toxic effects of antidepressants and mood stabilizers (see the section on ethnic psychopharmacology in Chapter 6.

Somatic interventions

Electroconvulsive therapy *Electroconvulsive therapy (ECT) is the use of electrically induced seizures for the safe and effective treatment of* severe depression. It is often the treatment of choice for the elderly, for those clients who have not responded to drug therapy, or for whom psychotropic medications are contraindicated. It is also appropriate for use with highly suicidal clients who, because of the therapeutic onset time lag, will not have sufficient symptom reduction benefit from antidepressants to decrease their suicidal risk. Although ECT is predominantly prescribed for adults with severe major depression, it is also used to treat acute mania and certain schizophrenic syndromes char-

The Nursing Process

MEDICATION TIPS

Mood Disorders

Clients Taking Antidepressants Need to Know That:

- It may take as long as 4 weeks before you feel the therapeutic effect of the antidepressant. Keep taking it even if there are no noticeable effects. If after 4 weeks there is no observable improvement, notify your nurse or doctor.
- Do not stop taking this medication abruptly. If you do, you may have symptoms such as headaches, dizziness, insomnia, or you may even feel depressed.
- Get up slowly from a sitting or lying down position. If you feel dizzy, sit quietly for a few minutes before moving to a standing position.
- Call your doctor or nurse immediately if you have any of the following symptoms: sore throat, fever, fatigue, severe headache, bruising easily, fast heart rate, difficulty urinating, rash, or hives.
- Do not drive or operate dangerous machinery if you experience drowsiness or dizziness. Sedation usually improves within a short period; give it a chance to decrease.
- Some people develop problems with sexual functioning when taking antidepressants (decreased desire for sex, difficulty having or maintaining an erection, impaired ejaculation, or orgasmic problems). If any of these occur, discuss the specific problem with your doctor or nurse. Changing the time of day you take your medication or switching to a different medication may or may not be helpful.
- Your skin may be more sensitive to sunburn; wear protective clothing, and use sunscreen.
- Many people taking antidepressants complain about having a dry mouth. If you do, carry a bottle of water or juice and take frequent sips. Chew citrus-flavored sugarless gum, or suck on ice chips or hard candy. Apply lip gloss or lip moisteners often. Brushing your teeth frequently also helps.
- If you experience constipation, increase your fluid, vegetable, and fiber intake as well as the amount and frequency of your exercise.

- Many antidepressants may cause some weight gain (Paxil, Prozac, and Zoloft may cause weight loss). If this is a problem for you, weigh yourself weekly, increase your exercise, and eat nutritious meals.
- Persons taking SSRI antidepressants (Paxil, Prozac, Zoloft) must take their medication in the morning (or may have trouble sleeping at night) and take it with meals (or may experience gastrointestinal upset).

Clients Taking Mood Stabilizers Need to Know That:

- Hand tremors usually decrease as your body becomes accustomed to the medication.
- Take with meals to decrease the chance of gastrointestinal upset.
- Maintain normal levels of dietary sodium.
- Daily fluid intake should range from 2,500 to 3,000 mL/day.
- Avoid high intake of caffeine, which increases urinary output.
- Report any episodes of excessive sweating, diarrhea, or increased urinary output to your doctor or nurse.
- Report any sudden weight gain and/or edema to your nurse or doctor.
- *Immediately* report any signs of lithium toxicity: persistent nausea and vomiting, severe diarrhea, difficulty walking or coordinating your muscles, blurred vision, or ringing in your ears.
- Remember to follow your doctor or nurse's instructions about how often and on which dates you will have a blood test to (1) monitor your lithium level or (2) check your blood count. Blood should be drawn after the last lithium dose.
- If you forget to take a dose, do the following: if it is within 2 hours of the next dose, do not take the missed dose. If you are taking sustained-release capsules, do not take the missed dose if it is within 6 hours of the next dose.

acterized by affective symptoms (Fitzsimons, 1995). ECT helps 80% of persons with severe impairments return home to resume more normal lives.

Risks and side effects The risks and side effects of ECT include the following:

1. During a seizure the brain has increased metabolic demands; without oxygenation and muscle relaxation, anoxia can occur. Oxygen (100%) is administered before the seizure to prepare the client for the period of apnea that will occur from the muscle relaxant and seizure.

The Nursing Process

2. Memory loss is a common side effect of ECT. Because depressed clients often have memory loss, it is difficult to differentiate between the memory loss attributable to depression and that which is attributable to ECT. Attempts to decrease memory loss and confusion have been effective when unilateral ECT is administered to the nondominant hemisphere in comparison with when it is administered bilaterally.

3. Medical complications such as laryngospasm, circulatory insufficiency, tooth damage, vertebral compression fracture, and prolonged apnea occur in one out of 1,300 to 1,400 treatments. Mortality for ECT is approximately one per 10,000 clients. The most common cause of death following ECT are complications of anesthesia and cardiac complications such as ventricular arrhythmias.

ECT is contraindicated for clients with severe cardiac conditions, severe hypertension, cerebral lesions such as tumors, or musculoskeletal injuries, especially of the spinal column. The presence of organic mental disorders is not a contraindication for ECT.

Pretreatment nursing actions   All clients who are candidates for ECT must undergo a complete physical assessment, including history, blood chemistries, urinalysis, EEGs, electrocardiograms (ECGs), and x-rays of the spine and chest.

Major aspects of the pretreatment stage are client and family education and obtaining informed consent. Client and family education involves:

1. Assessing the client and family anxiety level and ability to understand
2. Teaching the client and family about ECT and the rationale for its use in mood disorders
3. Individualizing the amount of information shared (e.g., treatment, post-ECT confusion, memory loss, etc.)
4. Assessing the client and family response
5. Providing an opportunity to express feelings about ECT
6. Providing time to discuss concerns and answer questions.
7. Instructing the accompanying adult in dealing with post-ECT effects (e.g., need to orient to TPP, fill in memory blanks, administer antiemetic, etc.)

The ECT treatment   A physician, a nurse, and an anesthesiologist or anesthetist (physician or nurse) are in attendance when ECT treatments are given. Most clients who are depressed receive between six to twelve ECT treatments (Valente, 1991; Kashka and Keyser, 1995). For each treatment, the client, who has received nothing by mouth, is usually premedicated with an anticholinergic (e.g., atropine) agent to prevent aspiration and cardiac dyshythmias. A fast, short-acting anesthetic is administered to the client lying supine on a stretcher in the treatment room. The client is prebreathing oxygen at 10 L for 1 to 2 minutes before the ECT. The ECT electrodes are applied by the physician, and a monitor strip is run to check electrode placement and functioning of the machine. Following administration of succinylcholine, 30 to 100 mg for muscle relaxation, a pharyngeal airway is placed. Ventilatory assistance with a positive pressure bag using 100% oxygen is in place throughout the treatment.

The ECT stimulus is applied unilaterally or bilaterally, with EEG and ECG monitors running. Concurrent with the passage of the electrical stimulus is a period of muscle contraction, followed by the tonic phase of the seizure. Last, the clonic phase occurs. Each phase is barely discernable because of the anesthesia and muscle relaxants that are administered. After the seizure, the client begins breathing spontaneously within 60 to 120 seconds. The client regains consciousness shortly thereafter (Fitzsimmons, 1995).

Posttreatment nursing actions   Posttreatment nursing actions include the following:

1. Monitor vital signs every 5 minutes until awake, every 15 minutes until alert
2. Suction as needed
3. Position on side until reactive
4. Remove airway when client breathes spontaneously
5. Monitor memory status
6. Orient to environment
7. Discharge to recovery room or by wheelchair to room or unit
8. Assist to ambulate
9. Offer analgesia or antiemetic as needed

Phototherapy   *Phototherapy involves client exposure to bright artificial light for a specified amount of time each day.* The use of bright light or full-spectrum light in the absence of natural morning sunlight, has been used effectively in the treatment of SAD, which typically recurs on a seasonal basis during the winter months.

Clients with SAD are exposed to bright artificial light several hours per day. Antidepressant effects are observed 4 to 5 days after therapy is initiated. Other clients

The Nursing Process

use devices like the Light Visor®, manufactured by Bio-Brite, Inc. Users of the "Light Visor" report that approximately 30 minutes of visor use in the morning produces similar improvement in mood, energy, and alertness. By the end of April, when outdoor light is sufficient to maintain good mood and normal energy levels, clients with SAD no longer need phototherapy.

Health Teaching

With the emphasis on reintegration of clients into the community, family members—the largest group of care providers for persons with serious neurobiological disorders—are increasingly responsible for the care provided. Families need and will continue to need concrete help from health professionals to overcome barriers such as denial and stress. Similarly, clients strive for stability through acquiring information and developing self-management skills. Nurses must address the specific needs of clients and families for education regarding mood disorders. Because major depression and bipolar disorder have a high recurrence rate, clients and families must be equipped with the knowledge necessary to manage these neurobiological disorders just as they would for any other physical illness (Badger, 1996; Pollack, 1995b; Van Hammond and Deans, 1995). A psychoeducation model provides health-relevant information, skills development, and psychosocial support in relation to:

- The client's mood disorder and its treatment (especially medication effects and side effects).
- Strategies related to self-management of depressed or manic symptoms, medication monitoring, problematic behavior patterns, and relapse prevention.
- Creating a collaborative atmosphere between families and professionals that encourages practical problem-solving, instills hope, decreases feelings of stigma, burden, and isolation, promotes a structured home environment to reduce stress, and encourages use of community resources such as those listed on p. 636.

The Teaching Points on p. 645 provide a list of topics that become the foundation for a psychoeducation plan that includes suggestions and strategies designed to assist family members in coping more effectively with mood disorders. It is essential that clients with mood disorders and their family members understand and recognize relapse triggers and symptoms so that a recurrence can be "nipped in the bud" if possible. For example, clients with bipolar disorder and family members need to know that the early symptoms occurring with mania (e.g., feeling too excited, losing one's temper easily, spending money too fast, having trouble finishing a task, having thoughts racing) may be the first sign of instability; that the disease is recurring (Murphy and Moller, 1993). Gaining control of symptoms and recognizing some positive response to medication and treatment promotes stability and increases hope for the future. Identifying triggers for manic symptoms is important in developing strategies for wellness self-management and actualization (Moller and Murphy, 1996b). Holidays and vacations; death of a significant other; getting too tired, stressed or anxious about money; or receiving negative feedback from others are triggers for some clients. Clients often become less and less sensitive to and interested in others. Family members need to know that this is a sign of the neurobiological disorder rather than a nonverbal statement of disaffection, as in the following example:

A 10-year-old boy whose father had bipolar I disorder attended a family psychoeducation session with his mother and was heard to describe his father's relapse pattern. "Usually Dad joins in with the rest of us in going to church and reading the bible and saying our prayers. But I get scared when he starts staying up late studying the bible and writing long passages word for word and wakes me up in the middle of the night to tell me about God. He talks real fast and loud and he sounds mad at me. No matter what I say, it's not okay. He keeps asking me questions and interrupting my answers; he just rambles and rambles about working on a special project for God."

By the end of the 12-session psychoeducation program, the whole family understood that this trigger occurred when the father stopped taking his lithium because the family funds were low. Strategies for coping with symptom management and relapse prevention included saving money by ordering a 3-month supply of a generic brand from a mail-order pharmacy, joining a support group sponsored by the local chapter of the National Depressive and Manic-Depressive Association, writing out a structured schedule that balances work and play, and developing assertiveness and limit setting skills.

Nearly 74% of Americans who seek help for depression or symptoms of depression will go to a primary care provider, physician or nurse practitioner, rather than a mental health professional. Unfortunately, the diagnosis of depression is missed in 50% of primary care cases, and when it is diagnosed, appropriate treatment is provided in less than 19% of the cases (Montano, 1994; Zung et al., 1993). Psychiatric nurses, especially advanced practice

The Nursing Process

TEACHING POINTS

Clients With Mood Disorders and Their Families

Teach the client, family, and significant others the following:

1. Teach about symptoms and the usual course of the particular mood disorder.

2. Explain the basics of neurotransmission, circadian rhythms, kindling, and other biological factors as they relate to the disorder and the prescribed medications.

3. Explain treatments for mood disorders including psychotropic medications, psychotherapies, and other treatments

4. Teach the labels for a wide range of normal emotional responsiveness, both pleasant and unpleasant. Teach clients to recognize and label their own emotions and their effect on others in different kinds of interactions.

5. Encourage clients to develop a list of strong emotions and for each one, identify at least one appropriate way to manage that specific feeling.

6. Collaborate with client and family in identifying problematic interaction patterns (e.g., oversensitivity, unresponsiveness, unrealistic expectations, meddling, manipulation, impulsivity, guilt, anger).

7. Teach stress management techniques, including assertiveness training.

8. Explain the importance of developing a structured activity plan for each day.

9. Collaborate with client and/or family to identify and/or plan specific activities at home that the client needs to accomplish to function adequately (e.g., ADLs, school/work/family responsibilities)

10. Coach the client in identifying a list of diversional activites the client can participate in at home (e.g., reading, cooking a meal, listening to music, attending a lecture or concert, playing a sport or game, going to the beach, attending a social gathering, going to the movies, working on a hobby).

11. Collaborate with the clients to create an activity schedule that includes both diversional and goal-oriented activities. Discuss the relationship between what a person does and how the person feels.

12. Teach clients and families (a) the symptoms of relapse, (b) how to recognize early signs of impending relapse, and (c) the value of having a "relapse action plan."

nurses, are well-equipped to develop and implement education programs for primary care nurses that address assessment, diagnosis, and treatment of depression in primary care settings (Krauss, 1993; Wells, Burnham and Camp, 1995). Such programs need to focus on the following:

- Criteria for assessing and diagnosing depression
- Psychopharmacological and psychotherapeutic treatment approaches
- Care coordination among multiple agencies and providers
- Referral resources
- Cultural and life cycle stage variations

More appropriate care for depression could improve outcomes and cost-effectiveness of care through reduc-

tion of inappropriate primary and specialty care visits for physical health problems that are actually undiagnosed symptoms of depression (Sturm and Wells, 1995).

Case Management

Because of the cyclical and recurrent nature of mood disorders, clients with major depression and bipolar disorder tend to have a high intensity in their use of mental health services. Case management is a useful approach to accessing and coordinating appropriate inpatient and outpatient physical and mental health services. Whether functioning as a case manager for an insurance company, for a health care system, or home care agency, psychiatric nurses are effective case managers. In the case of mood disorders, the nurse's knowledge base about physical as

The Nursing Process

well as mental health disorders is essential, as in the following example:

> By the time Martin D, age 50, had had his fourth episode of bipolar disorder (two episodes of major depression and two episodes of mania), he had lost his most recent job, his wife had divorced him, and he was homeless. When planning his discharge from his most recent hospitalization, the case manager had to collaborate with Martin to access and coordinate transition to a day-treatment program, residence in a group home, initiation of occupational and vocational therapy, securing of entitlement benefits including disability and Medicaid, and involvement in a NAMI community support group. The case manager collaborated with the health care providers or case workers in each of these settings to access, coordinate, monitor, and evaluate the appropriateness and effectiveness of each mental health service as well as the total treatment plan. In the role as case manager, the nurse revised the plan as Martin improved and could move on to new services that met his current needs while continuing to promote the goal of relapse prevention.

See Chapters 17, 21, and 38 for more information on case management.

Health Promotion and Health Maintenance

Despite its prevalence, public awareness is low about the signs and symptoms and treatments available for depression and bipolar disorder. Most persons who have depressive disorders do not seek treatment because they do not know that they have a treatable disease. To solve this problem, in 1988 the National Institute of Mental Health (NIMH) initiated a national education campaign called Depression/Awareness Recognition and Treatment (D/ART) about depressive disorders. References about NIMH D/ART community resource materials are listed in the box on p. 636. The campaign's goal is to increase health care provider and consumer awareness and reduce unnecessary suffering by encouraging persons with depressive disorders to obtain appropriate treatment (Reiger et al., 1988). National Depression Awareness Day, another nationwide campaign to increase public recognition about depression as a treatable disease, occurs annually in October. Nurses, other health professionals, and consumers participate in this education and screening program that directs people in need to appropriate treatment follow-up services.

Children of parents with affective disorders are a high-risk population for the occurence of a mood disorder (Zausniewski, 1994). These children describe themselves as having no one to talk to about what is happen-

ing in their family. They understand little about their parent's illness. They tend to cope with their distress by using avoidant coping mechanisms such as apathy, avoiding their parent, crying alone, and running away when things get tense. However, they may also exhibit aggressive, acting-out behavior (Gross et al., 1995). In addition, research findings also suggest that boys of more severely depressed mothers are more likely to have poorer social competence and more behavior problems than girls. Boys' behavior may be particularly distressing for mothers with depression, increasing the likelihood that these mothers will respond to and reinforce their sons' difficult behaviors.

Preventive intervention for children of parents with mood disorders can include the following:

1. Giving correct information about the parent's mental health problem to prevent harmful misconceptions
2. Suggesting age-appropriate pamphlets, books, or films for the child/children to read or to have read to them
3. Referring children to a support group, preventive intervention program, counselor, adult confidant, or other professional with whom the child can discuss the situation
4. Providing functional opportunities for parents and children to spend time to keep family relationships functional when hospitalization of a parent occurs

Chapters 18 and 38 provide in-depth discussion of health promotion, prevention, and maintanance intervention.

Evaluation

The effectiveness of nursing intervention for clients with mood disorders is determined by changes in the client's cognitive, affective, behavioral, and physiological functioning. The nursing care plan on p. 631 provides an example of outcomes related to cognitive restructuring. Other outcomes related to mood disorders include reduction of suicidal ideation, no self-harm, prevention of violence, decreased impulsivity, increased expression of feelings and concentration, setting realistic goals, improvement in grooming and hygiene, and restoration of a restful sleep pattern represent some of the short-term outcomes that indicate effective resolution of a major depressive or manic episode. Long-term outcomes that indicate potential for improved functional status, quality of life, and prevention of relapse are evident when the client does the following:

The Nursing Process

- Verbalizes understanding of the importance of taking medications daily and completing laboratory tests on schedule
- Identifies early warning signs of relapse and articulates a relapse action plan
- Knows where to seek assistance through use of community resources
- Attends a self-help community support group
- Attends a vocational rehabilitation program
- Maintains a clean living environment in group home
- Participates in recreational activities with family members

- Meets weekly with case manager to assess progress, discuss problems, and revise treatment plan according to current needs

Fortunately, mood disorders are treatable illnesses, and an effective treatment can be found for almost all clients. Recovery is the rule, not the exception and the goal of treatment is to get well and stay well. When clients with mood disorders are engaged in collaborative partnerships with care providers, their commitment to achieving the outcomes discussed above increases significantly.

THE CONSUMER'S VOICE

Bipolar Disorder

Pat Guerard

I am a woman with mental illness. My doctor cannot tell me the exact cause of my illness, nor can he tell me why the medications I take work. I am in recovery today; I can work and I enjoy my family life. When I was first told that I had a mental illness, I denied it. I told myself that I had a "nervous breakdown," whatever that means. It sounded better, almost normal, and certainly not a life sentence. It has taken me years to accept my diagnosis of manic depression, and just as long to find the correct medications that help stabilize me. I am also a recovering alcoholic. This is known as having a dual diagnosis. Before I sought help from a doctor, I knew something was wrong with me so I self-medicated with alcohol. I can no longer indulge in alcohol if I want my meds to work.

I have gone on and off my medications many times. I am more creative and inventive off my meds. But the people I love will not come near me. I have been divorced twice, and I have lost my son to this illness; he is currently in foster care. He chose not to live with me. This illness is devastating, not only to the person who has it, but to the whole family. On medication I can be predictable, reliable, and trusted. I have made a commitment to my daughter that we will live in the same place for at least 3 years so that she can graduate from high school with her friends. In the past, we moved almost every year.

Many people have experienced the psychiatric equivalent of the common cold. Who has not felt depressed at one time, thought they heard the door bell ring when it didn't, or rationalized a shopping spree they could not afford? The difference between them and me is that I cannot stop. When I have an episode, I lose control; I lose all my choices. I wind up in a hospital in restraints.

I have discovered several tools that are important to my recovery. First is communication. I am learning to communicate clearly what I mean. I am learning to actively listen, to be open-minded and willing to negotiate. For me, communication has been a bridge between the "normal world" and the world of clinical knowledge. I continue to learn as much as I can about this illness. My second tool came to me after a period of recovery—insight. I taught myself and my family about my illness. I looked for behavior cycles, and I now keep a journal to help me avoid "triggers," or situations that trigger me into an episode. The third tool is planning. I plan everything. Fridays and the fall season are my worst times, so I set up a crisis plan. I have a doctor, a social worker, and a hospital that all work together with me to get through a relapse or crisis episode.

Most importantly I own and take responsibility for my illness. I try to keep up with new theories and treatments. I am an active advocate in my local mental health association. With the help of our caregivers and a supportive health care climate, we, the psychiatrically disabled, can achieve our goals of wellness and independence.

KEY POINTS

- Mood disorders are the most common, yet challenging of the neurobiological disorders, affecting at least 10 to 15 million Americans at any given time. Of the 30,000 annual suicides in the United States, approximately 16,000 are associated with depressive disorders.
- Mood disorders generally involve a single or recurring depressive (unipolar) and/or manic (bipolar) episode but also occur with nonmood disorders and with physical health problems.
- Biological correlates of mood disorders include the neurotransmitter, neuroendocrine, and genetic hypotheses, as well as kindling and biological rhythms. Psychosocial correlates that explain the basis for mood disorders include psychodynamic theory, cognitive theory, the hopelessness, behavioral, and stress models.
- Clients with mood disorders are increasingly encountered by nurses in community-based settings such as day treatment, halfway houses, home care, group homes, and community mental health centers. Clients with severe depression and those who are manic, who are a danger to self and/or others and who have psychotic features, may be admitted to inpatient units for treatment stabilization. Nurses also encounter clients with mood disorders, especially depression in medical-surgical, primary care, and long-term care settings.
- Physiological, cognitive, affective, and behavioral changes are associated with depression and mania.
- Individualized application of the nursing process is crucial to formulating realistic and attainable outcomes.
- Milieu management with clients who are depressed, manic, or suicidal considers safety, low environmental stimuli, limit setting, and promotion of physical activity.
- Counseling interventions used with clients who are depressed, manic, or suicidal promote therapeutic use of self, expression of feelings, facilitation of self-esteem, cognitive restructuring, social skills development, and effective suicide postvention.
- Interventions that promote self-care enhance grooming, hygiene, nutrition, and sleep.
- Nurses collaborate with members of the mental health team in providing psychobiological intervention that includes psychopharmacological agents, ECT, and phototherapy.
- Interventions related to health teaching include psychoeducation programs
- Case management involving clients with mood disorders involves accessing and coordinating resources across treatment settings.

 CRITICAL THINKING QUESTIONS

Victor, age 35, had been working as a computer programmer in a large corporation for 6 years. His immediate supervisor was recently transferred and Victor was promoted to manager, in charge of 15 people in the department. He was flattered by the promotion but anxious about the increased responsibility of the new position. Shortly after Victor assumed his new position, his co-workers noticed a change. He had a great deal of energy and began working long hours. He began to talk loudly and rapidly, becoming hostile if his staff members did not immediately respond to his demands. Victor's wife noticed that he slept and ate very little. When she confronted Victor about a call from the bank indicating that the mortgage payment had not been received, he lost his temper and screamed at his wife, "Don't you meddle in my affairs! Mind your own business!" Because of his irritability at work, several staff members reported his behavior to the division manager. When the manager met with Victor to discuss his behavior, he lost control, shouting, cursing, and striking out at anyone nearby. The security officers restrained him and took him to the emergency room of the nearest hospital. He was detained in a crisis stabilization area until the staff decided whether he should be admitted to an inpatient unit. Victor had no history of mental illness. He was assigned an initial diagnosis of bipolar I disorder and was medicated with chlorpromazine (Thorazine) 50 mg intramuscularly stat, as needed and 50 mg by mouth, four times daily, and lithium carbonate 600 mg four times daily.

1. Which assessment data indicate that the diagnosis of bipolar I disorder is appropriate
2. Which assessment data will influence the decision to admit Victor to an inpatient unit rather than discharge him from the crisis stabilization area after 12 hours?
3. What are the priority nursing interventions for Victor?
4. What kind of health teaching would be appropriate for Victor?
5. Why was chlorpromazine administered in addition to lithium carbonate?
6. What is the nurse's role in managing Victor's lithium medication protocol?

• Mental health promotion and maintenance is accomplished through identification and screening of populations at risk for a mood disorder, preventive intervention programs, and psychiatric rehabilitation programs.

REFERENCES

Abrahamson, L.Y., Metalsky, G.D., and Alloy, L.B. (1989). Hopelessness depression: A theory-based subtype of depression. *Psychological Review, 96:* 2, 358-372.

Adams, D. (1992). Suicidal behavior and history of substance abuse. *American Journal of Drug Abuse, 18,* 343.

Affonso, D. (1992). Postpartum depression: A nursing perspective on women's health and behavior. *Image, 24:* 2, 215-221.

American Psychiatric Association. (1994a). *The diagnostic and statistical manual of mental disorders, fourth edition.* Washington, DC: Author.

American Psychiatric Association. (1994b). *Practice guideline for treatment of patients with bipolar disorder.* Washington, DC: Author.

Anderson, D.B. (1991). Never too late: Resolving the grief of suicide. *Journal of Psychosocial Nursing.*

Badger, T.A. (1996). Living with depression: Family members' experiences and treatment needs. *Journal of Psychosocial Nursing, 34:* 1, 16-20.

Bandura, A. (1977). *Social learning theory.* Englewood Cliffs, NJ: Prentice-Hall.

Beck, C.T. (1995). The effects of postpartum depression on maternal-infant interaction: A meta-analysis. *Nursing Research, 44:* 5, 298-304.

Beck, A.T. (1972). *Depression: Cause and treatment.* Philadelphia: University of Pennsylvania Press.

Beck, A.T. (1979). *The cognitive therapy of depression.* New York: Guilford Press.

Beck, A.T., Kovacs, M. & Weissman, A. (1979b). Assessment of suicidal ideation: The scale for suicidal ideation. *Journal of Consulting and Clinical Psychology, 47,* 343-352.

Beck, A., Ward, C., Mendelson, M., Mock, J., & Erbaugh, J. (1961). An inventory for measuring depression. *Archives of General Psychiatry, 4:,* 561-571.

Beck, A.T., Weissman, A., Lester, D., & Trexler, L. (1974). The measurement of pessimism: The hopelessness scale. *Journal of Consulting and Clinical Psychology, 42:* 861-865.

Beeber, L.S. (1996). Pattern integrations in young depressed women. *Archives of Psychiatric Nursing, X:* 3, 151-156.

Betrus, P.A., & Elmore, S.K. (1991). Seasonal affective disorder, part I: A review of the neural mechanisms for psychosocial nurses. *Archives of Psychiatric Nursing, V:* 6, 357-364.

Bourdon, K.H., Rae, D.S., Locke, B.Z., Narrow, W.E., & Regier, D.A. (1992). Estimating the prevalence of mental disorders in U.S. adults from the epidemiological catchment area survey. *Public Health Reports, 107:* 6, 663-668.

Bowlby, J. (1980). *Loss: Attachment and loss. Vol. 3,* New York: Basic Books.

Buchanan, D.M. (1991). Suicide: A conceptual model for an avoidable death. *Archives of Psychiatric Nursing, V:* 6, 341-349.

Bushnell, F.K.L., & DeForge, V. (1994). Seasonal affective disorder. *Perspectives in Psychiatric Care, 30:* 4, 21-25.

Campinha-Bacote, J. 1994. Transcultural psychiatric nursing: Diagnosis and treatment issues. *Journal of Psychosocial Nursing, 32:* 8, 41-45.

Campinha-Bacote, J. (1992). Ethnomusic therapy and the dual-diagnosis Afriican American client. *Holistic Nursing Practice, 6:* 3, 59-63.

Cardell, R., & Horton-Deutsch, S. (1994). A model for assessment of inpatient suicide potential. *Archives of Psychiatric Nursing, VIII:* 6, 366-372.

Carter, B., & McGoldrick, M. (1989). *The changing family life cycle: A framework for family therapy, 2nd ed.* Needham Heights, MA: Allyn and Bacon.

Cooper, C. (1995). Patient suicide and assault: Their impact on psychiatric hospital staff. *Journal of Psychosocial Nursing, 33:* 5, 26-29.

Cotton, D.H.G. (1990). *Stress management. New York:* New York: Brunner/Mazel, Publishers.

Derni, A.S., & Howell, C. (1991). Hiding and healing: Resolving the suicide of a parent or sibling. *Archives of Psychiatric Nursing, V:* 6, 350-356.

Derogatis, L. (1977). *SCL-90-R.* Baltimore: Johns Hopkins University Press.

DeVane, C.L. (1994). Pharmacogenetics and drug metabolism of newer antidepressant drugs. *The Journal of Clinical Psychiatry, 55:* 12, 38-47.

Endicott, J., & Spitzer, R. (1978). A diagnostic interview: The schedule for affective disorders and schizophrenia. *Archives of General Psychiatry, 35:,* 837-844.

Fitzsimons, L. (1995). Electroconvulsive therapy: What nurses need to know. *Journal of Psychosocial Nursing, 33:* 12, 14-17.

Freud, S. (1953). *Mourning and melancholia.* New York: Liveright Publishing Corporation.

Gitlin, M.J., Swendsen, J. Haller, T., & Hammen, C. (1995). Relapse and impairment in bipolar disorder. *American Journal of Psychiatry, 152:* 10, 1635-1640.

Glazenbrook, C.K., & Munjas, B.A. (1986). Sex roles and depression. *Journal of Psychosocial Nursing, 24,* 9-12.

Glod, C.A. (1991). Seasonal affective disorder: A new light? *Journal of Psychosocial Nursing, 29:* 3, 38-39.

Goodwin, W. & Jamison, K. (1990). *Manic depressive illness.* New York: Oxford University Press.

Gove, W.R. (1972). The relationship between sex roles, marital status, and mental illness. *Social Forces, 51:* 34-44.

Gross, D., Conrad, B., Fogg, L. Willis, L., & Garvey, C. (1995). A longitudinal study of maternal depression and preschool children's mental health. *Nursing Research, 44:* 2, 96-101.

Hamilton, M. (1968). A rating scale for depression. *Journal of Social and Clinical Psychology, 6:* 278-296.

Hayes, A. (1995). Psychiatric nursing: What does biology have to do with it?. *Archives of Psychiatric Nursing, IX:* 4, 216-224.

Hirschfeld, R.M.A. (1994). Guidelines for the long-term treatment of depression. *The Journal of Clinical Psychiatry, 55:* 12, 59-67.

Hoff. L.A. (1989). *People in crisis: Understanding and helping (3rd ed.).* Menlo Park, CA: Addison-Wesley.

Hulme, P.A. (1996). Somatization in Hispanics. *Journal of Psychosocial Nursing, 34:* 3, 33-37.

Jarrett, R.B., & Rush, A.J. (1994). Short-term psychotherapy of depressive disorders: Current status and future directions. *Psychiatry, 57:* 6, 115-129.

Jefferson, J.W., & Greist, J. H. (1994). Mood disorders. In *The american psychiatric press textbook of psychiatry* (2nd ed.). R. Hales, S. C. Yudofsky, & J.A. Talbott (Eds.). Washington, DC: American Psychiatric Press, 465-494.

Kaplan, H.I., Sadock, BJ., & Grebb, J.A. (1994). *Synposis of psychiatry (7th ed.).* Baltimore: Williams and Wilkins

Kashka, M.S., & Keyser, P.K. (1995). Ethical issues in informed consent and ECT. *Perspectives in Psychiatric Care, 31:* 2, 15-21.

Keltner, N.L., & Folks, D.G. (1991). Alternatives to lithium in the treatment of bipolar disorder. *Perspectives in Psychiatric Care, 27:* 2, 36-37.

Kessler, A. J., Barklage, N. E., & Jefferson, J.W. (1989). Mood disorders in the psychoneurologic borderland: Three cases of responsiveness to carbamazepine. *American Journal of Psychiatry, 146:* 1, 81-83.

Klein, M. (1975). *Love, guilt, and reparation and other works.* New York: Dell Publishers.

Krauchi, K., Wirz-Justice, A., & Graw, P. (1990). The relationship of affective state to dietary preference: Winter depression and light therapy as a model. *Journal of Affective Disorders, 20:* 1, 43-51.

Krauss, J.B. (1993). *Health care reform: Essential mental health services.* Washington, DC: American Nurses Publishing.

Kurlowicz, L.H. (1993). Social factors and depression in late life. *Archives of Psychiatric Nursing, VII:* 1, 30-36.

Lawson, W. (1989). Racial and ethnic differences in psychiatric research. *Hospital and Community Psychiatry, 37:* 50-54.

Lewinsohn, P., Youngren, M., & Grosscup, S. (1984). Reinforcement and depression. In R. Depue (Ed.), *The psychobiology of depressive disorders.* New York: Academic Press.

Lin, K., Poland, R., & Lesser, I. (1986). Ethnicity and psychopharmacology. *Culture, Medicine, and Psychiatry, 10,* 152-265.

Lindemann, E. (1944). Symptomatology and management of acute grief. *American Journal of Psychiatry, 101,* 141.

Lipson, J. G. (1992). The health and adjustment of Iranian immigrants. *Western Journal of Nursing Research, 14:* 1, 10-24.

Lowry, M. R. (1996). Don't settle: Augment antidepressants when improvement is less than 100%. *Psychopharmacology Update, 7:* 10, 1, 8.

Maynard, C.K. (1993). Comparison of effectiveness of group interventions for depression in women. *Archives of Psychiatric Nursing, 7:* 5, 277-283.

McCloskey, J.C., & Bulechek, G.M. (1996). *Nursing Interventions Classification (NIC). 2nd edition.* St. Louis: Mosby.

McEnany, G.W. (1990). Psychobiological indices of bipolar mood disorder: Future trends in nursing care. *Archives of Psychiatric Nursing, 4:* 1, 29-38.

McEnany, G. (1996a). Part I: Rhythm and blues revisited: Biological rhythm disturbances in depression. *Journal of the American Psychiatric Nurses Association, 2:* 1, 15-22.

McEnany, G. (1996b). Part II: Rhythm and blues revisited: Biological rhythm disturbances in depression. *Journal of the American Psychiatric Nurses Association, 2:* 2, 12-15.

McGoldrick, M. (1991). Echoes from the past: Helping families mourn their losses. In *Living beyond loss.* F. Walsh and M. McGoldrick (Eds.). New York: W.W. Norton & Company, 50-78

McGoldrick, M., & Walsh, F. (1991). A time to mourn: Death and the family life cycle. In *Living beyond loss.* F. Walsh and M. McGoldrick (Eds.). New York: W. W. Norton & Company, 30-49.

Mellick, E., Buckwalter, K.C., & Stolley, J.M. (1992). Suicide among elderly white men: Development of a profile. *Journal of Psychosocial Nursing, 30:* 2, 29-34.

Miller, T.W. (1988). Advances in understanding the impact of stressful life events on health. *Hospital and Community Psychiatry, 39:* 6, 615-621.

Moller, M.D., & Murphy, M.F. (1996). The three R's program: A wellness approach to the rehabilitation of neurobiological disorders. *The International Journal of Psychiatric Nursing Research.*

Montano, C.B. (1994). Recognition and treatment of depression in a primary care setting. *The Journal of Clinical Psychiatry, 55:* 12, 18-37.

Muecke, M.A., & Sassi, L. (1992). Anxiety among Cambodian refugee adolescents in transit and in resettlement. *Western Journal of Nursing Research, 14:* 3, 267-285.

Murphy M.F., & Moller, M.D. (1993). Relapse management in neurobiological disorders: The Moller-Murphy symptom management assessment tool. *Archives of Psychiatric Nursing, VII.*

National Institute of Mental Health Consensus Development Conference Statement. (1985). Mood disorders: Pharmacologic prevention of recurrences. *American Journal of Psychiatry, 142:* 3, 469-476.

Nemeroff, C.B. (1994). Evolutionary trends in the pharmacotherapeutic management of depression. *The Journal of Clinical Psychiatry, 55:* 12, 3-17.

Palmer-Erbs, V. (1996). Psychiatric rehabilitation: A breath of fresh air in a turbulent health-care environment. *Journal of Psychosocial Nursing, 34:* 9, 16-21.

Rahe, R. H. (1979). Life change events and mental illness. *Journal of Human Stress, 5,* 2-10.

Pollack, L.E. (1993). Do inpatients with bipolar disorder evaluate diagnostically homogeneous groups? *Journal of Psychosocial Nursing, 31:* 10, 26-32.

Pollack, L.E. (1995a). Treatment of inpatients with bipolar disorder: A role for self-management groups. *Journal of Psychosocial Nursing, 33:* 1, 12-16.

Pollack, L.E. (1995b). Striving for stability with bipolar disorder despite barriers. *Archives of Psychiatric Nursing, IX:* 3, 122-129.

Post, R.M. (1989). Introduction: Emerging perspectives on valproate in affective disorders. *Journal of Clinical Psychiatry, 50:* 3, 3-9.

Radloff, L. (1977). The CES-D scale: A self-report depression scale for research in the general population. *Applied General Measurement, 1:,* 385-401.

Regier, D.A. et al. (1988). The NIMH depression awareness, recognition, and treatment program: Structure, aims, and scientific base. *American Journal of Psychiatry, 145,* 1351.

Restak, R.M. (1989). The brain, depression and the immune system. *Journal of Clinical Psychiatry, 50:* 5, 3-9.

Rickelman, B.L., & Houfek, J.F. (1995). Toward an interactional model of suicidal behaviors: Cognitive rigidity, attributional style, stress, hopelessness, and depression. *Archives of Psychiatric Nursing, IX:* 3, 158-168.

Ruble, D., Greulich, F. Pomerantz, E., & Gochberg, C. (1993). The role of gender-related processes in the development of sex differences in self-evaluation and depression. *Journal of Affective Disorders, 29:,* 97.

Segal, S.P., & VanderVoort, D.J. (1993). Daily hassles of persons with severe mental illness. *Hospital and Community Psychiatry, 44:* 3, 276-277.

Seligman, M.P. (1975). *Helplessness.* San Francisco: W.H. Freeman.

Silk, A., & Shaffer, H. (1996). Dysthymia, depression, and a treatment dilemma in a patient with polysubstance abuse. *Harvard Review of Psychiatry, 3:* 5, 279-284.

Strickland, T., Rangarath, V., Lin, K., Poland, R., Mendoza, R., & Smith, M. (1990). Psychopharmacologic considerations in the treatment of black americans. *Psychopharmacology Bulletin, 27:* 4, 441-448.

Sturm, R., & Wells, K.B. (1995). How can care for depression become more cost-effective? *Journal of the American Medical Association, 273:* 1, 51-58.

Thase, M.E. et al. (1994). Response to cognitive-behavioral therapy in chronic depression. *Journal of Psychotherapy Practice and Research, 3:* 204-213.

Ugarriza, D.N. (1995). A descriptive study of postpartum depression. *Perspectives in psychiatric care, 31:* 3, 25-29.

U.S. Department of Health and Human Services. (1993). Depression in primary care: Detection, diagnosis, and treatment. *Journal of Psychosocial Nursing, 31:* 6, 19-28.

Valente, S.M. (1991). Electroconvulsive therapy. *Archives of Psychiatric Nursing, 5:,* 223-228.

Van Hammond, T., & Deans, C. (1995). A phenomenological study of families and psychoeducational support groups. *Journal of Psychosocial Nursing, 33:* 10, 7-12.

Wagnild, G. and Young, H.M. (1990). Resilience among older women. *Image: Journal of Nursing Scholarship, 22:* 4, 252-255.

Warren, B.J. (1994). Depression in African-American women. *Journal of Psychosocial Nursing, 32:* 3, 29-33.

Weissman, M. et al. (1993). Sex differences in rates of depression: Cross-national perspectives. *Journal of Affective Disorders, 29:,* 77.

Wells, K.B., Burnham, A., & Camp, P (1995). Severity of depression in prepaid and fee-for-service general medical and mental health specialty practices. *Medical Care, 33:* 4, 350-364.

Yeasavage, J., Brink, T., Rose, T., Lum, O., Huang, V. Adey, M., & Leirer, V. (1983). Development and validation of a geriatric depression screening scale. *Journal of Psychiatric Research, 17:* 37-49.

Young, R. C., Biggs, J.T., Ziegler, V. E., & Meyer, D.A. (1978). A rating scale for mania: Reliability, validity, and sensitivity. *British Journal of Psychiatry, 133,* 429-435.

Young, J.E., & Klosko, J.S. (1994). *Reinventing your life.* New York: Plume.

Zauszniewski, J.A. (1994). Potential sequelae of family history of depression: Identifying family members at risk. *Journal of Psychosocial Nursing, 32:* 9, 15-20.

Zung, W.K. (1965). A self-rating depression scale. *Archives of General Psychiatry, 12:* 63-70.

Zung, W., Broadhead, E., & Roth, M. (1993). Prevalence of depressive symptoms in primary care. *Journal of Family Practice, 37,* 337.

VIDEO RESOURCES

Mosby's Psychiatric Nursing Video Series:
   Volume 2: Major Depression
Mosby's Chronic Disease Self-Management Kits:
   Depression Video and Book Kit

Chapter 31

Delirium, Dementia, and Amnestic and Other Cognitive Disorders

Karen Howell Richardson
Anita Leach McMahon

LEARNING OUTCOMES

After studying and applying the concepts in this chapter, the learner will be able to:
- Discuss theories about the etiologic factors of delirium, dementia, and other cognitive disorders.
- Describe the differences between delirium and dementia.
- Differentiate between clients with symptoms of forgetfulness, dementia of the Alzheimer's type, and vascular dementia.
- Specify the symptoms of dementia, pseudodementia, and delirium.
- Communicate effectively with clients who have cognitive limitations.
- Apply the nursing process with clients who have cognitive impairments.
- Provide support to caregivers of clients with cognitive impairments.
- Discuss counseling, milieu therapy, self-care, and interventions for clients with cognitive disorders.
- Implement effective health teaching, health promotion, and case management strategies with clients experiencing symptoms of progressive dementia.

KEY TERMS

Acalculia
Agitation
Agnosia
Agraphia
Alexia
Amnestic disorder
Amyloid
Anomia
Aphasia
Apraxia
Astereognosis
Auditory agnosia

Confabulation
Conservatorship
Delirium
Dementia
Dementia of the Alzheimer's type (DAT)
Durable Power of Attorney (DPA)
Explicit memory
Forgetfulness
Guardianship
Iconic memory
Implicit memory

Living trust
Living will
Long-term memory
Palilalia
Paraphasia
Polypharmacy
Pseudodementia
Remotivation therapy
Reminiscence therapy
Semantic memory
Sundown syndrome
Will

One of the greatest challenges facing the health care delivery system today is the care of clients and caregivers of persons who live with cognitive disorders, particularly dementia of the Alzheimer's type (DAT). The term *dementia* literally means *without a mind.* DAT is a slow, as yet irreversible, process that affects a person's whole life and the lives of those closest to him or her. Clients experience the insidious loss of the essence of who they are at all levels of personhood. In general dementia is progressive and is characterized by the gradual decline of physical, emotional, social, cognitive, and spiritual dimensions of the self. It ultimately results in death. Delirium, however, involves disturbance of consciousness and a change in cognition that develops rapidly and is often of shorter duration than dementia. Amnestic disorder is a term used to describe memory impairment unrelated to other diseases.

There are over 3 million people in the United States who are afflicted by the devastating effects of cognitive disorders, and the number is growing. Extensive research is under way to determine the causes and find cures (or at the least, find a means to reverse the neurological damage that is done by these diseases). Treatment for the most dementing primary disease processes is at present palliative.

Delirium, dementia, and amnestic and other cognitive disorders are the classifications in the fourth edition of the *Diagnostic and Statistical Manual of Mental Disorders* (DSM-IV) (1994) that were formerly known as organic mental disorders. The predominant disturbance in these disorders is a clinically significant deficit in cognition or memory that results in significant changes in a client's level of functioning and disturbed behavior, caused by either reversible or irreversible effects, or dysfunction of the brain.

Personality, affective expression, ability to communicate, and social behavior are impaired. Clients' experiences of themselves, others, and the world are altered. If progressive deterioration occurs, then the client's awareness of past or present events changes, the ability to function independently and perform activities of daily living (ADLs) diminishes, and the ability to relate to significant others is lost. This awareness is emotionally painful when it is accompanied by a fleeting recognition that the disorder is one that will leave the client physically and mentally incapacitated. The burden of care falls on spouses and families, who provide the care personally or bear the financial burden of professional home care or nursing-home costs. The daily care required for the dementias eventually involves a 24-hour commitment.

The purpose of this chapter is to provide an understanding of persons who have delirium, dementia, and other cognitive disorders. Strategies for supporting family caregivers and the problems both clients and caregivers encounter are discussed. Factors associated with the development of cognitive disorders are identified and related to increased risk and preventive interventions. Particular attention is given to clients with progressive DAT, because it is the most common of the dementia disorders.

EPIDEMIOLOGY

The increased risk of dementia among this age group is a challenge for the health care system. Dementias, including DAT, have the fastest-growing incidence of any illness in the geriatric population, which is expected to total 5.5 million by 2030. Presently, about $58 billion is spent annually to care for the victims of DAT at home and in nursing care facilities. Seventy percent of the cost is provided by the families of victims. This figure is projected to rise to $750 billion by the year 2030. DAT is present in 60% of long-term residents and is the fourth leading cause of death in those over age 65, at 150,000 deaths per year. DAT is more common in females, and there is an increased incidence with advancing age (20% to 30% of those over age 85 are believed to be affected). Approximately 60% of all dementias, including DAT, are of the primary degenerative type. The second most common type of dementia is vascular dementia, formerly known as multi-infarct dementia, which is associated with cerebrovascular disease and accounts for 20% of all dementias. The remaining 20% include dementias caused by other disorders (Stolley, 1994).

Delirium, a more acute cognitive disorder, is common in hospitalized clients. Although delirium is more prevalent in the elderly, it occurs in all age groups. It is usually secondary to problems such as substance abuse, exposure to toxins, and hypoxia (lack of oxygen) and is often related to various disease processes. The frail elderly are highly susceptible to delirium. Approximately 10% of all hospitalized elderly have delirium, and 10% to 15% will develop delirium during the hospitalization. Unfortunately, delirium is often confused with dementia and goes untreated.

Age, family history, the presence of mental retardation in family members, head injury, ingestion of aluminum, and other chemicals and viral infections predispose individuals to dementia. Box 31-1 lists factors that contribute to symptoms of dementia and delirium.

THEORETICAL FRAMEWORK

Multiple theories exist to explain the course and progression of dementia and delirium. Some researchers attribute dementia and delirium to the destruction of brain tissue, and others assert that alteration in neurochemical processes causes symptoms. Still others attribute impairment to changes in brain structure and

BOX 31-1

Factors that Contribute to Symptoms of Delirium and Dementia

VOLATILE AGENTS

Gasoline, aerosols, glues, paint removers, solvents, lacquers and varnishes, dry-cleaning agents, home-cleaning products

HEAVY METALS

Lead paints, ceramic glazes, moonshine whiskey, mercury, arsenic, manganese

INSECTICIDES

Parathion, malathion

BRAIN TRAUMA

Concussion, contusion, hemorrhage, thrombosis, penetrating wounds, blast effects, electrical trauma, repeated courses of electroconvulsive therapy

DRUGS

Alcohol, barbiturates, opioids, cocaine, amphetamines, cannabis, hallucinogens, salicylates

INFECTIONS

Tuberculosis, fungal meningitis, viral encephalitis, neurosyphilis, Cruetzfeldt-Jakob disease, AIDS, Kuru

SPACE-OCCUPYING LESIONS

Tumors, subdural hematoma, subarachnoid hemorrhage, cerebral abscess

METABOLIC DISORDERS

Electrolyte imbalance, uremia, hepatic encephalopathy, hypoglycemia, hyperglycemia,

ENDOCRINE DISORDERS

Thyroid deficiency (myxedema), thyrotoxicosis (Grave's disease), adrenal dysfunction, pituitary deficiency

NUTRITIONAL DEFICIENCIES

Protein deficiency, vitamin C deficiency, folic acid deficiency, niacin deficiency, thiamine and B_{12} deficiency

HYPOXIA-ISCHEMIA

Cardiac failure, respiratory failure, carbon-monoxide poisoning

NEUROLOGICAL DISORDERS

Seizures, Huntington's chorea, Parkinson's disease, Pick's disease, DAT, transient ischemic attacks (TIAs)

---

circulation or to extrinsic causes such as head trauma, exposure to toxins, infectious agents, and abuse of substances. The following sections explore biological, environmental, and cognitive theories related to the development of symptoms of dementia, delirium, and the amnestic disorders.

Biological Correlates

Approximately 45% of individuals with symptoms of dementia are diagnosed with DAT. Currently, DAT remains a diagnosis of elimination; that is, testing eliminates all other explanation of a client's symptoms. Definitive diagnosis of DAT requires examination of brain tissue through biopsy or autopsy. By the time a person is diagnosed with DAT, the brain shows deterioration. The pathology of the disease is extremely complex and involves extensive loss of neurons, particularly in the cerebral cortex as well as the appearance of abnormal protein deposits (amyloid) within the neurons and in the neutrophils.

The following are research findings that attempt to explain causes of brain degeneration in clients with DAT. Clients with DAT exhibit signs of the following:

- Increased number of neurofibrillary tangles and plaques in the cerebral cortex; Color Plate 10 illustrates amyloid plaques
- Deterioration of temporal, parietal, and occipital regions of the cerebral cortex. Color Plate 13 presents the positron emission tomography (PET) scan of a client with DAT showing hypometabolism in these three regions
- Decreased levels of acetylcholine, norepinephrine, serotonin, and somatostatin
- Decreased corticotropin-releasing hormone (CRH)
- Inhibition of the hypothalamic-pituitary axes with subsequent disruption of hormone release
- Higher concentrations of aluminum in the brain
- *Amyloid* (*abnormal fibrous protein deposits*) accumulation in the center of plaques and in the walls of blood vessels of the brain (see Color Plate 10).

Structural changes in the brain

The symptoms of DAT vary as the disease progresses and as degeneration of the brain continues. Fig. 31-1 illustrates the atrophy and degeneration that occur in the course of the progressive downward spiral of symptoms that characterizes DAT. Table 31-1 lists brain regions af-

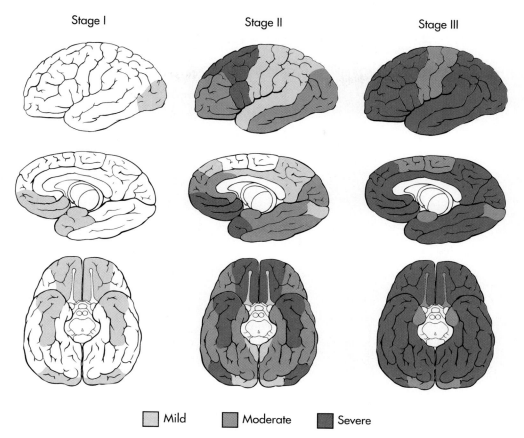

Stage I   Stage II   Stage III

☐ Mild   ☐ Moderate   ■ Severe

Fig. 31-1 Schematic drawings of the stages of brain deterioration related to Alzheimer's disease.

Haber fig 31-01

fected by progressive brain atrophy found in clients with DAT. Specific areas of the brain determine the exact manifestation of symptoms. Atrophy of the brain, widened cortical sulci, and enlarged cerebral ventricles are present in persons with DAT and may sometimes be visualized on PET scans, magnetic resonance imaging (MRI) scans, computed tomography (CT) scans, or pneumoencephalograms (Sounder et al., 1995). Color Plate 12 illustrates an MRI scan showing cortical atrophy in a client with DAT.

Another area of the brain that is implicated in DAT is the suprachiasmatic nucleus of the hypothalamus, which is the principle pacemaker of the circadian rhythm system. It is theorized that deterioration in the hypothalamus of clients with DAT disrupts timing of behaviors and sleep architecture and may be implicated in *sundown syndrome* (*increased agitation and confusion that occurs in late afternoon*) (Bliwise, 1994; Burney-Puckett, 1996).

Neurotransmitter theory

The amount of acetylcholine, the neurotransmitter important in learning and memory, is reduced in clients with DAT and possibly in the other cognitive disorders. Acetylcholine is produced in the basal nucleus of the brain, an area of nerve-cell deficiency in dementia. This deficit affects the temporal lobes, causing memory loss. It is believed that decreased levels of acetylcholine may allow a buildup of amyloid. The drug tacrine (Cognex) slows the natural breakdown of acetylcholine and has been effective in a small number of clients with DAT and those with amnestic disorders (Keltner, 1994).

Genetic Correlates

Of the many causes suspected, the only one generally regarded as having a degree of certainty suggests genetic predisposition in some individuals. The prevailing theory is that genetic factors combine with other variables to produce dementia. Chromosome 21 (the same one responsible for Down syndrome) contains the gene that makes beta-amyloid protein, the major substance in neuric plaques. The offspring of women who bear children before age 20 and after age 40 have an increased incidence of DAT. These same age groups

TABLE 31-1

Regions affected by atrophy of brain

BRAIN REGIONS AFFECTED BY ATROPHY	SYMPTOMS OF DAT
Hippocampus (limbic system)	Short-term and long-term memory deficit Depression occurs secondary to loss of memory and ability to learn
Cerebral cortex (temporal, parietal, and occipital regions)	Visual impairment Receptive and expressive **aphasia** *(impairment of ability to speak or understand spoken messages)* **Apraxia** *(impairment of ability to perform purposeful acts or manipulate objects)* Delusions Hallucinations **Agnosia** *(loss of ability to recognize familiar objects, places or persons)*
Prefrontal cortex	Apathy Poor judgment Concreteness Impaired insight Diminished problem-solving ability **Acalculia** *(inability to solve simple math problems)*
Motor cortex	Difficulty walking Difficulty swallowing Loss of sense of self in space

of mothers have increased risk for premature births and infants with Down syndrome. This suggests that children of older parents may have a chromosomal abnormality that makes them more susceptible to DAT (Mann, Neary, and Testa, 1994).

A genetic deficit allows production of beta-amyloid, which is deposited in greater amounts in the brains of clients with DAT. Apolipoprotein E (ApoE) genetic testing can be used to assist in the diagnosis of clients with symptoms of DAT and to help determine the best treatment (Weiner, 1991).

Infection

The viral theory proposes that a combination of prions (infectious agents smaller than conventional viruses), which cause subacute encephalopathy, and genetic factors may cause Kuru and Creutzfeldt-Jakob disease, which result in dementia. Tuberculosis, untreated syphilis, fungal meningitis, and viral encephalitis may also progress sufficiently to cause dementia.

Dementia caused by human immunodeficiency virus (HIV) commonly involves diffuse multifocal destruction of white matter and subcortical structures. Spinal cord fluid of clients with AIDS-related dementia have slightly elevated protein levels and a mild lymphocytosis. It has been suggested that alterations in the body's immune system that cause autoantibody production (antibodies that attack normal body tissue) may account for symptoms of dementia. Other theories suggest environmental toxins. Studies suggest that high levels of aluminum may possibly be related to development of DAT, delirium, and other cognitive disorders (Greutzner, 1988).

Memory

Many efforts have been made to understand how the memory functions. In clients with DAT, deterioration of memory is a gradual process. For those with delirium and amnestic disorders, the onset is more acute. Relevant structural elements of memory include iconic memory; primary, secondary, and remote memory; and semantic memory. Table 31-2 describes relevant implications for clients who exhibit memory loss as a result of primary dementia, delirium, or amnestic disorders.

TABLE 31-2

Structural elements of memory

DEFINITION	CLINICAL RELEVANCE
Iconic Memory	
First stage of information processing that includes the formation of short-term memory; *relatively large storage capacity for visual stimuli*	Clients have difficulty acquiring and retaining new information (short-term. memory deficit) Clients are unable to use new information in the here and now.
Primary Memory	
Involves situations in which material is maintained for 30 seconds or less; involves individuals' ability to process information related to task performance and attention	Clients have difficulty processing directions for complicated tasks. Clients are able to focus on one task at a time and may become confused if asked to perform more than one task. Impairment is evident even when one of the tasks involves motor performance rather than a mental activity.
Secondary Memory	
Involves the distinction between implicit and explicit memory; *implicit memory involves the extent to which prior exposure to similar events facilitates recognition and recall of new material;* *explicit memory* is the conscious recognition of personally experienced events.	Clients with dementia have a deficit in free recall, story recall that requires logical memory, paired association learning, pictorial recognition, and facial recognition. Encoding of information and ready retrieval of information is impaired in clients with dementia and delirium.
Remote Memory	
Sometimes referred to as *long-term memory, it includes information about the distant past.*	Clients with DAT apparently lose recent memory first and the more remote memory last. A law of regression suggests that the extent of memory loss is inversely related to the age of the memory. The vast stores of remote memory may allow persons with DAT to cover up loss of iconic or short-term memory or to use exaggeration and confabulation rather than actual factual memories.
Semantic Memory	
Concerns a person's knowledge of the world, including general principles, associations, and rules.	Clients have language function deficits. Expressive and/or receptive aphasia exists in some clients. Clients with dementia exhibit concrete thinking and cannot follow abstract commands.

The *Nursing Process*

Assessment

Delirium, dementia, and severe memory loss (amnestic disorder) are dysfunctional behavioral constellations. The degree of dysfunction depends on the length of time the client has exhibited symptoms and the intensity and persistence of those symptoms. The Nursing Process section of this chapter highlights the DSM-IV disorders of delirium and dementia, as well as the associated clinical manifestations of cognitive impairment, forgetfulness, pseudodementia, and severe memory loss. Attention is also given to the needs of caregivers of clients with progressive dementia.

Clinical Profiles

Delirium

Delirium *(acute confusion) is a disturbance of consciousness and a change in cognition that develops over a period of hours to days and tends to fluctuate during the course of the day.* For example, the person is oriented in the morning and by evening the same person is disoriented and combative. A major contributing factor is a disturbance in sleep architecture. Consciousness disturbances include a decrease in the clarity of awareness of the environment and an impairment in the ability to focus or maintain attention.

The DSM-IV classifies the following types of delirium:

- Delirium due to a general medical condition (Box 31-2)
- Substance intoxication delirium and substance withdrawal delirium (including the side effects of medications) (Box 31-3)
- Delirium due to multiple etiologies (for example, both a substance and a medical condition)
- Delirium not otherwise specified (a determination of the etiology is not made because there is insufficient evidence of a cause) (APA, 1994)

The causative factors of delirium are generally totally or partially reversible. Reversibility and acute onset differentiate delirium from dementia. The behavior of clients with delirium may range from restlessness to extreme hyperactivity and from sluggishness to extreme lethargy. Box 31-4 lists the cognitive, perceptual, behavioral, and affective symptoms of delirium.

A major cause of delirium in the elderly is ***polypharmacy***, *that is, the simultaneous taking of multiple prescribed and over-the-counter medications.* Polypharmacy is a serious concern. Many older persons see multiple primary care providers because of a variety of medical conditions. One or more of these providers may be unaware of the others. The result may be that the person is receiving and taking multiple prescriptions of the same medication. For example, a client may have one prescription labeled *Lasix* and the other labeled *furosemide.* A client may also be taking two or more medications that interact adversely with each other. Another problem is sharing medications with family members or friends without medical advice or follow-up examinations. For older clients the rate of drug absorption and excretion is decreased, and delirium may occur if dosages are not adjusted downward.

Emotional factors such as depression, fear, and loneliness, as well as malnutrition, dehydration, and other physical problems (see Box 31-1) may also contribute to the onset of delirium. Head injuries, infections, par-

---

Box 31-2

Diagnostic Criteria for Delirium due to a General Medical Condition

A. Disturbance of consciousness (i.e., reduced clarity of awareness of the environment) with reduced ability to focus, sustain, or shift attention.
B. A change in cognition (such as memory deficit, disorientation, language disturbance) or the development of a perceptual disturbance that is not better accounted for by a preexisting, established, or evolving dementia.
C. The disturbance develops over a short period of time (usually hours to days) and tends to fluctuate during the course of the day.
D. There is evidence from the history, physical examination, or laboratory findings that the disturbance is caused by the direct physiological consequences of a general medical condition.

NOTE: The name of the general medical condition is coded on Axis I (e.g., Delirium Due to Hepatic Encephalopathy; the general medical condition is also coded on Axis III).

Modified from American Psychiatric Association. (1994). Diagnostic and statistical manual of mental disorders, fourth edition, *Washington, DC: author.*

The Nursing Process

BOX 31-3

Diagnostic Criteria for Substance Withdrawal Delirium

A. Disturbance of consciousness (i.e., reduced clarity of awareness of the environment) with reduced ability to focus, sustain, or shift attention.

B. A change in cognition (such as memory deficit, disorientation, language disturbance) or the development of a perceptual disturbance that is not better accounted for by a preexisting, established, or evolving dementia.

C. The disturbance develops over a short period of time (usually hours to days) and tends to fluctuate during the course of the day.

D. There is evidence from the history, physical examination, or laboratory findings that the symptoms in Criteria A and B developed during, or shortly after, a withdrawal syndrome.

NOTE: This diagnosis should be made instead of a diagnosis of Substance Withdrawal only when the cognitive symptoms are in excess of those usually associated with the withdrawal syndrome and when the symptoms are sufficiently severe to warrant independent clinical attention.

Reprinted with permission from American Psychiatric Association. (1994). Diagnostic and statistical manual of mental disorders, fourth edition, *Washington, DC: author.*

BOX 31-4

Symptoms of Delirium

COGNITIVE

- Impairment of recent memory
- Disorientation to time and place but not usually self
- Language disturbances (any or all may occur)
  -Dysnomia (impaired ability to name objects)
  -Dysgraphia (impaired ability to write)

PERCEPTUAL

- Misinterpretation of sensory impact
- Illusions
- Hallucinations

BEHAVIORAL

Daytime
- Sudden movements
- Getting out of bed when unsafe
- Groping
- Picking at bedclothes

Nighttime
- Calling out
- Screaming
- Muttering
- Moaning
- Other sounds

AFFECTIVE

- Fear
- Anxiety
- Depression
- Anger
- Irritability
- Euphoria
- Apathy

ticularly those that cause high fever, and toxins or problems that cause brain hypoxia may cause delirium. Withdrawal from alcohol (see Chapter 26) and sensory deprivation caused by diminished sight and hearing are the most common causes of delirium. The following clinical example illustrates some of the symptoms of delirium:

> Anne R. is an 88-year-old woman who has been living in an adult congregate living facility (ACLF) for 3 years. She had been functioning well until about 6 months ago. She became withdrawn, and any attempt to help her socialize were met with anxious outbursts. The staff noted that she was unable to answer questions related to orientation, but she was able to state that she was confused. Plans were made to transfer Anne to a nursing home. A physical examination was required and revealed that she had bilateral cerumen impactions (ear wax) blocking both ear canals. Once the cerumen was removed, Anne demonstrated orientation and resocialization. Her anxiety decreased and she was able to remain at the ACLF.

Dementia

Dementia is an organic condition characterized by cognitive deficits including impairment of memory, abstract thinking, judgment, and higher cortical functions. Dementia may be progressive, static, or intermittent. The reversibility of dementia depends on the underlying physiological condition and the effectiveness of the interventions selected for resolving these impairments. Persons who have dementia experience decreased ability to retrieve memories. Those with DAT progressively and pervasively forget all memories of the immediate, recent, and remote past.

The Nursing Process

There are several types of dementia; each is differentiated based on physiological causation. Box 31-5 lists each of the types of dementia in the DSM-IV. The two most common types of dementia are DAT and vascular dementia.

Vascular dementia, caused by a lack of adequate brain blood supply, differs from DAT. Cognitive disturbances are similar, but physical symptoms are specific. Persons who have vascular dementia have a "patchy" loss of cognitive functioning that leaves some memories intact and others permanently lost. Focal neurological signs and symptoms (exaggerated deep-vein reflexes, extensor plantar response, pseudobulbar palsy, gait abnormalities, and extremity weakness) are present. Laboratory evidence indicating cerebrovascular disease is also evident. In either case, delirium and depression (pseudodementia) must be ruled out as the cause of symptoms. Color Plate 11 in Chapter 15 shows a PET scan of a 67-year-old man with vascular dementia.

Another form of dementia is directly related to HIV. It involves diffuse multifocal destruction of white matter and subcortical structure as a direct pathophysiological consequence of HIV. It is typically characterized by slowness, forgetfulness, poor concentration, and difficulties with problem-solving (APA, 1994). Other symptoms are similar to those of DAT. Of note is the fact that children born with HIV may also develop dementia. Symptoms in children include developmental delay, hypertoxia, microencephaly, and basal ganglia calcification.

Dementia of the Alzheimer's type

Alzheimer's disease, or *DAT, begins insidiously with mild levels of memory loss that may at first be mistaken for* *the normal forgetfulness of aging.* Box 31-6 lists the DSM-IV criteria for DAT. The deterioration of the client occurs in stages that can last from 3 to 20 years, but DAT usually averages 8 years. Progression through the stages and severity of symptoms vary with each individual.

The following stages illustrate the progression:

- *Early confusional stage:* characterized by forgetfulness, slow response times, personality changes, problems with social conversation, denial, early emotional problems, and change in abilities and actions
- *Late confusional stage:* characterized by memory problems, impaired judgments, deterioration of decision-making and financial management abilities, denial, risky behaviors such as unsafe driving, need for assistance with ADLs, disorientation to time and place, self-absorption, restlessness, irritability, impatience, and depression
- *Early dementia:* characterized by dependency, need for help to initiate most activity, memory gaps, extreme emotional reactions, diminished logic and reasoning, social withdrawal, and feelings of being overwhelmed by simple decisions
- *Middle dementia:* characterized by severe reactions (aggression, anger, depression, and withdrawal), delusions, hallucinations, repetitive behaviors, movement and coordination difficulties, the need for complete assistance with bathing and feeding, and loss of touch with events and experiences. Intellectual changes include:
- *Acalculia - inability to calculate*
- *Alexia - inability to read*
- *Agraphia - inability to write*

Comprehension is affected by:

- *Agnosia - inability to attach meaning to sensory impression*
- *Astereognosis - inability to recognize objects by touch*
- *Auditory agnosia - inability to recognize familiar sound or words.*
- *Late dementia:* characterized by loss of all cognitive abilities (speech, memory, and affect; loss of abilities to walk, sit, and smile; loss of bowel and bladder function; extreme eating difficulties; and finally stupor, coma, and death. In the late (severe) stage, memory is absent, and the client is totally dependent on the caregiver, bedridden, and usually mute. Infections and aspiration pneumonia are often the causes of death. Nursing research aimed at extracting and naming meaningful behavioral syn-

BOX 31-5

Types of Dementia

- DAT
- Vascular dementia
- Dementia due to the following:
  -HIV
  -Head trauma
  -Parkinson's disease
  -Huntington's chorea
  -Pick's disease
  -Creutzfeldt-Jakob disease
  -General medical conditions
- Substance-induced persisting dementia
- Dementia due to multiple etiologies

The Nursing Process

dromes in demented elders is found in the Research Highlight on p. 662.

The duration of each stage of dementia is not orderly, but rather is unique to each individual. The early and late confusional stages range from 2 to 4 years; the middle stages of dementia may be 2 to 10 years in duration; and the late stages of the disorder usually last 1 to 3 years.

Each of the progressive stages of DAT brings about more and more loss. Changes in language, behavior, sensory perception, and motor activity are observed as brain deterioration progressess. Table 31-3 lists several functional losses and changes and suggests explanations for each. The following clinical example depicts some of the symptoms of DAT.

> Jack S. is a 63-year-old man who comes to the Family Medicine Clinic for the first time because, as his wife Jane states, "He isn't walking right, and he sometimes forgets he has eaten. I think there's something wrong." During the admission history and physical, the advanced-practice nurse notes that Jack is disoriented to person and place (he thinks he's at the store). He repeats his wife's name, "Jane, Jane, Jane," whenever she is not directly in sight. He keeps asking, "Who are you?" even though the nurse explains who she is and what she is doing with each step of the examination.
>
> Jack's wife reports that over the last year she had to take away and hide the keys to the car. "He kept getting lost. Finally he couldn't remember how to start the car anymore." She reports that he often wanders at night, and once she had to call the police to help find him. They do not go out socially anymore, and they seldom entertain at home. Jack appears to be in good physical health. All his x-rays and blood work are normal. His CT scan shows generalized moderate brain atrophy consistent with his age. His wife states that he does not drink or smoke. Jane reports that she is frustrated with his behavior, has had numerous headaches lately, gets very little sleep, and has lost 15 pounds in the last 6 months. A diagnosis of progressive DAT is made.

Pseudodementia

Psuedodementia is a term used to describe a constellation of symptoms that include cognitive and memory impairments suggestive of dementia, but which are symptoms of depression. About 15% of persons thought to have dementia are later discovered to have a depressive disorder. The elderly (age 75 and older) are more often found to be depressed than younger persons. This increased incidence of depression contributes to a significant overlap between elderly persons who meet the criteria for pseudodementia and those who have early-onset symptoms of DAT or the other dementias. Another confounding factor is that during the early stages of dementia, people are commonly depressed in response to the loss of cognitive abilities (Hogstel, 1995).

Pseudodementia is a treatable and reversible condition, whereas DAT and the other progressive dementias

---

Box 31-6

Diagnostic Criteria for Dementia of the Alzheimer's Type

A. The development of multiple cognitive deficits manifested by both
  (1) Memory impairment (impaired ability to learn new information or to recall previously learned information)
  (2) One (or more) of the following cognitive disturbances:
    (a) Aphasia (language disturbance)
    (b) Apraxia (impaired ability to carry out motor activities despite intact motor function)
    (c) Agnosia (failure to recognize or identify objects despite intact sensory function)
    (d) Disturbance in executive functioning (i.e., planning, organizing, sequencing, abstracting)
B. The cognitive deficits in Criteria A1 and A2 each cause significant impairment in social or occupational functioning and represent a significant decline from a previous level of functioning.
C. The course is characterized by gradual onset and continuing cognitive decline.
D. The cognitive deficits in Criteria A1 and A2 are not due to any of the following:
  (1) Other central nervous system conditions that cause progressive deficits in memory and cognition (e.g., cerebrovascular disease, Parkinson's disease, Huntington's disease, subdural hematoma, normal-pressure hydrocephalus, brain tumor)
  (2) Systemic conditions that are known to cause dementia (e.g., hypothyroidism, vitamin B_{12} or folic acid deficiency, niacin deficiency, hypercalcemia, neurosyphilis, HIV infection)
  (3) Substance-induced conditions
E. The deficits do not occur exclusively during the course of a delirium.
F. The disturbance is not better accounted for by another Axis I disorder (e.g., Major Depressive Disorder, Schizophrenia).

From American Psychiatric Association. (1994). Diagnostic and statistical manual of mental disorders (4th Ed.). Washington, DC: author.

The Nursing Process

RESEARCH HIGHLIGHT

Kolanowski, A.M. (1995). Disturbing behaviors in demented elders: A concept synthesis. *Archives of Psychiatric Nursing, 11* (4), 188-194.

Summary

The purpose of this research was to systematically describe behaviors of clients with symptoms of dementia. Concept synthesis is used to group disturbing behavior symptoms into patterns of behavior or syndromes.

Concept synthesis was used to extract meaningful syndromes of disturbing behaviors exhibited by elderly clients with dementia. The data set included 586 nursing home residents from three nursing homes who were rated on the Disturbed Behavior subscale of the Psychogeriatric Dependency Rating Scale (PG-DRS). Standard definitions of behaviors were used during the rating process. Ratings were done by nursing staff most familiar with residents.

Three clusters of closely related behaviors were identified using factor analysis. Cluster One, labeled *agitated psychomotor behavior,* included motor and feeling components and was comprised active physical aggression and disruptive, restless, socially objectionable, and noisy behavior. Cluster Two was labeled *aggressive interpersonal communication* and included demanding, manipulative, verbally aggressive, and disruptive behavior. Cluster Three was labeled *expressive difficulty* and embodied problems with communication and speech content. Modification of the clusters resulted in five classifications. Verification of clusters found empirical support.

Five disturbing behaviors associated with dementia were described: (1) *aggressive psychomotor behavior,* an increase in gross motor movement that has the effect of harming or repelling another; (2) *nonaggressive psychomotor behavior,* an increase in gross motor movement without an apparent negative effect on others; (3) *verbally aggressive behavior,* vocalizations that have the effect of repelling others; (4) *passive behavior,* a decrease of gross motor movement accompanied by apathy and a lack of interaction with the environment; and (5) *functionally impaired behavior,* loss of ability to perform self-care, the expression of which may be aversive and burdensome.

Implications for Nursing Practice

- Standardized concepts may be used to facilitate development of consistent interventions or may be related to specific client profiles.
- Altering the psychosocial milieu of clients who are cognitively intact but depressed may help reduce verbal aggressions.
- Altering the physical environment of clients who are functionally intact but cognitively impaired facilitates safety of clients who are wanderers.
- Problematic aggressive behaviors in persons with dementia are often triggered by a response to the environment in which clients have little or no control. Use simple communication techniques and provide control whenever possible.
- Problematic behaviors may be a response to fear. Changing the clients' surroundings often calms clients.
- Provide structure and consistency for clients.

are not at the present time. For this reason, it is important that the diagnostic distinction be made and that appropriate interventions implemented. Nurses in inpatient settings have an important role in providing the documentation of the client's functioning over 24-hour periods that helps the team make an accurate diagnosis. The differences in the clinical picture of persons with pseudomentia and those with DAT and other progressive dementias are presented in Table 31-4.

The nurse must be alert to the contributing factors that lead to depression, such as losses and loneliness. The following clinical example illustrates this point.

Mary R. moved into an apartment building for senior citizens 1 year ago, after the death of her husband. During an appointment at the building health center for her 6-month check-up, she tells the nurse that she thinks she is becoming "senile" because she is so forgetful. When the nurse asks

The Nursing Process

TABLE 31-3

Major functional losses or changes of clients with dementia of Alzheimer's type

IMPAIRMENT	POSSIBLE CAUSE
Language Loss or Change	
Aphasia-loss of ability to use meaningful speech; loss of verbal comprehension	Atrophy of parts of brain responsible for cognitive function (see Color Plate 6 for an illustration of a PET scan showing glucose metabolism during cognitive tasks involving language)
Paraphasia-a form of aphasia characterized by the misuse of spoken words or word combinations	
Anomia-Inability to remember names of persons and objects	Decline in long-term and short-term memory
Apraxia-Inability to understand meaning of things	Receptive aphasia secondary to brain atrophy
Palilalia-pathological repetition of words	
Confabulation-Exaggerated or made up stories	Attempt to compensate for forgotten memories
Behavioral Loss or Change	
Pacing and wandering	Loss of familiarity with environment
Compulsive ritualistic behavior	Attempt to compensate for loss of cognitive abilities
Hoarding	
Poor hygiene	Recall of how to bathe, dress, and organize the environment deteriorates
Disorderliness	
Roaming at night	Disruption of sleep/wake cycle
Impulsivity in social situations	Loss of social inhibitions
Sensory/Perceptual Loss or Change	
Exaggeration of normal aging losses	Inability to independently make accommodation for losses
Hallucinations	Cognitive impairment altered perception of self, others, and the environment
Delusional thinking	
Paranoia	
Motor Loss or Change	
Difficulty carrying out intentional motor activity	Loss of memory of how and what to do; loss of sense of self in space
Exaggerated decreased stability and shuffling gait	

her what it has been like for her since she moved into the apartment from her home, she gives a detailed description of her loneliness, weight loss, lack of appetite, insomnia, and past difficult life.

Amnestic disorder

Amnestic disorder is characterized primarily by a disturbance in memory or amnesia (forgetfulness) that is due to the direct physiological effects of a general medical condition or the persisting effects of substance abuse or toxin exposure. Clients typically are unable to learn new information or are unable to recall previously learned information or past events. They have usually become socially withdrawn, and friends notice a decline in all levels of functioning (APA, 1994).

The memory deficit in clients with amnestic disorder is most apparent when they are required to spontaneously recall information. This request often leads to

The Nursing Process

TABLE 31-4

Differentiation between pseudodementia and DAT

PSEUDODEMENTIA (DEPRESSION)	DAT
Family history of affective illness	Family history of Alzheimer's disease (sibling or parent)
Posture stooped	Stands erect (early in disease process)
Refuses to undertake normal social activities, loss of interest	Gradually gives up shopping or attending social gatherings alone because of difficulty remembering how to get there and how to return home
Slow to answer questions	Answers questions spontaneously (early in disease process)
Answers question with one or few words	Answers with many words but not fluently
Answers to questions often vague, gives "I don't know" answers	Answers are not relevant to questions; uses confabulation; makes up answer rather than admits not knowing
When open-ended questions are asked, becomes attentive; gives long, detailed answers, indicating good concentration and attention	Short attention span; difficulty answering open-ended questions; responses do not fit the question
Understands what is asked: able to select appropriate words to convey relevant response	Does not comprehend questions; pathological, repetitious use of spoken words and phrases (palilalia) or misuse of words or word combinations (paraphasia)
Oriented to time and place	Disoriented to time and place; becomes lost in a familiar environment; exhibits "searching" or "wandering" behaviors
Is able to perform tasks that require the incorporation of new information	Is unable to perform tasks that require the incorporation of new information and repeatedly asks questions about what to do
Is able to follow a conversation between two people	Has difficulty following a conversation between two people and may interject irrelevancies or comments on a subject discussed previously.
Is able to recall recent events	Has difficulty recalling both personal and nonpersonal recent events
When asked to recall distant past, talks about memories of losses and disappointments	As disease progresses over time, forgetting increases, and past memories are erased
Exaggerates extent of mental impairment, is aware of some cognitive impairment, and complains about poor memory and concentration	Denies or underestimates mental impairment
Discrepancy between complaints and observable impairment of memory and attention	Absence of complaints is discrepant with observable impairment of memory and attention
Indecisive	Confused or sure, despite reality-based feedback to the contrary
History of depressive episodes	No history of depressive episodes
Presence of persistent, bizarre, and structured delusions	Delusions are sporadic, poorly structured, and tend to be paranoid
Hallucinations may occur	Hallucinations are rare

The Nursing Process

TABLE 31-4—cont'd

Differentiation between pseudodementia and DAT

PSEUDODEMENTIA (DEPRESSION)	DAT
Able to concentrate on ruminations about past helplessness, hopelessness, worthlessness, and regrets	Diminished concentration
Sleep problems: early morning awakening	Nocturnal confusion: awakens in the middle of night; is confused and behaves as if it were daytime
Loss of appetite	Appetite unchanged
Observably depressed affect	Affect shallow and labile
Insecure with others	Demanding of others
Relatively rapid onset and rapid progression	Insidious onset, gradual progression
Depression precedes dementia	Dementia present before depression; depression transitory
May be best at night in relation to functioning	Apt to be worse at night in relation to functioning
Temporary impairment of intellect that is restored when depression decreases	Deterioration of general intellect
Affective distress unchanged by location	Distress or anxiety less apt to occur in home surroundings and increase in unfamiliar environment
Spatial orientation intact	Impaired ability to recognize clues to negotiate a familiar or new area
Knows how to dress and undress	Does not remember how to put clothes on or take them off
Recognizes persons, places, objects, and their meanings	Fails to recognize persons, places, objects, and their meanings
No disoriented wandering	Wanders away from home or hospital because nothing seems familiar and is searching for the familiar
Retains social inhibitions	Reduced social inhibition

frustration, and clients may become impatient with themselves when they are asked. Some clients compensate for memory gaps by using confabulation, and they may exhibit the other common symptoms of dementia.

Joe K. was recently hospitalized for severe malnutrition, probably the result of an episode of acute pancreatitis and a lifelong pattern of heavy alcohol use. Despite his heavy drinking, Joe maintained a successful career until recently, when co-workers noticed frequent forgetfulness and a decline in his productivity. He has been frustrated and agitated more often, and his wife noticed that such feelings usually follow what he calls a "memory gap." Joe stopped playing poker with his friends 2 months ago, and he refuses to entertain at home, an activity he previously enjoyed. He appears apathetic and depressed, and he does not acknowledge that he is in the hospital.

A diagnosis of amnestic disorder may not always be appropriate since disturbances of memory occur on a continuum and include forgetfulness, pseudodementia, and dementia. *Forgetfulness is a universal phenomenon that involves putting memories out of consciousness. It involves ignoring, omitting, or overlooking things or people.* It is the experience of "drawing a blank" or letting something or someone "skip one's mind."

Forgetfulness occurs more often in older persons than it does in their younger counterparts. The changes in cognitive functioning that indicate forgetfulness include

The Nursing Process

alterations in attention, naming ability, and abstraction. In older adults memory remains intact, but there is a decrease in the speed with which thoughts are accessed. The reaction time for the initiation of information retrieval is slowed. They require more information before they act on new information. With time, minimal prompting, and sufficient information regarding the need to act, older adults are able to retrieve and recall immediate, recent, and remote stored memories and use this information appropriately and effectively (Cromwell and Phillips, 1995). The following clinical example illustrates the phenomenon of forgetfulness:

> Mr. Ambers is an 85-year-old man who lives alone. His eyesight is failing, but he remains cognitively alert and is able to carry out ADLs independently. He had recent outpatient cataract surgery to correct his failing eyesight. During the admission history and physical, he expressed concern that he might be "getting senile." He described forgetting his grandchildren's birthdays, mixing up their names, and taking a longer time to understand directions for cooking prepackaged foods. He often feels frustrated and embarrassed because he forgets where he leaves his eyeglasses. After careful assessment of mental status, the nurse reassured Mr. Amber, that he is experiencing forgetfulness, a phenomena normal for his age.

Caregivers

Family members are the primary caregivers of clients with cognitive impairments. Primary caregivers include spouses, adult children, grandchildren, and siblings. Although women have traditionally been the primary caregivers, men who care for their wives and middle-age sons caring for parents with cognitive impairments are on the increase.

Caregiving particularly for a client with progressive dementia eventually becomes a 24-hour commitment. Demands on time and physical energy are exhausting. The burden of caring for an impaired spouse or parent is inherently stressful and may have a negative impact on the caregivers' health and sense of well-being. The health problems encountered by caregivers include depression and anxiety, emotional distress, and multiple somatic problems (England, 1996). The spouse of an elderly client with dementia is often the primary caregiver. Dementia disrupts the couple's final stage of family development and their plans and fantasies related to retirement. The couple is often isolated, less aware of community resources, and less able to seek out these resources. They are reluctant to depend on adult children, or their children may be geographically remote from

them. Caregiving spouses may exist in a social limbo, feeling neither married nor single. The way love is given and received in the couple's relationship is altered. Sexual interactions are impaired. Lack of sexual interest; insensitivity toward the spouse without dementia; and incessant, inappropriate demands or aggressive behavior may occur.

Adult child caregivers often have to balance caregiving responsibilities with obligations to their own families. If unresolved anger toward a parent exists, physical abuse, abandonment, or overprotectiveness of the client with dementia may occur. Some adult child caregivers neglect their own children, a factor that may lead to family dysfunction.

The following example illustrates some of the issues involved in caring for a client with cognitive impairments:

> Mr. Bruce is a 79-year-old man who was admitted to the hospital after a fall at home that caused a fractured hip. His wife, Priscilla, who is 20 years younger, reports that he has been unsteady on his feet for the last year. The nurse notes that Mr. Bruce is disoriented. He is unable to feed himself and asks repeatedly where he is and when he can go home.
>
> Tests do not reveal any reason for Mr. Bruce's cognitive deficits, and a diagnosis of DAT is made. When told, Mrs. Bruce responds, "I thought so, but I was afraid he would have to go to a nursing home if I told anyone. I'm all alone with him; our children live out of state and haven't been for a visit since last year. They think everything has been okay. I haven't told them anything. They'll be upset now."

Focused Assessment

Assessment of clients with cognitive impairments is a multifaceted process that includes physical, cognitive, social, emotional, environmental, and behavioral components (Luggen, 1996). Physical assessment focuses on clients' oral health, nutrition, ability to chew and swallow, sleep and rest patterns, bowel and bladder function, gait and balance, and weight. Box 31-7 outlines diagnostic tests and procedures required to rule out the possibility of reversible problems or to make a diagnosis of dementia. Assessment of a client's ability to perform and carry out ADLs independently is paramount.

Cognitive assessment consists of a complete assessment of neurological function and includes tests for hearing, vision, taste, smell, and touch, as well as memory and orientation to person, place, and time. (Color Plates 11 and 13 illustrate PET scans of clients with DAT.) A standardized mental status examination is done (Fig. 31-2). Clients are observed for symptoms of sundown

The Nursing Process

Box 31-7

Diagnostic Tests and Procedures for Clients with Cognitive Impairment

Neurological assessment

Pharmacological assessment

Mental status examination

Chest x-ray and electrocardiogram

CT scan (rule out tumor, hydrocephaly, and subdural hematoma) and MRI (indicates structural changes)

Drug studies

Complete blood count with differential (identify infection, anemia)

Electrolyte studies (identify potassium, sodium, and glucose imbalances that might cause confusion)

Thyroid function studies (hypothyroidism mimics early dementia)

Blood cultures and liver function studies

Lumbar puncture

Vitamin B levels (deficiency of B vitamins implicated in delirium)

Instructions: Ask questions 1–10 in this list, and record all answers. Ask question 4A only if patient does not have a telephone. Record total number of errors based on 10 questions.

  +   −

____ ____ 1. What is the date today?_____

                                  Month/Day/Year

____ ____ 2. What day of the week is it? _____

____ ____ 3. What is the name of this place? _____

____ ____ 4. What is your telephone number? _____

____ ____ 4a. What is your street address? _____

                (Ask only if patient does not have a telephone)

____ ____ 5. How old are you? _____

____ ____ 6. When were you born? _____

____ ____ 7. Who is the President of the United States now? _____

____ ____ 8. Who was the President just before him? _____

____ ____ 9. What was your mother's maiden name? _____

____ 10. Subtract 3 from 20 and keep subtracting 3 from each new number, all the way down.

____ TOTAL NUMBER OF ERRORS

0–2 errors	Intact intellectual functioning
3–4 errors	Mild intellectual impairment
5–7 errors	Moderate intellectual impairment
8–10 errors	Severe intellectual impairment

Allow one more error if subject has had only a grade-school education.

Allow one less error if subject has had education beyond high school.

Fig. 31-2 Short Portable Mental Status Questionnaire (SPMSQ). (From Pfeiffer, E. (1975). A short portable questionnaire for assessment of organic brain deficits in elderly patients. *Journal of American Geriatric Society, 23,* 433-441.)

---

syndrome, disturbed perception, illusions, hallucinations, and motor behavior. The ability to communicate effectively and disturbances in language ability are noted.

The clients' level of social interaction and their coping ability and degree of exercise and activity are assessed. The ability to access the environment and to respond to its cues safely is noted. Problematic behavior such as wandering, misplacing things, or pacing are observed.

Careful assessment of affect and emotional states are solicited. Clients are assessed to rule out anxiety and depression. Family members are asked about agitated or aggressive behavior and whether catastrophic reactions have occurred. Table 31-5 suggests questions that may be used in a focused assessment of clients with cognitive impairment and gives examples of possible client responses. Table 31-6 lists selected formal assessment instruments used to gather additional essential needed data.

Data collection about the caregiver and the client's family is an essential part of the assessment and include the following:

- Relationship of caregiver to client
- Physical and mental health of caregiver
- Levels of depression, stress, burden, strain, or physical change since caregiving began
- Impact of caregiving responsibilities on family roles and client-caregiver relationships
- Amount of individual social support and availability

of community resources to caregiver and other family members

- Financial resources that support the caregiving role

Nursing Diagnosis

The DSM-IV diagnoses of dementia, delirium, amnestic disorder, and other cognitive disorders replace the label of *organic mental* disorders. Although dementia had historically been used to label a progressive or irreversible course, the DSM-IV label does not involve progress but is based on the pattern of cognitive deficits that develops over time. Reversibility is a function of the underlying pathological condition and effective treatment. Delirium

The Nursing Process

TABLE 31-5

Focused assessment for clients with cognitive impairment	
ASSESSMENT	**CLINICAL EXAMPLE**
Orientation	
Is the client oriented to time?	Perceives time passing rapidly; confused about whether it is spring or summer; perceives date as 10 years earlier.
Is the client oriented to place?	Believes that he is living in a resort and not a nursing home; goes to nurses' station asking for his bill because he wants to check the room-service charges.
Is the client oriented to person?	Does not recognize her children;
Does the client become more disoriented late in the day or at night? Does the client exhibit symptoms of sundown syndrome?	Becomes agitated, yelling at people as twilight approaches.
Thought Processes	
Is there evidence of forgetfulness that is creating problems or indicating potentially serious problems? Has the forgetfulness increased recently?	Puts pot of soup on to boil and forgets, resulting in burning pot and its contents; constantly misplacing things; goes to bed in clothes worn during the day and does not change into night clothes; increasing forgetfulness.
Is there evidence that the immediate, recent, or remote memory is impaired?	When shown how to put right arm in sleeve is unable to duplicate the action with left arm; shortly after meeting someone, asks who person is; appears to enjoy talking about childhood experiences with other clients.
Is the client able to follow verbal/written directions?	Begins asking where home is located; becomes more distractible; shortening attention span.
Is there evidence of "substitution behavior"?	When asked to get coat in preparation for a trip out to a mall, goes to the kitchen and begins cleaning the sink.
Is the client able to describe a situation (current/past) in a logical and coherent way?	Attempts to describe visit and dinner with family. Description is interspersed with incidents that occurred during a previous vacation; activities of ordering food, eating, and trip back to nursing home not presented in a logical time frame or exposition of ideas.
Is client able to engage in problem solving?	Inability to think about information logically impairs steps in problem-solving process.
Does the client exhibit symptoms that reflect dementia or pseudodementia?	Deficits in self-care hygiene; unable to button shirt until specific directions are provided; tells spouse lunch was delicious, but 1 hour later cannot recall having eaten or what was eaten at the meal.
Does the client exhibit deficits in calculating, using a fund of information, or learning new tasks?	When playing a simple game, client is told to pick up six chips and give three to partner; unable to count required chips.
Does the client exhibit language impairments? Is speech more impoverished than it has been in the past?	Cannot ask for eating utensils when they are missing; asks for a shovel and pitchfork instead of fork and spoon.
Does the client fail to recognize familiar objects?	Does not recognize a toothbrush or recall what it is used for.

The Nursing Process

TABLE 31-5—cont'd

Focused assessment for clients with cognitive impairment

ASSESSMENT	CLINICAL EXAMPLE
When the client is asked a question, does the response reflect confabulation?	When asked to explain the reason he put all his clothing in a bag outside his room, he tells the nurse that he is packing for a vacation and that a bus will be picking him up and driving him to Florida for the winter.
Affect and Mood	
Is there evidence of emotional lability or inappropriate affect, blunting, shallowness, unresponsiveness, euphoria, irrational anger, or sadness?	Little or no facial expression, affect flat; unresponsive toward family members when they visit; outbursts of tearfulness or exaggerated laughing in the absence of stimuli; cannot provide reason for emotional outburst.
Is there evidence that the client is/was involved in a grieving process?	Currently withdrawn, tearful, disheveled appearance; makes statements: "Why did this happen to me?" "I've lost myself" and "Where is my home?"
What is client's emotional response to the disease process: unlike or like responses to past crises?	Response has been characterized by irritability and hostility toward others, reflective of past behavioral responses to crises.
Sensory Perception	
Does the client exhibit delusional thinking or report illusions or hallucinations?	Complains often of people watching him, spying on him, and coming into his room at night and reorganizing it; misperceives spouse entering room at night as her daughter; tells nurse she hears angel voices talking to her.
Motor Activity	
Does the client exhibit motor impairments?	Unsteady gait, unable to use cane effectively, safer ambulation with walker; hyperactivity has been replaced with increasing retardation of motor activity.
Biological Rhythms	
Have there been changes in eating, sleeping, or other patterns recently? In the past year?	Nocturnal wandering has occurred recently. Now needs help feeding self. Asks for food in the early morning hours and after bedtime; needs to be encouraged to eat at mealtime even though there are complaints of not feeling hungry.
Self-Care	
Is self-care deteriorating?	Does not bathe unless supervised; disheveled appearance.
Behavior and Personality	
What changes in behavior have occurred during the past few months? past year?	Behavior had been very ritualistic last year; currently is disorganized.
Has there been evidence of social disinhibition?	Has begun undressing in public places.
What behavioral changes have occurred?	Initially very ritualistic; has become increasingly disorganized and agitated; wanders.
Is there evidence of personality changes that have been observed over time or described in behavioral terms by significant others?	Wife states that her husband had been an open, friendly, and trusting man but has become chronically suspicious.

The Nursing Process

TABLE 31-5—cont'd

Focused assessment for clients with cognitive impairment

ASSESSMENT	CLINICAL EXAMPLE
Is the client's judgment becoming unreliable or dangerous to self or others?	Withdrew large sums of money from the bank, asked for small bills, closed out his accounts, took money home, and hid it in his refrigerator and stove.
Have there been changes in the way the client manages interpersonal relationships?	Instigates fights with others; is intrusive; lacks respect for other clients' space and possessions; overbearing and demanding.
How would you describe the client's sociability?	Sociability is decreasing.
Are there changes in the client's behavior that violate social conventions and have potential for causing embarrassment or being labeled deviant?	Was observed voiding by a tree in the front yard.
What coping mechanisms is the client using to defend against awareness of the deficits?	Denies being lost and blames it on wife's moving to a strange town when environment becomes unfamiliar.
Is the client becoming isolated and withdrawing from social contact with others?	Chooses to sit alone in dining room; does not participate in group therapy; walks away when clients and staff attempt to talk with him.
Does the client exhibit impaired functioning in particular situations? What types of behavior occur? What types of situations elicit the dysfunctional behavior?	Becomes agitated and hostile when family members visit; is relatively calm at home alone with wife; appears disorganized by the noise and presence of others.
Does the client avoid situations that would expose the loss of memory or intellectual functioning?	Walked out of admission interview and refused to join other clients in group and recreational activities.
Do the client's deficits contribute to behavior that is a danger to others?	When rules are enforced, such as smoking in a designated area, he becomes combative.
Do the client's deficits require protection from self-injury?	Unable to use electric razor to shave; wife caught him attempting to rinse it under running water while it was plugged in.

may involve short-lived dementia and is used to describe a disturbance in consciousness and a change in cognition that develops over a short time. It is usually caused by the direct physiological consequences of a general medical condition. Clients with amnestic disorder have severe memory impairment but do not exhibit the symptoms of more extensive cognitive impairment.

The nursing diagnoses appropriate for clients with dementia, delirium, and amnestic disorder vary with the stage and severity of the clients' symptoms. Nursing diagnoses are used to describe symptoms related to cognitive impairment and disruptions in the client's ability to safely carry out ADLs, and his or her ability to relate to others, as well as to feel, choose, move, or engage in meaningful activity. Box 31-8 lists selected nursing diag-

noses that may be used with clients who have symptoms of dementia, delirium, and other amnestic disorders and for those who are their caregivers. The second part of the nursing diagnoses is developed to reflect each illness and the clients' individualized assessment data.

Outcome Identification

Outcomes for clients with acute dementia and delirium are usually short term and are related to physiological outcomes. The goal is to facilitate restoration of cognitive processes. On the other hand, outcomes for clients with progressive dementia are more long range. They reflect the stage of the disease, as well as the caregiver's ability to manage the progressive nature of symptoms indepen-

The Nursing Process

TABLE 31-6

Selected assessment instruments

INSTRUMENT	DESCRIPTION
Glascow Coma Scale	Quantitive measure of level of consciousness
Serum alcohol and drug levels (see Chapter 27)	Measures potential toxicity (delirium)
Mini Mental Status Examination (Folstein, et al., 1975)	Assesses client's cognitive state
Instrumental Activities of Daily Living (IADL) Scale (Lawton & Brody, 1969)	Measures self maintenance or instrumental ADLs (meal preparation, shopping, telephone use, transportation, medication compliance, housekeeping, laundry, and money management)
Short Portable Mental Status Questionnaire (SPMSQ) (Pfeiffer, 1975)	Objective measure of a client's level of cognitive impairment (see Fig 31-2)
Barthel Index of ADL (Mahoney & Barthel, 1965)	Measures functional status and rates self-care activities in areas of feeding, mobility, and bowel and bladder control
Geriatric Depression Scale (Yesavage and Brink, 1983)	Measures level of depression in older adults; essential for differentiating pseudodementia from progressive irreversible cognitive disorders
NIMH Dementia Mood Assessment Scale (Sunderland, et al., 1988)	Measures mood in clients who are cognitively impaired

Box 31-8

Nursing Diagnoses

DEMENTIA

Impaired environmental interpretation syndrome
Chronic confusion
Altered thought processes
Impaired memory
Risk for trauma
Risk for disuse syndrome
Impaired verbal communication
Impaired social interaction
Spiritual distress
Impaired physical mobility
Activity intolerance
Sleep pattern disturbance
Diversional activity deficit
Impaired home-maintenance management
Altered health maintenance
Self-Care deficit: feeding, bathing/hygiene, dressing/grooming, or toileting

DELIRIUM

Acute confusion
Risk for injury
Impaired verbal communication
Relocation stress syndrome
Anxiety

CAREGIVER ISSUES

Ineffective family coping: compromised
Decisional conflict
Fatigue
Caregiver role strain
Risk for caregiver role strain
Spiritual distress
Impaired social interaction

AMNESTIC DISORDER

Impaired memory
Altered thought processes

From NANDA (1994). Nursing diagnoses definitions and classifications 1995-1996, Philedelphia: Author

dently. Ultimate goals are aimed at providing physical and emotional comfort measures for the client; assuring physical, emotional, and social support for the caregiver; and preventing physical and emotional problems in the caregiver. Table 31-7 lists outcome criteria for clients and caregivers during each of the stages of progressive dementia. Learners should be aware that goals presented need to be modified with specific measurable outcome

criteria and time frames that reflect individual needs of clients (see Chapter 5).

Planning

Planning the care for clients and families dealing with reversible dementia or delirium involves both short-term

The Nursing Process

TABLE 31-7

Outcomes related to the stages of progressive dementia

CLIENT	CAREGIVER
Early Confusional	
Use "cognitive crutches" to facilitate memory	Plan with client for future legal and financial aspects of client care (power of attorney, wills, etc.)
Acknowledge need for companion when driving	Acknowledge memory and personality changes in client
Make decisions regarding long-term health, financial, and legal needs	
Maintain independence in all ADLs	
Late Confusional	
Acknowledge cognitive losses	Acknowledge that client has need of supervision when handling complex tasks
Accept support and supervision for complex tasks such as handling finances	Verbalize understanding of client's moods and depression
Use posted labels and signs to help name objects and locate rooms in the home	Acknowledge feelings of rejection and being unappreciated
Maintain physical health	
Relinquish driving privileges	
Early Dementia	
Accept help to initiate ADLs	Encourage the independence of client while maintaining client's safety
Maintain physical health	Utilize therapeutic communication to support emotional needs
Maintain orientation to environment	Restrain from doing everything for client
Comply with medications used to manage anxiety, agitation, paranoia, and sleeplessness	Request needed help and services from family and friends
Middle Dementia	
Follow planned structure and routine as often as possible	Maintain safe environment
Accept assistance with all ADLs	Assume full legal and financial responsibility for client
Wear identification bracelet at all times	Join caregiver support group
Accept care and attention of caregivers	Hire help at home or place client in nursing home
	Maintain social contacts in the community
Late Dementia	
Remain free of complications associated with late-stage dementia (pneumonia, fluid and electrolyte imbalance, choking, etc.)	Verbalize limitations of caregiving
	Meet challenges of acknowledging gradual loss and death of loved one
Remain free of ducubiti	Maintain contact (touch, loving words) with client even when he or she cannot reach out

The Nursing Process

and long-term preventive strategies. Planning the care of a client usually includes short-term care and is aimed at:

- Determining underlying cause of cognitive disorder
- Attending to physiological status
  -Fluid and electrolyte balance
  -Hypoxia
  -Anoxia
  -Diabetic problems
- Maintaining a low-stimulus environment
- Monitoring level of orientation
- Providing reality orientation and assurance
- Teaching the client to avoid underlying sources of problem (toxins, alcohol, etc.)

Planning the care of clients with irreversible progressive dementia is a complex, multifaceted process that requires interdisciplinary approaches. Clients with DAT progress through several stages, each of which requires clients and their caregivers to plan for immediate and long-term needs. The phases of DAT may progress rapidly or slowly. Clients diagnosed before age 60 usually progress through stages rapidly and die within 3 to 5 years. When onset begins at a later age, the disease progresses more slowly for 10 or more years. Care planning begins once the diagnosis is made. A care plan for a client with AIDS-related dementia is presented on p. 674.

Implementation

Implementation of planned care for clients with acute and chronic confusional states presents a challenge for nurses. The following sections apply standards of psychiatric-mental health nursing practice to the care of clients with dementia, delirium, and other cognitive impairments.

Counseling

Direct counseling of clients with cognitive deficits is generally supportive and directed at orienting clients to their surroundings. Interactions are directed at improving communication with clients and supporting caregivers. Maintaining meaningful communication between clients with progressive dementia and their caregivers is an essential component of the counseling process. In the early stages of dementia, signs, labels, and written messages reassure and comfort clients. As a client moves into the later stages of dementia, nonverbal communication, particularly touch, is helpful. It is important to teach significant others and caregivers to avoid talking as if the client were not there and to remember that the client needs affection. Affection is communicated with touch

or hugs. Helping the client communicate reduces frustration and prevents aggressive outbursts. Some strategies to help clients with dementia convey their messages include the following:

- Remain calm and supportive.
- Position self at eye level; smile and convey openness.
- Maintain eye contact and use touch to convey active listening and acceptance.
- Show interest in what is being said and in the affect being conveyed, even if it is difficult to understand.
- Exercise patience and understanding.
- Observe all nonverbal gestures, tone of voice, and other clues to emotion.
- Offer a guess when client cannot find the word.
- Provide feedback when you grasp meanings.
- Supply the correct word when a wrong one is used. Refrain from future corrections if client becomes upset.
- Offer comfort and reassurance.

Receptive aphasia is often a problem for clients with cognitive impairment. Using simple sentences facilitates understanding by clients and diminishes their confusion. The following example illustrates the use of one-step directions.

> Gloria M. is a 72-year-old woman with DAT. She comes to the day-care center each day so her 58-year-old daughter can work at her part-time job. Gloria's confusion has increased over the last several months. Her progressive memory loss requires the use of structured one-step directions for her to continue feeding herself: "Here is your lunch Gloria. I'll cut your meat and sit with you while you eat." Gloria's nurse chooses a quiet table alone with Mrs. M. She says, "Gloria, this is your napkin. Put it on your lap. Pick up your fork (she points to it). Put it in the meat. Lift it to your mouth (she guides Mrs. M's hand). Put it in your mouth. Chew the meat. Swallow the meat."

From the example, it is obvious that patience and a slow-paced approach are necessary to help Gloria maintain as much independence as possible. Cognitive stimulation strategies help maintain the client's orientation.

Reality orientation is useful counseling strategy that helps clients with dementia remain "in touch" with their environment. It is a therapeutic modality used within a group setting or in a therapeutic nurse-client relationship. It uses structured repetitive activities to orient individuals to time, place, and person. Box 31-9 lists interventions for promoting reality orientation in clients. On the other hand, validation therapy does not attempt to orient the client but rather is aimed at accepting, under-

The Nursing Process

 NURSING CARE PLAN

Dementia

NURSING ASSESSMENT DATA

Donald M. is a 39-year-old former business executive who was admitted to the medical unit of your hospital with pneumonia. *Subjective data:* He states, "Sometimes he doesn't remember who I am. He thinks I'm out to get him. His emotions are up and down." *Objective* Donald's partner of 15 years reports that he has had AIDS for the last 10 years. He is depressed and disoriented to place and person. His friend reports sleep disturbances, confusion, agitation, and extreme restlessness over the last 4 weeks. *DSM-IV diagnosis:* Dementia due to HIV

NANDA Diagnosis: Altered thought processes related to signs of dementia (secondary to AIDS)

Outcomes	Interventions	Rationale	Evaluation
Short term 1. Will sleep for 8 hours between 10 PM and 6 AM *after 3 days.* **Long term** 1. Client will demonstrate intellectual ability and judgment at present level of function for as long as possible. 2. Client will respond to simple concrete statements without experiencing frustration.	• Establish nonstimulating bedtime ritual. • Provide quiet and minimal light. • Administer benzodiazepines or antihistimines as ordered. • Promote awareness and comprehension of surroundings through use of cognitive stimulation. • Promote client's awareness of personal identity time and environment (Box 31-9) Reality Orientation • Use nonverbal communication techniques with client.	• Rapid eye movement (REM) sleep promotes rest. • Reduced stimuli promotes sleep. • Structure decreases confusion. • Reduced light and noise at regular intervals help readjust client's biological clock and reestablish circadian rhythms. • Intermediate-acting benzodiazepines (clorazepate, oxazepam, temazepam) promote sleep and are drugs of choice for clients with dementia. • Antihistamines are helpful if restlessness is also present (sedation is a side effect). • Cognitive stimulation promotes optimal memory function, orientation, and thought processes. • Clients with dementia have difficulty coping with changes in routine and memory loss. Consistent, structured routines support memory functions and orientation, reduce confusion, and prevent frustration. • Physical expressions of caring and affection (touch, hugs, etc.) promote calm in client.	**Short term** 1. *Partially met:* Client has been sleeping for 5 hours since routine began. Hours of sleep dose of benzodiazepine will be increased. Consider using antihistamine (decreases restlessness). **Long term** 1. *Met:* Client maintains orientation to person and place with prompting. Continue cognitive-stimulation exercises and reality-orientation strategies. 2. *Met:* Client is more calm. Nonverbal acknowledgment of significant other and primary nurse. No episodes of agitation for 1 week. Follows simple commands when dressing and eating.

The Nursing Process

NURSING CARE PLAN

Dementia—cont'd

Outcomes	Interventions	Rationale	Evaluation
	• Teach friend (caregiver) strategies to effectively communicate with client.	• Maintaining simple, direct communication reduces confusion and facilitates client understanding of meanings of message.	
	• Reduce competing distracting background noise when speaking to client. Use low lighting and soft colors.	• Reducing noise and environmental stimuli prevents sensory overload and diminishes agitation (central nervous system [CNS] stimulation) and confusion.	
	• Teach friend not to be alarmed when client experiences confusion and agitation and to remain calm and stay with client.	• Clients with dementia experience emotional lability from effects of disease in areas of brain that control mood and affect and from frustration and feelings of powerlessness.	
	• Administer medication as ordered. Monitor effects.	• Low dose antipsychotics (0.25-1 mg haloperidol [Haldol]) are recommended for management of suspiciousness, paranoia, and sundown syndrome.	

standing and validating whatever the client communicates to another.

Remotivation therapy is a form of structured group therapy used to stimulate communication among individuals who are uninvolved and confused. It consists of a specific number of sessions scheduled over 6 to 8 weeks. Structure includes introductions, reading about a specific topic, discussion of the topic, discussion of daily activities, and expressions of appreciation.

Reminiscence therapy is the process of facilitating recall of memories from the past and is helpful for clients with memory deficits associated with amnestic disorders and the memory loss associated with dementia. Reminiscence is usually used to encourage happy memories, but it may be painful for clients. For example, clients may be happy talking about their wedding day but be sad because their spouse of many years has died. Reminiscence therapy promotes the recall of past events, feelings, and thoughts. The process of using reminiscence therapy is outlined in Chapter 35. The use of music, art, poetry, photos, and pets may be used to facilitate recall.

Milieu Therapy

The care of clients with dementia may take place at home, in adult day-care programs, in sheltered assisted-living facilities, and in nursing homes. Clients with delirium and those with acute cognitive symptoms require hospitalization to restore physiological stability. Whatever the setting for care, the therapeutic milieu needs to provide structure and involvement of the client in his or her care for as long as possible. Box 31-10 suggests ways to provide a safe, therapeutic environment for clients with delirium. The most challenging aspect of milieu therapy for clients with dementia is maintaining the safety of the client while managing problematic behaviors such as wandering, night wandering, yelling or calling out, pilfering, and hoarding.

Some environmental adjustments that may be made are included in the following list:

• Provide adequate low-glare lighting.
• Remove potential dangers, such as throw rugs or small objects, from floors.

The Nursing Process

Box 31-9

Reality Orientation

DEFINITION

Promotion of patient's awareness of personal identity, time, and environment

ACTIVITIES

Use an approach that is consistent (e.g., kind firmness, active friendliness, passive friendliness, matter-of-fact, and no demands) when interacting with the patient and that reflects the particular needs and capabilities of that patient

Inform patient of person, place, and time, as needed

Avoid frustrating patient by quizzing with orientation questions that cannot be answered

Label items in environment to promote recognition

Provide a consistent physical environment and daily routine

Provide access to familiar objects, when possible

Dress patient in personal clothing

Avoid unfamiliar situations, when possible

Prepare patient for upcoming changes in usual routine and environmental before their occurrence

Provide caregivers who are familiar to the patient

Use environmental cues (e.g., signs, pictures, clocks, calendars, and color coding of environment) to stimulate memory, reorient, and promote appropriate behavior

Provide objects that symbolize gender identity (e.g., purse or cap)

Encourage use of aids that increase sensory input (e.g., eyeglasses, hearing aids, and dentures)

Remove stimuli, when possible, that create misperception in a particular patient (e.g., pictures on the wall and television)

Provide a low-stimulation environment for patient in whom disorientation is increased by overstimulation

Provide for adequate rest/sleep/daytime naps

Limit visitors and length of visits if patient experiences overstimulation and increased disorientation from them

Provide access to current news events (e.g., television, newspapers, radio, and verbal reports), when appropriate

Approach patient slowly and from the front

Address the patient by name when initiating interaction

Use a calm and unhurried approach when interacting with the patient

Speak to patient in a slow, distinct manner with appropriate volume

Repeat verbalizations, as necessary

Use gestures/objects to increase comprehension of verbal communications

Stimulate memory by repeating patient's last expressed thought

Ask questions one at a time

Interrupt confabulation by changing the subject or responding to the feeling or theme, rather than the content of the verbalization

Avoid demands for abstract thinking, if patient can think only in concrete terms

Limit need for decision making if frustrating/confusing to patient

Give one simple direction at a time

Use picture cues to promote appropriate use of items

Provide physical prompting/posturing (e.g., moving patient's hand through necessary motions to brush teeth), as necessary for task completion

Engage patient in concrete "here and now" activities (i.e., ADLs) that focus on something outside self that is concrete and reality oriented

Involve patient in a reality orientation group setting/class, when appropriate and available

Monitor for changes in sensation and orientation

From McCloskey, J.C., & Bulechek, G.M. (Eds.). (1996). **Nursing interventions classification (NIC). (2nd Ed.).** *St. Louis: Mosby.*

- Keep the environment and routine as consistent as possible.
- Schedule mealtimes consistently.
- Use cues such as calendars, pictures, clocks, holiday decorations, and drawings to facilitate orientation to current events, seasons, days of the week, and time of day.
- Remove mirrors if client is frightened by them.
- Decrease noise levels, avoid paging systems, and remember that radio and television may add to confusion and disorientation.
- Provide space for pacing and wandering.
- Label photos in large print with names of family or staff members.
- Provide boundaries such as stop signs, safety locks, or red or yellow tape on floor to prevent client from wandering and becoming lost.
- Use symbols or colors to help client locate rooms such as the bedroom or bathroom.
- Label clothing and objects such as chairs, tables, lamps, bookshelves, to promote name recognition of items. Use large block letters.

The Nursing Process

Box 31-10

Delirium Management

DEFINITION

Provision of a safe and therapeutic environment for the patient who is experiencing an acute confusional state

ACTIVITIES

Identify etiological factors causing delirium

Initiate therapies to reduce or eliminate factors causing the delirium

Monitor neurological status on an ongoing basis

Provide unconditional positive regard

Verbally acknowledge the patient's fears and feelings

Provide optimistic but realistic reassurance

Allow the patient to maintain rituals that limit anxiety

Provide patient with information about what is happening and what can be expected to occur in the future

Avoid demands for abstract thinking, if patient can think only in concrete terms

Limit need for decision making, if frustrating/confusing to patient

Administer PRN medications for anxiety or agitation

Encourage visitation by significant others, as appropriate

Recognize and accept the patient's perceptions or interpretation of reality (hallucinations or delusions)

State your perception in a calm, reassuring, and nonargumentative manner

Respond to the theme/feeling tone, rather than the content, of the hallucination or delusion

Remove stimuli, when possible, that create misperception in a particular patient (e.g., pictures on the wall or television)

Maintain a well-lit environment that reduces sharp contrasts and shadows

Assist with needs related to nutrition, elimination, hydration, and personal hygiene

Maintain a hazard-free environment

Place identification bracelet on patient

Provide appropriate level of supervision/surveillance to monitor patient and to allow for therapeutic actions, as needed

Use physical restraints, as needed

Avoid frustrating patient by quizzing with orientation questions that cannot be answered

Inform patient of person, place, and time, as needed

Provide a consistent physical environment and daily routine

Provide caregivers who are familiar to the patient

Use environmental cues (e.g., signs, pictures, clocks, calendars, and color coding of environment) to stimulate memory, reorient, and promote appropriate behavior

Provide a low-stimulation environment for patient in whom disorientation is increased by overstimulation

Encourage use of aids that increase sensory input (e.g., eyeglasses, hearing aids, and dentures)

Approach patient slowly and from the front

Address the patient by name when initiating interaction

Reorient the patient to the health care provider with each contact

Communicate with simple, direct, descriptive statements

Prepare patient for upcoming changes in usual routine and environment before their occurrence

Provide new information slowly and in small doses, with frequent rest periods

Focus interpersonal interactions on what is familiar and meaningful to the patient

From McCloskey, J.C., & Bulechek, G.M. (Eds.). (1996). Nursing interventions classification (NIC), (2nd Ed.). *St. Louis: Mosby.*

- Schedule regular rest times.
- Provide urinals and commodes at bedside and use a night light to help prevent night wandering.
- Label doors to bathroom, kitchen, and bedroom to promote orientation to places.
- Provide diversional activities and redirect behavior to prevent hoarding and pilfering.

Self-Care Activities

Monitoring the physical health and meeting basic needs of clients with progressive dementia is central to nursing management. Mealtimes, bathtimes, and other activities should be predictable. Changes in routine should be introduced slowly, so feelings of comfort and security are maintained.

Among the greatest challenges for caregivers are the problematic eating behaviors of clients with dementia. Table 31-8 lists problematic eating behaviors and suggests interventions for each. Nurses use these strategies directly or teach them to clients (Cohen, 1994; Ford, 1996). If it is not possible to maintain adequate nutrition, "tube feedings" may need to be considered. A permanent gastrostomy tube is the most convenient and least traumatic form of providing direct intergastric nutrition. However, for some families the insertion of a permanent tube may be viewed as an extraordinary means of sustaining life and may be prohibited by the client's living

TABLE 31-8

Problematic eating behaviors with interventions

EATING BEHAVIOR	INTERVENTION
Attention/concentration deficit	Verbally direct client through each step of the eating process. Place utensils in hand. Make food and fluids available and visible.
Combative, throws food	Identify the provocative agent and remove it. Stand or sit on nondominant side. Provide nonbreakable dishes with suction holders. Give one food at a time. Reward appropriate mealtime behavior.
Chews constantly	Tell client to stop chewing after each bite. Serve soft foods to reduce the need to chew. Offer small bites.
Eats nonedible things	Remove nonedibles from reach. Provide finger foods. Provide edible centerpiece or table decoration.
Eats too fast	Have client set utensils down between bites. Offer food items separately. Offer bulky foods that require chewing. Use smaller spoon or cup.
Eats too slowly	Monitor eating pace. Provide verbal cues, such as "chew" and "take a bite." Serve client first to allow more time Use insulated dishes to maintain proper food temperatures
Forgetful/disoriented	Provide simple routines. Maintain a constant environment. Assign seating. Minimize distractions. Limit choices.
Forgets to swallow	Tell client to swallow. Feel for swallow before offering next bite. Stroke upward on larynx.
Inappropriate emotional expression	Engage in conversation. Ignore emotional display. Provide quiet environment.
Paces	Sit beside client at table. Aerobic exercise before meals. Provide finger foods. Use cups with covers and spouts.
Shows paranoia	Provide structured routine. Present food in a consistent manner. Serve foods in closed containers. Do not put medicine in food.
Spits	Evaluate chewing and swallowing ability. Tell client not to spit ("Keep food in your mouth"). Place client away from others who would be offended. Provide mealtime supervision.
Will not go to dining room	Ask why. Change dining location. Provide a single dining partner versus a group. Serve meals in room.

The Nursing Process

will. Nurses need to consider the wishes of clients and caregivers during the decision-making process.

Psychobiological Interventions

Although there are no specific drugs that specifically treat dementia, the behavioral problems associated with the disorder sometimes respond to pharmacological treatment. Table 31-9 lists behaviors, selected drug treatments, and key monitoring factors for clients with symptoms of cognitive impairment. The goal is to use a single drug that can manage several symptoms. The principle is to find the least amount of drug to achieve the maximum effect.

Tacrine (Cognex) is a relatively new pharmacological agent used to treat dementia. It is a reversible cholinesterase that elevates acetylcholine concentrations in the cerebral cortex by slowing the breakdown of acetylcholine. Although it does not alter underlying dementia, it may boost memory in clients with mild to moderate DAT and amnestic disorders. Clients should be cautioned to report any side effects, especially twitching or eye spasms, which may indicate overdose. The drug should not be abruptly increased or decreased, and regular monitoring of hepatic function is recommended.

Pharmacologic treatment of delirium is aimed at restoring consciousness, calming and/or sedating the client, as well as preventing irreversible brain damage. The cause of symptoms will determine the choice of medication.

Health Teaching

Clients with cognitive impairments are often unable to participate successfully in the teaching-learning process because of their cognitive deficits. However, they can be helped to maintain previous levels of knowledge. Teaching is therefore aimed primarily at family caregivers. Many of the intervention strategies included in this chapter may be shared with family members or other at-home caregivers, as well as those who manage the care of clients in nursing homes and day-care settings.

Teaching topics aimed at caregivers include information about the disease process, ways to access support services, safety management, ways to maintain adequate nutrition, taking care of their own health, promoting sleep and rest in the client, and getting adequate rest themselves. Modifying the environment for safety often contributes to the caregiver's peace of mind. Of paramount importance is enhancing communication between clients and their caregivers. The Teaching Points at right lists suggestions for communicating with clients who are cognitively impaired.

Case Management

Case management of clients with dementia is challenging. Clients with dementia are high-intensity users of multiple services. Nurses who are case managers need to familiarize themselves with available resources and facilitate client and family access to them. Case management of clients with cognitive impairment is aimed at:

- Monitoring and maintaining the client's physical health
- Adapting the environment to provide safety and structure for the client
- Maintaining optimum communication between the caregiver and client
- Reality orientation
- Maintaining social interaction
- Promoting social interaction and self-esteem for clients and their caregivers

The home care of a person with dementia requires support for the family members and caregiver (see Chapter 21). Support may be instrumental or expressive. *Instrumental support* is the provision of tangible resources. Examples of instrumental support include legal,

TEACHING POINTS

Communicating With Persons Who Are Cognitively Impaired

- Keep confusion and distraction at a minimum.
- Approach person from the front, avoiding any sudden movement
- Get the person's attention.
- Begin each conversation by identifying yourself and addressing the person by name.
- Speak slowly and distinctly. Avoid shouting. Monitor tone in voice.
- Use short, simple, familiar words.
- Explain all actions clearly, simply, and one step at a time.
- Do not rush.
- Cover one point at a time.
- Use nonverbal communication and gestures to reinforce or enhance message.
- Treat the person with dignity and respect. Avoid talking down to him or her or using pet names, such as "honey" or "pops."
- Avoid complex and idiomatic language, such as "run up a bill" or "hop right over."
- Avoid use of negative directions, such as "do not."

The Nursing Process

TABLE 31-9

Pharmacological agents helpful in treatment of symptoms of cognitive impairment

SYMPTOM	MEDICATION/TREATMENT	MONITORING COMMENTS
Suspiciousness, paranoia, sundown syndrome	Low-dose antipsychotic: • Haloperidol (Haldol), 0.25-1 mg daily • Mesoridzine (Serentil), 10-50 mg daily	Correct any sensory impairment. Observe for drug interactions (parkinsonism, akathisias, sedation, and falls). Stop drug if pacing increases. Start low; go slow.
Anxiety	Treat underlying physical problems (pain, dyspnea, urinary urgency, and sensory impairment. Low-dose benzodiazepine: • Diazepam (Valium) Low-dose azaspirodecanedione: • Buspirone (BuSpar)	Avoid sedative-hypnotics, especially barbiturates and non-benzodiazepine agents. Observe for untoward effects.
Acute catastrophic reaction	Remove source of upset. Low-dose antipsychotics: • Haloperidol (Haldol), 2-5 mg intramuscular (IM) stat • Lorazepam (Ativan), 1 mg IM	Observe for desired effect of drug (sedation). Observe for untoward effect (increased anxiety).
Insomnia	If associated with confusion, use low-dose antipsychotic. If associated with depression, use: • Nortriptyline (Pamelor) or Trazodone (Desyrel) Intermediate-acting benzodiazepines: • Temazepam (Restoril) • Lorazepam (Ativan) • Oxazepam (Serax) Antihistamine: • Diphenhydramine (Benadryl)	Antianxiety agents may cause disinhibition or increased confusion. Rebound anxiety at the end of dosing interval may be a problem with chronic use. Antihistamines are particularly helpful if clients are experiencing restlessness, akathisia or extrapyramidal side effects of an antipsychotic.
Angry or violent outbursts	Use low dose antipsychotic: • Trazodone (Desyrel) if chronic pain is suspected cause Mood stabilizer may be helpful: • Carbamazepine (Tegretol) • Propranolol (Inderal), beta-adrenergic blocker	Disruptive or aggressive outbursts are Difficult to control with medication. Seizurelike brain activity may precipitate angry outbursts Assess if related to pain or other physiologic stimuli. Keep log of outbursts noting behaviors and stimuli observed immediately before episode.

The Nursing Process

financial, or home-repair assistance; sharing in the hands-on caregiving responsibilities that provide the primary caregiver with respite time; or financial support for the employment of people who help with the maintenance of the home and the provision of direct care. *Expressive support* involves emotional availability to the client and caregiver. Examples of expressive support include sending humorous cards; arranging surprise get-togethers; and providing meaningful exchanges among clients, caregivers, and family members.

Promoting optimum health for caregivers and providing short-term respite or relief is an essential component of case management of clients with progressive dementia and other cognitive disorders. Box 31-11 outlines activities involved in providing respite care to family members.

Early in the course of progressive dementia, particularly DAT and vascular dementia, it is vital that clients and their families obtain competent legal advice. Nurses in their role as advocates are in a position to recommend such action but ethically may not profit from it. Legal help is generally needed and can make the difference between economic survival and destitution, between dignity and indignity, and between preservation of individual rights or their erosion (Alzheimer's Association, 1991). The following documents may ease the care of clients and lessen present and future financial problems for caregivers:

- **Durable power of attorney (DPA):** *a document that allows clients to designate another person to act on their behalf.* A DPA may be broad and give power to control and manage everything, or it may be limited to specific assets or activities.
- **Living will:** *a document that allows the client's designee to make health care decisions.*
- **Living trust:** *a document that appoints a trustee to manage some or all assets that are placed in trust.* Such a trust helps avoid the costly and timely probate process. They are also used to protect an individual's assets or to hold money to pay for goods and services that a public benefits recipient (someone relying on Supplemental Security Income or Medicaid) might not otherwise receive.
- **Will:** *a document that specifies how assets are distributed at death.*
- **Conservatorship:** *the court appoints an individual to care for a client's assets when it is determined that an individual is no longer able to do so alone.* A conservatorship is monitored by the court in the best interest of the client.
- **Guardianship:** *a guardian may be appointed by the court when a client is no longer able to care for him- or herself.* A guardian may place the client in a nursing home if he or she cannot manage at home.

Other legal considerations include transfer of titles for property, filing of tax returns, and giving consent for treatment. Nurses need to direct clients to settle such matters early in the disease process. Case managers should also advise clients about entitlements such as Social Security Disability, Medicare, and Medicaid. Clients with dementia may be eligible for financial support and aid once the disease has progressed to its later stages.

Consideration of nursing-home placement may be the client's and caregiver's first contact with case-management services. Nurses become involved in assessing what is needed to maintain the client at home or assisting in the nursing-home or day-care placement decisions. Nursing homes and day-care facilities are becoming more aware of the needs of clients with Alzheimer's disease and their families. Many have developed specialty units or groups designed to manage the specific behaviors of each stage of the disease.

BOX 31-11

Respite Care

DEFINITION

Provision of short-term care to provide relief for family caregiver

ACTIVITIES

Establish a therapeutic relationship with patient/family
Monitor endurance of caregiver
Inform patient/family of available state funding for respite care
Coordinate volunteers for in-home services, as appropriate
Arrange for substitute caregiver
Follow usual routine of care
Provide care, such as exercises, ambulation, and hygiene, as appropriate
Obtain emergency telephone numbers
Determine how to contact usual caregiver
Provide emergency care, as necessary
Maintain normal home environment
Provide a report to usual caregiver on return

From McCloskey J.C., & Bulechek, G.M., (Eds.). (1996). Nursing interventions classification (NIC). *(2nd ed.). St. Louis: Mosby.*

The Nursing Process

Health Promotion and Health Maintenance

Health promotion and prevention of delirium are aimed at educating individuals and communities to avoid toxins and conditions that cause symptoms of delirium. Alcohol and drug education is a key component in this effort and is discussed at length in Chapter 27.

Health promotion for clients with dementia is aimed at maintaining the clients' independence for as long as possible and preventing health decline in caregivers. Caregivers of clients with dementia are a primary target of health-promotion interventions. Preventing illness in family members of caregivers is an overall goal. Several steps that facilitate effective caregiving can be taught to caregivers (Cohen & Eisdorfer, 1993):

- *Recognize and prioritize problems:* caregivers generally do not have a problem seeking and accepting help when problems with loved ones are acute. However, they do have difficulty when problems are insidious and progressive. Education is aimed at recognizing signs and symptoms of the progressive stages of dementia.
- *Overcome denial:* family members deny subtle changes in their loved one. It usually takes a critical event for family members to recognize the gradual losses that are occurring and to seek the necessary assistance.
- *Manage emotions:* caring involves emotions. Family members need to be taught to recognize their feelings and to seek counseling or attend a support group before issues become serious.
- *Build collaborative partnerships with health care providers:* family members are called on to deal with a whole set of problems that involve personal, social, and financial resources, as well as roles and relationships. Teaching families to establish partnerships in care with medical and legal professionals is an important nursing role.
- *Balance needs and resources:* caregivers need to be taught to balance competing obligations and responsibilities and to minimize disruptions in their own lives. Accepting help from outside the family may be a solution. Clients should be given information about agencies that supply companionship, skilled nursing care, home chore, or other needed services.
- *Learn to control and prevent crises:* Careful planning for future needs and for the progressive physical deterioration of the client alieviates having to make important decisions during a crisis.
- *Let go and move on:* Making the decision to institutionalize a parent or loved one in a nursing home or to employ full-time help at home is a difficult one. Nurses provide information and maintain a supportive attitude as families let go and evaluate the best course of action. Whenever possible, the client should be involved in the decision-making process.

Other means of promoting the health of caregivers involves helping them access the resources necessary to optimize and maintain the client's maximum level of functioning, as well as their own. Clients and their caregivers can be taught to access help through their health professionals and community mental health centers that provide specialized care for clients with dementia.

Not all communities have readily available services. Area Agencies on Aging (AAAs) are involved in developing resources that support the needs of the aging population in their local communities and can be a valuable information resource. Other organizations that provide resources for clients and caregivers coping with dementia are listed in the Community Resources box on p. 683.

Support groups have been considered a key resource for cognitively impaired clients and their families, particularly the groups sponsored by the Alzheimer's Association. They provide important information about formal local services as well as emotional support during the slow course of the disease. Other forms of support include respite care, adult care, home health care, legal services, outpatient geropsychiatric clinics, and psychiatric hospitals.

Evaluation

Evaluation of clients with delirium involves monitoring the client's level of orientation. Standardized assessment instruments should be used, and observations of clients should be carefully noted so progress toward goals can be evaluated. Physiological causes of increased confusion that are acute and reversible are carefully monitored.

Evaluation of clients with dementia is related to the length of time the client is able to maintain functional ability and the success with which clients and their families attain social supports. Modification of goals is an ongoing, long-term, multidisciplinary process that requires constant reevaluation and revision of comfort measure and treatments. The focus of care changes as clients and families move through the progressive stages of dementia.

The Nursing Process

 COMMUNITY RESOURCES

Alzheimer's Association
919 North Michigan Avenue
Suite 1000
Chicago, IL 60611-1676
(800)272-3900

Alzheimer's Disease International (ADI)
12 South Michigan Avenue
Chicago, IL 60603
(312)335-5777

American Association of Homes and Serves for the Aging (AAHSA)
901 E Street NW
Suite 500
Washington, DC 20004-2037
(202)783-2242

American Association of Retired Persons (AARP)
601 East Street NW
Washington, DC 20049
(202)434-2277

American Senior Citizens Association (ASCA)
P.O. Box 41
Fayetteville, NC 28302
(919)323-3641

American Society of Aging (ASA)
833 Market Street
Suite 512
San Francisco, CA 94103-1824
(415)882-2910

Association of Retired Americans (ARA)
9102 North Meridian street, Suite 405
Indianapolis, IN 46260
(317)571-6888

Beverly Foundation
70 South Lake Avenue, Suite 750
Pasadena, CA 91101
(818)792-2292

Center for the Study of Aging (CSA)
706 Madison Avenue
Albany, NY 12208
(518)465-6927

Children of Aging Parents (CAPs)
1609 Woodbourne Road
Suite 302A
Levittown, PA 19057
(800)227-7294

Gerontological Society of America (GSA)
1275 K Street Northwest
Suite 350
Washington, DC 20005-4006
(202)842-1275

National Institute on Aging (NIA)
Public Information Office
Federal Building, Room 5C27, Building 31
9000 Rockville Place
Bethesda, MD 20892
(301)496-1752

The Nursing Process

THE CONSUMER'S VOICE

Caregiver of a Person with Alzheimer's Disease

Anita Leach McMahon

My dad died November 4, 1995. My mom, his beloved Peggy, was there, as were some of my brothers and sisters, their spouses, and some of his grandchildren. I was some 1,200 miles away, a long-distance caregiver.

It has been said that I'm my father's daughter, a description that both pleases and frightens me. I am pleased because he was my dad, because he too was a psychiatric nurse and my role model in so many personal and professional ways. I am frightened because he died in the end stages of progressive dementia, a disease that stretches across generations of families to claim its victims.

As we gathered from all over the country later that Saturday evening to celebrate his life, we wept, laughed, and remembered a full, busy, rich, and giving life. We remembered the many years of fading: the funny things (like his hat), and the scary things (like climbing on the roof). We remembered his painfully slow journey into the dark night of unknowing.

We recalled the beginning of the end, the time when my mother was visiting my sister and broke her hip and we all became aware of how "old" he had become. He was 85 then and still driving! While Mom recovered, my parents both stayed with my sister, who used all her wonderful nursing skills and love to care for them. My brother recalled rescuing him after that when he wandered off. I wonder now if his stories of the old days were a kind of confabulation. I wonder too how aware he was that he was losing his memory. His brother and sister had also had dementia, and he often talked about them and wanting to return to Ireland to die as they had.

Over the next few years, there were more and more incidents of memory loss and confusion. He went over and over his "books," willing himself to remember his business affairs. There were the incidents of restlessness and night wandering and the subsequent installation of safety locks. There was the search for the "right" medication to help him sleep so Mom could get her rest. There was the frustration of untoward reactions to medications, and physicians who wouldn't hear what was happening. I felt powerless to stop what was happening to him as little by little the man he was vanished. I wondered about the meaning of such wasting of a brilliant mind and kind heart. It was during that time that I had my last lucid conversations with him and felt connectedness for the last times, saw the last smiles, made the last promises, and knew the last certain recognition he had of who I was.

The last year before Dad died was the hardest. It was difficult to watch him die "by inches." He lost his abilities to swallow, to talk intelligibly, to smile, to walk, and to get out of bed. There was no question of putting him in a nursing home. Mom cared for him and insisted he would be cared for at home. During the last months we had a full-time caregiver with Mom. I think having a stranger in her house was very difficult. It brought tears to my heart and a realization of the depth of her loss when she said one day, "Taking care of him is easy now."

My youngest sister and her husband became the mainstay of my parents' life during that time. I became a "frequent flyer," ostensibly to help out but mostly to meet my own need to do something. I clung to the

The Nursing Process

THE CONSUMER'S VOICE

Caregiver of a Person with Alzheimer's Disease—cont'd

hope of fleeting moments of recognition from him while I prayed that he was unaware of the wasting of his body, his mind, and his spirit. I pondered the suffering that he experienced and what my mother must be feeling. I spent many hours being Dad's nurse and his oldest daughter. I took comfort in his comfort and was able to give some relief to my sister, and loving care to my mom. I took care of some of the legal issues and health care finances. I wondered each time I left to return to my own home if it would be the last time I would kiss him good-bye.

We celebrated Dad's funeral, and I took comfort in the many friends, colleagues, and family members who

came to pay tribute to him. We remembered his intelligence and his gift for having a good time. We remembered stories about the psychiatric hospital where he was the "supervisor of male nurses." We remembered his Irish stories and his blue eyes and his smile. We remembered and told our stories about how strict he was when we were growing up and in later years how he was always there when we needed help. We remembered how much he valued each of us and how proud he was of our achievements. We remembered love.

CRITICAL THINKING QUESTIONS

Cheryl C. is a 66-year-old married woman with three grown children. She is admitted to the orthopedic unit after a fall at home that resulted in a fractured hip. On admission she is alert and oriented but states that she is in severe pain. She is medicated, and the pain is relieved within 1 hour. She denies any major health problems and states that she has never been in the hospital "except to have kids." Cheryl is placed in Bucks traction and scheduled for surgery in the morning. Her preoperative laboratory tests reveal elevated liver enzymes, bilirubin, and white blood cells (WBCs).

Two days after uneventful surgery, she is disoriented and agitated. The night nurse reported at one point that Cheryl experienced visual hallucinations. Her speech is incoherent and she often uses expletives, a behavior her husband states has occurred only once before, "a year ago the day after she had been drinking for a week and stopped." Her oldest daughter reports that her mother takes lots of medications and wonders if she is still getting all of them. A "brown-bag" assessment of her medications reveals three different prescriptions from three different doctors for pain medications (opioids) and a prescription for lo-

razepam (Ativan) from their family physician. Several over-the-counter medications were among those brought in by her husband. When Cheryl's son visited, he talked with the nurse and revealed that he has been a member of Alcoholics Anonymous (AA) for about a year, "I really had a heavy-duty drinking problem. I guess you know Mom drinks a lot, too." A tentative diagnosis of substance withdrawal delirium is made.

1. Which assessment data support the diagnosis of substance withdrawal delirium?
2. What other factors may contribute to Cheryl's symptoms?
3. What are the priority nursing interventions for Cheryl?
4. Were there any actions the nurse or treatment team could have taken to prevent Cheryl's behavior? If so, what would they be?
5. What is the recommended treatment protocol for Cheryl?
6. What is her prognosis?
7. What are some health promotion strategies considered appropriate for clients and families coping with substance withdrawal delirium?

KEY POINTS

- DAT affects approximately 4 million people. Approximately 10% of persons over age 65 and 50% of those age 85 or older are affected.
- DAT progresses through stages, reflecting gradual brain deterioration.
- Delirium, or acute confusion, is a disturbance of consciousness and a change in cognition that develops over a short time.
- Disturbances of memory occur on a continuum
- Pseudodementia is a term used to describe a constellation of symptoms that include cognitive and memory impairments suggestive of dementia, but which are in fact symptoms of depression.
- Short-term (iconic) memory involves the processing and recall of new or recent information. Long-term or remote memory involves the ability to recall information from the distant past.
- Sundowning describes the deterioration of a clients cognitive functions and an increase in agitation in late afternoon hours. It is believed that sundowning is associated with deterioration in the suprachiasmatic nucleus of the hypothalamus, the principle pacemaker of the circadian rhythm system.
- Nursing diagnoses and outcomes criteria should relate to the stage of a client's symptoms of dementia or the nature of symptoms of delirium.
- Caregivers of clients with progressive dementia need counseling, social support, and respite.
- Nursing interventions with clients who are experiencing symptoms of progressive dementia require a multidisciplinary approach.

REFERENCES

Alzheimer's Association. (1991). *Legal consideration for Alzheimer patients* (Pamphlet Ed. 2082). Chicago: Author.

American Psychiatric Association. (1994). *Diagnostic and statistical manual of mental disorders* (4th ed.). Washington, DC: Author.

Bliwise, D.L. (1994). Dementia. In M.H. Kryger, T. Roth, & W.C. Dement (Eds.), *Principles and practice of sleep medicine* (pp. 790-800). Philadelphia: Saunders.

Burney-Puckett, M. (1996). Sundown syndrome: Etiology & management. *Journal of Psychosocial Nursing, 34*(5), 40-43.

Cohen, D. (1994). Dementia, depression, and nutritional status. *Primary Care, 21*(1), 107-119.

Cohen, D., & Eisdorfer, C. (1993). *Caring for your aging parents: A planning and actions guide.* New York: Tarcher/Putnam.

Cromwell, S.L., & Phillips, L.R. (1995). Forgetfulness in elders: Strategies for protective caregiving. *Geriatric Nursing, 16*(2), 55-59.

England, M. (1996). Caregiver planning. *Image, 28*(1) 17-22.

Folstein, M.F., Folstein, S.E., & McHugh, P.R. (1975). Mini mental state: A practical method for grading the cognitive state of patients or the clinician. *Journal of Psychiatric Research, 12,* 189-198.

Ford, G. (1996). Putting feeding back into the hands of patients. *Journal of Psychosocial Nursing, 34* (5), 35-39.

Greutzner, H. (1988). *Alzheimer's: A caregiver's guide and sourcebook.* New York: Wiley.

Hogstel, M.O. (1995). *Geropsychiatric nursing* (2nd Ed.). St. Louis: Mosby.

Keltner, N. (1994). Tacrine: A pharmacological approach to Alzheimer's disease. *Journal of Psychosocial Nursing, 32*(3), 37-39.

Kolanowski, A.M. (1995). Disturbing behaviors in demented elders: A concept synthesis. *Archives of Psychiatric Nursing, 11* (4), 188-194.

Lawton, H.P., & Brody, E.M. (1969). Assessment of older people: Self-maintaining and instrumental activities of daily living. *Gerontologist, 9*(1), 179-186.

Luggen, A.S. (1996). *NGNA care curriculum for gerontologic nursing.* St. Louis: Mosby.

Mahoney, F.L., & Barthel, D.W. (1965). Functional evaluation: The Barthel index. *Maryland State Medical Journal, 14,* 61-65.

Mann, D.M., Neary, D., & Testa, H. (1994). *Color atlas and text of adult dementias.* London: Mosby-Wolfe.

McCloskey, J.C., & Bulechek, G.M. (1996). *Nursing interventions classification (NIC)* (2nd Ed.). St. Louis: Mosby.

North American Nursing Diagnoses Association (NANDA). (1994). *Nursing diagnosis definitions and classifications, 1995-1996.* Philadelpha: Author.

Pfeiffer, E. (1975). A short portable questionnaire for assessment of organic brain deficits in elderly patients. *Journal of American Geriatric Society, 23,* 433-441.

Souder, E, Saykin, A.J., & Alavi, A. (1995). Multi-modal assessment in Alzheimer's disease: ADL in relation to PET, MRI, and neuropsychology. *Journal of Gerontological Nursing, 21*(9), 7-13.

Stolley, J. (1994). When your patient has Alzheimer's disease. *American Journal of Nursing, 94*(8), 34-41.

Sunderland, T., Hill, J.L., Lawlor, B.A., & Molchan, S.E. (1988). NIMH dementia mood assessment scale (DMAS). *Pharmacology bulletin, 24* (4), 747-753.

Weiner, M.F. (1991). *The dementia: Diagnosis and management.* Washington, DC: American Psychiatric Press.

Yesavage, J.A., & Brink, T.L. (1983). Development and validation of a geriatric depression screening scale: A preliminary report. *Journal of Psychiatric Research, 17,* 37-49.

VIDEO RESOURCES

Mosby's Psychiatric Nursing Video Series: *Vol. 6. Alzheimer's Disease.*

Part Six

Populations at Risk

Chapter 32

Psychosocial Problems of Physically Ill Persons

Ann Robinette

LEARNING OUTCOMES

After studying and applying the concepts of this chapter, the learner will be able to:

- Discuss the impact that physical health problems impose on the emotional well-being of the individual, family, and society.
- Describe the stresses associated with the phases of illness and the different settings where the physically ill receive treatment.
- Identify selected clinical conditions and their specific psychosocial issues.
- Identify the particular biopsychosocial components of physical illness that should be assessed, and the tools for that assessment.
- Implement appropriate interventions through the nursing process to minimize the effects of psychosocial issues on health and maximize the individual's recovery and functioning.

KEY TERMS

Biopsychosocial	Psychophysiological	Psychosomatic
Pain	Psychosocial	Somatoform

"Life is complex." (Peck, 1993) This is not a new thought, but rather one particularly applicable to the issues involved in dealing with the emotional or psychosocial aspects of physical illness. *Psychosocial refers to aspects of social and psychological behavior* (e.g., the psychosocial development of a child). Only recently has it become clear that the mind-body interactions are part of a complex, interwoven system profoundly and continually affecting and influencing one another. To talk about the "mind-body" connection reflects the limits of the way this relationship can be conceptualized. It is discussed as if it is linear in nature and not the interwoven relationship it truly is.

Typically, medical-surgical nurses are the first to encounter these symptoms in their clients and therefore play a key role in addressing the psychosocial symptoms of clients with physical problems. For example, the home health nurse visiting a client in cardiac care might address the client's anxious feelings about having sexual relations for the first time after a heart attack. The surgical nurse on an inpatient unit identifies and deals with the body image issues of the client with a new below-the-knee amputation. The hospice nurse deals with the anger of an individual with terminal cancer. The psychiatric clinical nurse specialist is consulted about a client with symptoms of alcohol withdrawal in a busy inner city emergency room. These examples represent only a handful of the situations in which nurses deal with the complex emotional components of the client's physical illness. These clients clearly represent a population at risk whose psychosocial needs are as important as their physical needs.

The purpose of this chapter is to help students and practicing nurses learn how to identify and manage the psychosocial components of physical health problems. Explored in this chapter are common psychosocial issues and responses for all persons who face illness and which all nurses encounter regardless of specialty area or health care setting. This chapter's secondary focus is to acknowledge and address those illnesses known as psychosomatic illnesses. *Psychosomatic refers to a group of disorders whose etiologic factors, at least in part, are believed to be related to or directly caused by emotional factors.* The main domain of this chapter concerns ways to adequately meet the psychosocial needs of the physically ill.

ROLE OF THE NURSE

The practice of nursing is holistic in nature. A biopsychosocial model is the foundation for this holistic approach. In a *biopsychosocial model, the biological, psychological, and social aspects of a client's life are examined to provide a comprehensive approach to care.* There are two principles to this model: (1) most illness is influenced and determined by biological, psychological, and social occurrences; and (2) the predisposition, onset, course, and outcome of most illnesses are influenced by biological, psychological, and social phenomena (Cohen-Cole and Levinson, 1994).

The impact of these three components are not always equal. For example, in heart disease, it has been demonstrated that there is a significant biological component. Although there are social and psychological variables, the biological aspect will usually be the dominant one. The best nursing care comes from an assessment of all three spheres and interventions that address them all, particularly those symptoms in which all three domains intersect.

For example, an overweight homeless man with adult onset diabetes and foot sores comes to his local community clinic. The nurse triaging this client discovers the client's grandmother had diabetes, that his diet consists of an occasional nutritious meal at the local shelter, but more commonly is cheap wine and dumpster fodder, and that cleanliness and regular bathing are rare luxuries. If the nurse prescribes the textbook nursing interventions of following a diabetic diet and daily foot soaking and care, the client will be noncompliant. The challenge is to find ways to help this client, given his social, biological, and psychological situation (e.g., perhaps by obtaining vouchers for meals at a shelter and daily clinic visits with the original nurse for oral medication and foot care.

Basic Level of Practice

The responsibility for the implementation of the nursing process to manage psychosocial aspects of physical health problems is usually that of the registered nurse. This is a nurse who practices at the bedside in an acute care hospital; in a primary care setting, either public or private; in home care; at a school; at a homeless shelter; in an emergency room; in a skilled nursing facility, or wherever the physically ill are treated. All nurses are educated to meet the psychosocial needs of their clients and to address their coping abilities and their emotional needs. However, managing the complexity of the physiological and the psychosocial interactions that have been discussed may call for more expert intervention. Two additional options are available.

Advanced Practice Level

Psychiatric consultation-liaison nurse

One option would be for the registered nurse to consult with a psychiatric consultation-liaison nurse (PCLN). The PCLN is an advanced practice registered nurse (APRN) with a master's degree in psychiatric-mental health nursing and a second specialty interest in the medically ill. PCLNs, though traditionally based in the hospital, currently work in all practice settings. PCLNs function in direct care roles with clients about particular psychosocial aspects of their physical illness or in consultative roles to other nursing staff regarding the management of their clients' psychosocial issues. PCLNs make psychiatric and psychosocial diagnoses and implement a variety of interventions with clients and families. With the nursing staff, PCLNs offer education about these complex psychosocial or psychiatric issues, and psychosocial interventions for the nurses to include in their care to the clients and families.

Case management

A second option uses a case management system to address the needs of this population. A psychiatric-mental health nurse at the basic or advanced level could be the case manager. However, given the needs and diversity of this population, a psychiatric APRN would have the clinical expertise, clinical judgment, and leadership best suited to achieve quality client outcomes while maintaining appropriate use of scarce resources (Micheels, Wheeler, and Hays, 1995). In the role of case manager, the psychiatric-mental health APRN coordinates the treatment planning between all of the providers, makes referrals to appropriate resources (e.g., family therapy, psychotherapy, occupational therapy, physical therapy, day care programs, and others), and manages medications, as illustrated in the following example:

> In a home care agency, a psychiatric APRN evaluates a 68-year-old woman for depression who has had a stroke and has hemiplagia of her left arm and hand. In consultation with colleagues at the home care agency, the psychiatric APRN is made the client's case manager. As such, she works with the home care nurse, the home health aide, the physical therapist and the social worker to provide the necessary services for this client. The psychiatric APRN consults with the agency psychiatrist to prescribe anti-depressant medication for the client and the psychiatric APRN provides the appropriate psychotherapy to the client to help her work through her depression.

IMPACT OF PHYSICAL ILLNESS
Impact on the Individual

Physical illness has a profound effect directly on individuals, their families, and friends; and indirectly on society as a whole. Illness deprives a person emotionally and physically (LeMaistre, 1993). Illness, serious or not, affects a person's sense of well-being, sense of self, and identity. How one looks and feels, and what one is able to physically and mentally accomplish are all affected by physical illness. Persons with high self-esteem are self-accepting, enjoy respect and love both professionally and personally, and have a sense of control over their own

personal destiny. Illness and disability influence this sense of self. The more serious the illness, the more stressful it is for the person to try to maintain usual self-esteem. It may be harder for persons to be self-accepting when they are less physically intact. If job performance is compromised or if unable to work, the usual way of judging personal worth is lost. If goals have to be altered or if the body and its illness or disability now determine the schedule, a person may feel out of usual control. If a person has solid self-esteem to begin with, the ability to stabilize and adapt to the new situation is high. If self-esteem is shaky from the start, physical illness only stresses that further. (Gorman, Sultan, and Luna-Raines, 1989). Positive self-esteem facilitates the kind of adaptability called for in coping with physical illness.

Body image refers to how a persons sees herself or himself physically. It is an integral part of self-esteem and identity. Like self-esteem, body image fluctuates throughout the lifetime. If body image is poor, self-esteem is likely to be poor. Illness and disability have a major impact on a person's body image. This can be seen directly in the case of a woman who loses a breast to cancer or indirectly in how persons view themselves after illness, (e.g., the diabetic client who views his body as defective even though his blood sugar is controlled). An intact, strong, and realistic body image premorbidly (before illness) will help a person cope with these kind of changes.

The key issues of self-esteem and body image affect a person's competence and productivity, and in turn are affected by illness or disability. Guilt and powerlessness are feelings or responses that occur in the face of physical health problems. Losses and feelings of accompanying grief are also key issues. In addition to these key issues, the developmental stage of the individual affects how individuals deal with their physical health problems (see Chapter 7).

Impact on the Family

Sickness affects the whole family not just the client. Hermann and Carter (1994) conceptualize illness and its "reverberations" among the family using Dillon's (1990) concept of the "illness family." Shifts and breakdowns in interlocking obligations (e.g., no one in the family makes outside plans without checking with other family members first) and role reciprocities (e.g., wife takes care of home and children while husband works to financially support the family) causes the whole family system to get "ill" when one member becomes ill. If health care providers assess elements of that system independently, they run the risk of missing crucial information, which will inhibit the client from getting well. Therefore it is important to meet with the family whenever possible.

Features to look for at the time of assessment include (Dillon, 1990):

- Covert agendas among family members (EXAMPLE: A daughter needs her father to get well and not die because she uses him as a buffer between herself and her mother.)
- Hidden loyalties, subsystems, and secondary gains of the sick role (EXAMPLE: A wife with a past history of successfully treated cervical cancer often feels neglected by her husband and children. She has many incidents of unexplainable chest pain and fevers and her family spends much time accompanying her to emergency rooms or doctors' offices.)
- Idiosyncratic meanings of the illness and wellness as they affect the family identity and functioning (EXAMPLE: The father in an Italian immigrant family is diagnosed with tuberculosis. The entire family is ashamed and will not tell their neighbors his exact illness because they believe others will think his illness resulted from the family being "dirty" and "unclean.")

The implications for the health care providers are striking: the family of the client may need as much if not more care than the client. If their needs are not attended to (i.e., caregiver burnout or excessive stress), they may experience physical or mental illness, and the client's needs may be unmet. The acuteness or the chronicity of the illness dictates to a certain extent the repercussions of that illness in the family; the more chronic the illness, the more serious the disruption. At a minimum, family members experience disruption in child care, of school and work schedules, and of eating and sleeping schedules while they visit in the hospital or at home, or they may deal with the adjuvant therapy stage of the illness, as in the following example:

Sandra M. is 55 years old, has multiple myeloma, has had a bone marrow transplant, and is now in need of posttransplant follow-up care in a nearby apartment provided by the hospital. She needs around-the-clock care, and her 70-year-old husband John has agreed to be her caregiver. However, before her illness, Sandra had taken care of all domestic matters, and John had never shopped or prepared meals. While Sandra was in the hospital, John ate all his meals in restaurants. Now he is faced with learning these new domestic chores while being stressed by his wife's illness. In addition, he has poor eyesight and cannot see well enough to drive at night. If his wife has a medical emergency during the night, he would not be able to see well enough to drive her to the hospital.

The family is the largest provider of health care, not the hospital, home care agency, physician, or nurse. (Ellers, 1993), and although the family and the client may agree that family members are the optimal care providers, families often pay a high price for delivery of this care. For example, results from data collected during the Support to Understand Prognoses and Preferences for Outcomes and Risks of Treatment (SUPPORT) show that (1) one third of the 2,129 clients and/or surrogates surveyed needed considerable caregiving from the family; (2) in 20% of the cases a family member had to quit work or make another life change to provide for a seriously ill family member; and (3) 31% reported the loss of most or all of their life savings, whereas another 29% reported the loss of a major source of income (Covinsky et al., 1994). As the baby boomers age, the need for family caregivers will only increase.

Loss of Productivity

A 1994 issue of *Morbidity and Mortality Weekly Report* reported that "an estimated 35 [to] 40 million persons in the United States have a disability; estimated direct and indirect annual costs related to disability (including medical expenses and lost work days) total $170 billion." This statistic does not convey the personal meaning that diseases have on one's productivity and life, as shown in the following example:

Mr. H. is a 38-year-old married businessman with severe familial hyperlipidemia, who had coronary artery bypass surgery (four grafts) 6 months ago. Now two of the grafts are clogged shut. Although he runs his privately owned business out of his home, currently he is only able to work an hour and then must rest an hour. His wife has had to go to work at the local supermarket and can no longer provide child care for their 4-year-old son. The next medical step is a heart transplant, and there is no certainty that his body will accept the new heart.

Because productivity is a central aspect of most adults' self-esteem and self-image, its loss or decrease can initiate grieving especially when the loss is likely to continue and increase as with multiple sclerosis (MS) and AIDS; this is just the beginning. Managing the emotional aspects of physical health problems is not just a luxury. To not address these issues is to deny their profound effects on an individual's health and society's economy.

STRESSORS ASSOCIATED WITH COPING WITH PHYSICAL ILLNESS
Illness as a Crisis

Illness can usually be defined as a crisis, and generally, it is an unanticipated situational crisis (see Chapter 10).

Acute Illness

An acute illness is one caused by a disease that produces symptoms and signs soon after exposure to the cause, that runs a short course, and from which there is usually a full recovery or an abrupt termination in death

(Phipps, 1995). Not every acute illness is a crisis. The severity of that illness and how much it affects an individual's self-esteem, body image, sense of competence, productivity, sense of powerlessness, sense of loss and guilt, and the relationship with the family is important in calculating how stressful that acute illness will be to the client and family. Furthermore, how clients cognitively appraise (Lazarus and Folkman, 1984) the stressors also plays a large part in determining the impact on them of those stressors and how effectively they will be resolved (see Chapter 14).

Catastrophic Illness

Catastrophic illness is any sudden, often great, medical event that can end in a substantial or ruinous condition (i.e., death or even expense). When a person faces a medical disaster or emergency or is initially given a medical diagnosis such as metastatic cancer or MS, the most common initial reactions are shock, fear, and anxiety. The care team best responds to these reactions with succinct, authoritative, and consistent reassurance. Crisis interventions are appropriate here (see Chapter 10). If these measures prove inadequate, short-acting benzodiazepines can be used with caution; if the reactions escalate into panic or a psychotic loss of control, fast-acting antipsychotic medications used wisely can be helpful (Kaplan, Sadock, and Grebb, 1994).

Chronic Illness

Acute illness can become chronic illness. A chronic illness is one caused by disease that produces symptoms and signs within a variable period, that runs a long course, and from which there is only partial recovery. (Phipps, 1995). Chronic illness is on the rise. Although scientists have been unable to "cure" most illnesses today, technology has developed many treatments for diseases that were originally fatal. Cystic fibrosis is an example of a previously fatal pediatric disease, and although all persons with HIV still eventually die, acquired immunodeficiency syndrome (AIDS) is now considered a chronic condition because of the medications and treatments that have been developed since its inception. Furthermore, because the average age of the U.S. population continues to rise, a higher percentage of the population is now at risk for certain chronic diseases such as cancer (Phipps, 1995).

Generally, the stressors associated with having a chronic disease are much the same as previously mentioned: the impact on sense of self, competence and productivity, financial resources, and relationships with family and friends. However, there are some differences between a chronic and an acute illness: (1) Chronic illness involves the loss of a foreseeable future as well as the sense of immediate competency (LeMaistre, 1993);

and (2) chronic illness is usually progressive. In a chronic illness, a person's physical condition does not remain static. There are exacerbations and remissions, but overall, physical abilities tend to deteriorate. With each of these changes, the person must adjust psychologically. The severity and rapidity of these physical changes and losses can easily overwhelm one's coping ability, as in the following example:

Sam K. has had MS for 30 years; the progression initially was slow, but in the last few years, he has had few remissions and many exacerbations. One of his chief coping mechanisms is to continue to work and function as normally as possible.

He owns his own tire business, so he has been able to cope despite his illness. He has had to switch from a walker to a wheelchair and now has periods of incontinence. However, he refuses to stop working, even though it now takes his wife 2 to 3 hours to get him ready to go. His son who works with him often has to change him after he has an incontinent episode.

Recently, he suggested to his wife that they take a cruise together. When his wife tried to talk with him realistically about how difficult this would be for them both, Sam got upset, went to bed, and has refused to eat or get dressed for 1 week. He sleeps 22 hours a day.

Terminal Illness

Any acute or chronic illness can become terminal. A terminal illness ends in death, such as amyotrophic lateral sclerosis (ALS). Western culture is a death-denying culture. Terminal illness forces confronting the denial that somehow death will not occur. Facing a terminal illness primarily means facing grief and loss—the loss of everything one cherishes and holds dear, but mainly the loss of one's existence.

In Lindemann's 1944 classic work on grief, he described the normal symptoms of grief or an uncomplicated grief, that all persons might experience and the abnormal symptoms of grief or a morbid grief reaction that a few persons experience. The families and friends of an individual with a terminal illness grieve as well. Table 32-1 describes some of the grief processes, their characteristics, associated time frames, and special needs and tasks (see Chapter 30).

Generally, the more significant the loss, the more intense the grief feelings and the longer it will take to recover from such a loss. For example, parents whose 7 year old child dies from cancer may grieve more intensely, and take longer to recover than the 84-year-old wife whose husband dies in his sleep. However, as each person lives uniquely, each grieves uniquely. The times, stages, variety of symptoms, and intensity of one's grief vary. Although there is no right or wrong way to grieve, persons who exhibit a number of the abnormal symptoms of grief may need professional assistance to work through that reac-

TABLE 32-1

Grief processes

TIME	CHARACTERISTICS	SPECIAL NEEDS	TASKS
1 week-2 months	Cognitive confusion No full comprehension regarding significance of loss Like a bad dream Numbness, trance-likeness, blunting of feelings, yet sensitive to hurts	Support from loved ones, but not over-support; need emotional distance, and some solitude and privacy	Maintaining integrity of self Trying not to fall apart Carrying out day to day functions
6 months	Most difficult time Shock is diminished Support not available like earlier Aimlessness, depression, loneliness, frenzied activity, apathy, fatigue, loss of appetite, sleeplessness, poor memory, frequent weeping, feelings of craziness, self-pity, anger, guilt, resentment May experience hallucinations or presence of loved one	Desire to talk about deceased and details of death; need reassurance all was done to help the one who died Importance of support groups and individuals Begin to normalize life again.	Admit and accept reality of the loss See the experience in the perspective of one's past, present, and future. Renew relationships
6 months-1 year	Greater sense of peace and stability Regaining sense of a hopeful future Occasional painful memories Mourning process reaching completion	Putting "one's house in order" (financial, legal, and others) Move toward normalization	Seek work or activities to give life meaning Restoration of ego integrity Recognize value of faith

Based on data from Batler, L.R. (1983). Through the valley of shadow. *Frederick, MD: Hidden Valley Press.*

tion. Nurses are often in positions to recognize these problems and offer interventions or an appropriate referral.

Dying and death

Death is an event and a state (Martocchio and Dufault, 1991). Dying is a process of coming to an end. When asked what they feared most about dying, most persons responded that they were worried about being in pain, being alone, and not having "a death with dignity." Denial, anger, bargaining, preparatory depression, and acceptance are five stages a person may endure after receiving an initial diagnosis of a terminal illness. Moving from a position of relatively stable health to the diagnosis of a terminal illness may result not only in feelings of shock or denial but feelings of loneliness, conflict, guilt, and meaninglessness. The person may engage in bargaining with a higher power for a miracle cure or at a minimum, extra time to be present at a special event such as a child's graduation or wedding. Gradual realization that death is an inevitable consequence is often accompanied by preparatory depression that precedes movement toward acceptance. This stage is usually characterized by increased self-awareness and self-reliance as well as contact with others. There are highs and lows associated with this process; persons do not proceed in a linear fashion through these stages. As with grief, individuals have their own unique trajectories during these stages. There is no right or wrong way to die. Health care providers need to respect the ways in which persons do manage their dying. Box 32-1 lists some helpful interventions to use with dying clients and their families.

Joseph R. is a 64-year-old married man with end-stage, non-Hodgkin lymphoma. He does not wish to receive any more treatment and wants to die at home with his family. His wife works, and although she is in agreement with his wish to come home, she realizes that she cannot be his caregiver because it is too painful for her. He has two grown daughters who are willing to care for him at home.

A referral is made to their local hospice team by Joseph's oncologist. A hospice nurse makes the initial visit and assessment with the family and arranges for the addition of a

---

Box 32-1

Interventions For Use With Clients Who Are Dying

HELPING THE DYING PATIENT

- When you walk into the client's room, be prepared to sit and talk.
- Assess the client's understanding. Begin by asking their understanding of the situation.
- Listen for feelings. Do not assume clients fear what you fear.
- Encourage expression of feelings.
- Avoid "saccharine" reassurance or brutal confrontation.
- Let the client proceed at own pace and expect momentary reversals and inconsistencies.
- Treat comatose clients as if they were conscious.

HELPING THE FAMILY

- Get to know the family members.
- Listen carefully to feelings; encourage expression.
- Encourage family to share in the care of the client.
- Encourage communication between family and client.

HELPFUL STATEMENTS

- "Is there something you would like to talk about?"
- "How do you feel about being in (specify setting)?"
- "Tell me more about how you feel."
- "I'm sorry you have pain."
- "I'm sorry I can't change things for you,"
- "What has your physician told you about your condition?"
- "How do you understand your condition?"

---

home health aide to provide his physical care. She contacts the oncologist for additional pain medication to make Joseph more comfortable. She sets up a visit with the social worker to help arrange the family's financial affairs, and she suggests the involvement of the hospice priest to help Joseph's wife cope with her grief. The nurse provides support and encouragement to Joseph and his daughters; he died within three weeks of leaving the hospital. Joseph was grateful to die pain-free, in his own bed, surrounded by his family. The family was appreciative that they could give him the death he wanted and for the support of the hospice staff that allowed them to do this.

WHERE DO THESE CLIENTS PRESENT?

For persons with heart disease, cancer, cerebrovascular disorders, chronic obstructive pulmonary disease (COPD), pneumonia, influenza, diabetes mellitus, and HIV infections, the initial diagnosis and treatment is made by a primary care provider. These clients have presenting symptoms for treatment in a variety of settings: private offices, clinics, an emergency room, homeless shelters, and prisons. Following initial treatment, these clients may be followed by that initial primary care provider, referred to a specialist, admitted to the hospital, or followed closely by a home health care service (see Chapter 21).

Where a person is treated and cared for when he or she becomes ill can add another level of stress to the experience of being physically ill. Each setting has its own unique set of attributes, advantages, and disadvantages. Box 32-2 provides some strategies to prevent regression during hospitalization.

CLINICAL PROFILES

The health problems with a psychosocial component that will be developed in the clinical profiles section of this chapter will include psychophysiological disorders, HIV/AIDS, cancer and somatoform disorders.

Psychophysiological Disorders

Psychophysiological disorders refer to those physical disorders with etiologic factors that are related in part to emotional factors. These disorders are also known as psychosomatic disorders. They continue to be a controversial and puzzling group of disorders because it is hard to clearly differentiate the role played by heredity or other biological factors versus psychosocial factors. Predisposing hereditary factors and psychological personality features are implicated in the development of particular "diseases." Chronic, severe, and perceived stress also play a causative role in the development of many somatic diseases (Kaplan, Sadock, and

Box 32-2

Strategies to Prevent Regression During Hospitalization

Be aware that clients often react to hospitalization by regressing emotionally and behaviorally.

Allow clients as much control as possible:

a. When to do things, such as bathe, have a treatment, go for a test, rest
b. To refuse certain procedures or to question the necessity of certain hospital routines, such as routine vital signs during the night, a 5 AM bath
c. To wear own clothes when possible

Educate clients as much as they can manage, encourage questions about treatment choices so that they can be active participants in the treatment, not passive victims of it.

Address clients by their last name (e.g., Mr. Logan, not Bill) until you know the client better or are invited to become more familiar.

Do not talk to clients from a superior position such as standing over the bed; try to be at their level.

Grebb, 1994) (see Chapter 14). Consequently, an overweight 35-year-old woman, whose mother and grandmother had gall stones, finds herself having her first gall stone attack after eating a late lunch of a greasy cheese and refried bean burrito in the car after a long, stress-filled day on her new job.

Furthermore, the impact of psychosocial dynamics on the immune system has been shown to affect both health and illness. These psychosocial processes include one's life experiences, one's current life stressors, and one's personality traits. Two other factors have a role in this discussion:

- Physical illness itself can precipitate a variety of psychological states that have an adverse affect on the disease process and in some cases, can produce symptoms more threatening than the original one (Green, 1994). An example would be a suicidal depression in a client with advanced metastatic lung cancer.
- Compliance with the prescribed treatment regimen is influenced by issues within the unconscious, as well as sociocultural norms (Green, 1994). For example, a gay man with HIV who unconsciously feels guilty for his sexual preference often misses his prophylactic pentamidine (Nebupent) treatments because he "forgets" he has the appointment.

The *Diagnostic and Statistical Manual of Mental Disorders, Fourth edition,* (DSM-IV) (American Psychiatric Association [APA], 1994) has defined the category of

Psychological Factors Affecting a Medical Condition (PFAMC). This category specifies the influence of psychological processes on the initiation or exacerbation of physical illness. In the past, these conditions have been called psychosomatic or psychophysiologic and have included such disorders as tension headache, diabetes, angina pectoris, ulcerative colitis, and many others (Walker and Katon, 1994). The new category allows the provider to specify a wider variety of psychological stimuli and health problems. See Table 32-2 for examples of psychosomatic diseases, the current implicated predisposing factors, psychological factors, and treatment recommendations.

In thinking about the psychosocial components of physical illness, there are two other diseases and one category of disorders that are worthy of more explanation: HIV/AIDS, cancer, and the somatoform disorders.

HIV/AIDS

In October 1993, the Centers for Disease Control and Prevention (CDC) had documented 340,000 cases of AIDS in the United States with the projection that by the end of 1994, there would be more than 400,000 AIDS cases in the United States with more than 300,000 deaths. The number of people estimated to have the virus is more than 1,176,000 (CDC, 1993).

Generally persons with HIV are young:

- 21% are in their twenties
- 47% are in their thirties
- 21% in their forties

Originally, those infected with the virus were from socially stigmatized groups: homosexual men, intravenous (IV) drug users, and persons of color. Today however, adolescents, women, and heterosexuals have a growing incidence of the disease.

"The complexity and multiplicity of problems confronting people with HIV infection and the psychological fear it engenders affect every aspect of a person's life" (Flaskerud, 1995). No other public health problem has had such ramifications. Specific features of AIDS that contribute to the unique psychological, social, and psychiatric aspects of the disease are as follows:

- Those affected are young.
- The disease is incurable, demands significant behavioral changes, and threatens all intimate relationships.
- The disease may identify the person as being part of a stigmatized group.
- The stigma associated with the infection alienates most persons.
- The person with AIDS is often "blamed" for having the illness because of the moral implications of the illness.

TABLE 32-2

Clinical profiles of common psychosomatic disorders

PREDISPOSING FACTORS	PSYCHOLOGICAL FEATURES	TREATMENT
Gastrointestinal		
Peptic ulcers		
Genetically predisposed; preexisting organ damage; bacterial infectious agent, *Helico pylori* implications	Unconscious conflict; stress, anxiety	Medications-both to treat the excess acid and the bacteria, dietary restrictions, biofeedback, relaxation therapy, psychotherapy
Cardiovascular		
Hypertension		
Suspected familial genetic predisposition	Outwardly congenial, compliant, and compulsive; occurs in Type A personalities	Antihypertension medication; behavioral techniques (e.g., biofeedback, relaxation, meditation)
Coronary artery disease (CAD)		
Age, gender, race and family history, poor nutrition, obesity, cigarette smoking	Type A personality, stressful life	Medication: cardiac, anti-anxiety, pain; stress reduction techniques, supportive treatment
Cardiovascular-Musculoskeletal		
Migraine headaches		
Family history; women more than men, certain foods: chocolate, nuts, onions	Obsessional personality, overly controlled, perfectionistic, with severe nonspecific emotional stress or conflict	Cafergot, antidepressants, and analgesics; behavioral techniques and psychotherapy
Cluster headaches		
Alcohol, nitrates, begin in early adulthood and occur in middle-age men	Tension and stress	Narcotic analgesics, behavioral techniques to reduce tension
Tension headaches		
Fatigue and stress	Type A personality most prone; frequently associated with anxiety and depression	Nonnarcotic analgesics, behavioral techniques to deal with stress, antidepressants if appropriate, psychotherapy
Respiratory		
Asthma		
Genetic, allergic, infections; acute and chronic stress	No specific personality type, perhaps excessive dependency needs	Bronchodilators, antiinflammatory agents, preventing infections, avoiding environmental irritants; systematic desensitization and hypnosis
Autoimmune		
Inflammatory bowel disease		
Familial incidence, genetic factors are significant	Compulsive personality traits-neat, orderly, clean, punctual, hyperintellectual, timid, inhibited in expressing anger, nonspecific stress	Antiinflammatory medication, anticholinergic, antidiarrheal agents, supportive psychotherapy during exacerbations, interpretive during quiescent periods.
Lupus		
Genetic, infectious agents, environmental irritants, physical or emotional stress, exposure to ultraviolet B radiation, certain medication, women more than men	No specific personality type	Antiinflammatory medication, rest, exercise, stress management, support groups, support of psychotherapy.

TABLE 32-2—cont'd

Clinical profiles of common psychosomatic disorders

PREDISPOSING FACTORS	PSYCHOLOGICAL FEATURES	TREATMENT
Rheumatoid arthritis		
Hereditary, allergic, immunological	Psychological distress	Analgesics, antiinflammatory agents, rest, exercise, support groups, supportive psychotherapy
Integumentary		
Psychosomatic skin disorders (generalized psychogenic pruritus)		
External or internal causes (e.g., dermatoses or DM)	Emotional conflicts such as repressed rage or anxiety, strong needs for affection and frustration of that need	Medication for symptoms of pain and itching, psychotherapy
Neurological		
Multiple sclerosis		
Familial tendency resulting from common hereditary and environmental factors, women more than men, current theories implicate virus or autoimmunity as causation	Physical or emotional stress	Symptomatic; during acute phase controlling exacerbation; in remission, preventing exacerbation

- Uncertainty is the hallmark of this disease causing great psychological distress.
- Persons with HIV are vulnerable to feelings of guilt, self-hatred, rejection, and ostracism, as well as the fear, anxiety, depression, and anger that often occur with a life-threatening illness.
- Mental illness (including anxiety, depression and delirium) may be exacerbated by HIV, and mental illness may prompt behaviors that cause HIV; more than 80% of person with AIDS, have AIDS-related dementia (see Chapter 31). Virtually all persons with AIDS experience anxiety and/or depression generated by the sudden or gradual physical, cognitive, and social losses experienced by this client population as they inevitably move toward the terminal stage of their illness.
- The current health care system and providers dealing with those with HIV are overloaded by the demands of this illness for medical, psychological, and social resources.
- HIV has a high social and political profile that may be stressful to those with it and that may stir up the fears of the public.

Managing the care of those with HIV/AIDS is often overwhelming to everyone involved. Often cared for by significant others and family members, the reality of caregiver burden is a significant issue for nurses to address with caretakers. Providing continuing support, understanding, and an appreciation of all that persons with AIDS and their caregivers face is crucial.

Cancer

As the second leading cause of death in the United States, with one out of every three persons predicted to be diagnosed with some form of cancer, cancer is a widespread disease Everyone fears it, and everyone is vulnerable to it. Although definite causes are still unproven, many factors are implicated: genetics, high-fat and low-fiber diets, environmental exposures, and cigarette smoking to name a few. There are specific stresses associated with a cancer diagnosis in general, including the following (Lederberg, 1990):

- Cancer is universal, unpredictable, and often deadly.
- The characteristics of cancer treatments are stressful.
- Two out of the three major treatments, chemotherapy and radiation, are very dangerous and can cause serious, at times, life-threatening side effects. Bone marrow transplant can be called an "absurdly stressful" treatment. The third treatment, surgery, often causes pain and sometimes disfigurement as with head and neck cancer.
- Even the non–life-threatening side effects, nausea, vomiting, and hair loss are distressing and uncomfortable.
- Much of cancer treatment is palliative (supportive), not curative.
- There is much uncertainty about treatment decision making; this ambiguity is hard to tolerate and is easily interpreted as "experimentation."
- The pain from tumors or as a treatment side effect is a great fear for those with cancer.

Common initial reactions to a cancer diagnosis are shock, fear, dread, numbness, denial, and/or a sense of impending death. These reactions are in response to the above-mentioned stresses associated with the diagnosis. Although much progress has been made in the understanding and treatment of cancer, the historical view still has a powerful impact. Abhorrence and fear were the common reactions in the early part of the twentieth century (Holland, 1990). Some of that reaction lingers to color today's response and interferes with early detection.

Recurrence can bring the experience of acute emotional turmoil similar to that felt on initial diagnoses. However, Weisman and Worden (1986) found that those who expected recurrence experienced less distress than those who were surprised. Recurrence changes cancer from an awful, dreaded acute illness to a chronic illness that will probably end in death (Hindes et al., 1996).

Somatoform Disorders

Although strictly a psychiatric diagnosis (APA, 1994), the somatoform disorders are included in this chapter because they almost exclusively present as physical illness or symptoms in a medical or surgical setting. *Somatoform* disorders are *characterized by physical symptoms for which there is no adequate medical ex-*

TABLE 32-3

Somatoform disorders

WHERE PRESENT	CLINICAL PRESENTATION	MANAGEMENT STRATEGIES
Somatization Disorder Emergency rooms, general medical or surgical offices, hospitals	Multiple physical symptoms—recurrent and chronic; sickly by history	One primary caregiver Regularly scheduled brief visits at monthly intervals Hear complaints as emotional explanations of psychic pain
Conversion Disorder Emergency rooms, medical hospitals	One or more motor or sensory neurological symptoms (e.g., paralysis, parathesias, and/or blindness) with no identifiable physiological cause	Hypnosis Anxiolytics Behavioral relaxation Supportive or behavioral therapy
Hypochondriasis General medical office or clinic	Disease concern or preoccupation	Document symptoms Psychosocial review Stress reduction techniques Education re: coping with a chronic illness Group psychotherapy Regular physical examination
Body Dysmorphic Disorder Dermatologists, internists or plastic surgeons	Subjective feelings of ugliness or concern with body defect	Therapeutic alliance Stress management Psychotherapy Antidepressant medication
Pain Disorder General medical offices, emergency rooms	Pain syndrome simulated	Therapeutic alliance Redefine goals of treatment Antidepressant medication

planation (Kaplan, Sadock, and Grebb, 1994). The clients experience enough physical distress to impair everyday functioning. They convince medical staff to treat them either medically or surgically. However, the effects of these treatments are short-lived and need to be repeated or new treatments tried. Unfortunately, since the cause of the distress and dysfunctionality is psychologically based rather then physically, a "cure" is never achieved, unless these clients allow themselves to be treated for their psychiatric disorder. However, there is much resistance to this. Table 32-3 lists the five somatoform disorders and pertinent clinical features.

The Nursing Process

Assessment

Nurses always need to assess how the client and family are coping with the physical illness. Many disturbing feelings, responses, and experiences are associated with acute and chronic illness and the treatments they require. The psychosocial assessment needs to address not only the particular emotional response of the client, but also where that client is on the illness path:

- At the initial diagnosis of an acute illness
- After a period of adjustment (e.g., 3 to 4 weeks) to the illness
- After a recurrence of the initial illness or when it is clear that the acute illness is now a chronic one
- When the illness becomes terminal

Box 32-3 provides specific questions nurses can use to assess the psychosocial state of the client at each of these stages.

Clients and their families commonly experience: fear, anxiety, sadness, depression, anger, hope, grief, despair, courage, pride, love, helplessness, envy, and loneliness—any feeling that can be imagined possible when physically ill. The most common however are probably anxiety, depression, and grief or sadness over lifestyle and physical losses and changes.

Anxiety

Anxiety is a universal experience. It is a normal reaction to stress or threat. Anxiety occurs at any phase in the health-illness process. Since it is usually not in response to a discrete event, anxiety can be difficult to cope with. One of the main tasks of the nursing staff is to assess clients' anxiety. Excessive anxiety interferes with the ability to hear, process information, make decisions, and act in a logical way. Thus anxiety can interfere with daily functioning and can lead to nonadherence (see Chapter 22).

BOX 32-3

Assessment Questions

On initial diagnosis with a physical illness:
- What information do you have about the diagnosis?
- What kind of information would be helpful at this time?
- Do you understand the procedures, tests, and treatments?
- What other information do you need about them?
- How are you feeling about the diagnosis?
- What is most distressing about the diagnosis?
- What is helping you cope right now?
- How have you coped with difficult experiences like this in the past?
- Are there other supports you would find helpful right now?

After a period of adjustment to the illness:
- How much energy, fatigue, or pain are you experiencing?
- To what extent are you able to carry out your previous roles?
- What kind of help do you receive from your family and friends?
- To what extent has life returned to normal for you?

After an exacerbation of the illness:
- How are you feeling about the exacerbation?
- How surprised were you by it?
- How has your attitude been affected? Are you hopeful or discouraged?
- What information do you need at this point?
- What support are you getting, and is it adequate?

When the illness is terminal:
- How are you feeling physically and emotionally?
- What are you needing from your family now?
- What are you needing from your caregiver now?
- If you have any unfinished business, what do you need to take care of that business?

Adapted from Northhouse, L.L., & Lancaster, D. (1994). Coping. In J. Gross & L.B. Johnson (Eds.). Handbook of oncology nursing. (2nd ed.). Boston: Jones and Bartlett.

The Nursing Process

Depression

Depression in the medically ill is a well-documented fact. However, accurate diagnosis and treatment of that depression is less well-established. Many factors confound the accurate diagnosis and treatment of depression in the medically ill. Some nonpsychiatric providers do not distinguish *feelings* of depression, sadness, having "the blues," and normal grief reactions from the *disease* depression. Others do recognize the difference, but fail to recognize there are treatment possibilities for both, though they may differ in nature. Recognition of these differences and the nurse's own reaction to these feel-

TABLE 32-4

Phases of the transition model

PHASES	DESCRIPTION	TASKS/STRATEGIES
Endings-the old way is over	Assess what is lost, what has actually ended How much functioning is compromised? How are relationships actually affected? Are these things gone for good or merely a time?	Grieve for what is actually lost Mark the ending in some symbolic way, (e.g., a ceremony, plant something to commemorate the loss)
Neutral zone or wilderness—the place between the old and new	Two aspects: 1. An uncomfortable, confusing time, characterized by apathy, confusion, being "out of sorts", not very productive 2. A time of opportunity when "all bets are off" and new ways of being or relating can be tried here	Understand this aspect of transition and normalize the feelings Recognize the normal slump that's part of this phase Create temporary structures, responsibilities, ways of doing things—a set of "winter rules" Provide people with support and encouragement to endure, this phase will not last forever
New beginning	The new state of affairs Begins with a new idea or vision Needs the step-by-step details added to make the vision real Need multidimensional plan: communication, leadership, training, incentives and ritual	Maximize what can be in the new situation Acknowledge all it took and takes to be here What are new ways persons can now be involved? Are there models to pattern oneself after? Provide assistance for those who doubt they can handle the change; provide coaching or counseling Choose a symbol to celebrate the new identity

Adapted from Bridges, W. (1991). Managing transitions: Making the most of change. *Reading, MA: Addison-Wesley.*

The Nursing Process

ings facilitates an accurate assessment of the client's mood and affect. (See Chapter 30 for specific assessment questions for depression.)

Change, Loss, and Grief

In his book on managing transitions, Bridges (1991) talks about "change" as a discrete event that occurs, and the process that one goes through about each "change" is called *transition*. There are three phases to transition: endings, the neutral zone or wilderness, and beginnings. Persons cycle through these phases as they make changes in their lives. This model is helpful in looking at the changes brought on by physical illness and is shown in Table 32-4 with strategies for each phase.

Pain

Pain may be defined as "an unpleasant sensory and emotional experience associated with actual or potential tissue damage or described in terms of such damage" (International Association for the Study of Pain, Subcommittee on Taxonomy, 1979). The anatomy and physiology of pain have been studied extensively.

An individual's perception of pain and appreciation of its meanings are complex and involve psychological and emotional processes in addition to the neurological ones.

Pain commonly accompanies physical illness. Acute pain is usually temporary, has a sudden onset and subsides with or without treatment. Examples include an ordinary headache, or the pain of a traumatic injury or from a kidney stone. Chronic pain is ongoing, may start gradually, may persist or recur over time, may last more than 6 months, and is more difficult to manage. Examples include, severe rheumatoid arthritis, advanced cancer, or transmandibular joint (TMJ) pain. Each person is the authority on his or her own pain. Through education, growing numbers of health care providers understand this and base their treatment of pain on this belief. However, too many providers have outmoded ideas of addiction and stoicism and ineffectively manage their clients' pain. A structured assessment can help nurses focus on their patient's experience of pain rather than their own biases.

An initial evaluation of pain includes (Agency for Health Care Policy and Research [AHCPR], Guidelines, 1994):

- A detailed history, including an assessment of the pain intensity and character.
- A physical examination, emphasizing the neurological examination.

- A psychosocial assessment
- Appropriate diagnostic workup to determine the cause of the pain

Box 32-4 gives specific questions to ask during this initial assessment.

Ongoing pain needs assessment and documentation:

- At regular intervals after treatment has begun
- With each new pain reported
- At a designated time frame, after each pharmacological or nonpharmacological intervention (e.g., 15 to

Box 32-4

Questions for Pain Assessment
Pain Intensity and Character

ONSET AND TEMPORAL PATTERN

- When did your pain start?
- How often does it occur?
- Has its intensity changed?

LOCATION

- Where is your pain?
- Is it at more than one site?

DESCRIPTION

- What does your pain feel like?
- What words describe your pain?
- On a scale of 0 to 10, with 0 being no pain and 10 being the worst pain you can imagine, how much does it hurt right now? How much does it hurt at its worst? At its best?

AGGRAVATING AND RELIEVING FACTORS

- What makes your pain better?
- What makes it worse?

PREVIOUS TREATMENT

- What types of treatments have you tried to relieve your pain? How effective were or are they?

EFFECT

- How does the pain affect your physical and social functioning?

From Jacox, A., et al. (1994). Management of cancer pain. *Clinical practice guideline no. 9. AHCPR Publ No. 94-0592. Rockville, MD. Agency for Health Care Policy and Research, U.S. Department of Health and Human Services, Public Health Service.*

The Nursing Process

30 minutes after parenteral drug therapy and 1 hour after oral administration).

Delirium

Delirium is another common disorder in the physically ill, too often underrecognized and underdiagnosed in the medical setting (see Chapter 31).

Screening Tools

There are various tools available to the nurse or other health care providers to more accurately assess common responses to physical illness. These tools are adjuncts to the provider's interview, own personal observations of the client and/or the family, or findings on physical examination or diagnostic workup. Table 32-5 lists screening tools and their purposes.

Focused Assessment

In addition to the other specific assessment questions already proposed, the following questions are also helpful in a psychosocial assessment of the client and family or significant other.

1. How long have you been ill?
2. How are you feeling about being ill?
3. How has being ill changed your life?
4. How have you coped with these life changes?
5. How would you describe your quality of life?
6. Besides not being ill, what one or two things would you change to improve your quality of life?

Nursing Diagnosis

Many nursing diagnoses are applicable to the psychosocial components of physical illness. It is important to specify how the problem or diagnosis relates directly to the physical issue, (e.g., body image disturbance related to the loss of right leg following a motorcycle accident). A second example might be anxiety related to the experience of rigors as a side effect while receiving amphotericin B (Fungizone) during bone marrow transplant. Table 32-6 lists selected NANDA nursing diagnoses applicable to these populations and their families, correlated with the diagnostic criteria for psychological factors affecting medical conditions.

Outcome Identification

In the same way that nursing diagnosis needs to specifically relate to the particular psychosocial problem of the physical illness, so do the outcomes for the nursing interventions. In the example of the man who has a distorted body image, following a leg amputation, to say the outcome will be a restored body image is too global. Better choices for short-term goals are as follows:

- Being able to look at his wound
- Being able to dress his wound
- Being able to talk about the loss of his leg and what it means to him and how it will affect his daily life

Being realistic about what can be accomplished by who the client actually is, not the "ideal" client one reads

TABLE 32-5

Screening tools

TOOL	PURPOSE
Pain Management Log	Rates pain on an assessment scale
	Record of drug/non-drug pain interventions and response
Social Readjustment Scale	Measures impact of cumulative life events on a person
	Predicts susceptibility to illness
	Education tool for preventive measures
Life Orientation Scale	Measures optimism
	Could be useful in predicting hopefulness or hopelessness regarding illness and coping

The Nursing Process

TABLE 32-6

Selected NANDA nursing diagnoses correlated with DSM-IV criteria for psychological factors affecting medical conditions

DSM-IV DIAGNOSES AND CRITERIA*	NANDA DIAGNOSES†
. . . [Specified Psychological Factor] Affecting. . . [Indicate the General Medical Condition]	
A. A general medical condition (coded on Axis III) is present.	
B. Psychological factors adversely affect the general medical condition in one of the following ways:	
(1) the factors have influenced the course of the general medical condition as shown by a close temporal association between the psychological factors and the development or exacerbation of, or delayed recovery from, the general medical condition	
(2) the factors interfere with the treatment of the general medical condition	
(3) the factors constitute additional health risks for the individual	
(4) stress-related physiological responses precipitate or exacerbate symptoms of the general medical condition	
Choose name based on the nature of the psychological factors (if more than one factor is present, indicate the most prominent):	
Mental Disorder Affecting. . . *[Indicate the General Medical Condition]* (e.g., an Axis I disorder such as Major Depressive Disorder delaying recovery from a myocardial infarction)	Adjustment, impaired
Psychological Symptoms Affecting. . . *[Indicate the General Medical Condition]* (e.g., depressive symptoms delaying recovery from surgery; anxiety exacerbating asthma)	Anxiety (specify level)
Personality Traits or Coping Style Affecting. . . *[Indicate the General Medical Condition]* (e.g., pathological denial of the need for surgery in a patient with cancer; hostile, pressured behavior contributing to cardiovascular disease)	Coping, ineffective individual
Maladaptive Health Behaviors Affecting. . . *[Indicate the General Medical Condition]* (e.g., overeating; lack of exercise; unsafe sex)	Denial, ineffective
Stress-Related Physiological Response Affecting. . . *[Indicate the General Medical Condition]* (e.g., stress-related exacerbations of ulcer, hypertension, arrhythmia, or tension headache)	Hopelessness
Other or Unspecified Psychological Factors Affecting. . . *[Indicate the General Medical Condition]* (e.g., interpersonal, cultural, or religious factors)	Spiritual distress

*Reprinted with permission from American Psychiatric Association. (1994). Diagnostic and statistical manual of mental disorders, fourth edition. Washington, DC.
†From North American Nursing Diagnosis Association. (1994). NANDA nursing diagnoses: Definitions & classification, 1995-1996. St. Louis: Mosby.

The Nursing Process

NURSING CARE PLAN

Woman With Breast Cancer

NURSING ASSESSMENT DATA

Subjective: "I feel so bad; I thought I'd beat it. It's the worst thing that could have happened, but I'm sort of relieved. I know what's ahead. I just want as much time as I have left to be with my husband and kids." *Objective:* A 41-year-old, married woman, with two children, ages 11 and 8; status postmastectomy of right breast, followed by chemotherapy treatments. One year posttreatment, metastases diagnosed in right lung and bones. She is tearful, with wringing hands, sighing, and shaking foot. *DSM-IV diagnosis:* Adjustment disorder with mixed emotional features.

NANDA Diagnosis: Grieving, anticipatory, related to potential losses

Outcomes	Interventions	Rationale	Evaluation
Short term	• Develop nurse-client relationship.	• Developing trust and communication are prerequisites to assisting the client in meeting the outcomes of the master care plan.	**Short term**
1. Will begin to verbalize feelings about losses and potential losses with her clinic nurse *at weekly appointments.*			1, 2, 3. Met by the end of the current visit.
2. Client will assess with clinic nurse how sadness is impinging *on her immediate functioning.*	• Assess the effects of the client's mood on her ability to get home, immediately care for her children, attend to her immediate responsibilities.	• Unresolved or dysfunctional grieving interferes with functioning.	4. Met in 1 week.
3. Client will make appropriate, immediate plans to deal *with the results of that assessment.*	• Problem solve with the client on her immediate resources to help care for her and her family.	• Crisis intervention may be the necessary first step in supporting the client after hearing of her recurrence.	5. Met in 2 weeks.
4. Client will assess with clinic nurse how grief and/or increasing physical disability affect daily activities with family and her other responsibilities, *on the next clinic visit.*	• Will consult with members of multidisciplinary team to assess other resources available to the client.	• Coordinating communication and planning with other members of the multidisciplinary team are part of the nurse's overall and case management role, as well as his/her ethical/legal responsibility.	
5. On the next two clinic visits, client will plan strategies with clinic nurse to minimize the effects of her grief and declining physical functioning *on her daily activities.*	• Assess the client's coping skills and reinforce those that help her to function optimally; suggest other ways of managing for the times when she gets immobilized.	• Supporting the client's optimum independence and autonomy has been shown to increase one's ability to cope with difficult events.	
	• Will assess timing of long-term planning with client regarding ongoing grief work and plans for her death. Help client make plans so that she can process the data and its effect on her and her family (see Box 32-2).	• One's ability to deal with one's own death depends on many intrapsychic and interpersonal issues; each person deals with these as best they can in as timely a manner as they can. It is the nurses responsibility to understand and	

The Nursing Process

NURSING CARE PLAN

Woman With Breast Cancer—cont'd

Outcomes	Interventions	Rationale	Evaluation
Long term 1. Maintains maximum level of functioning for as long as possible. 2. Demonstrates increasing acceptance of the loss of her life and future. 3. Makes appropriate plans for the care of her children, her funeral, to deal with her unfinished business.		honor that intrapsychic timetable and not impose an external idea of "how one should die."	**Long-term** 1. Currently being met. 2. Partially met; client is reluctant to consciously feel much sadness (a) because she still feels really good physically and she is avoiding feeling bad until she has to, and (b) she is afraid it will upset her husband and children. Continue to gently explore anticipatory grief and remind client that family may be upset and afraid to talk with her. 3. Not met for reasons above and client's own denial about the terminal nature of her condition. Honor client's own defenses since they are not adversely affecting her seeking of treatment. Consult with team for other ideas.

about in nursing textbooks is a goal. The client and the nurse can both be successful in setting and reaching goals.

Planning

The plan of care reflects a variety of factors including the nature of the health problem—acute or chronic; the stage of illness—initial, recurring, or terminal; the client's age, family role, and coping skills; and available support systems. Where treatment of the health problem will occur is also a consideration. The nursing care plan beginning on p. 706 for a client with metastatic breast cancer

illustrates how many of the above factors are incorporated into the plan of care.

Implementation
Counseling

The goal of this strategy is to offer time-limited (1 to 25 sessions), focus-specific attention to a particular problem affecting the person's health. Cognitive therapy, for example, which focuses on how a person thinks about something and then how that thinking affects their feelings and actions, is an effective brief therapy model. If the person's thought are distorted, this distorted think-

The Nursing Process

ing will negatively affect feelings and behaviors. According to cognitive theory, changing the way we think about something, changes our feelings and behaviors.

Cognitive therapy involves four processes: (1) eliciting an automatic thought, (2) reality testing that automatic thought, (3) identifying underlying distorted assumptions, and (4) reality testing the validity of the distorted assumptions. For example, a client who had a transfusion reaction in the past becomes anxious about having another transfusion, believing, "the worst will happen, I'm sure I'll have another reaction, these kinds of things always happen to me." The nurse can suggest that the client "reframe" her expectation. To do so the client would have to counter the negative, defeatist thinking of "the worst will happen" to "that was just an isolated incident; I am sure this blood is fine and I will have an uneventful experience" (see Chapter 30).

Cognitive therapy is most helpful for persons who are anxious about specific treatment issues or who are depressed about their illness and the changes it has brought to their lives, as in the following example:

> A 38-year-old man was recently diagnosed with HIV. Currently, he is immobilized by fear that he is going to die soon. He has not been to work for 1 week. He feels his life is over and believes his current lover will leave him if told.
>
> Cognitive therapy can help him begin to plan realistic goals about managing his life, work, relationship, and medical status. Role playing would be helpful in practicing what to say to his partner, friends, and employer. He can practice thought stopping and reframing when the intrusive thoughts about dying surface. Diversion can be coupled with this to help reinforce the thought stopping and reframing, and to help him focus on something else. Homework assignments will help him realistically plan one day at a time as well as give him a place to write down his feelings and fears. Every time he accomplishes something on his goal list he is practicing self-reliance techniques and needs to give himself credit for this. Meditation and imagery will help him manage his anxiety and visualize a more optimistic picture of his life and how he wishes to be.

Crisis intervention may be necessary for the physically ill person or the family. Many situations can be perceived as a crisis: initial diagnosis; recurrence or exacerbation of the illness; a sudden "turn for the worst" that may be life-threatening; the death of the client, a close family member, or friend of the family while the client is ill; the loss of critical financial resources, and others. In these situations, the nurse or provider needs to assess the client's immediate needs, and follow this with another evaluation of the situation soon thereafter (see Chapter 10).

Supportive counseling can also be helpful to reinforce a client's coping abilities during a physical illness or with a disability. This is also true for those dealing with change, loss, grief, or lifestyle changes that accompany physical illness. Supportive counseling can take place on an individual basis or in a group. Disease-specific support groups are popular and helpful to support both the client and the family. These groups not only allow for emotional ventilation, but can also increase the coping skills of all involved.

- Man to Man—A prostate cancer support group
- I Can Cope—A breast cancer support group
- Sickle cell support group
- ALS support group
- MS support group

Insight-oriented group therapies and family therapies may also be appropriate interventions for certain people who wish more in-depth work.

Milieu Therapy

This intervention is often taken for granted or assumed to be understood. Many difficulties could be avoided by making aspects of this care explicit. Milieu management includes the following:

- Orientation of the individual and the family to the care setting
- How that setting functions
- What they might expect
- How best to get their needs met within the setting
- The creation of a safe environment, both in terms of the physical nature of that environment, but also in terms of trust in the caregivers in that environment
- The inclusion of the patient and family in treatment planning; this sounds obvious, but is often presumed to be
- The prerogative of the treatment team
- Consideration of culturally diverse responses to illness (See the Cultural Highlights box on p. 709)

If the treatment setting is the home, as is at present more prevalent, it is even more important for nurses to educate all family members on how to create a safe environment while still retaining the atmosphere of the home.

Self-Care Activities

The promotion of maximum independence in activities of daily living (ADLs) has always been part of the nurse's role regardless of setting or diagnosis. It is particularly important for clients with chronic or terminal illness to

The Nursing Process

CULTURAL HIGHLIGHTS

Assessment

Many cultures have strong beliefs in a folk health system which includes beliefs about illnesses, folk remedies, and in folk healers.

- *Curanderismo* is the general term for a folk healing system of Latin America and the curandero/curandera (male/female) is the folk healer (Campinha-Bacote, 1994).
- In the Navaho culture, there is the medicine man/woman or the shaman for the Indians of South America or Borneo.
- Herbal remedies are used for healing in many cultures and in particular to correct an imbalance of the "hot/cold" substances in the body (Maduro, 1983). Many Mexican-Americans and Asian-Americans embrace these beliefs.
- In a South-American Indian tribe, song is used to facilitate a difficult childbirth.

Clients from other cultures are therefore often reluctant to seek out modern medicine and view it as something trustworthy and helpful.

In addition, symptoms of culture-bound illnesses often have symptoms similar to or may mimic many medical conditions. For example, the symptoms of Voodoo illness (from the black Caribbean culture) include nausea, vomiting, diarrhea, convulsions, muscle weakness, and paralysis (Campinha-Bacote,1994).

Both of these phenomena complicate diagnosis and appropriate treatment planning if not understood and integrated into the plan of care.

Diagnosis

In addition to the traditional modern diagnostic tests one would normally order for differential diagnosis, the provider must carefully interview both clients and their families about the circumstances of their symptoms. Was there a frightening experience which produced "Susto," a culture-bound illness, with the symptoms of anorexia, listlessness, and apathy? Did the symptoms include an abruptly appearing fever, rashes, nervousness, or irritability? Has there been a profound conflict with another family member so that the person is suffering from "mal ojo" or evil eye for offending someone perceived to be stronger.

Clarifying the origin of the symptoms will help distinguish a medical illness from a culture-bound illness and from psychopathology.

Interventions

1. Incorporate the folk remedies, beliefs, and the folk healer into the treatment plan as much as possible without compromising care to facilitate compliance.
2. Incorporate the family as much as possible into the care, (e.g., in inpatient settings, Asian families often wish to provide much of the personal care to the client as well as provide the "appropriate" food.
3. Metabolic rates, clinical drug responses, and side effects vary significantly in differing ethnic groups. Medication management needs to take this into account (e.g., Hispanics need lower effective dose levels of antidepressants and have a lower threshold for side effects (Lawson, 1986).

maintain as much of their functional status and quality of life as possible. For example, a 43-year-old man with AIDS has had to stop working as director of social work at a university hospital as a result of the stress and pace of the job and his degree of fatigue. However, most days he feels pretty good and wants to do more than lie around the house. He would like to volunteer at a local homeless shelter 1 half-day per week and also travel some on the weekends, but he is not sure he can manage it. He plans to discuss this with his nurse at the outpatient clinic.

Nurses are also responsible for coordinating the support systems that facilitate that self-care. This is part of the overall nursing role or part of a case management function. Multidisciplinary team planning is crucial to optimize team planning and most frequently initiated by nurses.

Psychobiological Interventions

Psychobiological interventions include medication management, stress management techniques, nutrition and diet regulation, exercise and rest schedules, and interventions to manage the cognitively impaired, either delirium and/or dementia.

Medication management

Medication management addresses client symptomatology. Nurses need to know which medications are most helpful for what symptoms, the potential side effects and other drug interactions. Nurses also need to be aware of the client's other medications, their side effects and possible interactions. The complexity of the psychosocial and physical health problems makes medica-

The Nursing Process

tion management a complicated proposition. If the client is also elderly and on many medications with reactions that potentiate or confound one another, the situation is more complex. Knowledge of and education about medications are clearly an important function of the nurse.

Lorazepam (Ativan) (1-2 mg IV/episode), droperidol (Inaspine) (0.25-50 mg IV/episode), and diphenhidramine HCl (25-50 mg IV/episode) are commonly prescribed for nausea (e.g., from chemotherapy). Opiod and nonopiod analgesics are commonly administered orally, intramuscularly or intravenously for acute pain. In chronic pain, oral, nonopiod, analgesics, such as nonsteroidal anti-inflammatory drugs (NSAIDs) are more common. Tricyclic antidepressants (TCAs) are helpful in the treatment of chronic pain. The dosages needed are usually much less than those used to treat depression (e.g. nortriptyline [Pamelor] begun at 10-25 mg daily, or amitriptyline HCl [Elavil] 25-50 mg daily) given at bedtime, increased as needed over 3 weeks until the effective dose is reached. Placebos should not be given without the client's consent. Deceiving the client undermines the trust necessary for effective treatment to occur. The box below gives tips for pain medication.

Psychiatric APNs who are appropriately educated, ANA credentialed, and permitted by state law may prescribe medications as a routine part of their practice.

Stress management

Stress management strategies are important for all nurses to have as part of their repertoire of nursing interventions. They include systematic muscle relaxation, guided imagery, visualization, and affirmations; concrete problem-solving about managing the stresses in one's life should also be considered. If the nurse receives special training, hypnotherapy could also be included (see Chapter 14). These interventions are valuable in a variety of situations: for the anxious client, for clients with acute or chronic pain, or for clients having difficulties coping with their situation.

Health Teaching

Clients and their families need health-relevant information, skills development, and psychosocial support to handle the experience of illness and the rigors of medical treatment. The following strategies are designed to assist clients and families with:

 MEDICATION TIPS

Pain Medication (Nonopiod and Opiod)

1. The health care team believes your pain is real and you need to report any pain as soon as possible.

2. The primary goal is for you to be as pain-free as you can be.

3. It is crucial that you understand the nature of your pain, its treatment, and your role in controlling your pain.

4. You can prevent pain by taking your medication "around-the-clock" on a regular schedule. Do *not* wait until your pain is severe to take your pain medication. It is hard for the medication to "catch up" with your pain, if you do not take it around the clock.

5. Using narcotic pain medication does *not* automatically lead to addiction.

6. The health care team deals with any tolerance to your narcotic medication by increasing your dose.

7. It is helpful to time physical activities to the peak levels of your pain medication. Ask your provider when your specific medication has its peak level.

8. Be aware of the side effects of your pain medication and ways to control them (e.g., stool softener for constipation or not taking the medication on an empty stomach to avoid nausea and vomiting.

9. Do not suddenly stop taking this medication. There could be severe withdrawal reactions: anxiety, shaking, muscle twitching, confusion, hallucinations, and rarely seizures.

10. Learn about the nonpharmacological interventions for pain and how to use them to assist in your pain control.

11. Do not hesitate to discuss anything about your pain with your provider. The health care team cannot help you control the pain if you do not tell us your symptoms, fears, and concerns.

The Nursing Process

- Understanding as much as they can manage about their specific illness process and the tests, procedures, and treatments involved.
- Identifying the risk/benefit ratio of different treatments
- Remembering that psychological reactions to illness are also crucial aspects
- Normalizing responses to both physical and psychological reactions
- Coping with the changes the illness has imposed on their lives; this might involve restructuring roles, temporarily discontinuing activities, or managing the care of the client at home.
- Acquiring resources about community support systems. These resources may be educational, social, spiritual, for emotional support, or for financial help.

- Learning to advocate for more resources for their particular illness or disability. This can be a useful coping mechanism for them. Consequently, being aware of political or advocacy actions or groups specific to their situation is another way nurses can educate both clients and the public. See the Consumer Resources box below.

Ellers (1993) notes that clients "who participate in successful educational programs are more satisfied with their health care and express markedly less anxiety."

Educating about dying, death, and anticipatory grief can be a rewarding, though at times painful, experience. If the client and family are open to the information, this intervention can be enormously relieving to all, both by providing accurate information and the op-

 CONSUMER RESOURCES

Psychosocial Problems of Physically Ill Persons

American Cancer Society
1599 Clifton Road NE
Atlanta, GA 30329
(404) 320-3333

American Heart Association
7272 Greenville Avenue
Dallas, TX 75231-4596
(800) 642-1196
(214) 373-6300

Arthritis Foundation
1314 Spring Street, NW
Atlanta, GA 30309
(404) 872-7100
(800) 283-7800

I Can Cope (self-help group)
c/o American Cancer Society
1599 Clifton Road
Atlanta, GA 30329
(404) 320-3333

Look Good, Feel Better (LGFB)
American Cancer Society
(800) 395-LOOK

Lupus Foundation of America
4 Research Plaza, Suite 180
Rockville, MD 20850-3226
(800) 237-0590
(301) 670-9292

National Gay Task Force Crisis Hotline
(800)221-9044

National Hospice Organization
1901 North Moore Street, Suite 901
Arlington, VA 22209
(703) 243-5900

National Multiple Sclerosis Society
733 Third Avenue
New York, NY 10017
(212) 986-3240

Public Health Service AIDS Hotline
(800)342-AIDS

United Ostomy Association
36 Executive Park, Suite 120
Irvine, CA 92714
(714) 660-8624

The Nursing Process

TEACHING POINTS

Psychosocial Adjustment to an Acute Illness

Teach the client, family, and/or the significant others the following:

- Persons go through three stages in the cycle of health and illness: (1) the transition from health to illness, (2) the period of the "accepted" illness, and (3) convalescence.
- All feelings and reactions are "normal" at this time: shock, fear, anxiety, guilt, sadness, anger, and others.
- All persons regress in feelings and actions while ill; some of this allows you to heal by resting, eating specific diets, sleeping, following prescribed treatments. This stage is usually only temporary.
- How you coped before you were ill is also how you will cope now, although this coping does not always work as well when you are sick (e.g., if you were active as a way of managing stress, that is hard to do or contraindicated during an acute illness.
- Ask as many questions and find out as much information as you want from the members of your health care team. The better informed you can be, the faster your recovery may be.
- Tell all your health care providers what you need and how they can best help you. If you are dissatisfied or an-

gry with your caregivers, talk with them directly as soon as you can to avoid misunderstandings or the development of mistrust. If you are angry with one of the staff members, do not be afraid of retribution if you speak with them about your concerns. Clients often worry needlessly about this.
- Your role in the family or your relationships will change while you are ill; this is normal. What can help is talking about this openly and perhaps finding other ways to manage these changes. There are health care team members who can help with this.
- Illness is a stressful time for *all* family members, not just the client. The family or significant others need to make sure their needs are met during this period as well, or they will end up depleted and unable to help anyone else. This is not being "selfish"; it's actually in everyone's best interest.
- Think ahead to what you will need in terms of resources in the convalescent period. Talk with your health care providers about how these needs can be met.

portunity to talk about a difficult issue. The important thing for the nurse to attend to is the client's process and what he or she may want. "Following the client's lead" is the best approach. Teaching Points on psychosocial adjustment to an acute illness are presented above.

Health Promotion and Health Maintenance

As mentioned above, families and clients find involvement with community support and self-help groups a good coping mechanism. With so much focus on the illness, and reaction to that illness, promotion of normalcy and wellness in the individual and the family is primary. All family members need to take good care of themselves: eat moderately and well, exercise moderately, and get adequate rest. Each family member also needs to consciously decide how best to cope with the stress of the situation and to continue involvement in activities that are pleasurable and meaningful. These interventions may seem obvious, however, they are often the very activities that families abandon when a member is ill, either from lack of time, energy or guilt. Those providing

care in the home must also have regularly scheduled respite time away from that care. Too often, the needs of the caregiver are shoved aside by themselves or others; the inevitable outcome is a "burned-out" caregiver who serves no one.

Evaluation

Managing the biopsychosocial aspects of physical illness can seem like an overwhelming task. The interactions are intricate, complex, and numerous. Breaking down these interactions into component parts, rather than dealing with them globally, makes the task more manageable. This is also true for evaluating the outcomes of our interventions—the more specific and realistic the definition of the outcomes, the more measurable those outcomes will be.

KEY POINTS

- All physical illnesses have biopsychosocial components that need to be dealt with in addition to the physiological aspects.

CRITICAL THINKING QUESTIONS

Carlos A. is a 60-year-old, Hispanic, married man, with seven children, the youngest of whom is age 17. He recently retired from a 20-year career with the postal service where he was a mail carrier with a walking route. Carlos has enjoyed good health but recently visited his internist for persistent diarrhea and sharp, epigastric pain. His internist referred him to a gastroenterologist who suspected gall stones and performed an endoscopic retrograde cholangiopancreatography (ERCP) to diagnose and remove these stones.

During the outpatient procedure, Carlos developed unexpected, respiratory distress and was admitted to the intensive care unit (ICU) where it was necessary to place him on mechanical ventilation so he could breathe. He was in intensive care for seven days, and when he was extubated, he was very weak, disoriented, and somewhat confused. He was transferred to a general surgical unit to recover.

While on this unit, Carlos became less confused, regained his orientation, but began to express concerns and doubts about his gastroenterologist's partner who had also provided some of his care. Carlos began to tell the nurses that he believed this doctor was "evil, had put jigsaw blades in his neck, 'messed' with his private parts, all in an attempt to kill him so the doctor could marry his wife." Carlos also began to use foul language. The staff questioned his wife Maria about this behavior and found Carlos had no past psychiatric history or any episodes resembling this one. Maria also reported that Carlos had never used foul language before, since he is a lay minister and quite religious.

Carlos' attending gastroenterologist ordered a neurological consultation to rule out a stroke or another neurological event. The neurologist found no evidence of a stroke, but Carlos' electroencephalogram (EEG) was abnormal, showing evidence of seizure activity,

consistent with partial, complex seizures. A psychiatric consultation was ordered and their diagnosis was post-ictal psychosis.

Maria and the children were extremely upset over the entire affair. They often stated that Carlos had come in healthy for a simple outpatient procedure and now was a physically ill man "talking crazy." They believed all of this was the fault of the medical staff. Carlos refused to let his gastroenterologist's partner treat him and began to refuse certain medications and the hospital food, believing they had been contaminated. He said that everybody thinks he's crazy, but if they would look at the x-rays of his neck with him, it would prove once and for all who was right or wrong. Carlos is also having trouble sleeping and angry that the staff will not help him with this problem either.

1. Is the family right? Is Carlos' condition the fault of the medical staff? Why or why not?
2. How would you approach this family? What could you say to help them deal with this difficult situation.
3. How would you approach Carlos? How would his Hispanic background be playing a part in his beliefs? How would you help him get the nutrition that he needs and the medications he needs to take?
4. What precautions might be necessary to protect Carlos? Is he in danger as he believes?
5. How would you deal with Carlos' assertion that the staff thinks he is crazy? Is he crazy? What could you say to him or his family to help them make sense of this. Do you think looking at a neck x-ray with Carlos would benefit him? How?
6. Why is Carlos not sleeping at night? What interventions might you suggest to help with this?

- Physical illness takes a tremendous toll on the emotional well-being of individuals and their productivity.
- The burden of caring for physically ill persons places serious strains on the family and the physical and emotional health of family members.
- The kind of illness and the treatment setting places additional stressors on individuals and their families as they attempt to cope with these changes.

- The most common psychosocial problems seen are anxiety, depression and delirium.
- Untreated psychological reactions negatively affect one's health.
- Many interventions exist to deal with the psychosocial aspects of physical illness
- Nursing assessment and intervention are crucial aspects in facilitating the client's and family members' adjustments to the physical illness, regardless of setting.

REFERENCES

American Psychiatric Association. (1994). Diagnostic criteria for psychological factors affecting medical conditions. *Diagnostic and statistical manual of mental disorders IV, fourth edition.* Washington, D. C.: Author.

Batzler, L.R. (1983). *Through the valley of shadow.* Frederick, MD: Hidden Valley Press.

Bridges, W. (1991). *Managing transitions: making the most of change.* Reading, MA: Addison-Wesley.

Centers for Disease Control and Prevention. (October, 1993). *HIV/AIDS Surveillance Report.* (Third Quarter Edition), 5(3).

Centers for Disease Control and Prevention. (1994). Prevalence of disabilities and associated health conditions-United States, 1991-2. *Journal Of American Medical Association, 272*(22), 1735.

Cohen-Cole, S.A., & Levinson, R. M. (1994). The biopsychosocial model in medical practice. In A. Stoudemire (Ed.), *Human behavior,* (2nd ed.). Philadelphia: J.B. Lippincott.

Covinsky, K.E. et al. (1994). The impact of serious illness on patients' families. *Journal of the American Medical Association, 272,*(23), 1839-1844.

Dillon, C. (1990). Families, transitions, and health: Another look. In K. Davidson & S. Charlie (Eds.), *Social work in health care.* New York: Haworth.

Ellers, B. (1993). Involving and supporting family and friends. In M. Gerteis, S. Edgman-Levitan, J. Daley, & T. Delbanco (Eds.), *Through the patient's eyes.* San Francisco: Jossey-Bass.

Flaskerud, J. H. (1995). Psychosocial and psychiatric aspects. In J. H. Flaskerud & P. J. Ungvarski (Eds.), *HIV/AIDS* (3rd ed.). Philadelphia: W.B. Saunders.

Gorman, L. M., Sultan, D., & Luna-Raines, M. (1989). *Psychosocial nursing handbook for the nonpsychiatric nurse.* Baltimore: Williams & Wilkins.

Green, S.A. (1994). Supportive psychological care of the medically ill: a synthesis of the biopsychosocial approach in medical care. In A. Stoudemire (Ed.), *Human behavior.* Philadelphia: J.B. Lippincott.

Hermann, J.F., & Carter, J. (1994). The dimensions of oncology social work: intrapsychic, interpersonal, and environmental interventions. *Seminars in Oncology, 21,*(6), 712-717.

Hinds, P.S. et al. (1996). Coming to terms: Parents' response to a first cancer recurrence in their child. *Nursing Research, 45*(3), 148-153.

Holland, J. C. (1990). Fears and abnormal reactions to cancer in physically healthy individuals. In J. C. Holland & J. H. Rowland (Eds.), *Handbook of psychooncology.* New York: Oxford University Press.

International Association for the Study of Pain. (1979, updated 1982, 1986). Pain II. pain terms: a current list with defintions and notes on usage. Subcommittee on taxonomy. *Pain, 6,* 249-252.

Jacox, A. et al. (1994). Management of cancer pain. *Clinical practice guideline no.9,* AHCPR Publication No.94-0592.

Rockville, MD., Agency for Health Care Policy and Research, U. S. Department of Health and Human Services, Public Health Service.

Kaplan, H.I., Sadock, B.J., & Grebb, J.A. (1994). *Synopsis of psychiatry* (7th ed.). Baltimore: Williams & Wilkens.

Lazarus, R.S., & Folkman, S. (1984). *Stress, appraisal and coping.* New York: Springer.

LeMaistre, J. (1993). *Beyond rage: mastering unavoidable health changes.* Oak Park, IL: Alpine Guild.

Lederberg, M.S. (1990). Psychological problems of staff and their management. In J. C. Holland & J.A. Rowland (Eds.), *Handbook of psychooncology.* New York: Oxford University Press.

Lindemann, E. (1994). Symptomatology and management of acute grief. *American Journal of Psychiatry, 101, 141-148.*

Martocchio, B.C., & DuFault, K., Sr. (1993). Loss, dying, and death. In W.J. Phipps, B.C. Long, N.C. Woods, & V.L. Cassmeyer (Eds.), *Medical-surgical nursing,* (4th ed.). St. Louis: Mosby.

Micheels, T.A., Wheeler, L.M., & Hayes, B.J. (1995). Linking quality and cost effectiveness: Case management by an advanced practice nurse. *The Journal for Advanced Nursing Practice, 9*(2), 107-111.

North American Nursing Diagnosis Association (NANDA), (1992). *Accepted diagnoses,* 10th National Conference of NANDA.

Northhouse, L. L., & Lancaster, D. (1994). Coping. In J. Gross & B. L. Johnson (Eds.), *Handbook of oncology nursing.* (2nd ed.). Boston: Jones and Bartlett.

Peck, M.S. (1993). *Further along the road less traveled.* New York: Simon & Schuster.

Phipps, W. J. (1995). Chronic illness. In W.J. Phipps, J. Sands, M.K. Lehman, V. L. Cassmeyer (Eds.), *Medical-surgical nursing: Concepts and Clinical Practice* (5th ed.). St. Louis: Mosby.

Walker, E.A., & Katon, W. J. (1994). Psychological factors affecting medical conditions and stress responses. In A, Stoudemire (Ed.), *Human behavior.* Philadelphia: J.B. Lippincott.

Weisman, A.D., & Worden, J.W. (1986). The emotional impact of recurrent cancer. *Journal of Psychosocial Oncology, 3,* 5-16.

U.S. Department of Health and Human Services. (12/93). Vital and health statistics. Washington, DC: National Center for Health Statistics.

VIDEO RESOURCES

Mosby's Continuing Health Care Education Video Series:
AIDS Caregiving: Universal Precautions, Protections, and Psychosocial Issues.

Chapter 33

Infants and Children

Michele L. Zimmerman

LEARNING OUTCOMES

After studying and applying the concepts of this chapter, the learner will be able to:

- Describe the scope of emotional mental disorders of infants and children.
- Describe the complex interaction of psychological, genetic, biological, environmental, situational, and familial phenomena in the development of childhood psychiatric problems.
- Describe the vulnerable populations at risk for the development of childhood mental disorders.
- Explain the protective factors that foster resiliency in children.
- Discuss the roles of the nurse in providing prevention and intervention in childhood mental disorders.
- Appreciate the significance of attending to children's emotional needs to enhance the mental health of a society.
- Apply the nursing process to the basic care of children with emotional disorders.
- Identify psychopharmacological interventions for children and the responsibility of the nurse.

KEY TERMS

Anaclitic depression	Encopresis	Play therapy
Art therapy	Enuresis	Resiliency
Attachment theory	Information processing	Rumination disorder
Attention deficit/hyperactivity disorder (ADHD)	Mental retardation	Sand tray therapy
Autistic disorder	Oppositional defiant disorder (ODD)	School phobia
Cognitions	Pervasive development disorder (PDD)	Separation anxiety disorder (SAD)
Conduct disorder		Temperament
Disruptive behavior disorder (DBD)	Pica	Tics
		Tourette's disorder

hildren's mental health needs in the United States overwhelm available services. The children of the United States can be considered in crisis because of inadequate health services. Crime, poverty, violence, use of drugs and alcohol, lack of education, low self-esteem, lack of community and family values, and inadequate information are risk factors for children's physical and emotional health (Cassetta, 1994). Nurses who are advocates for children and families can make services more accessible through early identification of children at risk, as well as by providing prevention and intervention.

Children who are particularly vulnerable to the development of emotional and mental disorders are low–birth weight infants, homeless children, children with acquired immunodeficiency syndrome (AIDS) or with a parent who has AIDS, and victims of rape and sexual abuse. Children with untreated mental disorders experience self-esteem, school, family, and peer-relationship problems. Chronic underachievement, school dropout, substance abuse, and legal problems are consequences of these illnesses. There is a complex interplay of genetic, physiological, psychological, developmental, situational, familial, and environmental factors that interrelate to cause psychological and developmental difficulties. Nurses work with children who need psychiatric-mental health care in pediatric medical-surgical units, in shelters, in residential and group homes and psychiatric facilities, in the emergency room, at school, and during home-health visits. Unlike adults, children cannot refer themselves for help because of developmental issues and dependency on adults. Nor are children capable of determining their need for psychiatric intervention.

Nurses are uniquely prepared to make a significant contribution to children's emotional well-being and are able to skillfully assess physical and psychological development. Nurses at the basic level of preparation provide early primary-care intervention to children, effectively preventing later costly problems and assisting children with developing into mentally competent adults. Priorities in the national nursing research agenda that apply to child mental health issues focus on low birth weight infants and mothers, symptom management in children, women's health research related to family and child care, and outcome testing of therapeutic actions (Hinshaw, 1992). Advance practice nurses provide treatment and are skilled in the provision of several modalities of psychotherapy. They lead other members of the interdisciplinary team, do research, teach, consult, practice independently, and in some states where they have prescriptive authority, manage medication protocols.

The purpose of this chapter is to introduce readers to the scope of mental disorders in children. It is intended to familiarize nurses with available resources for intervention and treatment of childhood emotional disorders. Interventions focus on assessment, education, and referral of children and their families.

EPIDEMIOLOGY

Statistics estimating the prevalence of mental illness in the estimated 63 million American children reflect only a portion of the children actually in need of services. A study commissioned by the National Institute of Mental Health (NIMH) in 1989 found that 12% of children under age 18 (7.5 million) have at least one diagnosable mental illness, and that figure may be as high as 15%, or 9.5 million children. Approximately 5%, or 2 million children, receive mental health treatment in outpatient centers, and of those who do receive treatment, 70% to 80% do not receive appropriate services.

The number of children who are victimized by violence is underreported in crime statistics. Children's deaths resulting from maltreatment may be underestimated by as much as 85% (Cassetta, 1994). In 1993, 1,018,692 children were victims of abuse. Of that number, 26% were 3 years of age or younger and 51% were age 7 or younger (Krauss, 1993).

Parental psychopathology and other family factors, such as poor parenting, marital discord, and family dysfunction, increase risk for childhood psychiatric disorders. Millions of other children bear risk factors for developing emotional and mental problems.

THEORETICAL FRAMEWORK

There are numerous theories that explain the complex phenomena of mental disturbance in children. Usually, several theories must be used to understand the development of problems and to tailor nursing interventions.

Biological Correlates

Genetic factors

A prevalent biological theory implicates genetic transmission in the development of childhood emotional problems. Family and parental traits are passed on by genetic transmission, and genes influence the developmental environment, which influences fetal genetic material. Children inherit genetic material from both parents. Evidence of genetic susceptibility in childhood mental disorders has been found through twin, family, and linkage studies (Workman et al., 1993). Autism, affective disorders, specific reading disorders, attention-deficit/hyperactivity disorder (ADHD), and Tourette's disorder are childhood psychiatric disorders thought to have a genetic basis (Lombroso, et al., 1994).

Maternal health Maternal health status and health practices create the intrinsic factors that may affect a child's risk for developing psychopathological disorders. The developing fetus is affected by the intrauterine environment; carries genetic markers for particular traits and disorders; and is also vulnerable to environmental stress, substances, and intrinsic body toxins.

Maternal smoking and drug and alcohol use have been shown to irreversibly affect the fetus in ways predictive of behavioral difficulties and health problems immediately at birth. Maternal cocaine use often causes severe problems in affected neonates. Babies affected by cocaine are irritable and difficult to handle. Interactive behavior is diminished, and there is poor response to environmental stimuli. Babies affected by cocaine are also difficult to soothe, which interferes with bonding because the parent does not receive a reciprocal response from his or her attempt to comfort the infant. At birth, they show signs of tremulous muscular rigidity, growth retardation, tachycardia, tachypenia, diarrhea, and necrotizing enterocolitis.

Maternal alcohol use may cause organogenesis during the first trimester, increase the risk of spontaneous abortion during the second trimester, and exert a potential for intrauterine growth retardation (IUGR) during the third. There is no cure for children born impaired with fetal alcohol syndrome (FAS) or fetal alcohol effects. The damage is lifelong (see Chapter 27).

Children born to mothers who are addicted to heroin exhibited evidence of *neonatal abstinence syndrome,* characterized by small gestational age, gastrointestinal (GI) problems, central nervous system (CNS) problems that include hyperactivity and excessive crying, and several other complications. Poor maternal nutrition and maternal immaturity, such as adolescent pregnancy, also negatively impact the developing fetus.

Trauma

Early trauma is related to the development of a variety of psychiatric clinical syndromes. Children more readily experience somatic responses to trauma, which gives rise to a variety of psychophysiological disorders. As a result of early trauma children may suffer difficulties with information processing and memory storage, which may result in learned helplessness, poor tolerance of affection, inability to cope with stress, and fixation on the trauma. This disruption in information processing often leads to poor school performance and inability to learn from experience.

Children exposed to traumatic experiences may exhibit the symptoms of hyperarousal, heightened anxiety, thought intrusion (spontaneous thinking about the trauma or having invasive thoughts), and a "numbing" response (Rak and Patterson, 1996).

Hyperarousal reflects the persistent expectation of danger. Traumatic events may cause dramatic changes in behavior of children, such as mood swings, aggression, regression, dissociation, fearfulness and anxiety, poor concentration and learning, and failure to master developmental tasks. The long-standing experience of trauma in childhood has a direct impact on the devel-

opment of adult mental disorders. Psychiatric nurses often note the mention of a variety of traumatic experiences in histories of clients under their care. A great deal of societal denial still exists however around the issue of child abuse, particularly the sexual abuse of children. This is not a problem unique to the United States, and it crosses all cultures (DeMause, 1991). Fig. 33-1 shows a drawing of someone of the opposite sex by a 9-year-old girl who was sexually abused.

Resiliency Theory

***Resiliency** may be thought of as a child's invulnerability to risks in the environment.* As there are factors

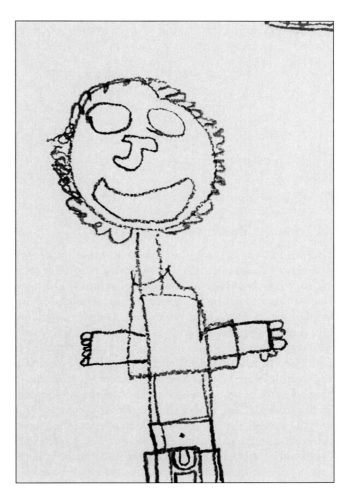

Fig. 33-1 Drawing by a 9-year-old girl who was sexually abused. The girl doing the drawing was abused by a 15-year-old boy. Note that the figure is transparent and has obvious male genitalia. It is unusual for latency-age children to draw genitalia if they have not been sexually abused. The figure is constructed in a primitive way, which indicates regression in the face of trauma.

that increase children's vulnerability to psychopathological disorders, there are also protective factors that reduce the risk of developing a psychopathological condition in children. Resiliency helps explain why some children develop disorders and others do not, even in similar or more adverse circumstances. Protective factors such as problem-solving ability, social competence, supportive adult role models, and average intellectual ability reduce the risk of psychopathological disorders in children who are exposed to adversity and help explain why children in similar circumstances have different outcomes (Krauss, 1993).

More attention must be given to the qualities and factors influencing resiliency in children, since fostering resilience is a form of preventive intervention. The resilient child may be conceptualized as showing signs of invulnerability and may exhibit any of the following behaviors:

- An uninvolved approach to the world with defenses of suppression, isolation, and distancing
- Leading a "charmed life," attributed to an overprotective mother with displays of self-centeredness, dependency, and avoidance behavior
- Becoming a "hero" in the midst of adverseness, behaving in a self-effacing, giving way
- Interpersonal skill with peers and adults with highly developed independent behavior
- Reflective control of feelings and impulsive behavior. They are described as "perfect" children.

Attachment Theory

Attachment theory suggests that the most significant affectional bond is between parent and child and that this bond is essential for healthy emotional bonding (see Chapter 7). Numerous situations contribute to infant and child attachment disruption. Box 33-1 lists factors that disrupt attachment.

Disturbance of attachment is positively correlated with later psychopathology. Erikson's (1950) conceptualization of basic trust refers to attachment operations. Bowlby (1994) saw attachment as essential to the survival of the species. Research indicates that infants who are able to securely attach are able to feel more optimal maternal care than those who are insecurely attached (Thompson, 1991). This theoretical formulation helps explain the higher incidence of child abuse directed toward infants born prematurely and who have spent prolonged periods separated from parents in hospitals, and the higher incidence of child abuse among adolescent mothers who are struggling with developmental issues of their own.

The child who is securely attached uses the attachment figure as a "safe base" or home, is able to increase

---

BOX 33-1

Factors Causing Disruption in Attachment

- Parental mental disorder
- Parental chemical dependency
- Parental absence (illness, death, abandonment, incarceration, migrancy, military deployment, refugee situations, foster home placement, termination of parental rights)
- Adopted child returned to birth parents
- Abduction, including abduction by a parent
- Prolonged hospitalization of parent or child
- Separation or divorce of parents

---

proximity to the primary attachment figure in strange situations or in the face of separation, misses the parent when separated, and is able to return to exploration and play when the parent is available (Weiss, 1995). Some characteristics of securely attached children are social competence, the ability to form good peer relations, empathetic ability, assertiveness, cooperativeness, ego strength, resiliency, self-esteem, self-reliance, and internal self-control.

Family Systems Theory

Infants and children are members of and live in families. Ideally families provide both roots and wings to children; the roots build a secure foundation and attachment to the family that endures over time, and the wings provide children with the ability to move away and fly on their own (Kersey, 1983). The greater the degree of dysfunction, the longer its duration, and the less support available to the child, the greater the potential for emotional harm.

Several familial factors, including the following, influence children.

- *Quality of the parental dyad.* The strength and functioning of the parental relationship significantly affects the child's psychological health or level of anxiety.
- *Parents' family-of-origin issues.* The children are affected in positive or negative ways when one or both parents are still dealing with the quality of their own relationships with parents and adult siblings.
- *Birth order.* Parents respond to their children according to their own birth order and according to the order in which the children are born. Parents who are second or third children themselves may look to their oldest child for leadership more than

first-born parents do. Parents who are oldest children may be competitive with their only or oldest children.

- *Stages of family life cycle.* First-born children often receive more parental attention, whereas children born late in life may be kept infantile. Children born around the time of a death or loss in a family may be unconsciously viewed as a replacement for the lost person.
- *Degree of anxiety.* Children learn how to deal with anxiety in response to the ways their parents respond to manifested anxiety.
- *Environmental and economic stresses.* Children respond to worries and stresses related to finances and jobs, and they are stressed by relocation, unemployment, separations, and other events.

Behavioral Theory

Behavioral theory forms the basis for behavioral interventions with children. Behavior is seen as connected to and in response to environmental interactions with key persons in the child's environment. Abnormal behavior that cannot be attributed to a brain dysfunction or chemical imbalance is believed to be produced in the same manner as healthy behavior. Behavioral theory underlines the ways parents facilitate cooperative, responsible behavior in children or raise unhappy, uncooperative, or delinquent children.

Behavioral theory rests on the assumption that most behavior develops and is maintained by the following types of learning:

1. *Respondent conditioning (Pavlov's dog).* This implies that people learn to respond to a stimulus in a particular manner based on previous experiences. An example of this is the child whose parent always criticizes schoolwork and never says anything positive. Eventually the child expects a negative reaction and begins to hide bad papers and grades. As he or she matures, the child hides everything from his or her parents.
2. *Operant conditioning.* This reflects the process by which behavior is modified by strengthening or weakening its consequences. In helping children be cooperative, parents set consequences for certain behaviors. This is the principle of reward and punishment. Finding something positive to say to a child on a regular basis has a tendency to increase cooperative and positive behavior. However, telling a child he or she is stupid or that no good will occur results in the child believing that and acting accordingly.
3. *Cognitive behavior modification.* This makes use of attributions, cognitions, expectations, and

beliefs to influence behavior and affect. A parent states, "I believe that you can do this task."
4. *Social learning.* This is observational learning that helps change behavior as a result of observing a model. Children imitate adults and role models. For example, if parents lie, their children learn to lie.

Cognitive Theory

Cognition refers to the way a person thinks about self and the world. *Thoughts or images of an event are cognitions. Meaning is assigned to these thoughts or images based on attitudes or assumptions derived from earlier experiences.* Cognitive or thinking distortions are involved in the development and maintenance of some psychopathology. Cognitive development theory describes and explains changes in children's mental representations of their physical and social worlds from birth to maturity. These internalized frames of reference are used by children to view and interact with their environment. Cognitive operations account for transforming self-perceptions, perception of events, self-organization, development of moral reasoning, emotional understanding, simultaneous, multiple feelings, and social response patterns.

According to cognitive theory, *information processing is the serial transformation from old to new information and involves memory. Information processing explains why children and adults remember catchy slogans, sayings, or jingles and why advertisers use this technique to help people remember their products.* Information processing techniques using behavioral therapy include the following:

- *Chunking* is consolidating or grouping information to help children learn. This is particularly effective in teaching numbers.
- *Imaging* involves coupling a picture with an idea to assist learning. This accounts for the alteration in sensory experience when someone who is traumatized sees a reminder of the event. Coupling a positive or soothing image with a traumatic memory can assist in overcoming the negative response and is an intervention used in relaxation training.
- *Rehearsal* is the repetition of a behavior to help achieve mastery of it. The nurse can help children rehearse during play simulations in preparation for anticipated events, such as hospitalizations.
- *Novelty* involves the introduction of something unusual, new, or different into the child's world that has the ability to attract attention (Frost, 1995). For example, introducing a child to a computer program may distract him or her from the trauma of his or her parents' divorce.

Developmental Correlates

It is essential for the nurse to have a complete understanding of normal child development. Children change rapidly, and there is a range of normal development in size and achievement of psychological, physical, intellectual, and cognitive milestones among children. The nurse must be fully cognizant of child development for both assessment and implementation of interventions with children. Chapter 7 discusses the developmental milestones of children that explain phenomena such as the child's readiness to learn certain behaviors or skills at specific times.

Temperament

Temperament comprises the features of a child's persona that reflect emotional disposition, behavior, feelings, and thoughts. It is an aspect of child development receiving increased attention due to advances in neuroscience and genetics. Contributions to an understanding of temperament include the following concepts:

- Basic dispositions influence the different way individuals react to the same objective events.
- Biological contributions to individual differences indicate a genetic component to temperament.
- Temperament is related to basic emotions and motivations and is distinct from cognitive abilities.
- Temperament can be observed in stable behavior patterns.
- The expression of temperament may change with development (Arcus, 1994).

The study of temperament explains the significance of child/parental "goodness of fit," that is, how well they interact with each other. The following are manifestations of children's temperament:

- *Activity*—how energetic, active, or passive the child behaves
- *Adaptability*—how the child deals with stress, change, and novelty
- *Intensity*—how the child approaches tasks, situations, and persons
- *Approach/withdrawal*—the child's response to social situations
- *Mood*—the child's optimism or pessimism, happiness or sadness
- *Attention/persistence*—how the child solves problems, learns, and deals with experience
- *Distractibility*—the child's ability to focus on tasks or become easily distracted
- *Rhythmicity*—how long the child takes to get going or settle down, best or worst time of day, child's need for sleep
- *Threshold of responsiveness*—how sensitive the child is to environmental changes

There is an interactional quality between the child and the parents' temperament, as well as between the child's temperament and the way he or she is perceived and dealt with in society. Temperamental qualities can have a protective role in mitigating difficult circumstances. For example, sociable, outgoing children are resilient in the face of multiple risk factors for dysfunction. Sociable children who are easily approached evoke positive feedback from other children as well as adults, so it is easier for such children to obtain support. On the other hand, inhibited children have greater risk for the development of anxiety disorders. Irritable children with "difficult" temperaments, in combination with parental conflict, are at great risk for later behavior disorders. Children with extreme ranges of difficult temperaments are much more likely to develop a clinical diagnosis in adolescence. Children who have good dispositions have some of the protective factors that help reduce the risk of developing a psychopathological disorder (Krauss, 1993).

MENTAL DISORDERS OF CHILDREN

As many as 17% to 20% (or 11 to 14 million) children have some type of diagnosable disorder (Krauss, 1993). There are several categories of childhood mental disorders, or disorders first diagnosed in childhood. DSM-IV disorders of infancy, childhood, and adolescence include mental retardation, learning disorders, motor skills disorders, communication disorders, pervasive developmental disorders (PDDs), tic disorders, attention-deficit and disruptive behavior disorders, feeding and eating disorders, and elimination disorders. Other disorders include separation anxiety disorder (SAD), autistic disorder, reactive attachment disorders, and stereotypic movement disorder (APA, 1994). Additionally, children may also experience symptoms of common adult disorders such as anxiety, schizophrenia, mood disturbances, the somatoform disorders, and adjustment disorders.

Mental Retardation

Mental retardation can coexist with other DSM-IV disorders. It is characterized by significantly subaverage intellectual functioning as measured by an intelligence quotient (IQ) of 70 or below, concurrent deficits in adaptive functioning, and onset before age 18.

Children who are mentally retarded are commonly kept in the community to maintain a normal environment for as long as possible. Education within the community is more available than in the past, when children who were mentally retarded were often sent to state schools distant from their homes. Mental retardation is caused by biomedical factors such as hereditary disorders, alterations of embryonic development, pregnancy problems, perinatal difficulties, and acquired childhood diseases (trauma, infections, cardiac arrest, and toxins).

Learning Disorders, Motor Skills, and Communication Disorders

The inclusion of learning disorders in psychiatric literature is controversial, because diagnosis and intervention usually take place within the school system. Learning disorders include mathematics disorder, written expression disorder, and reading disorder. The child with a learning disorder may have normal intelligence but develop low self-esteem with the belief that he or she is stupid because of difficulty mastering concepts in the classroom. Learning disorders may accompany other DSM-IV disorders, such as a disruptive behavior disorder.

Motor skills disorder describes a marked impairment in the development of motor coordination. It involves difficulties in coordination and achieving motor milestones. As children with this disorder grow, they are described as clumsy, they may perform poorly in sports, or they may exhibit poor handwriting. Parental disappointment in the children may contribute to associated sadness, low self-esteem, and poor socialization. Motor skill disorder may be associated with other childhood emotional disorders.

Communication disorders are those involving speech—both articulation and understanding. Stuttering is a communication disorder. The communication disorders may be compounded by associated anxiety and frustration. Children with communication disorders are helped with stress management and relaxation techniques or with treatment of underlying neurological deficits, such as hearing loss.

Pervasive Developmental Disorders

Pervasive developmental disorders (PDDs) are extreme neuropsychiatric diseases and include children diagnosed with autism, Rett's and Asperger's disorders, and childhood degenerative disorders. PDDs primarily affect verbal and nonverbal communication, social skills, and imaginative activity. Children with a PDD have severe impairment in basic psychological functions and are often mentally retarded as well. PDDs are usually diagnosed in the first few years of life and are chronic, permanent disabilities that heavily burden families. Children with a PDD often are institutionalized in long-term care facilities. Families are stressed by the unclear etiology and by developmental stresses that are exaggerated by the disorder. Other children in a family may be ignored and begin to act out in response to the parent's preoccupation with the affected child. The disorders classified as PDDs include autistic disorder, Rett's disorder, childhood disintegrative disorder, and Asperger's disorder.

Autistic disorder is an impairment in social interaction characterized by poor eye contact, fixed facial expression, posture, and social gestures. Peer relationships are usually absent, and there is a lack of interaction, sharing, or reciprocating with others. The child who is autistic does not approach the parent and is often described as being in his or her own world. Communication is severely impaired, and there may be an absence of social language, although idiosyncratic language may be present. Behavior is restricted, repetitive, and stereotyped. Children with autistic disorder may spin around constantly, flap their arms, or rock. They may collect pieces of lint or paper clips, or they may become wildly hysterical at a noise or any change in the environment.

Childhood disintegrative disorder is similar to that of the child with autistic disorder, except for the period of apparent normalcy disorder. The child with this disorder develops normally for the first 2 years and then loses previously acquired skills.

Rett's disorder affects only girls, and is characterized by early normal development followed by deceleration of head growth between 5 months and 4 years of age, loss of hand skills, loss of social engagement skills, poor coordination and gait disturbance, and impairment in receptive and expressive language. Asperger's disorder and severe psychomotor retardation are similar to autism. Children have impaired social interaction skills and restricted repetitive and stereotyped patterns of behavior. However, there are no apparent language or cognitive delays. It is believed by some that Asperger's disorder is a form of autism.

Disruptive Behavior Disorders and Attention-Deficit/Hyperactivity Disorder

Disruptive behavior disorders (DBDs) and attention deficit/hyperactivity disorder (ADHD) are marked by behaviors that disturb other people and are perceived as disruptive. ADHD, conduct disorder, and oppositional defiant disorder are discussed in the following sections.

ADHD is a common neuropsychiatric disorder affecting 6% to 9% of all children and extending into adulthood. Color Plate 7 in Chapter 15 presents a positron emission tomography (PET) scan of an adult with ADHD. ADHD refers to a cluster of problematic behaviors:

- Developmental inappropriateness, inattention/distractibility, and impulsivity
- Hyperactivity
- Comorbidity in 80% of children with learning disorders, language and communication disorders, conduct disorders, oppositional defiant disorders, anxiety disorders, mood disorders, Tourette's disorder, and chronic tics

Children with ADHD are impaired in multiple domains. They have poor peer, adult, and family relationships; school performance and leisure activites are problematic; and self-esteem, self-control, and obedience are lacking. Behavior manifested by children and adults with ADHD are listed in Box 33-2.

Parent-effectiveness training is used to help parents communicate and structure the child's environment in a predictable and organized manner. A key management strategy is stretching the child's attention span. Rewarding nonhyperactive behavior is the key to preparing a child for school. The child can be shown pictures in a book and be rewarded with praise if attentive. Reading stories with color pictures and playing games of gradually increasing difficulty, progressing to dominoes, card games, and dice games, may be helpful. Matching pictures is an excellent way to build up attention span and train memory. However, too many toys can be distracting. The Teaching Points below list guidelines for parents living with a child who is hyperactive.

Conduct Disorder

A diagnosis of *conduct disorder in children is made when there are persistent patterns of conduct in which basic rights of others and major rules and norms are violated.* It is a primarily psychogenic disorder, although there may be biological factors that compromise the child. Behaviors associated with conduct disorder are noted in Box 33-3.

Family dynamics of children with conduct disorder include frequent moving; ineffective, inconsistent parenting or shifting of parent figures; parental absence or al-

coholism; and a family known to multiple agencies. Sometimes children with conduct disorders have been physically or sexually abused, and their behavior is an attempt to master anxiety. They may first come to the attention of authorities because of a pattern of perpetrating violence on other, smaller children. The children and their parent figures usually need long-term treatment and medication management for the associated conditions. Medication management may include lithium, carbamazepine, and propranolol (see Chapter 15).

Oppositional Defiant Disorder

Oppositional defiant disorder (ODD) describes a pattern of negativistic, hostile, and defiant behavior without the serious violation of other people's basic rights seen in the child with conduct disorder. Children who have ODD defy adults and peers who are well-known to them—and justify their behavior. The externalizing symptoms of the child with ODD include arguing, not cooperating, deliberately annoying others, and spitefulness. Their problematic behavior is more severe than that seen in other children their age. The nurse in the primary care role is in a position to notice these children and provide management strategies to parents, as well as give them a referral for more intensive therapy. Medication for associated conditions, such as depression or hyperactivity, and structured community programs can be of benefit in symptom management and in the prevention of more serious difficulties.

Eating Disorders of Infancy or Early Childhood

Eating disorders that are not normally seen in adults include *pica, the eating of nonnutritive substances,* and *rumination disorder which is a syndrome charac-*

BOX 33-2

Symptoms Associated with ADHD

Easily distracted
Procrastination
Poor follow through
Difficulty with team sports
Outbursts of rage
Violent behavior
Impulsivity
Inattention
Distractibility
Loses possessions
Tantrums
Minipanic
Risk taking
Excessive talking
Can't wait turns
Disorganized
Somatic tension

TEACHING POINTS

10 Guidelines for Living with a Child Who is Hyperactive

- Accept the child's limitations.
- Provide outlets for the release of excess energy.
- Keep home life organized.
- Avoid fatigue.
- Avoid formal gatherings.
- Maintain firm discipline.
- Decrease distractions.
- Enforce discipline.
- Protect the child against any overreaction by the neighbors.
- Get away from the child from time to time.

terized by partially digested food being brought up into the mouth and ejected or chewed and reswallowed. Infants with rumination disorder often fail to gain weight. They are also at risk for abuse and attachment disorders because their caregivers are repulsed by their odor and frustrated by their behavior.

Tic Disorders

Children in the mental health system often experience tic disorders. *Tics are sudden, repetitive movements, gestures, or utterances mimicking some aspect of normal behavior.* Box 33-4 lists common movements associated with tics, which are commonplace among children and are sometimes associated with conditions such as Huntington's disease, multiple sclerosis and post-viral encephalitis. Tics cannot be controlled, but they can be suppressed for a time through the use of medication. Tics become worse when the child is stressed, fatigued, or excited (McSwiggan-Hardin, 1995). There may be anxiety as a result of social embarrassment, and depression is commonly associated with tic disorders.

Tourette's disorder is a specific and the most common, discrete tic disorder thought to be neuropathological in origin, that is, characterized by multiple tics usually of the head. The child with Tourette's has tics every day that may occur in clusters. These tics manifest as coughing, twitching, blinking, twisting, and sometimes cursing. There may be serious social impairment and associated depression. Pharmacotherapy can alleviate symptoms, and research is ongoing to discover a Tourette's-specific drug for treatment (Leckman and Cohen, 1991).

Elimination Disorders

Common childhood elimination disorders include enuresis and encopresis. *Enuresis is incontinence or voiding of urine during the day or night into the bed or clothes after the age of expected bladder control.* It is involuntary, but occasionally the child may void intentionally. Enuresis is classified as primary enuresis when continence has never been attained. Secondary enuresis occurs in children who have achieved a period of dryness (usually 1 year), which is followed by incontinence. It is common in children who are emotionally stressed. Nocturnal enuresis refers to nighttime voiding, and diurnal enuresis refers to daytime voiding of urine. Physical examination must rule out any organic cause, such as a urinary tract infection. Sometimes children who are enuretic are developmentally delayed (Mack, 1989).

Enuresis interferes with a child's self-esteem as well as socialization, since the child may be reluctant to go to camp or to visit friends or relatives. It also increases tension between parents and children. Children often become enuretic after a stressor, such as family discord, loss, or sexual trauma. Behavioral treatment, psychotherapy, parenting education, and psychopharmacology with clonidine are helpful. The nurse is a resource to parents and helps them select and comply with therapeutic regimens.

Encopresis is the repeated passage of feces into places not appropriate for that purpose, such as bedclothes or clothing, by children who have passed toilet-training age. Age 4 is the usual cut-off age. Some children who are encopretic have never been successfully toilet trained (*primary encopresis*), and some have been successfully trained and then begin soiling (*secondary encopresis*) (Sprague and McRae, 1990). Soiling in the clothing is a complex condition and presents a treatment challenge.

Elimination disorders may be first noticed in children when they are hospitalized for a physical or emotional health problem or when they first enter school. Encopresis is a condition that may also be noted in the primary care setting.

BOX 33-3

Signs and Symptoms of Conduct Disorder

- Physical aggression
- Cruelty to people and animals
- Property destruction, including setting fires
- Stealing (overt and covert)
- Lying and cheating
- School truancy and runaway behavior
- Use of tobacco, alcohol, or nonprescribed drugs
- Lack of empathy, guilt, or remorse, often blaming others
- Low self-esteem covered by bravado with low frustration tolerance, irritability, and recklessness
- Poor academic achievement

Box 33-4

Types of Movement Associated With Tics

Choreiformic—random, irregular, and nonrepetitive dancing
Dystonic—Slower twisting interspersed with prolonged states of muscle stiffness
Athetoid—Slow, irregular writhing, usually of fingers, toes, face, and neck
Myoclonic—Brief, shocklike muscle contractions
Hemiballismic—Intermittent course with large, unilateral movements
Synkinetic—involuntary movement that accompanies a voluntary one

The encopresis may be the result of a complex interaction of one or more etiological factors, such as coercive toilet training, lax toilet training, a faulty parent-child relationship, developmental delay, or trauma. Children who are encopretic usually soil their clothing continually, appear oblivious to the odor, hide their soiled clothing, and deny their encopresis. They may have infrequent, large, painful bowel movements.

Care is taken to rule out physical disorders first. The differential diagnosis must take into account recent stressors, other associated conditions such as developmental delays or retardation, and whether the child is attending to the signals to defecate.

Childhood Schizophrenia

The criteria for diagnosing childhood schizophrenia are the same as those for diagnosing schizophrenia in adults (see Chapter 29). Schizophrenia is now considered rare in children, although incidence increases steadily during adolescence. This disorder needs to be distinguished from one of the PDDs. The onset of schizophrenia, if the diagnosis is correct, before age 13 is referred to as very-early–onset schizophrenia (VEOS). Symptoms of schizophrenia, affective disorders with psychotic features, and possibly personality and dissociative disorders overlap.

Children with PDD may be misdiagnosed as having schizophrenia. Nonpsychotic symptoms such as idiosyncratic thinking and perceptions caused by developmental delays, exposure to traumatic events, or overactive imaginations in children are some of the causes of uncertainty. Cultural, developmental, and intellectual factors must also be evaluated to assess a child's report of possible psychotic symptoms.

Childhood Mood Disorders

Although diagnoses of childhood mood disorders are increasing, their existence is often overlooked. Just as childhood schizophrenia was overdiagnosed in the past, childhood depression was thought to be unusual and rare. However, there exists an earlier age of onset of mood disorder with each progressive decade since the 1940s (Carlson, 1995). A substantive body of research in the last several years validates the existence of depression in children, particularly among children in impoverished situations or where their needs are not met. There is a familial or genetic tendency in the development of depression.

The greatest risk factor for children is having a parent who is affectively disordered (Beardslee and Wheelock 1994), giving credence to the complex interrelationship of genetic, psychological, and environmental factors (see Chapter 30). Children of parents who are depressed are less securely attached, probably as a result of the depressed mother's inability to relate positively to the child; are spoken to less; and receive less structure and discipline. Overall, parents with depression relate less to their children than parents who are not depressed. Fig. 33-2 is a drawing by a 12-year-old girl depicting her family life. The perception is clear that the family is not there for her. This constitutes a form of emotional and often physical neglect.

Others at high risk for depression are children with chronic illness who are unable to participate in age-appropriate activities; children separated from parents, neglected, psychologically rejected, or abused children; and children experiencing chronic pain. ADHD, conduct disorder, specific developmental disorders, and chaotic home environment also predispose children to mood disorders (Weller and Weller, 1991).

Parents may note behavior changes, such as irritability, whininess, boredom, or difficulty sleeping. Children may also have vegetative symptoms of depression, such as evening insomnia, loss of appetite, or difficulty in motivation. Parents may interpret these symptoms as behavior problems or rebellion. In children, the symptom of failing to gain weight substitutes for weight loss. Somatic complaints, such as headaches or stomach aches, are quite common in children who are depressed. However, because of children's cognitive and developmental level, they may not appear listless and they may still play and interact with others. The symptoms may be evident in an inability to concentrate or an irritability and crankiness, and psychotic ideation may be present.

In preschool children, the association of depression with abuse or neglect suggests a psychobiological continuum with anaclitic depression. **Anaclitic depression** is a term used to describe the failure to thrive and

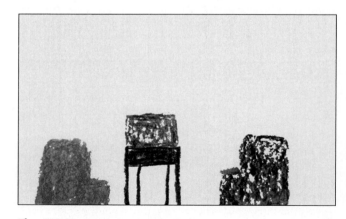

Fig. 33-2 Family portrait drawn by a 12-year-old child with depression. The family is absent, indicating a lack of nurturing and the emotional unavailability of parents and siblings.

unresponsiveness of children who are not touched or cuddled. Comorbidity of behavior and anxiety disorders with major depressive disorder in middle childhood occurs in over 75% of children with depression.

Anxiety Disorders

Children experience anxiety in many of the same ways as adults (see Chapter 22). Some variations are unique to children. They exhibit a high incidence of inhibited temperament and often have a parent with an anxiety disorder, depression, or alcoholism.

Separation anxiety disorder (SAD) in children is characterized by signs and symptoms of excessive anxiety. Symptoms develop to the point of panic after separation from a major attachment figure. Extreme psychophysiological distress when anticipating separation from a parent or outright refusal to attend school may bring these children to the attention of the health care system. They may verbalize worry that harm will befall an attachment figure and follow their parent around or refuse to be in a room by themselves. They may refuse to visit friends or spend the night, which interferes with self-esteem and socialization.

School phobia is a form of pathological shyness characterized by severe anxiety about attending school, often accompanied by psychophysiological symptoms. Failure to attend school has negative consequences for children. Families may unconsciously support the child's symptoms because of dysfunctional issues of their own, thus making them ineffective in helping children return to school.

Other phobias are common in children and include fear of the dark or of certain animals. Assessment must be made to differentiate phobias from children's normal anxiety, concern, shyness, and developmentally appropriate behavior. When the specific fear is associated with avoidance behavior and there is functional or social impairment, the behavior is usually of a serious nature and a psychiatric diagnosis is made.

Obsessive-Compulsive Disorder

Obsessive-compulsive disorder (OCD) in children is differentiated from normal ritualistic behavior of childhood because it causes significant impairment in functioning. For example, a young child may not like to have certain foods touching each other on his or her dinner plate, but a child with OCD may not eat because he or she has to compulsively count the strands of spaghetti after laying them out side by side on the plate. Pathological concern with bodily functions and obsessional worrying, along with rituals of cleaning, checking, and counting, are manifested by children with OCD. Parents often become involved in the child's rituals and reinforce the behavior.

Post-Traumatic Stress Disorder

Post-traumatic stress disorder (PTSD) occurs when an unusual event outside the normal human experience overwhelms the victim. It is common in children who are abused, are victimized, or who witness traumatic events. PTSD may occur after accidents or disasters, after neighborhood or school violence, in hostage situations, and during war. The child's ordinary coping strategies and defenses are overwhelmed, and he or she feels helpless and hopeless (see Chapter 24).

There is mounting evidence that PTSD is a neurophysiological disorder in which the microenvironmental milieu of the CNS is permanently altered. Experiences activate the neurosensory apparatus, changing the neuronal networks responsible for sensation, perception, and processing of information. These experiences may permanently modify the structures associated with sensitization, learning and memory, and in the developing brain, differentiation. The developing infant's or child's brain is exquisitely sensitive to stress and trauma. The syndrome's severity is proportional to the duration of the trauma and age of the child when the stressors began (Faller, 1993).

Contrary to popular misconceptions, children are susceptible to trauma and do remember trauma at some level. Because of their immaturity and lack of lived experiences, children are more vulnerable to traumatic events than adults. Children are dependent, physically smaller, not allowed to challenge adult authority, and are unable to survive without adult protection. Children who have been traumatized often reexperience the traumatic event through repetitive play in which themes or aspects of the trauma are reexperienced or reenacted. Fig. 33-3 is a drawing by a youngster with PTSD that depicts a chaotic family environment.

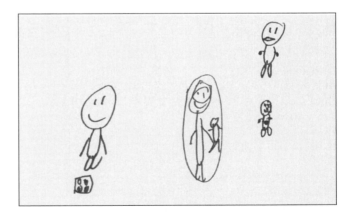

Fig. 33-3 Family drawing by a child with PTSD. The child is from a physically and sexually abusive, chaotic, and violent family. The father is in bed touching the victim's genitals. The brother is on the top right after beating the sister. The mother is in the kitchen ignoring the violence.

Terr (1990) treated a number of children who had been kidnapped and buried in a school bus in Chowchilla, California. She noted in the repetitive, ritual aspect of the children's play the unhappy themes of children being stolen and buried.

Children exposed to violence in families and in their environment often display symptoms of PTSD. They may lose recently acquired developmental skills, and they may have a belief that they will not live to be very old.

The day-to-day experience of violence in some communities has a bearing on the increase in violent behavior observed among children. The increase in physical, sexual, and emotional abuse of children continues and perpetuates a "world of abnormal rearing" (WAR). Children who have been traumatized have difficulty putting feelings into words, misperceive the environment, have problems calming themselves, and often lash out angrily at everything around them (Gallop et al., 1995).

In all 50 states, registered nurses are mandated reporters of suspected physical or sexual abuse. Some psychosocial indicators alerting the nurse that sexual abuse of a child may be occurring are found in Box 33-5. The nurse must also be knowledgeable about physical evidence of childhood sexual abuse (see Chapter 36).

Fig. 33-4 depicts a self-portrait drawing by a physically abused child.

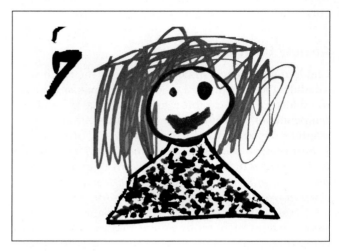

Fig. 33-4 Self-portrait drawing by a physically abused child. Note the heavy pounding marks on the body, as well as the scribbled hair (anxiety), lack of arms or hands (helplessness), lack of legs or feet (child can't escape), and distorted facial features (one eye larger or blackened and mouth smeared).

BOX 33-5

Psychosocial Indicators of Child Sexual Abuse

SEXUAL INDICATORS

- Statements indicating precocious sexual knowledge, often made inadvertently
- Sexually explicit drawings (not open to interpretation)—Child draws a picture of fellatio or ejaculation
- Sexual interactions with other people, such as younger children, or invitations for sexual activity made to adults by the child
- Sexual interactions involving animals or toys
- Masturbation is indicative of possible sexual abuse if:
  - Child masturbates to the point of injury
  - Child masturbates numerous times a day or can't stop
  - Child inserts objects into vagina or anus
  - Child makes groaning or moaning sounds while masturbating
  - Child engages in thrusting motions while masturbating
- Report to someone that they are being sexually abused.

NONSEXUAL INDICATORS IN YOUNG CHILDREN

- Sleep disturbances
- Enuresis and/or encopresis
- Regressive behavior
- Self-destructive or risk-taking behavior
- Impulsivity, distractibility, difficulty concentrating
- Refusal to be left alone
- Fear of the alleged offender
- Fear of people of a specific gender
- Firesetting (more characteristic of male victims)
- Cruelty to animals (more characteristic of male victims)
- Role reversal in the family or pseudomaturity

NONSEXUAL BEHAVIORAL INDICATORS IN ALL CHILDREN

- Problems relating to peers
- School difficulties
- Sudden noticeable changes in behavior

From Faller, K.C. (1993). Child sexual abuse: Intervention and treatment issues. U.S. Department of Health and Human Services. Administration on Children, Youth and Families. Washington, DC: National Center on Child Abuse and Neglect.

The *Nursing Process*

Identification of children in need of mental health services is a challenge to nurses who work in primary care settings, home care, and pediatric units. Many of these children are never treated in formal psychiatric settings. The shortage of child mental health services contributes to this phenomena.

Assessment

Assessment of children is a complex, multifaceted process that presents a challenge for nurses and for those who collaborate with them in the care of children. Multiple sources contribute to the assessment data needed to properly formulate psychiatric and nursing diagnoses.

Play is the primary method used for facilitating assessment of a child. The nurse observes and interacts with the child in a semistructured play interview. There should be a range of toys, including blocks and building materials such as Legos, dolls, dollhouses and furniture, drawing materials, puppets, toy telephones, games, toy soldiers, and other miniatures that the child can manipulate, as well as books. The environment should be child-friendly and nonthreatening. The nurse conveys an air of acceptance and unconditional positive regard for the child to enable development of a trusting relationship. The child should never be prevented from returning to a parent when the desire to do so is apparent.

Preschool and young school-age children are comfortable sitting on the floor, and the nurse should join the child. It is handy to interview the child in a carpeted room and to have cushions and low furniture or tables available.

During play time, the nurse assesses mental status that includes the child's motor skills, mannerisms, vocabulary, and fund of general knowledge. The nurse further notes overall appearance, including the presence of bruises or cuts; the level of anxiety; inattention; and mannerisms, such as chewing on a shirt collar, putting the fingers in the mouth or clutching the genital area. The nurse notes the child's gross motor coordination and whether the child is left- or right-handed, how he or she manipulates toys and crayons, and how the child follows instructions. Experience playing with children hones the nurse's skills in relating to and evaluating children's developmental and mental status.

Family Assessment

Informants who contribute to family assessment include parents, siblings, school officials, social school service workers, and the child. The primary informants are the parents. The nurse obtains the following information.

- *Health history,* including allergies, accidents, illnesses, hospitalizations, medications, and responses to medication
- *Developmental history,* which shows milestones and the mother's health during pregnancy, as well as circumstances of delivery
- *Brief genogram,* showing the child's position in the family, the ages of family members, divorces, deaths and causes, marital and other separations with dates, and interactions with parents and siblings
- *Family health issues,* including a history of psychiatric illness, the presence of alcohol and chemical dependency, and a perception of significant nodal events
- *Perception of child's school performance*
- *Child's ADLs,* such as appetite, sleep patterns, change in play patterns, and bowel and bladder habits
- *Method of discipline,* such as spanking, quiet room, scolding, or other
- *Social functioning,* including hobbies, organized activities such as sports, friendships, and interaction with pets
- *History of presenting problem,* including symptoms, duration, and parental reaction

Siblings are interviewed to obtain their perceptions of the child's behavior. Differences in information are explored during family meetings.

Child Interview

The interview with the child is structured in an age-appropriate manner and includes observation for symptoms, physical assessment, observation for age-appropriate competencies, observation of parental interaction, and mental status.

Child interviews may be videotaped for training or legal purposes, as well as to capture parent-child interactions. The child's behavior must be considered in the context of his or her developmental level, the family, the

The Nursing Process

child's living situation, his or her school situation, and other environmental factors. It is important to ascertain the child's level of social supports. The interview with the child should be alone, although some portions include the observation of parent-child interaction if the interview is done in a formal health care setting. An observation room with a one-way mirror is ideal for this purpose.

Children experience the same stressors as adults, but they often have fewer resources, including life experiences, wisdom, judgment, and coping skills. Stressed parents often unconsciously turn to their children for support, and in the process they parentify or adultify their children. Children are best assessed in a natural setting in which they are comfortable. Home visiting provides the ideal opportunity to evaluate a child's functioning. With health care moving from the hospital to the community, the psychiatric home health nurse's role increases in importance.

When determining whether the child's behavior deviates significantly from normative behavior, the nurse considers the child's overall functioning, the child's description in his or her own words of the way he or she feels, the parent report, the family history, the school report, and significant or recent life events. Developmental issues must be considered. For example, it is normal for a 3-year-old child to experience separation anxiety when his father drops him off at day care but not for a 9-year-old child going to school. The same 3-year-old boy may rub his genitals while riding in the car, but if the 9-year-old child did this, it could be cause for concern. The nurse keeps in mind that children often show transient behavioral regression and loss of recently acquired skills and competencies when under stress.

Feelings are an important component of assessment with younger children. Feelings charts portraying exaggerated faces with feelings are helpful in assisting children to express inner feelings. Children may not have the vocabulary to describe such feelings as overwhelmed, grief-stricken, terrified, or ecstatic, but they may be able to select their feelings from a chart.

The nurse assesses the child's affect, such as anxiety, depression, apathy, guilt, and anger. If depression is likely to be an issue, further evaluation of the child's feelings, level of sadness, self-esteem, and suicidal risk is essential. The child's ideation and vegetative symptoms must be evaluated. Often parents may be unaware of their child's depression, particularly if they are overwhelmed with their own current stressors. Children may not disclose feelings of sadness to parents for a variety of reasons, including a desire not to burden the parent, fear that the

parent will be angry, and emotional unavailability of the parent.

When assessing depression in children, the following questions are used:

- How do people treat you?
- Do you think people like you?
- Do you cry a lot?
- Do you feel sad or unhappy a lot?
- How does your teacher like you?
- Do you feel bad all the time?
- Do you ever think about dying?
- Do you feel like hurting yourself?

If these questions yield affirmative responses, the nurse gently probes further, asking the child to, "Tell me about this." Open-ended questions, as well as focused assessment, are particularly useful here.

Skills and strengths that may predict a child's ability to function as a healthy adult are also determined during an assessment. The following predictive abilities indicate strength in a child:

- Establishing closeness and trust in relationships
- Handling separation and making independent decisions
- Negotiating joint decisions and conflict
- Dealing with frustration and unfavorable events
- Celebrating good feelings and experiencing pleasure
- Delaying gratification
- Relaxing and playing
- Cognitively processing thoughts and words
- Establishing a sense of direction and purpose

School Interview

If the child is in school, assessment needs to include an interview with teachers. Teachers are interviewed about the child's behaviors during the month previous to the interview and about current function. Information obtained should include perception of the child's school performance, including reports of grades and teacher reports of behavioral issues and peer relationships. Parental consent is obtained to interview teachers. Generally, parents and teachers are better reporters about children's behavior, whereas children more accurately report their feelings.

Assessment Tools Used in Evaluating Children

Rating scales and checklists are useful to assess a child's level of function and to obtain a large amount of behavioral information in a rapid and economical way. Rating scales are also helpful to establish a data base for guiding interventions. Some examples of rating scales the nurse may encounter while giving services to children are found in Box 33-6.

The Traumatic Event Drawing Series is an assessment tool to evaluate a child's self-concept and view of a traumatic event, such as physical or sexual abuse, witnessing of a violent episode, or a natural disaster. The child is asked to make seven drawings with crayons while the examiner asks the child questions. Interviews using anatomically correct dolls are part of the focused assessment for suspected child sexual abuse. Interviewing to validate suspected sexual abuse in children should never be attempted by untrained persons (Lewin, 1995).

Nursing Diagnosis

Nursing diagnoses for children with mental disorders are formulated in ways that are similar to those for adults. However, selected North American Nursing Diagnosis Association (NANDA) nursing diagnoses pertain specifically to children. Examples of nursing diagnoses and associated DSM-IV diagnoses that may be used with children diagnosed with a mental disorder are found in Table 33-1. Related factors are added to the nursing diagnostic statement based on unique assessment characteristics of the child and family.

DSM-IV differentiates between adult and children on Axes II, IV, and V (see Chapter 5). Axis II assessment in children considers developmental impairment in cognitive, social, and motor skills, including mental retardation, whereas Axis II for adults refers to personality disorders.

Outcome Identification

Outcome identification for children involves focusing on specific changes that both the child and the parent want.

BOX 33-6

Evaluation Tools Used in Child Psychiatry

- Achenbach Child Behavior Checklist for Ages 4-18
- Conner's Parent and Teacher Scales
- Children's Attributional Style Questionnaire
- Moos Family Environment Scale
- Barkley Hyperactivity Parent/Teacher Checklists
- Traumatic Event Drawing Series

Outcomes do not rest with the child alone but are dependent on the interaction between the environment and the child. Outcomes with children need to be concrete and developmentally appropriate, have the support of the parent, and be achievable. Examples of realistic short-term outcomes for a child with ADHD might include:

- Sitting still in school for 15 minutes each hour
- Remaining calm during changes in the classroom
- Cooperating with others when asked
- Completing homework assignments within 1 hour
- Verbalizing positive attributes about the self daily.

Setting long-term outcomes for children with mental disorders is a somewhat unpredictable process. Children with multiple intrinsic and extrinsic risk factors are less likely to be symptom-free as adults than those children who exhibit signs of resiliency or possess skills that predict competency. The efforts of nurses and others who care for children are aimed at promotion of health for their adulthood and ultimately for society.

Planning

The treatment of children by the mental health care system has changed markedly in recent years. Children are admitted to acute inpatient services primarily only for crisis stabilization. The emphasis is on treating the child in the context of the family, rather than on fixing the child without any family involvement. Consequently, children who are more acutely ill are now being treated as outpatients.

Children do not refer themselves for services but come in contact with the mental health professionals usually after they cause problems for someone through disruptive behavior, or after they have been victims of abuse or violence. Children remain an underserved population because risk factors and vulnerability issues are on the increase.

Planning in inpatient settings involves setting short-term, achievable goals with maximum family involvement, referral to community agencies, and rapid discharge. Children miss the benefit of forming close attachments to nursing staff, which unfortunately replicates the often unstable transitional placements that the child may have experienced in the community.

Nurses assume an active role in the referral process. The goal of any plan for children with a mental disorder is to relieve symptoms, prevent reoccurance of a crisis, promote healthier functioning, rebuild a healthier network for the child, and promote the health or society through health promotion activities with children and their families.

The Nursing Process

TABLE 33-1

DSM-IV disorders of infancy, childhood, and adoleslcence with selected NANDA nursing diagnoses

DSM-IV DIAGNOSES*	NANDA DIAGNOSES†
Mental retardation	Risk for disorganized infant behavior
	Impaired verbal communication
	Self-care deficit
	Risk for altered parent/infant/child attachment
Learning disorders	Sensory-perceptual alterations
Motor skills disorders	Altered growth and development
	Diversional activity deficit
Pervasive developmental disorders	Impaired social interaction
	Potential for violence, self-directed
	Ineffective family coping: compromised
Autistic disorder	Impaired social interaction
	Impaired verbal communication
	Risk of altered parent/child attachment
Attention-deficit/hyperactivity disorder	Potential for violence, self-directed
	Potential for violence, directed toward another
	Family coping: disabling, ineffective
Feeding and eating disorders of infancy and early childhood	Altered nutrition
	Impaired home maintenance management
	Ineffective infant feeding pattern
Tic disorder	Powerlessness
	Body-image disturbance
	Ineffective management of therapeutic regimen, individual
	Social isolation
Conduct disorder	Risk for altered parenting
Oppositional defiant disorder	Ineffective management of therapeutic regimen, families
	Impaired social interaction
Elimination disorder	Bowel incontinence
Encopresis	Altered bowel elimination
	Ineffective denial
Enuresis	Incontinence
	Self-esteem disturbance
	Altered growth and development
Separation anxiety disorder	Anxiety
	Risk for altered parenting
	Risk for altered parent/child attachment

*From American Psychiatric Association. (1994). Diagnostic and statistical manual of mental disorders, (4th ed.). Washington, DC: author.
†From North American Nursing Diagnosis Association. (1994). NANDA nursing diagnoses: definitions & classification, 1995-1996. St. Louis: Mosby.

The Nursing Process

Implementation

The American Nurses Association Standards of Care (1994) guide the roles of nurses with clients who are mentally ill. Roles include counseling, milieu management, self-care activities, management of psychobiological interventions, health teaching, health promotion and disease prevention, and collaboration with other health professionals.

When intervening with children and their families, cultural diversity needs to be considered. The Cultural Highlights box below suggests several facts related to nursing process applications with children.

Counseling

Counseling children involves the use of play therapy, behavioral management, cognitive and management therapy, and family counseling. The use of counseling techniques facilitates rapport and mutual trust between the child and the nurse.

Play therapy

Play is the most commonly used modality with children. Play is used to foster trust and to facilitate a therapeutic relationship between a child and the nurse. ***Play therapy is an intervention defined as the purposeful use of toys and other equipment to assist a child in communicating his or her perception of the world and to help him or her master the environment.*** Play is one of the most important aspects of a child's day-to-day life and of his or her growth and development. Children's ability to express themselves through play compensates for their lack of sophistication with verbal and written language. Play is an ego function expressing the child's bodily and social processes as mediated through the self. It helps the child relax, release excess energy, master situations, resolve conflicts, and relieve anxiety. Play helps children to learn about themselves and their environment while helping them test out new behaviors and roles.

The opportunity to play is essential to children's optimal growth and development. This does not mean pro-

---

CULTURAL HIGHLIGHTS

Infants and Children

By the year 2000, children age 18 and younger from culturally diverse groups are expected to comprise one third of the U.S. and Canadian population (Andrews and Boyle, 1995).

1. Japanese culture is viewed as a nontouch culture, with much touch for infants but considerably less as the child matures (Giger and Davidhizar, 1995).

2. Many West Indian parents equate psychiatric care with removal of the child from the family for an extended time (Gopaul-McNicol, 1993).

3. The use of folk-medicine techniques, such as coining, cupping, burning, and pinching to treat illness among Southeast Asian cultures leaves marks on the child's body. The nurse needs to be able to explain that these practices are seen as abusive in the United States and to make every effort to help the family discontinue their practice. Reporting these practices is still mandatory, as is any intentional harm to a child, no matter what the motivation. Folk medicine practices may lead to infection, and their use may prevent a child from

receiving help that can provide symptomatic relief (Andrews and Boyle, 1995).

4. *Mal ojo,* or evil eye, is an affliction feared by people throughout the world. It is believed to be prevented by patting or touching a child when admiring him or her.

5. The Vietnamese belief is that touching a child's head takes away his or her spirit. Some Latino/Hispanic parents may have concerns about strangers touching their children. When in doubt, the nurse should ask the parents (Andrews and Boyle, 1995).

6. Many Vietnamese persons believe that American medicines are stronger than needed and often use only one half of the dose prescribed (Giger and Davidhizar, 1995).

7. West Indian families, confronted with their children's difficult behavior after sometimes waiting a long time to be reunited with them in the United States, may think that returning the children to the home island is the only option available to them.

The Nursing Process

viding the child with expensive, battery-operated toys but rather allowing the child to freely use imagination and creativity. The use the child makes of a toy is more significant than the toy itself. For example, a stick may be a magic wand, a fishing pole, a weapon to protect oneself, a king's scepter, a baseball bat, or a hockey stick.

Play therapy is a specialized skill used by child therapists to formulate diagnostic assumptions and implement interventions. Several techniques are used. These are listed in Box 33-7. The play therapy area should be a free and protected space with a variety of toys, games, and play materials. The therapist has goals for play therapy sessions.

Areas where children spend time, such as waiting rooms or clinics, should have a variety of age-appropriate play materials available. Play may consist of games, story telling, drawing, reading or play acting, or helping children design and manipulate a miniature world where they can express themselves and resolve problems. *Sand tray therapy* is a modification of play therapy. It combines play and art therapy. *Children are provided with trays of sand and other objects used to create scenes.* The sand allows the child to change the scene.

Art therapy is used extensively with children. Children are asked to draw their experience. Art provides information about the child's behavior, developmental level, and perceptions of an experience. Examples of the use of art in the treatment and assessment of children are found throughout this chapter.

BOX 33-7

Models of Play Therapy

STRUCTURED PLAY

Encourages children to express the unconscious
The therapist encourages the child to play or replay a
scene; anatomical dolls or other toys that help the child
express his or her experience may be used

MUTUAL STORY TELLING

A technique used to encourage children to express feelings or reenact a trauma or loss; puppets may be used

NONDIRECTIVE PLAY

Children are permitted to play without direction from
therapist

BEHAVIORAL PLAY

Play acting to teach a child new ways of behaving

Cognitive therapy

Cognitive strategies useful for children include use of mnemonics, imagery, role reversal, and novelty. These are incorporated into play therapy, psychodrama, story telling, and sand tray work. Frost (1995) uses cognitive therapy in story telling and slogan development to help children with information processing, a process advanced by Burgess in her work with children who have been traumatized (Burgess, 1988). Ellis' work in rational emotive therapy has particular usefulness in helping children stop negative self-talk and modify negative belief systems. Cognitive and behavioral therapy is discussed in Chapter 16.

Group counseling

Group intervention with children has the same curative effect as group intervention with adults and may be used for children with particular problems, such as impaired self-esteem or trauma (see Chapter 11). Self-esteem enhancement involves assisting a child to increase his or her personal judgment of self-worth. Group therapy for children who have been traumatized sexually has increased awareness of sexual trauma in the etiology of child problems. Nurses have developed a time-limited, inpatient group for children who have been sexually traumatized called *Superkids,* which deals with issues of shame, blame, anger, fear, trust, and love (Morris, 1994).

Groups can be potent forces in helping children of separated and divorced parents process anger, confusion, and loss; extrinsic risk factors or parental discord and instability may be processed with older children. Group therapy for children whose parents are alcoholics is helpful, particularly as a parallel process during their recovering parents' aftercare. Art-therapy groups are especially useful in assisting children to express concern and anxieties. Play therapy groups and psychodrama are also effective treatment modalities with children (Zimmermann, 1987).

Family counseling

Some believe that children cannot be treated unless the family is involved in the process. The child's presenting problem may be closely connected to parental behavior in abusive and violent families, in families with chemical dependency, and during separation and divorce. The child's diagnosis may stress the family system. Family therapy and family group or parenting classes are usually standard components of treatment when a child is hospitalized with a psychiatric diagnosis.

The nurse working in child and family settings must be aware of the availability of family treatment in the

The Nursing Process

community and should develop skills in presenting parenting classes. Parents look to the nurse to provide resources such as books and videos; to teach them about the stages of family development and various community resources such as ALANON family groups, Parents Without Partners, and divorce/separation groups. Pictures of families cut from magazines may be used by children in a group to facilitate expression of feeling about family relationships. The nurse also provides anticipatory guidance by teaching parenting classes and helping new parents. During a home visit the nurse can reinforce parental teaching that began in the hospital and model soothing strategies, as well as attend to other psychosocial needs of new parents.

Behavioral therapy

Behavioral interventions are most useful when implemented consistently in three arenas: in the home, in the classroom, and with the individual child. A nurse can teach parents about behavior management strategies. Parents are taught how to use "time out" for inappropriate behavior. Children may be taught self-control and relaxation techniques with use of behavior techniques. The use of parent-teacher behavioral checklists specify observable behavior, qualify successes or changes, and demonstrate positive changes for children and their families.

Behavioral therapists actively direct treatment. They may suggest out-of-session homework. Children and their parents may be given assignments, encouraged to read and attend specific support groups, or to start an exercise program. Treatment goals are mutually set between child, family, and counselor, and goal attainment is evaluated often. This approach is compatible with solution-focused, short-term treatment approaches.

An assumption of behavior therapy is that behavioral changes are instigated and maintained by involving key persons in the child's environment. The successful child therapist sees the parent as an ally, seeks parental support by helping with parenting modification, and encourages parental education to support the child's growth in treatment toward becoming a happy and effective human being.

Milieu Therapy

Parental involvement in the inpatient treatment of children is the strongest predictor of positive outcomes after discharge from treatment. Therapeutic visits of family when the child is an inpatient provide opportunities for participation in milieu strategies such as parent education, multifamily group therapy, and recreational activities. Family therapy is usually a mandatory component of the child's therapeutic environment. A school program must be provided as an adjunct to inpatient or day treatment. A multidisciplinary team approach involves close collaboration with all individuals involved in the children's care (Pizzello and Breitmayer, 1993).

Shortened lengths of hospital stay mean that most inpatient children's programs deal with acutely ill children in need of rapid stabilization. With a shift to day or partial-hospital approaches, residential care facilities provide long-term care only for children who cannot safely function in the community. Parental involvement in the child's care, family therapy, and the use of community resources are essential components in the delivery of mental health services to children.

Parenting education helps parents modify behavioral patterns and learn more effective ways of coping with their children. They also help parents of children who have experienced severe disruptions in attachment and have difficulty or are unable to bond in a healthy way. Studies demonstrate that developmental outcomes can be improved and the cost of hospitalization can be reduced if caregivers are assisted with interpreting infant behavior and instructed about developmentally appropriate responses. Parent education is critical for the parents of high-risk babies.

The therapeutic environment in child psychiatric nursing refers to people and all other social and physical environmental factors with which the child interacts, including the health and school systems, and provides a round-the-clock secure retreat for children. Nurses are the only professionals responsible for maintaining the therapeutic environment on a 24-hour basis. Principles of the therapeutic milieu that apply on the general psychiatric unit also apply on any children's units, whether in the acute care setting, child psychiatric unit, or a residential care setting (see Chapter 20). However, issues of safety appropriate to the need children have for adult supervision require more intensive staffing ratios.

In a therapeutic children's milieu, rules, expectations, and consequences should be clearly understood. Children earn or lose points and privileges as consequences of behavior. The object is to establish a sense of self-efficacy and develop responsibility for one's own behavior. The environment should closely convey a child-friendly, child-centered approach. A central day room with bedrooms opening off the room is less institutional than the corridor model and also provides for better supervision. Children show much variation in age, developmental needs, and abilities, thus challenging the resourcefulness and creativity of the nursing staff to establish an environment suitable to children.

The Nursing Process

Self-Care Activities

Children love to learn. They are curious and interested in novelty. They have active imaginations and enjoy playing games and receiving attention. This natural ability means children can be taught self-care techniques that will be helpful to them throughout life. Visualization, relaxation, guided imagery, and other stress-management techniques are useful for children. Identification of feelings, mastering anger outbursts, and assertive communication are all part of effective self-management.

Psychobiological Interventions

Developmental issues and the physiological differences of children complicate the understanding of pediatric psychopharmacology. Most psychotropic medications are high in fat solubility. Children's percentage of total body fat, which is a reservoir for lipid-soluble compounds, increases during the first year of life and then decreases until the prepubertal increase. Children at different ages have different volumes of deep storage of fat, which affects the overall residual time that medicine remains in the body after discontinuation of treatment (Hughes & Peskorn, 1994). Another difference is the proportion of liver size to overall mass. Children have bigger livers than adults, and because the liver detoxifies drugs and other substances, children clear drugs more rapidly than adults. The onset of puberty also causes changes in hepatic activity as a result of the increased circulation of sex hormones.

The use of multiple psychotropic agents to treat childhood mental disorders is becoming an increasingly common practice. Some of the conditions in which combinations of medications are used include ADHD, depression, bipolar disorder, anxiety, psychosis, tic disorders, and aggression and conduct disorders (Wilen et al., 1995). ADHD responds well to stimulants, nonstimulants, and tricyclic antidepressants, but this practice may be a source of concern for parents. Stimulants such as dextroamphetamine (Dexedrine) and methylphenidate (Ritalin) are used almost exclusively to treat children. Dosages are determined by the child's weight. Medication Tips for working with children are shown at right.

Nurses working with children need to be familiar with the actions, interactions, and side effects of all the pharmacological agents prescribed for the child's medication regimen. Medications are similar to those discussed in Chapter 15. However, children who experience rapid clearance may need more frequent dosing, although total drug doses are less than for adults and are related to the child's body size. Children are more likely to experience drug withdrawal symptoms (Sylvester and Kreuci, 1994). Adequate observation and documentation must occur to distinguish between withdrawal symptoms, side effects, and effects of the disorder. Coordination of care between children's psychiatric and primary health care providers is essential. However, there are differences in the use of psychopharmacological agents with children (Box 33-8).

Health Teaching

Health teaching is an essential component in the nurse's care of children with emotional disorders (see Chapter 16). Children's social competence depends on skills training in family, extended family, schools, and neighborhoods. During childhood, successful interaction is learned by developing friendships and interactional skills. Later, as adults, children with poor peer relationships suffer a higher degree of emotional disturbance than those who established satisfactory friendships. Therefore it is important that children have the chance to develop friendships and the ability to socialize. Social competency involves behaviors that can be taught. Successful social skills learning may help offset other negative experiences.

For the child to maintain gains made during inpatient hospitalization or as a result of outpatient therapy, it is critical that parents comprehend and support the child's recovery. Parents who admit a child to a facility often believe they have failed, whether their actions contributed to the illness or not. It is essential for the nursing staff to

 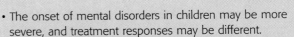

MEDICATION TIPS

- The onset of mental disorders in children may be more severe, and treatment responses may be different.
- Children often differ in response to a medication's main and side effects.
- Children may metabolize and eliminate medications more rapidly.
- When medicating children, start slow, titrate carefully, and use the lowest effective dose.
- The final dose may be higher than in adults because of metabolic and organ differences.
- Clinical observations of effects are essential because of the absence of carefully controlled studies of pharmacotherapy in children.
- The same medicine is used for children as for adults in many cases, although variations in dosing considers difference in size, metabolism, and desired action.
- Combined pharmacotherapy is being used safely with children.

The Nursing Process

provide family support and encourage involvement in the child's care. Parenting education is essential.

Case Management

Nurses work with others who have interest in the emotional and mental well-being of children. Nurses further the agenda for children's mental health by becoming involved as case managers at all levels—in neighborhoods, religious institutions, schools, and professional associations, and through political activity. As experts in the science of caring and psychiatric well-being of children, nurses can serve as a resource to others. Computerization can facilitate this coordination of care by allowing rapid access to medical records. Nurses have opportunities to promote the development of creative programs geared to meet specific community needs. A key to the success of case management strategies involves forming partnerships with parents and the agencies they need to access.

Health Promotion and Health Maintenance

Health promotion and prevention of the residual effects of childhood emotional disorders is a major role of nurses who work with children. Nurses promote the health of children by becoming involved in national and local organizations that are concerned with the health of children. Community Resources are listed below. Another means of promoting children's health is through the use of audiovisual materials. Children's books and videos portray positive role models.

Promoting a child's self-esteem employs numerous health-promoting strategies. Table 33-2 lists strategies used by nurses to promote children's self esteem. Strategies are employed by the nurse and taught to significant individuals in the child's environment.

Recent emphasis on child abuse, neglect, and violence requires the nurse to coordinate prevention efforts with other agencies and professionals. The U.S. attorney general has said the following:

No child should die from malnutrition, but they do. We may not be able to prevent every abuse-related death of a child,

COMMUNITY RESOURCES

Children's Mental Health

American Academy of Pediatrics
141 Northwest Point Boulevard
Box 927
Elk Grove, IL 60609-0927
(800) 433-9016

American Professional Society on the Abuse of Children
407 S Dearborn, Suite 1300
Chicago, IL 60605
(312) 554-0166

Association of Child and Adolescent Psychiatric Nurses
1211 Locust Street
Philadelphia, PA 19107
(800) 826-2950

Child Welfare League of America
440 First Street, NE
Suite 310
Washington, DC 20001-2085
(202) 638-2952

Clearinghouse on Child Abuse and Neglect Information
Box 1182
Washington, DC 20013
(703) 385-7565

BOX 33-8

Medicating Children

- Antihistamines lower the seizure threshold and cause delirium and worsening of tic disorders.
- Lithium is cleared rapidly by children, so they may require higher doses to stabilize a mood disorder
- Valproate (Depakote) carries the risk of hepatotoxicity in children under age 10.
- The dietary restrictions and attendant risks with monoamine oxidase inhibitors (MAOIs) makes their use problematic with a pediatric population.
- Children both metabolize neuroleptics rapidly and are more sensitive to their main effects.
- Stimulants are the first line of treatment in the treatment of ADHD. It is becoming a more universal practice to continue this treatment through adulthood.
- The SSRIs are a safe and effective treatment for depression in children.
- Buspirone (Bu Spar) may be helpful in managing aggression and agitation in children with mental retardation or a PDD.

The Nursing Process

but we can try. We can make sure that no child who dies in this country is laid to rest without our knowing how and why he or she died. This will enable us to design programs that teach parents how to properly supervise and care for their children and to learn when and how to intervene effectively before these tragedies occur (US Attorney General Janet Reno, February 16, 1994).

Family preventive intervention is helpful to parents of high-risk or low–birth weight infants who remain hospitalized for a long time. The nurse facilitates bonding and helps alleviate parental fears and anxieties. Because low–birth weight babies are at higher risk for abuse and disrupted attachment, the nurse is a key figure in evaluating parents for risk and providing counseling. Conduct disorder, a childhood condition that is often a precursor to violence and adult criminal activity, is another area on which to focus primary prevention efforts with families (Fischel, 1990).

Poor prenatal care is positively associated with dysfunctional lifestyles. In their role as primary mental health care providers, nurses can be powerful advocates for family prenatal care. Furthermore, the possible savings that result from improved parent-child interaction have not yet been measured. As care shifts from acute care to ambulatory and home settings, the role of early intervention by nurses may well expand dramatically. The nurse as an activist for children and families at risk can assist in making services more accessible, provide support, and identify pregnant women in need of care.

Evaluation

The successful outcome of interventions with children is dependent to a large extent on the ability of parents to maintain and cooperate with the treatment plan for the child. It is generally believed that as parents become better able to meet their own needs, the child will have more success managing his or her symptoms.

Ongoing evaluation of outcomes for individual children and for the world community of children is an important component of the nursing process because successful interventions are an investment in the children's future. Preventing mental disorders in children and diagnosing and treating them accurately facilitates a happier and more hopeful future for them. The planning and successful implementation of effective prevention and early intervention programs can only be achieved with ongoing evaluation of the outcome of interdisciplinary efforts.

TABLE 33-2

Enhancing a child's self-esteem

TARGETED AREA	STRATEGY
Caregiver expectations	Describe expectations for the child
	Assess anticipated developmental milestones
	Review family patterns and influences
Personal value	Communicate confidence in the child
	Structure situations to promote success of the child
	Implement effective ways of praising the child
	Be a role model of valuing self
Communication	Listen attentively
	Encourage openness to feelings
	Avoid using judgmental statements
	Elicit different points of view
Discipline	Use effective methods of limit setting
	Discuss and implement appropriate consequences
	Review problem-solving techniques
	Discourage use of physical punishment
Guidance	Encourage open exchange with the child
	Know the child's activities away from home
	Express interest in school events
	Become familiar with the child's friends
Autonomy	Demonstrate respect for the child
	Promote the child's responsible decision making
	Expect reciprocal respect

Modified from Sieving, R. & Ziebel-Donisch, S. (1990). Journal of Pediatric Health Care, 2(4), 290.

KEY POINTS

- Crime, poverty, violence, use of drugs and alcohol, lack of education, low self-esteem, lack of community and family values, and inadequate information are among the risk factors affecting children's physical and emotional health.
- Resiliency is the child's invulnerability to environmental risks. It explains why some children develop mental disorders and others do not.
- Disturbance in the affectional bond between parent and child (attachment) is positively correlated with development of later psychopathological disorders.
- The study of temperament explains the significance of child/parent "goodness of fit." It is manifested in the child's activity, adaptability, intensity, approachability, mood, distractibility, persistence, rhythmicity, and threshold of responsiveness.
- Disorders listed in the DSM-IV that are first diagnosed in childhood include mental retardation, learning, motor skills, and communication disorders; PDDs; attention-deficit and disruptive behavior disorders; and eating and elimination disorders.
- Assessment of children is a complex multifaceted process that presents a challenge for nurses and those who collaborate with them in the care of children.
- Play is the primary method used for facilitating assessment of a child.
- Multiple informants contribute data needed to formulate nursing diagnoses and establish realistic outcomes of the nursing interventions.
- Play therapy is the most commonly used intervention with children. It is the purposeful use of toys and other equipment to help children communicate their perceptions of the world and to help them master the environment.
- Interventions with children include family counseling, play therapy, use of pharmacological agents, case management, use of behavioral modification strategies, parent effectiveness training, and stress management strategies.
- Involvement of parents in the care of their children is a key component in the planning and achievement of successful outcomes.

REFERENCES

American Nurses Association. (1994). *Statement on psychiatric mental health clinical nursing practice and standards of psychiatric mental health nursing practice.* Washington, DC: Author.

American Psychiatric Association. (1994). *Diagnostic and statisical manual of mental disorders, Fourth edition.* Washington, DC: Author.

 CRITICAL THINKING QUESTIONS

Sallie Prince is a 29-year-old single mother working as a cashier in a building supply store. She receives a minimum amount of child support, and her exhusband who is alcoholic is several months behind on payments. He has stopped picking up Amanda, the 10-year-old child, because of the arguments around money. Amanda believes she is somehow to blame for the family's economic stress. She misses her father, believes she can't make her mother happy, and worries about ways she can change things. Amanda prepares the evening meal and must deal with the landlord and utility company calling about overdue bills. When this does not go well, Amanda's mother blames Amanda. Amanda also tries to comfort her mother when she complains about her job and Amanda's father. Amanda is well liked by her teachers, and she is an outgoing child who gets along well with others. The family is referred to the psychiatric home health nurse by the school counselor, who notes Amanda's sadness and concern about her mother.

1. What do you think about Amanda and her mother?
2. How does Amanda fit into the vulnerable populations for emotional problems?
3. What factors foster resiliency with Amanda?
4. What are important points for the nurse to cover during a home visit?
5. What are the most important differences between assessment in a hospital setting and the home?
6. What other community support services might be helpful to this family?

American Professional Society on the Abuse of Children. (1990). *Guidelines for the psychosocial evaluation of suspected sexual abuse in children.* Chicago: Author.

Andrews, M.M., & Boyle, J.S. (1995). *Transcultural concepts in nursing care.* Philadelphia: J.B. Lippincott.

Bowlby, J. (1994). *Attachment.* New York: Basic Books.

Cantwell, D. (1995). Attention deficit hyperactivity disorder and stimulant therapy. In *Frontiers in clinical pediatric psychopharmacology.* Key West, FL: American Academy of Child and Adolescent Psychiatry.

Carlson, G. (1995). Mood Disorders. In *Frontiers in clinical pediatric psychopharmacology.* Key West, FL: American Academy of Child and Adolescent Psychiatry.

Cassetta, R. (1994). Children: A community in crisis. *The American Nurse.* November/December, 1-21.

Donovan, J. (1994). Major theoretical frameworks for psychiatric nursing. In C. Houseman (Ed.), *Psychiatric certification review guide for the generalist and clinical specialist in adult, child, and adolescent psychiatric and mental health nursing* Potomac, MD:Health Leadership Associates.

Faller, K.C. (1993). *Child sexual abuse: Intervention and treatment issues.* U.S. Department of Health and Human Services: Administration for Children and Families, Administration on Children, Youth and Families. Washington, DC: National Center on Child Abuse and Neglect.

Fishel, A.H. (1990). A community-based program for emotionally disturbed children and youth. *Journal of Child and Adolescent Psychiatric and Mental Health Nursing, 3*(4), 128-133.

Geissler, E.M. (1994). *Cultural assessment.* St. Louis: Mosby.

Giger, J.N., & Davidhizar, R.E. (1995). *Transcultural nursing: Assessment and intervention.* St. Louis: Mosby.

Gopaul-McNicol, S. (1993). *Working with West Indian families.* (2nd ed.). New York: Guilford.

Hallowell, E.M. & Ratey, J.J. (1994). *Driven to distraction: Recognizing and coping with attention deficit disorder from childhood through adulthood.* New York: Simon and Schuster.

Hinshaw, A.S. (1992). Nursing research: Weaving the past and the future. In L. Aiken, & C. Fagin (Eds.), *Charting nursing's future.* Philadelphia: J.B. Lippincott.

Kersey, K. (1983). *The art of sensitive parenting.* Washington, DC: Acropolis.

Krauss, J. (1993). *Health care reform: Essential mental health services.* Washington, DC: American Nurses Association.

Leckman, J.F., & Cohen, D.J. (1991). Clonadine treatment of Tourette's syndrome. *Archives of General Psychiatry, 48,* 324-328.

Lewin, L. (1995). Interviewing the young child sexual abuse victim. *Journal of Psychosocial Nursing, 33*(7), 5-10.

Lombroso, P.J. et al. (1994). Genetic mechanisms in childhood psychiatric disorders. *Journal of the American Academy of Child and Adolescent Psychiatry, 33,* 921-938.

Mack, A. (1989). *Dry all night.* Boston: Little, Brown.

McBride, A.B. (1988). Coming of age: Child psychiatric nursing. *Archives of Psychiatric Nursing II, 2,* 57-64.

McClellan, J., & Werry, J. (1994). Practice parameters in the assessment of children and adolescents with schizophrenia. *Journal of the American Academy of Children and Adolescents, 6*(94), 616-635.

McSwiggan-Hardin, M.T. (1995). Tic disorders. In B. Johnson, (Ed.), *Child, adolescent and family psychiatric nursing* (pp. 285-286). Philadelphia: J.B. Lippincott.

Morris, P.A. (1994). Superkids: Short-term group therapy for children with abusive backgrounds. *Journal of Child and Adolescent Psychiatric Nursing, 7*(1), 25-31.

Offord, D.R., & Bennett, K.J. (1994). Conduct disorder: Long-term outcome and intervention effectiveness. *Journal of the American Academy of Child and Adolescent Psychiatry, 10*(94), 1069-1078.

Pizzello, L., & Breitmayer, B.J. (1993). Evaluation of treatment integrity on a child psychiatric unit: An illustration. *Journal of Child and Adolescent Psychiatric and Mental Health Nursing, 6*(3), 16-17.

Rak, C., & Patterson. (1996). Promoting resilience in at-risk children. *Journal of Counseling and Development, 74*(4), 368-373.

Reno, Janet (1994, February 16). Presentation. Washington, DC.

Sprague-McRae, J.M. (1990). Encopresis: Developmental, behavioral and physiological considerations for treatment. *The Nurse Practitioner, 15*(6), 8-24.

Steving, R. and Ziebel-Donisch, S. (1990). Enhancing self-esteem in children. *Journal of Pediatric Health Care, 4*(2) 290.

Sylvester, C.E., & Kruesi, M. (1994). Child and adolescent psychopharmacotherapy: Progress and pitfalls. *Psychiatric Annals, 24*(2), 83-89.

Thompson, R. (1991). Attachment theory and research. In M. Lewis (Ed.), *Child and adolescent psychiatry: A comprehensive textbook* (p. 103). Baltimore: Williams & Wilkins.

Wilens, T.E., Spencer, T., Biederman, J., Wozniak, J., & Connor, D. (1995). Combined pharmacotherapy: An emerging field in pediatric psychopharmacology. *Journal of the American Academy of Child and Adolescent Psychiatry, 34*(1), 110-112.

Workman, et al. (1993). Human genetics. In Kenner, et al. (Eds.), *Comprehensive neonatal nursing.* Philadelphia: W.B. Saunders.

Zimmerman, M.L., et al (1987). Art and group work: Interventions for multiple victims of child molestation. Part II. *Archives of Psychiatric Nursing, 1*(1), 40-46.

Chapter 34

Adolescents

Jeanne Ryan Botz
Sharon Bidwell-Cerone

LEARNING OUTCOMES

After studying and applying the concepts of this chapter, the learner will be able to:
- Differentiate between normal adolescent turmoil and psychiatric symptoms of adolescents.
- Respond therapeutically to dysfunctional behaviors with developmentally appropriate interventions.
- Apply the nursing process to selected adolescent behaviors.

KEY TERMS

Acting out	Gangs	Resilience
Acting up	Juvenile delinquency	"Roid rage"
Attachment	Kleptomania	Sensitive periods
Binding dynamics	Limit setting	Suicide contagion
Cults	Moralistic self-righteousness	Temperament
Delegating dynamics	Omnipotent authoritarianism	Tricholillomania
Expelling dynamics	Pyromania	Vulnerability

Adolescence is a transitional developmental phase that occurs somewhere between the ages of 10 and 20, although there is striking variability in terms of when individuals cross the great divide between childhood and adulthood. Adolescence seems like one long holding pattern for those who experience it in western culture. However, it is in fact a dynamic time characterized by three main types of development. The first is *physical,* which starts with puberty and ends with completion of growth. The second is *cognitive,* which is the intellectual maturation that makes adolescents more skilled than children in the use of logic and reason. The third is *psychosocial,* which is integral to the first two. Relating to parents with new independence, to friends with new intimacy, to society with new commitment, and to oneself with new understanding ideally results in adolescents finding the answer to the question: "Who am I?" This chapter will discuss common mental health issues prevalent during adolescence. Nursing interventions that address specific adolescent needs will be discussed.

EPIDEMIOLOGY

The prevalence of mental illness in adolescence is comparable to that in adulthood. In the United States, where adolescents comprise approximately 11% of the population, this developmental stage is widely regarded as difficult. While no time in life is problem-free or accurately defined by only its problems, adolescence retains a persistent reputation as a period ripe for behavior disturbance. A series of recent studies suggests that the prevalence of significant mental illness among teen-agers ranges from 17% to 22%, however, 12% is the conservative estimate more often cited. Of these teen-agers with symptoms, nearly half are deemed severely disabled. This figure exceeds 20% in the inner cities where extreme adversity is the norm (IOM, 1994). In fact the major cause of disability among adolescents is mental disorders. The *Healthy People 2000 Review* reports that the U.S. Public Health Service's goal is to reduce to less than 10% the prevalence of mental illness in this age group (U.S. Public Health Service, 1993).

Risk Factors

Nurses have been concerned with how persons interact with particular environments since Nightingale wrote, "What nursing has to do…is to put the patient in the best condition for nature to act upon him." Identifying personal vulnerabilities and environmental influences (risks) on mental health can be useful for understanding troubled adolescents and implementing effective strategies to help them.

Adolescents with risk factors have rates of mental illness that exceed those in the general population. Rates increase in proportion to the number of risk factors that are experienced. Risk factors shown by research to be associated with mental disorders in adolescence are listed in Box 34-1.

Vulnerability refers to potentially debilitating personal factors that may influence mental health. Each of these factors increases the chance of mental illness and may occur in combination. Inborn and acquired vulnerabilities shown by research to be associated with adolescent mental disorders are listed in Box 34-2.

Resilience refers to protective factors that shield individuals from mental illness. These factors can be inferred when no mental dysfunction is found in adolescents, even though their lives contain the same risks and vulnerabilities known to cause mental illness in others. An important research goal is to determine the mechanisms by which these factors provide protection (Jessor, 1993). Resilience factors that have been scientifically documented are listed in Box 34-3.

THEORETICAL FRAMEWORK

Theorists view humans from a variety of perspectives, but they all seek to provide frameworks for explaining behavior. One theory alone is too limited to explain the

---

BOX 34-1

Risks for Adolescent Mental Disorders

- Poverty
- Crowded inner-city neighborhoods
- Racial inequality
- Large family size
- Unstable families
- Marital discord
- Inconsistent caretakers
- Prolonged parent-child separation
- Foster care
- Maternal mental illness
- Paternal criminality
- Depressed parents
- Parents with substance abuse disorders
- Rejection by parents
- Physical, sexual, emotional abuse
- Homelessness
- Catastrophic events
- Bereavement
- Aberrant peer groups
- Models for deviant behavior

diversity of any phase of human development. An eclectic perspective that considers many theories simultaneously is the approach favored by most nurses caring for adolescents.

Biopsychosocial Model

Recent advances in biology and genetics indicate that a multidisciplinary theoretical perspective provides the most satisfactory explanation for symptoms of adolescent mental disorders. This approach broadly acknowledges the interaction of risk, vulnerability, and resilience. Adolescents have the same neurobiological basis for symptoms, as their adult counterparts. However, the physiological hormonal turmoil that is normal in adolescence does make teen-agers more vulnerable to exacerbation of symptoms. This gives rise to the idea of **sensitive periods.** Sensitivity period theory focuses on *times of physical development during which persons are particularly susceptible to events such as sensory deprivation, malnutrition, and exposure to toxins.* The powerful role parents play in meeting infant developmental needs affects mental health during adolescence (see Chapter 33).

Temperament *refers to differences in emotions, activity, and arousal that are biologically determined and present at birth.* An association has been shown between difficult infant temperament and later behavior disturbance. The degree of temperamental "fit" between parent and child is known to influence relatedness and emotional connectedness.

Attachment *refers to the emotional bond that develops between infants and their special caregivers.* This bond is thought to be biological in nature and to have evolved to support survival of the species. Infants who do not attach to their caregivers fail to accomplish developmental tasks, which leaves them as adolescents with poor communication skills and an inability to form peer relationships.

Developmental Theories

Adolescence is a time during which complex changes in biological, social, and emotional development occur. The rapidity of change challenges adolescents to cope effectively or to regress and display dysfunctional behaviors. Various developmental theories explain adolescent behavior and norms. The application of these theories to adolescent behaviors enhances the nurse's ability to assess and care for this population. In any case, developmental theory defines the expected tasks of adolescence (see Chapter 7).

Family Theory

Family theory focuses on the importance of viewing the family as a whole rather than examining the difficulties of an identified individual. For example, the stealing behavior of an adolescent may be interpreted as a problem with communication or rigid rules in the family rather than a personality flaw of the child. Families remain the most meaningful frame of reference for adolescents despite the fact that peers and the community acquire relatively more emphasis than held during childhood. Therefore appraisal of the family unit is integral to a comprehensive assessment of adolescents. Families with ef-

---

BOX 34-2

Vulnerabilities for Adolescent Mental Disorders

- Low birth weight
- Prematurity
- Early difficult temperament
- Developmental disabilities
- Mental retardation
- Brain damage
- Epilepsy
- Chronic illnesses
- Physical disabilities
- Low perceived life chances
- Low self-esteem
- Risk-taking propensity
- Poor school performance

BOX 34-3

Resilience to Adolescent Mental Disorders

- Easy temperament
- Good problem-solving abilities
- High intelligence
- Supportive family
- Caring adults outside the home
- Compensatory experiences outside the home
- Models for conventional behavior
- Neighborhood resources
- Supports for coping and values
- Intolerance of deviance
- Values on achievement
- Values on health
- Good schools
- Good school performance
- Involvement in church and school clubs

fective interpersonal relationships are inherently growth-producing (see Chapter 12).

Separation dynamics

Families that have difficulty promoting growth demonstrate problems with separation dynamics. Separation is a fundamental issue for adolescents and their families. Teen-agers need to move toward increasing independence and decreasing dependence on families, while parents need to "let go" and facilitate their offsprings' independence. Dysfunctional family dynamics that are separation-related include delegating, expelling, binding, omnipotent authoritarianism, moralistic self-righteousness, and peerlike parent-adolescent relationships.

Delegating dynamics are forces within the family that influence adolescents to act as proxies for their parents, which is done at the expense of teen-agers' growth and development. Conflict occurs between the parents. They wish to consolidate their relationship with the adolescent and with each other and to be rid of the adolescent. They send conflicting messages such as, "Leave, but don't leave because we need you." They assign the adolescent to missions as proxies for themselves, while at the same time hold on to them. Adolescents incorporate this ambivalence and unconsciously fulfill the assigned mission. There are four types of missions that adolescents carry out to serve the needs of parents, which are presented in Table 34-1 with clinical examples.

Expelling dynamics are forces that result in premature separation of adolescents from their families. They alter family structure in ways that interfere with the sense of belonging and connection, creating internal desires in the adolescents to put distance between themselves and their families. Isolation and loneliness result and are acted out with running away behavior and distancing tactics such as alcohol or drug abuse.

Binding dynamics are forces within the family that interfere with the permeability of boundaries. The unspoken assumption is that the needs of the members can only be met within the family unit. The outside world is viewed as dangerous and unsatisfying, which colludes to conspire to keep members inside. This dynamic fulfills some needs for security, support, and nurturing, but it does so at the expense of individual ideas, feelings, experiences, and behavior. When members are prevented from separating and individuating, their potential for self-actualization is reduced. The binding process corrals the members affectively, cognitively, and by challenging their loyalty. The adolescent, in response to covert and overt messages from parents not to leave the family, becomes excessively dependent on it and is blocked from becoming independent except in dysfunctional ways, which is then seen as rebellion.

TABLE 34-1

Delegating dynamics

DYNAMIC	DEFINITION	EXAMPLE
Helping	Adolescent assumes parental role.	Meghan, a 13 year old, is the primary care-giver of her 3-year-old sister on weekends while their single mother works.
Fighting	Adolescent is the mediator or physical protector.	Craig, a 16 year old, recently came to school with a black eye that resulted from a physical confrontation with his alcoholic father, who was beating Craig's mother.
Scouting	Adolescent acts out parent's unconscious fantasies.	Kristen, a 13-year-old seventh grader, is permitted to date a sexually active 17-year-old junior.
Preserving	Adolescent is the main glue keeping the family together.	Peter is a 15 year old whose parents are both chronically physically ill and depend on him to do major household tasks after school. This prevents him from being involved in sports and other activities.

Omnipotent authoritarianism

Omnipotent authoritarianism is characterized by parental proclamations such as, "You do it this way, because I told you to." This behavior pattern *occurs when parents defend their status as authorities and attempt to preserve their self-concept as all-knowing adults with the privilege of seniority.* Authority is maintained by devaluing the viewpoints, activities, and accomplishments of adolescents. As a result, adolescents are not empowered, because the needs of their parents take precedence. This generates frustration, depression, anxiety, regression, and helplessness. Some adolescents in this situation opt out of identity formation completely and view suicide as a solution. Others exhibit rebellious behavior that is counterproductive to resolving developmental tasks.

Moralistic self-righteousness

Moralistic self-righteousness is characterized by moralizing, preaching, and a "holier than thou" attitude with the aim to elicit respect and submission. Obedience to parental directives extends to areas where adolescents should otherwise be increasing autonomous problem solving and decision making such as choosing friends. However, the dilemma is the choice between rebellion (which is bad) and conformity (which is perceived as good). Either course results in derailment of self-development and a reduced sense of belonging to peer groups.

Peerlike parents

Parents who characterize themselves as "friend" or "pal" and project the image of being "in tune" demonstrate unreserved understanding and acceptance of behavior that is overpermissive, sets few limits, and is supported by rationalization. These parents identify with the ideal parents they would have liked to have had, and they have a need to remain young. They may dress and act more like teen-agers than their offspring do. Their regressive enactment of the teen-age role deprives the actual adolescents of empathic and helpful authority figures and violates generational boundaries. Peerlike parents obstruct the expression of developmentally necessary parent-adolescent conflict, the absence of which interferes with identity formation.

MENTAL DISORDERS OF ADOLESCENCE

Certain behaviors are so severe or persistent that they significantly interfere with normal functioning. Once they reach this point, they are regarded as mental disorders that require the services of a wide range of health care professionals in inpatient and outpatient settings. This section presents a brief overview of some of the conditions experienced by adolescents with an emphasis on their unique responses to them. Table 34-2 lists the DSM-IV disorders commonly diagnosed during adolescence. The learner should note that the same disor-

TABLE 34-2

DSM-IV disorders diagnosed during adolescence

DSM-IV CLASSIFICATION	GENERAL FEATURES	SIGNIFICANCE TO ADOLESCENCE
Disruptive behavior disorder	Persistent pattern of behavior that disregards social rules, norms, and rights of others or consistent negativistic, defiant, and hostile behavior	Adolescent-onset develops between the ages of 10 and 16; at risk to develop antisocial personality disorder and substance-related disorders; impairment in social, academic, and occupational achievements
Separation anxiety disorders	Excessive anxiety concerning separation from home or individual	Occurs after a life stress; adolescent reluctant to engage in independent activities (e.g., going away to college or to a friend's home)
Cognitive disorders	Disturbance in conciousness; memory impairment with or without change in cognition	Diagnosed in adolescence; most likely due to substance use, head trauma, poor nutrition, or medical problems (e.g., HIV, meningitis, or other infections)
Somatiform disorder	History of multiple physical complaints, motor or sensory dysfunction, preoccupation with pain, physical deficit, or medical condition	Initial symptoms are often present in adolescents (e.g., menstrual difficulties, increase in school absence, or increase in health clinic visits)

Continued.

TABLE 34-2—cont'd

DSM-IV disorders diagnosed during adolescence

DSM-IV CLASSIFICATION	GENERAL FEATURES	SIGNIFICANCE TO ADOLESCENCE
Dissociative disorders	Disruption in the integrated function of memory, identity, consciousness, or perception of the environment	Disorders result from severe trauma or extremely stressful events; may be gradual, transient, or chronic; amnestic and dissociation identity disorder may be seen in adolescents evidenced by impaired school work and poor peer relationships
Sexual and general identity disorders	Recurrent, intense sexual urges, fantasies, or behaviors involving unusual objects, activities, situations, or strong, persistent cross-gender identification	Paraphilias and cross-gender identification disorders often develop during adolescence and are often kept secret, decrease in sexual development, and isolation are noted in the teen-ager
Adjustment disorder	Emotional or behavioral symptoms in response to an identified stressor	May occur during adolescence as a response to a stressor such as going to a new school, divorce, or natural disaster
Sleep disorders	Abnormality in sleep-wake generating or timing mechanism	Primary insomnia, hypersomnia, sleepwalking, sleep terror disorder, and nightmares can occur in adolescence and impair school work, school attendance, and physical health
Impulse-control disorders	Failure to resist an impulse drive; temptation to perform or act, characterized by an arousal, gratification, and relief	Age of onset of *kleptomania (stealing) and pyromania (fire starting)* have not been identified, but compulsive behavior such as *trichotillomania (pulling out one's hair),* gambling, and explosive disorder have either childhood or adolescent onset and can lead to legal problems or isolation from peers

ders occur in adulthood, therefore general features of the disorders and symptoms unique to the adolescent population are also addressed.

Mood Disorders

Depression

Adolescents normally experience fluctuating moods. This does not signal a problem unless their mood shifts are intense and persistent and interfere with normal functioning. Depression is the single most powerful symptom that determines whether adolescents are referred to mental health services. Unfortunately depression often goes unrecognized unless symptoms are flagrant, even though 8% of adolescents suffer from it.

Core characteristics of major depression are the same for all age groups, although some characteristics change or are more evident with different ages. The mood may be irritable rather than sad in adolescent depression. Also, psychomotor retardation, hypersomnia, and delusions are more common in adolescents than in children (APA, 1994). Although not part of the criteria for depression, poor academic performance, substance abuse, antisocial behavior, sexual promiscuity, truancy, and running away may be more indicative of depression in this age group (Kaplan, Sadock, and Grebb, 1994). Chapter 30 discusses the criteria for major depression. Screening for depression in adolescents is a key preventive measure. The most commonly used screening instrument is the Adolescent Depression Form (Shaffer and Fisher, 1994).

Mania

Depression can be accompanied by mania, which is a hyperactive physical and mental state with elevated mood. Mood swings ranging from depression to mania is a condition called *bipolar disorder.* Although it is generally diagnosed in adults, it can also appear in adolescents. Approximately 10% to 15% of adolescents with recurrent major depression develop bipolar I disorder. Mixed episodes appear to be more common in adolescents than in adults (APA, 1994). Symptoms of mania in adolescents may be more developmentally related and include symptoms of substance abuse, suicide attempts, fighting, academic problems, somatic preoccupation, brooding, and other antisocial behaviors. Core characteristics of bipolar disorder I or II are similar for adults and adolescents and are discussed in Chapter 30.

Suicide

The assessment of suicidal ideation in the adolescent is critical. Suicide is on the increase. The adolescent rate increased 200%, while the general population rate increased 17%. Suicide is the third leading cause of death among 15 to 19 year olds. Surveys indicate that 6% to 13% of teen-agers have attempted suicide at least once in their lives. The vast majority do not seek or receive mental health care (Garland and Zigler, 1993).

Psychological profiles of adolescents who have committed suicide reveal the following risk factors:

- Depression or mania
- Antisocial or aggressive behavior
- Family history of suicidal behavior
- Availability of firearms

The Teaching Points below address other behaviors that may indicate suicidal thoughts in adolescents and may be used as a teaching guide for peer-to-peer or peer counseling recognition of suicidal teen-agers.

Incarcerated youths are at extreme risk for suicide. Their rates of suicide have been reported to be as high as 2,041 per 100,000 juveniles incarcerated in adult jails. Completed suicide is often precipitated by a shameful or humiliating experience (e.g., arrest, failure at school, rejection, interpersonal conflict, sexual or physical assault, or conflicts over sexual orientation) (Garland and Zigler, 1993).

Some adolescent suicides are the result of social imitation where taboos against suicidal behavior are lowered. This **suicide contagion** effect is not confined to geographical areas near the original suicide, because newspaper and television coverage can create "copycats." Box 34-4 reveals strategies that were originally adopted to help media dampen suicide contagion. Health care providers need to keep these strategies in mind when interacting with teen-agers (CDC, 1994).

Psychotic Disorders

Schizophrenia

Symptoms of schizophrenia are the most severe psychiatric problems adolescents can have, and they are not rare. It is estimated that approximately 50,000 cases of schizophrenia exist at any given time, although no epidemiological studies of its prevalence during the teenage years exist. The mean age of onset for schizophrenia is 19 years, which indicates that many adolescents develop symptoms earlier. Chapter 29 presents a detailed discussion of the symptoms of schizophrenia.

The most common early symptom of schizophrenia in adolescents is acute hypochondriasis. It is often accompanied by strange fears, school phobia, insomnia, agitation, and concrete and paranoid thinking. Intelligence and orientation to the environment are normal at the onset, but these traits may rapidly deteriorate to complete disorganization. In such cases, hospitalization is required. Most adolescents with schizophrenia are subsequently stabilized and treated on an outpatient basis. These teen-agers need simple, practical, and concrete support in order to manage the stress associated with meeting normal developmental tasks. They char-

TEACHING POINTS

Signs of Suicide

- Change in grades
- Giving away possessions
- Decreased interest in after-school activities
- Few friends
- Breakup with girlfriend or boyfriend
- Pressure by family to stop dating an exclusive person
- Wearing black
- Listening to morose or violent music
- Drug and/or alcohol use
- Discussing suicide
- Self-mutilation

BOX 34-4

Strategies to Reduce Suicide Contagion

- Avoid simplistic explanations for suicide.
- Do not engage in repetitive discussion of the recent suicide event.
- Do not provide graphic descriptions of suicide.
- Do not present suicide as a means for accomplishing an end.
- Do not glorify suicide or persons who commit it.
- Focus on deceased's nonsuicide characteristics.

acteristically have difficulty making good choices and sound judgments when several options are available. They will always need special assistance, because a full cure is generally not possible.

Conduct Disorders

Conduct disorders affect 6% to 8% of adolescents and account for 30% to 70% of psychiatric hospital admissions for this age group. The condition shows a high degree of persistence from childhood to adolescence to adulthood; however, it rarely begins after age 18. Unfortunately the prognosis is poor. Little information is available in the literature that describes effective therapies. The high rate of hospitalization reflects frustration with failed outpatient therapies (Lock and Strauss, 1994).

Substance Abuse

Alcohol and drug use are major health problems for U.S. adolescents, because initiation to substance use peaks among 16 to 18 year olds. All socioeconomic groups are affected, but males outnumber females considerably. Although total substance abuse by teen-agers declined during the 1980s, current rates are still unacceptably high. Recent increases in marijuana and inhalant use among eighth graders are disappointing considering the drug-resistance programs that are now part of most elementary and junior high school curriculums. In fact the use of nicotine, considered a gateway drug among adolescents, has doubled since 1992.

Substance abuse affects four groups of adolescents. First are those who have parents with substance abuse disorders. Of this group, a higher than average number will become users or abusers themselves. Second are teen-agers who are users to varying degrees, for various reasons, and with varying results. Third are adolescents who deal drugs, but who may or may not use them. The fourth group consists of adolescents who are not users, but who are indirectly affected because of contact with peers who do use (Bailey, 1992).

Experimentation with alcohol and drugs does not necessarily mean that serious mental dysfunction will occur. Yet substance abuse can precipitate behaviors that did not exist before, such as depression, anxiety, suicide, violence, conduct disorders, school failure, and short-term and long-term memory loss.

Teen-agers with pre-existent psychiatric, social, and physical problems are more likely to be attracted to substance abuse in the first place. Social relationships are often shallow and restricted to others who use or supply drugs or alcohol. Learning slows or comes to a virtual halt. Adolescents, like their adult counterparts, deny the extent of their problems by stating, "I can stop anytime I want. I just don't want to." Many teen-agers eventually enter rehabilitation programs, but relapse rates are high. Criminal convictions are often what propels them into these programs.

It is unlikely that adolescents will come to health care providers with chief complaints of substance abuse (see Chapter 27), but parents may take them for help. It is, however, one of the most commonly missed diagnoses in young people, which contributes to an average 18-month gap between onset of problematic substance use and detection of abuse (Bailey, 1992).

Anabolic steroids are a relatively new substance of abuse. Males who aspire to be athletes are mainly involved as they seek to increase muscle strength and reduce time between workouts. This practice is associated with use of other dangerous substances: cocaine, alcohol, marijuana, cigarettes, and smokeless tobacco. Needle sharing is common practice with steroid use, which increases the chances of HIV infection. Reports are increasing regarding *serious behavior problems that accompany anabolic steroid use, such as violence* (**"roid rage"**), psychosis, mania, hypomania, and depression (Franklin, 1994).

Eating Disorders

Adolescence is the time of onset of eating disorders. Pressures to be thin, athletic, and physically attractive are generally the early motives for limiting eating, binging, and purging. If the adolescent is predisposed to eating dysfunction and the behavior persists, serious consequences occur (see Chapter 28 for a complete discussion of eating disorders). Adolescent girls are particularly vulnerable to the development of eating disorders and should be routinely assessed for symptoms even when eating behaviors are not the focus of intervention.

The $\mathcal{N}$*ursing* $\mathcal{P}$*rocess*

Assessment

Distinguishing expected adolescent behaviors from those that are detrimental to mental health or those that represent symptoms of psychiatric disorders is a challenge for nurses. Among the issues that represent mental health problems for adolescents are risk taking, acting out, acting up, sexual activity, violence, gang and cult membership, running away, and school performance problems. Clinical profiles for each are discussed to facilitate nurses' identification of symptom clusters.

Clinical Profiles

Risk taking

Adolescents engage in a significant number of dangerous activities. In 1988 injuries were the leading cause of death in the United States among persons age 13 to 19, 42% of which were caused by motor vehicle accidents. Impaired driving accounted for most of those accidents. The National Adolescent Student Health Survey (1988) revealed that 17% of adolescents used alcohol while driving, boating, or swimming during the preceding year.

Another survey revealed that 25% of 12 to 13 year olds had engaged in at least one health risk behavior such as failure to wear safety belts, fighting, or tobacco and alcohol use (JAMA, 1994). This same survey determined that teen-agers who were out of school (i.e., truants, dropouts) uniformly engaged in more risky behaviors than those who were in school.

A number of explanations have been offered for why adolescents participate in dangerous activities. First is adolescent egocentrism, a personal fable, or unrealistic thinking that makes teen-agers think nothing harmful can happen to them. Second it is believed that biochemical alterations in the brain neurotransmitter monoamine oxidase (MAO) may account for especially severe sensation-seeking behaviors. Third is the theory of modular cognitive separation that proposes the adolescent has an inability to see connections between cause and effect. Fourth is a psychoanalytical explanation that looks at risk-taking behaviors as a function of poor self-concept and diminished parental availability. Teen-agers who are not valued by their families do not, in turn, value themselves. Involvement in dangerous activities can be viewed as a continuum ranging from recklessness (a way to become socially involved with peers) to severe sensation-seeking behavior (with elements of self-destructiveness).

Concern about adolescent risk-taking behavior is valid because adolescents experience adverse mental health outcomes as a result (Eggart et al., 1994). Acting-out and acting-up behaviors are the most frequent set of behaviors that the nurse has to deal with in various care settings.

Acting out

Acting-out behavior is impulsive, pathological, antisocial, and dangerous. It is primarily a behavioral manifestation of poor coping in the presence of anxiety and depression. Adolescents who act out are unconsciously choosing antisocial behavior over depression. They are governed by mistrust, which may be the result of abusive and dysfunctional family situations. When their many needs are not met, they engage in defensive lashing-out behaviors. Ironically this makes it even more difficult for their needs to be met. Adolescents who act out create chaos with sullen, argumentative, and demanding behavior. This behavior may seem predictable in the sense that it consistently challenges rules, regulations, and authority figures and that it entails physical violence and aggression.

Acting up

Acting-up behavior is primarily the manifestation of poor impulse control and inability to tolerate frustration. High levels of testosterone may contribute to a biological propensity for impatience, irritability, aggressiveness, and destructiveness in male adolescents. This behavior may also reflect inadequate socialization in which parents have role-modeled impulsivity. Adolescents who act up overreact to limits and rules. They lack the ability to accept responses such as "later you can…" or "not now because…." They live in a here-and-now world. Their demanding behavior is predictable in the sense that it regularly occurs when there are obstacles to immediate gratification.

Sexual activity

Since the 1970s sexual activity has increased among adolescents in the United States, and the age at which sexual activity begins has dropped. At the same time, rates of unintended pregnancies and sexually transmitted dis-

The Nursing Process

eases (STDs) have increased. All this means that many teen-agers are engaging in sexual activity long before they are emotionally ready, and they are exposing themselves and others to serious physical harm. The Centers for Disease Control and Prevention (CDC) surveyed adolescents across the United States in grades 9 to 12 and revealed that 70% reported being currently sexually active, 20% reported having intercourse with four or more partners in their lifetime, 77% reported using contraception only occasionally, and only 46% reported using a condom at last intercourse (CDC, 1993a).

Pregnancy rates have increased, derailing normal development by cutting off experiences that prepare adolescents for adulthood. Children born to teen-age parents run the triple risk of being unwanted, poor, and exposed to inadequate parenting. STDs among adolescents have reached epidemic proportions. One in seven teen-agers is thought to have one or more STDs at any given time, twice the rate for adults in their 20s. Of special concern is the fact that sexual activity is now accompanied by the threat of HIV and AIDS.

Sexual relations with many casual partners may be symptomatic of underlying depression and anxiety. Adolescents who exhibit such behavior are usually frantically seeking love and affirmation of their identities. The negative opinions of others concerning their sexual activities reinforce their own negative self-concept. Adolescents may be unable to break the pattern even though such behavior only aggravates their depression and anxiety. Teen-agers exhibiting promiscuous behavior may have been exposed to parents with multiple sexual partners or have been sexually abused.

Homosexuality is a sexual orientation rather than a mental disorder. Nevertheless there are mental health concerns associated with same-sex orientation. For example shame, embarrassment, and fear often inhibit disclosure of homosexuality to parents and peers, which results in social isolation and lack of meaningful social support. When gender-role nonconformity becomes known it may result in exclusion from peer groups. Either way, gay and lesbian youth, who usually become aware of their sexual orientation during adolescence, face more than their share of emotional stress. Many adolescents experiment sexually with same-sex partners, but this should not be confused with permanent sexual orientation.

The more benign sexual experimentation that sometimes occurs during adolescence may be labeled deviant by their families. Labels such as "whore" and "queer" may become self-fulfilling prophecies where the adolescent reasons, "If I am accused no matter what I do, I might as well do it."

Violence

Many adolescents do not master the skills necessary for resolving interpersonal conflicts and resort to violence. Surveys indicate that teen-agers experience two-and-a-half times more assaults than persons over the age of 20.

Homicide or lethal violence is the second leading cause of death among this age group nationally. Almost half of all murder victims are either related to (12%) or acquainted with (35%) their assailants, and 29% of homicides are the result of an argument (Durant et al., 1994). The broad dimensions of adolescent violence suggest that it should be viewed as a public health problem.

Juvenile delinquency is a broad term used to describe adolescents who break the law. The definition of juvenile delinquency is to some degree culturally determined. The concept has no precise psychiatric definition and is laden with value judgments. These adolescents generally lack a moral code accepted by broader society, a well-developed conscience, or any consideration of the consequences of delinquent behavior.

Gangs and cults

Adolescents who feel alienated and who have not internalized societal norms are at risk for aligning themselves with *deviant subcultures or gangs.* *Gangs are the more common of these groups and offer an instant family that provides companionship, loyalty, identity, and status. Members claim a geographical area and spend a great deal of time together.* Gangs tend to be primarily male, but it is thought that female gangs are on the rise. Factors shown to be associated with gang membership include members of same gender and same ethnic group, high tendency for violence, defiant parental behavior, truancy, substance abuse, failure to experience guilt, low self-esteem, lack of positive role models, poor academic performance, dysfunctional family life, and low levels of parent education.

Cults are specialized gangs organized around a belief system that is expressed through ceremonies and rites. They are usually led by charismatic authority figures who say that they possess special powers. These leaders create an atmosphere of awe so as to impress prospective members and secrecy to hide undesirable aspects of the cult. The cohesiveness of the group is maintained by shared allegiance to the belief system, the associated rituals, and the leader. Unlike other gangs, cults do not generally attract members who have otherwise been involved in antisocial activities. However, cults are antisocial by nature, because they reject prevailing social norms. They can also be dangerous to the physical and emotional health of members, who are usually seeking direction for uncertain and confused lives.

The Nursing Process

An increasing number of adolescents are involved in Satanism or devil worship. Satan is viewed as all-powerful and able to extend his power to cult members if they choose him as their supreme being. Adolescents become involved in cults because they are desperate, angry, and alone. They seek structure, mastery, and a sense of control, and experience strong needs to "belong."

Running away

It is difficult to know how many runaways are in the United States, but national studies estimate that there are 500,000 of them (mostly adolescents) at any given time. The largest subgroup of runaways are *situational runaways* who leave home for a day or two after a disagreement with parents. They usually return within a few days, perhaps as part of a behavior pattern to manipulate or avoid conflicts with parents. Adolescents who run away but stay close to home usually have fantasies of punishing their parents for real or imagined injustices. They envision scenarios in which their parents are regretful, welcome them home, and treat them in special ways. Circumstances associated with situational runaways include the following:

- Eldest daughters seeking relief from major household responsibilities
- Adolescents who have been used as pawns in parental conflicts
- Parents trying to obstruct the normal adolescent separation process
- Reunion fantasy causing adolescents to run away as a ploy to pull parents together

A small percentage of the 500,000 runaways are departure runaways. For them escape from their families is a genuine survival tactic. These runaways are more chronic in that they usually travel to distant metropolitan areas and do not return voluntarily. They are depressed and angry about their treatment at home and hungry for affection and a sense of belonging. Throwaways are youth who are asked to leave home and who usually endure lifestyles similar to departure runaways. It is estimated that there are approximately 127,000 throwaways in the United States. Circumstances associated with departure runaways and throwaways include the following:

- Parental criminal activity, alcoholism, and addiction; overall chaotic home environment
- Physical, emotional, and sexual abuse and neglect
- Conflicts over same-sex orientation

Departure runaways and throwaways move from struggles to survive at home to similar struggles on the streets. They are usually totally on their own with no employable skills. Social service support is unavailable, because runaways and throwaways lack addresses, legal guardians, or social security numbers. As homeless street people, runaways and throwaways steal, panhandle, push drugs, and turn to heterosexual or homosexual prostitution in order to buy food and shelter. They are vulnerable to predators such as pimps, pornographers, and drug dealers. Most become substance abusers in an attempt to escape the pain of life on the streets. This population of adolescents is at the highest possible risk for rape, assault, homicide, suicide, overdose on drugs, unwanted pregnancies, inadequate nutrition, poor hygiene, sleep deprivation, and STDs including HIV/AIDS and other communicable diseases.

School performance problems

School performance problems are both the cause and effect of other difficulties in the lives of adolescents. For example, developmental disabilities render adolescents vulnerable to academic failure. Teen-agers with a disability are likely to experience persistent failure and the ridicule, frustration, and low self-worth that goes along with it. Unrecognized developmental disabilities may cause adolescents to be mislabeled as unintelligent or as behavior "problems." Developmental disabilities may also impair the moral judgment that is crucial to normal adolescent development.

School performance problems may be the consequence of emotional problems that begin in childhood and persist through adolescence. For example, school phobia is usually associated with shy and withdrawn individuals who start avoiding school as youngsters. A frightening or humiliating incident can bring the trauma back during adolescence and produce quiet, compliant "loners" whose lifestyles are out of the normal teen-age mainstream.

Separation from parents often provokes phobic behavior. Parents may foster this response for reasons that meet their own emotional needs. They may characterize the outside world as dangerous and relationships with nonrelated adults and peers as disloyal.

Rebellious adolescents are usually disengaged from learning, because their mental energy is occupied with emotional distress. When in school they tend to exhibit disruptive and aggressive behavior and a know-it-all facade that covers up low self-esteem and feelings of inadequacy. Absenteeism may occur gradually as they become disenchanted with learning, or it may occur precipitously when substance abuse or deviant subgroups enter the picture. Lack of learning at this key developmental stage places adolescents at a serious disadvantage later in life when they seek employment. Faced

The Nursing Process

with reduced employment options, they are at greater risk for leading nonproductive lives.

Focused Assessment

Nurses must understand normal adolescent behavior before they can differentiate it from abnormal or pathological behavior. In Chapter 5 the general principles of psychiatric nursing assessment were discussed. Assessment of the adolescent with troubled behaviors must address some specific issues that include developmental as well as current perceptions and behaviors. Box 34-5 lists components that need to be included in an adolescent assessment in all treatment settings.

Assessment of adolescents does not occur in isolation from their families. Including the assessment of the family when formalizing treatment planning is imperative to formulating treatment plans and setting outcomes and goals. The assessment of the family must include the following:

- Perceptions of the problems
- Past and current family-offspring relations
- Separation processes of parents from their own families or origin
- Understanding of normal adolescent behavior and developmental tasks

BOX 34-5

Adolescent Assessment Components

- Developmental history (prenatal, infancy, and early childhood milestones and difficulties)
- School performance and learning problems
- Abuse and neglect (verbal, physical, and sexual)
- Use of substances by teen-ager, family, significant others; by mother during pregnancy
- Behavior manifestation (running away, impulsivity, gangs, cults, sexual activity)
- Psychiatric symptoms (past history of depression, suicide attempts, cutting self, psychosis, or anxiety)
- Perceptions of problem by client and family
- Ability to communicate thoughts, feelings, and events
- Past and present prescribed medication use
- Over-the-counter medication use
- Degree of involvement in activities outside of school and home (extracurricular)
- Family history (adolescents' perception of family function or dysfunction and level of support)

- Ideas about what they think will resolve the adolescent's situation

Chapter 5 presents the outline for a focused assessment. Chapter 12 describes the components of family assessment. Table 34-3 lists selected standardized tests that are used to ascertain additional information about adolescents and their families. Intelligence and personality testing are essential to differentiate normal adolescent behavior from symptoms that indicate a serious mental disorder.

Nursing Diagnosis

Assessments of troubled adolescents and their families typically generate many nursing diagnoses. Table 34-4 contains selected nursing diagnoses common to teenagers who have problems serious enough to warrant intervention. These diagnoses are accompanied by corresponding client outcomes that reflect therapeutic goals in both the hospital and outpatient setting. Nursing diagnoses for adolescents should also reflect family issues. Inclusion of altered parenting skills is imperative to changing a dysfunctional family situation.

Outcome Identification

Outcome criteria for adolescents need to be concrete and attainable within a short period of time so that the teen-ager receives frequent and consistent feedback. Outcomes must first address immediate short-term and crisis issues and gradually work toward more long-term and multifaceted goals. Peer, community, and educational goals also need to be addressed, particularly in outpatient and home settings. Family-and parental-focused outcomes must be easily attainable, as dysfunctional family systems are frequently inconsistent and have problems with problem solving.

Planning

Multidisciplinary care planning for adolescents includes extensive communication among the treatment team, family, and school and in some situations representatives of the court system and legal guardians. Case management (see Chapter 17) becomes essential to effective comprehensive ongoing care of adolescents and their families. Planning is aimed at melioration of acute symptoms and behaviors, as well as at the prevention of relapse and prevention of chronicity.

The development of a strong united clinical treatment team is assisted by the creation of agency clinical protocols and standards of nursing care for treatment of ado-

The Nursing Process

TABLE 34-3

Selected psychological tests for adolescents

TEST	TYPE	AGE	DESCRIPTION
Wechslor Intelligence Scale for Children-Revised (WISC-R) (Psychological Corporation)	IQ test	6-16	Intelligence (IQ) test assesses individual's ability to understand and act intelligently. Has standard scores for verbal performance and full scale IQ.
Stanford-Binet (Riverside Publishing Company)	IQ test	2-23	Test scores total IQ, verbal, abstract, visual and quantitative reasoning, short-term memory, and standard age.
Woodcock-Johnson Psychoeducational Battery (DLM/Teaching Resources)	Achievement tests	K-12	Test scores adolescent's ability. They yield scores in reading, math, and written language and give grade and expected age based on responses.
Vinland Adaptive Behavior Scales (American Guidance Service)	Adaptive behavior scale	0-19	Test measures adaptive behavior, communication, daily living skills, and socialization. Instrument has separate scores that indicate adolescent disabilities.
Rotter Incomplete Sentences Test (Psychological Corporation)	Projective personality test	Adolescent	Test measures psychological responses. It yields qualitative analysis of psychological state.
Millon Adolescent Personality Inventory (MAPI) (National Computer Systems)	Personality test	13-18	Computerized test that yields broad standard scores for personality styles and adolescent concerns. It is useful for ascertaining appropriate treatment modalities and activity plans.
Holstead-Reitan Neuropsychological Test Battery for Older Children (Neuropsychology Press)	Neuropsychological test	9-14	Test includes cognitive, perceptual motor tests for suspected brain damage.
Bender Visual-Motor Gestalt Test (American Orthopsychiatric Association)	Neuropsychological test	5-adult	Test assesses visual-motor deficits. It yields visual-figure retention scores with age equivalents.

The Nursing Process

TABLE 34-4

Nursing diagnoses and related outcome criteria common for troubled adolescents

NURSING DIAGNOSIS	HOSPITALIZATION OUTCOME CRITERIA	OUTPATIENT OUTCOME CRITERIA
Risk for violence related to history of assaultiveness, poor impulse control, illegal activities, and gang participation	Client will refrain from contacting gang members while in hospital.	Client will follow family contract rules.
	Client will verbalize acceptance of responsibility for assaultive behavior by end of two group sessions.	Client will complete anger-management course.
Self-esteem low, related to negative feedback and lack of positive affirmation	Client will identify strengths daily and use them to accomplish daily goals while in the hospital.	Client will make daily and weekly goals and keep journal to address compliance.
Impaired social interaction related to cult participation	Client will abstain from wearing cult dress or drawing cultlike symbols while in hospital.	Client will not associate with cult members for 1 week.
		Client will begin to verbalize understanding of destructiveness of cult.
Altered growth and development related to poor school attendance	Client will attend all classes while in hospital.	Client will acknowledge that absenteeism will impair future achievement.
	Client will make plans to complete unfinished class work by end of week.	Client will make plan to complete high school.
Altered parenting related to delegating dynamics of family	Parents will verbalize need for taking responsibility for care of younger children in family group by end of first family meeting.	Parents will make schedule that allows teen-ager to engage in peer activities by time of next session.

lescents. This also helps staff with conflicts that may arise from countertransference or projection. It prevents staff member's personal experiences from contaminating the goals of the treatment team. For example, a nurse who has a 15-year-old teen-ager at home runs the risk of projecting angry feelings toward adolescents on the unit after an argument at home concerning curfews.

Including parents in treatment planning for adolescents is imperative. First, the parents are the legal guardians of their children, and thus their consent for treatment must be obtained. Second, parental considerations such as values and cultural views need to be included in the treatment plan. Third, treatment planning must also include outcomes and interventions specific for parents and families. Changes in the family and parental system must be achieved in order for the adolescent to make progress.

Implementation

Adolescents are an underserved population. Recent efforts to address the mental health needs of children and adolescents have been promoted by psychiatric nurses with specialty preparation to care for children and adolescents.

To provide comprehensive care to adolescent clients, multiple community services need to be available. Inpatient and outpatient facilities, foster care services, family support groups, school-based mental health services, in-home therapy services, psychological testing, and supervised after-school programs are but a few of the needed, but scarce resources.

Nurses at the basic level intervene in all settings by providing needed counseling, teaching about and supervising self-care activities, overseeing psychobiological treatments, leading psychoeducation programs, provid-

The Nursing Process

ing case management, and engaging in community health promotion programs.

Counseling

Individual, group, and family counseling are all effective interventions for adolescents (see Chapters 9, 11, and 12). Adolescents, like adults, engage in therapeutic nurse-client relationships.

In working with adolescents it is important for nurses to engage the teen-ager early in the therapeutic process. Authoritative and challenging positions will interrupt the therapeutic process and are not helpful. Once the teen-ager is engaged in the relationship, introducing family therapy is important in making long-term changes in behavior. Goals for therapy should focus on what the adolescent believes needs changing. Therapeutic assignments need to be concrete and easily attainable, and should have short time frames (e.g., teen-ager will keep curfew for the next 3 days).

Counseling is frequently short-term, secondary to the increase of adolescents in managed care programs, which puts added importance of engaging the teen-ager quickly, setting goals, and collaborating with family and school. The mneumonic DWARF (see Table 9-2 in Chapter 9) can help nurses more effectively through the phases of the therapeutic relationship. Designing (D) the relationship with an adolescent requires establishing trust before moving to facilitate change. Boundaries for therapeutic meetings are firm but need a more casual approach with teen-agers. For example, meeting with the adolescent client while sharing a soda or while playing ping-pong would be appropriate in the design and warming up (W) phases.

Contracting with the adolescent, or agreeing (A), requires outcome determination by the client and parents. This is an important intervention for increasing personal control. Contracts entail a written document, with clients retaining a copy while another is placed in the chart. Contracts are effective to the extent that they are consistently used and outline meaningful restrictions. Contracts can be used in the hospital or on an outpatient basis. Suicide, nutrition, and impulsiveness are the most frequent behaviors for which contracts are written with adolescents.

The working or rehabilitation (R) phase with adolescents involves responding to their resistant behaviors in a therapeutic way. Table 34-5 addresses resistant behaviors, dynamics, and possible interventions that may be used with adolescents in all settings. Terminating or finishing (F) the therapeutic encounter with an adolescent often precipitates defensive and regressive be-

haviors. The finishing process for the adolescent may produce feelings that are similar to past parental abandonment or may duplicate dependent-independent conflicts with parents.

Adolescents tend to progress more quickly in group therapy, probably because of the importance of peer influence and teen-agers' tendency to reject adult and parental authority. Promising programs that are built on this premise are peer counseling programs, which have been incorporated in many schools. Peer groups facilitate the learning of relationship skills and enhance adolescents' self-esteem by offering feedback from others adolescents know and trust. Group themes among adolescents include dating, sex, embarrassment about symptoms, experimentation with drugs, violence, and conflict with parents. Groups may be established to deal with adolescents who have homogeneous issues such as teenage pregnancy and participation in gangs and cults or to prevent involvement in the use of alcohol and drugs.

Family counseling is generally routine treatment when an adolescent is the client. Family intervention with teenagers is appropriate when the adolescent's problems involve dysfunctional relationships with parents or siblings. It is part of the long-range planning for an adolescent, because parents must give consent to the treatment plan. Chapter 12 suggests several therapeutic family interventions that may be used in counseling adolescents.

Milieu Therapy

The adolescent may be treated in a variety of milieus. Interventions may include working in a foster home to help foster parents manage troublesome behaviors in a day-treatment center, or during acute hospitalization. The milieu of the adolescent also includes school and other places where there is interaction with peers.

Hospitalization results when adolescents become unmanageable in their normal settings. Requests for admission for inpatient treatment can come from many sources such as schools, courts, primary health care providers, outpatient mental health programs, psychiatrists, or parents. The normally challenging task of establishing therapeutic relationships with adolescents is even greater in hospital settings, because they are usually there against their will. On one hand, certain teen-age characteristics facilitate good relationships. For example, they are typically curious about themselves and others and appreciate constructive, caring feedback. They are concerned about how others see them and generally have an interest in the future. On the other hand, adolescents tend to be skeptical about adult advice and solutions, and they resist activities that hint at domination

The Nursing Process

TABLE 34-5

Treatment-resistant behaviors of adolescents and appropriate interventions

ADOLESCENT'S BEHAVIOR	MESSAGE	DYNAMICS	NURSING INTERVENTION
Acts like junior therapist	"I act like you, so I'm not sick or crazy, and I don't need treatment."	Identification with the aggressor	Give client feedback about use of behavior to avoid dealing with own problems.
Move to develop a peer (social) relationship with the nurse by asking personal questions (e.g., "Have you ever used pot?" or "Do you have a boyfriend?")	"If I can prove that you are no better than me, then you have nothing to offer me."	Leveling	Explore with client how this information would be useful to the treatment process. Point out that the purpose of therapy is for the client to use time to talk about self and own problems.
Acts flirtatious or seductive	"If I can seduce you, then you are not perfect or strong enough to help me."	Counterphobic way of dealing with sexual impulses that are frightening	Encourage client to talk about beliefs, values, feelings, fears, and fantasies about sex.
Oversubmissiveness	"I'm being good and you disapprove, so you want me to be bad. If you want me to be bad, you cannot help me."	Beat adults at their own game	Express doubt and disbelief that anyone could be in specific situations and not feel angry or wish to rebel.
Persistent avoidance: daydreaming, refusal to participate in group therapy or group activities, pseudo seizures	"I will provoke you to retaliate."	Prove that adults hate, hurt, and reject	Persist with patience; offer firm limits that are consistently enforced without anger. Explore what it must feel like to stay out and just watch what is happening.
Manipulates a more disorganized peer to act out and calls nurse to help the "sick" peer	"See how sick that person is; he or she needs you more than I."	"A scapegoat will divert the nurse's attention from me. No one understands or can help me."	Continue to give attention to clients who seek help for other clients or provoke the latter to act out.
Tells peer rather than therapist about details of problems	"I can divide and conquer." "If I divide and conquer, then you can't be relied on to help."	Transference and splitting divert the nurse's attention from me; no one understands or can help me."	Direct client to discuss problems with appropriate team members. Maintain clear, open communication with other team members.
Acts with craziness and pseudostupidity	"I'm sick; don't trust me, but help me."	Ward off or protect staff from self-perceived dangerousness	Acknowledge client's fears; encourage exploration of strengths.

The Nursing Process

TABLE 34-5—cont'd

Treatment-resistant behaviors of adolescents and appropriate interventions

ADOLESCENT'S BEHAVIOR	MESSAGE	DYNAMICS	NURSING INTERVENTION
Engages in intellectual or artistic activities that exclude interactions with others	"See how productive I am."	Avoid dealing with feelings	Limit solitary activities. Talk about how difficult it is to interact. Acknowledge how difficult it is to talk about feelings, but how it is necessary to resolving problems.
Organizes or joins a disruptive peer group	"We are more powerful than you."	"It's 'us' against 'them.'" "If our gang can disrupt your work, you can't help."	Firmly enforce preestablished limits. Exercise consistent patience. Confront client on avoidance of work in therapy. Deal with each adolescent as an individual.

by or dependence on adults. Nurses who are primarily perceived as authority figures have difficulty establishing therapeutic relationships with teen-agers.

Teen-agers may enter the hospital skeptical that anyone there can understand or help them. Adolescents with long-standing problems with their parents may anticipate that the staff will treat them in a similar manner. Consequently they may set up a replay of the dysfunctional parent-child dynamic with their nurses and expect punitive retaliation. Adolescent clients often test the limits, break the rules, and threaten destruction of property and physical harm so as to provoke the staff. Nurses and other staff members may eventually impose punitive limits if pressed long and hard enough. Unfortunately perceptions of "injustice" usually provoke further client turmoil, because punitive staff responses support their low expectations of adults.

The staff may feel guilty about emotional responses to adolescent clients. Unfortunately guilty feelings can render nurses vulnerable, because their "rejection" of adolescents may mimic behavior parents have exhibited. Younger nurses are more likely to identify with adolescents because of their developmental proximity. They may cast the family in the "bad role" and underestimate the negative contributions of the client. The opposite may occur with older nurses who are more removed from adolescence and likely to be parents. Still other nurses experience an unconscious need to provoke adolescents to act out antisocially and, thereby, receive vicarious gratification for their inhibited antisocial wishes. This dynamic may result in transfer of "disruptive" clients

to more "appropriate" units while staff members are unaware of their own contributions to the disruption.

Limit setting

Effective management of behavior and expression of emotions are major therapeutic issues with adolescents. Many of them act before they think and get into trouble because of impulsivity. Increased personal control is a function of social learning and affective regulation. Thoughtful use of limit setting helps teen-agers learn how to behave in socially appropriate ways. *Limit setting involves consistent enforcement of rules and policies without exception. When violations occur, consequences result.* This may entail restriction of activities, quiet time, restraints, or seclusion. These strategies are not punishments but may be perceived as such. On the contrary, they must be used in order to de-escalate out-of-control behavior and to provide clients with therapeutic opportunities to thoughtfully examine their behavior.

Self-Care Activities

Adolescents seem to be at opposite extremes of health and hygiene issues. They will spend hours getting ready for a date, drying their hair, and changing, but their messy rooms are often a source of constant arguments with parents. Despite all this grooming, an adolescent's appearance may remain disheveled.

Interventions to promote proper hygiene and health habits must consider the trends of adolescents versus the

The Nursing Process

comfort of others and the mores of their families and communities. More recently tattooing and body piercing may need to be addressed by the nurse. Setting limits on the dress of those adolescents involved in cults and gangs may also be part of the treatment plan.

Sexuality issues were addressed earlier in this chapter. However, nursing interventions in this area also must involve pregnancy and STD prevention. These interventions must again take family and community values into consideration. Education is a key element in managing the sexual issues of adolescence.

Psychobiological Interventions

Medications that are most commonly used in psychiatric treatment settings are discussed in detail in Chapter 15. The Medication Tips below present important points that must be considered in the medication management of adolescents. All drugs classes and subgroups of psychotropic medication are effective in treating adolescents with symptoms. Some drugs are restricted, however, because they are specifically approved only for adults or have not been studied in adolescents younger than age 16.

Dosages of psychotropic medications need to be adjusted according to height, weight, motivation level, and

 MEDICATION TIPS

Adolescent Psychopharmacology

- Adolescents are more susceptible to extrapyramidal side effects.
- Adolescents have poor fluid intake, which makes them susceptible to constipation, dry mouth, and urinary retention.
- The nurse should monitor vital signs to evaluate hypotension.
- Drowsiness may interfere with school.
- The nurse should monitor medications for signs of abuse, which include selling medication at school, especially antianxiety or sympathomimetic agents.
- The adolescent, family, and school professionals should be taught about indications, side effects, response criteria, interactions, and compliance issues to facilitate proper adjustment of medication dosages.
- The nurse should assist the client, the family, school professionals, and other mental health professionals to have reasonable expectations of medications.
- The nurse should monitor for potential overdose when client is experiencing suicidal thoughts.

side effects. This is particularly important in prescribing antipsychotics, as teen-agers have a higher rate of extrapyramidal side effects. Adolescents diagnosed with mania and placed on lithium need close monitoring of lithium levels, as teen-agers tend to have a poor fluid intake, which could cause toxicity. Adolescents who had been diagnosed with ADHD and are on stimulants need close monitoring, as these drugs have become drugs of abuse. The selective serotonin reuptake inhibitors (SSRIs) are slowly becoming the most commonly prescribed medications for depression and do have fewer side effects than the tricyclic antidepressants.

In general, medication in conjunction with psychotherapy is the best combination in treating teen-agers. Care needs to be taken that they fully understand the need for the medication. For many adolescents there may be initial shame. But as positive results occur as a result of taking medication and the teen-ager experiences relief from painful symptoms, compliance becomes the norm.

Health Teaching

Health teaching of adolescents involves educational efforts in a number of arenas. Health care professionals as well as school officials, parents, and those who manage after-school activities need to learn about risk behaviors and the subtle symptoms of depression and psychosis (see Chapter 16).

The care of the at-risk adolescent must include the primary caregiver, whether that is a parent, grandparent, or other caregiver. Parent education strategies that relate to the adolescent can be found in Box 34-6. These parental interventions can be included in care plans in all settings and are the basis for nursing health teaching to assist families in changing a dysfunctional system.

Case Management

Nursing care of adolescents involves collaboration among health, education, recreation, and occupation professionals. Multidisciplinary treatment plans provide the best opportunities for exchange of information and perspectives. Case management activities facilitate the most holistic and comprehensive treatment approach. Areas of collaboration that are important to the care of adolescent clients include the following:

- Use of a consistent therapeutic approach
- Development of outcome criteria and interventions that contribute to resolution of problems stated in the multidisciplinary treatment plan
- Monitoring and documenting problems and changes related to care

The Nursing Process

• Notifying other care providers when problems can be anticipated and participating in problem solving

The addition of other supports in the community, such as recreational programs, Big Brother/Big Sister programs, or other mentorship programs, are especially important for teen-agers. Many local churches have programs for teen-agers that offer support. Encouraging after-school activities such as sports or clubs that are usually available for both middle school and high-school students can be facilitated by nurses in the case management role. Further discussion of case management interventions can be found in Chapter 17.

Health Promotion and Health Maintenance

In today's cost-conscious society, the necessity of disease prevention has become critical. In the adolescent age group, the prevention of mental health problems and mental illness has become the domain of the school system. For example, health education classes have focused on the prevention of drug and alcohol abuse and are implemented from kindergarten through 12th grade. Many high schools have included sex education in their curriculums. Programs to keep pregnant teen-agers and single teen-age mothers in school are growing. These programs combine education and parenting skills by encouraging teen-age mothers to bring their children to school. Roles in these programs challenge nurses to integrate multiple specialties.

In this more and more violent culture, schools have begun to include gang-resistance classes in the curriculum. On campus, health clinics have become an integral part of linking the school and community by offering health and social services to both groups. School personnel have had to become more informed

---

BOX 34-6

Parent Education: Adolescent

DEFINITION

Assisting parents to understand and help their adolescent children

ACTIVITIES

Ask parents to describe the characteristics of their adolescent child

Discuss parent-child relationship during earlier, school-age years

Discuss disciplining of parents, themselves, when they were adolescents

Teach normal physiological, emotional, and cognitive characteristics of adolescents

Identify developmental tasks or goals of the adolescent period of life

Identify defense mechanisms used most commonly by adolescents, such as denial and intellectualization

Address the effects of adolescent cognitive development on information processing

Address the effects of adolescent cognitive development on decision making

Have parents describe methods of discipline used before adolescent years and their feelings of success with these measures

Describe the importance of power/control issues for both parents and adolescents during adolescent years

Teach parents essential communication skills that will increase their ability to empathize with their adolescent and assist their adolescent to problem solve

Teach parents methods of communicating their love to adolescents

Explore parallels between school-age dependency on parents and adolescent dependency on peer group

Reinforce normalcy of adolescent vacillation between desire for independence and regression to dependence

Discuss effects of adolescent separation from parents on spousal relationships

Share strategies for managing adolescent's perception of parental rejection

Facilitate expression of parental feelings

Assist parents to identify reasons for their responses to adolescents

Identify avenues to assist adolescent to manage anger

Teach parents how to use conflict for mutual understanding and family growth

Role-play strategies for managing family conflict

Discuss with parents issues over which they will accept compromise and issues over which they cannot compromise

Discuss necessity and legitimacy of limit setting for adolescents

Address strategies for limit setting for adolescents

Teach parents to use reality and consequences to manage adolescent behavior

Reprinted with permission from McCloskey J.C., & Bulechek, G.M. (Ed.). (1996). Nursing interventions classification (NIC). (2nd ed). St. Louis: Mosby.

The Nursing Process

on various mental health issues in adolescents, as they are often the ones who identify problems and suggest referrals to guidance counselors or health clinics for testing. Consumer resources and agencies that offer health promotion materials to those who work with adolescents are listed in the Consumer Resources box below.

Evaluation

Evaluating nursing outcomes should focus on adolescent behaviors that either reflect accomplishment or continued problem behaviors. The treatment plan should be gradually revised, incorporating more complex goals as the adolescent accomplishes previous goals. The evaluation process should address which goals are met, not met, or partially met. Frequent and concise feedback as-

sists teen-agers to evaluate their own behavior and encourages them to become a part of, rather than work against, the team. The majority of adolescents have difficulty with abstract concepts, and thus teaching critical-thinking skills must be tempered to this premise.

KEY POINTS

- Adolescence is not necessarily a tumultuous and negative developmental stage. However, teen-agers have emotional problems that render them unique compared to children and adults.
- Adolescent mental health and behavior problems primarily stem from the interaction of risk, vulnerability, and resilience. Adverse social influences, inadequate coping resources, and dysfunctional parenting are particularly important. These factors

 COMMUNITY RESOURCES

Adolescents

Boys' and Girls' Clubs of America
771 First Avenue
New York, New York 10017
(212) 351-5906

Children's and Youth Emotions Anonymous
P.O. Box 4245
St. Paul, MN 55104
(612) 647-9712

Federation of Families for Children's Mental Health
1021 Prince Street
Alexandria, VA 22314-2971
(703) 684-7710

National Clearinghouse for Alcohol and Drug Information
P.O. Box 2345
Rockville, MD 20847-2345
(800) 628-1696

National Resource Center on Child Sexual Abuse
107 Lincoln Street
Huntsville, AL 34801
(205) 534-6868

Alateen (Children/Teen-agers of Alcoholics)
(800) 344-2666

Covenant House Nineline
(800) 999-9999

National Runaway Hotline
(800) 231-6946

National STD Hotline
(800) 227-8922

National Youth Crisis Hotline
(800) HIT-HOME

National Youth Suicide Hotline
(800) 621-4000

Pregnancy Hotline
(800) 238-4269

Rainbows
(Children grieving loss such as divorce or death)
(708) 310-1880

Students Against Drunk Driving (SADD)
(508) 481-3568

CRITICAL THINKING QUESTIONS

Janice is a 16-year-old girl who was brought to the office by her mother and stepfather. She complains of hypersomnia, irritability, mood swings, weight loss, inability to concentrate on school work, and difficulty with activities of daily living (she frequently refuses to shower or change clothes.) She has been hospitalized twice for similar behaviors. Janice has recently refused to go to school after obtaining Fs and Ds. This is her second high school in one semester. Her mother was recently hospitalized for an overdose of lithium carbonate. Janice's natural father lives in another state, sends child support, but does not want custody of Janice. Her stepfather is supportive but overwhelmed and discouraged by the recent hospitalization of his wife and Janice's psychiatric and school problems.

1. How are the various theories of psychiatric nursing relevant to this case study?
2. What are the key points that the nurse must assess at the initial meeting with Janice and her family?
3. How can the various family dynamics be used to understand this family system and influence outcomes?
4. What are nursing diagnoses that relate to DSM-IV criteria that could be addressed during the first 72 hours of inpatient treatment?
5. Which treatment alternative should be considered for Janice and her family? Give short- and long-term goals for each.
6. What referral sources in your own community could help address the various needs of this client and her family?

interfere with the progress teen-agers make toward a positive, adult self-concept and identity.

- A multidisciplinary and eclectic theoretical perspective provides the most satisfactory theoretical explanation for adolescents' mental health problems.
- Adolescents tend to hide their depression and anxiety so as to protect themselves from feelings of vulnerability and dependency. Problem behaviors are the symptoms of their inner conflicts.
- Nursing care in adolescent psychiatric treatment settings needs to address the problems of both teen-age clients and their families. Separation dynamics are commonly at the root of dysfunctional families.

- Therapeutic relationships are typically resisted by adolescents if nurses provoke feelings of domination or dependence or exacerbate preexisting problems with authority figures.

REFERENCES

American Psychiatric Association (APA). (1994). *Diagnostic and Statistical Manual of Mental Disorders* (4th ed.). Washington, DC: Author.

Bailey, G.W. (1992). Children, adolescents, and substance abuse. *Journal of the American Academy of Child and Adolescent Psychiatry, 31*(6), 1015-1017.

Broge, D.G. (1995). Adolescent depression: A review of the literature, *Archives of Psychiatric Nursing, 9*(1) 45-55.

Centers for Disease Control (CDC). (1992). Unintended childbearing: Pregnancy risk assessment monitoring system—Oklahoma, 1988-1991. *MMWR, 41*(59), 933-937.

Centers for Disease Control (CDC). (1993a). Teenage pregnancy and birth rates—United States, 1990. *MMWR, 42*(38), 733-737.

Centers for Disease Control (CDC). (1993b). Violence-related attitudes and behaviors of high school students, New York City, 1992. *MMWR, 42*(40), 773-777.

Centers for Disease Control (CDC). (1994). Suicide contagion and the reporting of suicide: Recommendations from a national workshop. *MMWR, 43*(6), 13-17.

Clark, C.M. (1994). Clinical assessment of adolescents involved in satanism. *Adolescence, 29*(11), 461-467.

D'Angelo, J., Brown, R., English, A., Hein, K., & Remafedi, G. (1994). HIV infection and AIDS in adolescents. *Journal of Adolescent Health, 15*(5), 427-435.

Durant, R.H., Pendergrast, R.A., & Cadenhead, C. (1994). Exposure to violence and victimization and fighting behavior of urban black Americans. *Journal of Adolescent Health, 15*(4), 311-318.

Franklin, J.E. (1994). Addiction medicine. *JAMA, 271* (21), 1650-1651.

Garland, A.F., & Zigler, E. (1993). Adolescent suicide prevention. *German Psychologist, 48*(2), 169-182.

Hammond, W.R., & Yung, B. (1993). Psychology's role in the public response to assaultive violence among young African-American men. *American Psychologist, 48*(2), 142-154.

Institute of Medicine (IOM). (1994). *Research on children and adolescents with mental, behavioral, and developmental disorders.* Washington, DC: National Academy Press.

Jessor, R. (1993). Successful adolescent development among youth in high-risk settings. *American Psychologist, 48*(2), 117-126.

Kaplan, H., Sadock, B., & Grebb, J. (1994). *Synopsis of Psychiatry* (7th ed.). Baltimore: Williams & Wilkins.

Keltner, N., & Folks D. (1997). *Psychotropic drugs* (2nd ed.). St. Louis: Mosby.

Lock, J., & Strauss, G.D. (1994). Psychiatric hospitalization of adolescents for conduct disorders. *Hospital and Community Psychiatry, 45*(9), 925-928.

Morgan, I.S. (1994). Recognizing depression in the adolescent. *MCN, 19*(3), 148-155.

National Adolescent Student Health Survey. (1988). *A report on the health of America's youth.* Oakland, CA: Third Party Publishing.

Roye, C.F. (1995) Breaking through to the adolescent patient. *American Journal of Nursing, 95*(12), 19-23.

Stanton, B., Li, X., Black, M., Ricardo, I., Galbraith, J., Kaljee, L., & Feigelman, S. (1994). Sexual practices among preadolescent and early adolescent low-income urban African-Americans. *Pediatrics, 93*(6), 966-973.

U.S. Public Health Service. (1993). *Healthy people 2000: National health promotion and disease prevention objectives.* Washington, DC: U.S. Government Printing Office.

Chapter 35

Elderly Persons

Anita Leach McMahon

LEARNING OUTCOMES

After studying and applying the concepts in this chapter, the learner will be able to:
- Describe theories that explain the aging process.
- Describe issues common to the aging population that contribute to the development of mental disorders.
- Discuss losses experienced in late life that contribute to the development of emotional distress.
- Describe how dysfunctional bereavement, suicide, isolation, and loneliness contribute to the onset of depressive symptoms in the elderly.
- Identify manifestations of anxiety in the elderly.
- Assess elderly persons who are clients in the mental health care system.
- Use counseling, self-care, milieu, psychobiological, and case management interventions with elderly persons who are clients in the mental health care system.
- Develop health promotion and health teaching approaches that are appropriate for use with the elderly.

KEY TERMS

Autoaggression	Legacy	Reminiscence therapy
Bereavement	Life care community	Reunion fantasy
Benign suicide	Life review therapy	Short-term memory
Creativity	Loneliness	Silent suicide
Dysfunctional bereavement	Long-term memory	Thinking
Geropsychiatric nursing	Masked depression	Translocation crisis
Hypochondriasis	Psychogenic mortality syndrome	

s the population grows older, issues related to the mental health of the elderly become more apparent. Growing old does not eliminate the possibility of mental illness, nor is it implied that disabling mental disorders exist just because of the aging process. The well-adjusted older adult carries into late life the capacity to maintain self-esteem, self-confidence, purpose in life, and a satisfying sense of personal identity and social role, despite the losses that may occur throughout the aging process.

On the other hand, it should be pointed out that the existence of mental disorders and distress in the elderly are complex phenomena compounded by a lifetime of events. The extremes of any diagnosis of a mental disorder in the elderly are relatively easy to recognize, but differentiating symptoms from normal aging can be difficult. Nurses need to be aware of normal aging processes, as well as of those phenomena that mask themselves as mental dysfunctions.

The elderly have traditionally been underserved by the mental health care system. Factors that have contributed to this lack of care include the following:

- Misperception that the elderly do not benefit from mental health services
- Failure of elderly persons to seek help because of the stigma associated with having symptoms of a mental disorder and distrust of services
- The myth that mental disorders in old age are expected
- Inaccurate diagnoses of behavioral problems in the elderly
- Bias among health care professionals who view elderly clients as unable to change
- The complexity of emotional disorders in the elderly and the lack of professionally prepared experts in the subspecialties of geropsychiatry and geropsychiatric nursing
- The inability of the elderly to pay for services and a general lack of public funding to pay for them
- Lack of services that are accessible to a population with mobility problems and lack of transportation

The mental health issues of older adults are not unlike those of the general population. Persons who have symptoms of a mental disorder in their younger years continue, although in less acute ways, to be clients of the mental health care system. Some may have the characteristics of persons with severe and persistent mental illness (see Chapter 38), whereas others may have experienced a single episode that never reoccurs. Some people, however, do not become a part of the mental health care system until they are in the later stages of their lives. Severe loneliness and isolation, hypochondriacal preoccupations, depression and suicide, paranoid reactions, dementia, delirium, and substance abuse are among the most common mental health problems of the aging population.

Nurses are poised to assume leadership in this growing field. *Geropsychiatric nursing, a subspeciality of psychiatric nursing, is aimed at providing care to elderly consumers.* The role requires an understanding of the physical and developmental characteristics of the elderly, as well as specialized counseling skills. Geropsychiatric nurses blend specialized psychobiological milieu management and self-care intervention abilities with case management strategies to serve the multifaceted needs of elderly clients in the mental health care system. Emphasis is placed on maximizing independence in the activities of everyday living and on promoting, maintaining, and restoring mental health and physical well-being.

The purpose of this chapter is to discuss explanations of the aging process. Emphasis is placed on application of the nursing process with elderly clients who are manifesting symptoms of emotional distress.

EPIDEMIOLOGY

The fastest growing segment of the population is the elderly portion. In 1990 it was estimated that by the year 2030, about one fifth of the total population will be age 65 or older (U.S. Bureau of Census, 1991). The elderly population has generally been getting older and is expected to continue doing so for the next several decades because of longer life spans and improved quality and availability of health care.

Of the elderly, 95% are community-based. The remaining 5%, or approximately 1.3 million, are in nursing homes or related facilities. Approximately 65% of these residents have a mental disorder. Elderly with earlier mental impairments who survive into late adulthood represent an increasing number of these individuals. It is estimated that 25% are referred to the mental health system for disruptive behavior, whereas general confusion accounts for 10% of referrals (AARP, 1997).

Women experience a higher prevalence of anxiety and depression, whereas the mental disorders that are more prevalent in men are addictions and personality disorders. Prevalence rates of depression in the elderly range from 13% to 31%, and the elderly are disproportionately represented among those who commit suicide. Of completed suicides, 25% are persons over age 65, and noncaucasian men over age 80 comprise the highest rate of suicide of any group. The overall percentage of deaths caused by suicide among the elderly is on the rise.

Estimates of the prevalence of alcoholism in the elderly range from 2% to 15%. Isolation and diminished social contact make an accurate estimate a difficult task. Medication misuse in the elderly accounts for 15% of acute drug reactions observed in any age group. The Cultural Highlights box below presents epidemiological data of elderly persons from different cultures.

THEORETICAL FRAMEWORK
Biological Correlates

Multiple biological theories abound that attempt to explain why people grow old. A dominant belief is the *neuroendocrine control theory,* which suggests that aging is one phase of a life-span regulatory program that begins at fertilization and continues until an individual's death. The theory suggests that at a given time that is uniquely and genetically determined in each individual, the hypothalamic-pituitary-thyroid (HPT), hypothalamic-pituitary-adrenal (HPA), and the hypothalamic-pituitary-gonadal (HPG) pathways exert a declining influence on the immune system and organ tissues (see Chapter 13). Exactly what physiological mechanism signals the decline is unknown. Skeletal muscle is directly influenced by similar signals from the hypothalamus, whereas smooth and cardiac muscles and skeletal-motor systems respond via the autonomic nervous system. The biological theories may be summarized simply by stating that aging is a universal, progressive, intrinsic, and selective slowing down of physiological processes.

Sensory processes play a major role in the mental health of elderly persons. The senses are the means by which people experience the world outside themselves, as well as their internal functions. Vision allows experience of color, intensity, distance, and field angle. Impaired hearing is common in elderly persons, who generally have more difficulty hearing both high-pitched sounds and sounds of low intensity. Elevated taste thresholds, that is, a need for a more intense stimulus to taste things, may also occur. On the other hand, there seems to be no change in an elderly person's sense of smell. Sensitivity to touch increases with age, but elderly persons appear to be less sensitive to pain.

Loss of vision, hearing, or any other sense can be partly compensated for by increased use of another sense, but when several senses decline simultaneously, as happens with many elderly persons, adaption to the environment becomes a serious problem. Individuals often become increasingly isolated, lonely, and depressed because of the decrease in sensory input.

Another theory implicates the *immune system* in the aging process. Cells in the immune system become increasingly diversified with age and begin a progressive loss of self-regulation. A process known as **autoaggression** is set in motion. *Cells normal to the body are misidentified as alien and are attacked, while simultaneously there is impaired surveillance by antibody cells.* Decreased efficiency of the immune system increases vulnerability to disease, particularly infections, cancer, adult-onset diabetes, and autoimmune problems. Amyloidosis, the accumulation of a waxy, starchlike glycoprotein (amyloid) in tissues and organs, of the brain is also known to occur (Wayne, et al., 1990).

Other theories include somatic error and transmission hypotheses and the idea of programmed cell behavior as explanations for the aging process. Free-radical, cross-link, and wear-and-tear theories have also been considered.

Developmental Correlates

Mentally healthy elderly persons are those who have adjusted to their life stage and situation. They have positive self-concepts, a capacity to view themselves as unique beings, an ability to communicate effectively, a sense of belonging, relative independence and freedom, privacy

CULTURAL HIGHLIGHTS

- Use of alternate healing methods and maintaining independence of the family and their involvement in an elderly person's care are key components of eastern cultures (Evans and Cunningham, 1996).
- Persons of color (persons of African-American, Hispanic, Native American, and Asian/Pacific Islander ancestry) are a rapidly growing segment of the population. By the year 2050, it is expected that they will represent 33% of the population (American Society on Aging [ASA] 1992).
- The life expectancy of Native Americans is shorter than that of all other U.S. races at 65 years, compared with 73.3 years for persons who are not of Native American

ancestry. American Indian elderly persons have the poorest health status of any ethnic group (ASA, 1992).
- During the last 3 decades there has been a 400% increase in the number of Asian/Pacific Islander elderly (AARP, 1987).
- Fifty-seven percent of elderly African-Americans and 52% of Hispanic elderly report limitations in activities of daily living (ADLs) produced by common conditions, compared with 44% of older caucasians (ASA, 1992).
- Sweden is the country with the oldest population. Of the population, 23% is over age 60.

that includes space to call their own, a sense of themselves as whole people, and recognition of themselves as loving and valued human beings. Mentally healthy older adults are persons with the following characteristics: a sense of control over their destinies; strong religious and cultural traditions that include a belief in an afterlife; strong kinship, social network, and extended family bonds; the ability to use and contribute to community resources; ownership of property; and a sense of autonomy and independence. (See Chapter 7 for a full discussion of developmental issues of older adults.)

In a classic work about the mental health of elderly persons, Butler and Lewis (1982) state that the major developmental tasks of the elderly are clarifying, deepening, and finding use for what has already been attained through a lifetime of learning and adapting. They state that elderly persons must teach themselves to conserve their strength and resources and to adjust to those changes and losses that occur as part of aging.

Cognitive Correlates

Cognitive processes do not decline simply because of the aging process. There are apparent cognitive changes in the elderly, but these are generally caused by malfunction of the circulatory or neurological systems rather than by the aging process itself. Intelligence, learning, memory, thinking, and creativity are the mental processes of greatest concern to mental health practitioners. Researchers have found that there are no significant differences in spatial relationships, verbal skills, or psychomotor skills, all of which are components of intelligence. Elderly persons are sometimes deficient or slower during learning, need more time to store and retain new information, and have overall slower retrieval times for stored information, but they do not experience any significant change in intelligence.

Learning capacity for elderly persons continues well into their eighties and beyond. They may be either impeded or helped by earlier learning, and it is known that they need more time to learn new tasks. Practice, particularly of new tasks, greatly improves performance. When the material to be learned is meaningful, and when they can control the pace and rate of learning, elderly persons learn as well as their younger counterparts of equal intelligence.

Memory is linked to learning in older individuals. Many elderly persons complain that they have difficulties with their memory. They are generally referring to **short-term memory**, *the ability to remember the recent past*. Misplaced keys, dentures, and eyeglasses are commonly the concern voiced to the nurse. Forming a habit of always putting these items away in the same place usually solves the problem. Many older people have excellent **long-term memory**, *the ability to recall*

the distant past (see Chapter 31 for a full discussion of correlates of memory).

Thinking *is defined as the process of developing new ideas.* Thinking helps put order into multiple data by differentiating and categorizing the data into concepts. Studies show that, as age increases, a person's ability to form concepts declines. However, observation indicates that elderly persons may remain adept at concept formation but simply become set in their ways because of personality or environmental factors.

Creativity *is problem solving that is unique, original, and inventive.* The ability to be creative does not come to an abrupt halt when a person becomes older; rather, there is a gradual decline in creative effort. A crucial issue in the creativity of older people is the presence or absence of social supports for creative efforts. For older adults to continue being creative, encouragement is needed from others in their environment. Often, increased leisure time facilitates a person's discovery of some previously unknown creative talent.

Familial Correlates

Longevity is probably genetically determined and characterizes individual families' rates of aging. The dynamics created in the family with elderly members are not unlike those discussed in Chapter 12. However, there are shifts in the roles each family member assumes, as well as shifts in family triangles. The couple relationship becomes a focal point for older adults. Elderly couples are usually characterized by a high degree of interdependence and caring. Marital satisfaction is a central factor in overall life satisfaction, but older couples, like their younger counterparts, may experience marital discord and even divorce. Approximately 15,000 couples over age 65 are granted divorces each year.

The sexual intimacy of older people reflects their physical capacity; their emotional needs; and their cultural, social, and religious norms. It is usually physically possible for sexual intimacy to continue into the later years, provided the couple have established a pattern of sexual intimacy in their middle years.

When one spouse dies, widowhood occurs. Widowhood is felt throughout the entire family system. Personality disorganization, yearning for the bereaved spouse, changed economic resources, and increased contact with adult children are among the more obvious shifts.

In a family's later years, triangles realign as adult children assume increasingly significant roles in the lives of their aging parents. Early discharge from hospitals and the emerging phenomenon of the four-generation family have been responsible for the assumption by adult children, many of whom are themselves in their middle and late years, of caregiving roles with their aging parents. When elderly adults recognize adult children as individuals with their own rights, needs, limitations, and unique life histories, and when the adult children are mature and secure, satisfactory relationships develop. However, a number of stressors are associated with caring for aging parents. These include financial problems; competing responsibilities for family, spouse, and work; unresolved parent-child conflicts; changes in family roles; and uncertainty about the future. Even for persons who ordinarily have effective coping skills, the intensity of family relationships caused by an elderly parent who is ill may lead to guilt, depression, loneliness, avoidance, withdrawal, loss of identity, role uncertainty, anger, and loss of power or control.

An increasingly significant role in the lives of families with older adults is grandparenting. Of elderly persons in the United States, 75% are grandparents or great-grandparents, and about 7% of all households headed by elderly persons include grandchildren (AARP, 1997). The role of valued grandparent is achieved rather than automatically ascribed and is based on the personal qualities of the elderly person. Contributions of grandparents to families include roles as surrogate parents, providers of income, homemakers, baby-sitters, support persons in times of crisis, teachers, confidants, and reservoirs of family wisdom and history.

The *Nursing Process*

Assessment
Clinical Profiles
Depression in older adults

Depressive disorders in adults of all ages are usually the result of a combination of biological, physical, psychosocial, and cultural factors. However, it is estimated that 10% to 15% of elderly persons living in the community will at some point in later life experience some sadness and 5% will experience serious depression. Prevalence is higher among the elderly in hospitals and nursing homes. Depressive episodes are viewed on a continuum from episodes of temporary sadness to moderate depression, severe depression, and suicide. Depression in the elderly may be the result of physical, cognitive, social, and affective losses; alteration in self-image; or decrease in sensory activity. Depression is also associated with the physical disorders common in the elderly, especially those ailments that cause incapacitation or pain. Drugs, particularly antihypertensives, sedatives, hypnotics, and alcohol, cause depression in elderly persons (Rosen and Buschmann, 1996).

Depression in the elderly may be *masked and exhibited with physical symptoms* **(masked depression).** Apathy, preoccupation and "staring into space," reduced eye contact, overactivity, extreme annoyance with others, sleep disturbances, confusion, fatigue, constipation, slowing of movements and speech, withdrawal, and irritability are symptoms of depression that may be overlooked and attributed to the aging process. Elderly persons with depression are characterized as having a greater incidence of weight loss and preoccupation with somatic complaints than younger clients. There is a complex interrelatedness between symptoms and signs of

depression and those of physical illness or other mental disorders (Cohen et al., 1996). In the elderly, sorting out symptoms and signs caused primarily by the affective disorder from those that have an organic basis presents a major challenge. Depression coexists with dementia in one third of outpatients and in about one half of persons in nursing homes (Hogstel, 1995). Depression is so often misdiagnosed that pseudodementia is used to label clients with reversible or partially reversible impairments of cognitive function caused by depression (see Chapter 31).

Dysfunctional bereavement　*Bereavement, the process of grieving, is a form of depression and sadness that few older adults escape, and it may lead to suicidal thoughts and behavior.* **Dysfunctional bereavement** *is problematic if it lasts for more than 1 year, is accompanied by deterioration of health, is characterized by extreme guilt and hopelessness, and is accompanied by suicidal ideation.* **Reunion fantasies,** *wishes to join a deceased loved one in the afterlife,* are a form of suicidal ideation. Elderly persons are at greatest risk for suicide for the first day or two after the death of a spouse and for the first year. Anniversaries of the loss, wedding anniversaries, and birthdays of the spouse are also vulnerable times. Alcohol abuse further increases the risk of suicide after the death of a spouse.

Suicide　Undiagnosed depression may lead to an elderly person's suicide. One fourth of all reported suicides in the United States are committed by persons age 60 and older. The highest rate of suicide occurs in noncaucasian men in their eighties, and the majority of the

The Nursing Process

elderly who commit suicide do so with a firearm. In persons over age 65, 50% of those who attempt suicide succeed, compared with 10% of the general population. Unsuccessful attempts in elderly persons are accounted for by impaired judgment, coordination, or cognition. Severe loss is believed to be the major cause of suicide in the elderly. The wish to control the circumstances, timing, and method of one's own death is another motivation, particularly among the terminally ill. Suicide pacts between spouses are also common among the elderly.

Silent suicide, the intention to kill oneself by passive means through self-starvation or noncompliance with essential medical treatment, is prevalent among the elderly. Silent suicide may go unrecognized because of the absence of overt psychiatric symptoms, the presence of real medical complaints, or recent personal losses that are valid reasons for overwhelming sadness.

- Ben Z. continues to smoke and overeat despite the fact that he has had three heart attacks.
- Margo S. stops taking her insulin because she decides she can no longer live without her husband, who died recently.

The personal belief systems of health care providers and family members may lead to the false conclusion that a client's physical decline is "failure to thrive," a label often attributed to the frail elderly and the institutionalized "old old" who are showing signs of becoming progressively weaker. Also known as *psychogenic mortality syndrome, or the giving-up complex, failure to thrive results when an elderly person no longer makes self-initiated efforts to maintain life.* Staff need to determine that a client's ominous physical decline is not depression or passive suicide. Other elderly persons may choose "benign" suicide and be thought of as making "rational" end-of-life decisions. *Benign suicide is an active decision to end one's life prematurely by not following a recommended treatment regimen.* Nurses are challenged to differentiate a client's seemingly benign, passive suicidal course from a choice that involves the right to a dignified death.

Loneliness and isolation

Feelings of isolation, loneliness, and hopelessness are thought to be among the major emotional problems faced by elderly persons, affecting between 12% and 40% of the population over age 65. If *loneliness* is defined as *a reactive response to separation from persons and things in which people have invested themselves,* then it is likely that all elderly persons experience some degree of loneliness. Some examples of losses that precipitate loneliness and environmental isolation in the elderly are the death of a spouse; a shrinking peer group; the death, relocation, or physical illness of a significant other; a geographic move; a language barrier; lowered energy levels; immobilizing pain; changes in body image; and economic changes, such as the loss of a pension or large debts as a result of medical bills.

Loneliness is often difficult to diagnose, because many elderly people do not admit that they feel lonely. For others, the lonely feelings occur only at certain times (usually at night) and are not readily observed by caregivers. Still others, because of their personalities or because of a need to project an image of a "picture of health," fail to recognize their loneliness and isolation. They unconsciously disguise or overcompensate for their symptoms.

Anxiety

Elderly persons worry about many things, are often anxious, and may even experience panic disorder. Many of the symptoms of panic are somatic and may be unrecognized when the client is an older adult (National Institutes of Health [NIH], 1994). (See Chapter 22 for a discussion on panic symptoms.) If nurses focus solely on physical symptoms rather than explore the affectual dimension of clients, they may fail to recognize anxiety. Factors to assess in older adults with symptoms of anxiety include precipitating events or issues, recent changes, degree of neglect of ADLs, presence of physical signs of anxiety, and degree of anxiety.

Obsessive-compulsive disorder (OCD) is another common form of anxiety (see Chapter 22). OCD is composed of obsessive symptoms (persistent intrusive thoughts), as well as compulsive symptoms (repetitive behavior that is performed in an attempt to reduce anxiety). Some of the ritualistic routines of older adults may be manifestations of OCD.

Extreme anxiety may also be a factor in hypochondriasis. *Hypochondriasis, or somatoform disorder, is overconcern with one's physical and emotional health, accompanied by various bodily complaints for which there is no physical basis.* The person with hypochondriasis has usually spent years pursuing attention for many illnesses. Families and friends are generally burnt out from years of dealing with complaints. Persons with hypochondriacal complaints are vulnerable because if they do develop a "real" illness, they may not be taken seriously. For some, hypochondriacal complaints begin later in life and stem from a person's sense of defectiveness and deterioration. Somatic complaints may become a pattern of interaction, and as

The Nursing Process

such, they may be a means of overcoming loneliness. The somatic complaint provides the elderly person with something to talk about and guarantees communication with family members, other elderly persons, and health care professionals. It may provide the person with an organizing purpose to his or her day. Taking pills, going to doctors, attending therapy sessions, and generally complaining are often signs that a person's life lacks purpose or meaning. Older people who have multiple psychosomatic complaints may also be identifying with decreased family members and friends or displacing anxiety about other concerns.

Cognitive and perceptual impairment
Dementia and delirium and amnestic disorders are the leading causes of cognitive impairment in elderly persons. An extensive discussion of dementia and delirium is found in Chapter 31. Some elderly clients may at first appear to have symptoms of dementia, but they may in reality be responding to severe stress. Other causes of cognitive symptoms must first be ruled out. The mnemonic **DEMENTIA** found in Box 35-1 helps the nurse recall the list of problems that must be considered before a diagnosis of cognitive impairment is considered.

Paranoid reactions are common responses to extreme stress. Stressors such as relocation, social isolation, and deafness create perceptual problems in older adults. Newly institutionalized residents of a nursing home often experience some paranoid ideation. Individuals who use the defense of projection throughout life are those clients most likely to have paranoid reactions. Resentment, anger, delusions of grandeur, ideas of reference, ideas of persecution, and suspiciousness are common symptoms of paranoia.

BOX 35-1

Dementia Mnemonic

Causes of Cognitive Impairment

D—Drugs
E—Emotional disorders
M—Metabolic or endocrine dysfunction
E—Eye and ear dysfunction
N—Nutritional deficiencies
T—Tumor and trauma
I—Infections
A—Arteriosclerotic complications (myocardial infarction [MI], congestive heart failure [CHF]; alcohol)

The relationship between loss of vision, deafness, and paranoid reactions is well documented (Dellasega, 1991). When several senses decline simultaneously, as happens with the elderly, accurate perception of the environment is impaired. Persons with diminished sensory input may develop paranoid thinking and become isolated, lonely, and depressed. The sensory-impaired elderly person creates a new inner world to fill the void created by the loss of sensory contact with the real world. At first the new inner world created by increasing silence is threatening, unknown, and hostile, causing suspiciousness. Misinterpretation of auditory stimuli results. Decreasing self-esteem is projected onto others. Ideas of reference develop, and active delusions of persecution may occur.

Elderly clients who had a diagnosis of schizophrenia as younger adults do not outgrow their symptoms. Rather, symptoms and the treatment of them are complicated by the aging process. Elderly persons are less likely to continue to experience hallucinations, but instead flat affect and poverty of speech prevail. Chapter 29 in this book has a complete discussion of schizophrenic symptoms, and Chapter 38 describes the client with severe and persistent symptoms.

Substance-related disorders
Overuse of alcohol and drugs is a major way that the elderly cope with stress and depression. When genetic vulnerability exists, substance disorders may develop. Chapter 27 discusses the behaviors associated with substance-related disorders. Patterns of misuse and abuse may also exist in the elderly and include overuse, underuse, and erratic use.

The most common pattern of erratic use is taking the prescribed medication only when severe or acute symptoms occur, rather than on a regular basis as prescribed. Teaching Points aimed at helping older clients comply with medication schedules and avoid medication misuse are presented on p. 768.

Illicit drug use in the elderly is growing. As the population grows older, a person who has had previous drug problems may continue abuse into late life. Late-onset abuse of illicit or prescribed drugs occurs most often as a reaction to loss or a changed social environment. The rate of alcohol abuse among older adults is similar to the rate for the general population, but the rate appears to be on the rise. The most commonly reported factors associated with alcoholism in the elderly are loss, loneliness, and physical illness. Elderly persons drink to ease the psychogenic pain of loss, to facilitate coping with social isolation and loneliness, and to self-medicate inexpensively (Leach McMahon, 1993). Elderly persons who

The Nursing Process

 TEACHING POINTS

Ways to Avoid Medication Misuse

- Use large block letters to label medications.
- Use a pill box to keep track of daily doses.
- Color code pill bottles to avoid confusion among pills.
- Avoid over-the-counter drugs unless suggested by prescriber.
- Inform health care professional about drug, alcohol, nicotine, and tobacco use.
- Use only one pharmacy to fill prescriptions.
- Never share drugs with a friend.

abuse alcohol may be divided into the following three categories:

- Chronic, early-onset group, who have abused alcohol throughout life
- "Reactors," who begin drinking in response to an adverse event associated with aging
- Intermittent users, who drink in response to stress or for the depressant effects on the central nervous system (Leach McMahon, 1993)

Alcoholism is a problem of older persons that is often unrecognized. It is commonly confused with age-related problems such as dementia and social isolation. It accounts for a high incidence of accidents, particularly falls. The hidden nature of the problem is propagated by family members who protect a parent or spouse. Others hid the problem because they feared the stigma of being labeled alcoholic. Some of the elderly experience spontaneous remission of alcohol dependence because their bodies' responses to alcohol are unpleasant and because they fear dying prematurely.

Some diagnostic clues that an elderly person is drinking too much are insomnia, impotence, uncontrolled gout, multiple unexplained bruises, rapid onset of confused states, uncontrollable hypertension, and unexplained falls. However, each of the symptoms mentioned may also indicate other impaired physiological processes.

Focused Assessment

Persons with mental disorders age at different rates and in unique ways. In addition to the behavioral manifestations of their symptoms, the assessment needs to differentiate the normal aging process from deviations in that process, so an accurate data base can be acquired. Elderly persons often have multiple symptoms that confuse or mask their underlying problems. The client's lifestyle of coping with health problems, functional capacity, ability to cope with ADLs, social support system, living situation, economic well-being, and recent life events are all factors that need to be included in a comprehensive assessment of an elderly client.

Assessment for elderly persons requires integration of the cognitive, affective, social, and behavioral data gathered by the nurse. The systems principle—that any change in any aspect of a person's life affects all the other facets—becomes evident when working with the multifaceted issues of the elderly. When assessing elderly persons, the nurse is guided by the following principles:

- *Establish a rapport with the elderly client.* Nurses are often much younger than their clients. Treating the elderly with respect involves awareness of one's own feelings about aging, accepting older persons as they are, being knowledgeable about the aging process, and treating the person as an intelligent and feeling adult.
- *Assessment takes longer.* Interviews, examinations, and testing should be unhurried and relaxed. The complete assessment is divided into short sessions and should take place at a time of day when the older person is most alert. Soliciting information in short segments facilitates the process and prevents tiring the elderly client.
- *A person's impaired hearing may present a problem with the assessment.* Box 35-2 lists interventions that are useful when assessing clients with hearing deficits. Additionally, nurses should experiment with the pitch of their voices, because some elderly persons hear low-pitched voices more readily.
- *Persons who have had a stroke have difficulty with communication.* The nurse should approach clients who have had a stroke on the unaffected side. For clients with aphasia, nurses need to be patient with their struggle to speak. Words are supplied only when absolutely necessary. An audiovisual aid such as a writing pad, blackboard, or typewriter can be used for asking questions and receiving answers. Clients are always treated as intelligent and worthwhile people.
- *The nurse assesses not only an elderly person's basic health but also the changes in health status that have evolved over the life span.* A thorough physical assessment is essential because it forms the basis for determining or ruling out an organic basis for psychiatric problems such as dementia or depression. Table 35-1 includes assessment instruments commonly used with older adults to obtain the necessary data base, to assess the presence or absence of the common mental

The Nursing Process

Communication Enhancement: Hearing Deficit

DEFINITION

Assistance in accepting and learning alternate methods for living with diminished hearing

ACTIVITIES

Facilitate appointment for hearing examination, as appropriate

Facilitate use of hearing aids, as appropriate

Teach patient that sounds will be experienced differently with the use of a hearing aid

Keep hearing aid clean

Check hearing aid batteries routinely

Give one simple direction at a time

Listen attentively

Refrain from shouting at patient with communication disorders

Use simple words and short sentences, as appropriate

Increase voice volume, as appropriate

Do not cover your mouth, smoke, talk with a full mouth, or chew gum when speaking

Obtain patient's attention through touch

Use paper, pencil, or computer communication, when necessary

Facilitate location of resources for hearing aids

Facilitate location of telephone for the hearing impaired, as appropriate

Reprinted with permission from McCloskey, J.C., & Bulechek, G.M. (1996). Nursing interventions classification (NIC) (2nd ed.). St. Louis: Mosby.

health problems of the elderly, and to determine level of function (Lueckenotte, 1996).

• *Assessing achievement of life purpose is an essential component of an elderly person's data base.* Assessing a person's philosophical perspective on life and observing whether the "life review" process has begun provides important information about the individual's acceptance of inevitable death. The role of religious and cultural practices is a highly significant facet of an elderly person's ability to cope with the end-stage of life. Some questions that nurses use to assess the philosophical dimensions of a person's life include the following:

–What are your life dreams?

–What was your greatest life accomplishment?

–What things in your life do you wish you could change?

–How do you feel about dying?

–What are your beliefs about life after death?

–What is your religion? How do your family's religious beliefs influence your view of death?

–What are your cultural beliefs about death and growing old?

• *Assessment of the elderly person's degree of social support facilitates the determination of family and caregiver needs.* The level of social support for elderly persons is a key factor in their ability to maintain their independence.

Nursing Diagnosis

Elderly clients have DSM-IV diagnoses that are similar to those of their younger counterparts. However, it is common to see elderly persons with several modifiers, particularly those that indicate chronicity. Axis III diagnoses, indicating the presence of a medical condition, are also prevalent. The most common DSM-IV diagnoses for elderly clients are dementia, delirium (see Chapter 31), and depression (see Chapter 30).

Nursing diagnoses for clients usually reflect the interrelationship of physical, affective, behavioral, and cognitive factors. Because of the elderly person's already diminished reserves, new stresses often create problems that are not easily diagnosed or distinguished from dysfunctional behavior. Examples of nursing diagnoses that commonly occur in elderly clients are listed in Box 35-3.

Planning

The development of a realistic plan of care for the elderly is a collaborative multidisciplinary effort. Planning varies depending on whether clients reside at home, in a nursing home, or in another type of treatment facility. Case management of elderly clients is a key component in facilitating the planning process and achieving positive outcomes. Interventions are aimed at the ultimate goal of maintaining quality of life rather than at restoration of health. Outcome criteria should be realistic and consider the strengths and weaknesses of the client, environmental limitations, and the availability of family caregivers or community resources. Care plans throughout this text may be modified to meet the unique needs and functional status of elderly clients.

Outcome Identification

Outcomes of the care of elderly persons need to be realistic and reflect the interrelationship among the physical, affective, cognitive, social, and behavioral aspects of

The Nursing Process

TABLE 35-1

Selected assessment instruments for use with the older adult

INSTRUMENT	TYPE OF ASSESSMENT	SPECIFIC AREAS OF ASSESSMENT
FANCAPES (Mnemonic device used to recall areas of assessment) (Ebersole and Hess, 1994)	Assess functional ability, basic needs, and the extent to which assistance is necessary	**F**luids, **A**eration, **N**utrition, **C**ommunication, **A**ctivity, **P**ain, **E**limination, **S**ocial skills, and perception of death
Short Portable Mental Status Questionnaire (SPMSQ) (Phieffer, 1975)	Standardized questionnaire designed to measure the mental status of elderly persons	Yields a score that indicates an elderly person's level of disability
Geriatric Depression Scale (GDS) (Yesavage and Brink, 1983)	Nurse-administered standardized questionnaire that provides a rating for the severity of depression in the elderly	Degree of depression (normal, mild, moderate, or severe)
Michigan Alcoholism Screening Test (MAST)	Self-administered questionnaire that screens for alcoholism	Provides scores that indicate possible or definite alcoholism
Barthel Index (Mahoney and Barthel, 1965)	Rates level of independence with self-care activities	Feeding, moving from wheelchair to bed, toileting, transfer on and off toilet, bathing, walking on a level surface, propelling a wheelchair, and ascending and decending stairs
Instrumental Activities of Daily Living Scale (IADL) (Lawton and Brody, 1969)	Measures adeptness with complex ADLs of elderly persons living in the community	Using the telephone, shopping, food preparation, housekeeping, doing laundry, transportation, taking medication, and handling finances

the client. Outcomes should be concrete and short term, and include elderly persons' needs for assistance to accomplish the stated goal. For example, an outcome criterion for a young adult who is depressed may be *independent maintenance of self-care activities* as evidenced by improved grooming and clean clothes. For an elderly person, the analogous outcome criterion may be *to accept interdependence* as evidenced by cooperation with a health care aide who performs certain daily grooming activities.

Implementation

Caring for elderly clients and their families requires all of the nurse's physical, psychosocial, and spiritual energy. The management of care of elderly persons is a holistic multidisciplinary process that requires not only a commitment to the elderly and their unique needs, but specialized counseling, health teaching, and milieu management skills. The elderly need high levels of assis-

tance with self-care activities, and pharmacological management of symptoms requires sophisticated knowledge of each person's individual needs. Case management is of paramount importance and focuses on coordination of the multiple services needed to promote and maintain the mental health of elderly persons.

Counseling

Nurses need to be adept at establishing individual therapeutic relationships with clients and at managing group and family support intervention strategies. As with any nurse-client relationship, rapport must first be established. Principles for establishing a therapeutic relationship with clients and proceeding through it are discussed in Chapter 9. Goals of the therapeutic relationship with elderly clients include the following:

- Recognition of self as a valuable human being capable of coping with stress

The Nursing Process

Examples of Nursing Diagnoses Common in Elderly Clients

BEHAVIORAL

Risk for injury related to motor and sensory deficit
Relocation stress syndrome related to impaired
   psychosocial health status

AFFECTIVE

Social isolation related to depressed affect
Dysfunctional grieving related to death of spouse
Spiritual distress

COGNITIVE

Impaired environmental interpretation syndrome
Chronic confusion
Altered thought process related to translocation crisis

FAMILY/SOCIAL

Caregiver role strain
Altered role performance
Decisional conflict related to indecision about nursing-
   home placement of spouse

• Awareness of emotional reactivity to stressful
  events or illness
• Development of coping resources that are age-
  appropriate
• Collaboration in planning strategies that maximize
  recovery and independence

Several barriers to therapeutic communication with the elderly may exist. Depression may be present, or clients may be experiencing diminished contact with reality because of medication effects, physical discomfort, or pathological conditions. There may be environmental noise and distractions, cultural differences, language difficulties, or information overload. The most common communication difficulty occurs because of visual or hearing deficits. Box 35-4 lists strategies for enhancing communication with individuals who have diminished vision. See Box 35-2 for strategies for helping clients who have diminished hearing understand messages better.

Many specific group strategies are effective for intervening with elderly clients and their families (Clark and Vorst, 1994). These include groups for older adults with specific disorders such as depression or anxiety, exercise groups, poetry and music groups, cooking groups, assertiveness-training groups, caregiver support groups, widow/widower support groups, and chronic-illness adaptation groups. Chapter 11 includes a full dis-

Communication Enhancement: Visual Deficit

DEFINITION

Assistance in accepting and learning alternate methods for
   living with diminished vision

ACTIVITIES

Identify yourself when you enter the patient's space
Note patient's reaction to diminished vision
   (e.g., depression, withdrawal, and denial)
Accept patient's reaction to diminished vision
Assist patient in setting new goals to learn how to
   "see" with other senses
Build on patient's remaining vision, as appropriate
Walk one or two steps ahead of the patient, with patient's
   hand on your elbow
Describe environment to patient
Do not move items in patient's room without informing
   patient
Read mail, newspaper, and other pertinent information to
   patient
Identify items on food tray in relation to numbers on a
   clock
Fold paper money in different ways for easy identification
Inform patient where to locate radio or talking books
Provide a magnifying glass or prism eyeglasses, as appro-
   priate, for reading
Provide Braille reading material, as appropriate
Initiate occupational therapy referral, as appropriate
Refer patient with visual problems to appropriate agency

Reprinted with permission from McCloskey, J.C., & Bulechek, G.M. (1996). Nursing interventions classification (NIC) (2nd ed.). St. Louis: Mosby.

cussion of the purpose of groups and gives examples of activities common in each.

Other counseling strategies that are particularly therapeutic with the elderly include reminiscence therapy and life review therapy. ***Reminiscence therapy***, *also called oral history, autobiography, and milestoning, is the recall of past events, feelings, and thoughts to facilitate adaptation to present circumstances* (Haight and Burnside, 1993). Reminiscence is a useful strategy for maintaining a client's orientation to reality, improving quality of life, and when used in a group setting, increasing socialization.

Life review therapy *is based on reminiscing techniques and is both an assessment tool and a therapeutic technique. This comprehensive review of all aspects of one's life* is intended to prepare elderly persons to plan for the remainder of their existence (Butler and Lewis,

The Nursing Process

1982). Remembering is guided by the nurse and is usually characterized by feelings of nostalgia, regret, or pleasure. Extreme emotional pain, despair, depression, guilt, obsessive rumination, and panic may complicate the process. Life review techniques should be used only with clients who can manage such reactions. The expected outcomes of the life review are atonement, serenity, constructive reorganization, and creativity. Both reminiscence therapy and life review therapy may occur in group settings, however life review is more comfortable for clients when it occurs in the context of an individual counseling session. Some methods used to stimulate recall of memories include use of photo albums or scrapbooks, construction of family trees, use of old newspapers, magazines, or musical records, and the writing of letters to old friends.

Family counseling is also important when working with older clients. Families need financial as well as emotional and social support if they are expected to negotiate the task of caregiving without undue stress. Planning for the care of an elderly relative and sharing the responsibility with other siblings when the elder is a parent helps diminish caregiver stress. Family supportive therapy, discussion groups, education groups, respite care, volunteer short-term recreational and homechore programs, and adult day care programs are among the supportive programs in place to prevent caregiver stress in family members. Nurses are in key roles to assess family needs and to make appropriate referrals for family therapy (see Chapter 12).

Milieu Therapy

Managing the milieu is a significant and far-reaching intervention. The environment of elderly persons includes their personally significant space and territory, as well as the larger geographical environment. The concept of personal space has to do with the need for privacy, solitude, and anonymity. Elderly persons need more light, less noise, and warm, bright colors in their physical environment. Nurses are in a position to educate clients and families about providing these needs.

A geropsychiatric unit in the hospital is generally planned with older, physically limited clients in mind. Hand rails, bedside rails, softly padded chairs with fairly high seats, bright colors, large-print signs, hazard-proof appliances, nonskid floors, special mattresses, and an up-to-date orientation board are among the features found there.

An elderly person's place of residence is often his or her symbol of independence—or lack of it. A lack of finances with which to maintain a home of many years or an unwanted move to smaller, more convenient housing

after the death of a spouse is often at the root of an elderly person's psychosocial problems. Elderly persons feel lost and become anxious when forced to leave a place that has been the focal point for family gatherings and memories. Adult children may visit less often after the home in which they grew up has been sold, contributing further to the family's collective sense of loss or depression. Even couples who plan and look forward to a move to a retirement community are faced with what is known as a *translocation crisis, a crisis related to the experience of moving to a new place.*

Some elderly persons who have lived their middle years in relatively safe urban areas find themselves in deteriorating and unsafe neighborhoods, which may precipitate fear, loneliness, and isolation. Still other elderly persons are unable to find suitable, safe, and affordable housing. Severe grief reactions and depression follow or accompany a translocation crisis or concern about a place to live. Displaying a picture of the former home in a place of prominence and openly discussing the move facilitates adjustment to the new milieu.

When clients move to a new place it is important that they have their own personal space or territory. The elderly, like persons of any age, may maintain a sense of personal space by cluttering, by gathering environmental props (which are usually significant personal items), and by behaving in a possessive manner. A need for personal territory accounts for such behavior as the hoarding of string, newspapers, or greeting cards, as well as being rigid about a particular seat at the table or in a group, having favorite furniture, and being possessive about personal items such as pictures or religious articles. Possessive traits tend to escalate in direct proportion to a person's loss of control over environmental circumstances.

For clients who remain in the community, lack of transportation is a major source of crisis. Causes include declining eyesight, which impairs ability to drive an automobile; limited access to public transportation; declining physical health; geographical location that limits accessibility to public transportation; limited economic resources; and geographically distant adult children. Nurses may suggest that elderly clients take advantage of public transportation services available in their communities.

Self-Care Activities

Maintaining functional independence and the physical well-being of clients are primary goals of self-care interventions for the elderly. Meeting the spiritual needs of elderly persons is a key self-care intervention. As death approaches, people are called on to transcend the ordinary events of life and to perceive commonplace happenings

The Nursing Process

in entirely new ways. Finding meaning in the later years and accepting death are major developmental tasks of the elderly. Personal meaning and self-fulfillment have as many varied expressions as there are people. Some people actualize themselves through mystical or religious experiences, whereas others leave artistic legacies or express themselves through objects, deeds, crafts, progeny, or autobiographical statements. Some people view life as having only death at its end. For these people, transcendent expression of self includes developing and enhancing the virtues of hope, wisdom, courage, humor, faith, and idealism. A sense of duty, prestige, secularism, and pragmatism are more practical expressions of life's meaningfulness.

Religious practices, dreams, symbols, fantasies, daydreams, and visions are all expressions of the spiritual dimension of the self. Religious practice has been found to be positively correlated with feelings of happiness, usefulness, and personal adjustment and to be a support system for those in failing health. Nurses need to learn about, understand, and facilitate access to the religious-practice needs of the elderly.

An important component of actualizing the self for elderly clients is a *legacy,* or *bequeathing part of the self to others.* Some legacies are formal and managed by the legal system, whereas others are as simple as leaving part of oneself. In a living legacy, a person donates his or her body or body parts to science for transplants. Spatial legacies involve written or verbal autobiographical accounts of a person's environment. Physical legacies may include property, assets, and personal possessions. Human legacies include children, grandchildren, and other descendants.

Persons who have found meaning for their lives by facing the inevitability of death as the beginning of an afterlife specify their legacies in concrete and vibrant ways. They have in a sense discovered the secret of immortality. Nurses become active listeners and often strong advocates to secure legacies left by their clients. Elderly clients in the mental health system often have few physical or human legacies and find peace—even joy—in the smallest token of themselves that they can give to others. Helping them write or artistically express themselves helps facilitate this end.

Psychobiological Interventions

The use of pharmacological agents to treat the symptoms of mental disorders common to the elderly may be as problematic as it is therapeutic. Several physiological changes associated with aging are responsible. Altered gastrointestinal absorption related to a decrease in stomach acid, increased body fat, decreased muscle mass, and decreased total body water affect the distribution and elimination of drugs in elderly persons. A decrease in hepatic metabolism and hepatic blood flow affects the rate of metabolism of the psychotropic drugs and further complicates the process of safely medicating elderly clients.

Drug-drug interactions, drug-food interactions, and noncompliance are other issues that have an impact on psychopharmacological treatment of elderly persons. One half of all over-the-counter drugs are purchased by the elderly, and approximately 25% of prescribed drugs are used by them. These factors and multiphysician use by elderly clients make the potential for untoward interactions high. Dosages need to be adjusted based on rates of metabolism and potential interactive effects.

Noncompliance with medication and treatment regimens is common among older adults, particularly those for whom long-term medication regimens have been prescribed. Consequences of the noncompliance are unpredictable, with a wide range of possible outcomes, including return to the hospital (see Chapter 15). Factors that contribute to noncompliance in the elderly include living alone, adverse effects of treatments or medication, the cost of medication, the type of illness, confounding medical illness, the relationship to the prescriber, complexity of the treatment, and cognitive or sensory impairment. Medication Tips to be considered when psychotropic medications are prescribed for elderly clients are presented below.

 MEDICATION TIPS

Administration of Psychotropic Drugs to the Elderly

- Antipsychotics (phenothiazenes) in combination with diuretics increase the incidence of hypotension, confusion, and incontinence.
- Tardive dyskinesia and other extrapyramidal reactions are common occurrences in the elderly clients.
- Hypnotics may lower body temperature to dangerous levels in elderly persons prone to hypothermia.
- Psychoactive drugs increase intraocular pressure and reduce visual accommodation. Clients with glaucoma should avoid their use.
- Elderly persons are more vulnerable to lithium and tricyclic toxicity because of slowed renal filtration and clearance.
- Elderly persons experience paradoxical reactions to psychotropic agents more often than younger individuals.

The Nursing Process

Health Teaching

Education of elderly clients and their families includes strategies that aim to maintain clients' present level of function, assist clients and their families with self-medication, and support and promote independence. Although the elderly learn at a slower pace, they remain willing and eager students of new and practical information. Learning stimulates interest, fosters socialization, enhances coping, and promotes self-esteem. Chapter 16 discusses strategies that facilitate effective health teaching and learning.

Older adults learn best in one-on-one situations and large groups. Smaller groups of peers are also effective. Because of diminished vision and hearing, larger print is needed for written materials and audiovisuals, and care needs to be taken to be sure verbal material is heard. Health promotion topics include exercise, diet, stress management, retirement preparation, and information about Social Security benefits. Secondary prevention topics may focus on management of loss and grief, prevention of abuse and neglect, medication management, screening for anxiety, depression, substance abuse, physical problems, and the signs and symptoms of the major mental disorders. Information about community resources, hospice care, taking medications safely, and placement issues are helpful for critically ill elderly clients and their families.

Case Management

Case management is the coordination of a specific group of resources and services that facilitate the development and implementation of individualized care plans to improve the quality of care provided to elderly persons (see Chapter 17). Examples of services that nurses in their role as case managers may suggest to elderly clients and their families include transportation, escort services, chore services, business and financial counseling, nutrition programs, telephone counseling, shelter for elderly homeless persons, retired senior volunteer programs, housing and social support activities. Outreach services help identify clients who are mentally ill and needy. Peer counseling and peer helper programs provide support and assistance to elderly persons coping with developmental crises. "Young old," or newly retired elderly, reach out to support the "old-old" or frail individuals. Self-help groups lend support for problems such as medication compliance, behavioral change, or retirement adjustment.

The major benefits of a case management approach include maintenance of the elderly person at home, shorter hospital stays, reduction of confusion for the client, family, and involved agencies, elimination of duplication of services, and the prevention of emergencies by planning for crisis situations.

Health Promotion and Health Maintenance

Health promotion and health maintenance for the elderly is aimed at maintaining independent function for as long as possible and at minimizing the effects of long-term treatment. The elderly are a high-risk group, since their symptoms are often compounded by socioeconomic stressors and failing physical health and functional ability. Participation of elderly clients in their care and in decisions related to where they will reside and be treated promotes their well-being and self-esteem.

Services needed by elderly persons to maintain psychosocial well-being include access to information and referral; financial aid, particularly Social Security services; banking and financial access; recreation; and leisure activities and transportation. *Life care communities, places individuals enter when they are healthy, provide the needed services at the wellness level and continue them through skilled nursing-home care.* Other supportive services include home delivery meals, homemaker services, foster care, telephone reassurance, psychiatric home care, day treatment, and hospice care. Organizations that serve the needs of the elderly are presented in the Community Resources box on p. 775.

Evaluation

Evaluation of outcomes planned for elderly persons who have been treated for symptoms of mental disorders should demonstrate a decrease in symptoms and achievement of a level of independence comparable with previous physical and functional ability. Achievement of outcomes fosters self-esteem and is evidenced by the clients' realistic acceptance of the aging process and the limitations imposed by symptoms.

KEY POINTS

- Elderly persons who are healthy carry into late life the capacity to maintain self-esteem, self-confidence, purpose in life, a satisfying sense of personal identity, and a social role, despite losses that occur as part of the aging process.
- Depressive disorders in the elderly may be masked and exhibited with physical symptoms such as weight loss and multiple somatic complaints.
- The highest rate of suicide occurs in non-caucasian men over age 80. Silent suicide prevails among the elderly.
- Feelings of isolation, loneliness, and hopelessness are thought to be the major emotional problem faced by elderly persons, affecting between 12% and 40% of the population over age 65.

The Nursing Process

COMMUNITY RESOURCES

The Elderly

American Association of Retired Persons (AARP)
601 E. Street NW
Washington, DC 20049
(202) 434-2277

American Society on Aging (ASA)
833 Market Street, Room 516
San Francisco, CA 94103-1824
(415) 882-2910

Gerontological Society of America (GSA)
1275 K Street NW, Suite 350
Washington, DC 20005-4006
(202) 842-1275

National Association of Area Agencies on Aging
1112 16th Street NW, Suite 100
Washington, DC 20036
(202) 296-8130

National Institute on Aging
Public Information Office
Federal Building
Room 5C27, Building 31
9000 Rockville Parkway
Bethesda, MD 20892
(301) 496-4000

Social Security Administration
6325 Security Boulevard
Baltimore, MD 21207
Medicare Hotline (800) 2345-SSA

• Symptoms of anxiety in the elderly include somatic complaints, repetitive behavior, and hypochondriasis.
• Overuse and abuse of alcohol and drugs are the major ways in which the elderly cope with stress and depression. The signs of alcoholism in the elderly may not be distinguishable from symptoms associated with the aging process.
• Assessment for the elderly requires integration of the cognitive, affective, social, and behavioral data gathered by nurses.
• Planning for elderly persons with symptoms of mental disorders is aimed at maintaining functional status and independence with activities of daily living.

CRITICAL THINKING QUESTIONS

Mr. Forte is a 67-year-old man who has been admitted to the geropsychiatric unit in an acute state of confusion. His wife reports that he has been apathetic, sits in his chair all day, and eats only when she insists on it. She reports he consumes a six-pack of beer daily and has done so for several years. He becomes angry if she suggests he not drink, so she does not ask him anymore. Last month, Mr. Forte had a complete physical examination, and except for hypertension he was in good health. His physician prescribed a diuretic and low sodium diet. There appear to be no other stressors in the family, although Mrs. Forte states, "He's been like this since he retired 2 years ago. He has always been quiet and a bit of a loner." He has no previous history of mental problems. A policy on the unit is to withdraw clients from their medication and to keep them drug-free for at least 1 week after admission. By the end of 1 week, Mr. Forte has improved dramatically. His earlier confusion has been replaced by anger at the staff for keeping him on the unit. A diagnosis of depression was made, and he was referred for outpatient counseling. Alcoholics Anonymous (AA) and a support group for retirees were recommended. He was placed on a low dose of paroxetine (Paxil). He agreed to take the medication but refused any other support.

1. What nursing diagnoses are appropriate for Mr. Forte on admission? What nursing diagnoses are more appropriate on discharge?
2. What teaching would you do with Mr. Forte's wife about the suggested follow-up procedure?
3. Why was Mr. Forte diagnosed with depression rather than dementia?
4. How does Mr. Forte's drinking impact his life and his symptoms?
5. How do you feel about elderly clients who drink?
6. What feelings do you have about Mr. Forte's refusal to accept treatment? How would you handle the situation if you were his nurse?

• The management of care of the elderly is a holistic multidisciplinary process that requires not only a commitment to the elderly and their unique needs but specialized counseling, health teaching, and milieu management skills.
• The elderly need high levels of assistance with self-care activities and skillful pharmacological management.

REFERENCES

American Association of Retired Persons. (1987). *A portrait of older minorities.* Washington, DC: Author.

American Association of Retired Persons. (1997). *A profile of older Americans: 1996.* Washington, DC: Author.

American Society on Aging. (1992). *Serving elders of color: challenges to providers and the aging network.* (Report of National Low Income Minority Elder Initiative to Department of Health and Human Services). Washington, DC: Author.

Burnside, I. (1994). *Nursing care of the aged.* St. Louis: Mosby.

Clark, W., & Vorst, V. (1994). Group therapy with chronically depressed geriatric patients *Journal of Psychosocial Nursing, 32*(5), 9-13.

Dellasega, C. (1991). Meeting the mental health needs of elderly clients. *Journal of Psychosocial Nursing and Mental Health Services, 29*(21), 10-14.

Ebersole, P., & Hess, P. (1994). *Toward healthy aging* (4th ed.). St. Louis: Mosby.

Evans, C.A., & Cunningham, B. (1996). Caring for the ethnic elder. *Geriatric Nursing, 17*(3), 105-110.

Haight, B.K., & Burnside, I. (1993). Reminiscence and life review: Explaining the differences, *Archives of Psychiatric Nursing, 7*(2), 91-98.

Lawton, H. P., & Brody, E. M. (1969). Assessment of older people: Self maintaining and instrumental activities of daily living. *Gerontologist, 9*(2) 179-186.

Leach McMahon, A. (1993). Substance abuse among the elderly. *Nurse Practitioner Forum, 4*(4), 231-238.

Lueckenotte, A.G. (1996). *Gerontologic nursing,* St. Louis: Mosby.

Mahoney, F., & Barthel, D.W. (1965). Functional evaluation: The Barthel index, *Maryland State Medical Journal, 14,* 61-65.

Phieffer, E. (1975). A portable mental status questionnaire for the assessment of organic brain deficit in elderly patients. *Journal of American Geriatrics Society, 23*(10), 433-441.

Rossen, E.K., & Buschmann, M.T. (1995). Mental illness in late life: The neurobiology of depression. *Archives of Psychiatric Nursing, 9*(3), 130-136.

U.S. Bureau of Census. (1991). *Statistical abstract of the United States: 1991.* (111th ed.). Washington, DC: U.S. Government Printing Office.

Wayne, S.J., Rhyne, R.L., Garry, P.J., & Goodwin, S.A. (1990). Cell mediated immunity as a predictor of morbidity and mortality in subjects over 60. *Journal of Gerontology, 45*(2), 45.

Yesavage, J.A., & Brink, T.L. (1983). Development and validation of a geriatric depression screening scale: A preliminary report. *Journal of Psychiatric Research, 17,* 37-39.

Chapter 36

Victims and Victimizers

Carole A. Shea

LEARNING OUTCOMES

After studying and applying the concepts of this chapter, the learner will be able to:

- Define physical, psychological, and sexual abuse, neglect, and exploitation as clinical conditions that require compassionate nursing care.
- Document clinical evidence of abuse, neglect, and exploitation of clients across the life span.
- Identify persons at risk of becoming victims or perpetrators of family and domestic violence, using epidemiological information and theories about victimization and aggression.
- Formulate nursing diagnoses and outcome criteria for victims and perpetrators of family and domestic violence using assessment data.
- Select interventions that enhance the client's self-esteem, promote safety, and instill hope.
- Develop a nonjudgmental manner that is sensitive to clients' autonomy, dignity, and rights.
- Evaluate the effectiveness of nursing interventions with victims, family members, and perpetrators of family and domestic violence.
- Advocate with public groups to decrease society's tolerance of violence as a response to conflict situations and stressful living conditions.

KEY TERMS

Abuse	Intrafamilial sexual abuse	Psychological abuse
Exploitation	Perpetrator	Psychological neglect
Extrafamilial sexual abuse	Physical abuse	Sexual abuse
Family and domestic violence	Physical neglect	Victim
Incest		

The purpose of this chapter is to identify and define the types of abuse, neglect, and exploitation that occur in society; provide a historical, epidemiological, and psychiatric diagnostic picture of these problems; examine the circumstances in families, community-based facilities, and institutional settings associated with abuse and neglect; and describe the clinical profiles of victims and perpetrators. Theories that explain the occurrence of abuse, neglect, and exploitation and guide nursing intervention are discussed and applied through the nursing process.

OVERVIEW OF VIOLENCE

Family and domestic violence is a major public health problem. Interpersonal violence extends beyond the boundaries of the home to include neighborhoods, day care centers, nursing homes, and other long-term care facilities. The victims of violence experience physical, psychological, and sexual trauma that may result in injuries, physical illness, or psychological conditions requiring compassionate nursing care. A history of family violence is often a component of psychiatric disorders such as multiple personality disorder (MPD) and post-traumatic stress disorder (PTSD) (Glod, 1993; APA, 1994). Violence and abuse are also believed to exacerbate other psychiatric conditions such as anxiety, depression, schizophrenia, and substance abuse (Muenzenmaier, Meyer, Struening, and Ferber, 1993; Ross, Anderson, and Clark, 1994; Weitzman, Knickman, and Shinn, 1992).

Family and domestic violence is a maladaptive pattern of human interactive behavior that results in intentional abuse, neglect, or exploitation of a family member or intimate acquaintance. Victims of violence may also be abused by a neighbor, friend, community member, or care provider with whom they have a relationship. Nurses commonly encounter clients with various clinical conditions in inpatient psychiatric units, emergency departments, and pediatric clinics who have been traumatized by a family member or intimate acquaintance. Nurses in basic practice are responsible for making comprehensive assessments; listening carefully to the client's story; collecting data to document abuse and neglect; providing compassionate care, crisis intervention, counseling, and education; and reporting abuse as required by law.

Psychiatric nurses in advanced practice (APNs) may be involved in treating clients who manifest the long-term psychological effects of family violence. Sometimes APNs are called upon to intervene in a family's current cycle of interpersonal violence and abuse as part of crisis intervention. They provide psychotherapy and other mental health services for victims and perpetrators in community mental health centers, HMOs, VA hospitals, schools, forensic institutions, and other clinical agencies.

The *victim of family violence may be a spouse, child, sibling, elderly family member, or intimate acquaintance or other unrelated member of the household who has suffered harm inflicted by another family member or authority figure.* In abusive, neglectful, and exploitive situations, the victims are vulnerable and often powerless to care for or protect themselves. The neglect and trauma they experience have long-standing consequences. Victims are found among all sectors of society—rich and poor, females and males, young and old, and all races and nationalities (Gelles and Straus, 1988). Families are at greater risk for violence when they must live with psychological, economic, and other forms of environmental stress (Brasseur, 1995). However, some populations are overrepresented in *reported* cases of family violence, conveying to the public the mistaken impression that family violence is only a problem for poor and minority families (Asbury, 1993).

The *perpetrator of family violence is the person who inflicts intentional harm or makes the victim suffer by deliberate acts, circumstances, or conditions.* The perpetrator acts from a motive to exert power and control over the victim. The perpetrator exhibits a disregard for social expectations and legal codes that dictate how persons should behave toward one another and respect one another's personal well-being. Women are more likely to be the perpetrator of child abuse and neglect, but men inflict more *serious* injuries on children (Gelles & Straus, 1988). Men are also more likely to inflict serious injuries on women, even though women engage in various violent actions (e.g., pushing and hitting) about as often as men. The most frequent occurrence of family violence takes place between siblings. Elders are more likely to be abused, neglected, or exploited by family caretakers (Criner, 1994).

EPIDEMIOLOGY

Several problems influence the availability and accuracy of statistics about the prevalence and incidence of abuse, neglect, and exploitation. Family and domestic violence is a "hidden secret." Despite mandatory reporting laws for professionals, underreporting continues to be a problem. This underreporting suggests that available statistics barely reveal the extent of the problem among those who seek medical treatment. Therefore estimates of the prevalence of abuse and neglect among the general population, or those who do not seek any treatment, are almost impossible to forecast accurately (Gelles, 1993).

Another factor influencing statistics is the lack of consensus on the definitions of abuse and the signs and symptoms of abuse. There is, however, increasing research-based evidence to help in discriminating between accidental injury and deliberately inflicted trauma. This ability to discriminate may facilitate the identification of more victims in the future (Bourne, Chadwick, Kanda, and Ricci, 1993).

Child Abuse and Neglect

Estimates of child abuse and neglect indicate that there are about 3 million suspected cases reported per year. More than half the cases involve neglect of basic needs. About 50% of abused children were born prematurely or had low birth weight. Children are more likely to be abused if they are under age 3 or perceived as being different (i.e., physical or mental disability) or difficult (i.e., persistent crying or hyperactivity). Recent figures indicate that the major cause of death of children in the first year of life is traumatic injuries caused by neglect or abuse. More than 1,000 children die each year because of abuse or neglect (Devlin and Reynolds, 1994).

Sexual Abuse

The prevalence and incidence of child sexual abuse in the general population vary widely, with estimates from 6% to 62% for girls and 3% to 31% for boys (Conte, 1993). Some professionals in the field suggest that approximately 30% of all women have suffered some form of sexual abuse before reaching adulthood (Holz, 1994). One study of women found that 16% had been sexually abused by a relative before age 18, with 4.5% in the abused subsample molested by their fathers (Russell, 1986). The incidence of a history of sexual abuse among psychiatric populations is higher than among the general population (Doob, 1992), with figures for this population in the 40% to 50% range (Urbancic, 1987).

Spousal Abuse

Spousal abuse or domestic violence is a health care problem that affects victims, perpetrators, and the children who are observers or co-victims of abuse. Estimates suggest that about 30% of all women have been abused at some time by their male partners (Sampselle, 1991). Battering is the single most common cause of injury to women (Moss, 1991). A federal survey (Bachman, 1994) reported that women experience more than 10 times as many incidents of violence by an intimate partner as compared to men. The survey also indicated that women were more likely to suffer serious injury when abused by an intimate partner than when victimized by a stranger. Further, they were less likely to report being victimized by an intimate partner than by a stranger.

Despite these alarming statistics, a comparison of domestic violence rates measured in 1976 and 1985 (Gelles and Straus, 1988) reveal that violence against women and the rate of severe violence men committed against women *decreased* during that time period; and the rate of violence against men *increased* by a significant amount. The researchers point out that while women subjects reported committing a greater number of violent acts, the nature of the violence inflicted by women was less severe than that inflicted by men. Studies of domestic violence show that relationships of gay and lesbian couples also may be characterized by abuse (Fishwick, 1995). These relationships have not been studied extensively.

A special case of violence by intimate partners directed toward women occurs during pregnancy. Studies vary from 3% to 8% in the reported percentage of abuse during pregnancy. A recent large study of clients attending prenatal clinics found that one in six pregnant women experienced physical abuse (Parker, McFarlane, Soeken, Torres, and Campbell, 1993). Nurse researchers noted that, of those who suffered abuse, more teenagers (21.7%) experienced physical or sexual abuse during pregnancy than adults (15.9%).

Elderly Abuse

It is estimated that between 1 to 2 million elderly may suffer some form of abuse, neglect, or exploitation each year. Yet few incidents are actually reported to the authorities (Lachs and Pillener, 1995). One study indicated that 4% of all clients over age 65 who were treated in an emergency department showed signs and symptoms of abuse (Fulmer, McMahon, Baer-Hines, and Forget, 1992). Two trends may significantly affect elderly abuse. The first is the increasing life span. By the year 2000 there will be 30.6 million persons over the age of 65; this number of elderly persons will double by 2020 (Criner, 1994). Elderly persons have an increased risk of chronic illness and debilitation, depletion of financial resources, and dependence on aging children or grandchildren. Currently about 20% of elderly persons are dependent on family members for care, and only 5% live in institutions (All, 1994). The second trend is the decline in the birth rate of the population available to care for very old elderly persons. Also society's resources are becoming increasingly strained as the number of dependent elderly, especially those over age 85, continues to grow. With the projected decrease in government-sponsored entitlement programs such as Social Security and Medicare, elderly persons in the 21st Century will be at risk even more. Younger generations will be left struggling to support the infirm elderly. The economic and social pressures brought to bear on the smaller size families may increase the risk of stressful living conditions, substance abuse, and family violence (Gelles, 1993).

THEORETICAL FRAMEWORK

A variety of concepts and theories have been proposed to explain abuse, neglect, and exploitation. No one of these theories adequately explains the victimization phenomenon, but each contributes to an understanding of its possible origins and perpetuation.

Popular Conceptions of Victims and Violence

The concept of victimology helps to explain the universal blaming and rejection of victims. There appears to be resistance to believing the innocence of victims. Persons feel helpless and vulnerable when exposed to senseless violence and need to find rational explanations for the incident (Moss, 1991). Blaming the victim helps by providing a reason for why the victim was attacked. For example, "she should have known better than to go out alone at night dressed like that. . . ." Persons also have an irrational fear of contamination by the victim. Rejecting the victim becomes a self-protective maneuver. For example, "If I become friends with her, everyone will think they can take advantage of me, too."

Another popular explanation for abuse is the "cycle of violence" (Walker, 1984). In family life, tensions build up, the perpetrator explodes, the perpetrator then "makes up" with the victim, who seems to ignore the consequences of the violent behavior in order to avoid further conflict. At the next stage, the unresolved conflict and angry feelings go underground, and tensions begin to build up again. This cycle is repeated and the violence escalates with each repetition. The repercussions of the cycle are that violence is afflicted on other family members who then become predisposed to commit violent acts themselves as adult survivors of abuse.

Theories substantiated by research that provide guidance in the application of the nursing process include biological, interpersonal, family, and social perspectives of the dynamics of domestic and family violence. Theories about the occurrence of abuse and neglect of clients in institutions are also discussed.

Biological Perspectives

The last decade of research on the brain has increased the knowledge about the neurological basis for aggression, violent behavior, and response to repeated traumatic abuse. The fight-or-flight response is an adaptive mechanism for survival. However, over time it loses its effectiveness when it is invoked too often or for too long, such as happens with families trapped in a cycle of violence.

Aggression is mediated by the limbic system, the frontal lobe, and the temporal lobe, where the release of neurotransmitters aggravate or inhibit aggressive behavior (Harper-Jaques and Reimer, 1992). A surplus or deficit of the neurotransmitters, namely acetylcholine, dopamine, serotonin, and gamma-aminobutyric acid, singly or in combination, affects the cognitive, emotional, and motor processes of the brain. Alterations in the functioning of the brain structures or the biochemical communication links between the cognitive and emotional centers can result in inaccurate perceptions of stimuli, faulty storage or retrieval of memories, and misinterpretations of information. For individuals in a stressful interaction, these neurological alterations may be manifested as either an aggressive or submissive response, depending on the meaning attributed to the context of the situation. Over time the potentially useful fight-or-flight reaction to trauma becomes ineffective, as the arousal threshold set point becomes lower. This leaves individuals in a state of hyperarousal and more vulnerable to subsequent stress (Mackey, Sereika, Weissfeld, Hacker, Zender, and Heard, 1992).

Impairments from schizophrenia, Alzheimer's disease, head injury, vitamin deficiencies, and temporal lobe epilepsy may also contribute to sudden acts of aggression (Torrey, 1994). Even less serious cognitive impairments may play a role in the violent behavior of some undiagnosed individuals. It is not known to what extent some perpetrators of family violence may suffer neurological conditions or similar structural dysfunctions (Harper-Jaques and Reimer, 1992).

Substance abuse, another condition that impacts on neurological functioning, is frequently implicated in all types of family violence (Hayes and Emshoff, 1993). Most researchers agree that chemical dependence is a contributing factor to family violence, lowering individuals' inhibitions that might keep them from acting upon violent or aggressive impulses. It is not clear to what extent substance abuse causes violence, results from violence, or is used as an excuse for violence in the family. However, many studies show that the perpetrator was an alcoholic or was drinking at the time of the victimization.

Studies of memory and its relation to traumatic experiences are fertile areas of research (see Chapter 25). Victimization involves traumatic events as stressors that overwhelm the body's systems for managing stimuli associated with abuse. Various memory and learning patterns develop after experiencing abuse, which lead to reenacting the trauma, repeating the trauma as either victim or perpetrator, or displacing the aggression associated with the trauma (Burgess, Hartman, and Clements, 1995). Trauma is also hypothesized to alter structural development of the cortex in both hemispheres of the brain, making new behaviors difficult to learn.

Another phenomenon associated with brain function is "numbing." In the midst of an abusive situation, as the level of arousal increases, the victim becomes immobilized as endorphins flood the brain to bring relief from the inflicted pain. In the numb state, the victim then disconnects (dissociates) the thoughts and feelings that are engendered by the perpetrator's abusive actions. However, even after the event is over, the victim's activating system may fluctuate between hyperarousal and numbing, rather than returning to the baseline. This prolonged activation causes cellular changes in the central nervous system, leading to dysfunction and maladaptive growth and development (Burgess, Hartman, and Clements, 1995).

Other disruptions to biological systems include the sleep-wake and rest-activity cycles in victims of abuse. It is hypothesized that trauma affects the circadian rhythms that affect sleep-wake and rest-activity patterns (Glod, 1992). Two natural pacemakers, the X oscillator and the Y oscillator, are believed to regulate REM (rapid eye movement) sleep and activity. When these internal rhythmic regulators are disrupted by traumatic events, they become "out of sync." This results in clinical conditions in which sleep disorders figure prominently, such as PTSD, depression, and anxiety, or in maladaptive activity such as delinquency, impulsivity, and substance abuse. The impact of trauma on the brain and other biological systems is only beginning to be understood.

Interpersonal Perspectives

At the heart of many theories about the psychobiology of victimization is the concept of power. In this context, *power* refers to the interpersonal dynamic in which one person influences, controls, or coerces another through physical force or threat to change the victim's behavior. Common elements in all abusive, neglectful, and exploitive situations are the perpetrator's exercise of power to control, coerce, seduce, trick, deprive, or use the victim to satisfy needs (or for financial gain) and the victim's sense of powerlessness (Gelles and Straus, 1988). Powerlessness may be a physical and developmental reality, or it may be based on the victim's belief that actions will have no effect on the perpetrator, the victimizing circumstance, or its outcome. Important principles of power that relate to victimization and its prevention and resolution include the following:

- Power may be real or attributed.
- Power may be exerted without action.
- Power exists to the extent that it is accepted.

The powerlessness experienced by victims often involves their inabilities to recognize the following:

- The legitimacy of their self-interest and their right to protect themselves from harm
- The legitimacy of their perceptions, feelings, and preferences
- Their ownership of their bodies and their right to allow or disallow others to touch them

- Their right to make age-appropriate choices and decisions free from undue influence
- The legitimacy of their expectations for support, nurture, respect, and empathetic treatment by other family members or caretakers
- Their own strengths and value
- That adults and persons in authority are not entitled to violate their rights

There are three types of power relevant to abusive, neglectful, and exploitive situations: personal, positional, and coercive. *Personal power* is embedded in the victim-perpetrator relationship. The perpetrator's personal power is derived from the victim's admiration, respect, love, loyalty, or commitment to the relationship and the perpetrator's predisposition to take advantage of the victim's feelings and values for personal ends. *Positional power* is derived from the perpetrator's higher social status or age in relation to the victim and the victim's recognition and acceptance of this power differential. *Coercive power* is based on fear and is derived from the perpetrator's ability to reward or punish the victim.

A dimension of the perpetrator's use of personal and positional power is the perceived or real imbalance between the perpetrator's and the victim's knowledge and competence. This perceived or real imbalance is used as a source of power. Victims are especially susceptible to trickery when they believe incorrectly that such a knowledge imbalance exists and that they are disadvantaged. Their incapacity to correctly assess their own strengths and weaknesses and those of the perpetrator puts them at great risk for abuse.

Perpetrators who use either personal or positional power often do so in conjunction with power derived from coercion. They use rewards of attention, love, money, or caretaking. They inflict punishments such as withdrawal of rewards or deprivation of resources needed to meet needs, humiliation or shame, and physical or psychological pain or harm. Victims of sexual abuse may be coerced through the use of manipulation or threats that they or their loved ones will be physically harmed or killed if they resist or if they report the incident. Coercive power requires the perpetrator to have the capacity to use physical force or higher status to compel the victim's compliance, or it requires the victim's belief that the abuser can inflict the punishment or withhold the reward.

The Stockholm syndrome is another manifestation of the power dynamic that has similar features to domestic violence. This syndrome is characterized by a paradoxical psychological response between hostage victims and their captors (Moss, 1991). The behavior pattern of the captor includes terrorizing actions followed by varying degrees of kindness. The victimized hostages' behavior pattern is characterized by the development of a fondness for their captors. These victims become apathetic about escaping from the abusive situation. They are also apathetic toward those who plot escape from their abusers and those who attempt to rescue them, even in life-threatening situations. They appear immobilized by their situation: a cycle of abuse followed by token kindness. A similar captor-hostage relationship pattern has been identified in domestic violence between spouses, cohabitating adults, parents and children, and adult offspring and their elderly parents. The one who exhibits abusive behavior enacts the captor role, while the victim of the abuse enacts the hostage behavior (Moss, 1991).

Family Perspectives

Family abuse and neglect may become intergenerational problems. Research suggests that about 30% of abused children grow up to become abusive adults (Gelles, 1993). The use of violence and scapegoating to manage distressing feelings and resolve conflicts is learned and transmitted from one generation to the next. When abuse and neglect are family patterns, the situation will probably persist into future generations unless there are interventions that alter the pattern (Robinson, Wright, and Watson, 1994).

Violation of personal boundaries is a major factor in abuse among family members. Impaired boundary management is reflected in a lack of respect for individual members' integrity, right to safety, privacy, and ownership of their bodies, feelings, thoughts, and personal space. Physical, psychological, and sexual abuse are tolerated as accepted violations of the victim's person and personal space in these families.

Physical, psychological, and sexual abuse occur in both highly structured and disorganized and chaotic families. In the highly structured family, control of members is exerted by the perpetrator, and there may be little involvement between the family members and persons outside the home. Young victims tend to view the physical abuse as deserved discipline. Sometimes, sexual abuse is rationalized by the male perpetrator as his right to procreate and satisfy needs (Gelles and Straus, 1988).

Often the abusive and neglectful family is disorganized and chaotic. This type of family is characterized as having no respect for personal boundaries, little or no predictability in the home environment for meeting needs, inappropriate control and ventilation of feelings and emotions, impulsive and manipulative exchanges with members, and a tendency to escalate conflict situations. In these families, parents may exert little or no control, and older siblings may victimize the younger children. Violent destructive incidents may be related to alcohol or drug abuse. Usually a pattern of violence and abuse is established and continues until either the victim or perpetrator leaves home or is killed (Blau, Dall, and Anderson, 1993).

The defensive coping style of abusive parents tends to include triangling, projection, displacement, passive-aggressive behavior, and denial. When projection or scapegoating occurs, one or all of the children in a family may become the recipients of physical abuse. In this instance the family maintains its dynamic equilibrium by focusing and projecting the negative and difficult aspects of living on the scapegoated victim (see Chapter 12). Family factors that increase the risk of parental abuse include an adolescent pregnancy, an unwanted pregnancy, a child with a birth defect or mental retardation, a single parent with an inadequate support system, serious mental illness in a parent or spouse, poverty, substance abuse, and social stressors such as unemployment and geographical mobility that prevent the development of meaningful and supportive friendships within the community (Gelles and Straus, 1988).

Abuse of elderly persons may occur when their adult children have failed to resolve the stage of adolescent rebellion toward their parents. Consequently old conflicts reemerge when the adult child is responsible for the care of the dependent elderly parent. In some instances the adult child is retaliating for a time when the elderly parent was the abuser and the adult child was the victim (All, 1994). There are also situations in which the adult child caretaker's abuse is symptomatic of a mental illness or substance abuse disorder (Boudreau, 1993). The physical and emotional demands and the role reversal with the elderly parent generate stress and frustration and compound the caretaker's family life-cycle stress.

Elderly persons who must care for their incapacitated spouses also experience physical and emotional burdens. Nursing research suggests that the level of stress experienced by husbands and wives who are the primary providers of care to their infirm spouses is related to several factors: the amount of assistance needed by the client-spouse in the performance of activities of daily living (ADLs), the negative behavior exhibited by the client-spouse, the hours required to give the care, and the tangible and affective support available from others in providing care (Criner, 1994). High levels of stress, the absence of support, and the dependence of the infirm spouse have potential for overwhelming the provider-spouse, contributing to abuse and neglect of the client-spouse.

Social Perspectives

Family and domestic violence is an outcome of social forces that promote a culture that glorifies violence, institutionalizes oppression, and devalues certain members of society such as women, gays and lesbians, elderly, and persons with disabilities (Hiday, 1995). America is the most violent country of the developed nations. There are more than 12,500 murder victims in the United States each year, compared with less than 100 in Great Britain and even fewer in other European countries with similar cultural roots. Firearm accidents, criminal assaults, and deliberate attempts at vengeance or self-protection (particularly in the case of family violence) take a very high toll. The media play a big role in promoting violence through the "heroes" portrayed on television and the movie screen. This is a particular concern in the case of television shows aimed at children. Research consistently finds that watching violence—at home, on television, or in the movies—desensitizes children and adolescents to violence and stimulates aggressive behavior (Gelles, 1993; Singer et al., 1995).

Feminists and others have given voice to the persistent and deliberate oppression of women, children, and other minorities perpetrated by a male-dominated society (Campbell, 1992; Sampselle, 1991). When the basic inequality of any social group is legitimized, a fundamental imbalance permeates society and leads to the misuse and abuse of power. This sets the stage for personal, interpersonal, and family dynamics of abuse. Social norms and cultural beliefs that endorse power, dominance, and many of the so-called "traditional family values," such as the father is the head of the household, help to reinforce the idea that family violence and abuse are acceptable ways to behave toward family members and to resolve family conflicts, or at least that they must be tolerated as necessary evils.

Other social forces that have a direct impact on family violence are poverty, unemployment, racial discrimination, overcrowding, homelessness, environmental pollution, geographical mobility, social isolation, and disintegration of community. These conditions increase stress and decrease supports and resources for families, which make them more vulnerable to conflict and violence.

Institutional Perspectives

Children or those who have a serious illness or disability requiring institutionalization are especially vulnerable to the interpersonal and sociocultural forces of violence and abuse. Emotional linking, an important factor in caregiver abuse, is the development of a close relationship between caregivers and clients in long-term settings. These relationships involve characteristic emotional ties that can generate strong feelings. The closeness of the caregivers and clients in the relationship, the dependence of the clients, and the inadequacy of emotional support for the caregivers in both the work setting and the home situation all heighten the negative or inappropriate feelings of caregivers toward their clients. The caregivers may single out the clients they abuse and neglect for reasons unique to the relationship (Powers, Mooney, and Nunno, 1990; Weiler and Buckwalter, 1992). Their unresolved conflicts may be revived and reenacted with their clients.

Those who abuse and neglect their clients tend to be immature, impulsive, aggressive, and dissatisfied with their jobs or status in society and have inadequate coping resources. The abuser's inadequate coping mechanisms and limited impulse control increase the risk of abusive outbursts. The demands made by the active child, the confused incontinent person, or the hostile client tax their ability to provide empathetic care. The mismanagement of stress in their personal lives also contributes to their frustration. Abusive caregivers focus their anger and frustration on the vulnerable client, who then becomes the victim. Other factors that increase the risk of neglect and abuse in long-term care facilities include understaffing, changes in working conditions that generate caretakers' dissatisfaction, a lack of opportunities for staff to advance or increase their earnings, and the absence of a sense of accomplishment when clients make no progress or deteriorate (Morrison, 1994).

Some abusive caregivers experienced extreme physical discipline and neglect as children; therefore they are likely to view physical punishment as normal behavior. Caregivers who are unable to turn to others for support when they are distressed are likely to vent their frustration on vulnerable clients or abuse drugs and alcohol, which decreases their impulse control and increases the risk of both abusive and neglectful behaviors (Powers, Mooney, and Nunno, 1990). Patterns of abuse of those who are institutionalized are preventable when nurses act as advocates for their clients and take steps to ensure their own healthy work and personal lifestyles.

CLINICAL ISSUES: CONSPIRACY OF SILENCE

While the media expose sensational stories of family violence, such as the O.J. Simpson case, the daily suffering of countless "average" families in the privacy of their homes often goes unrecognized. A conspiracy of silence, imposed by cultural traditions and social stigma, keeps the full impact of this human tragedy from the public's awareness and prevents sustained action from being taken by the health care community.

Victims tend to feel isolated and different from others and perceive themselves to be at fault for the abuse. Therefore they have difficulty initiating discussion about their predicament. Factors that inhibit disclosure and reinforce their continued silence include shame, embarrassment, humiliation, self-blame, feeling responsible for the problems in the family, and past experiences when they tried to disclose abuse and were cut off, ignored, or accused of lying (Campbell, et al., 1994). Some victims are too young and cannot describe their victimization. Others may fear retribution if they reveal the person who abused them. Conversely, victims may worry about what will happen to the perpetrator if the law is strictly enforced or the perpetrator is removed from the household (Fishwick, 1995; Hoff, 1990).

Victims also fear that no one will believe them. Tragically this fear is often realized, particularly for the victims who accuse a family member or a respected member of the community of sexual abuse. In many instances the credibility of child victims is questioned. Relatives and health care providers often cannot accept that parents, spouses, caretakers, and important members of the community have been perpetrators of violence and abuse. This lack of validation and empathy by caregivers is more trauma for victims (Briggs, 1992; Campbell, 1994; Doob, 1992).

The Nursing Process

Assessment
Definition of Abuse

Abuse is the maltreatment of a person. The maltreatment or serious threat of harm, inflicted by the perpetrator, is intentional and can be distinguished from the victim's other social, economic, and health problems. To determine whether abuse has occurred, a knowledge of different ethnocultural patterns of behavior and relationships is necessary (Asbury, 1993; D'Antonio, Darwish and McLean, 1993). The Cultural Highlights on p. 785, present an example of how family violence is viewed according to Chinese culture.

Abusive actions represent a violation of legal codes that prohibit criminal behavior such as assault, battery, and rape. Health care professionals and others are mandated to report reasonable suspicions of child, elderly, and dependent-adult maltreatment in all 50 states. Those who make such reports have immunity from any prosecution (Brasseur, 1995; Weiler and Buckwalter, 1992).

The types of violence and abuse experienced by victims and inflicted by perpetrators include physical and psychological abuse, physical and psychological neglect, sexual abuse, and exploitation.

Clinical Profiles

Physical abuse and neglect

Physical abuse involves deliberate aggressive actions that inflict pain and/or nonaccidental injury that may cause temporary or permanent disfigurement or death. The perpetrator causes deliberate and intentional physical injury to or impairment of body parts, organs, or functions through the use of hands, feet, or objects (Sheridan, 1993). Definitions of physically abusive acts vary according to gender, beliefs, experience, and social context (Harper-Jaques and Reimer, 1992). Experts in the field contend that even mild forms of physical discipline, such as slapping, pushing, or spanking, should be considered abusive, because these acts would be illegal if directed toward adults or strangers (Burgess, Hartman, and Kelley, 1990; Gelles and Straus, 1988).

The clinical profile of victims of physical abuse includes evidence of traumatic injuries that are inconsistent with the descriptions of how the injuries occurred and descriptions that are vague, contradictory, or bizarre (Bourne, Chadwick, Kanda, and Ricci, 1993; Sheridan, 1993). Examples of physical abuse and the clinical evidence suggestive of traumatic physical abuse are presented in Box 36-1.

Physical neglect is the deprivation, nonprovision, or withholding of the basic necessities of life and societally available resources. The perpetrator of physical neglect deliberately withholds food, water, rest, clothing, shelter, or medications or refuses to provide a sufficient level of resources compared with what is provided to others in a similar socioeconomic situation. The consequences of this deprivation include impairment of physical and psychosocial development and functioning (All, 1994).

The clinical profile of victims of physical neglect reflects unmet physiological, safety, love, affiliative, and self-esteem needs. The behavioral characteristics and symptoms of physical neglect vary with the person's stage of development and ability to provide self-care.

Psychological abuse and neglect

Psychological abuse is the deliberate and willful destruction or significant impairment of a person's sense of competence and self-worth. This type of abusive behavior is less visible and more insidious than physical assault, but it is very devastating to the victim (Fishwick, 1995). The perpetrator inflicts psychological abuse through behaviors that instill fear, increase dependency, and damage self-esteem (Murphy and Cascardi, 1993). Verbal and nonverbal communication and the deliberate withholding of quality interactions (e.g., giving

Assessment

Traditionally men are the center of most Chinese families, assuming responsibility for the whole family. A marriage does not signify the creation of a new family; it is the continuation of the man's family line (Shon and Ja, 1982). Under this patriarchal system the status of the wife is lower than that of her husband, of her husband's parents, and of her husband's older siblings (Shon and Ja, 1982). The Chinese culture educates women to obey and respect their fathers when they are children, their husbands when wives, and their oldest sons when widows. When a Chinese man does not perceive obedience and respect from his children and wife, he may feel he is not fulfilling the traditional requirements of the husband and father role. This causes conflict within the family. He may displace his feelings of frustration and anger onto his children or his wife, inflicting physical and psychological abuse.

Wife battering is more likely to occur in Chinese families with less education, lower occupational status, and less income. Arguments over children, pregnancy, money, questions about the wife's fidelity, sexual problems, husband's alcohol use, and whether or not the wife will work outside the home have been identified as catalysts for specific violent episodes. When wives are hit, they are reluctant to tell persons outside their families because of a strong sense of shame for the family (Asbury, 1993).

Most Chinese parents love their children dearly. They expect to have total authority of their children, considering it their right and duty to scold or "spike" (hit) their children. They consider "spiking" an effective way to educate children as they grow and mature. Their disciplinary action is not expected to cause great physical harm. Spiking, however, may be considered physical abuse by Western standards, but it is not abusive by Chinese standards.

Sexual abuse is not reported because of shame and the stigma attached. Child sexual abuse within a family is unethical in the Chinese eyes. When incest does occur, the family experiences extreme guilt. Once they are exposed, not only the perpetrator but also the victim are regarded as guilty and dirty.

Elderly abuse is not common among Chinese; most children respect their parents very much and think that it is their responsibility to support their parents. Usually the parents hold the highest position within a family (Shon and Ja, 1982).

Today the status of Chinese women has improved, with more women getting an education and being more economically independent from their husbands. But the traditional viewpoints are still deeply rooted, especially in less-educated families and those who come from less-developed areas. In these families, women rarely realize that they have the right to seek legal protection, even when they are suffering in their marriage. Chinese society discourages divorce. So many women try to keep the family as a union, because they think divorce is very harmful to their children and brings great shame on the family (Shon and Ja, 1982).

Diagnosis

The symptoms of abuse in Chinese families are similar to those experienced by Western families (Asbury, 1993). However, many Chinese do not label abuse or neglect as family problems. Those who realize there is a problem feel too much shame to speak of the problem to an outsider or health care provider. It would mean that the father, mother, or both have failed the family. Therefore problems of family violence are not reported when clients seek health care.

The typical Chinese client rarely verbalizes feelings or psychological problems (Spector, 1991). The only indication that there may be a problem is subtle behavioral cues such as an untouched food tray or prolonged silence. Insomnia, inability to concentrate, sadness, unexplained physical trauma, and difficult family living conditions are helpful cues of abuse of family members. The victim's relatives may be valuable information sources, if they speak English. The Chinese language with its many dialects may be a major barrier during the assessment process (Asbury, 1993).

Typically child abuse in Chinese families is physical abuse. Child abuse may be easy to detect, because many Chinese parents speak freely about punishing their children not realizing that what they are doing is considered abuse by health care providers.

Intervention

Careful observations and sensitive questions to detect family violence can help the nurse to make a diagnosis and treatment plan. Because Chinese have different points of view about family violence, it is difficult for them to accept the diagnosis of abuse. The nurse must question the parents about their beliefs and actions with sensitivity to avoid offending them or causing them to lose face or feel shame. Special attention should be paid to the intent and context of the parents' behavior. Client explanations are needed, emphasizing respect for women's and children's rights and their autonomy as human beings but showing respect for the traditional parental roles. Education about expectations for children's behavior based on normal growth and development and effective parenting skills should be provided.

Mandatory interventions may be needed to stop wife battering and child abuse. Education emphasizing respect for one another should precede any attempt to remove the victims from the household unless lives are in jeopardy. Nurses can involve members of social associations from the Chinese community to protect victims' safety.

The Nursing Process

Box 36-1

Behaviors and Clinical Evidence of Physical Abuse

PHYSICAL ABUSE BEHAVIORS	CLINICAL EVIDENCE OF PHYSICAL ABUSE
• Slapping, kicking, or punching • Striking with an object • Shaking the victim violently • Inflicting blows that traumatize the head, face, abdomen, genitals, or limbs • Inflicting wounds with sharp instruments such as razors or knives • Whipping with belts, ropes, or electrical cords • Dislocating arms, shoulders, or legs • Fracturing limbs, ribs, or skull • Pulling hair out at the roots • Inflicting burns with lighted cigarettes, chemicals, or appliances such as a stove, iron, or curling iron • Immersing in scalding water • Throwing victim to the floor, down stairs, against furniture, or out of a window • Tying the victim to a bed, crib, or chair using cords, ropes, or chains • Locking the victim in a dark closet, cellar, or small bare room for extended periods • Attempting to drown or hang victim • Administering an excessive dose of prescribed medications	• Bruises around eyes or in the form of a hand on the face or body at various stages of resolution; thumb and finger marks on neck; striped bruises or lacerations on back, buttocks, chest, legs, or arms; rectangular, linear, or round bruises on body • Burns at various stages of resolution, particularly those inflicted by a cigarette, curling iron, or iron • Scalding water burns of hands, feet, buttocks, or perineum; chemical burns on face or throat • Fractured jaw, split lip, or chipped, loose, or missing teeth • Lacerated ears, nose, or throat; bite marks • Torsion fractures of the extremities or dislocated shoulder in child victim • History of multiple, old, treated and untreated injuries (scars or healed fractures) • Injuries on body parts that are usually covered by clothing • Long delay between injury and time treatment is sought • Seemingly accident-prone victim • Sedation from overmedication • Denial of obvious injury

the "silent treatment") are the major mechanisms of psychological abuse. Abusers use words and gestures that ridicule, harass, degrade, and humiliate their victims. They may say or behave in ways that deprecate victims' self-worth by convincing them that they—the victims—are stupid, crazy, bad, unwanted, or unlovable. They may act in a jealous manner or prevent victims from engaging in social interactions with family and friends. They may threaten harm to self or others or destroy victims' personal possessions. They may also distort victims' view of reality and ability to accurately perceive self, others, and situations. This type of abuse has a negative impact on victims' overall psychosocial development and ability to perform ADLs and maintain needed social relationships.

Psychological neglect is characterized by psychosocial unavailability and a cold, unfeeling style of relating. The perpetrator of psychological neglect exhibits a lack of warmth, empathy, sensitive personalized attention, and sociability toward the victim. As a caretaker or intimate partner, the perpetrator may intentionally fail to recognize the victim's dependence needs, respond to the victim's physical or developmental limitations, or acknowledge the victim's verbal and nonver-

bal expressions of need, desire, and distress (Hoff, 1990; Weiler and Buckwalter, 1992).

The victim's phobic fears of nonthreatening objects, persons, places, or situations may also suggest psychological abuse or neglect (Glod, 1993).

Sexual abuse

Sexual abuse occurs when the perpetrator uses the victim to satisfy needs for power, control, or sexual gratification, and the victim does not consent to this sexual activity or is incapable of resisting when it occurs. This type of abuse involves sexual contact that is coercive, developmentally inappropriate, and/or a violation of the victim's basic right to privacy. Sexual abuse is often accompanied by physical and psychological abuse (Glod, 1993; Kelley, 1995).

Abusive sexual contact can be categorized as intrafamilial or extrafamilial abuse. *Intrafamilial sexual abuse refers to acts of molestation or rape against the victim by someone who is a relative.* *Extrafamilial sexual abuse refers to acts of molestion or rape against the victim by someone who is an unrelated adult authority figure or a person who is known to the victim.*

The Nursing Process

Intrafamilial victims are members of the nuclear or extended family. *Sexual abuse is labeled* **incest** *when the perpetrator and the victim are close blood relatives* (e.g., father and daughter). Incest violates the ancient social taboo against sexual relations among family members. Victims of incest experience both short-term and long-term psychological effects. Research suggests the younger the victim, the more profound the effects of incest (Conte, 1993). Adult survivors of childhood incest constitute a significant group of clients who seek treatment for various psychological and physical problems (Doob, 1992; Glod, 1993).

Extrafamilial sexual abuse occurs when an unrelated adult authority figure, or powerful person who is known to the victim, engages in sexual acts with a child or adult who is incapable of consenting to or resisting the activity. The perpetrators may be employers, teachers, clergy, sports coaches, child care providers, or long-term caregivers. The victims of extrafamilial sexual abuse include children in day care facilities, schools, camps, and youth groups, and both adults and children who are institutionalized (Kelley, 1990).

Sexual harassment is another form of extrafamilial sexual abuse. Sexual harassment is abusive behavior in which a person, often in an authority position, makes unwanted sexual advances and physical contact, requests sexual favors, and behaves in other sexually explicit and implicit verbal and nonverbal ways that are offensive to the victim. The purpose of sexual harassment is to intimidate the victim or to create a hostile environment, usually in the workplace—a business office, hospital unit, factory, or academic setting (Kaye, Donald, and Merker, 1994). Workers may fear losing their jobs or being denied a promotion, so they tolerate the harasser's abusive behavior as in the following example:

> At the annual holiday party in a community health center, a male physician gave a female nurse a piece of sexy lingerie as a "grab-bag gift." The nurse was very embarrassed when she opened the "gift" in the presence of the other providers on the unit, especially because she was the only one who received such a personal, intimate item. She felt she could not confront the physician, who was also the director of the center, about his offensive gift without jeopardizing her job. When she investigated this incident further with her supervisor, she discovered that the physician had a pattern of this type of behavior with other young women who worked on the unit. His behavior could be construed as sexual harassment.

Laws against sexual harassment give victims the means to address this problem through legal action.

It is important to note that research suggests only a small proportion of child victims have genital findings or sexually transmitted diseases (STDs) (Frasier, Barchman, and Alexander, 1992). Therefore detection of sexual abuse may depend on evaluation by a special multidisciplinary team.

Exploitation

Exploitation *is the use of the victim for selfish purposes and/or financial profit.* The elderly are particularly vulnerable to exploitation (All, 1994; Fulmer, McMahon, Baer-Hines, and Forget, 1992). This type of victimization most commonly involves the use of coercion, deception, and/or fraud to gain access to the victim's money and property. The perpetrator violates the victim's personal rights to self-determination and freedom of choice. Family caregivers and members who are financially dependent on an elderly member may exploit the elderly person's vulnerability for personal gain. Examples of exploitation and clinical evidence suggestive of this type of victimization are presented in Box 36-2.

Undocumented immigrants are another prime target for exploitation by employers and those seeking to take advantage of the immigrants' vulnerability to deportation (Aroian, 1993). Children and adolescents, both boys and girls, may also be exploited through their involvement in child pornography, prostitution, and trafficking for sexual purposes (Drake, 1994; Sherman 1992). The advent of child pornography on the Internet and anonymous solicitations for sexual activity with children and adolescents by E-mail and electronic bulletin boards pose significant threats that sexual exploitation will become even more widespread. Children unknowingly provide sexual services, which may be photographed or videotaped, out of fear or in exchange for money or love and attention (Burgess, Hartman, and Kelley, 1990). They may also be kidnapped, chained, drugged, beaten, seduced, knifed, and threatened (Finkelhor and Korbin, 1988).

Assessment of the Victim

Nurses are often in an ideal position to make assessments of abuse and to influence change in the family system. The care of the victims of violence requires that nurses remain empathetic and objective. Awareness of legal obligations and the rights of victims is essential.

The nurse must take into account that the assessment of victims of abuse, neglect, and exploitation is often hampered by factors that interfere with victims' abilities to disclose their situations. Young children and institu-

The Nursing Process

Box 36-2

Behaviors and Clinical Evidence of Exploitation

EXPLOITIVE BEHAVIORS

- Coercively or manipulatively influencing a will change, naming perpetrator as beneficiary
- Coercively or manipulatively gaining control of real estate, bank accounts, stocks, or bonds
- Forcing a marriage or divorce that provides perpetrator with access to money or property
- Using children or adults, who cannot or do not give consent, for production of pornography, sexual gratification, or prostitution
- Employing immigrant workers for very low wages, imposing "sweat shop" labor conditions

CLINICAL EVIDENCE OF EXPLOITATION

- Pays exorbitant fees for goods and services provided by family members, caretakers, friends, or employers
- Transfers large sums of money, property, or stocks to caretakers, lawyers, bankers, or a friend on whom victim depends for performance of ADLs
- Adds names of persons victim depends on for performance of ADLs to bank accounts, deeds, stock portfolios, or wills
- Experiences recent loss of large sums of money
- Does not receive own mail, which is sent to someone else's address
- Does not participate in decision to move in with adult children, or decision is a function of physical or mental incapacity
- Is mentally competent but family member, lawyer, or friend seeks power of attorney
- Is mentally competent but is excluded from decisions about own health, welfare, and lifestyle, or options are misrepresented
- Works excessively long hours for very low wages

Box 36-3

Beliefs of Victims

- I have caused or contributed to the abuse and consequently feel total or partial responsibility, shame, and guilt.
- If I were more compliant, made fewer mistakes, and tried to please [the perpetrator], the abuse would stop.
- I am "bad" and deserve the abuse.
- If I tell anyone about the abuse/neglect/exploitation, I would be disloyal toward my family. I might lose my family.
- If I tell anyone about the abuse/neglect/exploitation, it would be humiliating to me and my family.
- I can't tell, because no one would believe me.
- There is no one who could or would help me. I am helpless, hopeless, powerless, and worthless.
- If I tell, there will be retaliation that might be worse than what I am experiencing [may be reality-based fear].

ical examination. Asking direct questions about abuse within the context of a comprehensive history is recommended for all clients, whatever the setting. However, nurses should ask about abuse *before* conducting the examination so that they can be especially sensitive to the client's response to touch and invasive procedures, if necessary (Furniss, 1993). The questions should be framed with regard for developmental appropriateness and cultural sensitivity to the client. Sometimes the victim may try to tell a plausible story about the injuries. If the nurse accepts these descriptions at face value, the abuse may not be identified or treated.

The Abuse Assessment Screen developed by the Nursing Research Consortium on Violence and Abuse is a useful tool to identify the client's self-report of physical, psychological, and sexual abuse, particularly in women. Other instruments may be used to collect research and evaluation data or track patterns of abuse and severity over time. Examples include: TRIADS of Abuse Checklist (abuse of children), Conflict Tactics Scale (partner abuse), the Index of Spouse Abuse (includes physical and psychological subscales), and the Danger Assessment Screen (measures the potential risk for homicide).

In addition to asking direct questions, nurses must rely on observations made during the interview and examination. Indirect clues are verbal behaviors such as the client's fearful, evasive, or inconsistent replies and nonverbal behaviors such as the client's flinching when approached or touched. Observation and examination of

tionalized victims may lack the verbal skills or physical capacity to describe the events and circumstances of their victimization. This is particularly true in the case of children who have been sexually abused. Older children, adolescents, and adult victims may be inhibited from disclosing their abuse because of beliefs that influence their perception of their situation. Examples of these beliefs are presented in Box 36-3.

The assessment of clients when abuse is suspected includes a health history, interview, observations, and phys-

The Nursing Process

BOX 36-4

Guidelines for Interviewing Abuse Victims

Explore the circumstances of the injuries or evidence of neglect to elicit detailed descriptions.
- Ask direct questions about abuse and neglect: Tell me about how you got hurt? What else was going on when this happened? Who else was there or saw what happened?
- Use play to allow a young child to describe the physically or sexually abusive event: I am going to give you this doll, and I want you to make believe that the doll gets hurt the same way as you did. Show me how the doll got hurt.

Explore the victim's perceptions and beliefs about being able to prevent the abuse.
- What are your ideas about what you could do to prevent your being hurt by (perpetrator) again?
- Looking back at what happened this time, what do you think you could have said or done to prevent or stop it from happening?
- Have you ever tried to do this in the past? Did it work?
- Why did you think that it might work this time?

Explore whether the abuse is an isolated incident or a long-standing pattern.
- Has anything like this ever happened before?
- Tell me about other times that you have been hurt.
- What kinds of hurts or injuries did you have?
- Which of those times did you go to a hospital?

Examine whether or to what degree the client has lost control of decisions that affect his or her life and property.
- You said your son takes care of your business; tell me more about this.
- Was there a time when you signed papers that gave your son the right to take care of your business?
- If you decided you wanted to live somewhere other than with your son, how could you do this?
- If you wanted to go to a store to buy something such as a new dress, do you have money to do this, or do you have to ask your son for money?

Explore the type and extent of physical neglect by inquiring about how basic needs are met in the current living situation and what factors contribute to the failure to meet these needs.
- Tell me what your home is like.
- Where do you sleep?
- What is it like living in your home?
- If I went to your home and opened the refrigerator door, what would I find?
- If I went to your home and opened a closet door, what would I find?
- If I were cold in your home, what would you do?

Exchange information with other providers involved in the client's care and discuss the evidence of suspected or actual abuse, neglect, or exploitation.

Interview accompanying family members, caretakers, or police for corroboration or resolution of suspicions about whether abuse, neglect, or exploitation has occurred.

Obtain and examine charts of prior admissions for evidence of previous treatment for physical trauma, sexual abuse, or neglect.

Explore the ways persons interact in the current living situation to identify patterns of relating and messages that are demeaning or threatening and how communication contributes to psychological abuse and neglect.
- When your (mom/dad/spouse) talks to you, what kinds of things are said?
- Tell me one thing your (mom/dad/spouse) says a lot to you.
- If you were really happy about something and you walked in the front door of your home, what would you do? Which person would you tell?
- If you were really scared or upset, what would you do? Which person would you tell?

Contact the local registry for abuse cases for reports of previous incidents, because there is a tendency to use different health care agencies for treatment when there is a pattern of abuse.

Use multiple sources of data to identify a pattern of abuse or neglect.

Report suspected abuse to authorities as mandated by law.

behaviors and clinical evidence presented earlier in this chapter contribute to an assessment database and documentation of abuse. In addition, the observation that the client is being cued, silenced, or threatened by an accompanying family member or caretaker provides evidence of abuse. Guidelines for conducting an assessment interview when abuse is suspected is presented in Box 36-4.

The Nursing Process

Assessment of the Perpetrator

The rehabilitation of perpetrators can reduce the likelihood of subsequent victimization. It is therefore important that nurses and other health care professionals encourage and facilitate perpetrators' participation in treatment (Prentky and Burgess, 1990). Intrafamilial abusers include parents, older siblings, and extended family members (biological, adoptive, step, foster), as well as spouses. Extrafamilial abusers include cohabitants, caretakers, friends, neighbors, babysitters, scout leaders, teachers, physicians, and clergy.

There is no single clinical profile for persons who victimize others (Isaac, Cochran, Brown, and Adams, 1994). These persons do, however, tend to have impaired self-esteem; strong, unrealistic dependence needs; immaturity; self-absorption; and a lack of respect and empathy for others. A history of sexual abuse during childhood and greater incidence of psychopathology than would be expected in the general population has been noted in perpetrators of abuse. Some perceive their victims to be their property. Their "ownership" conception of an intimate relationship leads these perpetrators to believe that they are entitled and have the right to use and abuse their victims in whatever way they please. Those who use physical force also employ psychological abuse to control their victims. They manipulate their victims by mixing pleasurable behaviors with abusive ones as necessary to keep their victims emotionally bonded to them (Moss, 1991).

Providing nursing care to perpetrators who have inflicted pain and destruction on their victims is one of the most difficult responsibilities in nursing. The nurse should begin by observing the client-abuser's verbal and nonverbal behavior toward the victim, looking for evidence of hostility or lack of empathy and caring that is incongruent with the client's predicament. Behavior toward staff should be observed for evidence of hostility, avoidance, evasiveness, or defensive or aggressive posturing. Observations of behavior directed toward silencing or controlling the victim's responses to staff questions should also be made. Observations of physical evidence of violent interactions on the abuser—bruises, scratches, disheveled appearance—are also appropriate. The focus of an interview with the client perpetrator is on the client's perception of the victim's predicament, their relationship, current life stressors, as well as helping the client explore feelings related to the victim.

Nursing Diagnosis

In cases of abuse, neglect, and exploitation, the victims and perpetrators may have mental health problems re-

lated to the circumstances of the victimization. The DSM-IV designates diagnoses for problems related to abuse or neglect according to the focus for clinical attention.

The psychiatric diagnoses applied to victims address their response to abuse, neglect, and exploitation and the psychobiological and psychosocial dysfunctions that stem from the victimization.

Nursing Diagnoses Applied to Victims

Nursing diagnoses used with victims of abuse, neglect, and exploitation encompass almost all aspects of personal, family, and social functioning and well-being. Diagnoses are based on assessment data and X-ray and laboratory findings and are influenced by family, social, cultural, and economic factors, as well as genetics and general health.

Victims who have been abused, neglected, or exploited or who have lived with domestic violence exhibit a variety of physical and psychosocial symptoms that have been associated with PTSD (Fishwick, 1995; Glod, 1992, Kelley, 1992). They are at high risk for emotional and behavioral difficulties, low self-esteem, an irrational lack of self-confidence, low academic or work achievement, and social incompetence. They tend to be more isolated than their peers and have fewer peer contacts. Their emotional distress may be manifested by somatic complaints such as chronic headaches, sleep problems, abdominal pain, facial tics, and gastrointestinal irritability. In their relationships with others, some may be unusually eager to please, gain approval, and receive attention. Others act out in negative ways such as lying, stealing, being aggressive, being promiscuous, and abusing alcohol and drugs (Paone, Chavkin, Willets, Friedmann, and Des-Jarlais, 1992). They may even try to provoke abusive behavior from others as a way of replicating a familiar style of relating and meeting some of their needs. The acting-out, substance abuse, school or employment problems and provocative and self-destructive behavior may mask underlying anxiety and depression (Sherman, 1992). Also, STDs, pregnancy, and/or abortions in young girls may suggest sexual abuse. A list of relevant nursing diagnoses for victims is presented in Box 36-5.

Nursing Diagnoses Applied to Perpetrators

Nursing diagnoses used with perpetrators of abuse and violence are related to the client-abuser's control issues, potential for and reality of aggressive behavior, history of abusive experience, and difficulties in communication and getting needs met. For many, because their childhood experiences may be similar to those of the victims

The Nursing Process

BOX 36-5

Nursing Diagnoses for Victims

- Altered nutrition: less than body requirements related to parents' depriving child of adequate food
- Urinary retention related to abusive sexual activity inflicted by older relative
- Risk for trauma related to father's pattern of physically abusing family members when he has been drinking
- Altered protection related to an elder's being kept in restraints for long periods of time
- Impaired social interaction related to husband's limiting spouse's access to family and friends
- Altered parenting related to lack of knowledge about children's normal growth and development
- Sexual dysfunction related to experiences of sexual abuse as a child
- Altered family processes related to incest of daughter by her stepfather
- Parental role conflict related to mother's physical neglect of two preschool children
- Defensive coping related to severe physical abuse of sons by their father
- Ineffective family coping: disabling related to long-standing pattern of physical and psychological abuse by family members
- Decisional conflict related to wife's reluctance to leave abusive husband for fear of retaliation
- Fatigue related to wife's constant belittling of husband in front of children and outsiders
- Sleep pattern disturbance related to fear of physical and sexual abuse
- Altered growth and development related to deprived early childhood
- Self-esteem disturbance related to older brother's bullying behavior
- Powerlessness related to inability of mother to prevent father from severely beating children
- Chronic pain related to repeated episodes of trauma inflicted by spouse
- Post-trauma response related to experience of psychological and sexual abuse by family's clergy
- Rape-trauma syndrome: Silent reaction related to fear of stigma and ostracism by college friends
- Fear related to boyfriend's threat to harm her if girlfriend tells police about his abuse of her
- Hopelessness related to inability to "reform" spouse's abusive behavior and have a loving relationship

Adapted from McFarland, G.K., & McFarlane, E.A. (1993). Nursing diagnosis & intervention: Planning for patient care (2nd ed.). St. Louis: Mosby.

BOX 36-6

Nursing Diagnoses for Perpetrators

- Risk for injury related to potential retaliation by victim
- Impaired verbal communication related to feelings of guilt and shame about abusive behavior
- Social isolation related to inability to trust others
- Altered role performance related to unrealistic expectations of role partner's behavior
- Caregiver role strain related to elderly parent's physical care needs
- Altered sexuality patterns related to desire to dominate and humiliate sexual partner
- Impaired adjustment related to lack of remorse for the consequences of abusive behavior
- Relocation Stress Syndrome related to restraining order prohibiting living at or visiting the family home
- Chronic low self-esteem related to physical and psychological abuse in family of origin
- Altered thought processes related to discontinuing prescribed antipsychotic medication
- Risk for violence: Directed at others related to perceived need to control behavior of others
- Anxiety related to inability to control the behavior of self and others
- Helplessness related to perceived inability to control own aggressiveness

Adapted from McFarland, G.K., & McFarlane, E.A. (1993). Nursing diagnosis & intervention: Planning for patient care (2nd ed.). St. Louis: Mosby.

---

of violence, the resulting psychobiological and psychosocial effects of their traumatic background may be similar to those of the victims'. Therefore they may also suffer from anxiety, depression, PTSD, and so on (Gondolf, 1993; Scheela and Stern, 1994). Examples of nursing diagnoses used with perpetrators who are treated within a psychiatric setting are presented in Box 36-6.

Outcome Identification
Outcomes for Victims

Outcomes of intervention for victims of abuse, neglect, and exploitation need to reflect an end to the victimization, empowerment of the victim, and the initiation of a healing process. Outcomes for children and dependent adults may not be achieved unless the perpetrator is simultaneously involved in and accepting of treatment, or the victim is removed from the perpetrator's care and influence.

The Nursing Process

The following are realistic examples of outcomes for a victim of violence:

- Reports decreased symptoms of anxiety
- Verbalizes that he or she is not responsible for the violent abusive episodes
- Makes a specific plan to increase personal safety
- Requests admission to a shelter or safe house, if necessary
- Explores relationship with own parents and developmental issues that may be related to abuse
- Requests information about services and self-help organizations
- Uses support of family and institutional and community resources in managing the multiple repetitive stressors that have contributed to abusive situations
- Learns conflict-resolution skills and new coping behaviors
- Reports no new episodes of abusive behavior according to the timetable of the plan

Outcomes for Perpetrators

Outcome criteria for intervention with clients who have been perpetrators need to reflect an end to their abusive, neglectful, and exploitive behavior, resolution of the factors that have contributed to their behavior, and initiation of a healing process that involves recognition of the pain and harm they have inflicted. The following are examples of outcomes for a perpetrator:

- Explores the influence of family's violent patterns of interaction on own abusive behavior
- Describes a connection between abusive behavior and an inability to engage in satisfying personal relationships with other adults and use of sexualized relationships to meet love and belonging needs
- Acknowledges responsibility for the consequences of own violent behavior
- Relates newly acquired knowledge about children's growth and development to previously held unrealistic expectations and frustration when children could not perform as expected
- Acknowledges relationship between abusive behavior toward victim and feeling out of control when victim pursued friendships, activities, and employment outside the home
- Uses support of family and institutional and community resources in managing the multiple repetitive stressors that have contributed to abusive and exploitive behavior

- Exhibits appropriate parenting behavior toward children based on newly acquired knowledge about children's growth and development
- Learns conflict-resolution skills and new coping behaviors
- Reports no new episodes of abusive behavior according to the timetable of the plan

Planning

Planning care for victims of family violence involves all that are concerned, including the victim, co-victims (children and others living in the household), and the perpetrator. The nurse should develop a nursing care plan in conjunction with the client-victim that is validating, respectful, and empowering (Campbell, 1992; Fishwick, 1995). The nursing care plan is most effective when it is comprehensive and attentive to the immediate care needs of the client, as well as future prevention measures.

In planning care, the nurse must anticipate the need to document trauma and collect evidence of abuse. Special protocols, techniques, and equipment are necessary to collect and preserve specimens that may be used in future civil or criminal trials (Nathan and Williamson, 1993; Tilden and Shepherd, 1987). Providing adequate privacy and sufficient time to conduct a compassionate interview must also be anticipated. It may be necessary to obtain additional personnel to enhance security for the client as well as professional staff, if the perpetrator gives evidence of aggressive or retaliatory behavior. Administrative personnel or a designated team of specialists may have to be notified of the suspected abuse, as well. The documentation and legal issues, resources and referral for services, and follow-up care must all be considered in the nursing care plan. A nursing care plan for a family in which the mother and child are victims of the father's violent behavior is presented on pp. 793-794.

Implementation
Interventions for Victims

Victims need to explain their abuse to someone who can help them and in some instances protect them from the perpetrator (Sheridan, 1993). Nurses are a potential source of help for victims when they are knowledgeable about the signs and symptoms of abuse, neglect, and exploitation and the factors that contribute to victims' silence. It is crucial for nurses to invest the time and demonstrate the concern and empathy necessary for the development of a therapeutic relationship. When this relationship provides a safe and supportive environment,

The Nursing Process

NURSING CARE PLAN

Family Violence

NURSING ASSESSMENT DATA

Subjective: "I'm so clumsy. I dropped a pot of hot water, and it splashed all over my arms and legs." *Objective:* Hand is red and blistered symmetrically to 2 inches above the wrists; feet and ankles are reddened. Husband refuses to leave the examining cubicle after bringing his wife to the emergency room. *DSM-IV diagnosis:* Physical abuse (focus on adult victim) and physical abuse (focus on adult perpetrator).

NANDA Diagnosis: Altered protection related to husband's attempt to punish his wife for talking too long on the phone by scalding her hands and feet in hot water

Outcomes	Interventions	Rationale	Evaluation
Wife, short term 1. Will describe her experiences of injury and physical abuse *within 1 week.* 2. Will follow prescribed regimen to heal burns *within 1 week.* 3. Will make a plan to increase safety of herself and children *within 2 weeks.* 4. Will verbalize that she is not responsible for husband's loss of control or actions *within 4 weeks.* **Husband, short term** 1. Will support wife's need for health care *within 1 week.* 2. Will examine consequences of his aggressive behavior *within 1 week.* 3. Will explore alternatives to control his temper *within 4 weeks.* **Wife, long term** 1. Will join a self-help group for abused spouses *within 1 month.* 2. Will report decrease in anxiety and fear of	• See Box 36-7. • Elicit from client and family members their patterns of relating and interacting. • Teach client and family about normal development and family stages. • Teach client how to care for burns. • Identify family strengths and adaptive coping mechanisms. • Practice active listening. • Maintain confidentiality to the extent allowed by law. • Develop a safety plan within the context of options to maximize well-being of wife and children. • Give a list of places and persons to contact in the community. • Report potential or actual abuse according to agency protocols and state laws.	• Research-based interventions provide effective standardized care. • The nurse facilitates the client's and family's expression of needs, feelings, preferences, and wishes to reinforce their legitimacy. • Breaking the code of silence enables the nurse to validate the client's suffering and perception of abusive events. • Education about normal growth and development tasks helps to correct unrealistic expectations about behavior. • Care for physical injury is necessary before client can address psychological issues. • Research shows that interpreting client's symptoms of distress as expected responses to trauma helps client make the link between distress and trauma and decreases guilt and shame. • Well-being of wife and children must be answered in case of future physical abuse. • Nurse must adhere to agency and state requirements	**Wife, short term** 1, 2. Met in 1 week. 3. Met in 2 weeks. 4. Partially met. At follow-up visit, wife verbalized that she knows she is not responsible for her husband's actions, but she related examples of trying to please him so that he would not beat her. Review dynamics of interpersonal behavior and concept of only being able to control one's own behavior. **Husband, short term** 1, 2. Met in 1 week. 3. Met in 1 month. **Wife, long term** 1, 2, 4. Met in 6 months. 3. Partially met in 6 months. Client gives examples of sharing decisions about small matters (e.g., what to buy at the grocery store) but does not feel free to voice dissenting opinion about child-rearing issue. Review interventions to empower client, teach assertiveness skills, and

The Nursing Process

NURSING CARE PLAN

Family Violence—cont'd

Outcomes	Interventions	Rationale	Evaluation
trauma *within 6 months*. 3. Will describe relationship with husband as one between equals *within 6 months*. 4. Will relate an example of using skills to resolve conflict with husband *within 6 months*. **Husband, long term** 1. Will acknowledge responsibility for aggressive behavior *within 1 month*. 2. Will join a self-help group for abusive spouses *within 1 month*. 3. Will relate one example of relinquishing control of wife's relationship with her friend *within 6 months*. 4. Will describe relationship between his childhood abuse and his own style of parenting *within 6 months*.	• Empower wife by respecting her autonomy in making decisions about her life (e.g., whether to report abuse to authorities, whether she should leave the home). • Look for subtle clues and indirect signs that abuse is a pattern of family behavior. • Ask questions directly about abuse and neglect. • Draw a genogram to assess the potential for history of family violence. • Teach conflict-resolution skills to solve problems and mediate differences. • Assess for stressful factors such as unemployment or illiteracy. • Teach assertiveness skills to communicate needs appropriately. • Establish a mechanism for continued follow-up care. • Refer to interdisciplinary team for long-term care and appropriate community services. • Assess family for resurgence of violent episodes.	• Wife needs to feel empowered to feel in control of her actions and decisions. • Clients may deny experience of abuse because of fear of retaliation, abandonment, and others. • Patriarchal dominance, traditional values, and patterns of strict discipline may put families at risk for abuse. • Training in conflict resolution, assertiveness, and empathy teaches self-awareness and responsibility for one's actions and consequences • External stressors deplete resources and strain adaptive responses. • Family violence may take months or years to treat, but each health care incidence is an opportunity to reinforce progress and increase safety	instill hope that progress is being made. **Husband, long term** 1. Partially met. Client acknowledges some personal responsibility, but he still believes others make him lose his temper and go out of control. Review contract for handling frustration and aggressive feelings. Make modifications to contract to increase probability of achievement of goals. 2. Not met within 6 months. Client refuses to join self-help group because "they are a bunch of criminals." Reframe group treatment as a means to learn about marital relations and parenting skills. Make referral to appropriate therapist. 3, 4. Met in 6 months.

victims can break the silence and begin the healing process. The nurse may choose to follow all or some of the interventions for abuse protection listed in Box 36-7, in providing care for victims of violence.

The nursing care plan should be implemented according to the priorities inherent in the clinical situation. For example, if life-threatening physical signs and symptoms are present, the nurse must attend to them first, such as stopping bleeding, dressing wounds, and medicating pain. In the absence of overt evidence of physical or sexual abuse, psychological signs and symptoms should be the main focus of the nurse's careful listening, sensitive questioning, and empathetic concern.

Interventions should be directed toward increasing the client's sense of self-worth, empowerment, and autonomy. Instilling hope and fostering self-determination are key components to building self-esteem. Nurse-client interactions that communicate respect, genuineness, and empathy foster the client's growth along these dimensions and support the development of appropriate ways to satisfy personal needs and function effectively in social roles. Victims have to regain an appreciation of their own intrinsic worth as a sound basis for meeting love and belonging needs in intimate relationships. Through the nurse-client relationship clients can learn about their strengths and potential for growth.

The Nursing Process

BOX 36-7

Abuse Protection

DEFINITION

Identification of high-risk, dependent relationships and actions to prevent further infliction of physical or emotional harm

ACTIVITIES

Identify adult(s) with a history of unhappy childhoods associated with abuse, rejection, excessive criticism, or feelings of being worthless and unloved as children

Identify adult(s) who have difficulty trusting others or feel disliked by others

Identify whether individual feels that asking for help is an indication of personal incompetence

Identify level of social isolation present in family situation

Determine whether family needs periodic relief from care responsibilities

Identify whether adult at risk has close friends or family available to help with children when needed

Determine relationship between husband and wife

Determine whether adults are able to take over for each other when one is too tense, tired, or angry to deal with a dependent family member

Determine whether child/dependent adult is viewed differently by an adult based on gender, appearance, or behavior

Identify crisis situations that may trigger abuse, such as poverty, unemployment, divorce, or death of a loved one

Monitor for signs of neglect in high-risk families

Observe a sick or injured child/dependent adult for signs of abuse

Listen to the explanation on how the illness or injury happened

Identify when the explanation of the cause of the injury is inconsistent among those involved

Encourage admission of child/dependent adult for further observation and investigation, as appropriate

Record times and duration of visits during hospitalization

Monitor parent-child interactions and record observations, as appropriate

Monitor for underreactions or overreactions on the part of an adult

Monitor child/dependent adult for extreme compliance, such as passive submission to hospital procedures

Monitor child for role reversal, such as comforting the parent, or overactive or aggressive behavior

Listen attentively to adult who begins to talk about own problems

Listen to a pregnant woman's feelings about pregnancy and expectations about the unborn child

Monitor new parent's reactions to infant, observing for feelings of disgust, fear, or unrealistic expectations

Monitor for a parent who holds newborn at arm's length, handles newborn awkwardly, or asks for excessive assistance

Monitor for repeated visits to a clinic, emergency department, or physician's office for minor problems

Monitor for a progressive deterioration in the physical and emotional care provided to a child/dependent adult in the family

Monitor child for signs of failure to thrive, depression, apathy, developmental delay, or malnutrition

Determine expectations adult has for child to determine whether expected behaviors are realistic

Instruct parents on realistic expectations of child based on developmental level

Establish rapport with families who have a history of abuse for long-term evaluation and support

Help families identify coping strategies for stressful situations

Instruct adult family members on signs of abuse

Refer adult(s) at risk to appropriate specialists

Inform the physician of observations indicative of abuse

Report any situations where abuse is suspected to the proper authorities

Refer adult(s) to shelters for abused spouses, as appropriate

Refer parents to Parents Anonymous for group support, as appropriate

Reprinted with permission from McCloskey J.C., & Bulechek G.M. (Eds.). (1996). Nursing interventions classification (NIC), *(2nd ed.). St. Louis, MO: Mosby-Year Book.*

Society is not responsive or sympathetic to victims who do not leave the situation in which they endure repeated acts of violence. The circumstances that compel battered women and men to stay in a violent relationship are poorly understood by the public and health care providers. Concern for the children; economic dependence; lack of education, resources, and marketable skills; feelings of shame; social stigma; fear of reprisal; and a perceived or real lack of alternatives are some of the reasons victims choose to remain in the home (Campbell

The Nursing Process

and Humphreys, 1993). Some victims do not leave, because they take responsibility for being abused. They believe that they provoke their partners' unpredictable rages or that they should be able to control their partners' behavior (Moss, 1991). Some are too "numbed" by the trauma to mobilize the energy necessary to flee the situation (Burgess, Hartman, and Clements, 1995). Nurses need to recognize that the victim's response to empowerment interventions may take considerable time before the client can achieve the desired outcomes. Examples of community agencies and organizations that provide information and services for victims are presented in the Community Resources box below.

Most adult victims, however, try many different strategies to avoid abuse or leave the situation (Campbell, 1992; Fishwick, 1995; Moss, 1991). Children, dependent adults, and chronically ill elderly persons lack the basic resources to leave an abusive or neglectful environment. Without support and outside assistance, the family con-

flict may end only with the death of the child, wife, husband, elderly person, or unrelated household member victim, given the escalating nature of the cycle of violence. Therefore the nurse, through the therapeutic alliance, should continue to build on the client's strengths and coping skills, even if the client is unable to leave the abusive situation.

Nurses who care for abused, neglected, and exploited clients are at risk of becoming overwhelmed by the enormity of the inflicted trauma and the emotional pain experienced by these victims (Briggs, 1992; Crothers, 1995; Rew and Christian, 1993). The systematic maltreatment of children, women, elderly persons, and those who are institutionalized engender heartfelt sympathy toward these victims and intense rage toward the perpetrators of abuse and neglect (Gallop, McKeever, Toner, Lancee, and Lueck, 1995). However, the development of a therapeutic relationship must move beyond sympathy if the nurse wishes to help clients shed their role as victims, re-

 COMMUNITY RESOURCES

Abuse, Neglect, and Exploitation

All 50 states have toll-free hotline numbers for reporting abuse. Check the local directory or call the National Child Abuse Hotline at (800) 422-4453 for assistance and information.

AYUDA Clinica Legal Latina
1736 Columbia Road, NW
Washington, DC 20009
(202) 387-0424

Center to Prevent Handgun Violence
1225 Eye Street, NW, Suite 1100
Washington, DC 20005
(202) 289-7319

Family Violence Prevention Fund
383 Rhode Island Street, Suite 304
San Francisco, CA 94103-5133
(415) 252-8900

Men's Anti-Rape Resource Center
P.O. Box 73559
Washington, DC 20056

National Center for Health Education
72 Spring Street, Suite 208
New York, NY 10012-4019
(212) 334-9470

National Center on Women and Family Law
799 Broadway, Suite 402
New York, NY 10003
(212) 674-8200

National Coalition Against Domestic Violence
P.O. Box 34103
Washington, DC 20043-4103

National Coalition on Television Violence
P.O. Box 2157
Champaign, IL 61825
(810) 439-3177

Parents Anonymous
5 Foothill Boulevard, Suite 220
Claremont, CA 91711

Victim Assistance Network
Mt. Vernon Center
8119 Holland Road
Alexandria, VA 22306

The Nursing Process

solve past traumas, and move toward effective decision making and coping. Prevention and effective intervention must focus on identifying persons at risk, deescalating conflicts at an early stage, and teaching new ways to communicate and relate as a family (Harrington and Dubowitz, 1993). Useful Teaching Points to emphasize with clients are presented below.

A therapeutic nurse-client relationship with a child has potential for enhancing the child's safety, preventing long-term assault, and developing a healthier sense of self. The first step is to establish trust as a foundation for disclosure of the abuse. The transition to focusing on the abuse itself is facilitated by interventions that address the child's guilty feelings about causing the abuse and creating problems for the abusive parent or adult. The child's ability to participate in a therapeutic relationship is also enhanced by the nurse's communication, which gives credibility to the information provided by the child (Kelley, 1995).

Elderly who are victims of abuse, neglect, and exploitation tend to present themselves as frightened, ashamed, hopeless, and powerless (Boudreau, 1993). They may avoid eye contact and seem inhibited from speaking freely, watching for cues from their family members or caretakers before answering questions (Criner, 1994). It is crucial that the nurse take time and have the patience to explore the elderly person's feelings and perceptions of options. The goal should be to ensure safety, promote autonomy, and respect the elderly person's dignity as the nurse works with the family or institutional caregivers. Prevention of elderly abuse is the ideal. Raising the consciousness of health care professionals about normal aging and the risk factors inherent in elderly abuse, linking family caregivers to support and respite services, and providing counseling and other resources to troubled families are methods of preventing elderly abuse.

Institutionalized victims who are vulnerable to abuse and neglect usually have serious physical and/or mental disabilities. Institutionalized children, adults, and elderly who are mistreated by their caretakers may be physically, psychologically, and sexually abused or neglected (Groze, 1990). Victims' dependence on others for the performance of ADLs generates frustration in both victims and perpetrators. The risk of abuse increases if the potential victims are also unable to communicate their needs and wishes. Nurses have a responsibility for monitoring and evaluating the care provided by caregivers in institutions. Monitoring, intervention, and evaluation activities should be focused on the quality of the physical and psychological care of institutionalized clients (see Chapter 19).

Interventions for Perpetrators

Perhaps the greatest challenge for nurses is developing a therapeutic relationship with a perpetrator. A nurse's self-awareness, sensitivity, and empathy are crucial for helping perpetrators to make a commitment for treatment and recognize and accept responsibility for the victimization they have caused. The task is difficult but necessary for the sake of the victim as well as the perpetrator.

Some nurses find that it helps to focus on the fact that perpetrators may have a history of themselves being victims of abuse, neglect, and exploitation and a special vulnerability to aggressive behavior. Interpersonal family aggression may have been transmitted from their family of

TEACHING POINTS

Victims of Abuse, Neglect, or Exploitation

Teach the client, family, and/or significant others the following:
- To understand the dynamics of stress, power, control, and aggressive, violent behavior
- To recognize psychobiological effects such as sleep disorders, the "numbing" effect on memory and other cognitive functions, and a heightened state of arousal and other altered autonomic nervous functions that may persist after experiencing a traumatic event as the body's way of coping with severe distress
- To develop a safety plan for potentially violent situations
- To identify personal, interpersonal, and social factors that put families at risk for a cycle of violence
- To understand normal growth and development of children and developmental tasks of families across the life span
- To develop assertiveness and conflict-resolution skills
- To perceive vulnerability in others and respond with empathy
- To access community resources for support (e.g., Parents Anonymous, women's shelters, church groups, social associations, and law enforcement agencies)
- To identify personal and family strengths and adaptive coping mechanisms
- To appreciate fundamental rights and responsibilities of human beings

The Nursing Process

origin, where they became more vulnerable to learning to provoke violence, tolerate violence, and seek aggressive partners (Capell and Heiner, 1990). Some perpetrators may take on the role of abuser as a way of mastering their own trauma. One explanation is that they learn dysfunctional ways to ventilate anger and frustration, to control others and their environment, from those who abused them as children (Robinson, Wright, and Watson, 1994). Perpetrators—those who abuse, neglect, or exploit others—need to understand the dynamics and circumstances that contribute to their dysfunctional behavior so that they can develop more effective ways of controlling their own behavior and relating to others. While perpetrators too deserve nonjudgmental care, they must still be held accountable for their abusive actions and the consequences.

Interventions for perpetrators include building a therapeutic alliance, setting limits on aggressive behavior, teaching new coping and conflict-resolution skills, and making contracts for acceptable social behavior. The process of rehabilitation of perpetrators has been compared to "remodeling" (Scheela and Stern, 1994) where the person goes through stages of falling apart, taking on responsibility, tearing out the damaged parts, rebuilding and reconstructing the self, doing the upkeep or maintenance, and finally moving on to a life beyond treatment. This model or metaphor of recovery helps to explain the tremendous variation in the way and the extent to which different perpetrators respond to treatment.

Collaborative Interventions

Nursing care of victims and perpetrators in abusive, neglectful, and exploitive situations involves collaboration with other professionals. For example, school health nurses have a responsibility for helping educate teachers and school administrators about the signs of child abuse and for working with them in the identification of victims and implementation of protective services.

Nurses employed in settings that provide health care to children and adults collaborate with other caregivers to identify clients whose injuries or infections suggest physical or sexual abuse. Through collaboration caregivers can assemble an assessment database to use in assisting clients to recognize their need for help and to enlist the support of child welfare protective services. When the victims of abuse are children, nurses collaborate with other caregivers and interface with social services, child welfare authorities, mental health services, and the judicial system to report suspected abuse and provide a safe environment for victims (Kellogg, Chapa, Metcalf, Trotta, and Roderiquez, 1993).

Effective collaboration in helping victims of abuse, neglect, and exploitation involves six steps:

1. The immediate treatment of injuries and sexually transmitted infections
2. Initiation of interagency cross referrals that involve health, welfare, refuge, and judicial protective services
3. Joint case conferences for collaborative care planning
4. Collaborative decision making regarding the allocation of responsibilities for implementing the plan of care
5. Simultaneous treatment of victims and perpetrators based on the collaborative plan
6. Formal periodic reassessment of the plan's implementation and its effectiveness and revision of the plan as needed to prevent treatment breakdown (Baglow, 1990)

Evaluation

Evaluation of the effectiveness of the nursing care plan and the achievement of the identified outcomes for victims and perpetrators is determined according to the clients' response to treatment and nursing interventions. An example of the outcomes that were met, partially met, and not met for clients who experienced family violence are noted in the nursing care plan on pp. 793-794. The cycle of family violence is often a well-established pattern of behavior, sometimes spanning many generations. Therefore the nurse may need to develop and change the nursing care plan over time as the family members learn new ways of relating and meeting their needs.

KEY POINTS

- Violence is one of the major health problems in western society.
- The types of violence experienced by victims and inflicted by perpetrators include physical and psychological abuse, physical and psychological neglect, sexual abuse, and exploitation.
- Common elements in all abusive, neglectful, and exploitive situations are the perpetrator's use of power to control, coerce, seduce, trick, or deprive and/or use the victim for financial gain, as well as the victim's sense of powerlessness.
- The victim is not to blame for the abuse; the perpetrator must be held accountable for the abuse and its consequences.

CRITICAL THINKING QUESTIONS

Bobby P., 20 months old, was admitted to the observation unit of the emergency department (ED) at 11:30 AM, with a concussion and broken clavicle. He cried vigorously during assessment and treatment of his shoulder injury. Now he is dozing on his mother's lap. She states that he fell out of the grocery cart as she was reaching for a cereal box. Her older son Tommy, age 6, stands close to her side, looking very fearful. He gives single word answers to your questions about how he is doing. His mother appears nervous as she asks, "When can I take Bobby home? His dad is going to be really upset about what happened to him today."

1. How would you assess for the possibility of child abuse or neglect in this case? What observations would you make? What questions would you ask the mother? What questions would you ask Tommy?

2. How would you differentiate accidental injury from intentional abuse or neglect in this case? Which of Bobby's clinical signs and symptoms, laboratory tests, and X-ray results would give you a strong suspicion of abuse or neglect? Are there some signs and symptoms that provide conclusive evidence of child maltreatment?

3. Bobby's mother seems anxious. Using therapeutic communication techniques, give three responses to her question about going home and Bobby's father's reaction. Provide a rationale for each response. Discuss the mother's likely reply to each communication.

4. If maltreatment was suspected by the ED team, what would be the steps to take in reporting this case to the authorities? Who should make the report? What are the ethical and legal issues involved in mandatory reporting of child abuse and neglect? How would you tell the mother about the report?

5. What steps would you take to prevent further injury to Bobby? What would be the focus of your teaching plan for Bobby's mother? Would you involve the father in the plan? Why or why not? Would you plan an intervention for Tommy? Why or why not?

6. What kind of follow-up care does Bobby need? To whom would you make a referral? What behaviors by the mother and other family members would indicate good clinical outcomes?

- Factors that inhibit the victim's disclosure of abuse, neglect, and exploitation include shame, misplaced self-blame, loss of self-esteem, a sense of powerlessness, an impaired sense of trust, misplaced loyalty, fear of retaliation, and the physical or developmental inability to verbalize and describe the experiences.

- Abuse and neglect may have long-lasting effects that result in mental health problems and serious psychiatric conditions such as PTSD.

- No one theory explains all situations of violence, but research suggests that psychobiological, interpersonal, family, and sociocultural dynamics all contribute to family violence.

- Nurses have a professional and civic responsibility to comply with mandatory reporting laws in cases of suspected child, elderly, and dependent-adult abuse and neglect.

- Violence prevention is possible through education and advocacy for programs that decrease social oppression and empower persons to assert their human rights to respect and autonomy.

REFERENCES

All, A.C. (1994, July). A literature review: Assessment and intervention in elder abuse. *Journal of Gerontological Nursing*, 25-32.

American Psychiatric Association (APA). (1994). *Diagnostic and statistical manual of mental disorders* (4th ed.). Washington, DC: Author.

Aroian, K.L. (1993). Mental health risks and problems encountered by illegal immigrants. *Issues in Mental Health Nursing, 14*(4), 379-397.

Asbury, J. (1993). Violence in families of color in the United States. In R. Hampton, T. Gullotta, G. Adams, E. Potter III, & R. Weissberg (Eds.), *Family violence: Prevention and treatment.* Newbury Park, CA: Sage Publications.

Bachman, R. (1994). *Violence against women: A national crime victimization survey report.* Washington, DC: U.S. Department of Justice.

Baglow, L.J. (1990). A multidimensional model for treatment of child abuse: A framework for cooperation. *Child Abuse and Neglect, 14*(3), 387-395.

Blau, G.M., Dall, M.B., & Anderson, L.M. (1993). The assessment and treatment of violent families. In R. Hampton, T. Gullotta, G. Adams, E. Potter III, & R. Weissberg (Eds.), *Family violence: Prevention and treatment.* Newbury Park, CA: Sage Publications.

Boudreau, F.A. (1993). Elder abuse. In R. Hampton, T. Gullotta, G. Adams, E. Potter III, & R. Weissberg (Eds.), *Family violence: Prevention and treatment.* Newbury Park, CA: Sage Publications.

Bourne, R., Chadwick, D.L., Kanda, M.B., & Ricci, L.R. (1993, February). When you suspect child abuse. *Patient Care, 22*-26, 28-29, 34, 37-38, 40, 46-48, 51-54.

Brasseur, J.W. (1995, July/August). Child abuse: Identification and intervention. *Clinician Reviews,* 83-85, 89-90, 93-95, 97-100, 103.

Briggs, K. (1992). Breaking the silence. *Nursing Times,* 88(40), 50-52.

Burgess, A.W., Harman, C.R., & Clements, P.T. (1995). Biology of memory and childhood trauma. *Journal of Psychosocial Nursing, 33*(3), 16-26.

Burgess, A.W., Hartman, C.R., & Kelley, S. (1990). Assessing child abuse: The TRIADS checklist. *Journal of Psychosocial Nursing, 28*(4), 7-14.

Campbell, J.C. (1992). Ways of teaching, learning, and knowing about violence against women. *Nursing & Health Care, 13*(9), 464-470.

Campbell, J.C., & Humphreys, J. (1993). *Nursing care of survivors of family violence* (2nd ed.). St. Louis: Mosby.

Campbell, J.C., & Parker, B. (1993). Battered women and their children. In J.J. Fitzpatrick, R.L. Tauton, & A.K. Jacox (Eds.), *Annual review of nursing research, Vol. 10* (pp. 77-94). New York: Springer.

Campbell, J.K., Pliska, M.J., Taylor, W., & Sheridan, D. (1994). Battered women's experiences in the emergency department. *Journal of Emergency Nursing, 20*(4), 280-288.

Capell, C., & Heiner, R.B. (1990). The intergenerational transmission of family aggression. *Journal of Family Violence, 5*(2), 135-152.

Celano, M.P. (1990). Activities and games for group psychotherapy with sexually abused children. *International Journal of Psychotherapy, 40*(4), 419-428.

Conte, J.R. (1993). Sexual abuse of children. In R. Hampton, T. Gullotta, G. Adams, E. Potter III, & R. Weissberg (Eds.), *Family violence: Prevention and treatment.* Newbury Park, CA: Sage Publications.

Criner, J.A. (1994). The nurse's role in preventing abuse of elderly patients. *Rehabilitation Nursing, 19*(5), 277-280, 297, 322.

Crothers, D. (1995). Vicarious traumatization in the work with survivors of childhood trauma. *Journal of Psychosocial Nursing, 33*(4), 9-13.

D'Antonio, I.J., Darwish, A.M., & McLean, M. (1993). Child maltreatment: International perspectives. *Maternal Child Nursing Journal, 21*(2), 39-52.

Devlin, B.K., & Reynolds, E. (1994). Child abuse: How to recognize it, how to intervene. *American Journal of Nursing, 94*(3), 26-31.

Doob, D. (1992). Female sexual abuse survivors as patients: Avoiding retraumatization. *Archives of Psychiatric Nursing, 6*(4), 245-251.

Drake, R.E. (1994). Potential health hazards of pornography consumption as viewed by psychiatric nurses. *Archives of Psychiatric Nursing, 8*(2), 101-106.

Finkelhor, D., & Korbin, J. (1988). Child abuse as an international issue. *Child Abuse and Neglect, 12*(1), 3-23.

Fishwick, N. (1995). Getting to the heart of the matter: Nursing assessment and intervention with battered women in psychiatric-mental health settings. *Journal of the American Psychiatric Nurses Association, 1*(2), 48-54.

Frasier, L.D., Barchman, V., & Alexander, R.C. (1992). Physical and behavioral signs of sexual abuse in infants and toddlers. *Infants and Young Children, 5*(2), 1-12.

Fulmer, T., McMahon, D., Baer, M., & Forget, B. (1992). Abuse, neglect, abandonment, violence, and exploitation: An analysis of all elderly patients seen in one emergency department during a six-month period. *Journal of Emergency Nursing, 18*(6), 505-510.

Furniss, K.K. (1993). Screening for abuse in the clinical setting. *AWHONN's Clinical Issues in Perinatal and Women's Health Nursing, 4*(3), 402-406.

Gallop, R., McKeever, P., Toner, B., Lancee, W., & Lueck, M. (1995). The impact of childhood sexual abuse on the psychological well-being and practice of nurses. *Archives of Psychiatric Nursing, 9*(3), 137-145.

Gelles, R. (1993). Family violence. In R. Hampton, T. Gullotta, G. Adams, E. Potter III, & R. Weissberg (Eds.), *Family violence: Prevention and treatment.* Newbury Park, CA: Sage Publications.

Gelles, R., & Straus, M. (1988). *Intimate violence.* New York: Simon and Schuster.

Glod, C.A. (1992). Circadian dysregulation in abused individuals: A proposed theoretical model for practice and research. *Archives of Psychiatric Nursing, 6*(6), 347-355.

Glod, C.A. (1993). Long-term consequences of childhood physical and sexual abuse. *Archives of Psychiatric Nursing, 7*(3), 163-173.

Gondolf, E.W. (1993). Male batterers. In R. Hampton, T. Gullotta, G. Adams, E. Potter III, & R. Weissberg (Eds.), *Family violence: Prevention and treatment.* Newbury Park, CA: Sage Publications.

Groze, V. (1990). An exploratory investigation into institutional mistreatment. *Children and Youth Services Review, 12*(3), 228-241.

Hanrahan, P., Campbell, J., & Ulrich, Y. (1993). Theories of violence. In J. Campbell, & J. Humphreys (Eds.), *Nursing care of survivors of family violence.* St. Louis: Mosby.

Harper-Jaques, S., & Reimer, M. (1992). Aggressive behavior and the brain: A different perspective for the mental health nurse. *Archives of Psychiatric Nursing, 6*(5), 312-320.

Harrington, D., & Dubowitz, H. (1993). What can be done to prevent child maltreatment? In R. Hampton, T. Gullotta, G. Adams, E. Potter III, & R. Weissberg (Eds.), *Family violence: Prevention and treatment.* Newbury Park, CA: Sage Publications.

Hayes, H.R., & Emshoff, J.G. (1993). Substance abuse and family violence. In R. Hampton, T. Gullotta, G. Adams, E. Potter III, & R. Weissberg (Eds.), *Family violence: Prevention and treatment.* Newbury Park, CA: Sage Publications.

Hiday, V.A. (1995). The social context of mental illness and violence. *Journal of Health and Social Behavior, 36*(2), 122-137.

Hoff, L. (1990). *Battered women as survivors.* New York: Routledge.

Holz, K.A. (1994). A practical approach to clients who are survivors of childhood sexual abuse. *Journal of Nurse Midwifery, 39*(1), 13-18.

Isaac, N.E., Cochran, D., Brown, M.E., & Adams, S.L. (1994). Men who batter: Profile from a restraining order database. *Archives of Family Medicine, 3*(1), 50-54.

Kaye, J., Donald, C.G., & Merker, S. (1994). Sexual harassment of critical care nurses: A costly workplace issue. *American Journal of Critical Care, 3*(6), 409-415.

Kelley, S.J. (1990). Parental stress response to sexual abuse and ritualistic abuse of children in day care centers. *Nursing Research, 39*(1), 25-29.

Kelley, S.J. (1992). Child maltreatment, stressful life events, and behavior problems in school-aged children in residential treatment. *Journal of Child and Adolescent Psychiatric and Mental Health Nursing, 5*(2), 5-13.

Kelley, S.J. (1995). Child sexual abuse: Initial effects. In J.J. Fitzgerald, & J.S. Stenenson (Eds.), *Annual review of nursing research, vol. 13,* (pp. 63-86). New York, Springer.

Kellogg, N.D., Chapa, M.J., Metcalf, P., Trotta, M., & Rodriguez, D. (1993). Medical/social evaluation model: A combined investigative and therapeutic approach to childhood sexual abuse. *Journal of Child Sexual Abuse, 2*(4), 1-17.

Kempe, C.H., Silver, F., Steele, B., Droegemueller, W., & Silver, H. (1962). The battered child syndrome, *Journal of American Medical Association, 181*(1), 17-24.

Lachs, M.S., & Pillener, K. (1995). Abuse and neglect of elderly persons. *New England Journal of Medicine, 332*(7), 437-443.

Mackey, T., Sereika, S.M., Weissfeld, L.A., Hacker, S.S., Zender, J.F., & Heard, S.L. (1992). Factors associated with long-term depressive symptoms of sexual assault victims. *Archives of Psychiatric Nursing, 6*(1), 10-25.

McCloskey, J.C., & Bulechek, G.M. (Eds.). (1996). *Nursing interventions classification (NIC).* (2nd ed.) St. Louis: Mosby.

McFarland, G.K., & McFarlane, E.A. (1993). *Nursing diagnosis & intervention: Planning for patient care* (2nd ed.). St. Louis: Mosby.

Morrison, E. (1993). Toward a better understanding of violence in psychiatric settings: Debunking the myths. *Archives of Psychiatric Nursing, 7*(6), 328-335.

Morrison, E.F. (1994). The evolution of a concept: Aggression and violence in psychiatric settings. *Archives of Psychiatric Nursing, 8*(4), 245-253.

Moss, V.A. (1991). Battered women and the myth of masochism. *Journal of Psychosocial Nursing, 29* (7), 19-23.

Muenzenmaier, K., Meyer, I., Struening, E., & Ferber, J. (1993). Childhood abuse and neglect among women outpatients with chronic mental illness. *Hospital and Community Psychiatry, 44*(7), 666-670.

Murphy, C.M., & Cascardi, M. (1993). Psychological aggression and abuse in marriage. In R. Hampton, T. Gullotta, G. Adams, E. Potter III, & R. Weissberg (Eds.), *Family violence: Prevention and treatment.* Newbury Park, CA: Sage Publications.

Nathan, R., & Williamson, S. (1993). Sexual assault documentation tool. *Journal of Emergency Nursing, 19*(5), 458-461.

Neisen, J.H., & Sandall, H. (1990). Alcohol and other drug abuse in a gay/lesbian population: Related to victimization? *Journal of Psychology and Human Sexuality, 3*(1), 151-168.

Paone, D., Chavkin, W., Willets, I., Friedmann, P., & Des-Jarlais, D. (1992). The impact of sexual abuse: Implications for drug treatment. *Journal of Women's Health, 1*(2), 149-153.

Parker, B., McFarlane, J., Soeken, K., Torres, S., & Campbell, D. (1993). Physical and emotional abuse in pregnancy: A comparison of adult and teenage women. *Nursing Research, 42*(3), 173-178.

Powers, J.L., Mooney, A., & Nunno, M. (1990), Institutional abuse: A review of the literature. *Journal of Child and Youth Care, 4*(6), 81-95.

Prentky, R., & Burgess, A.W. (1990). Rehabilitation of child molesters: A cost-benefit analysis. *American Journal of Orthopsychiatric Association, 60*(1), 108-116.

Rew, L., & Christian, B. (1993). Self-efficacy, coping, and well-being among nursing students sexually abused in childhood. *Journal of Pediatric Nursing 8*(6), 392-399.

Robinson, C.A., Wright, L.M., & Watson, W.L. (1994). A nontraditional approach to family violence. *Archives of Psychiatric Nursing, 8*(1), 30-37.

Ross, C.A., Anderson, G., Clark, P. (1994). Childhood abuse and the positive symptoms of schizophrenia. *Hospital & Community Psychiatry, 45*(5), 489-491.

Russell, D. (1986). *The secret trauma.* New York: Basic Books.

Sampselle, C.M. (1991). The role of nursing in preventing violence against women. *Journal of Obstetric, Gynecological, and Neonatal Nursing, 20*(6), 481-487.

Scheela, R.A., & Stern, P.N. (1994). Falling apart: A process integral to the remodeling of male incest offenders. *Archives of Psychiatric Nursing, 8*(2), 91-100.

Sheridan, D.J. (1993). The role of the battered woman specialist. *Journal of Psychosocial Nursing, 31*(11), 31-37.

Sherman, D.J. (1992). The neglected health care needs of street youth. *Public Health Reports, 107*(4), 433-440.

Shon, S.P. & Ja, D.Y. (1982). Asian families. In M. McGoldrick, J.K. Pearce, & J. Giordano (Eds.), *Ethnicity and family therapy* (pp. 208-228). New York: The Guilford Press.

Singer, M.I., Anglin, T.M., Song, L., & Lunghofer, L. (1995). Adolescents' exposure to violence and associated symptoms of psychological trauma. *Journal of American Medical Association, 273*(6), 477-482.

Spector, R.E. (1996). *Cultural diversity in health and illness* (4th ed.). Norwalk, CT: Appleton & Lange.

Surrey, J., Swett, C., Michaels, A., & Levin, S. (1990). Reported history of physical and sexual abuse and severity of symptomatology in women psychiatric outpatients. *American Journal of Orthopsychiatry, 60*(3), 412-417.

Tilden, V.P., & Shepherd, P. (1987). Increasing the rate of identification of battered women in an emergency department: Use of a nursing protocol. *Research in Nursing and Health, 10,* 209-215.

Torrey, E.F. (1994). Violent behavior by individuals with serious mental illness. *Hospital and Community Psychiatry, 45,* 653-662.

Urbancic, J.C. (1987). Incest trauma. *Journal of Psychosocial Nursing, 25*(7), 33-35.

Walker, L.E. (1984). *The battered woman syndrome.* New York: Springer.

Weiler, K., & Buckwalter, K.C. (1992). Geriatric mental health: Abuse among rural mentally ill. *Journal of Psychosocial Nursing, 30*(9), 32-36.

Weitzman, B.C., Knickman, J.R., & Shinn, M. (1992). Predictors of shelter use among low-income families: Psychiatric history, substance abuse, and victimization. *American Journal of Public Health, 82*(11), 1547-1550.

Zierler, S., Feingold, L., Laufer, D., Velentgas, P., Kantrowitz, G.I., & Mayer, K. (1991). Adult survivors of childhood sexual abuse and subsequent risk of HIV infection. *American Journal of Public Health, 81*(5), 572-575.

Chapter 37

Homeless Persons

Pam Price-Hoskins

LEARNING OUTCOMES

After studying and applying the concepts of this chapter, the learner will be able to:
- Respond effectively to the needs of homeless persons with mental illness.
- Relate mental illness to homelessness.
- Analyze the variables that maintain a condition of homelessness.
- Apply the facets of the nursing role with homeless persons with mental illness.

KEY TERMS

Assertive case management	Family dissolution	Houselessness
Deinstitutionalization	Homelessness	Situational homelessness

Homelessness *is a condition of being without a consistent dwelling place most of the time, as well as being without a support system, so that it becomes difficult to meet basic needs.* **Houselessness** *is being without a consistent dwelling place but having a good support system.* Houselessness and homelessness are conceptualized on a continuum, with homelessness being a more severe condition.

The social cost of homelessness is great. The United State's shame is the number of homeless persons—particularly children, persons who are mentally challenged, and elderly persons. The loss of personal income, taxable income, and personal productivity is great. The toll on personal physical and mental health of homeless persons is great as well. Because of exposure to the elements and the vulnerability to violence, personal health is more difficult to maintain. Even something as simple as a toothbrush for dental hygiene or a private place to defecate and something to clean with are difficult to obtain. Homeless persons, sooner or later, end up in the health care system with advanced illness, costing more money to manage than the cost of prevention. Homeless persons are diverted to institutions such as hospitals and jails, again costing considerable taxpayer dollars that could be spent in more humane, rehabilitative ways.

Nursing has been and will continue to be in the forefront in serving persons wherever they live in the community. One of the exciting and most challenging sites of nursing practice is in the community with homeless individuals and families. The purpose of this chapter is to explore the social phenomenon of homelessness and its effects on the health and illness of persons with mental illness in the United States.

EPIDEMIOLOGY

The homeless population is heterogenous, that is, composed of different ethnic groups, ages, genders, marital statuses, and health statuses. The largest segments of homeless persons are women, children, families, veterans, persons with severe and persistent mental illness, and persons with substance abuse disorders.

Knowing that the statistics are very rough guesses, it is thought that there are about 2.3 million adults in the United States who have no place to sleep or keep their belongings at any one time. Depending on the area of the country, 2.4% to 43% are 65 years or older (Harper and Lacey, 1993). Of the homeless population, 80% are men and 20% are women. About 42% of the homeless men are veterans (Winkleby and Fleshin, 1993). Half of the women are accompanied by children. Families make up about 34% of the homeless population (Scott, 1993). On any one night it is estimated that 100,000 children are without shelter. Those children are ordinarily accompanied by homeless, single mothers, many of whom have

mental illness and/or drug addiction and/or alcoholism. However, many families are on the streets because of marginal employment, recent loss of job, family violence, and *family dissolution, dissolving the family through abandonment, divorce, or death.*

About one third of all homeless men are mentally ill or chemically dependent; about 90% of homeless women are mentally ill (Virgona, Buhrich, and Teesson, 1993). Persons who have both mental illness and substance abuse disorders constitute 10% to 20% of homeless persons (Drake, Osher, and Wallach, 1991).

About 5% of homeless persons are teen-agers, 13 to 19 years old. The younger teen-agers are either under the supervision of a homeless adult or they are runaways, while the 16 to 19 year olds are independent of adult supervision, whether or not they have run away (Wright, 1991). The homelessness issue is alive and thriving in every country around the world.

THEORETICAL FRAMEWORK

Theories relevant to the creation of homelessness are also known as risk factors. Risk factors related to homelessness, sometimes called "pathways to homelessness," have economic roots, health roots, and sometimes both. Among the factors most commonly cited include the following:

- Deinstitutionalization
- Economic factors such as unemployment, poverty, and shortage of affordable housing
- Social problems such as nonaccommodation by relatives or friends, or marital disharmony
- Discharge from a primary health care facility to the streets
- Intentional homelessness, which makes up about 4% of all homeless persons choosing shelter and street living
- Chronic alcoholism

The following concepts are used to analyze causes of homelessness (Breakey and Fischer, 1985):

- Severe and persistent mental illness—About one third of the homeless population has severe and persistent mental illness. The research to date leaves the relationship between homelessness and mental illness unclear. Some clinicians and researchers believe that homelessness causes mental illness (Hamid, Wykes, and Stansfeld, 1993), while others believe that mental illness causes homelessness. What is clear is that there is a 20% to 40% relationship between the two; therefore nurses must assist some clients with mental illness with their housing needs. And some homeless persons may need assistance in accessing resources for severe mental disorders. Factors associated with both mental illness and homelessness are poor social support systems, difficulty in accessing public and private support systems, difficulty finding and maintaining employment, and confusion.

- Deinstitutionalization—Deinstitutionalization is a factor cited in homelessness. ***Deinstitutionalization is the transfer of persons with severe and persistent mental illness from hospitals for the treatment of their disorders back into the community.*** The assumption, when this movement began in the early 1960s, was that the community resources needed to support persons with severe and persistent mental illness would be readily funded by communities. With community support, clinicians and attorney advocates believed that persons with severe and persistent mental illness could survive and improve the quality of their lives. The unfortunate aftermath of these naive beliefs was the number of persons with severe and persistent mental illness who could not be maintained in homes and apartments or even single-room-occupancy dwellings (SROs); they may be found on the streets and under bridges and in cardboard boxes over exhaust grates.
- Substance abuse—Chemically dependent "Bowery bums" is the stereotype of homeless persons, with the societal prejudice embracing weakness, sin, unwillingness to help themselves, and unworthiness of any assistance from others. The statistics belie the stereotype, but for those, mostly men, who are chemically dependent, they have a particularly difficult time with homelessness. The toll the addictions take on human life is discussed in Chapter 27. The homeless person who is addicted has truly lost everything: home, job, ability to make a living, self-respect, family support, friends, often faith in a good God. The disease has rendered them powerless over the addictive substance and has stolen life and livelihood.
- Economic disadvantage—***Situational homelessness is the lack of stable housing because of economic or social factors, which could be relatively simply remedied.*** Twenty-five percent of U.S. children live below the poverty level. Many of these children live with single mothers; fathers have long since disappeared from the family's life. Women and their children are at particularly high risk for homelessness due to poverty; once homeless, locating affordable housing becomes exceedingly difficult (Hagen, 1990).
- Abuse—Physical and sexual abuse place women, their children, and disaffiliated adolescents in a vulnerable position in relation to homelessness (Hagen, 1990). Though it is difficult to leave a family residence (see Chapter 36), a parent, most often a mother, may only be able to save her life and the lives of her children by choosing homelessness.

The *Nursing Process*

Assessment

Factors included in the assessment of homeless persons include clinically relevant profiles, tools used by providers to measure homelessness and its ramifications, and assessment specifically focused on the issues of homelessness. Each of these will be explored in this section.

Clinical Profiles

Several groups are large enough among the homeless population to warrant special emphasis. These groups include youth, veterans, women, families, and persons with various illnesses and functional levels.

Youth

There are approximately 750,000 to 2 million new runaways per year, and about 500,000 are separated from their families and living on their own. Homeless runaway youth are more likely to come from female-headed, single-parent, or reconstituted families with many children, particularly step-siblings. Dysfunction in the family, family instability, and growth of single-parent and reconstituted families are closely related to running-away behavior (Shane, 1991). Youth are not accurately accounted for in the overall statistics of homeless persons, because they are "invisible," that is, not allowed in shelters or other places that adults are found and therefore are difficult to count.

The Nursing Process

Veterans

Veterans make up about 42% of the homeless men. However, veteran status does not seem to be a primary cause of homelessness but rather only a relationship. What causes the relationship is unclear. In one study, 1 veteran out of every 42 said their homelessness was due directly to their military service. Of the 10 veterans making that claim, nine had been exposed to combat, and all nine had severe injuries to the head, back, or extremities (Winkleby and Fleshin, 1993). Thus their ability to earn a livelihood may have been compromised.

Women and families

When women are undomiciled, 90% are severely mentally ill and/or alcohol/drug dependent. Diagnostically women tend to be psychotic, usually with schizophrenia, or have depression and personality disorders. In addition to psychosis, 7% to 9% of homeless women are addicted to alcohol or drugs (Bassuk, Rubin, and Lauriat, 1986).

Of women who are homeless 10% are on the streets because of situational problems. Women and their children are homeless primarily due to family difficulties such as divorce, eviction, and abuse.

Homeless women, compared with men who are homeless, are more likely to have young children in their custody. They tend to be younger than men who are homeless, more likely to be members of a minority group, and more often dependent on welfare. They have less frequent histories of substance abuse, incarceration, and felony convictions than men.

Families now comprise approximately 20% of the homeless population, with increasing numbers of families expected to join the ranks (Basler, 1986). One study found that of the children under 5 years of age, 47% showed at least one developmental delay, and 33% more showed two or more delays.

Screening Tools/Focused Assessment

Tools used by members of the multidisciplinary team to measure various aspects of homelessness are found in Table 37-1. These tools are useful for clinical measurement and for research purposes.

A focused assessment for homeless persons with mental disorders is found in Table 37-2. The assessment questions along with rationale for each question or set of questions are included.

Nursing Diagnosis

Nursing diagnoses for persons who are homeless and have mental disorders cover physical, mental, emotional, and spiritual health, as well as issues of relationships and roles. A few of the nursing diagnoses seen among this population are found in Table 37-3, along with related outcomes.

Because one third of the homeless population has chemical dependency or severe and persistent mental illness, all medical diagnoses are found among this population. Schizophrenia, bipolar disorder, organic mental

TABLE 37-1

Selected measurement tools used with homeless persons

Community-Based Inventory of Current Concerns (CICC) (Nyamathi and Flaskerud, 1992)	A 31-item questionnaire used with minority women to measure current living concerns. Factors included competency, personal instability/despondency, survival, and drug-related and parenting concerns.
Life Events Questionnaire (LEQ) (Masten, Neemann, and Andenas, 1991)	Questionnaire that assesses recent life stressors. It includes discrete and chronic stressors, events that vary in the amount of control the person can exert over the stressor.
Brief Symptom Inventory (BSI) (Derogatis and Melisaratos, 1983)	This tool includes 53 questions derived from the Symptom Check List-90. It is a self-report psychological symptom scale, rated from 0 to 4.
Scale for Level of Functioning/Homeless Persons (SLOF) (Lovell, Barrow, and Struening, 1992)	This is a 50-item scale based on interviewer observation. It measures social acceptability, work skills, personal care, interpersonal skills, and physical functioning.

The Nursing Process

TABLE 37-2

Focused assessment for homeless persons with mental illness

QUESTION/OBSERVATION	RATIONALE
Demographic Profile	
Gender and age	Demographics assist to identify issues that may be relevant in planning care and referral to community resources. Resources may be available only to certain groups such as veterans.
Age	
Culture	
Race	
Veteran status	
Religion/spirituality	
Continuum of Homelessness	
Who do you call in an emergency?	These questions help determine houselessness or homelessness, the strength of the support system, and its use. There may be a pattern of the use of resources by time of year or weather; patterns help to plan referrals.
Who are the other persons you keep in contact with? What is usually happening to you when you contact them?	
When the weather is bad, where do you stay?	
Where have you stayed in the last 7 days? In the past month, what other places have you stayed? In the past 6 months? In the past year?	
Family	
Who do you consider your family? What are the names, ages, and gender of each person? Where are they now? What are your hopes for the future in relation to your family?	Knowing who and how many persons need to be included, and at what level of planning, increases the plan's effectiveness. Homeless persons have opinions about what is most helpful to them and will undermine any plan that does not address their assessments of their own needs. Increasing the integrity of the family, whenever possible, strengthens the resources of the family as a whole and nurtures the individual members.
If family is with the homeless person, where are they staying? What accommodations have been most helpful to them? What interferes with their ability to be a family? What would be a good family solution to their homelessness?	
Basic Needs	
When was the last time you and your family ate? What did you eat? Where do you usually get your food?	These questions cover food, safety, violence and crime, income and employment, and illness symptoms and management. The nurse should be prepared to respond to needs that are assessed. Just being asked questions and getting no answers is frustrating to a person who has to scramble every day to survive. Nurses should not be surprised if homeless persons are mercenary in their attitudes toward them. At this level of poverty, the person is looking only for a way to meet basic needs. Every minute counts, and if the nurse cannot help, the person needs to know immediately. The person can then choose whether to spend time with the nurse.
What dangers do you face today? How do you handle them? What would help you to decrease those dangers?	
Have you been assaulted recently? What kind of help did you get for those assaults? What kind of help do you need now? (Make a visual inspection of any visible wounds.)	
Have you been violent toward anybody else recently? What happened? What danger are you in because of this action? What danger is the other person in because of you? How could this situation be resolved besides through violence?	

Continued.

The Nursing Process

TABLE 37-2—cont'd

Focused assessment for homeless persons with mental illness

QUESTION/OBSERVATION	RATIONALE
How do you get money to live each day? Are there any things you trade to get what you need? How do you keep your money safe? How much money do you need to live each week?	
What about work? What kind of work can you do? What do you need to be able to perform that work? What gets in the way of you keeping a job?	
What skills do you use to take care of yourself? Some persons act tough and mean, some find a group to hang with. What do you do?	
Illness Management	
What illnesses do you have? Which ones require medicine? How do you get your medicine? Any problems taking your medicine as your health care provider suggested? What symptoms do you have now that bother you? What symptoms do you have that bother other persons but do not bother you?	Assessment of all ailments—physical, mental, spiritual, and relational—need to be assessed here. There may be something that bothers the person that is not an illness but is frightening nevertheless. There may be other conditions that are obvious to the nurse, but the person has no awareness or concern about them. Some persons have symptoms that are self-protective and that they are unwilling to give up. There are other, very complex problems, and there is no point in pursuing issues the homeless persons with mental disorders want left alone.

disorder, chemical dependency, depression, and posttraumatic stress disorder (PTSD) are also seen.

Antisocial personality is another DSM-IV diagnosis found among the homeless population. Questions have been raised about the validity of this diagnosis, because the characteristics of homelessness overlap the characteristics of antisocial personality. However, in one study it was found that the characteristics of antisocial personality preceded homelessness; therefore it is a valid medical diagnosis and not a reflection of culture and life situation (North, Smith, and Spitznagel, 1993).

Outcome Identification

Quality of life is poor in several areas for persons with severe and persistent mental illness who are also homeless, (Lehman et al., 1995), as indicated with the following quality-of-life issues. Each of these is addressed in terms of outcomes for this population.

- Basic needs—No matter what other needs exist, until one has basic nutritional needs, hygiene,

clothing, and rudimentary shelter, no other needs can emerge as a priority. Simple hygiene items such as a toothbrush, soap, and sanitary pads are luxuries to homeless persons. Toothpaste, shampoo, and deodorant are almost beyond imagination. A place to receive mail and take a shower offers valuable services. Engaging homeless persons in any kind of relationship is founded on the helper's concern about the basic needs for food, clothing, shelter, housing, employment and entitlements, and health care (Dennis et al., 1991). If basic needs are not given priority by the nurse, the homeless person is not willing to be in the relationship.

- Safety—Predators, both homeless persons and others looking for vulnerable persons, prey on those without stable homes and support systems. Homeless persons learn to fear police officers, because they may evict them from the library or the public park and may want to know more about them than they are willing to divulge. Therefore homeless persons do not count on police for help.

The Nursing Process

TABLE 37-3

Selected NANDA nursing diagnoses and outcomes used with homeless persons who have severe and persistent mental illness

NANDA DIAGNOSIS	OUTCOME
Risk for infection related to inadequate, inconsistent skin cleaning and disorganized thinking	Client will develop no rash, scabies, or infestation of the skin while living in the shelter.
Risk for altered body temperature related to poor judgment about dressing for the weather and lack of adequate clothing	Client will maintain an oral temperature between 97.6 and 98.6 degrees during the winter months.
Caregiver role strain related to paranoia and homelessness	Client will meet food and clothing needs of self and children and will meet the requirements of the shelter in order to remain a maximum of 3 months.
Fatigue related to command hallucinations and unsafe living conditions	Client will sleep typical night's sleep of 6 hours and feel energetic enough to serve breakfast in the shelter 4 days in a row.
Ineffective management of therapeutic regimen (individual) related to dual diagnoses of drug addiction and bipolar disorder and homelessness	Client will have negative urine drug screen and will maintain therapeutic lithium level for 2 months while in the Community Work Placement Program.

Homeless persons band together in loosely knit groups. However, they come and go readily from the group and are wise not to trust all members of the group with everything. The group may or may not defend another group member, but there is at least some safety in numbers.

Solitary women quite often find a man to be her protector in exchange for sexual favors. She may engage in prostitution to make money for the two of them. This kind of affiliation decreases the vulnerability to rape and beatings from strangers.

• Residential stability—Housing is extremely important. Housing can be classified in three types: emergency shelter; transitional accommodations such as time-limited hostels and SROs, and long-term supportive residence arrangements in the community (Baxter and Hopper, 1984). However, many persons, particularly those with severe and persistent mental illness, may not be able to remain in one residence for a long period of time (Bachrach, 1992), hence the usefulness of three types of housing accommodations.

Because of the extent to which alcoholism and drug addiction are found among homeless persons, alcohol- and drug-free housing is essential to support and maintain recovery from these illnesses (McCarty, Argeriou, Huebner, and Lubran, 1991). For teen-agers, housing must have a strong emotional support component, although teen-agers may be difficult to form a relationship with (Angenent, Beke, and Shane, 1991).

Some researchers and clinicians have advocated for the availability of housing for clients who cannot or will not maintain sobriety, simply because housing may have to precede freedom from mood-altering chemicals (Caton, Wyatt, Felix, Grunberg, and Dominguez, 1993). Some homeless persons may never be drug-free. Is that a reason to deny them supported housing?

One study indicated that admission to residential treatment seemed to be the strongest determinant of clinical engagement of homeless persons with mental illness (Rosenheck and Gallup, 1991). In other words, a stable housing arrangement that was therapeutic in nature increased the likelihood of persons (in this study, veterans) being involved in psychiatric treatment.

A large majority of homeless persons placed in group and independent housing are able to remain housed and to avoid homelessness. They continue to use inpatient services at a high rate (Dickey et al., 1996). In other words, having stable housing does not decrease the recidivism of severe and persistent mental illness. However, treatment for mental illness does help persons to remain housed.

• Finances and employment—Persons who are homeless and have mental illness may have difficulty ef-

The Nursing Process

fectively handling job-related stress. Volunteering, job coaching and mentoring, job placement programs, and sheltered workshops are useful ways to address employment stressors and the difficulty in obtaining and maintaining employment. This is addressed in more detail in Chapters 20 and 38.

- Treatment outcomes—Research indicates that homeless men are more likely to be discharged against medical advice; to have had less than adequate discharge planning, particularly in relation to living arrangements, aftercare, and finances; and to have triple disorders of schizophrenia, substance abuse, and antisocial personality disorder (Caton, 1995). Engagement in the treatment process, adequate discharge planning, and attention to the medical issues plaguing clients are all intimately related to nursing care.

Treatment Outcomes

The following are common treatment outcomes:

1. Reduction of psychiatric symptoms—Homeless clients with mental disorders, especially those being discharged to the streets, need to be free of psychiatric symptoms that make them vulnerable to danger, such as inability to care for themselves, suicidal and self-mutilation thoughts, and hallucinations and delusions that interfere with an accurate perception of reality. Symptoms that may serve them well, and therefore may be considered functional behaviors, are paranoia, homicidal ideations, bizarre behaviors, and loud and obnoxious communication that keeps persons at a distance. Clinicians have difficult decisions to make and are often thwarted by clients when they want to treat the symptoms that may actually serve as survival skills on the streets. Careful negotiation must occur between clients and providers to agree on treatment outcomes that they can live with and that providers can, in good conscience, treat and leave untreated. For example, clients may be unwilling to take neuroleptics for thought disorders, because they are too sluggish to defend themselves. They also may not be able to afford them. On the other hand, how does the clinician treat hallucinations and delusions?

2. Improvement of social functioning—The social strata in which the homeless person with mental illness needs to function is with other street people and/or with other shelter or long-term residence occupants. They must also be able to re-

spond to hourly employment demands and to fill out entitlement forms, keep appointments. Skills such as assertiveness may not be nearly as useful as aggressiveness, and making eye contact and giving accurate information may be detrimental to survival on the streets. Ability to care for oneself in a variety of circumstances is the social functioning needed; the client is the person best able to define the skills needed to survive.

3. Improvement of social networks—Persons with severe and persistent mental illness have difficulty maintaining relationships. Homelessness is defined by the absence of social supports, while houselessness is defined by the presence of social supports. For houseless persons, including their support systems in planning and implementation of care actually strengthens the support. The support persons themselves often need supplemental, or respite, care. This care needs to be part of the care for the client, because it would actually assist to maintain the current houseless status.

   For clients without a support system, some semblance of a support system may be created. This usually starts with the case manager and resources mobilized on behalf of the client, such as a residence manager or a buddy assigned by the local chapter of the National Alliance for the Mentally Ill (NAMI).

4. Increased use of appropriate services, including entitlements—Overall, homeless clients with mental illness use mental health services at a high rate until the year they become homeless (North and Smith, 1996). This finding indicates that once persons are homeless, their use of mental health services decreases. Homeless persons use inpatient services much more than outpatient services, and their inability to pay is a major factor. A person is always admitted to inpatient treatment in crisis, and crisis is often precipitated by nonutilization of services and no medications, both problems of inadequate income. The vicious cycle of poverty, homelessness, and utilization of inpatient services is clear. An answer to this cycle is appropriate use of outpatient services, which includes entitlements to assist with the cost of ongoing treatment and medication.

   The Community Support Program, supported by National Institute of Mental Health, has been the most systematic response to date to the issues of persons with severe and persistent mental illness, some of whom are homeless. Services that are nec-

The Nursing Process

essary for mentally ill homeless persons include the following (Dennis et al., 1991):

- Outreach and engagement in nontraditional settings
- Intensive, long-term case management (small caseload, increased frequency of contact, and provision of services wherever they may be needed)
- Mental health treatment and rehabilitation services
- Staffing and operation of supportive living programs
- Management and administrative activities to link the above services together

Planning

Planning for the needs of homeless persons with mental illness can be overwhelming. Probably the simplest, most effective approach is to work with individuals on what they define as their immediate priorities. If those immediate priorities can be met, a rapport may be established, allowing further work on life needs, health issues, and quality of life.

While a dozen scenarios could be presented for comprehensive nursing care planning related to homeless persons who are also severely and persistently mentally ill, one has been presented here on pp. 812-813. It is a plan for Molten, the name the client has given herself. She spends her days in the day center with a blanket over her head and spends her nights across the street at the Emergency Shelter for Women.

While there are no interdisciplinary treatment plans or protocols for homeless persons at this time, a prototype of a continuum of services has been developed. The continuum requires interdisciplinary cooperation, collaboration and support, and policy making, public-funding support, and advocacy for homeless persons at every level of governmental, regulatory, and health services agencies. The continuum synthesizes all the needs of homeless persons, rather than dealing with only one or two issues separately (Kaufman, 1984). This continuum is a three-tiered approach and consists of the following:

- Emergency responses: food, shelter, financial services
- Transitional services: housing assistance, employment assistance, and health, mental health, and social services
- Stabilization: permanent housing in either independent or supported environments and supplemental services as required

In addition to the continuum, Kaufman indicates that case management and prevention of homelessness is the context within which the continuum would have maximum use. Individualization through case management services is especially important in the first two phases to provide the foundation for stabilization. The Evolving Consumer Households, implemented by the Massachusetts Mental Health Center, is an example of this continuum (*"Group living . . .", 1994*).

Standardized interventions are found in all clinical chapters of this text. When individualized for the homeless condition, they are appropriate for homeless persons with mental illness.

Implementation

All the nursing roles have important applications when working with homeless clients with severe and persistent mental illness. While the role of case management has been explored earlier in this chapter, additional information about the role is added here.

Counseling

Homeless clients who are mentally ill expect to be misunderstood and their circumstances absurdly simplified by mental health professionals. They expect professionals to hold the same stereotypes the lay public holds and therefore expect to be lectured, told what to do, and left to make things happen for themselves. On the other hand, if a professional jumps in to take over, and the solutions are not perceived as beneficial, the relationship is fractured, and the client may not be seen again. The counseling role must be handled sensitively. Rapport must occur first and hardly ever occurs in the traditional ways. Setting up an appointment or setting aside time for the client to come to a certain place is out of the question. Clients who have reasons to remain anonymous do not arrive at a predetermined time and place; the paranoia about the professional's intentions is too great. Rapport is developed by listening, by helping, by being available, by giving a light for a cigarette, by providing a soda or a sandwich, or by giving a cup of cold water. Saving a seat, cutting out a newspaper article of interest to the client, or bringing favorite cookies goes a long toward establishing rapport. These are all considered violations of the traditional boundaries between therapist and client. The methods used to establish rapport may be shared with colleagues and the treatment team for input to make certain objectivity is not lost and personal boundaries are truly not violated. However, new ways must be tried, because traditional methods of rapport

The Nursing Process

NURSING CARE PLAN

Homeless Person With Severe and Persistent Mental Illness

NURSING ASSESSMENT DATA

Subjective: Fearful, lonely, and isolated, Mary M. "Leave me alone. Ain't nobody gonna hurt me again." Sits on a chair in the day center around the corner from the main gathering hall, by the Director's office. A wool, army green, grimy blanket covers her head and is draped over her whole body. She has it arranged so that enough light can illuminate a magazine in her lap. She leans over in a way that she can see the magazine and any feet that pass her way without having to move. *Objective:* Unresponsive to verbal inquiries from any "feet" she does not recognize. If the other person is persistent, she becomes verbally threatening. Will answer "feet" she recognizes only after months of standing in front of her and then only after a full minute of waiting for a response to a question. *DSM-IV diagnosis:* Paranoid personality disorder.

NANDA Diagnosis: Risk for loneliness related to social isolation

Outcomes	Interventions	Rationale	Evaluation
Short term 1. Will continue to communicate with the two sets of "feet" she has chosen. **Long term** 1. Will increase the number of persons and the ways she recognizes them.	• The two persons already known to client should use their names when approaching her. "These shoes belong to Jeanna." • Known person should walk up to client and stop far enough away that she is unable to see the shoes. Person should ask her to guess who has come to visit with her. Person should have a magazine for her if she answers in any way, hostile or not. • Known person should introduce a new pair of shoes with name to client when the usual contact will be gone for awhile. Person should explain in front of client about her interest in magazines. Have the new person talk with client about some of his or her favorite magazines and ask client one question about the kinds of magazines she prefers.	• The nurse should use the relationships already established to broaden client's experience of them: She has indicated a willingness to relate to these two. • Client should be able to recognize the voice and may be willing to say the person's name. Person should continue to do this once a day until she responds. • The known person should make the transition to an unknown person. The reason should be authentic, and the introduction of a new person should show concern for client and her need for reading material and human contact while the regular person is away. This affirms client's human need for contact with another human being, without forcing her to acknowledge the need. The new relationship should be developed on the basis of a safe topic and one of client's interests: magazines.	**Short term** • Met. Though more verbally aggressive, client continued to respond to the two persons she was used to. **Long term** • Met. The client included two new people, whom she recognized by voice, shoes, and hands.

The Nursing Process

NURSING CARE PLAN

Homeless Person With Severe and Persistent Mental Illness—cont'd

Outcomes	Interventions	Rationale	Evaluation
	• Person should bring a different magazine each day, according to client's expressed interests. Person should become acquainted with the magazine and able to comment on an article, for example, "I will be interested to see what you thought of the article on the President's daughter." Then follow up the next day on her perceptions. "What did you think of the pictures of his daughter? She looked young and vulnerable to me."	• High expectation/low demand is important in the beginning of the relationship. Person should expect client to respond, but not demand that she do so. Person should not be disappointed when she does not respond. Sometimes she will, sometimes she will not, and sometimes she may be hostile and belligerent. Continuing approaches and consistency will be disconcerting, because her strange behavior is not scaring nurse away.	
	• When she responds, person should be very gentle in answer. Nurse should act as though her response was expected, which it was. At the end of the conversation, nurse could state that he or she was glad to hear her opinion, or some other affirming but nonthreatening response.	• The first response should not be treated as the beginning of a marathon conversation. It takes a great deal of courage to risk saying more than the usual cursory statement or to venture an opinion. Affirming her effort without saying so directly is nonthreatening and encourages further verbalization. Person should remain with a high-expectation/low-demand attitude throughout the course of the relationship. Mary owes the nurse nothing, not even a "good morning." "Good morning" must be a gift freely and caringly given.	

building have been notoriously unsatisfactory.

While building rapport, the client's basic needs must be addressed. Problem solving is the core of the nursing/counseling role with all clients, and it is absolutely essential with homeless clients with mental illness. Their needs are too immediate and too great to deal with other than the here-and-now.

Milieu Therapy

Milieu therapy focuses on safety and meeting needs. Homeless persons need a place to sit and rest, to talk and eat, and to get out of the weather. They may need medication for a fever, shampoo for lice, and debridement of maggot infestation or frostbite. They may need to be around other persons so they will not get beaten and

The Nursing Process

their few possessions stolen. They may need a place with low demand where they can get a decent meal and be treated with dignity.

Day centers

Day centers screen clients for tuberculosis so that other clients will not be exposed. This is one way that safety is established for all members of the homeless community. Persons who are interested in being tested for HIV or hepatitis can get a ride to the local health department for counseling and screening. Some day centers provide this kind of testing onsite. Someone who is physically ill may need to sit or lie down. Volunteer nurses often provide basic screening and comfort measures for guests of day centers. These kinds of services tell the guests that their reality is acknowledged and their needs, at least some of them, can be met in this place.

Low demand means that persons are expected to maintain decency and respect for each other, but beyond that, a wide range of behavior is tolerated. Persons are asked to sign in but do not have to prove their real identity. They are welcomed, shown around if they have not been to the center before, and told about basic rules such as no spitting or voiding on the floor, no yelling in anger, no hitting or any other aggressive acts, and no weapons. Persons may store their belongings or keep them. They often are grateful to have a place to check their belongings that does not cost money and where they will not be stolen.

Persons are expected to sign in for showers and access to the clothing room, for day care for their children, for food stamps they receive through the center, and so forth. Usually showers and new clothing can be accessed only once a week, because there are so many in need. However, if there is an emergency, a job interview, or an unusual circumstance, the rules can be changed to respond to the individual's need.

Educational groups, spiritual groups, medication groups, and therapy groups such as music or art are often offered by groups of students or staff. Unlike a hospital or treatment center, guests are not required to attend any of these. Incentives may be offered, but guests have the right to choose.

Domiciles

The most difficult self-management activity for homeless persons is getting adequate rest. Places that provide sleeping quarters focus on safety and cleanliness for their residents. Certainly sexual assault, assault and battery, weapons, or aggressive behavior disrupts the sense of safety that all guests need to have to be able to sleep.

Beds and bedding must be disinfected, and bedding should be warm. Beds must be far enough apart in a dormitory-style domicile that boundaries are clearly established. Many fights occur among residents because of personal-space violation. They have so little of their own that a temporary sleep space is a luxury that is loudly defended.

Self-Care Activities

The second most difficult self-management activity for a homeless person is self-care. In particular, activities of daily living (ADLs) are difficult to implement. Homeless persons have sponged off in sinks in public restrooms, dried off with paper towels, and skipped brushing their teeth, combing or washing their hair, and using deodorant, because they do not have the equipment needed. Creativity abounds, however. A paper towel with hand soap, when either can be found in a public restroom, can be used to brush teeth and wash hair. Fingers raked through the hair provides some semblance of neatness and gets out grass or other foreign material.

Sexual activity is another issue of some difficulty for homeless persons who are also mentally ill. Sometimes the problem is finding a partner, sometimes it is finding a private place, and sometimes it is getting rid of an unwanted partner in a secluded place. Homelessness brings with it loneliness and isolation; sexual activity is a way to temporarily address these conditions. However, homeless persons who are mentally ill very rarely address the need for protection from sexually transmitted diseases or pregnancy. The sense of helplessness and passivity, pervasive particularly among women, increases their vulnerability. Giving clients condoms and presenting scenarios to problem solve their use would be effective in preventing these problems.

Psychobiological Interventions

Obtaining and taking medications is an almost impossible task for homeless persons with mental disorders for several reasons. Compliance may be a problem, because medication takes away protective symptomatology, mentioned earlier. Medications may be too expensive to take regularly if at all. If a client can afford to purchase medications or medications are given as part of an entitlement program, the problem is being able to keep them in one's possession. Medication tips useful when working with homeless persons with mental disorders are presented on p. 815.

The Nursing Process

MEDICATION TIPS

Working With Homeless Persons With Mental Illness

- Clients must choose whether to buy medication or other necessities. If other necessities are supplied, they are more likely to take their medication.
- If clients are provided with their prescribed medication, they must decide whether they need the medications more or the money they would make if they were to sell the medication. The decision depends on how much they know about their disease and the medication, how much money they need at the moment, and how much money they can get for the medication.
- Clients who are prescribed mood-altering, addictive medications take them very inconsistently because of the money they can make on the streets with those drugs.
- If adherence to the medication regimen is the client's goal, the nurse must be willing to problem solve the many logistics that mitigate against compliance, such as eating with meals, taking the medication at certain times, or the side effects that may jeopardize the client's safety.
- The nurse must be willing to go out and locate the client if medication, such as neuroleptics, is to be given monthly by injection. The client may have great difficulty remembering and keeping a clinic appointment for receiving medications. The streets are unsafe for the nurse to be seen giving an injection and hence carrying needles and syringes. Therefore a place that meets both therapeutic and safety needs must be found. Often the client has a good suggestion.

TEACHING POINTS

Homeless Persons With Mental Illness

- The nurse should develop rapport and listen for a long time before attempting to teach.
- The nurse should only answer questions and give information; the nurse should not provide unsolicited advice.
- When asked for advice, the nurse should acknowledge the complexity of the problem, then assess the problem, including what the client has already tried or thought of.
- The nurse should teach by example; clients may or may not learn, but they will certainly have more opportunity if they see the lesson in action.
- The nurse should offer to do something with the client, rather than simply tell the client what to do.
- The nurse should remember that the way he or she solves problems may not work for a homeless person. The nurse needs to think through or try a solution before offering it to someone with fewer resources.
- The nurse should be willing to extend beyond clinical norms, with faculty member's or supervisor's approval. The nurse should be sure to be comfortable with the extension. If uncomfortable, the nurse will feel manipulated and exploited, which will hinder the relationship and sabotage the gift the nurse is giving.

Health Teaching

Learning from other homeless persons is an excellent resource for groups. Homeless persons often talk among themselves in informal groups and share solutions. Encouraging this kind of sharing builds self-esteem but most of all it is practical problem solving at its best. If nurses listen in on these sessions, they can become much wiser and better prepared to help other homeless persons who are mentally ill. Teaching Points for homeless persons with mental illness are found above.

Case Management

Research suggests that about 60% of homeless persons have no idea where to seek help or advice (Stark et al., 1989). Therefore case management that both connects persons with resources and teaches persons how to access and negotiate for their own resources is needed. Assertive case management, in a variety of forms, is one way to deliver this level of care. *Assertive case management is a process targeted at persons with severe and persistent mental illness who have a high rate of rehospitalization and consists of active resource utilization and mobilization on behalf of the client.* The role of case management with homeless persons with mental illness includes about 60% support activities and about 40% crisis work and counseling (Breakey, 1987). See Chapter 18 for more information about this role.

The Nursing Process

Health Promotion and Health Maintenance

As mentioned earlier, testing for communicable diseases among the homeless population is strategic to public health efforts. Testing for sexually transmitted diseases, hepatitis, HIV, and tuberculosis are quite common now, because this population is especially vulnerable to all these diseases. Health care professionals working with homeless persons assist by encouraging testing and by performing tests in such a way that they can be read, results reported, and treatment instituted when needed.

Today's reinvented government with a more conservative approach looks to public and private joint ventures to encourage, publicize, spearhead, and fund health prevention and promotion efforts. These ventures are working best at the local and state levels, where the monies can be targeted to specific population needs and community concerns and where accountability is tightly controlled.

Churches and philanthropic groups define their missions as assisting communities in promoting a safe, healthy environment, whether they focus on spiritual, environmental, or human issues. The Warren Foundation, for instance, has given millions of dollars to the study of schizophrenia and other brain disorders. The Robert Woods Johnson Foundation continues to fund new, innovative efforts to provide health care in cost-effective ways. Churches are active locally in funding and staffing soup kitchens, day centers, emergency shelters, food and clothing banks and in providing emergency funds for near-homeless persons. Nurses can encourage these efforts by giving specific ideas for meeting the needs of homeless persons, by providing opportunities for persons to get up-close and personal with homeless persons who are mentally ill, and by providing leadership in the efforts of clusters of individuals and organizations to get involved in their community's health problems.

Two other organizations concerned with homelessness are listed in the Consumer Resources box above. These organizations are excellent resources and are also good referral sources to other organizations serving the homeless community and those who work with homeless persons.

Evaluation

The outcomes for persons who are homeless and mentally ill include a stable residence and resources that assist the person to remain in stable housing. These resources may include entitlements, employment, reduction of symptoms of mental illness, improvement of general health, and increase in support systems. See the nurs-

CONSUMER RESOURCES

Homeless Persons

National Data Resource Center on Homelessness and Mental Illness
262 Delaware Avenue
Delmar, New York 12054
1-800-444-7415

Homeless Health Care Program, c/o National Association of Community Health Centers (NACHC)
1330 New Hampshire Avenue NW, Suite 122
Washington, DC 20036
(203) 659-8008

ing care plan on pp. 812-813 for the evaluation of specific outcomes developed for a specific client.

KEY POINTS

- The most pressing needs of homeless persons include food, clothing, shelter, safety, and opportunities to care for basic hygiene and ADLs.
- Needs that must be addressed to change a homeless person's health condition include stable housing, a steady source of income, and a support system.
- Persons with severe and persistent mental illness have, in addition to the above needs, need for ongoing case management, medications, and therapy that addresses their current situations and their own personal goals.
- Mental illness may cause homelessness, and homelessness may cause mental illness. The two are found together in about 20% to 40% of homeless persons, depending on the area of the United States.
- Outcomes for homeless persons with mental illness include meeting basic needs including saftey, residential stability, finances and employment, and treatment outcomes.
- Treatment outcomes for homeless persons with mental illness include reduction of psychiatric symptoms, improvement of social functioning, improvement of social networks, and increased use of appropriate services, including entitlements.

CRITICAL THINKING QUESTIONS

Richard, a 43-year-old man was thrown out of his residence where he lived with his wife and 14-year-old daughter after 20 years of nonstop drinking and bouts of severe depression. His wife told him, "You are doing yourself no good, and I cannot continue to raise our daughter under the influence of the alcohol. It's time you do something about your problem. In the meantime, you may not live here anymore." He asked his daughter to intercede for him, but she agreed with her mother. Richard has been on the streets for 4 months now, and it is winter. He has been admitted to your inpatient unit for a suicide attempt.

1. Richard receives $300 per month. Help him decide how to spend this money and include his basic needs. He spends all the money on alcohol at this time.

2. Go with another person in your clinical group to a local shelter for the homeless to which you would refer Richard. Take a city map with you. Outline a 1-mile radius around the shelter on the map and do a community assessment of the area. What resources are available within that radius? What, specifically, does Richard need that is and is not in that area?

3. Go into a place within that radius where you can buy food that does not require cooking or refrigeration. Write down the prices for basic staples, then compare those prices with your usual place to shop. What are the similarities? The differences? What can you buy that does not have to be cooked or refrigerated?

4. Plan a 3-day menu for Richard based on what you can buy in the 1-mile radius of the shelter. Spend less than 1 dollar per meal, average. Determine the nutritional value and calories you are able to purchase with that money.

5. Assess the accommodations of the shelter. What would it take for you to spend 3 nights there without going home? What changes would you need to make in your lifestyle? Which of your needs would have to be met differently? What changes would Richard need to make?

• All the nursing roles defined in psychiatric-mental health nursing's *Standards* have unique application in work with homeless persons with mental illness. Because of the complexity of the condition of homelessness, combined with the devastation of severe and persistent mental illness, each role is effectively applied when clients define the goals and the nurse willingly steps out of the "professional" position to help clients meet their needs.

REFERENCES

Angenent, H.L.W., Beke, B.M., & Shane, P.G. (1991). Structural problems in institutional care for youth. *Journal of Health and Social Policy, 2*(4), 83-98.

Bachrach, L.L. (1992). What we know about homelessness among mentally ill persons: An analytical review and commentary. *Hospital and Community Psychiatry, 43*(5), 453-464.

Basler, B (1986, Jan. 12). Homeless families to double. *New York Times,* p. 20.

Bassuk, E.L., Rubin, L., & Lauriat, A. (1986). Characteristics of sheltered homeless families. *American Journal of Public Health, 76,* 1097-1101.

Baxter, E., & Hopper, K. (1982). The new mendicancy: Homeless in New York City. *American Journal of Orthopsychiatry, 52,* 393-408.

Baxter, E., & Hopper, K. (1984). Shelter and housing for the homeless mentally ill. In H.R. Lamb (ed.). *The homeless mentally ill.* pp. 103-139. Washington, DC, American Psychiatric Association.

Blankertz, L.E., Cnaan, R.E., & Freedman, E. (1993). Childhood risk factors in dually diagnosed homeless adults. *Social Work, 38*(5), 587-596.

Breakey, W.R. (1987). Treating the homeless. *Alcohol Health and Research World, 11,* 42-46, 90.

Breakey, W.R., & Fischer, P.J. (1985, June). Down and out in the land of plenty. *Johns Hopkins Magazine,* 16-24.

Castaneda, R., Lifshutz, H., Galanter, M., & Franco, H. (1993). Age at onset of alcoholism as a predictor of homelessness and drinking severity. *Journal of Addictive Diseases, 12*(1), 65-77.

Caton, C.L.M., Wyatt, R.J., Felix, A., Grunberg, J., & Dominguez, B. (1993). Follow-up of chronically homeless mentally ill men. *American Journal of Psychiatry, 150,* 1639-1642.

Dennis, D.L., Buckner, J.C., Lipton, F.R., & Levine, I.S. (1991). A decade of research and services for homeless mentally ill persons: Where do we stand? *American Psychologist, 46,* (No. 11), 1129-1138.

Derogatis, L., & Melisaratos N. (1983). The brief symptom inventory: An introductory report. *Psychological Medicine, 13,* 595-605.

Dickey, B., et. al. (1996). Use of mental health services by formerly homeless adults residing in group and independent housing. *Psychiatric Services, 47* (2), 152-158.

Drake, R.E., Osher, F.C., & Wallach, M.A. (1991). Homelessness and dual diagnosis. *American Psychologist, 4*(11), 1149-1158.

Fischer, P.J., & Breakey, W.R. (1991). The epidemiology of alcohol, drug, and mental disorders among homeless persons. *American Psychologist, 46*(11), 1115-1128.

Grella, C. (1994). Contrasting a shelter and day center for homeless mentally ill women: Four patterns of service use. *Community Mental Health Journal, 30*(1), 3-16.

Group living that fosters autonomy for homeless mentally ill persons: Significant achievement awards (1994). *Hospital and Community Psychiatry, 45*(11), 1135-1136.

Gurland, B.J., et. al. (1977). The comprehensive assessment and referral evaluation (CARE): Rationale, development, and reliability. *International Journal of Aging and Human Development, 8,* 9-42.

Hagen, J.L. (1990). Designing services for homeless women. *Journal of Health and Social Policy, 1*(3), 1-16.

Hamid, W.A., Wykes, T., & Stansfeld, S. (1993). The homeless mentally ill: Myths and realities. *The International Journal of Social Psychiatry, 38*(4), 237-254.

Harper, M.S., & Lacey, B.M. (1993). Mental health/mental illness of the elderly who are homeless. *The ABNF Journal, 4*(2), 45-49.

Kaufman, N.K. (1984). Homelessness: A comprehensive policy approach. *Urban and Social Change Review, 17,* 21-26.

Lehman, A.F., Kernan, E., DeForge, B.R., & Dixon, L. (1995). Effects of homelessness on the quality of life of persons with severe mental illness. *Psychiatric Services, 46*(9), 922-926.

Lovell, A.M., Barrow, S.M., & Struening, E.L. (1992). Between relevance and rigor: Methodological issues in studying mental health and homelessness. In R.I. Jahiel (Ed.). *Homelessness: A preventive approach.* Baltimore: Johns Hopkins University Press.

Masten, A.S., Neemann, J., & Andenas, S. (1991). *Life events and adjustments in adolescents: A study of confounded measures and mediating processes.* Unpublished manuscript. Referred to in Masten, A.S., et al. (1993). Children in homeless families: Risks to mental health and development. *Journal of Consulting and Clinical Psychology, 61,* 335-343.

McCarty, D., Argeriou, M., Huebner, R.B., & Lubran, B. (1991). Alcoholism, drug abuse, and the homeless. *American Psychologist, 46*(11), 1139-1148.

Memmott, R.J., & Young, L.A. (1993). An encounter with homeless mothers and children: Gaining an awareness. *Issues in Mental Health Nursing, 14,* 357-365.

Mobray, C.T., Bybee, C., & Cohen, E. (1993). Describing the homeless mentally ill: Cluster analysis results. *American Journal of Community Psychology, 21*(1), 67-93.

North, C.S., & Smith, E.M. (1993a). A comparison of homeless men and women: Different populations, different needs. *Community Mental Health Journal, 29*(5), 423-431.

North, C.S., & Smith, E.M. (1993b). A systematic study of mental health services utilization by homeless men and women. *Social Psychiatry and Psychiatric Epidemiology, 28,* 77-83.

North, C.S., Smith, E.M., & Spitznagel, E.L. (1993). Is antisocial personality a valid diagnosis among the homeless? *American Journal of Psychiatry, 150*(4), 578-583.

Nyamathi, A.M., & Flaskerud, J. (1992). A community-based inventory of current concerns of improverished homeless and drug-addicted minority women. *Research in Nursing and Health, 15,* 121-129.

Robins, L.N., Helzer, J.E., Croughan, J., & Ratcliff, K.S. (1981). National institute of mental health diagnostic interview schedule. *Archives of General Psychiatry, 38,* 381-389.

Rosenheck, R., Frisman, L., & Gallup, P. (1995). Effectiveness and cost of specific treatment elements in a program for homeless mentally ill veterans. *Psychiatric Services, 46*(11), 1131-1139.

Rosenheck, R., & Gallup, P. (1991). Involvement in an outreach and residential treatment program for homeless mentally ill veterans. *Journal of Nervous and Mental Disease, 179*(12), 750-754.

Rosenheck, R., & Koegel, P. (1993). Characteristics of veterans and nonveterans in three samples of homeless men. *Hospital and Community Psychiatry, 44*(9), 858-863.

Rosenthal, D., Moore, S., & Buzwell, S. (1994). Homeless youths: Sexual and drug-related behaviours, sexual beliefs and HIV/AIDS risk. *AIDS Care, 6*(1), 83-94.

Rossi, P., et. al. (1987). The urban homeless: Estimating composition and size. *Science, 235,* 1336-1341.

Scott, J. (1991, July). Resettlement unit or asylum? Paper presented at the Royal College of Psychiatrists, Brighton, England.

Scott, J. (1993). Homelessness and mental illness. *British Journal of Psychiatry, 162,* 314-324.

Shane, P.G. (1991). An invisible health and social policy issue: Homeless/runaway youth. *Journal of Health and Social Policy, 2*(4), 3-14.

Shane, P.G. (1991). A sample of homeless and runaway youth in New Jersey and their health status. *Journal of Health and Social Policy, 2*(4), 73-82.

Shuler, P.A., Gelberg, L., & Brown, M. (1994). The effects of spiritual/religious practices on psychological well-being among inner city homeless women. *Nurse Practitioner Forum, 5*(2), 106-113.

Smith, E.M., North, C.S., & Spitznagel, E.L. (1993). Alcohol, drugs, and psychiatric comorbidity among homeless women: An epidemiologic study. *Journal of Clinical Psychiatry, 54*(3), 82-87.

Stark, C., et al. (1989). A survey of the "long stay" users of DSS resettlement units: A research report. London: Department of Social Security.

Starrfield, J.H., Avnon, M., Starrfield, W., Rabinowitz, J., & Heifetz, S. (1995). Effects of psychosocial rehabilitation for hospitalized mentally ill homeless persons. *Psychiatric Services, 46*(9), 948-950.

Susser, E.S., Lin, S.P., Conover, S.A., & Struening, E.L. (1991). Childhood antecedents of homelessness in psychiatric patients. *American Journal of Psychiatry, 148*(8), 1026-1030.

Susser, E.S., Struening, E.L., & Conover, S. (1987). Childhood experiences of homeless men. *American Journal of Psychiatry, 144,* 1599-1601.

Taylor, C.S. (1993). Answers: What goals and interventions are important for psychiatric nurses to use when working with homeless chronically mentally ill? *Journal of Psychosocial Nursing, 3*(4), 35-37.

Virgona, A., Buhrich, N., & Teesson, M. (1993). Prevalence of schizophrenia among women in refuges for the homeless. *Australian and New Zealand Journal of Psychiatry, 27,* 405-410.

Wenzel, S.L., et. al. (1993). Indicators of chronic homelessness among veterans. *Hospital and Community Psychiatry, 44*(12), 1172-1176.

Whitbeck, L.B., & Simons, R.L. (1993). A comparison of adaptive strategies and patterns of victimization among homeless adolescents and adults. *Violence and Victims, 8*(2), 135-152.

Winkleby, M.A., & Fleshin, D. (1993). Physical, addictive, and psychiatric disorders among homeless veterans and nonveterans. *Public Health Reports, 108*(1), 30-36.

Wright, J.D. (1991). Health and the homeless teenager: Evidence from the national health care for the homeless program. *Journal of Health and Social Policy, 2*(4), 15-35.

Zlotnick, C., & Robertson, M.J. (1996). Sources of income among homeless adults with major mental disorders or substance use disorders. *Psychiatric Services, 47*(2), 147-151.

Chapter 38

Persons With Severe and Persistent Mental Illness

Pam Price-Hoskins

LEARNING OUTCOMES

After studying and applying the concepts of this chapter, the learner will be able to:
- Analyze the elements of severe and persistent mental illness that complicate the management of mental illness.
- Refer clients with severe and persistent mental illness to the community supports they need.
- Develop nursing care plans that consider and include the strengths of persons with severe and persistent mental illness
- Specify case management objectives for working with persons with severe and persistent mental illness.

KEY TERMS

Chronic mental illness	Family burden	Severe and persistent mental
Custodial care	Impairment	illness (SPMI)
Disability	Institutionalization	Social skills training
Disadvantage	Quality of life	Stigma
Dysfunction	Self-reliance	

Severe and persistent illness, physical and mental, continues while medical researchers aggressively look for preventions and cures. The good news is that although persons may suffer from severe and persistent mental disorders, they may live productive, satisfying lives, given the skills and supports necessary to do so.

Chronic mental illness is defined as deviations from health that are persistent, leave residual disability, are caused by nonreversible neurobiological alteration, and require special training of the client for rehabilitation. Severe and persistent mental illness (SPMI) is characterized by diagnosis, duration, and disability (Bachrach, 1988). The diagnoses of schizophrenia and chemical dependence are considered chronic, or persistent. Duration is defined as a history of 2 years; disability may include inability to work full-time or to live independently.

The image of the unkempt, ill-clad man rummaging through trash barrels for his next meal is the stereotype of a person with SPMI. In fact this image fits only about 30% of clients with SPMI. Clients with SPMI are found in all sectors of society, maintaining a wide variety of lifestyles. Most clients with SPMI, however, are severely disabled in their daily functioning and have suffered with brain disorders for years. Quality of life is a constant struggle for families as well as for persons with SPMI.

Nurses with associate degrees and diplomas usually work with clients with SPMI in inpatient or day-treatment settings and in residential treatment. Nurses with bachelors degrees often work with these clients in day-care, day-hospital, residential-treatment, outpatient, and home settings. Usually nurses with masters degrees in psychiatric-mental health nursing work as case managers and provide individual, family, and group therapy to these clients. Nurses at various levels work together to provide clients with SPMI with comprehensive nursing across the continuum of care (see Chapter 1). SPMI offers a variety of challenges for prevention, promotion, and maintenance of health (see Chapter 18); nurses are involved at every level of these endeavors, from basic research to interventions to promote mother-baby bonding. The purpose of this chapter is to delineate guidelines for nursing care for clients with SPMI.

EPIDEMIOLOGY

Estimates of the number of persons with chronic mentally illness range from 1.7 million to 2.4 million in the United States. Of this number, 350,000 to 800,000 are severely and persistently mentally ill (Krauss, 1994). 700,000 persons are considered moderately disabled. The primary diagnoses represented in SPMI are schizophrenia (500,000 to 900,000 persons), senile dementia (600,000 to 1,250,000 persons), and chronic and severe depression (600,000 to 800,000 persons) (Kaplan and Sadock, 1994). However, almost all psychiatric diagnoses can be severe and persistent. See chapters dedicated to specific disorders for further epidemiological characteristics.

A large number of persons with SPMI live in institutions, mental hospitals, special care facilities, and nursing homes. They may also live with families, in boarding homes, in community residential facilities, in single-room-occupancy dwellings (SROs), or on the streets (see Chapter 20). About one third of all homeless persons are mentally ill; approximately 90% of homeless women are severely and persistently mentally ill (see Chapter 37).

HISTORY OF TREATMENT EFFORTS

In earlier years clients with SPMI were placed in asylums and were provided with *custodial care, treatment focused on safety and cleanliness,* rather than with therapeutic intent. The mental health revolution of the 1950s and 1960s moved treatment efforts to the community. Particularly the developments in psychotropic medication treatment made it possible for deinstitutionalization of clients to less-restrictive environments than the supervised 24-hour environment of the hospital. Currently clients live in a variety of settings, the goals being to achieve maximal functional status and to support clients in the environment in which they choose to live (Anthony, 1993).

However, even with advancement in treatment and community support, stigma continues to take its toll on the opportunities offered to clients with SPMI. *Stigma is the disgrace or shame assigned to a person or a family because of the presence of a mental disorder.* In ancient times a stigma was a mark burned into the skin of a slave or criminal, a sign of infamy or reproach. Although persons with SPMI do not have physical scars to communicate their illness, mental illness does carry social stigma. Persons with mental illness are treated as if they have earned and deserve their disease and as if the illness itself is a disgrace and a reproach. Stigma is not part of the illness; it is an additional, independent cost assigned by society and over which society has control.

THEORETICAL FRAMEWORK

Theories relevant to SPMI focus attention on ways in which clients are impacted. These include continuum of negative impact, quality of life, and institutionalization.

Continuum of Negative Impact

The continuum of negative impact of severe mental illness is presented in Table 38-1. The stages are impairment, dysfunction, disability, and disadvantage (Anthony, 1993). Each has its own symptoms and interventions.

TABLE 38-1

The negative impact of severe mental illness

STAGES	DEFINITIONS	EXAMPLES	INTERVENTIONS	RELATIONSHIP TO TREATMENT
Impairment	*Any loss or abnormality of psychological, physiological, anatomical structure or function*	In physical disabilities (diabetes is an impairment in physiological function.)	Treatment with medication to moderate glucose metabolism; neuroleptic medication to moderate symptoms	Treatment could moderate an impairment.
Dysfunction	*Any restriction or lack of ability to perform an activity or task in the manner or within the range considered normal for a human being*	In psychiatric disabilities (delusions, hallucinations, paranoia in psychological functioning) In psychiatric disabilities-demonstration of minimal proficiencies in the areas of self-care, social adjustment, and/or work skills	Implementation of a rehabilitation program	Treatment may modify the effects of dysfunction.
Disability	*Any restriction or lack of ability to perform a role in the manner or within the range that is considered normal for a human being*	Severity of disability is defined within the sociocultural context-unemployment, underemployment, homelessness.	Implementation of a rehabilitation program	Treatment will not change a disability.
Disadvantage	*A lack of opportunity for an individual that limits or prevents the performance of an activity or the fulfillment of a role that is normal (depending on age, sex, social, cultural factors) for that individual*	In psychiatric disabilities stigma and assumptions about rehabilitation potential	Implementation of a societal rehabilitation/education program on stigma and discrimination	Individual treatment will not change a disadvantage.

Quality of Life

Improved quality of life has become an important outcome of treatment. This is important with persons with SPMI because quality of life is intimately related to, but not determined by, severity of illness. Persons can have very little illness, yet have poor quality of life. On the other hand, persons can have SPMI yet have a high quality of life. One's ability to function is related to quality of life, but many other factors are also included. In other words, ability to function is necessary but not sufficient for high quality of life. While quality of life is important to everybody, it is expounded upon here because it can be affected by the interventions of health care professionals working with the client.

Quality of life is an individual's perception of his or her position in life in the context of the culture and

TABLE 38-2

Quality of life measures

TOOL	DESCRIPTION
Functional Living Index (Morrow, Lindke, and Black, 1992)	Developed for use with cancer clients, tool uses a subjective scale that yields quantitative data
Health-Related Quality of Life (Padilla, 1992)	Developed for use with cancer clients, scale measures physical well-being (general functioning, disease, and treatment-specific attributes), interpersonal well-being (social support and social and role functioning), and psychological well-being (affective and cognitive responses, coping ability, meaning of pain and cancer, feeling of accomplishment).
Quality of Life Index (QLI)	Scale quantifies quality of life in terms of health and functioning family life, socioeconomic status, and psychological/spiritual functioning (satisfaction with life, happiness, satisfaction with self, achievement of goals, peace of mind, personal appearance, and faith in God).
Quality of Well-Being Scale (QWB)	Objective scale yielding quantitative data related to well-being (mobility, physical activity, and social activity).
RAND Health Survey (Hays, Sherbourne, and Mazel, 1993)	Subjective scale, made up of 36 items, that quantifies physical function, pain, role performance, emotional well-being, social functioning, energy, and general health perceptions).

value systems in which he or she lives and in relation to his or her goals, expectations, standards, and concerns. Six domains of quality of life have been identified. They include the following:

- Physical health
- Psychological state
- Levels of independence
- Social relationships
- Environmental features
- Spiritual concerns, including personal beliefs

The client determines the evaluation of the quality of life. Health care providers follow the lead of the client in choosing and intervening in the variables needing improvement. Tools measuring quality of life have proliferated recently. Table 38-2 lists some of the available measures.

Institutionalization

Until the 1950s, persons were hospitalized for long periods of time. As a result clients became institutionalized. *Institutionalization is defined as becoming socialized to living in a highly structured, bureaucratic environment and comfortable with making very few personal choices.*

When phenothiazines became a prominent treatment modality and clients' behavior improved, the in-stitutionalized behaviors of passivity, inability to make choices, and lack of personal identity, meaning, purpose, and goals became apparent. Clients were much improved medically or psychiatrically but did not have the skills required to live in the community. The very skills that made clients successful in an institutional setting kept them from successfully transitioning to the community. In many ways the onus of this problem fell to nurses, because the client's social skills had not been maintained.

FAMILY MEMBERS' MENTAL HEALTH ISSUES

Family members are a major source of support for persons with SPMI. Clients may live with family members, which increases the amount of objective (measurable tasks to be accomplished) and subjective family burden experienced. *Family burden is the amount of objective and subjective responsibilities that are difficult to bear emotionally.* For clients who are unable to function independently or who have not been taught social skills the following objective burdens exist for family members (Jones, Roth, and Jones, 1995):

- Grooming
- Monitoring medication
- Performing housework
- Shopping

- Providing transportation
- Managing money
- Caring for client's children
- Managing time

Family burden is measurably decreased when clients have case managers. The family is relieved of the burden of identifying and coordinating services, making and accompanying clients to appointments, and intervening in crises. The family is an integral part of the care and treatment of the client and in many ways also receives care from the case manager (see Chapter 17).

Psychoeducation support groups have been useful for families of persons with SPMI. They provide psychosocial support, skill development, and health-relevant information. They are empowered to normalize their lives and to work collaboratively with health care professionals. They discover, through relationships with other families, that they can control certain elements in their lives and that they are important in the provision of care for their loved ones (Hammond and Deans, 1995). Nurses can augment families' coping by providing formal and informal ways for families to provide mutual support (Solomon and Draine, 1995).

The *Nursing Process*

Assessment

To plan client-relevant care a thorough assessment of the client must be completed. A general assessment, found in Chapter 5, and the disease-specific assessment, found in the relevant clinical chapter(s), must be completed. In addition, assessments related to the experience of SPMI, quality of life, and clinical profiles specific to the client need to be completed.

Clinical Profiles

For clients with SPMI there are six clinical profiles that need some explanation. These are dual diagnosis, demand/energy, denial, positive symptoms, negative symptoms, and self-reliance.

Dual diagnosis
Persons with more than one diagnosis of SPMI have much higher relapse rates. In fact about half of clients with SPMI also abuse substances or become dependent on alcohol or drugs at some time in their lives. It may be that using drugs and alcohol is a form of self-treatment, found not to work by those without addiction. However, those who have signs of dependence at first assessment must learn to manage their addiction as well as their other SPMI disorders (Bartels, Drake, and Wallach, 1995).

Demand/energy
The population with SPMI may be divided into three main categories: low-energy/low-demand, high-energy/high-demand, and high-functioning/high-aspiration. Low-energy/low-demand clients have SPMI, have been in

treatment since childhood, and are comfortable with the passive, dependent, traditional client role.

High-energy/high-demand clients are not comfortable with their illness, are difficult to engage in treatment, and arrive for help only when in crisis. They can be very demanding and often reject the help they demand.

High-functioning/high-aspiration clients accept and take responsibility for managing their disorders. They engage in collaborative relationships with caregivers. These clients have chronic mental disorders but their illnesses are not considered severe and persistent.

Denial
As with most chronic illness, clients with mental disorders often have great difficulty accepting their illness. The implications of having SPMI are vast and far-reaching. Acceptance of SPMI requires mourning, loss, change of lifestyle, commitment to managing the disorder, making adjustments in lifestyle and relationships, and finding meaning and purpose in and beyond the illness. Coming to terms with the presence of a SPMI is rarely a simple process. Taking and refusing to take medication, developing alternate explanations for the presence of symptoms, and treating the symptoms without medications are just a few of the symptoms of denial, as in the following example:

Ralph, a handsome, tall, 22-year-old African-American man was brought to the Trauma Emergency Center after he wandered off from the family home ill-clad and disoriented. After some discussion with the nurse, he began yelling, "You don't understand! This racist psychiatrist was jealous of me. I was in college on a scholarship and doing well. I just had

The Nursing Process

a few problems, and he gave me medication that kept me from thinking clearly. He said it was supposed to help, but I think it made me sick. Now I can't get that medication out of my system. I just want to purify my body so I can have a normal life." At that point he began to sob and fell into the nurse's arms like a child. "Please help me. I want my normal life back. I can't be sick and not be able to finish college and be an engineer and have a good life. Please help me!"

Positive symptoms

Positive symptoms of SPMI include the major symptoms of mental illness: hallucinations, delusions, suspiciousness, and disorganized speech. The overwhelming treatment of choice is psychotropic medication. The quality of life is negatively related to medication side effects, so assisting clients in managing side effects is essential to the goals established for persons with SPMI. The four side effects most bothersome to clients are akathisia, sedation, sexual side effects, and derealization or feeling like a zombie (Sullivan, Wells, and Leake, 1992).

Negative symptoms

Negative symptoms of SPMI include the following:

- Emotional withdrawal
- Motor retardation
- Unchanging facial expression
- Poverty of expressive gestures
- Poor eye contact
- Lack of vocal inflection
- Poverty of speech
- Poverty of content of speech
- Blocking
- Delay in vocal response
- Ambivalence
- Poor motivation

These symptoms are described by clients, families, and clinicians as the most troublesome to live with in that they impair functioning, impair quality of life, and reinforce stigma. They are also the most difficult to treat. The novel antipsychotics are more effective in decreasing negative symptoms than the traditional antipsychotic medications (Decina et al., 1994). The speech functions are influenced more than the motor functions. Because these symptoms are neurologically based (see Chapter 15) they are difficult to modify; however, they can be influenced with self-awareness, training, and habit formation. Poor motivation is a particularly devastating issue for the client and the family and can be discouraging to the nurse. An intervention protocol is provided in Box 38-1.

Self-reliance

Self-reliance is confidence in oneself to act. Persons with SPMI have difficulty trusting themselves to act appropriately on their own behalf. However, each person has areas of strengths and can trust themselves to act wisely in those areas; they may need encouragement, as in the following example:

> Carol has found that she can remember the smallest details; she has been encouraged to use her great memory to develop and maintain friendships. She has enjoyed remembering birthdays, anniversaries, and other special events and sending cards. She makes phone calls to follow up on information given to her, which has enhanced her friendship network. She is learning to allow these persons to respond to her needs as well.

Box 38-2 provides interventions to facilitate self-responsibility.

Focused Assessment

The assessment of persons with SPMI focuses on wanted and needed social skills and environmental supports. The domains for assessment of clients with SPMI are housing, physical health, mental health, income and finances, education, job status, friends, family, leisure time, spiritual life, legal problems, and drug-related problems (Corrigan, Buican, and McCracken, 1995).

Strengths and deficits

Strengths include client skills and interests, as well as the environmental supports available. Strengths provide the basis for building new skills and can help clients see that their situation has positive aspects. Clients' strengths may include (1) education, (2) job skills, (3) hobbies or nonvocational skills, (4) special aptitudes or resources, (5) intellectual abilities, (6) organizational skills, (7) aesthetic sensitivity, and (8) ability to form and maintain relationships.

Deficits include physical limitations that restrict mobility. Deficits also include the positive and negative signs and symptoms, listed above, that threaten to inhibit quality of life and functional status.

Family relationships

Relationships with family members is significantly related to clients' quality of life (Sullivan, Wells, and Leake, 1995). Perceived criticism from family members is difficult for persons with SPMI to handle. A mistake often made by family members is to give advice when a person is feeling defeated, guilty, or defensive. Although the advice may be well-meaning, it is perceived as criticism and

The Nursing Process

Box 38-1

Increasing Motivation

DEFINITION

Stimulating a specific action

ACTIVITIES

Ascertain in concrete, behavioral terms that client knows what is expected to be done (i.e., "Brush your teeth, next to your cheeks, next to your tongue, and where the teeth touch each other").

Ask client what is preventing the desired action. Assure the provision of any equipment or supplies that are needed.

Dialogue with client about the benefits to be immediately and personally derived by carrying out the expected activity (e.g., "Your mouth will taste better, you will have more moisture in your mouth, and your breath will smell better to other persons"). This is more useful if client can describe the benefits rather than being told what they are.

Assess whether client knows how or remembers how to do the expected action. Some clients have never started a dishwasher, done their own laundry, or brushed their own hair to someone else's satisfaction. Demonstrate the expected action and ask for a return demonstration.

Assess whether client knows what to do: when to start, when to finish, and how to judge the quality of the action. For instance, when to brush teeth and how long. (There are toothbrushes that play music for as long as the toothbrushing should last.) How does client judge the quality? Scraping those teeth hardest to reach with a fingernail and seeing if white comes off is a test for toothbrushing.

Ask client why the expected action will not work (meet the intended objective). Listen to the explanation; ask for suggestions to meet the objective in other ways. Problem

solve and negotiate with client adequate compromises and alternatives.

Give concrete, honest, accurate feedback about alternatives client suggests (e.g., "Using toilet bowl cleaner instead of toothpaste will cause sores in your mouth and stomach and is poison to your body. It *might* clean your teeth, but nobody has tried it and lived. Any other ideas?"). There are things such as baking soda and kitchen spices that could be used for tooth cleaning. The test for effectiveness and any side effects are how the client and nurse can decide.

Ask client what has to be done before the expected action can be accomplished. Problem solving around ritual behaviors and setting priorities can then be addressed.

Ask client what rewards or consequences would make the expected action worth accomplishing. The client may say, "Who cares about my breath? Nobody gets close enough to me to notice." The consequence, then, might be to arrange with a significant other for a breath test and possibly a hug for nice-smelling breath.

Find an acceptable way to acknowledge successful performance of the expected action. A simple, "thank you" may be an ample consequence.

Ask client what might happen if expected action were performed on a regular basis. The client may lose more than gain through regular performance. For instance, the client may receive less verbal exchange from significant others (even though the verbal exchange might take the form of nagging).

Based on data from Fournies, F.F. Why employees don't do what they're supposed to do and what to do about it. New York: Liberty Hall Press, 1988.

---

judgment (Covey, 1989) and therefore is not useful at that time.

Another common issue among family members of persons with SPMI is known as "high-emotional expression/low-emotional expression (EE)." Explained in more depth in Chapter 29, a high level of emotional expression creates disharmony: loud talking, emotionally laden words, lots of gestures, and criticism. Low-emotional expression is more conducive to the client's ability to process and act appropriately on the information provided. Low-emotional expression includes quiet discus-

sion, comfortable silence, use of neutral words, few gestures, and lots of emotional support. Caregiver burden is a constant concern for caregivers, clients, and the mental health team. Caregiver burden is further discussed in Chapter 35.

Nursing Diagnosis

Particularly for clients with SPMI, it is necessary to consider both the strengths and deficits of clients in their interactions with themselves, their families, and their sup-

The Nursing Process

Box 38-2

Self-Responsibility Facilitation

DEFINITION

Encouraging a patient to assume more responsibility for own behavior

ACTIVITIES

Hold patient responsible for own behavior

Discuss with patient the extent of responsibility for present health status

Determine whether patient has adequate knowledge about health care condition

Encourage verbalizations of feelings, perceptions, and fears about assuming responsibility

Monitor level of responsibility that patient assumes

Encourage independence, but assist patient when unable to perform

Discuss consequences of not dealing with own responsibilities

Encourage admission of wrongdoing, as appropriate

Set limits on manipulative behaviors

Refrain from arguing or bargaining about the established limits with the patient

Encourage patient to take as much responsibility for own self-care as possible

Assist parents in identifying age-appropriate tasks for which child could be responsible, as appropriate

Encourage parents to clearly communicate expectations for responsible behavior in child, as appropriate

Encourage parents to follow through on expectations for responsible behavior in child, as appropriate

Assist patients to identify areas in which they could readily assume more responsibility

Facilitate family support for new level of responsibility sought or attained by patient

Assist with creating a timetable to guide increased responsibility in the future

Provide positive feedback for accepting additional responsibility and/or behavior change

Reprinted with permission from McCloskey J.C., & Bulechek G.M. (ed.) (1996). Nursing interventions classification (NIC), *(2nd ed.) St. Louis: Mosby.*

port networks. Knowledge of both strengths and deficits keeps the nurse from developing unrealistic client outcomes that may prove overwhelming to some clients (Lamb, 1994).

In an acute, highly structured treatment setting nursing diagnoses most commonly focus on the client's deficits and challenges. When the client is more stable and living in the community, nursing diagnoses that focus on strengths and growth potential are more common. A nursing care plan that addresses a client's concerns about quality of life, growth potential, and strengths is presented on pp. 828-829.

Outcome Identification

The nursing goal is to work with the client to formulate diagnoses and a treatment plan that is truly individualized. Client outcomes are the measurable statements about what the client, family as appropriate, and treatment team want to achieve in a specific time frame.

In working with a client with SPMI, long- and short-term goals and accompanying outcomes need to be set. The outcomes should be realistic and should reflect rea-

sonable expectations. Ineffective patterns of interaction between the client and the environment were created over time, and multiple physical, cognitive, affective, behavioral, and social factors were involved. Even minor changes are major gains; the nurse who can appreciate the personal pain and risk required to take the smallest step is able to work well with persons with SPMI. For instance, no longer saying "Hello, bitch" and learning to say just "Hello" took one young woman with schizophrenia 7 months.

With mental illnesses, even so-called short-term goals may involve a longer time than would ordinarily be considered appropriate. Thus a short-term goal for an acutely ill or recovered person, such as joining a self-help group, may be a long-term goal for a person with SPMI; and achieving several other short-term goals may be required before the client can actually join the group. The other short-term goals may consist of learning the art of social conversation, controlling spontaneous jerking of limbs, choosing a group, finding out what the membership qualifications are, arranging transportation, role-playing anxiety-producing situations, and identifying and overcoming barriers the client personally feels would hinder the outcome.

The Nursing Process

NURSING CARE PLAN

Client With Severe and Persistent Mental Illness

NURSING ASSESSMENT DATA

Subjective: Mary Ann, 39 years old, is tired of repeated hospitalizations. She says her quality of life is "lousy," and she wants to, in her words: "Use my education, take care of my family, and get off the roller coaster that is my life." *Objective:* Diagnosed 13 years ago with bipolar disorder, client has had repeated emergency hospitalizations and stabilizations when discontinuing medication. She has a masters degree in city planning, four children, and a supportive husband. *DSM-IV diagnosis:* Bipolar disorder I.

NANDA: Altered role performance related to ineffective management of therapeutic regimen (individual)

Outcomes	Interventions	Rationale	Evaluation
Short term 1. Will obtain an interview in her field for a position she would like to have *within 3 months.* 2. Will attend PTA meetings, be involved in supportive roles at her children's schools, and spend 1 hour with each child per week *starting next week.* 3. Will experience life on an even keel, with a sense of control over her responses to situations *within 3 months.* **Long term** 1. Will obtain part-time employment in her field *within 6 months.* 2. Will state comfort with the time spent and the quality of interaction with each of her children. Client will develop a plan for improving relationships that are not yet satisfactory, *within 6 months.* 3. Will describe her life as even, with enough excitement to keep her	• Assist client to make a written commitment to take valproic acid as ordered for a minimum of 6 months to determine its efficacy in helping her with role performance and functional capacity. • Have client complete an objections letter concerning her medication, the side effects, and her perceptions of how her life has been adversely affected. • Explore remedies and reframe irrational beliefs about client's objections to the medication. • Develop a lifestyle plan with client, addressing a balance in activity-rest, work-leisure, nutrition, and exercise. Develop a phase-in plan suitable for her current level of functioning in each area. • Encourage client to develop contacts in her field, join her professional association, and subscribe and read her profession's journals. Encourage client to take refresher courses and continuing education offerings to increase her currency in her field.	• Medication is the pillar of the stability client needs with her disorder in order to obtain her goals. Her attempts to live without medication have failed. • Identification of objections client has experienced acknowledges the validity of her experience. Her experience must be effectively dealt with in order to achieve commitment to long-term medication compliance. • Validating client's experiences and finding solutions enables her long-term goals. • A healthy lifestyle is the best platform to support management of a chronic disorder. Controlling factors that one can control increases one's ability to influence factors not totally in one's control. • Increasing comfort and decreasing anxiety enhances one's opportunity to experience success.	**Short term** 1. Met. Obtained an interview within 1 month but had an anxiety attack and had to cancel. Obtained a second interview she successfully completed within 2 months. 2. Met. Was elected class mother for one of her children. Turned down two other opportunities, concerned that she would overextend herself. Assisted in one holiday celebration for each of the children during the school year. Began spending 1 hour per week with each child the next week and continues to do so 6 months later. Children indicate they appreciate the time, even though they sometimes don't get along with Mom. 3. Not met. Has had difficulty taking control over choices and emotions. Has not felt a sense of control during this period, al-

The Nursing Process

NURSING CARE PLAN

Client With Severe and Persistent Mental Illness—cont'd

Outcomes	Interventions	Rationale	Evaluation
interested, but feeling overwhelmed less than once per month, *starting after 3 months.*			though she describes life as "more tranquil." **Long term** 1. Met. Has enjoyed a part-time position in her field for the past 7 months. Glad she decided to do part-time because of the commitments to her children, her husband, and her home. 2. Met. She has thoroughly enjoyed her time with each of her children and has begun a journal for each of them, focusing on their gifts and special achievements during this time. 3. Met. Client describes an enjoyment of life but misses the frantic pace and the great sense of accomplishment she experienced during her highs.

Planning

Planning for clients with SPMI requires a treatment framework, psychiatric rehabilitation, and outcome identification, standards of care, and other nursing interventions. Failure to provide adequate nursing services can in part be blamed on inadequate planning and inadequate adaptation of the nursing care plan to the client's specific goals, strengths, and disabilities.

Treatment Plans

Comprehensive planning for the various needs exhibited by clients with SPMI includes concern with quality of life.

A case manager coordinates the efforts of various disciplines and services, both for efficiency and effectiveness. While coordination is needed for all clients, it is mandatory for clients with SPMI simply because of the lifelong nature of the illness, the amount of resources needed to support the client and the family, and the variety of resources needed. Cooperation and collaboration among team members is best exemplified in the treatment planning and follow-through of that plan.

Intervention protocols useful for persons with SPMI include the development of social skills and relapse prevention. While several are applicable to clients with specific illnesses, these two are particularly pertinent.

The Nursing Process

Social skills

Social skills training *is the systematic inculcation of specific task completion related to appropriate relations with others.* Social skills training significantly improves clients' social behavior and self-perception and reduces their social anxiety (Benton and Schroeder, 1990). Studies indicate that social skills training affects the negative symptoms of schizophrenia and other chronic mental disorders. However, the effects of social skills training deteriorate over time if not reinforced (Dobson et al., 1995). Nurses make a major contribution to clients' social adjustment by teaching and reinforcing social skills. Clients with SPMI have particular difficulty with the social skills of interpersonal skills, money management, job interviewing, assertiveness, expression of thoughts and feelings, use of community agencies, activities of daily living, and medication management.

Relapse prevention

Fifty-three percent of rehospitalizations are related to substance abuse and medication noncompliance (Haywood et al., 1995). Therefore prevention efforts focused on these two areas would greatly diminish relapse. Relapse prevention focuses on the following:

- Identification of triggers for relapse
- Management of triggers
- Intervention plans to prevent exposure and diminish response to triggers
- Contracting with support system members to provide honest, loving feedback about behavior indicative of relapse
- Emergency plans developed with the client, primary care provider, and support system to end relapse as soon as possible

For example, one client was able to describe her four stages of relapse (Lovejoy, 1989). The stages she identified included the following:

- Estrangement from self and environment
- Cloudiness, fear, and confusion; frenzy of activity to exert control
- Clarity of problem: others are trying to make me crazy
- Chaos and decompensation

Assisting clients who have repeatedly relapsed, a characteristic of SPMI, to develop insight into their own stages of relapse is difficult but rewarding. Equipped with this information, clients, families, and support persons can stop a relapse before hospitalization is necessary and before damage has been done to family roles and support networks.

A large part of relapse is noncompliance related to medications. Assisting the client to manage the side effects of medications and maximize the positive effects is an important part of the nurse's role. Often persons will ask about drug holidays, or abstinence from their medications for a period of time. Literature indicates that persons may be able to take drug holidays; however, relapse greatly increases. The recommendation, based on a thorough review of the literature, is to slowly taper medication to the lowest effective dosage rather than to abstain from medication completely (Gilbert et al., 1995).

Implementation

Included in this section are roles defined in psychiatric-mental health nursing's *Standards* (ANA, 1994) that are specifically applicable to working with persons with SPMI and that have not been covered elsewhere in this chapter. The roles are counseling, milieu therapy, health teaching, health promotion and maintenance, case management, and management.

Counseling

Collaboration with clients is absolutely necessary in assisting them to attain their goals through counseling and the development of problem-solving skills. Support and option development are key components of the counseling/problem-solving intervention (Palmer-Erbs and Anthony, 1995). Group therapy and insight-oriented psychodynamic treatment are not productive. Concrete focus on everyday problems, social skills training, and psychoeducation are effective counseling efforts for persons with SPMI.

Milieu Therapy

Clients live in a variety of environments, all of which can be harnessed on behalf of the client. For clients with SPMI, there are slight variations to consider in the hospital, in the day-treatment setting, and in the community.

Hospital milieu

Clients with SPMI need small groups or individual work that is focused on skills the client needs and wants to develop. However, until symptoms subside enough to allow the client to focus, support and a high-expectation, low-demand attitude toward activities are helpful. Clients and families may define the need for hospitalization as fail-

The Nursing Process

ure. Redefining hospitalization as an opportunity to develop more skills in an intense environment may decrease negative feelings. Hospitalization is a time to identify and build on the client's strengths and is part of the nursing care plan.

Day-treatment milieu

Day-treatment milieu that is highly structured improves the client's symptomatology, particularly the negative symptoms of SPMI. For clients with SPMI the inclusion of a choice of structured activities including supportive discussion groups, exercise groups, and activity groups improve the client's affect, behavior, and conversation (Dobson et al., 1995).

Community milieu

Healthy communities are able to support healthy community services. Characteristics of successful community services include the following (Kaplan and Sadock, 1995):

- Services developed specifically for persons with SPMI, not just services modified for the population
- Acute services as a part of the totality of services needed to manage SPMI
- Lifetime access to a range of comprehensive services
- Availability of hospitalization when needed
- Integrated psychosocial, pharmacological, and family support interventions
- A focus on the development of survival skills
- A true community support system that ensures continuity of care by case management or resource linkage
- Use of skilled personnel trained to work with SPMI
- Culturally relevant with the use of a wide variety of religious, racial, and other community resources (see Chapter 6)
- Acceptance of accountability for outcomes of services provided
- Evaluation of the effectiveness of program goals

In addition to the above factors, the importance of psychobiological interventions in the community cannot be overemphasized. Clients' medications are very expensive, and clients often have to forego social activities, new clothes, or other "luxuries" in order to pay for their medications. Understanding in the community for the needs of clients with SPMI is shown through services such as having thrift shops in accessible locations, churches with clothes closets, free or discount passes to movies, parks, and other forms of recreation.

Health Teaching

Persons with SPMI learn best when information is concrete and applied to their particular situations. The opportunity to actually perform or use the information, rather than to hear or read the information, is best.

Topics include the social skills and relapse prevention mentioned earlier. Specific information about the disease, relapse symptoms, and the phases of relapse equips clients and their families to manage their illness effectively.

Impromptu psychoeducation and 1-hour group psychoeducation are common approaches to psychoeducation of clients and their families. In addition, a structured program of several interrelated modules is useful. One structured modular program focused on medication and symptom self-management, coping with anxiety and depression, social skills, living skills, and leisure skills. Outcomes were improved community functioning, quality of life, and decreased severity of psychopathology (Halford, Hayes, and Varghese, 1989).

Psychoeducation is not limited to the client. Family members and significant others benefit from understanding the client's illness and the management required. Relationships with family members greatly influence the client's quality of life and probably the family members' as well (Sullivan, Wells, and Leake, 1992) and deserves a major focus from the nurse (see Chapters 12 and 16).

Case Management

For clients with SPMI, a particular form of case management has been developed: assertive community treatment. This model is effective in keeping clients out of the hospital and in improving quality of life (Burns and Santos, 1995). *The characteristics of this model are multiservice teams, 24-hour service availability, small caseloads that do not vary in composition, ongoing and continuous services, assertive outreach (direct help, out-of-office visits, and monitoring), in-vivo rehabilitation (working with the client in the home), brokerage (referral to other agencies), counseling and assessment, and monitoring (assessing client's current status, including health, accommodations, and legal status, and ensuring that services are being received).*

Of these characteristics, those found to be related to clients' quality of life were assertive outreach, brokerage, counseling and assessment, and monitoring (Huxley & Warner, 1992). Direct help is the most useful to clients with SPMI and includes working with clients in their homes, providing transportation, delivering medications to their homes, active monitoring of physical health, fre-

The Nursing Process

quently contacting family members, and attending social activities with clients.

An exciting recent development is the inclusion of a peer specialist on the intensive case management team. When consumers or peers are included, paid or voluntary, clients demonstrate gains in several areas of quality of life and an overall reduction in the number of major life problems experienced. The greatest gains have been

found in self-image and outlook and social support (Felton et al., 1995).

Health Promotion and Health Maintenance

Much of what happens to a client because of a psychiatric disorder cannot be controlled. However, the client can manage the neurobiological disorder most easily

 COMMUNITY RESOURCES

Clients With Severe and Persistent Mental Illness

Center for Psychiatric Rehabilitation
Boston University
930 Commonwealth Avenue
Boston, MA 02215
(617) 353-3549

Community Support Network News
(newsletter)
The Center for Psychiatric Rehabilitation
Boston University
930 Commonwealth Avenue
Boston, MA 02215
(617) 353-3549
Subscription charge of $20/year

Evaluation Center
The Human Resources Institute (HSRI)
2336 Massachusetts Avenue
Cambridge, MA 02140
(617) 876-0426

International Association of Psychosocial Rehabilitation Services (IAPSRS)
10025 Gov. Warfield Parkway
Colombia, MD 21044
(410) 730-7190

***The Key,* National Mental Health Consumers' Self-Help Clearinghouse (newsletter)**
Community Support Programs of the Center for Mental Health Services, Substance Abuse, and Mental Health Services Administration
311 South Juniper Street, Suite 1000
Philadelphia, PA 19107
(800) 553-4539
Subscription charge of $15/year

National Alliance for the Mentally Ill (NAMI)
200 North Glebe Road
Suite 1015
Arlington, VA 22203-3754
(703) 524-7600

National Empowerment Center
20 Ballard Road
Lawrence, MA 01843
(800) POWER-2-U

National Mental Health Consumers' Self-Help Clearinghouse
Community Support Programs of the Center for Mental Health Services, Substance Abuse, and Mental Health Services Administration
311 South Juniper Street, Suite 1000
Philadelphia, PA 19107
(800) 553-4539

National Stigma Clearinghouse
275 Seventh Avenue, 16th Floor
New York, NY 10001

***Rehab Brief: Bringing Research into Effective Focus* (newsletter)**
Conwal Inc.
510 Washington Street Suite 200
Falls Church, VA 22046
Charge for subscriptions

from the platform of a healthy lifestyle. Nurses can teach healthy lifestyle, assess health behaviors and status, and reinforce healthy behaviors. The focus of the nurse on the client's control over lifestyle choices cannot be overestimated. It is a powerful tool for the client. A healthy lifestyle promotes health and sometimes prevents disease.

Many client advocacy groups have sprung from the disappointment in society's ability to garner adequate research funds, measurably impact the stigma of mental illness, and provide information and support for clients and their families. Some of the groups available for consumers and others concerned about the prevention of mental illness and the promotion of mental health are listed in the Community Resources box on p. 832.

Evaluation

Areas of evaluation include the goals, or measurable outcomes, set in collaboration with the client and often their significant others. Goals that are of great concern to persons with SPMI are reduction of symptoms, prevention of relapse, number of hospital admissions, length of stay in inpatient settings, level of functioning, and quality of life (Drake and Burns, 1995). Level of functioning relates to social skills and is directly influenced by nursing care, as are quality of life issues such as family relationships and impact of medication upon the person's lifestyle. See the nursing care plan on pp. 828-829 for an example of evaluating client outcomes.

KEY POINTS

- The negative impact of SPMI includes impairment, dysfunction, disability, and disadvantage.
- With SPMI, quality of life is a major issue. Quality of life is ultimately defined by the client and may include physical health, psychological state, level of independence, social relationships, environmental features, and spiritual concerns.
- Families are the most consistent support a client with SPMI has, and they must be helped in decreasing the burden of providing ongoing care if they are to sustain support over the years.
- Clinical profiles often seen among clients with SPMI are dual diagnosis, demand/energy, denial, positive symptoms, negative symptoms, and self-reliance.
- A well-developed care plan considers the client's goals, strengths and limitations, social skills, and support systems.
- A focused assessment of clients with SPMI includes housing, physical health, mental health, income and finances, education, job status, friends, family, leisure time, spiritual life, legal problems, and drug-related problems.

 CRITICAL THINKING QUESTIONS

The Graysons were an average family with three children and two pets. Jayne, the oldest child, was athletic and outgoing. John, the only son, was tall, good-looking, quiet, and thoughtful. He enjoyed art, good books, and meaningful conversation. Joy was 2 years younger than John and was quite playful with many friends. She made good grades without trying and spent the bulk of her energy organizing groups of peers to join clubs, make lemonade stands, and collect funds for the local children who needed transplants.

John did well until his sophomore year in college, when he became isolative and secretive. He maintained adequate grades, but his clothing and behavior became eccentric. He was diagnosed that year with paranoid schizophrenia and moved home with his parents. He graduated from the local junior college and learned drafting. He tried several times to live on his own but ended up in financial trouble and with neighbors making complaints about the condition of his apartment. John has held a full-time job in a small drafting company where he does assignments requiring little interaction with other persons and a great amount of skill with interactive computer networks.

John is now 40 years old. His parents are 65 years old and ready to retire. They have been able to save some money and are wanting to travel, maybe build a small cabin in a warmer state, and spend some time in "retirement." The problem is, what to do with John? John is oblivious to this issue, comfortable living at home and assuming life will continue as it always has.

1. What are the issues related to John's quality of life that need to be addressed with his parents' retirement?
2. What are the issues related to the parents' quality of life that need to be addressed, keeping John's needs in mind?
3. Who needs to be involved in the problem-solving process related to the divergent needs of John and his parents?
4. Where would you start in identifying the issue in a way in which all parties involved could relate?
5. What options for living would you suggest to John? What options would you want him to suggest? Knowing his strengths, mentioned above, what ways would you choose to inform John of his options?
6. What would you predict would be the greatest family burden for John's parents?

- A well-integrated comprehensive treatment plan developed in conjunction with the client and other disciplines, overseen by a case manager, and implemented into the foreseeable future is most likely to help the client with SPMI to maintain a good quality of life.
- Nurses can make a major impact on the population of clients with SPMI by addressing medication compliance and drug abuse.

REFERENCES

Aaronson, N.K., et al. (1992). International quality of life assessment (IQOLA) project. *Quality of Life Research, 1*(5), 349-351.

American Nurses Association (1994). A statement on psychiatric-mental health clinical nursing practice and standards of psychiatric-mental health clinical nursing practice. Washington, DC: American Nurses Publishing.

Anthony, W.A. (1993). Recovery from mental illness: The guiding vision of the mental health service system in the 1990s. *Psychosocial Rehabilitation Journal, 16,* 11-24.

Anthony, W.A., Cohen, M., & Farkas, M. (1990). Psychiatric rehabilitation. Boston: Center for Psychiatric Rehabilitation.

Bachrach, L.L. (1988). Defining chronic mental illness: A concept paper. *Hospital and Community Psychiatry, 39,* 383-388.

Bachrach, L.L. (1995). The chronic patient: Recurring themes and a tribute. *Psychiatric Services, 46*(6), 553-554, 557.

Bartels, S.J., Drake, R.E., & Wallach, M.A. (1995). Long-term course of substance use disorders among patients with severe mental illness. *Psychiatric Services, 46,* 248-251.

Benton, M.K., & Schroeder, H.E. (1990). Social skills training with schizophrenics: A meta-analytic evaluation. *Journal of Consulting and Clinical Psychology, 58,* 741-747.

Bergner, M., Bobbitt, R., Pollard, W., Martin, D.P., & Gilson, B.S. (1976). The sickness impact profile: Validation of a health status measure. *Medical Care, 14*(1), 57.

Burns, B.J., & Santos, A.B. (1995). Assertive community treatment: An update of randomized trials. *Psychiatric Services, 46*(7), 669-675.

Corrigan, P.W., Buican, B., & McCracken, S. (1995). The needs and resources assessment interview for severely mentally ill adults. *Psychiatric Services, 46*(5), 504-505.

Covey, S.R. (1989). *The 7 habits of highly effective people: Powerful lessons in personal change.* New York: Fireside, published by Simon and Shuster, pp. 40, 81-88.

Decina P., et al. (1994). Adjunctive trazodone in the treatment of negative symptoms of schizophrenia. *Hospital and Community Psychiatry, 45*(12), 1220-1223.

Dobson, D.J., et al. (1995). Effects of social skills training and social milieu treatment on symptoms of schizophrenia. *Psychiatric Services, 46*(4), 376-380.

Drake, R.E., & Burns, B.J. (1995). Special section on assertive community treatment: An introduction. *Psychiatric Services, 46*(7), 667-668.

Eakes, G.G. (1995). Chronic sorrow: The lived experience of parents of chronically mentally ill individuals. *Archives of Psychiatric Nursing, 9*(2), 77-84.

Ellison, M.L., et. al. (1995). Characteristics of mental health case management: Results of a national survey. *Journal of Mental Health Administration, 22,* 101-112.

Felton, C.J., et al. (1995). Consumers as peer specialists on intensive case management teams: Impact on client outcomes. *Psychiatric Services, 46*(10), 1037-1044.

Ferrans, C., & Powers, M. (1992). Psychometric assessment of the Quality of Life Index. *Research in Nursing and Health, 15*(1), 29-38.

Gilbert, P.L., Harris, J., McAdams, L.A., & Jeste, D.V. (1995). Neuroleptic withdrawal in schizophrenic patients: A review of the literature. *Archives of General Psychiatry, 52,* 173-188.

Halford, W., Hayes, I., & Varghese, F. (1989). Do social skills matter? The relationship between social skills, social functioning, and quality of life in schizophrenic patients. Paper presented at the 24th Annual Convention of the Association for the Advancement of Behavior Therapy, San Francisco. Cited by D.J. Dobson, et al, 1995.

Hamera, E.K., et al. (1992). Symptom monitoring in schizophrenia: Potential for enhancing self-care. *Archives of Psychiatric Nursing, 6*(6), 324-330.

Hammond, R.V., & Deans, C. (1995). A phenomonological study of families and psychoeducation support groups. *Journal of Psychosocial Nursing and Mental Health Services, 33*(10), 7-12.

Hays, R.D., Sherbourne, C.D., & Mazel, R.M. (1993). The RAND 36-item health survey 1.0. *Health Economics, 2*(3), 217-227.

Haywood, T.W., et al. (1995). Predicting the "revolving door" phenomenon among patients with schizophrenic, schizoaffective, and affective disorders. *American Journal of Psychiatry, 152,* 856-861.

Hoffman, H., Wyler, A., & Kupper, Z. (1995). Age as a factor in identifying young adult chronic patients who are difficult to treat. *Psychiatric Services, 46*(4), 404-406.

Huxley, P., & Warner, R. (1992). Case management, quality of life, and satisfaction with services of long-term psychiatric patients. *Hospital and Community Psychiatry, 43*(8), 799-802.

Jones, S.L., Roth, D., & Jones, P.K. (1995). Effect of demographic and behavioral variables on burden of caregivers of chronic mentally ill persons. *Psychiatric Services, 46*(2), 141-145.

Kaplan, H.I., & Sadock, B.J. (1994). *Comprehensive textbook of psychiatry, VI.* Baltimore: Williams and Wilkins.

Krauss, J. (1994). *Health care reform: Essential mental health services.* Washington, DC: American Nurses Publishing.

Lamb, H.R. (1994). A century and a half of psychiatric rehabilitation in the United States. *Hospital and Community Psychiatry, 45,* 1015-1020.

Lovejoy, M. (1989), cited by Kaplan and Sadock, *Comprehensive textbook of psychiatry, V.* Baltimore: Williams and Wilkins, pp. 2092-2093.

Mannion, E., Mueser, K., & Solomon, P. (1994). Designing psychoeducational services for spouses of persons with serious mental illness. *Community Mental Health Journal 30*(2), 177-190.

Morrow, G.R., Lindke, J., & Black, P. (1992). Measurement of quality of life in patients: Psychometric analysis of the Functional Living Index-Cancer (FLIC). *Quality of Life Research, 1*(5), 287-296.

Padilla, G.V. (1992). Validity of health-related quality of life subscales. *Progress in Cardiovascular Nursing, 7*(1), 13-20.

Palmer-Erbs, V.K., & Anthony, W.A. (1995). Incorporating psychiatric rehabilitation principles into mental health nursing: An opportunity to develop a full partnership among nurses, consumers, and families. *Journal of Psychosocial Nursing, 33*(3), 36-44.

Polak P., & Warner, R. (1996). The economic life of seriously mentally ill people in the community. *Psychiatric Services, 47*(3), 270-274.

Quinlivan, R., et al. (1995). Service utilization and costs of care for severely mentally ill clients in an intensive case management program. *Psychiatric Services, 46*(4), 365-371.

Ryan, R.M. (1992). Treatment-resistant chronic mental illness: Is it Asperger's Syndrome? *Hospital and Community Psychiatry, 43*(8), 807-811.

Santos, A.B., et al. (1993). Intensive outpatient intervention reduces need for inpatient care for patients with chronic psychotic disorders: Pilot data. *American Journal of Psychiatry, 150,* 501-504.

Solomon, P., & Draine, J. (1995). Adaptive coping among family members of persons with serious mental illness. *Psychiatric Services, 46,* 1156-1160.

Stocks, M.L. (1995). Personal accounts: Perspectives on chronicity. *Psychiatric Services, 46*(1), 13-14.

Sullivan, G., Wells, K.B., & Leake, B. (1992). Clinical factors associated with better quality of life in a seriously mentally ill population. *Hospital and Community Psychiatry, 43*(8), 794-798.

Swett, C. (1995). Symptom severity and number of previous psychiatric admissions as predictors of readmission. *Psychiatric Services, 46*(5), 482-485.

Taube, C.S., et al. (1990). New directions in research on assertive community treatment. *Hospital and Community Psychiatry, 41,* 642-647.

Tessler, R., & Gamache, G. (1994). Continuity of care, residence, and family burden in Ohio. *Milbank Quarterly, 72*(1), 149-169.

Trigoboff, E. (1996). Through patients' eyes: Medication teaching to reduce psychiatric recidivism. (Special feature). *Capsules and Comments in Psychiatric Nursing, 3*(1), 9-13.